W9-BFS-559

NOTICE TO THE READER

Publisher does not warrant or guarantee any of the products described herein or perform any independent analysis in connection with any of the product information contained herein. Publisher does not assume, and expressly disclaims, any obligation to obtain and include information other than that provided to it by the manufacturer.
The reader is expressly warned to consider and adopt all safety precautions that might be indicated by the activities herein and to avoid all potential hazards. By following the instructions contained herein, the reader willingly assumes all risks in connection with such instructions.
The Publisher makes no representation or warranties of any kind, including but not limited to, the warranties of fitness for particular purpose or merchantability, nor are any such representations implied with respect to the material set forth herein, and the publisher takes no responsibility with respect to such material. The publisher shall not be liable for any special, consequential, or exemplary damages resulting, in whole or part, from the readers' use of, or reliance upon, this material.

Cover and Text Design: Charles Cummings Advertising/Art Inc.

Milady Staff:
President: Susan Simpfenderfer
Executive Editor: Marlene McHugh-Pratt
Acquisitions Editor: Pamela Lappies
Developmental Editor: Elizabeth Tinsley
Executive Marketing Manager: Donna Lewis
Marketing Coordinator: Tammy Race-Holmes
Editorial Assistant: Elizabeth Keller
Team Assistant: Lisa Borkowski
Project Editor: NancyJean Downey
Art and Design/Production Coordinator: Rich Killar

Printed in the United States of America
6 7 8 9 10 XXX 03 02 01

For more information, contact:
Milady, 3 Columbia Circle
PO Box 15015
Albany, NY 12212-0515
or find us on the World Wide Web at
http://www.Milady.com

Online Services

Milady Online
To access a wide variety of Milady products and services on the World Wide Web, point your browser to:
http://www.milady.com

Delmar Online
To access a wide variety of Delmar products and services on the World Wide Web, point your browser to:
http://www.delmar.com
or email: info@delmar.com

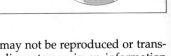

Internet

Printed in the United States of America
6 7 8 9 10 XXX 03 02 01

Library of Congress Cataloging-in-Publication Data
Milady's standard textbook of cosmetology.
p. cm.
Includes bibliographical references and index.
ISBN: 1-56253-466-1 (hc.)
1. Beauty culture. I. Milady Publishing Company.
TT957.M553 1999
646.7'2_dc21
99-19654
CIP

Milady's STANDARD

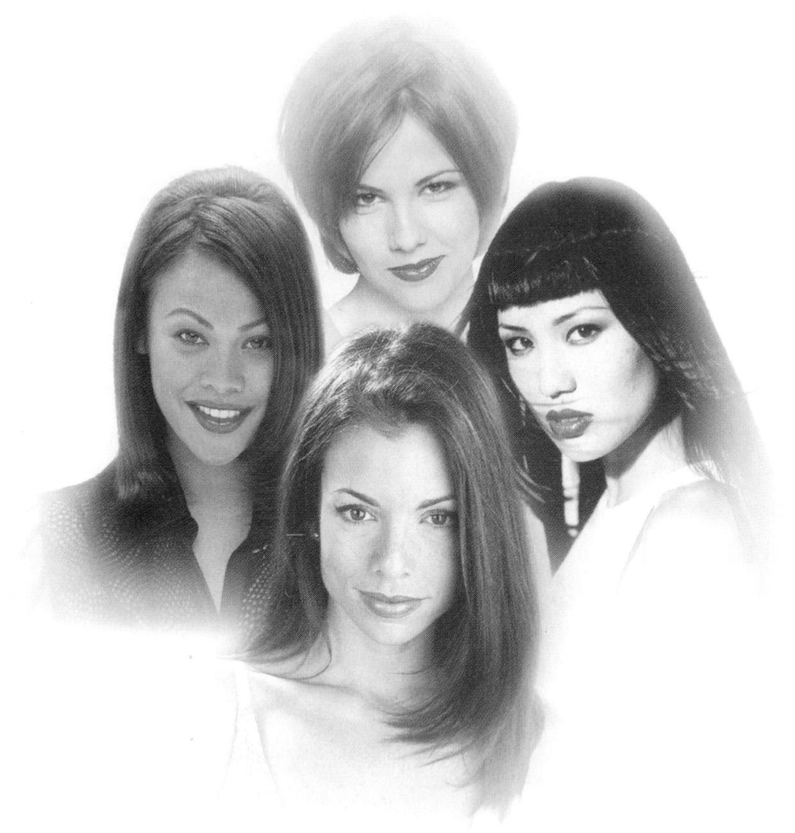

TEXTBOOK *of* COSMETOLOGY

CONTENTS

CHAPTER 11
PERMANENT WAVING

CHAPTER 12
HAIRCOLORING

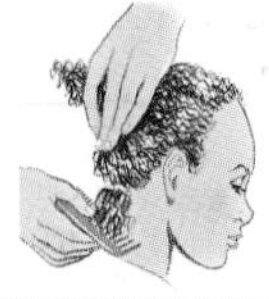

CHAPTER 13
CHEMICAL HAIR RELAXING AND SOFT CURL PERMANENT

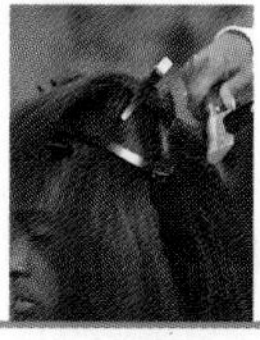

CHAPTER 14
THERMAL HAIR STRAIGHTENING (HAIR PRESSING)

CHAPTER 15
THE ARTISTRY OF ARTIFICIAL HAIR

CHAPTER 16
MANICURING AND PEDICURING

CHAPTER 17
THE NAIL AND ITS DISORDERS

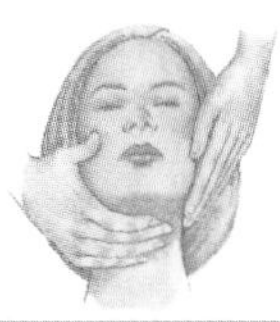

CHAPTER 18
THEORY OF MASSAGE

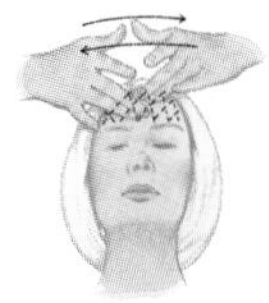

CHAPTER 19
FACIALS

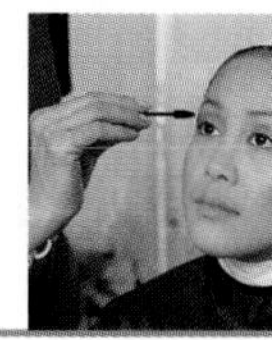

CHAPTER 20
FACIAL MAKEUP

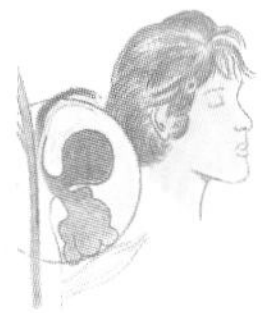

CHAPTER 21
THE SKIN AND ITS DISORDERS

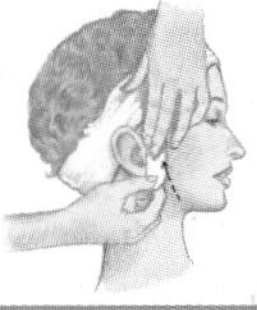

CHAPTER 22
REMOVING UNWANTED HAIR

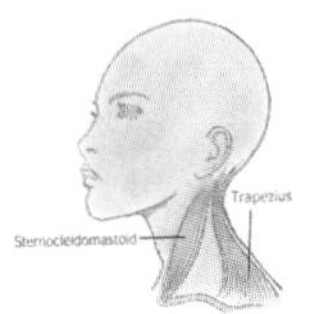

CHAPTER 23
CELLS, ANATOMY, AND PHYSIOLOGY

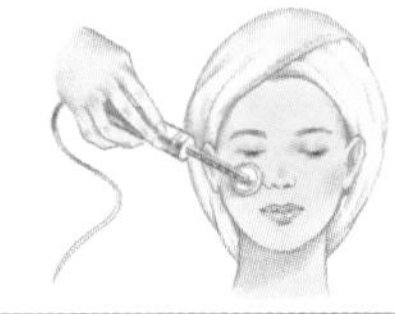

CHAPTER 24
ELECTRICITY AND LIGHT THERAPY

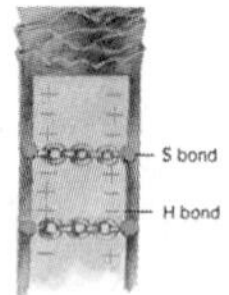

CHAPTER 25
CHEMISTRY

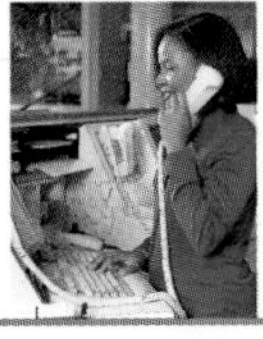

CHAPTER 26
THE SALON BUSINESS

PREFACE

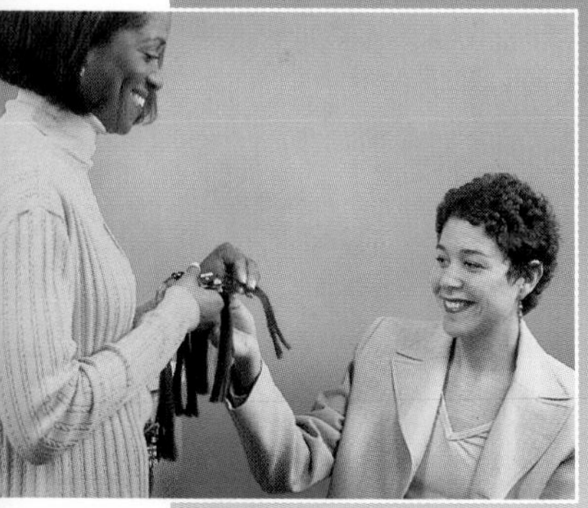

Congratulations! You are about to embark on a journey that can take you in a variety of directions and holds the potential to make you a confident, successful professional in cosmetology. As a graduate, you will have a diversity of jobs open to you, including hairstylist, colorist, nail technician, educator, platform artist, or makeup artist. You may choose to work in an independent salon, a spa salon, a national franchise, or an independent chain. You may specialize in salon management or massage. You may even team up with chemists to develop and market your own product line.

Whatever path you choose, you will play an important role in the lives of your clients. They will come to you for advice and professional expertise, and you will share with them your artistic vision in an environment that is soothing and relaxing. As a cosmetologist, you will become a trusted professional, the person your clients will rely on to provide them with ongoing service that enables them to look their best, and consequently feel their best. You will become as personally involved in your clients' lives as their physicians or dentists are, and with study and practice, you can be as much in demand as a well-regarded medical provider.

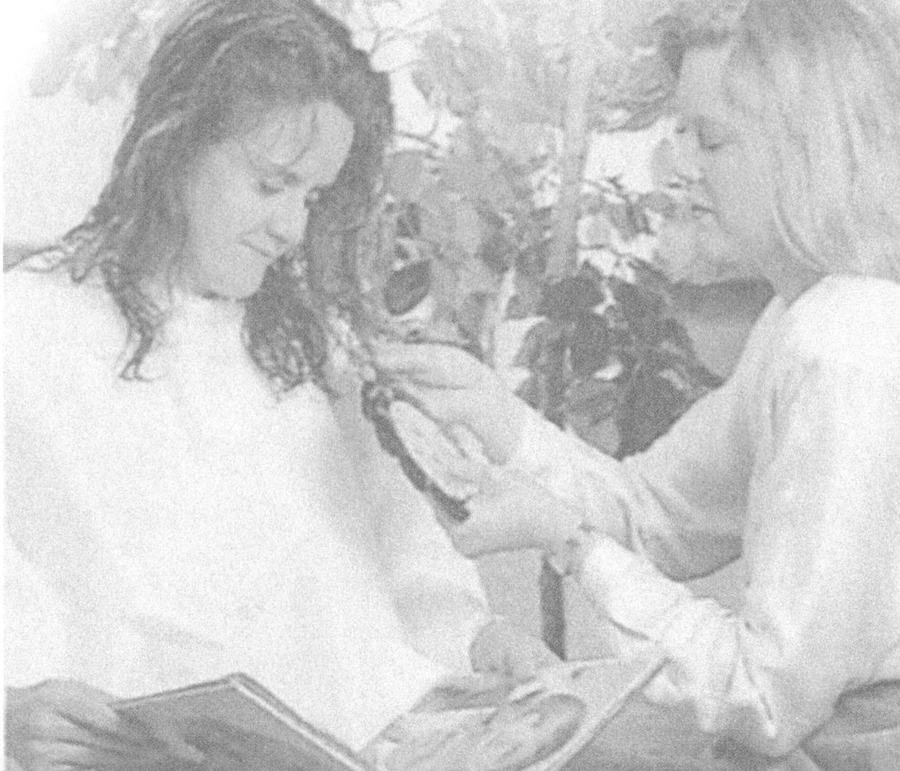

COSMETOLOGY'S EVOLUTION

Cosmetologists today have the potential for enormous growth and success, more so than at any time in history. Throughout the 1900s, the domain of the cosmetologist changed dramatically. From the advent of permanent waving to the development of nail enhancements, new skills and tools transformed and expanded the role of cosmetologists, requiring them to know even more and making continuing education a necessity.

Today you are entering upon a career that will demand a lot from you. You must be not only a talented hairstylist and nail technician, for example, but also a personal service expert, a businessperson, a self-promoter, as well as a poised and well-groomed salesperson. You must understand and practice sanitation and safety precautions and know how to recognize physical conditions that should prevent you from performing a service on a client. You must consult, advise, and listen carefully to your clients, recording information for future reference and considering the unique needs and lifestyles of each one. In addition, your clients will expect you to have a current knowledge of styles, techniques, and products. You will be asked to do much more than your counterparts at the beginning of the twentieth century!

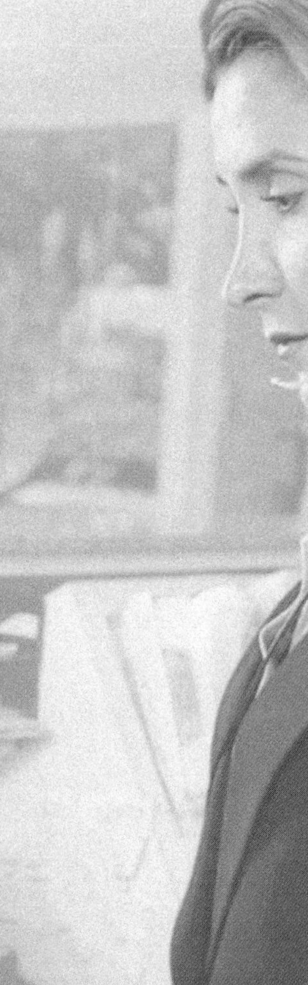

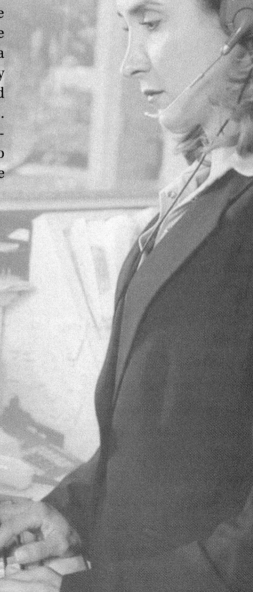

THE FUTURE OF COSMETOLOGY

With each advance in technology, cosmetologists must provide more and more services of a higher quality. New techniques in chemical services, haircolor, nail technology, and hair removal have expanded the salon menu, which now offers products and services to suit all types of clients. This means you will see each client more often, and that makes the relationship you develop with him or her all the more important. More than ever before, good business and communication skills are as necessary as good technical skills. Developing skills such as client consultations, retail sales, and client follow-ups, just to name a few, is now as important as learning the skills of hairstyling, manicuring, and esthetics. By learning and using the tools in this text along with other resources and your teachers' instruction, you will develop the abilities you need to build a loyal and satisfied clientele.

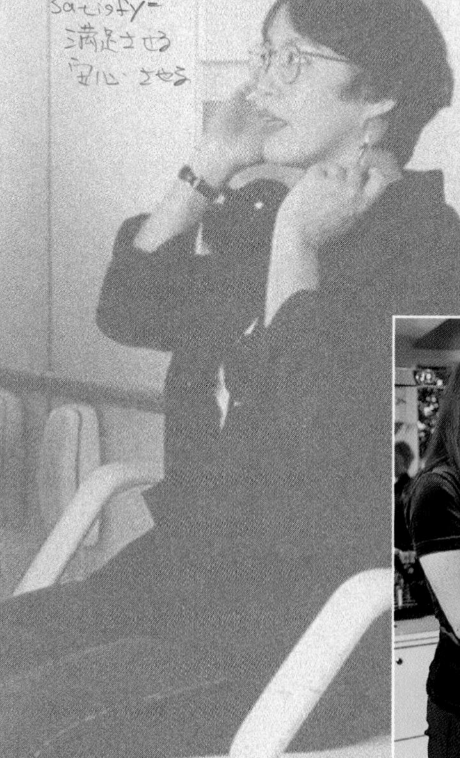

THE INDUSTRY STANDARD

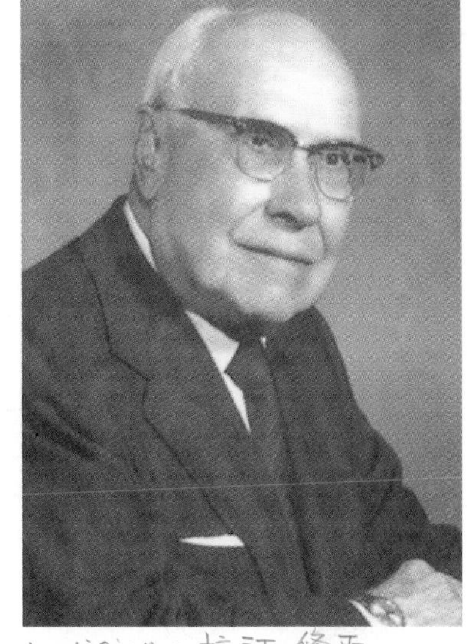

Milady's Standard Textbook of Cosmetology was the creation of **Nicholas F. Cimaglia**, founder of Milady Publishing Company. Initially published in 1938, it has been the first textbook choice of cosmetology educators for more than half a century and has seen many revisions. Throughout its lifetime, it has consistently been the most-used cosmetology textbook in the world. With the many changes in the field of cosmetology, new editions of the text are needed periodically, and Milady will uphold its commitment to quality education by continuing to revise the text to ensure its accuracy and to keep it current.

This new edition of *Milady's Standard Textbook of Cosmetology* provides you with the latest information you will need to pass the board exams as well as the concepts that will ensure your success once you're on the job. Before beginning the revision, we surveyed educators from every type of cosmetology school to determine exactly what material needed to be changed, added, or deleted. Then we went to the experts in that field to rewrite or revise the indicated chapters. Finally, we sent the finished manuscripts to yet more subject matter experts to ensure the accuracy and thoroughness of the new material. What you hold in your hands is the result.

The text now contains new and more comprehensive information on many subjects, including sanitation and disinfection, haircutting, haircoloring, and much more, as you'll see in the pages that follow. As a part of your cosmetology education, it will serve as a valuable reference, and you'll refer to it again and again throughout your career.

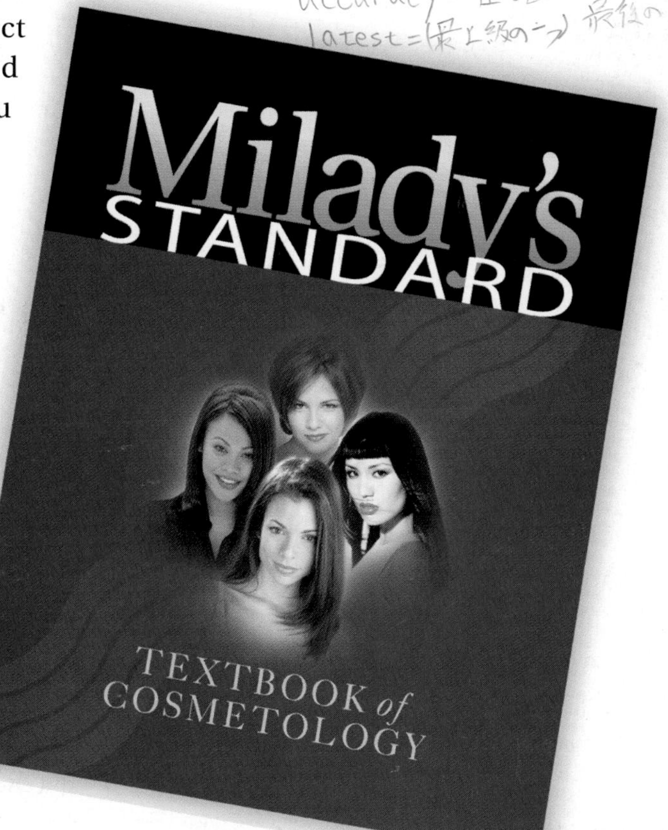

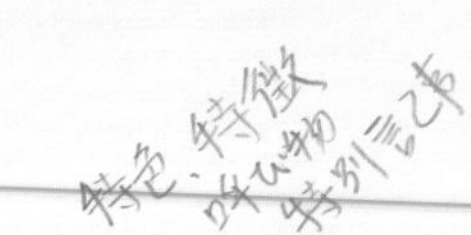

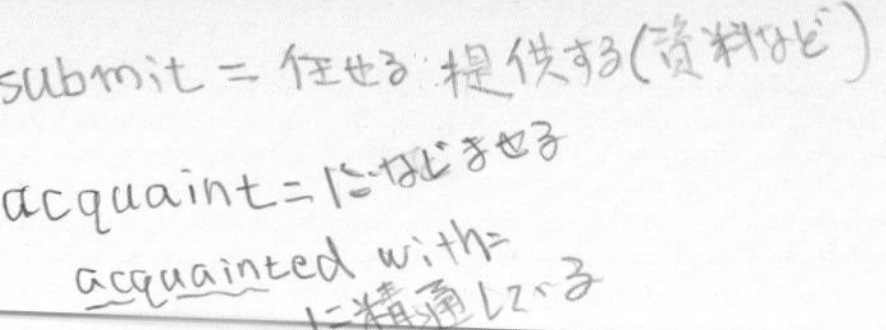

FEATURES

NEW FEATURES OF THIS EDITION

In response to the suggestions of the many cosmetology educators who reviewed the *Standard* and to those submitted by the students who use this text, this revision includes many changes, some of them dramatic. Getting acquainted with this book and its features now will put you on the path to a successful school experience.

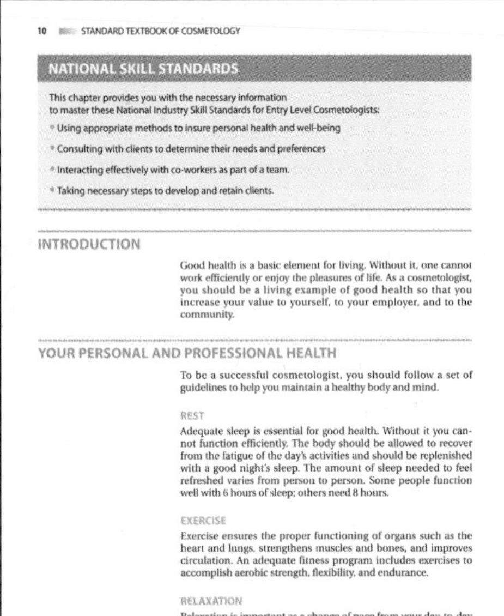

10 STANDARD TEXTBOOK OF COSMETOLOGY

NATIONAL SKILL STANDARDS

This chapter provides you with the necessary information to master these National Industry Skill Standards for Entry Level Cosmetologists:

- Using appropriate methods to insure personal health and well-being
- Consulting with clients to determine their needs and preferences
- Interacting effectively with co-workers as part of a team.
- Taking necessary steps to develop and retain clients.

INTRODUCTION

Good health is a basic element for living. Without it, one cannot work efficiently or enjoy the pleasures of life. As a cosmetologist, you should be a living example of good health so that you increase your value to yourself, to your employer, and to the community.

YOUR PERSONAL AND PROFESSIONAL HEALTH

To be a successful cosmetologist, you should follow a set of guidelines to help you maintain a healthy body and mind.

REST

Adequate sleep is essential for good health. Without it you cannot function efficiently. The body should be allowed to recover from the fatigue of the day's activities and should be replenished with a good night's sleep. The amount of sleep needed to feel refreshed varies from person to person. Some people function well with 6 hours of sleep; others need 8 hours.

EXERCISE

Exercise ensures the proper functioning of organs such as the heart and lungs, strengthens muscles and bones, and improves circulation. An adequate fitness program includes exercises to accomplish aerobic strength, flexibility, and endurance.

RELAXATION

Relaxation is important as a change of pace from your day-to-day routine. Going to a movie or a museum, reading a book, watching

NATIONAL SKILLS STANDARDS FOR ENTRY-LEVEL COSMETOLOGISTS

The National Skills Standards for Entry-Level Cosmetologists offer useful guidelines to review as you prepare to enter the cosmetology field upon graduation. Developed by the Cosmetology Advancement Foundation, these standards are helpful in identifying your strengths and weaknesses in relation to the requirements for success after you complete school. Because these standards include some skills that can't be measured on state board exams but are nevertheless extremely important to your professional success, they are not intended to replace or refute the requirements for licensure. Rather, they are guidelines for success in the cosmetology field.

To make it easy to find the related material in the textbook that addresses these skills, we have listed at the beginning of each chapter the skills addressed in that chapter. You may find the same skill listed at the start of several chapters.

LATEST INFORMATION ON DECONTAMINATION AND INFECTION CONTROL

Chapter 3, *"Decontamination and Infection Control,"* has been revised and updated to reflect the latest OSHA and EPA standards for disinfection in the salon. Specific safety measures to prevent the transmission of HIV and other diseases are emphasized.

4 CLEANERS, EQUIPMENT, AND DISINFECTANTS

heated to 325°F (approximately 163°C) for at least 30 minutes. Effective disinfection can occur only if the entire implement, including the handle, is submerged in an EPA-registered disinfectant solution.

SANITATION

The lowest level of decontamination is called ***sanitation*** or ***sanitization***. These words are also frequently misused and misunderstood. Sanitation means to "significantly reduce the number of pathogens found on a surface." Salon tools and other surfaces are sanitized by cleaning with soaps or detergents. Sanitized surfaces may still harbor pathogens or other organisms. Removing hair from a brush and washing the brush with detergent is considered sanitation. Putting antiseptics on skin or washing your hands is another example of sanitation. Your hands may be very clean when you are finished, but they are covered with microorganisms found in the tap water and on the towel.

The Professional Image

Sanitation should be a part of everyone's normal routine. In this way, you and your co-workers can maintain a professional image. Following are some simple guidelines that will help keep the salon looking its best.

1. Floors should be swept clean after each client service.
2. Hair, cotton balls, etc. should be picked up immediately.
3. Deposit all waste materials in a metal waste receptacle with a self-closing lid.

NEW INFORMATION ON HAIR LOSS TREATMENT

In Chapter 4, *"Properties of the Scalp and Hair,"* the latest information on hair loss, its causes, its emotional impact on male and female clients, and various treatment options, both medical and nonmedical, are discussed at length. Included are new photographs depicting stages of hair loss.

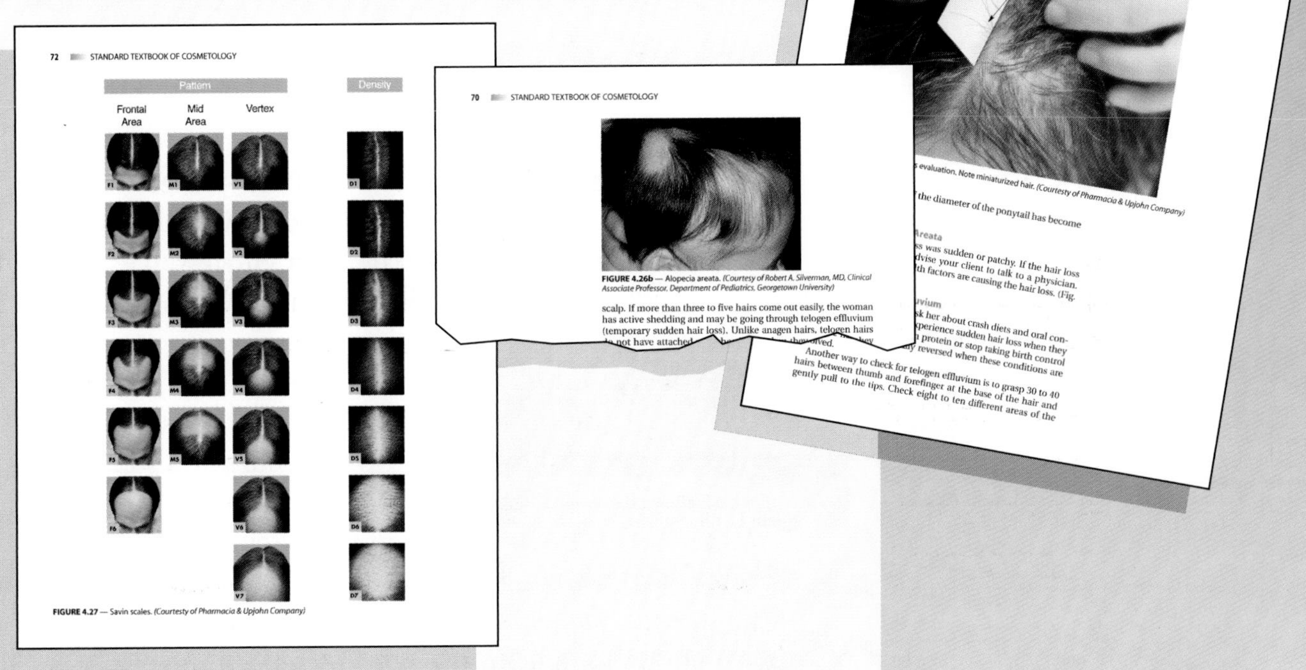

CHAPTER 4 PROPERTIES OF THE HAIR AND SCALP 69

...s evaluation. Note miniaturized hair. *(Courtesy of Pharmacia & Upjohn Company)*

...f the diameter of the ponytail has become

...Areata

...s was sudden or patchy. If the hair loss ...dvise your client to talk to a physician. ...th factors are causing the hair loss. (Fig.

...vium

...sk her about crash diets and oral con-...xperience sudden hair loss when they ...n protein or stop taking birth control ...ly reversed when these conditions are ...olved.

Another way to check for telogen effluvium is to grasp 30 to 40 hairs between thumb and forefinger at the base of the hair and gently pull to the tips. Check eight to ten different areas of the

72 STANDARD TEXTBOOK OF COSMETOLOGY

FIGURE 4.27 — Savin scales. *(Courtesy of Pharmacia & Upjohn Company)*

70 STANDARD TEXTBOOK OF COSMETOLOGY

FIGURE 4.26b — Alopecia areata. *(Courtesy of Robert A. Silverman, MD, Clinical Associate Professor, Department of Pediatrics, Georgetown University)*

scalp. If more than three to five hairs come out easily, the woman has active shedding and may be going through telogen effluvium (temporary sudden hair loss). Unlike anagen hairs, telogen hairs do not have attached ...

EXPANDED COVERAGE OF HAIRCUTTING AND HAIRSTYLING

Chapter 7, *"Haircutting,"* has been greatly expanded and updated, with many more color photos to illustrate different cutting techniques. Several technicals have been included not only to demonstrate cutting methods but to illustrate how to create basic styles.

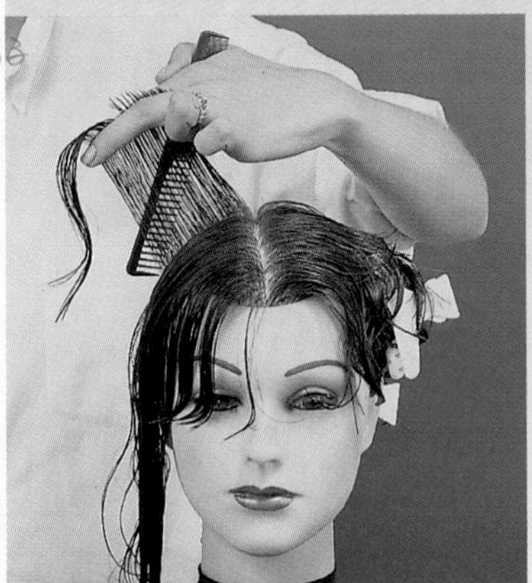

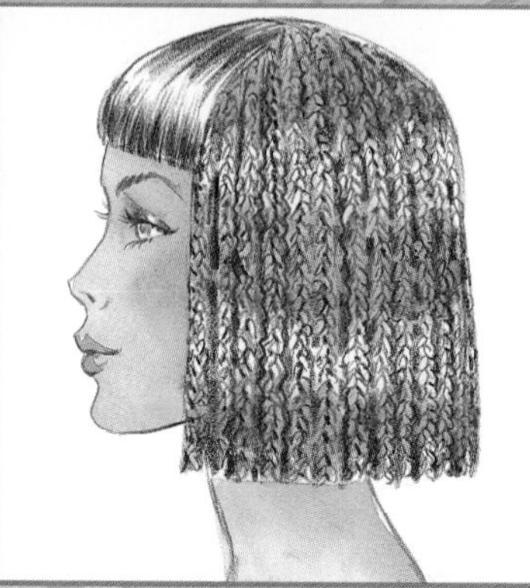

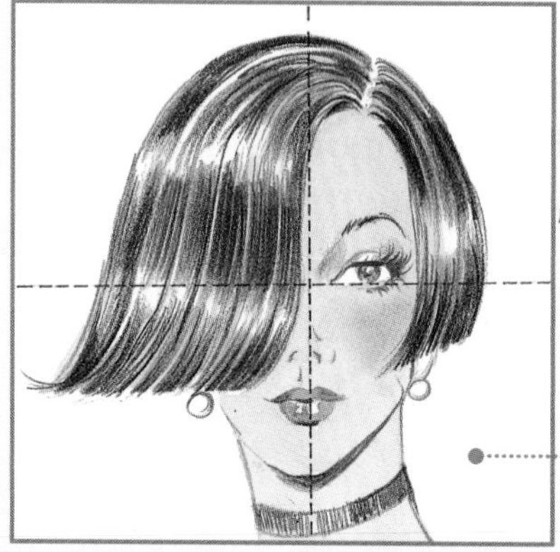

Chapter 8 becomes *"Artistry in Hairstyling"* in this new edition and is devoted solely to the principles of art and hair design, particularly as they relate to facial structure, hair type, and other factors.

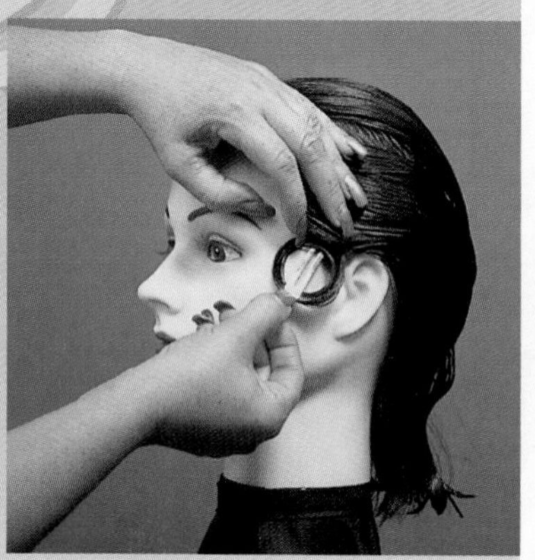

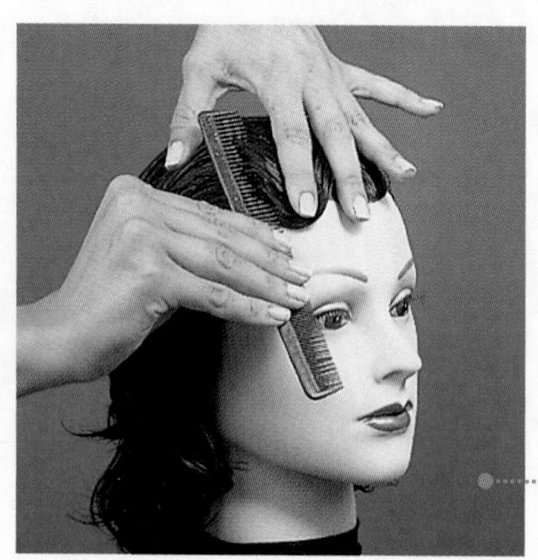

Chapter 9, *"Wet Hairstyling,"* now includes a section on finger waving (Chapter 8 in the previous edition) and revised material on styling with pin curls and rollers.

INCREASED HAIRCOLORING COVERAGE

Chapter 12, *"Haircoloring,"* has been updated to keep pace with such changes in the haircoloring industry as new products, new classifications of haircolor, and new techniques for working with unpigmented hair. Reviewed by the education committee of the International Haircolor Exchange, the chapter was reorganized and updated to make instruction easier and more logical.

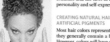

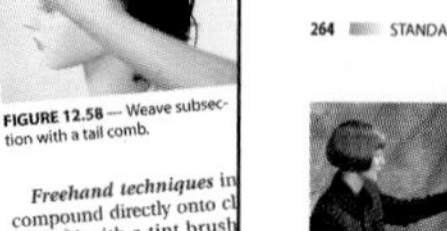

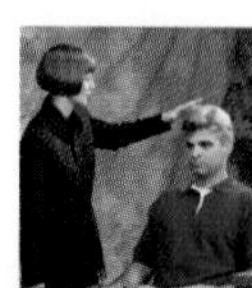

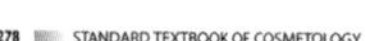

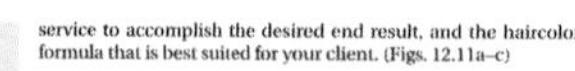

FIGURE 12.1a, b — There are many reasons clients choose to color their hair. To cover unpigmented hair is one.

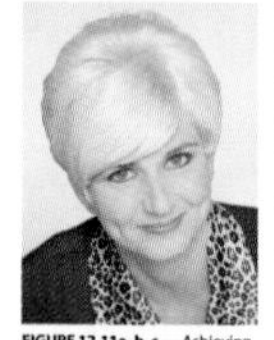

FIGURE 12.2 — Haircoloring is a popular service for male clientele today.

278 STANDARD TEXTBOOK OF COSMETOLOGY

service to accomplish the desired end result, and the haircolor formula that is best suited for your client. (Figs. 12.11a–c)

ENHANCING THE CLIENT'S NATURAL COLORING

The key to maintaining harmony is creating a balanced relationship which is a pleasing visual blend between hair, skin, and eye colors. Natural harmony can be achieved by recreating the relationship between hair, skin, and eye colors that nature created, although the colors may be lighter than the original.

Consider how tones change with maturity. Many clients initially want to return to the color of their youth. They do not realize that the pigment of their skin is aging in a process similar to that of the hair. To tint the hair back to the natural color of their youth creates a severe contrast that can be harsh. Generally, a color of a similar tone but lighter level will be more flattering.

There will always be clients who break these rules. Many do so with great success. Attractiveness is a quality that incorporates esthetics and the laws of art and balance, along with the client's personality and self-expression.

CREATING NATURAL HAIR COLORS USING ARTIFICIAL PIGMENTS

Most hair colors represent a balance of colors, which means that they generally contain a balance of each of the primary colors. However, colors will have a predominant base and a level of lightness or darkness that must be identified before formulating a tint for the hair.

Oxidation tints are identified by the predominant base tone and the level of color formulated by the manufacturer. Most manufacturers provide literature that identifies the level and base tone for you. You may identify the level and base tone of the client's hair by comparing it to the manufacturer's color identification chart (as a guide, not an absolute). Determining the tone in the eyes and skin will help you identify youR client's natural base tone. The Natural Category will indicate the intensity of pigmentation.

All colors—warm, cool, or neutral—can be formulated in tones that range from the lightest blonde to the darkest black, using the basic theory related to the Law of Color.

USING LEVEL, TONE, AND INTENSITY IN SELECTING A COLOR

When you have decided on the haircoloring products to use, you will next find the correct level, tone, and intensity to achieve your desired result. In many manufacturer's product lines, you will find more than one color tone at each level. Each of these shades will create a different tonality. Choose the one closest to what you

FIGURE 12.11a, b, c — Achieving natural haircolors with the Level System.

A NEW LOOK

More than 250 new color photographs and 150 new illustrations enhance the fresh new text design of this edition. Each chapter begins with *Learning Objectives*, which are "checked off" as they are covered in the chapter. *Review Questions* appear at the end of each chapter, with answers at the back of the book.

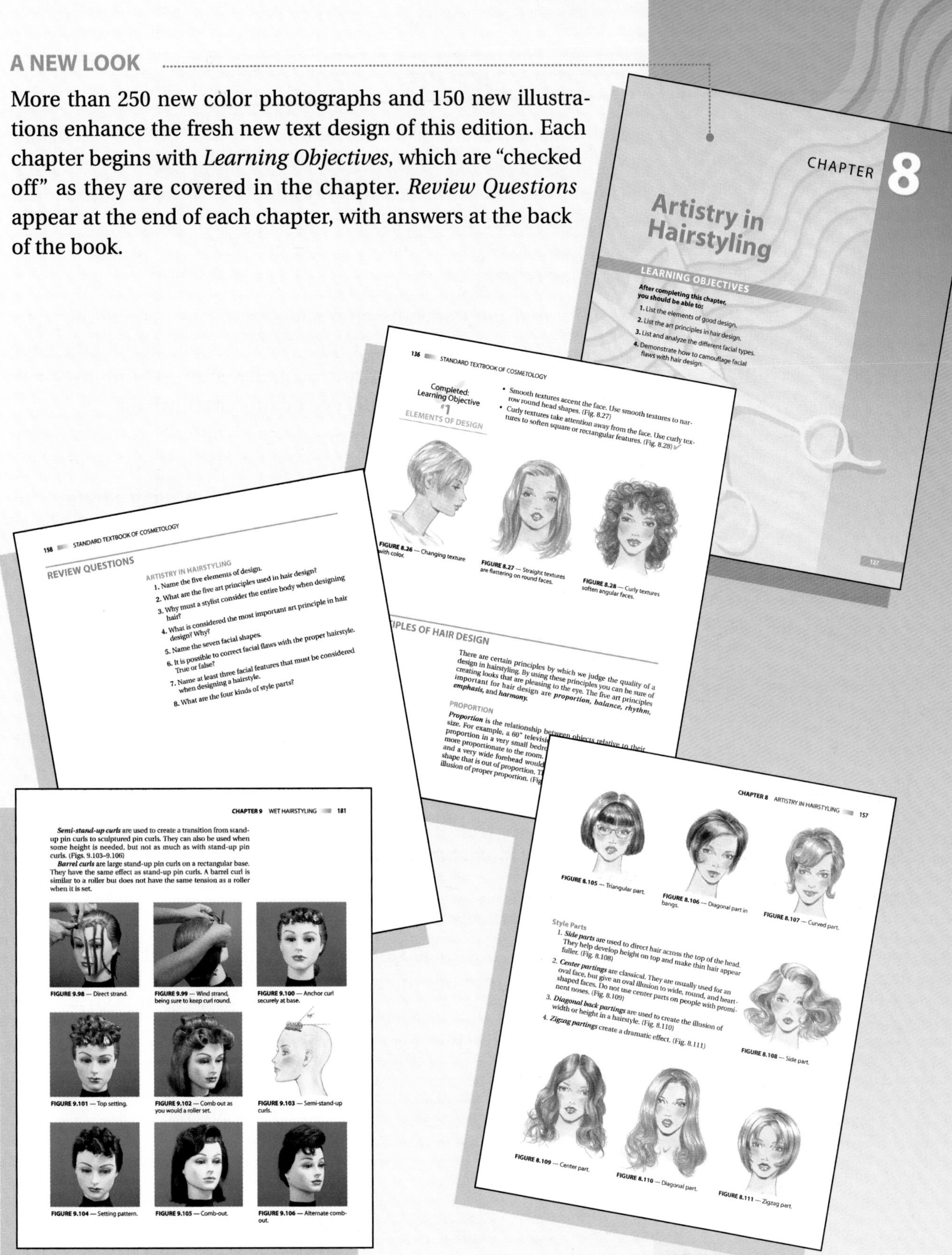

CHAPTER 8

Artistry in Hairstyling

LEARNING OBJECTIVES

After completing this chapter, you should be able to:

1. List the elements of good design.
2. List the art principles in hair design.
3. List and analyze the different facial types.
4. Demonstrate how to camouflage facial flaws with hair design.

127

136 STANDARD TEXTBOOK OF COSMETOLOGY

Completed: Learning Objective #1

ELEMENTS OF DESIGN

- Smooth textures accent the face. Use smooth textures to narrow round head shapes. (Fig. 8.27)
- Curly textures take attention away from the face. Use curly textures to soften square or rectangular features. (Fig. 8.28)

FIGURE 8.26 — Changing texture with color.

FIGURE 8.27 — Straight textures are flattering on round faces.

FIGURE 8.28 — Curly textures soften angular faces.

...IPLES OF HAIR DESIGN

There are certain principles by which we judge the quality of a design in hairstyling. By using these principles you can be sure of creating looks that are pleasing to the eye. The five art principles important for hair design are ***proportion, balance, rhythm, emphasis,*** and ***harmony.***

PROPORTION

Proportion is the relationship between objects relative to their size. For example, a 60" televisi... proportion in a very small bedro... more proportionate to the room. ... and a very wide forehead would... shape that is out of proportion. T... illusion of proper proportion. (Fig...

158 STANDARD TEXTBOOK OF COSMETOLOGY

REVIEW QUESTIONS

ARTISTRY IN HAIRSTYLING

1. Name the five elements of design.
2. What are the five art principles used in hair design?
3. Why must a stylist consider the entire body when designing hair?
4. What is considered the most important art principle in hair design? Why?
5. Name the seven facial shapes.
6. It is possible to correct facial flaws with the proper hairstyle. True or false?
7. Name at least three facial features that must be considered when designing a hairstyle.
8. What are the four kinds of style parts?

CHAPTER 9 WET HAIRSTYLING 181

Semi-stand-up curls are used to create a transition from stand-up pin curls to sculptured pin curls. They can also be used when some height is needed, but not as much as with stand-up pin curls. (Figs. 9.103–9.106)

Barrel curls are large stand-up pin curls on a rectangular base. They have the same effect as stand-up pin curls. A barrel curl is similar to a roller but does not have the same tension as a roller when it is set.

FIGURE 9.98 — Direct strand.

FIGURE 9.99 — Wind strand, being sure to keep curl round.

FIGURE 9.100 — Anchor curl securely at base.

FIGURE 9.101 — Top setting.

FIGURE 9.102 — Comb out as you would a roller set.

FIGURE 9.103 — Semi-stand-up curls.

FIGURE 9.104 — Setting pattern.

FIGURE 9.105 — Comb-out.

FIGURE 9.106 — Alternate comb-out.

CHAPTER 8 ARTISTRY IN HAIRSTYLING 157

FIGURE 8.105 — Triangular part.

FIGURE 8.106 — Diagonal part in bangs.

FIGURE 8.107 — Curved part.

Style Parts

1. ***Side parts*** are used to direct hair across the top of the head. They help develop height on top and make thin hair appear fuller. (Fig. 8.108)
2. ***Center partings*** are classical. They are usually used for an oval face, but give an oval illusion to wide, round, and heart-shaped faces. Do not use center parts on people with prominent noses. (Fig. 8.109)
3. ***Diagonal back partings*** are used to create the illusion of width or height in a hairstyle. (Fig. 8.110)
4. ***Zigzag partings*** create a dramatic effect. (Fig. 8.111)

FIGURE 8.108 — Side part.

FIGURE 8.109 — Center part.

FIGURE 8.110 — Diagonal part.

FIGURE 8.111 — Zigzag part.

OTHER FEATURES

Helpful sidebars appear throughout the text, offering information on a variety of topics. The material in the sidebars has been taken from Milady professional products and will help you learn to consider real-life use of material you are learning.

PROFESSIONAL PREP

Professional Prep sidebars offer suggestions for making the transition from school to salon. Topics include ideas for looking your best, presenting yourself professionally, and learning to speak and act in a manner that will keep clients coming back.

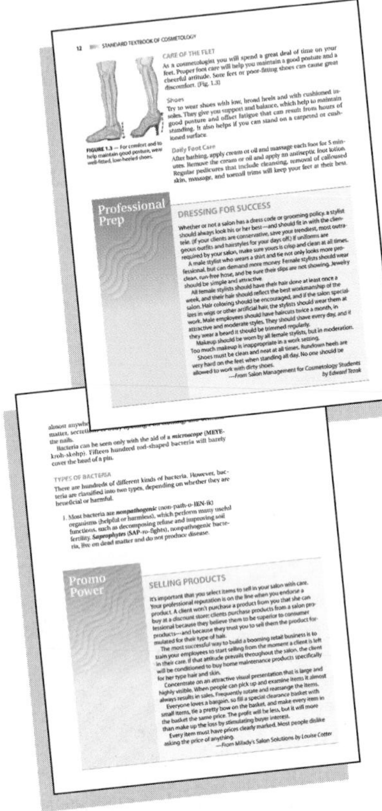

12 STANDARD TEXTBOOK OF COSMETOLOGY

CARE OF THE FEET
As a cosmetologist you will spend a great deal of time on your
feet. Proper foot care will help you maintain a good posture and a
cheerful attitude. Sore feet or poor-fitting shoes can cause great
discomfort. (Fig. 1.3)

Shoes
Try to wear shoes with low, broad heels and with cushioned insoles. They give you support and balance, which help to maintain
good posture and offset fatigue that can result from hours of
standing. It also helps if you can stand on a carpeted or cushioned surface.

Daily Foot Care
After bathing, apply cream or oil and massage each foot for 5 minutes. Remove the cream or oil and apply an antiseptic foot lotion.
Regular pedicures that include cleansing, removal of calloused
skin, massage, and toenail trims will keep your feet at their best.

FIGURE 1.3 — For comfort and to help maintain good posture, wear well-fitted, low-heeled shoes.

Professional Prep

DRESSING FOR SUCCESS
Whether or not a salon has a dress code or grooming policy, a stylist
should always look his or her best—and should fit in with the clientele. (If your clients are conservative, save your trendiest, most outrageous outfits and hairstyles for your days off.) If uniforms are
required by your salon, make sure yours is crisp and clean at all times.
A male stylist who wears a shirt and tie not only looks more professional, but can demand more money. Female stylists should wear
clean, run-free hose, and be sure their slips are not showing. Jewelry
should be simple and attractive.
All female stylists should have their hair done at least once a
week, and their hair should reflect the best workmanship of the
salon. Hair coloring should be encouraged, and if the salon specializes in wigs or other artificial hair, the stylists should wear them at
work. Male employees should have haircuts twice a month, in
attractive and moderate styles. They should shave every day, and if
they wear a beard it should be trimmed regularly.
Makeup should be worn by all female stylists, but in moderation.
Too much makeup is inappropriate in a work setting.
Shoes must be clean and neat at all times. Rundown heels are
very hard on the feet when standing all day. No one should be
allowed to work with dirty shoes.
—From Salon Management for Cosmetology Students
by Edward Tezak

almost anywhe...
matter, secreti...
the nails.
Bacteria can be seen only with the aid of a ***microscope*** (MEYE-
kroh-skohp). Fifteen hundred rod-shaped bacteria will barely
cover the head of a pin.

TYPES OF BACTERIA
There are hundreds of different kinds of bacteria. However, bacteria are classified into two types, depending on whether they are
beneficial or harmful.

1. Most bacteria are ***nonpathogenic*** (non-path-o-JEN-ik)
organisms (helpful or harmless), which perform many useful
functions, such as decomposing refuse and improving soil
fertility. ***Saprophytes*** (SAP-ro-fights), nonpathogenic bacteria, live on dead matter and do not produce disease.

Promo Power

SELLING PRODUCTS
It's important that you select items to sell in your salon with care.
Your professional reputation is on the line when you endorse a
product. A client won't purchase a product from you that she can
buy at a discount store; clients purchase products from a salon professional because they believe them to be superior to consumer
products—and because they trust you to sell them the product formulated for their type of hair.
The most successful way to build a booming retail business is to
train your employees to start selling from the moment a client is left
in their care. If that attitude prevails throughout the salon, the client
will be conditioned to buy home maintenance products specifically
for her type hair and skin.
Concentrate on an attractive visual presentation that is large and
highly visible. When people can pick up and examine items it almost
always results in sales. Frequently rotate and rearrange the items.
Everyone loves a bargain, so fill a special clearance basket with
small items, tie a pretty bow on the basket, and make every item in
the basket the same price. The profit will be less, but it will more
than make up the loss by stimulating buyer interest.
Every item must have prices clearly marked. Most people dislike
asking the price of anything.
—From Milady's Salon Solutions by Louise Cotter

PROMO POWER

The *Promo Power* sidebars help you in selling retail products to clients. Successful stylists know how important this is. Clients want to know what products to use to keep their hair and skin looking their best, and salon owners will tell you what a difference retail sales can make to the financial success of their business.

CAREER PATH

The *Career Path* sidebars present professional employment options open to you once you are a licensed cosmetologist. While some may require additional schooling, all stem from basic cosmetology training. You'll be surprised at what you will be qualified to do in addition to working in a salon.

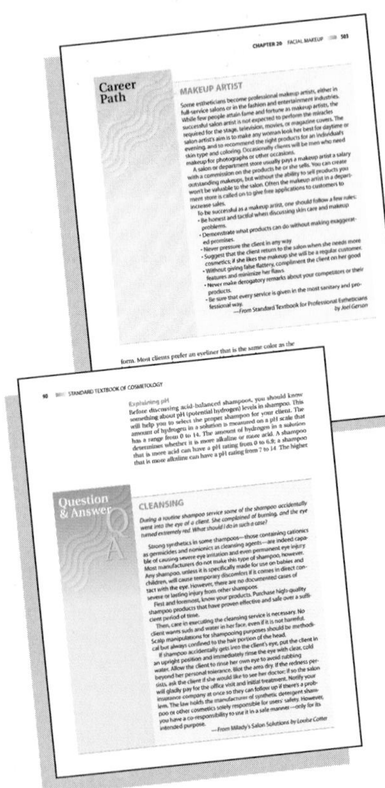

CHAPTER 20 FACIAL MAKEUP 503

Career Path

MAKEUP ARTIST
Some estheticians become professional makeup artists, either in
full-service salons or in the fashion and entertainment industries.
While few people attain fame and fortune as makeup artists, the
successful salon artist is not expected to perform the miracles
required for the stage, television, movies, or magazine covers. The
salon artist's aim is to make any woman look her best for daytime or
evening, and to recommend the right products for an individual's
skin type and coloring. Occasionally clients will be men who need
makeup for photographs or other occasions.
A salon or department store usually pays a makeup artist a salary
with a commission on the products he or she sells. You can create
outstanding makeups, but without the ability to sell products you
won't be valuable to the salon. Often the makeup artist in a department store is called on to give free applications to customers to
increase sales.
To be successful as a makeup artist, one should follow a few rules:
• Be honest and tactful when discussing skin care and makeup
problems.
• Demonstrate what products can do without making exaggerated promises.
• Never pressure the client in any way.
• Suggest that the client return to the salon when she needs more
cosmetics; if she likes the makeup she will be a regular customer.
• Without giving false flattery, compliment the client on her good
features and minimize her flaws.
• Never make derogatory remarks about your competitors or their
products.
• Be sure that every service is given in the most sanitary and professional way.
—From Standard Textbook for Professional Estheticians
by Joel Gerson

form. Most clients prefer an eyeliner that is the same color as the

90 STANDARD TEXTBOOK OF COSMETOLOGY

Explaining pH
Before discussing acid-balanced shampoos, you should know
something about pH (potential hydrogen) levels in shampoo. This
will help you to select the proper shampoo for your client. The
amount of hydrogen in a solution is measured on a pH scale that
has a range from 0 to 14. The amount of hydrogen in a solution
determines whether it is more alkaline or more acid. A shampoo
that is more acid can have a pH rating from 0 to 6.9; a shampoo
that is more alkaline can have a pH rating from 7 to 14. The higher

Question & Answer

CLEANSING
*During a routine shampoo service some of the shampoo accidentally
went into the eye of a client. She complained of burning, and the eye
turned extremely red. What should I do in such a case?*

Strong synthetics in some shampoos—those containing cationics
as germicides and nonionics as cleansing agents—are indeed capable of causing severe eye irritation and even permanent eye injury.
Most manufacturers do not make this type of shampoo, however.
Any shampoo, unless it is specifically made for use on babies and
children, will cause temporary discomfort if it comes in direct contact with the eye. However, there are no documented cases of
severe or lasting injury from other shampoos.
First and foremost, know your products. Purchase high-quality
shampoo products that have proven effective and safe over a sufficient period of time.
Then, care in executing the cleansing service is necessary. No
client wants suds and water in her face, even if it is not harmful.
Scalp manipulations for shampooing purposes should be methodical but always confined to the hair portion of the head.
If shampoo accidentally gets into the client's eye, put the client in
an upright position and immediately rinse the eye with clear, cold
water. Allow the client to rinse her own eye to avoid rubbing
beyond her personal tolerance. Blot the area dry. If the redness persists, ask the client if she would like to see her doctor; if so the salon
will gladly pay for the office visit and initial treatment. Notify your
insurance company at once so they can follow up if there's a problem. The law holds the manufacturer of synthetic detergent shampoo or other cosmetics solely responsible for users' safety. However,
you have a co-responsibility to use it in a safe manner—only for its
intended purpose.
—From Milady's Salon Solutions by Louise Cotter

QUESTION & ANSWER

The *Question & Answer* sidebars appear throughout the book and raise questions about the real-life application of the surrounding text. Topics range from what to do when shampoo gets into a client's eye to the best way to blow-dry long hair.

EXTENSIVE TEACHING/LEARNING PACKAGE

While the *Standard Textbook of Cosmetology* is the centerpiece of the program, Milady offers a wide range of supplements to aid students and educators in using it. All supplements have been revised and updated to complement the new edition of the textbook and new technology-delivered supplements have been added.

STUDENT SUPPLEMENTS

Theory Workbook

Designed to reinforce classroom and textbook learning, the *Theory Workbook* contains chapter-by-chapter exercises on theory subjects. Included are fill-in-the-blank exercises, multiple-choice questions, matching exercises, and labeling of illustrations, all coordinated with material from the text. Each workbook chapter begins with a study tip and ends with a list of vocabulary words from the corresponding textbook chapter. More than 30 pages of final review examinations to prepare students for testing are included at the end of the workbook.

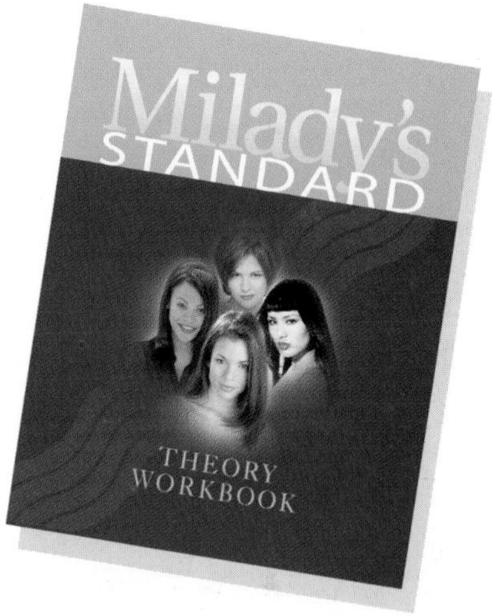

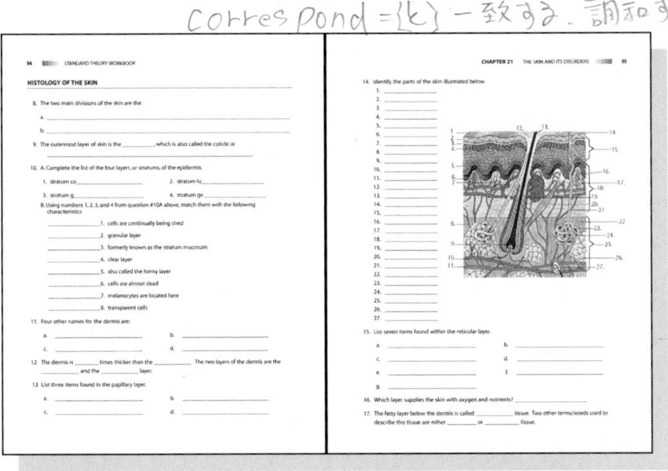
94 STANDARD THEORY WORKBOOK

HISTOLOGY OF THE SKIN

8. The two main divisions of the skin are the:
 a. ____
 b. ____
9. The outermost layer of skin is the ____, which is also called the cuticle or ____
10. A. Complete the list of the four layers, or stratums, of the epidermis.
 1. stratum co____ 2. stratum lu____
 3. stratum g____ 4. stratum ge____
 B. Using numbers 1, 2, 3, and 4 from question #10A above, match them with the following characteristics.
 ____ 1. cells are continually being shed
 ____ 2. granular layer
 ____ 3. formerly known as the stratum mucosum
 ____ 4. clear layer
 ____ 5. also called the horny layer
 ____ 6. cells are almost dead
 ____ 7. melanocytes are located here
 ____ 8. transparent cells
11. Four other names for the dermis are:
 a. ____ b. ____
 c. ____ d. ____
12. The dermis is ____ times thicker than the ____. The two layers of the dermis are the ____ and the ____ layer.
13. List three items found in the papillary layer.
 a. ____ b. ____
 c. ____ d. ____

CHAPTER 21 THE SKIN AND ITS DISORDERS 95

14. Identify the parts of the skin illustrated below.
 1. ____ through 27. ____
15. List seven items found within the reticular layer.
 a. ____ b. ____
 c. ____ d. ____
 e. ____ f. ____
 g. ____
16. Which layer supplies the skin with oxygen and nutrients? ____
17. The fatty layer below the dermis is called ____ tissue. Two other terms/words used to describe this tissue are either ____ or ____ tissue.

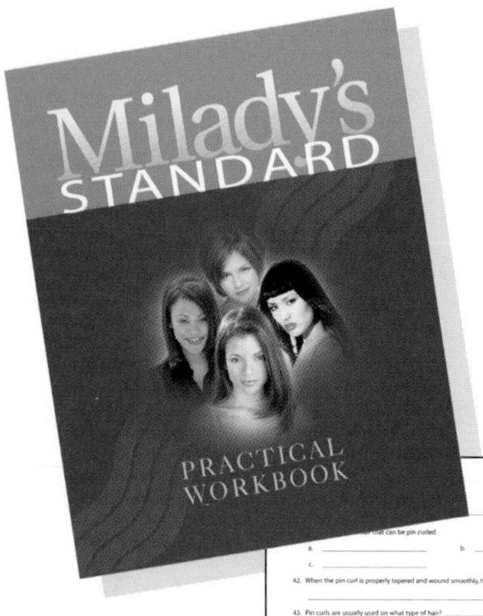

Practical Workbook

The 300-plus pages of the *Practical Workbook* help students to master the techniques, procedures, and product usage needed for licensure as covered in the textbook. Using fill-in-the-blank, matching, multiple-choice, and labeling exercises, students will benefit from the reinforcement of practical applications. Tests that emphasize essential facts and word reviews for each chapter are also included.

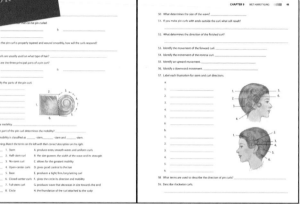

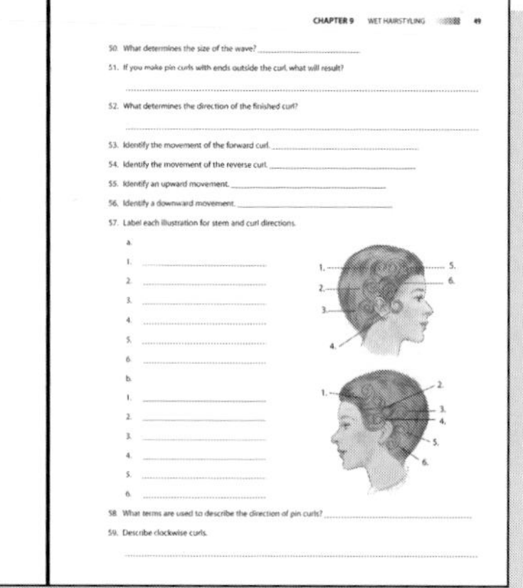

Exam Review

The *Exam Review* contains chapter-by-chapter questions in a multiple-choice format to help students prepare for the state board exam. While not intended to be the only form of review offered to students, it aids in overall classroom preparation. The *Exam Review* has been revised to eliminate obvious answers and give-away answers to other questions, making it more valuable for the student and the instructor. The questions in the *Exam Review* are for study purposes only and are not the exact questions students will see on the board exams.

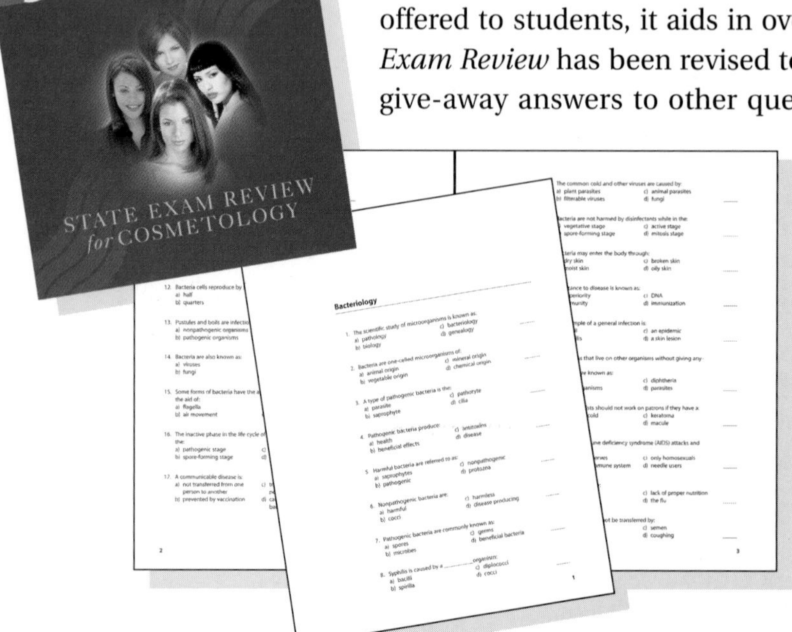

Milady's Standard Study Guide: The Essential Companion

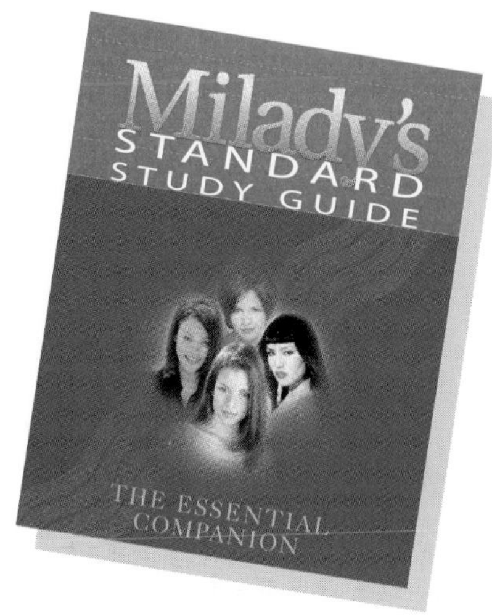

Milady's Standard Study Guide: The Essential Companion is designed to help students recognize, understand, and retain the key concepts presented in each chapter of the textbook. It provides six easy-to-follow features for each chapter—Essential Objectives, Essential Subjects, Essential Concepts, Essential Experiences, Essential Review, and Essential Notes—to enable students with various learning styles to comprehend and remember the important points and engage them in the theory and practical aspects so important to their licensing and professional success. Answers to *The Essential Companion* are supplied in *Milady's Standard Study Guide: The Essential Companion Answer Key.*

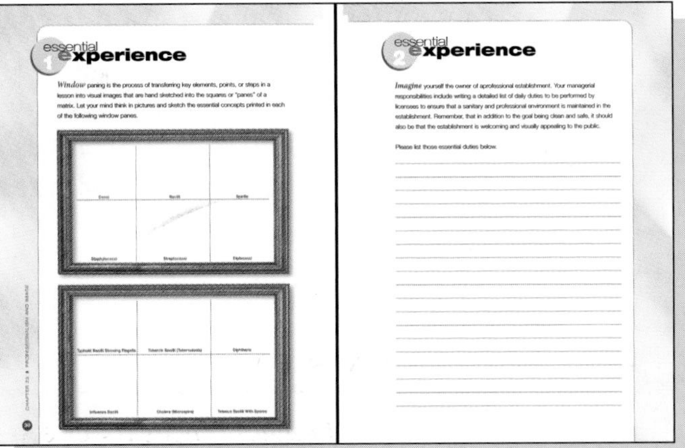

Milady's Standard Fundamentals of Cosmetology CD-ROM

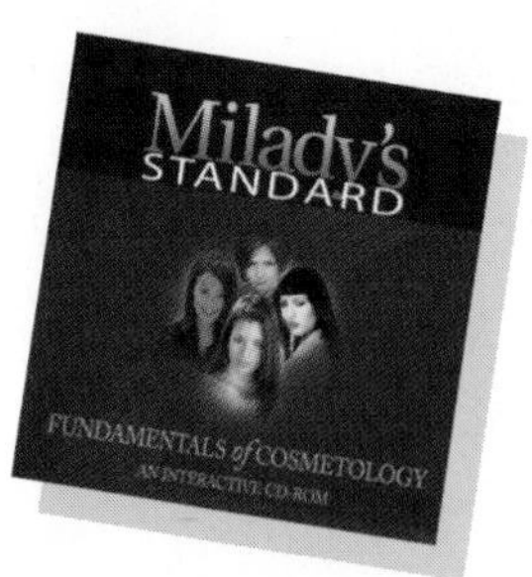

Milady's Standard Fundamentals of Cosmetology CD-ROM is an interactive student product designed to reinforce classroom learning, stimulate the imagination, and aid in preparation for board exams. Featuring more than 100 helpful video clips and graphical animations to demonstrate practices and procedures, it also contains a test bank with more than 1,300 chapter-by-chapter multiple-choice and matching questions to help students study for the exam. Other features are the game bank, which offers games to strengthen knowledge of terminology for each chapter, and a glossary that pronounces and defines each term.

ONLINE LEARNING TOOLS

Milady also offers online learning tools to make learning more interactive and help students study in a variety of different ways at any place and any time. All online tools can be previewed at www.MiladyOnline.com.

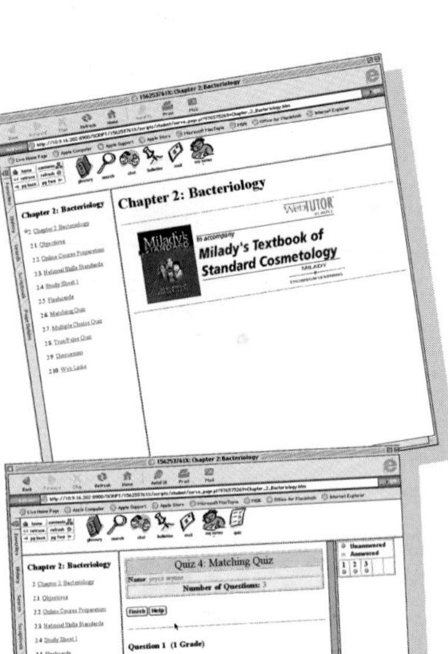

Milady's Standard Textbook of Cosmetology Web Tutor

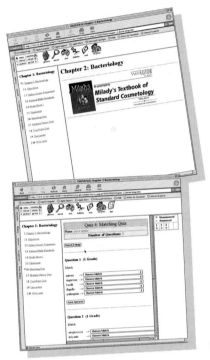

Designed to complement the textbook, *Milady's Standard Textbook of Cosmetology Web Tutor* is a content-rich, Web-based learning aid that reinforces and clarifies complex concepts. Web Tutor presents information in a new and different way, making it easier to understand as well as allowing easier management of time, progress checks, exam preparation, and organization of notes. Available on either the WebCT or Blackboard platform, it includes a course calendar, chat, e-mail, threaded discussions, and Web links, and offers objectives, study sheets, flashcards, discussion topics, three types of quizzes and more for each chapter.

Milady's Online Licensing Preparation: Cosmetology

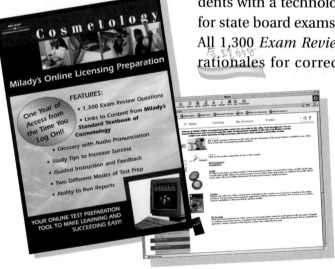

Milady's Online Licensing Preparation: Cosmetology provides students with a technology study alternative to better prepare them for state board exams, whether taken on a computer or on paper. All 1,300 *Exam Review* questions for cosmetology appear with rationales for correct and incorrect choices, and the correct answer links to the portion of the textbook in which the information is given. By using this tool, students will gain familiarity with a computerized test environment as they prepare for licensure.

EDUCATOR SUPPLEMENTS

Milady offers a full range of products created especially for cosmetology educators to make the classroom preparation and presentation simple, effective, and enjoyable.

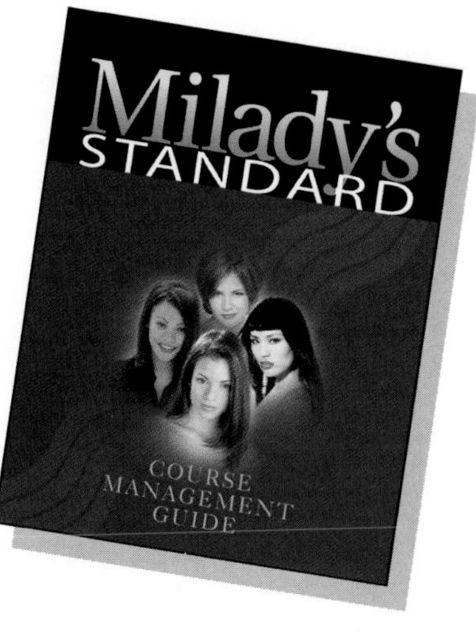

Course Management Guide (Printed Binder or CD-ROM)

Offered for the first time with this edition of the *Standard Textbook*, the *Course Management Guide* contains all the materials educators need in one three-ring binder or one CD-ROM. This innovative instructional guide is written with cosmetology educators in mind and is designed to make exceptional teaching easy. With formatting that provides easy-to-use material for use in the classroom, it will transform classroom management and dramatically increase student interest and understanding. Below are some of its many features:

Preface: Information on how to use this guide for more effective classes and improved student retention.

Lesson Plans: The lesson plans in the *Course Management Guide* are completely new and provide in-depth, comprehensive material for instructors to use in classroom presentations, written in a chapter-outline format that makes referencing the textbook easy. Lesson plans contain these features:

- Objectives
- Materials Needed
- Time Needed
- Prior Assignment
- Class Sign-in Sheet
- Learning Motivation
- In-Depth Notes (information to share during presentation)
- Teaching Tips
- Summary and Evaluation
- Learning Reinforcement Ideas and Activities
- Tests
- Transparencies
- Subject Outline (follows text)

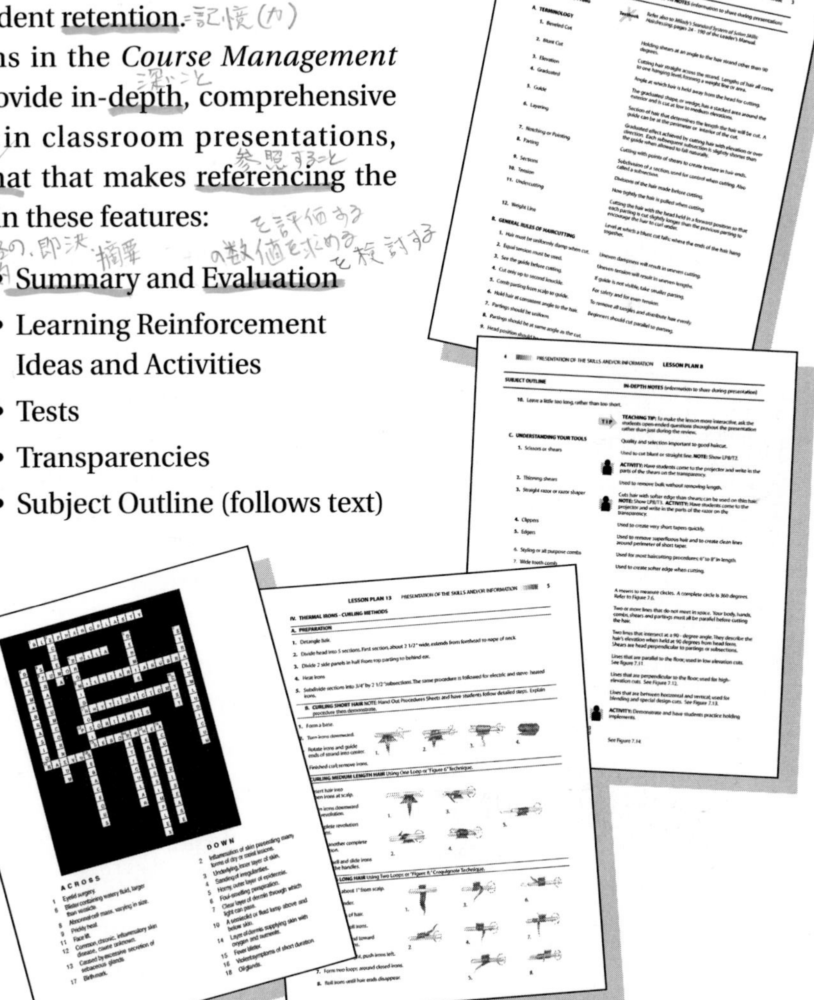

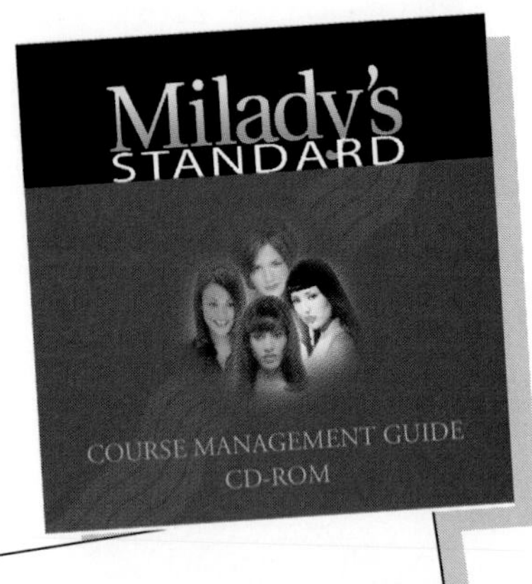

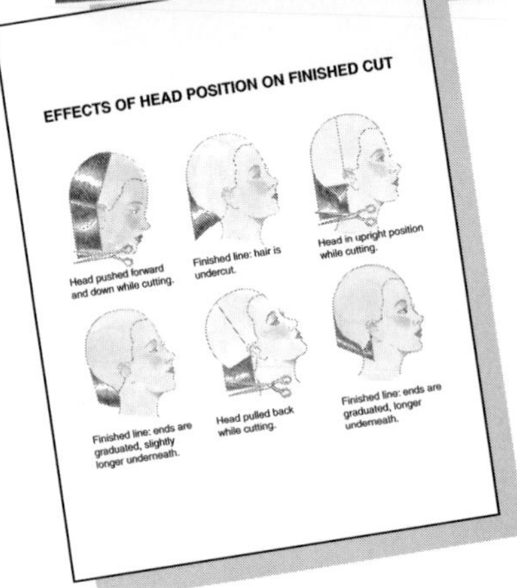

Workbook Answers: The answers to the *Theory Workbook* and *Practical Workbook* are included in this comprehensive new guide.

Resource Kit: A valuable store of transparencies, activities, and resources for educators to draw upon is included in this section of the *Course Management Guide*. Included are names, addresses, and Web sites for industry organizations and associations as well as the names of related books and magazines.

Added features you will find on the CD-ROM version:

- Every page from the *Course Management Guide* can be printed to appear exactly like the page from the printed binder:
- A Computerized Testbank contains all the *Exam Review* questions, which instructors can use to create random tests from a single chapter or the whole book, and answer keys are automatically created. A gradebook feature to track students' progress is also included.
- An Image Library of 500 photos and illustrations from the *Standard Textbook* can be added to PowerPoint presentations or printed onto paper or acetate for overheads. They can even be imported into other documents.

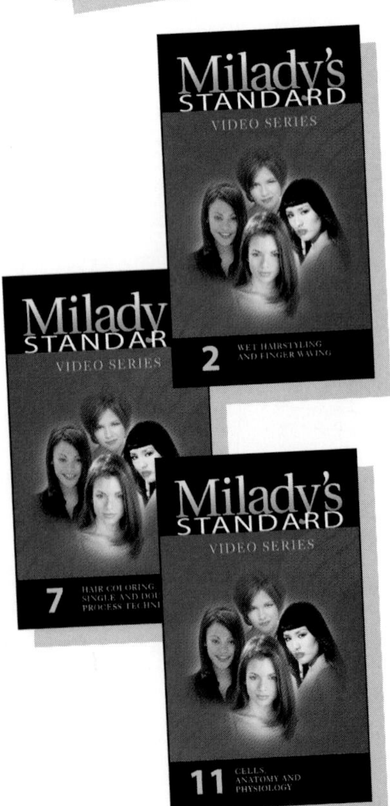

Video Series

The newly revised *Standard Videotape Series* contains twelve videos featuring complete coverage of the practical applications of the textbook. With new footage showing current styles and techniques, this series will enhance classroom learning and is essential for remedial work and individual learning. Tapes included are:

1 - Haircutting
2 - Wet Hairstyling
3 - Thermal Hairstyling and Thermal Hair Straightening
4 - Permanent Waving Theory and Techniques
5 - Chemical Hair Relaxing and Soft Curl Permanent
6 - Haircoloring Theory and Single-Process Technique
7 - Haircoloring: Double-Process Technique
8 - Manicuring and Pedicuring
9 - The Nail and Its Disorders
10 - The Skin and Its Disorders
11 - Facials and Makeup
12 - Cells, Anatomy, and Physiology; Chemistry

ACKNOWLEDGMENTS

Many cosmetologists and educators have contributed to the development of this book over the years since its initial publication in 1938. *Milady's Standard Textbook of Cosmetology* owes its creation to the lifetime dedication of Nicholas F. Cimaglia, founder of Milady Publishing Company. Mr. Cimaglia was also one of the founders of the National Association of Accredited Cosmetology Schools and the Teachers' Education Council, and helped form the National Accrediting Commission for Cosmetology Arts and Sciences.

The standard set by Mr. Cimaglia has been carried on in the beauty education industry by his son, Thomas Severance, and by two gentlemen whose tireless efforts have established the success of *Milady's Standard Textbook of Cosmetology*: Jacob Yahm, the father of accreditation in our industry and a driving force behind the National Interstate Council of State Boards of Cosmetology; and Arnold DeMille, founding editor of the *National Beauty School Journal* (now *Beauty Education*) and continuing education specialist.

Milady Publishing recognizes with gratitude and respect the many professionals who have offered their time to contribute to this edition of the *Standard Textbook*. The Adam Broderick Salon and Spa in Ridgefield, CT, was the setting for two important photo shoots. Colleen Hennessey and other staff members deserve our special thanks for their invaluable assistance, as does our photographer, Stephen Ciuccoli. The current staff of Milady surveyed many instructors as they shaped and refined this edition of the textbook. They held focus groups, solicited written critiques, and reviewed drafts of the book with industry experts. Milady Publishing wishes to extend enormous thanks to the following people who have played a part in this edition as well as previous editions:

Contributors to this edition

Brian Bartholomew
Pharmacia & Upjohn Company
Bridgewater, NJ

Gerri Cevetillo
Ultronics
Mahwah, NJ

Thia Spearing
Matrix Evaluation Salon
Solon, OH

Kenneth Young
Hot Heads Salon
Oklahoma City, OK

Reviewers of this edition

Gloria Andres
F.A.C.E.S.
Fremont, OH

Christy Collins
Michigan College of Beauty
Ida, MI

Jennifer Conley
Xenon International School of Hair Design
Wichita, KS

Linda Cottrell
Shampoo Academy of Hair
Oklahoma City, OK

R. DeMaio
Advanced Institute
Linden, NJ

Elaine Dock
Central Technical School
Drumright, OK

Carol Fugeve
Josef's School of Hair Design
Fargo, ND

Charlotte Henderson
Cannella School of Hair Design
Chicago, IL

Brenda Hildreth
Pawtucket School of Hair Design
Pawtucket, RI

Orie Hutchins
Santa Fe Community College
Sante Fe, NM

Ruth Ann Lewis
Maryland Community College
Spruce Pine, NC

Dr. Edward Tony Lloneau
Kizure Products
Compton, CA

Karen Marple
La James College
Iowa City, IA

Sharon Mawhorter
Hacienda La Puente Adult Education
City of Industry, CA

Julie Mead
EQ School of Hair Design
Omaha, NE

Lisa Miller
Mr. John's School of Cosmetology
Decatur, IL

Nancy Rapaport
Springfield Technical Community College
Springfield, IL

Carolyn Rigsby
Tri County Vocational School
Pleasant Shade, TN

Marilyn Sharp
Merrell University of Beauty
Jefferson City, MO

Phyllis Sippel
Trend Setters College of Cosmetology
Bradley, IL

Michael Vanacore
Learning Institute for Beauty Sciences
Brooklyn, NY

Mary Lou Williams
Transitions School of Cosmetology
Flint, MI

Reviewers of previous editions

Dr. Howard Adcock
Pizzaz Beauty School
Memphis, TN

Gary Ahlquist
Tensorlon
San Diego, CA

Kenneth Anders
Kenneth's Design Group
Columbus, OH

Jan Austin
Austin Beauty School
Albany, NY

Emma Ayala
Emma's Beauty School
Mayaguez, PR

Giselle Bahamonde
Austin Beauty School
Albany, NY

Linda Balhorn
Chicago, IL

Mark Beck
Cooperative Training Systems
Fort Collins, CO

Olive Lee Benson
Olive's
Boston, MA

Kathleen Bergant
Milwaukee Area Technical College
Milwaukee, WI

Karen Bilbo
Creative Hairdressers Inc.
Falls Church, VA

Charlotte Blanchard
Austin Beauty School
Albany, NY

Jan Bragulla
Creative Nail Design, Inc.
Carlsbad, CA

Doris Brantly
South Carolina State Board of Cosmetology
Columbia, SC

Ann Briggs
IHE Education Committee
Port Arthur, TX

Sam Brocato
Brocato International Lockworks USA
Baton Rouge, LA

Burmax Co.
Hauppauge, NY

Sheldon R. Chesky
Clarkson Valley, MO

Clairol/Logics
New York, NY

Margaret Clevinger
Columbine Beauty Schools
Wheatridge, CO

Denise Corbo
Manassas Park High School
Manassas Park, VA

Louise Cotter
Adrian Creative Images
Orlando, FL

Van Council
Van Michael Salon
Atlanta, GA

Isabel Cristina
Teaneck, NJ

Nina Curtis
International Dermal Institute
Marina del Rey, CA

Joseph Dallal, M.Sc.
Zotos International, Inc.
Darien, CT

Elizabeth Daniels
Total Beauty Enterprises
Hempstead, NY

Wendy Davis
DeKalb Beauty College
Stone Mountain, GA

Darla Del Duca
South Vocational Technical High School
Pittsburgh, PA

Michael Dick
Santa Cruz Beauty College
Santa Cruz, CA

Peggy Dietrick
Laredo Beauty School
Laredo, TX

Karen Donovan
Jean Madeline Education Center
Philadelphia, PA

Janice Dorian
Mansfield Beauty School
Quincy, MA

Nancy Dugan
Plastic Surgery Center
Montclair, NJ

Rosalyn Duncan
Debbie's School of Beauty Culture
Houston, TX

Leslie Edgerton
Nu-Tech Hair Salons
Fort Wayne, IN

Mary Eiring
Moraine Park Technical College
Fond Du Lac, WI

Frederick Ford
Career Beauty School
Florissant, MO

Wadad Frangie
Austin Beauty School
Albany, NY

Anne Fretto
Career Academy
Seal Beach, CA

Balmer Galindez
Bronx, NY

Ray Gambrell
South Carolina State Board of Cosmetology
Greenwood, SC

Linda Gately
IHE Education Committee
Tremont, PA

Lavonne Gearheardt
Ohio State Board of Cosmetology
Columbus, OH

Dennis Gebhardt
IHE Education Committee
Montclair, CA

Joel Gerson
New York, NY

Fino Gior
Advanced Electrolysis Center
Great Neck, NY

Pat Goins
Pat Goins Beauty School
Bossier City, LA

Jerry Gordon
J. Gordon Designs
Chicago, IL

Aurie Gosnell
National Interstate Council
Aiken, SC

Barbara Griggs
Creative Nail Design
Pasadena, MD

Darleen Hakola
IHE Education Committee
Portland, OR

Scheryl Hanson
Lancaster School of Cosmetology
Lancaster, PA

Victoria Harper
Kokomo, IN

Juanita Harris
International Beauty Schools
Cumberland, MD

Michael Hill
Arkansas State Board of Cosmetology
Fayetteville, AR

Linda Howe
Pittsburgh, PA

Harvey Huth
Albany, NY

International Haircolor Exchange
Haircolor Education Committee
Eagan, MN

Evelyn Irvine
Virginia Board for Cosmetology
Newport News, VA

Sandra Isaacs
Chino, CA

Charlote Jayne
Garland Drake International
Newport Beach, CA

Dan Jeans
Ritter/St. Paul Beauty College
St. Paul, MN

Glenda Jemison
Franklin Beauty Schools
Houston, TX

Michele Johnson
Tipton, MI

Jonathan R. Jones
Jean Madeline Education Center
Philadelphia, PA

Janit Kangas
South Carolina State Department of Education
Columbia, SC

Tama Kieves
Denver, CO

Lenny La Cour
Chicago, IL

Barbara Lane
Sheridan Vo-Tech
Hollywood, FL

Carole Laubach
San Jacinto College
Pasadena, TX

Dee Levin
IHE Education Committee
Philadelphia, PA

Linnea Lindquist
Minneapolis Technical College
St. Paul, MN

Dottie Lineberry
Chantilly High School Cosmetology Center
Chantilly, VA

Marc London
Pasadoula Beauty Acadeny
Moss Point, MS

L'Oreal
New York, NY

Rhonda Lyon
Gi Gi Laboratories
City of Commerce, CA

Rocky Lyons
Lyons Salons
Miami, FL

Charles Lynch
International Beauty School
Lancaster, PA

Lois Dorian Malconian
Mansfield Beauty School
Quincy, MA

Thomas Marks
Southern Nevada Vo-Tech
Las Vegas, NV

Cal Martini
IHE Education Committee
Phoenix, AZ

Thia Masciana
IHE Education Committee
Torrance, CA

Geri Mataya
Uptown Hair Design
Pittsburgh, PA

Adele McNiven
Kelowna, British Columbia

Victoria Melesko
Clairol Incorporated
New York, NY

Damien Miano
La Dolce Vita Salon
New York, NY

Carol Micciche
Lancaster Beauty School
Lancaster, PA

Lynn Mills
Don's Beauty School
San Mateo, CA

Beth Minardi
Carmine Minardi
Minardi Minardi Image Makers
New York, NY

Vincent and Alfred Nardi
Nardi Salon
New York, NY

Florence A. Neblett
National Institutes of Cosmetology
Washington, DC

Stanley K. Nielson
Sevier Valley Technical School
Richfield, UT

James K. Nighswander
Sangamon State University
Springfield, IL

Pat Nix
Indiana State Board of Cosmetology Examiners
Booneville, IN

André Nizetich
IHE Education Committee
San Pedro, CA

Debra Norton
Arkansas State Board of Cosmetology
Little Rock, AR

Patricia Oberhausen
Richland Northeast High School
Columbia, SC

Joe O'Riorden
East Coast Salon Owner's Association
Marlboro, MA

Larry Oskin
Marketing Solutions
Fairfax, VA

Mark Padgett
West Columbia, SC

Lynn Parentini
Esthetic Research Group
Long Island City, NY

Susan L. Peña
Reading, PA

Alfonso Peña-Ramos
Reading, PA

Carol Phillips
Herndon, VA

Stan Campbell Place
Maybelline
Gahana, OH

Renée Poignard
Kennesaw, GA

Patrick Poussard
Brooklyn, NY

Horst Rechelbacher
Aveda Corporation
Minneapolis, MN

Redken
Canoga Park, CA

Richard B. Rosenberg
RBR Productions Inc.
Teaneck, NJ

Tom Ross
Ohio State Board of Cosmetology
Columbus, OH

Thelma Ruffe, RN
Old Bridge, NJ

Margaret Ruffin
Derma-Clinic Academy of Skincare
Atlanta, GA

Sue Sansom
Arizona State Board of Cosmetology
Phoenix, AZ

Maura T. Scali-Snipes
Florida Community College
Jacksonville, FL

Douglas Schoon
Vista, CA

Nikki Schwartz
American Beauty Academy
Houston, TX

Schwarzkopf
Culver City, CA

Paul Scillia
Roman Academy of Beauty Culture
Hawthorne, NJ

Serge
Bruno Dessange
New York, NY

Joan Sesock
Austin Beauty School
Albany, NY

Keiko Shino
Garland Drake International
Newport Beach, CA

Lois Shirley
IHE Education Committee
Houston, TX

Gianni Siniscalchi
Gianni Hair and Skin Care
Montclair, NJ

Heather Slack
Arts of Nails and Beauty Academy
Winter Haven, FL

Tom Sollock
Hot Heads Salon
Oklahoma City, OK

Patricia Spencer
Riverside Community College
Riverside, CA

Rosemary Steffish
Lancaster Beauty School
Lancaster, PA

Judith Stewart
PJ's College of Cosmetology
Carmel, IN

Michael Stinchcomb
Yves Claude Salon
New York, NY

Jack Storey
Scruples Inc.
Lakeville, MN

Stephanie Tebow
Pro-Tech College
Carterville, IL

Edward Tezak
Warren Occupational Technical Center
Golden, CO

The Wella Corporation
Englewood, NJ

Alma Tilghman
North Carolina State Board of Cosmetology
Beaufort, NC

Veda Traylor
Arkansas State Board of Cosmetology
Mayflower, AR

Peggy Turbyfill
Mike's Barber and Beauty Salon
Hot Springs, AR

Judy Ventura
North Providence, RI

Martha Weller
University of New Mexico–Gallup
Gallup, NM

A. Dan Whitley
Sangamon State University
Springfield, IL

Lois Wiskur
South Dakota Cosmetology Commission
Pierre, SD

Sheila Zaricor
IHE Education Committee
Memphis, TN

Arnold Zegarelli
Zegarelli Inc.
Pittsburgh, PA

Zotos Corporation
Darien, CT

Introduction

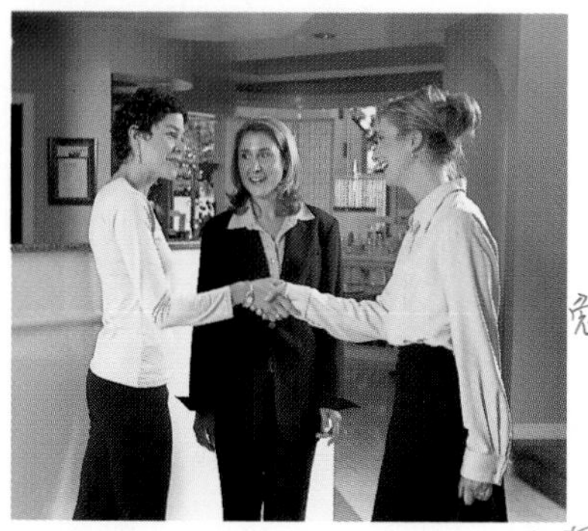

Welcome to the cosmetology profession.

Here you are at the threshold of opportunity. You have a chance for glamour, excitement, and other untold rewards. Welcome to the world of cosmetology! Apply yourself and there are no limits to the possibilities. Your license to practice cosmetology is an unlimited passport to the world.

Whether you like working with hair, skin, or nails, your certification provides you with the opportunity to select a career path to suit you. To get the most out of your passport, make the most of your education. Every lesson has something to teach you, something that may start you on your way. Your license unlocks countless doors, but it is what *you learn* that can really launch your career.

THE WORLD OF COSMETOLOGY

As you begin your journey, you may not know whether you prefer working with hair, skin, or nails. Even if you do have something in mind, leave yourself open to other possibilities. Let your learning guide you. Enter each classroom with an open mind and a wholehearted desire to learn as much as you can.

Some of the most well-known people in the beauty world began just as you are beginning. A broad beauty education gave them the chance to enthusiastically explore different avenues of cosmetology until they found the path that suited them. Why not give yourself that chance as well? You have so many possibilities. Here are just some of the many vocations that you may be tempted to try upon graduation. No matter what area interests you, take the time to read the following sections. Each one has helpful information suggested by some of the most accomplished professionals in the beauty world today.

MAKEUP ARTIST

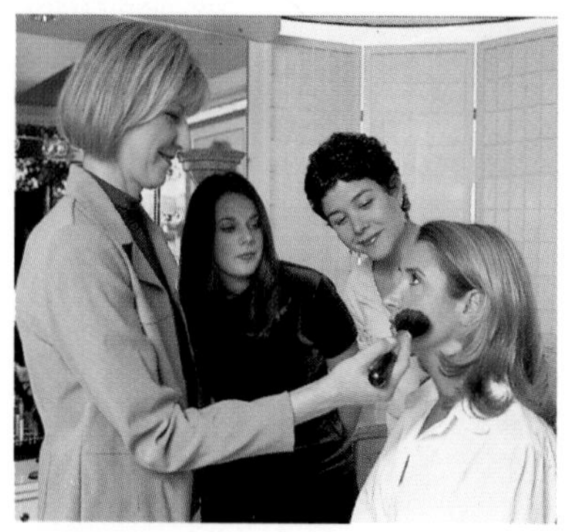

Makeup artist.

Are you artistically inclined? Do you like blending, shading, creating? A makeup artist "paints faces," explains one top artist in the field. "He or she brings out beauty without making it look like a disguise." Makeup artists most frequently apply cosmetics to enhance a client's appearance, but they can create *any* image a particular job calls for.

As a makeup artist, you can establish yourself in a salon with a private clientele, become makeup director for a prestigious department store, represent a line of cosmetics, work in television and movie production, find a position with a fashion magazine, or work behind the scenes in theater production. You can operate as an independent freelancer, which allows you to create your own schedule, or you can find full-time employment with one company.

Advice from the Experts

"Makeup artistry is so much more than just fashion and taste. It's a lot of training," advises a top talent in the field. "If you don't learn as much as you can, eventually it corners you." Pay strict attention in *all* your classes. Concentrate on chemistry and anatomy.

After beauty school, consider continuing your education in the fine arts, with an emphasis on drawing and painting courses. Theater experience will also prove helpful, especially a study of stage lighting.

Work in a salon for at least six months after school. Consider volunteering your services to community theaters, fashion shows, and department stores in your area. Volunteer work will afford you experience and help you build a resume as well as contacts, that is, people you meet who may be important to your career. Start to develop a portfolio that you can present to potential employers. In this portfolio, compile before and after photographs of makeovers you have performed, along with any awards or certificates you may have earned.

SKIN CARE SPECIALIST/ESTHETICIAN

Are you drawn by the allure of a radiant complexion and the secrets of different creams and lotions? An ***esthetician*** offers treatments to perfect the look and health of skin.

As an esthetician you can work in a salon, teach, travel throughout the world giving demonstrations at beauty shows, or become a consultant to a cosmetic company. You can work exclusively for one company or you can be a freelancer.

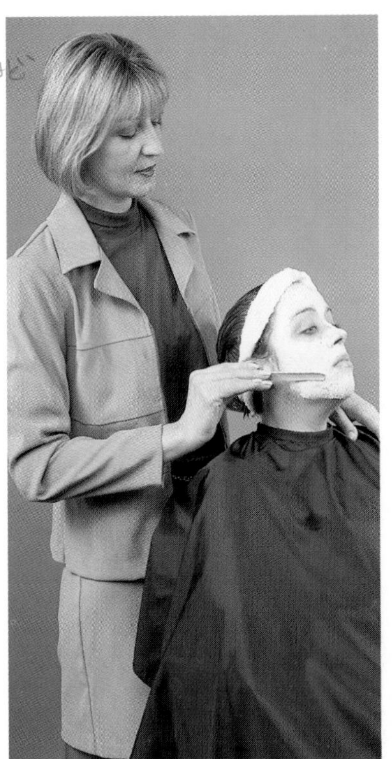

Skin care specialist/esthetician.

Advice from the Experts

Consider attending a beauty school that specializes in or emphasizes facial treatments. "Devote yourself to your training," advises an esthetician who lectures worldwide. "It's such a short training period and once you start work, it's difficult to get away to take classes."

Read as much as you can about skin care. "Since I was always reading, I could sound authoritative when I spoke to clients," continues the skin care expert. Attend seminars where you can meet and learn from the specialists in your area of interest. Subscribe to professional publications that list events and classes you can participate in to supplement your education. Study the different skin care products on the market so that you understand what they are supposed to do and how you can use them.

COSMETIC CHEMIST

Are you curious and creative? Do you like experimenting? Cosmetic chemists supply the beauty world's expanding needs by creating new products through research and experimentation. "Every business has its tools," explains one cosmetic chemist. "I help make the tools that cosmetologists use." He continues, "I get a profile from the marketing company that shows what type of product they want to market. Then I go through my mental and physical library to bring together that product."

As a cosmetic chemist you can work for a cosmetic manufacturer or become a consultant to several companies.

Advice from the Experts

Learn everything you can in cosmetology school. "I draw from everything I've studied," confirms one highly paid cosmetic chemist. Pay close attention to your marketing courses. An understanding of the commercial marketplace will help to direct your scientific exploration. It is also important to acquire a chemistry education in addition to what you learn in beauty school. You should consider continuing your education in a college.

After completing your schooling, apply for an internship with a cosmetic company working on a panel that studies new products. If you can't get into a company this way, apply for a position in the manufacturer's marketing department.

PUBLISHING

Do you like to write? You can use your cosmetology license to enter the publishing world. With a beauty background, you can write articles, books, brochures, columns, educational manuals—even produce videos. "You get to wear the latest, trendiest hairstyles, clothes, and accessories *and* you get to do what you love," says one cosmetologist turned beauty writer.

As a writer with a cosmetology license, you can work for a publishing company, freelance, travel and review major beauty shows, or develop a lifestyle that combines it all.

Advice from the Experts

Master the technical basics of cosmetology. "You need to really understand *why* a certain procedure works better in order to write about it," explains one cosmetology editor with a major publishing firm. "It's a way to open doors. Then, you can go on to let your creativity out."

Fine-tune your writing skills by taking writing courses and reading as much as possible to see how things are written.

Keep current with what's happening in your industry by attending seminars. "You can use this knowledge to determine what to write, because you'll know what's needed," advises the publishing expert. "Be up on the latest information because you can bet your audience will be."

Practice networking; create contacts by being open and friendly with other people. These contacts might have a hot tip for you or remember your name when a position opens.

HAIRCOLORIST

Do you have an exacting eye for pigment? Do flattering shades jump out at you? A haircolorist picks out the best color and process to enhance a client's hair. The colorist mixes the dye, applies it, and evaluates the resulting shade.

"Haircoloring is such a creative part of the industry," says one noted haircolorist. "There's so many different ways to arrive at a color. It's not like haircutting where there's only one way."

As a haircolorist you can establish a specialized color department within a salon, become a color trainer (teaching at salons), work for a haircolor manufacturer, or become a ***platform artist***, demonstrating your technique at national and international shows.

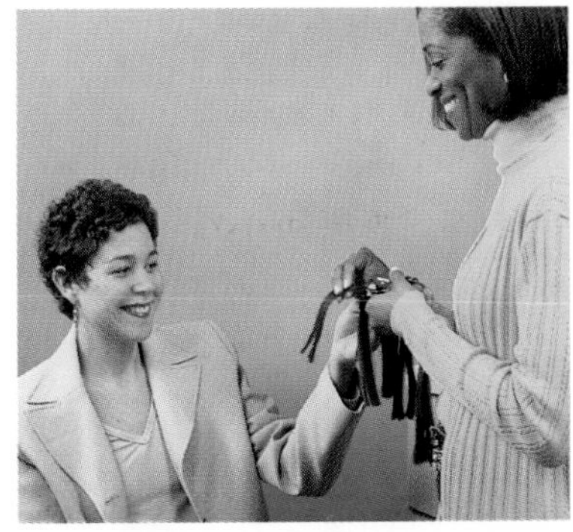

Haircolorist.

Advice from the Experts

Persevere and pay attention in beauty school. Take advantage of opportunities to work with your teachers. For example, ask if you can assist with a coloring. Observe other teachers or students doing color as often as you can. Attend classes and shows in your area. Most important, keep practicing. "Don't be afraid to make mistakes," advises one haircolorist. "You're going to make mistakes. It's the first ten thousand that are the toughest. Just keep going."

SALON OWNER

Do you have great ideas for how things *should* be done? Do you like varied responsibilities and challenges? Running your own salon allows you to set a standard for the quality of service you bring to the marketplace. You can choose the products and services to provide, and establish the level of skill you demand from your staff. You can exercise creativity, versatility, and independence in this position if you don't mind making decisions and putting in long hours.

Advice from the Experts

In beauty school you must learn everything you possibly can, paying particular attention to sales courses. When you graduate, take a job as a cosmetologist. "Never come right out and own a salon," says one salon owner of eighteen years. "A school environment is totally different from a salon. You absolutely need to work for a while first."

Owning a salon means assuming responsibility for paying bills, payrolls, and taxes as much as it means doing nails and giving haircuts and perms. You must develop business skills beyond what you learn in beauty school. Attend college business classes or seminars. You might even want to attend business school. You should also contact your local small business bureau and obtain literature about businesses in your area. Talk to local salon owners and learn what you can from their experience.

In addition to business expertise, you need people skills to run a salon. You will be in the public's eye and you will be managing a staff of employees. Take some courses that build upon your social skills and suggest successful techniques for resolving conflicts.

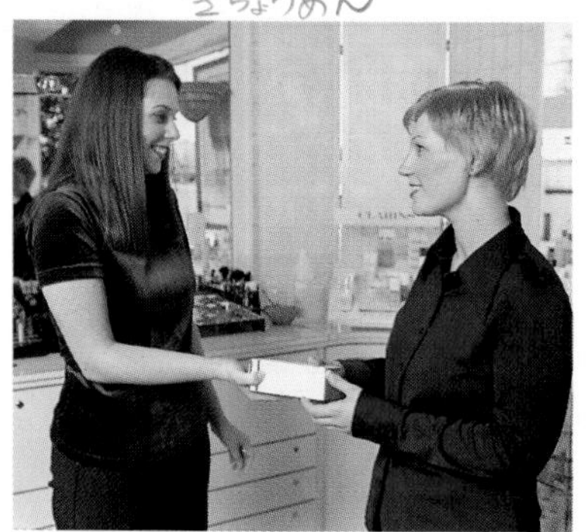

Retail specialist.

RETAIL SPECIALIST

Do you have a flair for selling? Do you communicate well and enjoy working with people? With a cosmetology license, you can become a retail specialist working with salons and manufacturers to promote their products' sales. "Retailing is nothing more than good communication," explains one retail specialist who lectures nationwide. "All you need to do is understand people enough to sell your product, your service, and yourself."

As a retail specialist, you can work in a salon, spa, or department store as a product manager handling the merchandising of inventory. Retail specialists also work as trainers, honing the sales techniques of a particular cosmetic company, or traveling throughout the country presenting general sales seminars. "Being a retail specialist is a great security," advises a self-made retail specialist. "Even as a stylist, every salon will want to hire you. You know a lot about sales, and salons today have to focus on sales."

Advice from the Experts

Get the best technological understanding you can at beauty school. To really sell a product, you need to know how to work with it and why it stands out as a product you recommend.

Work for a salon after beauty school. Time "in the trenches" gives you the experience you will need to market yourself to companies as an authority whom they can trust. Read about selling strategies. Spend time observing people. "If you don't understand people, you don't understand the business," advises one retail specialist, who recommends drawing from past work experience and practicing people skills daily.

COMPETITION CHAMPION

Are you a perfectionist? Do you get excited working toward a goal and winning? Competition champions compete for prizes and prestige in various cosmetology world championships. Here, "the best" display their individual talents and techniques. You must have dedication, good work habits, and utmost skill to enter this honored realm that holds so many rewards.

"The commitment reflects on your everyday lifestyle," explains one champion who has competed for years. "As you train to be a winner, you bring back that attitude to the salon. You have no limit to what you can do."

Competition champions often establish their own salons. Their reputation as distinguished artists attracts a following and adds to the prosperity of their business endeavors. Champions can also work as trainers, coaching the next generation of competitors.

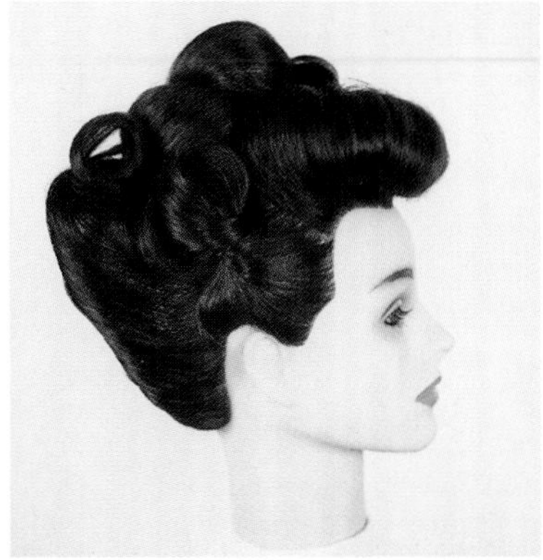

Competition winner.

Advice from the Experts

In beauty school, make sure you cultivate your styling skills as perfectly as possible. Pay close attention to details. Make sure everything is balanced and immaculate. "Your combing should be spotless," advises one champion who now trains competitors. "Walk around the client and look at your work from different angles."

To enter competitions, you may need to hire a world champion trainer, spend time creating and perfecting your skills, and search for the right model. But for those dedicated to the path, the reward can be exhilaration and prestige.

EDUCATIONAL SPECIALIST

Do you like to teach? Do you enjoy seeing people grasp new information? The beauty industry abounds in teaching opportunities. For example, an educational consultant who works for a product manufacturer might conduct seminars for a salon staff, demonstrating how to use various products. Other consultants work for manufacturers of ingredients that are sold to cosmetic companies. They give presentations to the marketing departments of cosmetic companies to demonstrate how an ingredient can improve or enhance a product.

Other educational specialists write curriculums and training manuals that teach consultants to teach. As an educational specialist, you might work for a major manufacturer or travel around the country training industry professionals to teach.

Advice from the Experts

Concentrate on all your courses in beauty school. "All skills become cumulative," explains one educational specialist on board with a major manufacturer. "You may not like to do manicures, but it's always another skill you can pose to an employer to get your foot in the door of a job you want." Since marketing goes hand in hand with the educational specialist's objectives, consider adding some business courses to your training.

Yet another way to begin your career is by working in a major department store training sales clerks to demonstrate and sell

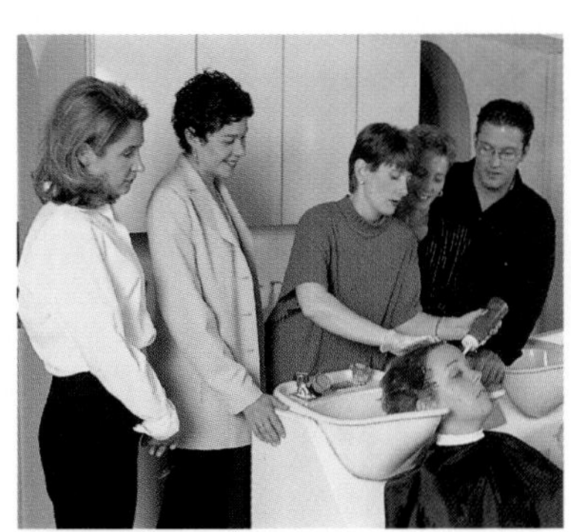

Educator.

cosmetics. Then, prepare your resume and mail it to every manufacturer you can think of, outlining your skills, experience, and the type of position you are seeking.

The list of career opportunities is endless. The beauty industry continues to grow in order to accommodate the vivid imaginations and abilities of the artists. Welcome to this wonderful world of possibilities where, if you can imagine your ideal career, with a little perseverance, you can probably spend your life doing it!

CHAPTER 1

Your Professional Image

LEARNING OBJECTIVES

After completing this chapter, you should be able to:

1. Demonstrate guidelines to maintain a healthy body and mind.
2. List the qualities of effective physical presentation.
3. Define personality.
4. List the qualities of effective communication.
5. Demonstrate good human relations and a professional attitude.
6. Define professional ethics.

NATIONAL SKILL STANDARDS

This chapter provides you with the necessary information to master these National Industry Skill Standards for Entry-Level Cosmetologists:

- Using appropriate methods to insure personal health and well-being
- Consulting with clients to determine their needs and preferences
- Interacting effectively with co-workers as part of a team
- Taking necessary steps to develop and retain clients

INTRODUCTION

Good health is a basic element for living. Without it, one cannot work efficiently or enjoy the pleasures of life. As a cosmetologist, you should be a living example of good health so that you increase your value to yourself, to your employer, and to the community.

YOUR PERSONAL AND PROFESSIONAL HEALTH

To be a successful cosmetologist, you should follow a set of guidelines to help you maintain a healthy body and mind.

REST

Adequate sleep is essential for good health. Without it you cannot function efficiently. The body should be allowed to recover from the fatigue of the day's activities and should be replenished with a good night's sleep. The amount of sleep needed to feel refreshed varies from person to person. Some people function well with 6 hours of sleep; others need 8 hours.

EXERCISE

Exercise ensures the proper functioning of organs such as the heart and lungs, strengthens muscles and bones, and improves circulation. An adequate fitness program includes exercises to accomplish aerobic strength, flexibility, and endurance.

RELAXATION

Relaxation is important as a change of pace from your day-to-day routine. Going to a movie or a museum, reading a book, watching television, or dancing are ways for you to "get away from it all." When you return to work, you will feel refreshed and eager to attend to your duties.

NUTRITION

What you eat affects your health, appearance, personality, and performance on the job. The nutrients in food supply the body with energy and ensure proper body functions. A balanced diet should include a variety of foods so that you obtain important vitamins and minerals. Drink plenty of water daily. Try to avoid sugar, salt, caffeine, and fatty or highly refined and processed foods and "fast" foods.

PERSONAL HYGIENE

Personal hygiene is the daily maintenance of cleanliness and healthfulness. The basics include daily bathing or showering, using deodorant, brushing your teeth and using mouthwash to freshen your breath during the day, and having clean and well-groomed hair and nails.

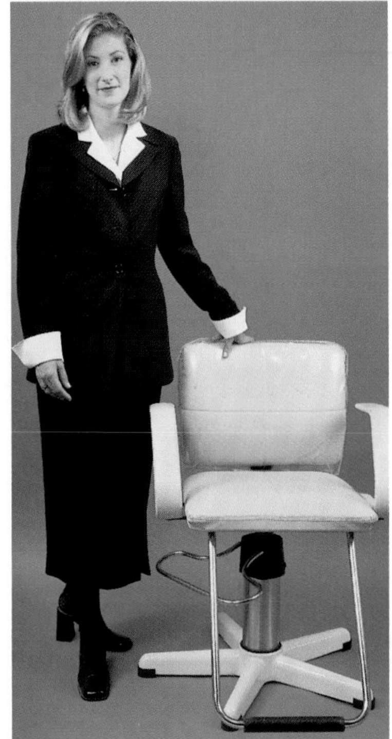

FIGURE 1.1 — A well-groomed female cosmetologist.

PERSONAL GROOMING

Personal grooming is an extension of personal hygiene. A well-groomed cosmetologist is one of the best advertisements for a salon. If you present a poised and attractive image, your client will have confidence in you as a professional. Many salon owners and managers consider appearance, personality, and poise to be as important as technical knowledge and manual skills. To begin, wear fresh undergarments daily and a freshly laundered, well-tailored uniform. Some salons do not require standard uniforms, but they may have a specific dress code. For example, some salons require that all their personnel wear the same color clothing. Select your outfits so that you reflect the image of the salon. Avoid obtrusive or excessive jewelry. A wristwatch will help you keep to your schedule.

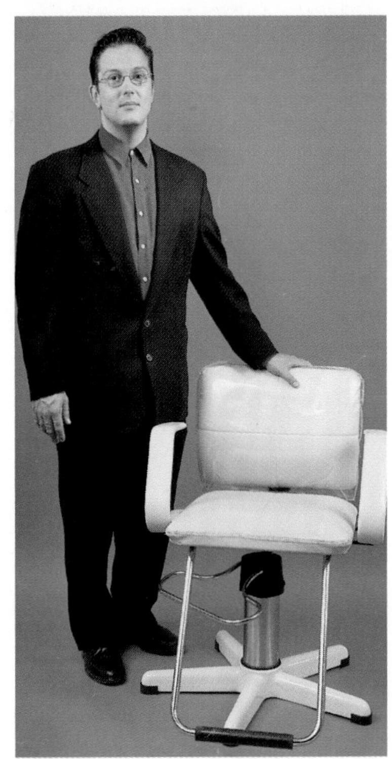

FIGURE 1.2 — A well-groomed male cosmetologist.

The Female Cosmetologist

The female cosmetologist should wear stylish shoes that fit and are still comfortable at the end of a long day. Your makeup should be flattering and suited to the environment of your salon. (Fig. 1.1)

The Male Cosmetologist

In addition to the general guidelines discussed, the male cosmetologist should keep facial hair neatly trimmed and groomed. (Fig. 1.2)

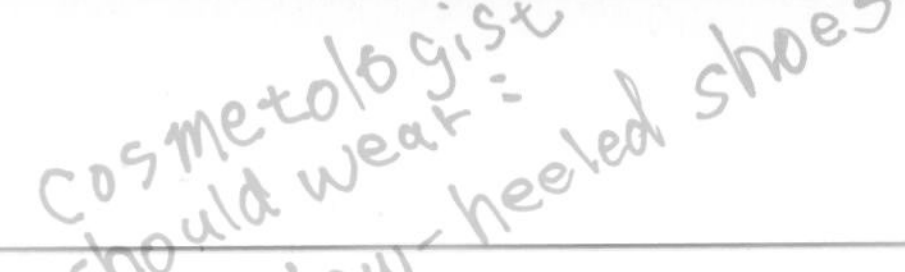

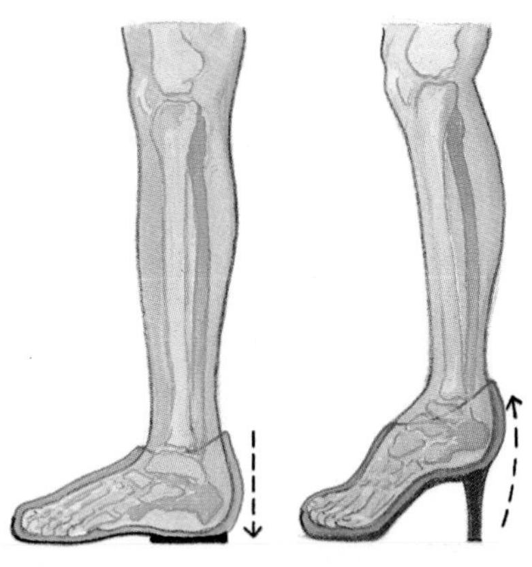

FIGURE 1.3 — For comfort and to help maintain good posture, wear well-fitted, low-heeled shoes.

CARE OF THE FEET

As a cosmetologist you will spend a great deal of time on your feet. Proper foot care will help you maintain a good posture and a cheerful attitude. Sore feet or poor-fitting shoes can cause great discomfort. (Fig. 1.3)

Shoes

Try to wear shoes with low, broad heels and with cushioned insoles. They give you support and balance, which help to maintain good posture and offset fatigue that can result from hours of standing. It also helps if you can stand on a carpeted or cushioned surface.

Daily Foot Care

After bathing, apply cream or oil and massage each foot for 5 minutes. Remove the cream or oil and apply an antiseptic foot lotion. Regular pedicures that include cleansing, removal of calloused skin, massage, and toenail trims will keep your feet at their best.

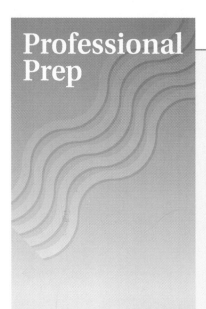

DRESSING FOR SUCCESS

Whether or not a salon has a dress code or grooming policy, a stylist should always look his or her best—and should fit in with the clientele. (If your clients are conservative, save your trendiest, most outrageous outfits and hairstyles for your days off.) If uniforms are required by your salon, make sure yours is crisp and clean at all times.

A male stylist who wears a shirt and tie not only looks more professional, but can demand more money. Female stylists should wear clean, run-free hose, and be sure their slips are not showing. Jewelry should be simple and attractive.

All female stylists should have their hair done at least once a week, and their hair should reflect the best workmanship of the salon. Hair coloring should be encouraged, and if the salon specializes in wigs or other artificial hair, the stylists should wear them at work. Male employees should have haircuts twice a month, in attractive and moderate styles. They should shave every day, and if they wear a beard it should be trimmed regularly.

Makeup should be worn by all female stylists, but in moderation. Too much makeup is inappropriate in a work setting.

Shoes must be clean and neat at all times. Rundown heels are very hard on the feet when standing all day. No one should be allowed to work with dirty shoes.

—*From* Salon Management for Cosmetology Students
by Edward Tezak

When your feet ache, podiatrists recommend that you soak your feet alternately in warm and cool water. See a podiatrist if corns, bunions, ingrown toenails, or other foot disorders exist.

HEALTHY LIFESTYLE

You should practice stress management through relaxation, rest, and exercise and avoid substances that can negatively affect your good health, such as cigarettes, alcohol, and drugs.

Completed: Learning Objective #1

MAINTAINING A HEALTHY BODY AND MIND

PHYSICAL PRESENTATION

Your posture, walk, and movements all make up your physical presentation. People form opinions about you by the way you present yourself. Do you stand straight or slouch; do you walk confidently or do you drag your feet? Your physical presentation is part of your professional image.

GOOD POSTURE

Good posture not only improves your personal appearance by presenting your figure to advantage and creating an image of confidence, it also prevents fatigue and many other physical problems. (Figs. 1.4, 1.5) Because you will be spending most of your time on your feet when working as a professional cosmetologist, good posture should be developed as early as possible through regular exercise and self-discipline.

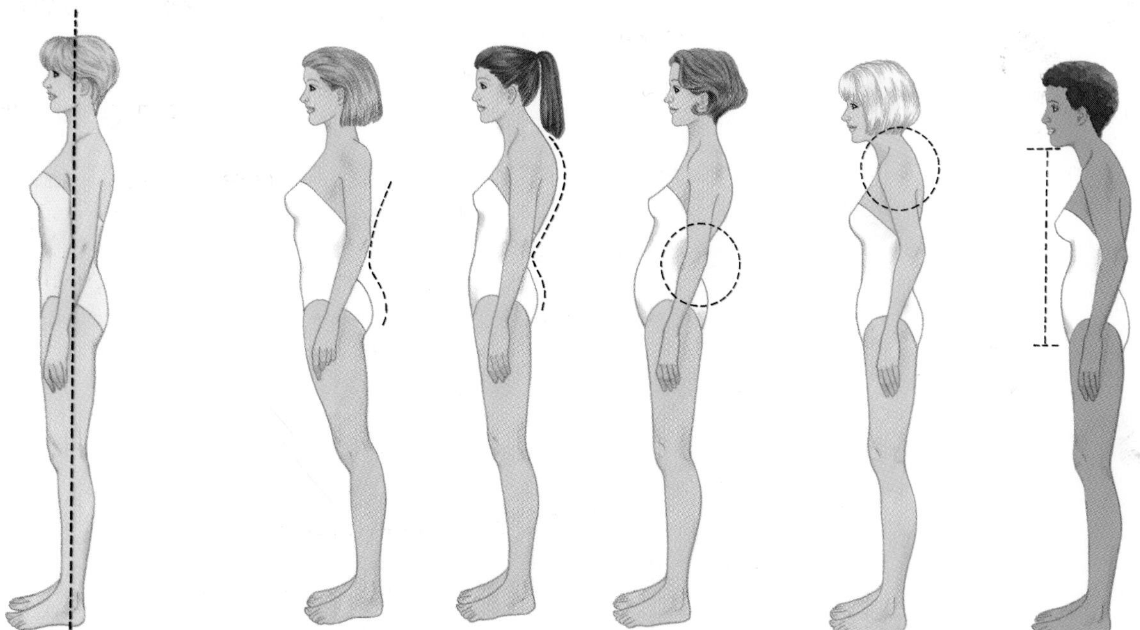

FIGURE 1.4 — Good posture.

FIGURE 1.5 — Five defective body postures.

PHYSICAL PRESENTATION ON THE JOB

To prevent muscle aches, back strain, discomfort, fatigue, and other problems and to maintain an attractive image, it is very important to practice good physical presentation while performing work activities. (Figs. 1.6, 1.7)

Checkpoints of Good Posture

- Crown of head reaching upward while chin is kept level with the floor.
- Neck is elongated and balanced directly above the shoulders.
- Chest up; body is lifted from the breastbone.
- Shoulders are level, held back and down, yet relaxed.
- Spine is straight, not curved laterally or swayed from front to back.
- Abdomen is flat.
- Hips are level (horizontally) and protrude neither forward nor back.
- Knees are slightly flexed and positioned directly over the feet with the ankles firm.

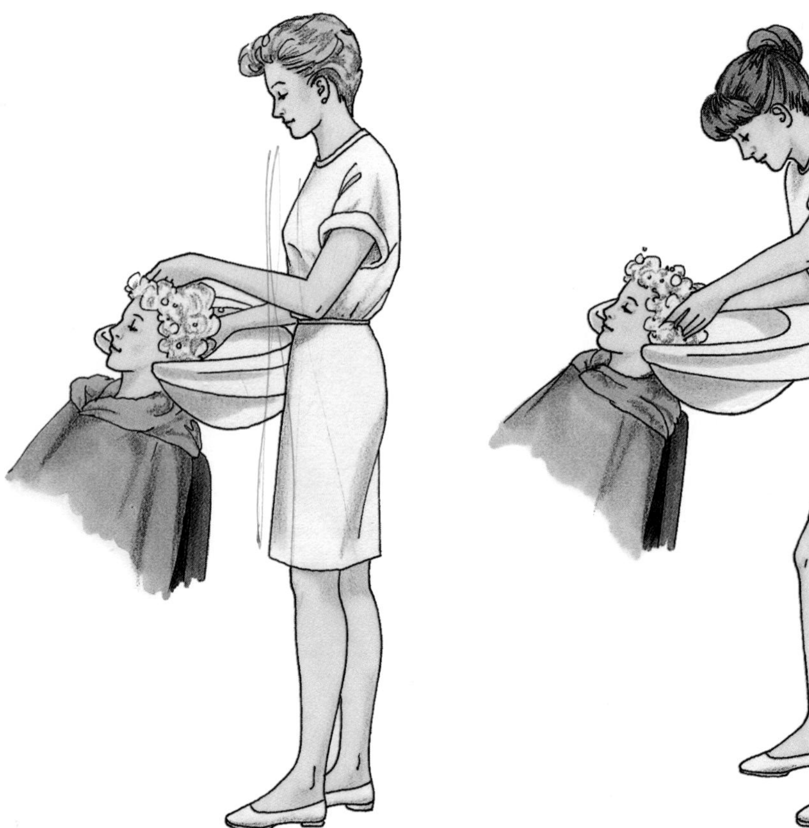

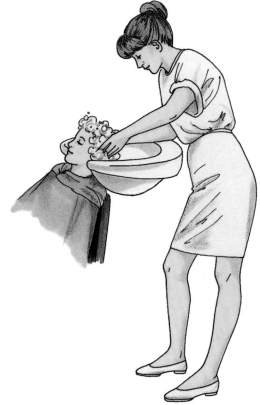

FIGURE 1.6 — To avoid back strain, maintain good posture when giving a shampoo.

FIGURE 1.7 — Poor posture.

Basic Stance for Women

- Place most of your weight on your right foot and point your toes straight ahead in a straight line.
- Place your left heel close to the heel or instep of your right foot and point the toes slightly outward.
- Bend your left knee slightly inward. (Fig. 1.8)

Basic Stance for Men

- Place your feet apart, but not wider than your shoulder width.
- Distribute your weight evenly over both feet.
- Your knees should be neither rigid nor bent.
- Your toes should point straight ahead or one or both feet should point slightly outward.
- For a more relaxed stance, bend one knee slightly while shifting some of your weight to the opposite foot. (Fig. 1.9)

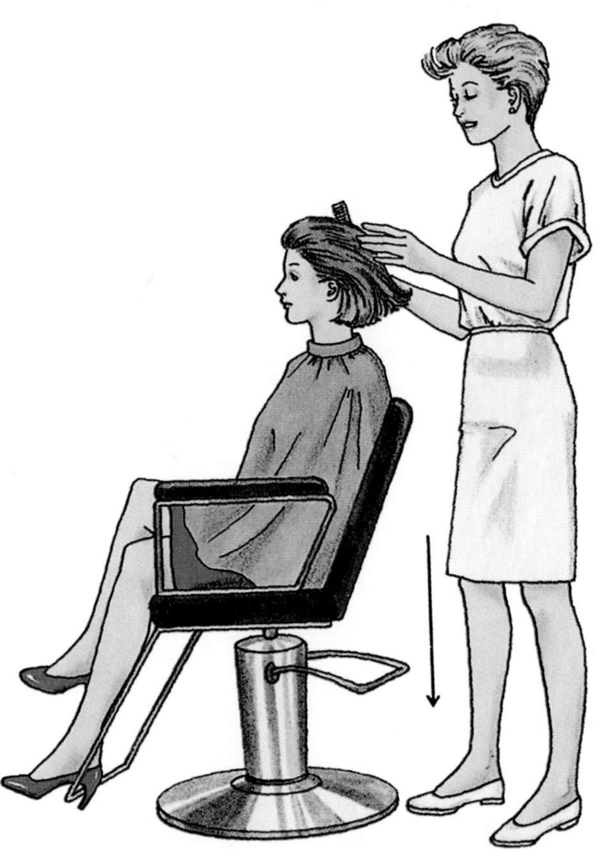

FIGURE 1.8 — Basic stance for the female cosmetologist, and the correct chair position for working on a client comfortably.

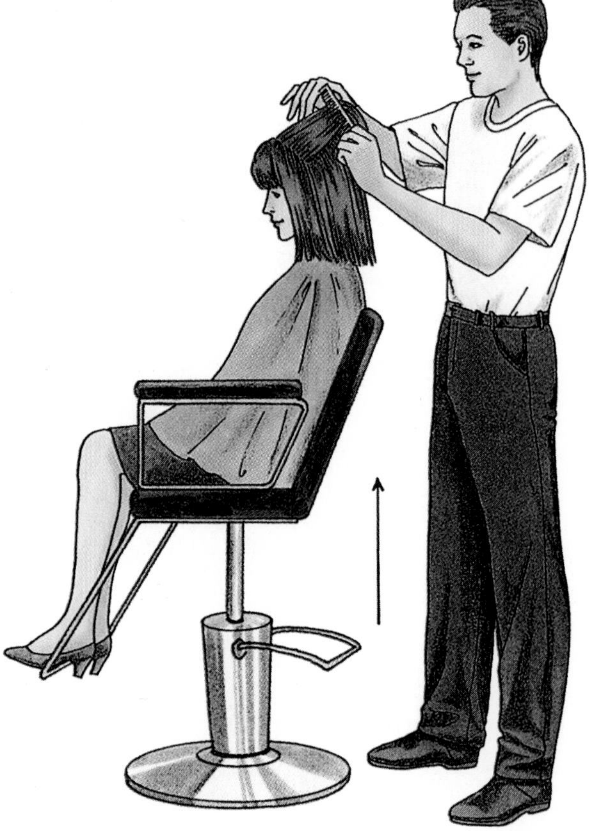

FIGURE 1.9 — Basic stance for the male cosmetologist, and the correct chair position for working on a client comfortably.

CORRECT SITTING TECHNIQUE

To sit attractively, use your thigh muscles and support from your hands and arms to lower your body smoothly into a chair. Do not fall or flop into a chair. When lowering your body, keep your back straight. Do not bend at the waist or reach with the buttocks. When seated, slide to the back of the chair by placing both hands on the front edge of the chair at the sides of your hips. Raise your body slightly and slide back. Do not wiggle or inch back.

When giving a manicure, assume a correct sitting position. Sit with the lower back against the chair, leaning slightly forward. If a stool is used, sit on the entire stool. Keep your chest up and rest your body weight on the full length of your thighs. (Figs. 1.10, 1.11)

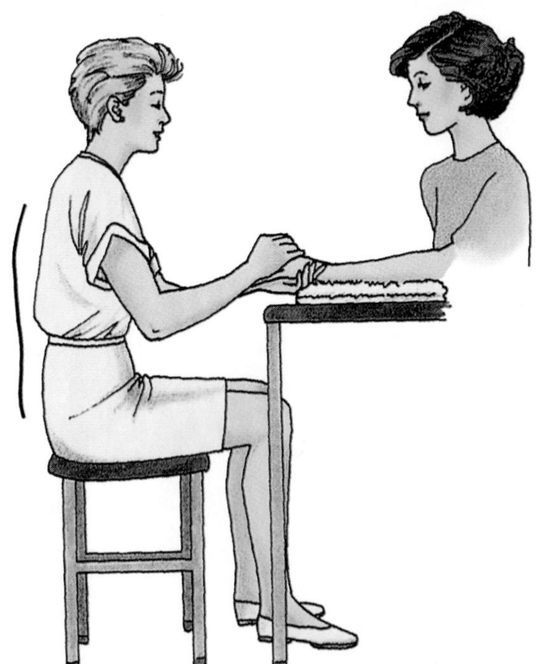

FIGURE 1.10 — Good sitting posture.

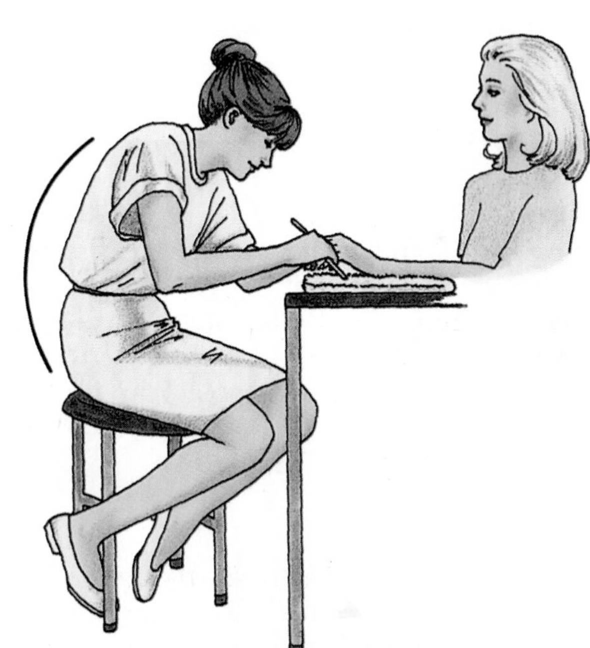

FIGURE 1.11 — Poor sitting posture.

Tips for a Proper Sitting Position

1. Keep your feet close together.
2. Keep your knees close together.
3. Place your feet out slightly farther than your knees.
4. Do not push your feet under the chair.
5. Keep the entire sole of your foot on the floor.

Completed: Learning Objective #2

EFFECTIVE PHYSICAL PRESENTATION

PERSONALITY

Your personality plays an important part in your personal and professional life. Personality can be defined as the outward reflection of your inner feelings, thoughts, attitudes, and values. Your personality is expressed through your voice, speech, and choice of words, as well as through your facial expressions, gestures, actions, posture, clothing, grooming, and environment. It is the total effect you have on other people.

DESIRABLE QUALITIES FOR EFFECTIVE CLIENT RELATIONS

Emotional Control

Learn to control your emotions. Discourage and do not reveal negative emotions such as anger, envy, and dislike. An even-tempered person is always treated with respect.

Positive Approach

Be pleasant and gracious. A smile of greeting and a word of welcome should be ready for each client and co-worker. A good sense of humor is also an important part of maintaining a positive attitude. A sense of humor enriches your life and cushions the disappointments. When you are able to laugh at yourself, you will have gained the ability to accept and deal positively with difficult situations.

Good Manners

Good manners reflect your thoughtfulness of others. Saying "thank you" and "please," treating other people with respect, exercising care of other people's property, being tolerant and understanding of other people's shortcomings and efforts, and being considerate of those with whom you work all express good manners. Courtesy is one of the keys to a successful career.

Bad Manners

Gum chewing and nervous habits such as tapping your foot or playing with your hair and personal items detract from your effectiveness. Yawning, coughing, and sneezing should be concealed when in the presence of others. Control body language that reveals negative communication, for example, sarcastic or disapproving facial grimaces. Pleasant facial expressions and attractive gestures and actions should be your goal.

Completed:
Learning Objective
#3
PERSONALITY

EFFECTIVE COMMUNICATION

Communication includes your listening skills, voice, speech, manner of speaking, and conversational skills. Your ability to communicate will have a great influence on your effectiveness as a cosmetologist. A cosmetologist needs good communication skills for the following reasons:

- To make contacts
- To meet and greet clients
- To understand a client's needs, likes, dislikes, and desires (Fig. 1.12)
- To be self-promoting
- To sell services and products (Fig. 1.13)
- To build business
- To talk on the telephone
- To carry on a pleasant conversation
- To interact with the salon staff

Completed: Learning Objective #4 EFFECTIVE COMMUNICATION

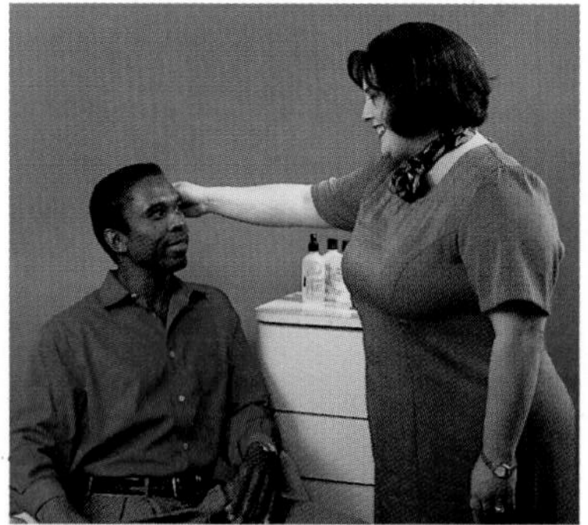

FIGURE 1.12 — Cosmetologist communicating with client.

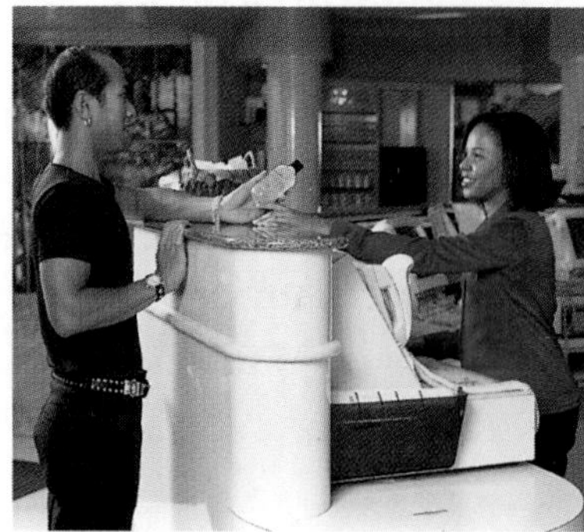

FIGURE 1.13 — The cosmetologist as salesperson.

HUMAN RELATIONS AND YOUR PROFESSIONAL ATTITUDE

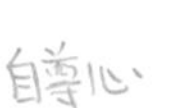

Human relations is the psychology of getting along well with others. Your professional attitude is expressed by your own self-esteem, confidence in your profession, and by the respect you show others.

Good habits and practices acquired during your school training lay the foundation for a successful career in cosmetology. The following are guidelines for good human relations that will help you to gain confidence and deal successfully with others.

1. Always greet a client by name, with a pleasant tone of voice. Address a client by his or her last name (Mrs. Smith, Mr. Jones, Miss Allen) unless the client prefers first names and it is customary to use first names in your salon.
2. Be alert to the client's mood. Some clients prefer quiet and relaxation, others like to talk. Be a good listener and confine your conversation to the client's needs. Never gossip or tell off-color stories.
3. Topics of conversation should be carefully chosen. Friendly relations are achieved through pleasant conversations. Let your client be the guide in the topic of conversation. In a business setting it is best to avoid discussing controversial topics such as religion and politics, topics that relate to your personal life such as personal problems, or subjects relating to other people such as another client's behavior, poor workmanship of fellow workers or competitors, or information given to you in confidence.
4. Make a good impression by looking the part of the successful cosmetologist, and by speaking and acting in a professional manner at all times.
5. Cultivate self-confidence, and project a pleasing personality.
6. Show interest in the client's personal preferences. Give your undivided attention. Maintain eye contact and concentrate totally on your client.
7. Use tact and diplomacy when dealing with problems you may encounter.
8. Be capable and efficient in your work.
9. Be punctual. Arrive at work on time and keep appointments on schedule. Plan each day's schedule so that you manage your time effectively.
10. Develop your business and sales abilities. Use tact when suggesting additional services or products to clients.
11. Avoid saying anything that sounds as if you are criticizing, condemning, or putting down a client's opinions.
12. Keep informed of new products and services so you can answer clients' questions intelligently.
13. Continue to add to your knowledge and skills.
14. Be ethical in all your dealings with clients and others with whom you come in contact.
15. Always let the client see that you practice the highest standards of sanitation.
16. Avoid criticizing your competitors.
17. Deal with all disputes and differences in private. Take care of all problems promptly.

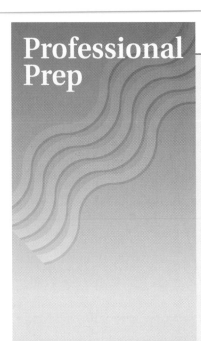

HONING YOUR PEOPLE SKILLS

Every business that provides services to people must deal with clients who are rude, pushy, upset, angry, hostile, selfish, deceitful, critical, and manipulative. These people all fall into a category labeled "difficult." How can you deal effectively with difficult people? Here are some tips:

Accept people as they are. Remember, you can't change another person's behavior. What you can change is the way you react to that person. Stop allowing other people's behavior to affect or influence you.

Ask questions to clarify and summarize. Only after the upset or angry person has had a chance to get the problem off his or her chest, calmly ask open-ended questions.

Refrain from becoming emotional. No matter what, you can't allow yourself to be drawn into the emotional part of the problem. You must remain cool and calm, pleasant and professional. You must think objectively, not emotionally.

Work on feeling good about yourself. People with low self-esteem are more vulnerable to difficult people and their tactics. Concentrate on being positive and upbeat. Think positive thoughts and make positive statements.

—*From* Communication Skills for Cosmetologists *by Kathleen Ann Bergant*

TO BE SUCCESSFUL...

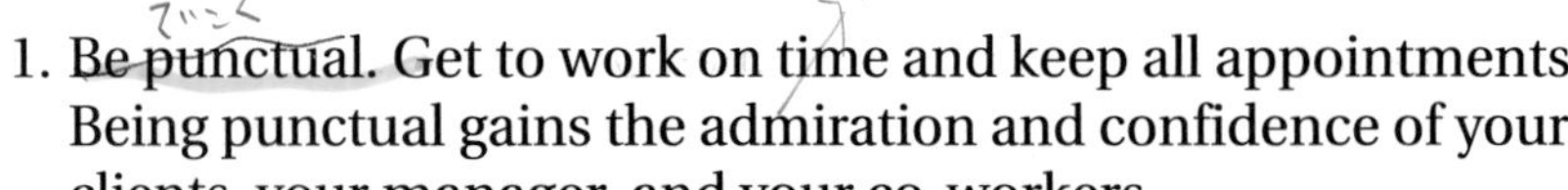

1. Be punctual. Get to work on time and keep all appointments. Being punctual gains the admiration and confidence of your clients, your manager, and your co-workers.
2. Be courteous. Courtesy plays an important part in bringing clients to the salon and in keeping them as regular customers.
3. Set a good example for your profession. Your own neat, attractive, and fashionable appearance expresses your pride in yourself and your profession. Clients have confidence in the cosmetologist who looks the part.
4. Be efficient and skillful. Practice your skills so that you can give services efficiently and gently. Clients appreciate the cosmetologist who cares about their comfort and is skillful when giving services.

5. Practice effective communications. Speaking well of others and being able to give sincere compliments will be an asset in your career as a professional cosmetologist. Being a good listener and being efficient and courteous when speaking on the telephone or with clients during the service will help you build a successful business.

To be successful, you should extend courtesy to all with whom you come in contact. This includes state board members and inspectors, who are contributing to the higher standards of cosmetology.

To be successful, you must know the laws, rules, and regulations that govern cosmetology, and you must comply with them. By complying, you are contributing to the health, welfare, and safety of your community.

Completed:
Learning Objective
#5
GOOD HUMAN RELATIONS AND PROFESSIONAL ATTITUDE

PROFESSIONAL ETHICS

Ethics is defined as the study of standards of conduct and moral judgment. Codes of ethics for various professions are established by boards or commissions. In cosmetology, each state has a board or commission that sets standards that all cosmetologists who work in that state must follow. However, ethics goes beyond a set of rules and regulations. In the field of cosmetology, ethics is also a code of behavior by which you conduct yourself. Much of what was discussed in the previous section is directly related to an informal code of ethical standards.

Ethics deal with proper conduct and business dealings with employers, clients and co-workers, and others with whom you come in contact. Ethical conduct helps to build the client's confidence in you. Having your clients speak well of you to others is the best form of advertising and helps you build a successful business. The following are rules of ethics you should practice:

1. Give courteous and friendly service to all clients. Treat everyone honestly and fairly; do not show favoritism.
2. Be courteous and show respect for the feelings, beliefs, and rights of others.
3. Keep your word. Be responsible and fulfill your obligations.
4. Build your reputation by setting an example of good conduct and behavior.
5. Be loyal to your employer, managers, and associates.
6. Obey all provisions of the state cosmetology laws.

7. Practice the highest standards of sanitation to protect your health and the health of your co-workers and clients.
8. Believe in the cosmetology profession. Practice it faithfully and sincerely.
9. Do not try to sell your clients a product or service they do not need or want.
10. As a student:
    - Be loyal to, and cooperate with, school personnel and fellow students.
    - Comply with school and clinic rules and regulations.

Questionable practices, extravagant claims, and unfulfilled promises violate the rules of ethical conduct and cast an unfavorable light on cosmetology. Unethical practices affect the student, the cosmetologist, the school or salon, and the entire industry.

Completed:
Learning Objective
#6
PROFESSIONAL ETHICS

REVIEW QUESTIONS

YOUR PROFESSIONAL IMAGE

1. List the guidelines you should follow to maintain a healthy body and mind.
2. Define physical presentation.
3. Define personality.
4. What does communication consist of?
5. Define good human relations.
6. How is your professional attitude expressed?
7. What is professional ethics?

CHAPTER 2

Bacteriology

LEARNING OBJECTIVES

After completing this chapter, you should be able to:

1. List the various types and classifications of bacteria.
2. Describe how bacteria grow and reproduce.
3. Describe the relationship of bacteria to the spread of disease.
4. Define AIDS and provide brief overview of AIDS.

NATIONAL SKILL STANDARDS

This chapter provides you with the necessary information to master this National Industry Skill Standard for Entry-Level Cosmetologists:

- Conducting services in a safe environment, taking measures to prevent the spread of infectious and contagious disease

INTRODUCTION

Bacteriology (bak-teer-ee-**OL**-o-jee), ***sterilization*** (ster-il-ih-**ZAY**-shun), and ***sanitation*** (san-ih-**TAY**-shun) are subjects of practical importance to you as a cosmetologist, because they have a direct bearing on your well-being as well as on your clients' welfare. To protect individual and public health, every cosmetologist should know when, why, and how to practice good disinfection and sanitation procedures.

In order to understand the importance of sanitation, disinfection, and sterilization, a basic understanding of how ***bacteria*** (bak-**TEER**-ee-ah) affect our daily lives is most helpful.

BACTERIOLOGY

Bacteriology is the science that deals with the study of ***microorganisms*** (meye-kroh-**OR**-gah-niz-ems) called bacteria.

As a cosmetologist, you should understand how the spread of disease can be prevented and what precautions you must take to protect your health and your clients' health. Once you have an understanding of the relationship between bacteria and disease, you will understand the need for school and salon cleanliness and sanitation.

State boards of cosmetology and state departments of health require that a business that serves the public must follow certain sanitary precautions. Contagious diseases, skin infections, and blood poisoning are caused either by infectious bacteria being transmitted from one individual to another, or by the use of unsanitary implements (such as combs, brushes, hairpins, clippies, rollers, manicure implements, esthetic tools, etc.). Dirty hands and fingernails are other sources of infectious bacteria.

Bacteria are minute, one-celled vegetable microorganisms found nearly everywhere. They are especially numerous in dust, dirt, refuse, and diseased tissues. Bacteria are also known as ***germs*** (**JURMS**) or ***microbes*** (**MEYE**-krohbs). Bacteria can exist almost anywhere: on the skin of the body, in water, air, decayed matter, secretions of body openings, on clothing, and beneath the nails.

Bacteria can be seen only with the aid of a ***microscope*** (**MEYE**-kroh-skohp). Fifteen hundred rod-shaped bacteria will barely cover the head of a pin.

TYPES OF BACTERIA

There are hundreds of different kinds of bacteria. However, bacteria are classified into two types, depending on whether they are beneficial or harmful.

1. Most bacteria are ***nonpathogenic*** (non-path-o-**JEN**-ik) organisms (helpful or harmless), which perform many useful functions, such as decomposing refuse and improving soil fertility. ***Saprophytes*** (**SAP**-ro-fights), nonpathogenic bacteria, live on dead matter and do not produce disease.

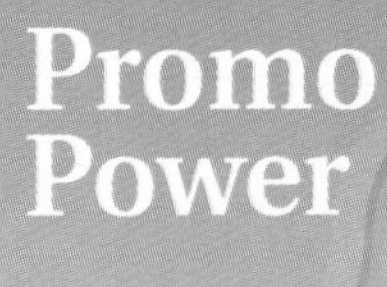

SELLING PRODUCTS

It's important that you select items to sell in your salon with care. Your professional reputation is on the line when you endorse a product. A client won't purchase a product from you that she can buy at a discount store; clients purchase products from a salon professional because they believe them to be superior to consumer products—and because they trust you to sell them the product formulated for their type of hair.

The most successful way to build a booming retail business is to train your employees to start selling from the moment a client is left in their care. If that attitude prevails throughout the salon, the client will be conditioned to buy home maintenance products specifically for her type hair and skin.

Concentrate on an attractive visual presentation that is large and highly visible. When people can pick up and examine items it almost always results in sales. Frequently rotate and rearrange the items.

Everyone loves a bargain, so fill a special clearance basket with small items, tie a pretty bow on the basket, and make every item in the basket the same price. The profit will be less, but it will more than make up the loss by stimulating buyer interest.

Every item must have prices clearly marked. Most people dislike asking the price of anything.

—*From* Milady's Salon Solutions *by Louise Cotter*

2. ***Pathogenic*** (path-o-**JEN**-ik) organisms (microbes or germs) are harmful, and although in the minority, produce disease when they invade plant or animal tissue. To this group belong the ***parasites*** (**PAR**-ah-sights), which require living matter for their growth.

It is because of pathogenic bacteria that beauty schools and salons must maintain certain sanitary and cleanliness standards.

PRONUNCIATIONS OF TERMS RELATING TO PATHOGENIC BACTERIA

Singular	*Plural*
coccus (**KOK**-us)	cocci (**KOK**-si)
bacillus (bah-**SIL**-us)	bacilli (ba-**SIL**-i)
spirillum (speye-**RIL**-um)	spirilla (speye-**RIL**-a)
staphylococcus (staf-i-lo-**KOK**-us)	staphylococci (staf-i-lo-**KOK**-si)
streptococcus (strep-to-**KOK**-us)	streptococci (strep-to-**KOK**-si)
diplococcus (dip-lo-**KOK**-us)	diplococci (dip-lo-**KOK**-si)

CLASSIFICATIONS OF PATHOGENIC BACTERIA

Bacteria have distinct shapes that help to identify them. Pathogenic bacteria are classified as follows (Fig. 2.1):

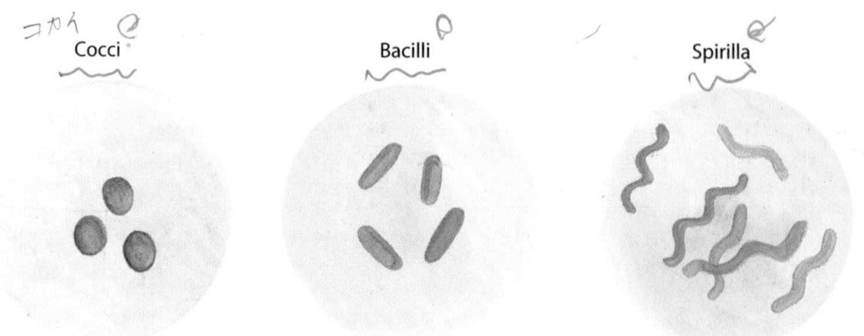

FIGURE 2.1 — General forms of bacteria.

1. ***Cocci*** are round-shaped organisms that appear singly or in the following groups (Fig. 2.2):
   a) ***Staphylococci:*** Pus-forming organisms that grow in bunches or clusters. They cause abscesses, pustules, and boils.
   b) ***Streptococci:*** Pus-forming organisms that grow in chains. They cause infections such as strep throat.
   c) ***Diplococci:*** They grow in pairs and cause pneumonia.

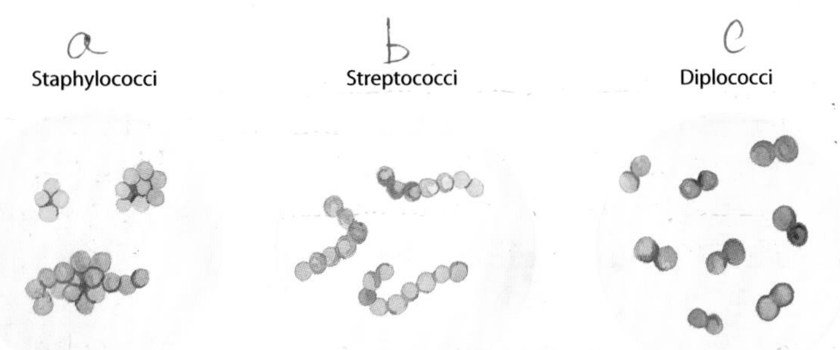

FIGURE 2.2 — Groupings of bacteria.

2. ***Bacilli*** are short rod-shaped organisms. They are the most common bacteria and produce diseases such as tetanus (lockjaw), influenza, typhoid fever, tuberculosis, and diphtheria. (Fig. 2.3)
3. ***Spirilla*** are curved or corkscrew-shaped organisms. They are subdivided into several groups. Of chief concern to us is the ***treponema pallida*** (trep-o-**NE**-mah **PAL**-i-dah), which causes ***syphilis*** (**SIF**-i-lis).

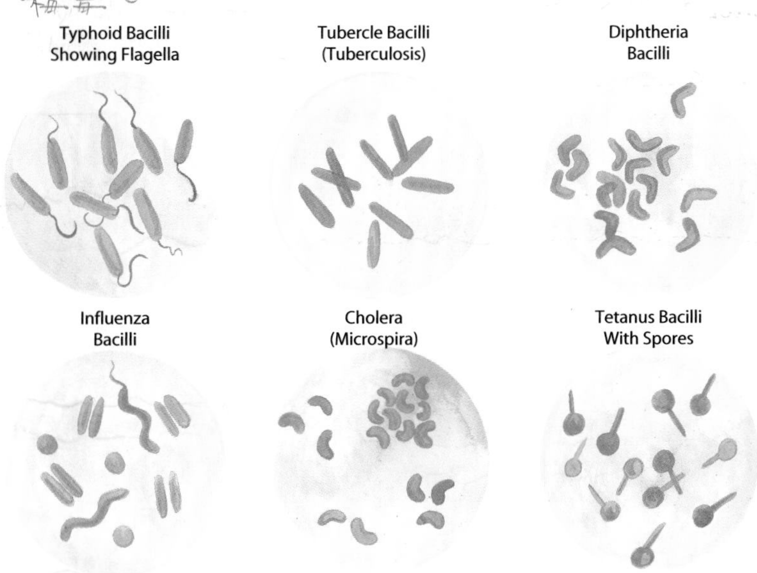

FIGURE 2.3 — Disease-producing bacteria.

Movement of Bacteria

Cocci rarely show active ***motility*** (self-movement). They are transmitted on the air, in dust, or in the substance in which they settle. Bacilli and spirilla are both motile and use hairlike projections, known as ***flagella*** (flah-**JEL**-ah) or ***cilia*** (**SIL**-ee-a), to move about. A whiplike motion of these hairs propels bacteria about in liquid.

Completed:
Learning Objective
#1
TYPES AND CLASSIFICATIONS OF BACTERIA

BACTERIAL GROWTH AND REPRODUCTION

Bacteria generally consist of an outer cell wall and internal ***protoplasm*** (**PROH**-toh-plaz-em), material needed to sustain life. They manufacture their own food from the surrounding environment, give off waste products, and grow and reproduce. Bacteria have two distinct phases in their life cycle: the ***active*** or ***vegetative stage***, and the ***inactive*** or ***spore-forming stage***.

Active or Vegetative Stage

During the active stage, bacteria grow and reproduce. These microorganisms multiply best in warm, dark, damp, or dirty places where sufficient food is available.

When conditions are favorable, bacteria grow and reproduce. When they reach their largest size, they divide into two new cells. This division is called ***amitosis***. The cells formed are called ***daughter cells***. When conditions are unfavorable, bacteria die or become inactive. (See chapter on cells, anatomy, and physiology.)

Inactive or Spore-Forming Stage

Certain bacteria, such as the anthrax and tetanus bacilli, form ***spherical spores*** with tough outer coverings during their inactive stage. The purpose is to be able to withstand periods of famine, dryness, and unsuitable temperatures. In this stage, spores can be blown about and are not harmed by disinfectants, heat, or cold.

When favorable conditions are restored, the spores change into the active or vegetative form, then grow and reproduce.

Completed:
Learning Objective
#2
HOW BACTERIA GROW AND REPRODUCE

BACTERIAL INFECTIONS

There can be no infection without the presence of pathogenic bacteria. An infection occurs when the body is unable to cope with the bacteria and their harmful toxins. A ***local infection*** is indicated by a boil or pimple that contains pus. The presence of ***pus*** is a sign of infection. Bacteria, waste matter, decayed tissue, body cells, and living and dead blood cells are all found in pus. Staphylococci are the most common pus-forming bacteria. A ***general infection*** results when the bloodstream carries the bacteria and their toxins to all parts of the body, as in syphilis.

A disease becomes ***contagious*** (kon-**TAY**-jus) or ***communicable*** (ko-**MYOO**-ni-kah-bil) when it spreads from one person to another by contact. Some of the more common contagious diseases that prevent a cosmetologist from working are tuberculosis, common cold, ringworm, scabies, and viral infections.

The chief sources of contagion are unclean hands and implements, open sores, pus, mouth and nose discharges, and the common use of drinking cups and towels. Uncovered coughing or sneezing and spitting in public also spread germs.

Pathogenic bacteria can enter the body through:

1. A break in the skin, such as a cut, pimple, or scratch.
2. The mouth (breathing or swallowing air, water, or food).
3. The nose (air).
4. The eyes or ears (dirt).

The body fights infection by means of:

1. Unbroken skin, which is the body's first line of defense.
2. Body secretions, such as perspiration and digestive juices.
3. White cells within the blood that destroy bacteria.
4. Antitoxins that counteract the toxins produced by bacteria.

Infections can be prevented and controlled through personal hygiene and public sanitation.

OTHER INFECTIOUS AGENTS

Filterable viruses (**FIL**-ter-a-bil **VEYE**-rus-es) are living organisms so small that they can pass through the pores of a porcelain filter. They cause the common cold and other respiratory (**RES**-pi-rah-torh-ee) and gastrointestinal (digestive tract) (gas-troh-in-**TES**-ti-nal) infections.

Parasites are organisms that live on other living organisms without giving anything in return.

Plant parasites or ***fungi*** (**FUN**-ji), such as molds, mildews, and yeasts, can produce contagious diseases, such as ringworm and ***favus*** (**FAY**-vus), a skin disease of the scalp.

Animal parasites are responsible for contagious diseases and conditions, such as head lice. For example, the itch mite burrows under the skin, causing ***scabies*** (**SKAY**-beez), and infection of the scalp by lice is called ***pediculosis*** (pe-dik-yoo-**LOH**-sis).

Contagious diseases and conditions caused by parasites should never be treated in a beauty school or salon. Clients should be referred to a physician.

IMMUNITY

Immunity (i-**MYOO**-ni-tee) is the ability of the body to destroy bacteria that have gained entrance, and thus to resist infection. Immunity against disease can be natural or acquired and is a sign of good health. ***Natural immunity*** means natural resistance to disease. It is partly inherited and partly developed through hygienic living. ***Acquired immunity*** is something the body develops after it has overcome a disease, or through inoculation.

A human disease carrier is a person who is personally immune to a disease yet can transmit germs to other people. ***Typhoid*** (**TEYE**-foid) ***fever*** and ***diphtheria*** (dif-**THEER**-i-a) can be transmitted in this manner.

Bacteria can be destroyed by disinfectants and by intense heat achieved by boiling, steaming, baking, or burning, and ultraviolet rays. (This subject is covered in the chapter on sterilization and sanitation.)

Completed: Learning Objective #3

THE RELATIONSHIP OF BACTERIA TO THE SPREAD OF DISEASE

ACQUIRED IMMUNE DEFICIENCY SYNDROME (AIDS)

You may already know that HIV-1 (Human Immunodeficiency Virus) is passed from person to person through blood and other body fluids, such as semen and vaginal secretions. A person can be infected with HIV-1 for up to 11 years without having symptoms. Sometimes people who are HIV-positive have never been tested and do not know that they are infecting other people.

HIV is the virus that causes AIDS (the disease). AIDS attacks and destroys the immune system. The AIDS Virus is transmitted through unprotected sexual contact, IV drug users sharing needles, and accidents with needles in healthcare settings. The virus can enter the bloodstream through cuts and sores and can be transmitted in the salon by a sharp implement. For example, if you accidentally cut a client who is HIV-positive and you continue to use the implement without cleaning and disinfecting it, you risk puncturing your skin (or cutting another client) with a contaminated tool. Likewise, if you're shaving a client's neck with clipper blades and body fluid is picked up from a blemish or open sore, transmission is possible.

Recent changes in state cosmetology board regulations have forced cosmetologists to practice proper infection control procedures in the salon. Disinfectants that are used in hospitals are now the standard for salon use. Used properly, these disinfectants provide optimum protection against HIV-1, Hepatitis B Virus, and even bacterial infections. Proper disinfection protects today's cosmetologists and the clients they service.

Completed: Learning Objective #4

AIDS OVERVIEW

REVIEW QUESTIONS

BACTERIOLOGY

1. Why is bacteriology necessary?
2. Define bacteriology.
3. What are bacteria?
4. Where can bacteria exist? Give examples.
5. Define two types of bacteria.
6. What are parasites and saprophytes?
7. Name and define three forms of bacteria.
8. Name and define three types of cocci bacteria.
9. How do bacteria multiply?
10. Describe the active and inactive stages of bacteria.
11. How do bacteria move about?
12. Name two types of infection and define each.
13. What is a contagious or communicable disease?
14. How can infections be controlled or prevented?
15. Name two diseases produced by a) plant parasites and b) animal parasites.
16. Define immunity. Name two types.
17. How can bacteria be destroyed?

CHAPTER 3

Decontamination and Infection Control

LEARNING OBJECTIVES

After Completing This Chapter, You Should Be Able To:

1. Explain and understand the importance of decontamination.
2. Explain the difference between sanitation, disinfection, and sterilization.
3. Discuss how to safely handle and use disinfectant products.
4. Describe which cleaners, equipment, and disinfectants are useful for salons.
5. Define universal precautions and discuss your responsibilities as a salon professional.

NATIONAL SKILL STANDARDS

This chapter provides you with the necessary information to master this National Industry Skill Standard for Entry-Level Cosmetologists:

- Conducting services in a safe environment, taking measures to prevent the spread of infectious and contagious disease

INTRODUCTION

Clients love to see a clean salon. It gives them a feeling of confidence in both you and your special training. Clean and orderly salons make a positive statement. There is no better way to make a good first impression.

However, there is more to keeping the salon clean than sweeping the floor and vacuuming the rugs. If proper care is not taken you could contribute to the spread of diseases.

Controlling infection and disease is an important part of the salon industry. Clients depend upon you to ensure their safety. Protecting against the spread of infectious germs and other organisms is also required by federal and state regulations and for good reason. One careless action could cause injury or serious illness. Being a salon professional can be fun and rewarding, but it is also a great responsibility.

Disease-causing germs will be one of your biggest enemies in the salon. Fortunately, preventing the spread of dangerous diseases is easy, if you know how.

PREVENTION AND CONTROL

CONTAMINATION

Take a moment to look around you. What do you see? No matter where you are, you will always see a surface of some sort. The surface of the table, the wall, the floor, your hand...most things have a surface. No matter how clean these surfaces look, they are probably ***contaminated***.

Surfaces of tools or other objects that are not free from dirt, oils, and microbes are contaminated. Any substance that causes contamination is called a ***contaminant***. Many things can be contaminants. Hair in a comb or makeup on a towel are contaminants.

Tools and other surfaces in the salon can also be contaminated with bacteria, viruses, and fungi. Even tools that look clean are usually covered with these microorganisms.

DECONTAMINATION

It would be impossible to keep the salon free from all contamination, nor is it necessary to try. However, it is your responsibility as a salon professional to be on constant alert for disease-causing microorganisms.

Removing pathogens and other substances from tools or surfaces is called ***decontamination***. There are three main levels of decontamination: sterilization, disinfection, and sanitation. However, only sanitation and disinfection are required in the salon.

Completed:
Learning Objective
#1
DECONTAMINATION

STERILIZATION

Sterilization is the most effective type of decontamination against microbes. Sterilization completely destroys all living organisms on a surface. Sterilization even kills bacterial spores, the most resistant form of life on Earth.

The ***steam autoclave***, the most popular method of physical sterilization and the most preferred due to its proven history of sterilizing, is like a pressure cooker. When steam is injected into a chamber at high pressure, it is possible to raise the temperature above that of boiling water. If something is left in the autoclave long enough, the high pressure and high heat will penetrate into all of the object's nooks and crannies. This will eventually kill all living organisms, including bacterial spores.

Another physical method of sterilization is the use of dry heat, a method more like an oven than a pressure cooker. Objects are placed into an ovenlike chamber and baked until all forms of life are dead.

Sterilization is the highest of the three levels of decontamination. It is a multi-step, time consuming, and difficult process. It is unnecessary, impractical, and virtually impossible to sterilize tools and surfaces in the salon.

Sterilization is used by dentists and surgeons. Their tools are critical instruments and are designed to break and penetrate the skin barrier. For this reason, it is necessary for estheticians to sterilize needles and probes used to lance the skin. A simpler and safer alternative would be to use disposable lancets or needles.

The word "sterilize" is often used incorrectly. For example, some practitioners tell clients that they are "sterilizing the nail plate or skin." This is impossible! Sterilizing the skin would quickly kill it and would destroy the nail plate, as well. We can only sterilize nonporous surfaces, such as metal implements. In short, sterilization is impractical and unnecessary in salons.

DISINFECTION

If sterilization is not practical and sanitation alone is not enough, what can you do to prevent the spread of dangerous organisms? Proper disinfection is the answer! ***Disinfection*** controls microorganisms on nonporous surfaces such as cuticle nippers and other implements. Disinfection is a higher level of decontamination than sanitation. It is second only to sterilization.

Disinfection provides the level of protection needed in the salon by killing most organisms, with one exception. Disinfection does not kill bacterial spores, but this is not necessary in the salon environment. It is important only in hospitals and other health care facilities where "critical" instruments are used to penetrate/cut skin. (Note: The only "critical" instruments used in the salon are needles for electrolysis and permanent makeup. Disposable needles are recommended for this purpose.)

Disinfectants are substances that kill microbes on contaminated tools and other nonporous surfaces. **Disinfectants are not for use on human skin, hair, or nails.** Never use disinfectants as hand cleaners. Any substance powerful enough to quickly and efficiently destroy pathogens can also damage skin. Always remember, disinfectants are serious, professional-strength products.

Completed: Learning Objective #2

SANITATION, DISINFECTION, AND STERILIZATION

Read Before Using

Manufacturers take great care to develop safe and highly effective systems. However, being safe does not mean they cannot be dangerous. Any professional salon product can be dangerous if used incorrectly. Like all tools, disinfectants must always be used in strict accordance with manufacturer's instructions.

Important Information

All disinfectants must be approved by the Environmental Protection Agency (EPA) and each individual state. The disinfectant's label must also have an ***EPA registration number***. Look for this number when choosing a disinfectant. It is the only way to ensure that the product is effective against certain organisms, and that the EPA has this test data on file. The product label will also tell you which organisms the disinfectant has been tested for, such as HIV-1 and the Hepatitis B Virus. Likewise, if a disinfectant has *not* been tested for a specific organism, it will *not* appear on the label. (Fig. 3.1)

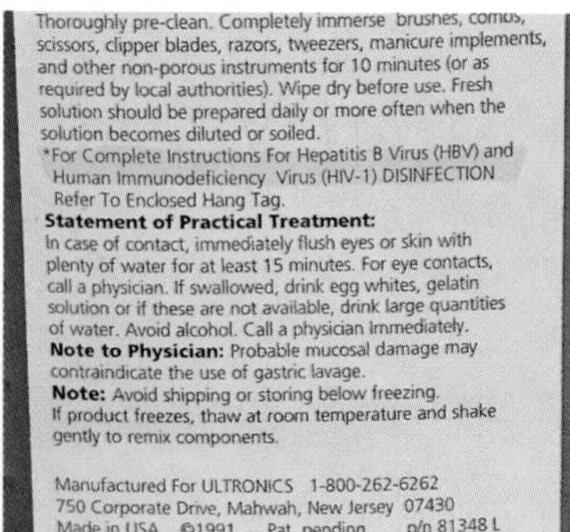

Thoroughly pre-clean. Completely immerse brushes, combs, scissors, clipper blades, razors, tweezers, manicure implements, and other non-porous instruments for 10 minutes (or as required by local authorities). Wipe dry before use. Fresh solution should be prepared daily or more often when the solution becomes diluted or soiled.
*For Complete Instructions For Hepatitis B Virus (HBV) and Human Immunodeficiency Virus (HIV-1) DISINFECTION Refer To Enclosed Hang Tag.
Statement of Practical Treatment:
In case of contact, immediately flush eyes or skin with plenty of water for at least 15 minutes. For eye contacts, call a physician. If swallowed, drink egg whites, gelatin solution or if these are not available, drink large quantities of water. Avoid alcohol. Call a physician Immediately.
Note to Physician: Probable mucosal damage may contraindicate the use of gastric lavage.
Note: Avoid shipping or storing below freezing.
If product freezes, thaw at room temperature and shake gently to remix components.
Manufactured For ULTRONICS 1-800-262-6262
750 Corporate Drive, Mahwah, New Jersey 07430
Made in USA ©1991 Pat. pending p/n 81348 L

FIGURE 3.1 — Efficacy claims must appear on the product label.

Besides the EPA registration number, federal law requires manufacturers to give you other important information, such as directions for proper use, safety precautions, a list of active ingredients, and an important information sheet called a ***Material Safety Data Sheet*** (MSDS).

Take the time to read all of this vital information. Then you will be certain that you are protecting yourself and your clients to the best of your ability!

> **CAUTION**
>
> *Disinfectants are too harsh for human skin or eye contact. Always wear gloves and safety glasses to prevent accidental exposure when mixing chemicals with water.*

OSHA

The Occupational Safety and Health Administration (OSHA) was created as part of the U.S. Department of Labor to regulate and enforce safety and health standards in the workplace. Regulating employee exposure to toxic substances and informing employees of the dangers of the materials used in the workplace are key functions of the Occupational Safety and Health Act of 1970. This act established the Hazard Communication Rule, which requires that chemical manufacturers and importers assess the hazards associated with their products. Material Safety Data Sheets and labeling are two important results of this law.

Material Safety Data Sheets provide all pertinent information on products, ranging from content and associated hazards, to combustion levels and storage requirements. These sheets should be available for every product used in the cosmetology school or salon, and may be obtained from the product's distributor and/or manufacturer. (Fig. 3.2)

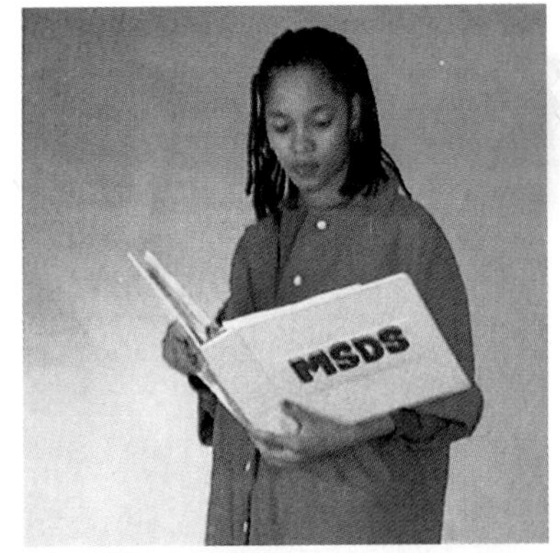

FIGURE 3.2 — Read your Material Safety Data Sheets (MSDS).

The standards set by OSHA are important to the cosmetology industry because of the nature of the chemicals used, for instance, the mixing, storing, and disposal of chemicals; the general safety of the workplace; and, most important, the right of the cosmetologist to know what is contained in the products he or she uses.

Hospital Disinfectants

To use a disinfectant properly, it is necessary to read and follow the manufacturer's instructions. Implements must be completely submerged for proper disinfection. (Fig. 3.3)

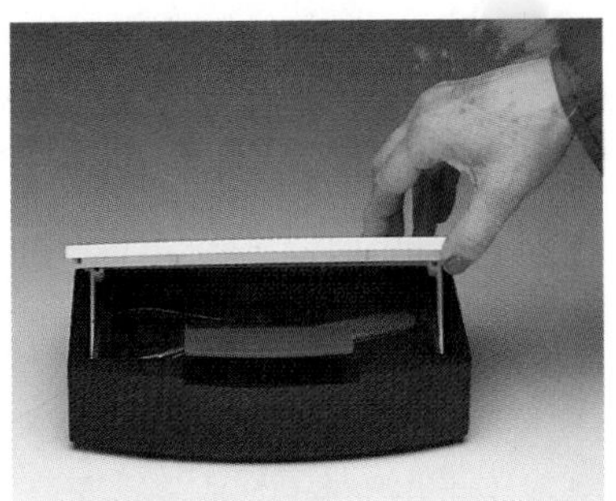

FIGURE 3.3 — Submerge implements completely in a disinfecting tray.

The product label will explain what the disinfectant has been tested for. To meet salon requirements, a disinfectant must be effective against bacteria, fungi, and viruses. A disinfectant that is "Formulated for Hospitals and Health Care Facilities," or a "Hospital Disinfectant," must also be pseudomonacidal (**SUE**-dough-mon-a-**SIDE**-l) in addition to being bactericidal (back-teer-a-**SIDE**-l), fungicidal (fun-gi-**SIDE**-l), and virucidal (vie-rus-

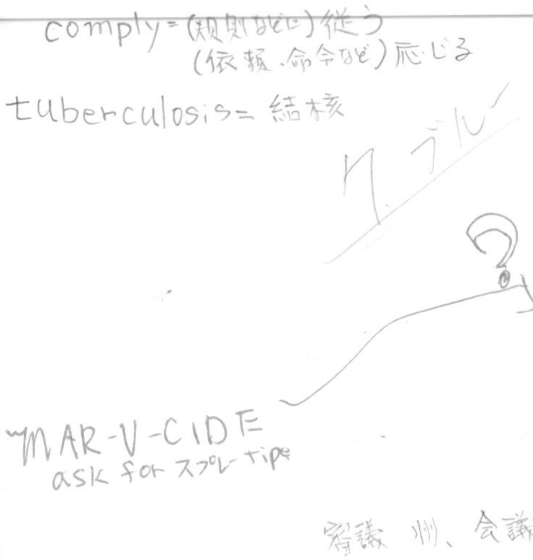

SIDE-l). If a disinfectant has been tested for additional organisms such as HIV-1, it will be stated on the label.

On February 28, 1997, OSHA (Occupational Safety and Health Administration) issued a new policy stating that, in order to comply with OSHA's Bloodborne Pathogens Standard, the use of an EPA-registered tuberculocidal (too-**BERK**-you-low-**SIDE**-l) disinfectant *or* an EPA-registered disinfectant labeled as effective against HIV and HBV is required. For this reason, when salon implements accidentally come into contact with blood or body fluids, they should be cleaned and completely immersed in an EPA-registered disinfectant that kills HIV-1 *and* Hepatitis B Virus or in a tuberculocidal disinfectant. The National Interstate Council of State Cosmetology Boards (NICS) now follows this standard for testing as well.

Proper Use of Disinfectants

Even the best disinfectants won't work very well if used incorrectly. All implements should be thoroughly cleaned before soaking to avoid contaminating the disinfecting solution. Hair, nail filings, creams, oils, and makeup will lessen the effectiveness of the solution. Besides, a dirty jar of disinfectant wouldn't give your clients much confidence in your abilities.

Jars or containers used to disinfect implements are often incorrectly called ***wet sanitizers***. Of course, the purpose of these containers is not to sanitize, but to disinfect. The disinfecting soak solution must be changed daily unless otherwise directed by the manufacturer's instructions. (Fig. 3.4)

Completed: Learning Objective #3

USE AND SAFETY OF DISINFECTANT PRODUCTS

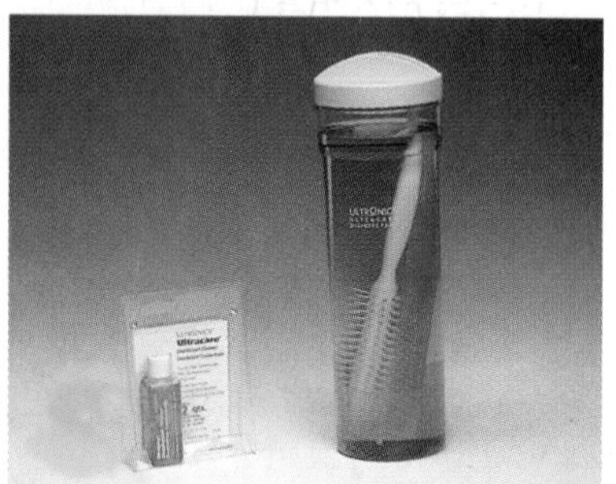

FIGURE 3.4 — Follow manufacturer's instructions when using any disinfectant system.

CAUTION

Because blood can carry many pathogens, you should never touch a client's open sore or wound. Insist that clients with open sores have a doctor certify they are not contagious. (Note: Blood spills occur when you or a client are accidentally cut with a sharp instrument. Apply antiseptic and/or liquid or spray styptic as necessary. Cover with Band-Aid or bandage as required to prevent further blood exposure.) Be sure to properly clean and disinfect any implement that comes in contact with a cut or open sore in an EPA-registered, hospital disinfectant that kills HIV-1 and Hepatitis B Virus or a tuberculocidal disinfectant. Also, seal contaminated wipes or cotton balls in a plastic bag before disposing, then wash your hands with an antibacterial soap.

APPEARANCE CAN BE A SELLING POINT

Of course you're scrupulous about sanitizing and disinfecting in your salon. In an era when the public is more aware than ever of the spread of disease, practicing safety in the salon—whether it's a full-service salon, a nail salon, or a skincare salon—is absolutely essential.

But you can follow every rule about making your equipment and environment germfree, and it still may not be enough to convince your clients that your salon is "really clean." For the layperson with no training in sanitation, appearances are everything. The key is to make your salon *look* sparkling clean, even in areas where the danger of germs being spread is minimal. First impressions are always important and if a client walks in and sees dingy curtains or stained walls, the immediate thought will be, "This place is not clean."

Here is a checklist to make sure your first impression is a good one:

- Windows and drapes should be cleaned at least once a week.
- Doors should be clean and easy to open.
- Wall displays should be easy to clean and easy to change regularly.
- The reception desk should be neat and well organized.
- The reception area should contain ashtrays in smoking areas (if you allow smoking).
- Walls within the styling area should be easy to clean and freshly painted or covered.
- Rest rooms, mirrors, floors, and counter space around each work area should be kept clean.
- Floors should be made of a nonporous substance that is long wearing and easy to clean.
- The exterior of the salon should be well maintained and well lit.
- Let your clients know that you are using hospital disinfection for their safety and well-being. Marketing tools, such as window decals and display cards for your station, are available free of charge from most disinfectant manufacturers. Call the manufacturer whose product you are using to request them. Telephone numbers usually appear on the product label, or you can call information.

TYPES OF DISINFECTANTS

Quats

There are several types of salon disinfectants. ***Quaternary ammonium compounds (quats)*** (**KWAH**-ter-nah-ree ah-**MOH**-nee-um **KOM**-pownds [***KWATS***]) are one type. Quats are considered to be very safe and fast acting. Older formulas relied on only one quat and were not very effective. Newer products (called super quat formulas) use blends of several different quats that dramatically increase effectiveness.

Most quat solutions disinfect implements in 10 to 15 minutes. Leaving some tools in the solution for too long may damage them. Long-term exposure to any water solution or disinfectant may damage fine steel.

With today's modern formulas, corrosion of metal surfaces can be easily avoided, especially if you keep implements separated from each other while disinfecting. Metal implements such as scissors and nail clippers should be oiled regularly to keep them in perfect working order.

Quats are also very effective for cleaning table and counter tops.

Phenols

Like quats, ***phenolic*** (fee-**NOH**-lick) ***disinfectants (phenols)*** have been used for many years to disinfect implements. They too can be safe and extremely effective if used according to instructions. One disadvantage is that certain rubber and plastic materials may be softened or discolored by phenols. Phenols are used mostly for metal implements.

Extra care should be taken to avoid skin contact with phenols. Phenolic disinfectants can cause skin irritation, and concentrated phenols can seriously burn the skin and eyes. Also, take care to keep phenols out of the reach of children as some are poisonous if accidentally ingested.

Alcohol, Bleach, and Commercial Cleaners

The word ***alcohol*** is often misunderstood. There are many chemical compounds that may be classified as alcohol. The three most widely used are ***methyl*** (**METH**-il) ***alcohol*** (methanol), ***ethyl*** (**ETH**-il) ***alcohol*** (ethanol or grain alcohol), and ***isopropyl*** (eye-so-**PROH**-pil) ***alcohol*** (isopropanol or rubbing alcohol).

In the salon, ethyl and isopropyl alcohol are often used for disinfecting implements. To be effective, the strength of ethyl alcohol must be no less than 70%. Isopropyl alcohol's strength must be 99% or it is ineffective. Since alcohol is not an EPA-registered disinfectant, it is not permitted for use with implements in states requiring hospital disinfection.

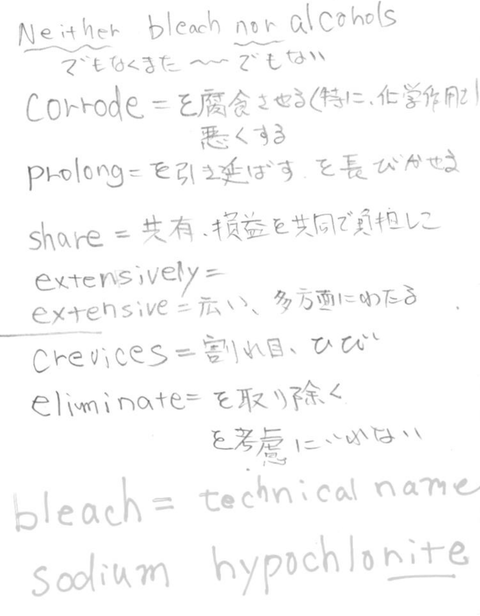

There are many disadvantages to using alcohols. They are extremely flammable, evaporate quickly, and are slow-acting, less-effective disinfectants. Alcohols corrode tools and cause sharp edges to become dull. The vapors formed upon evaporation can cause headaches and nausea in high concentrations or after prolonged exposure.

Household bleach (***sodium hypochlorite***) (**SOH**-dee-um high-poh-**KLOR**-ite) is an effective disinfectant, but shares some of the same drawbacks of alcohols. Neither bleach nor alcohols are professionally designed and tested for disinfection of salon implements. These may have been used extensively in the past, but have since been replaced by more advanced and effective technologies.

Although quats are perfectly suitable for cleaning any surface (unless otherwise specified in the manufacturer's directions), you may wish to clean floors, bathrooms, sinks, and waste receptacles with a commercial cleaner such as Lysol® or Pine-Sol®. Both are very effective disinfectants, but should not be used on salon implements. They are general, "household level" disinfectants and are not designed for professional tools.

Ultrasonic Cleaners

Ultrasonic baths or cleaners are useful when combined with disinfectants. Ultrasonic baths use high-frequency sound waves to create powerful, cleansing bubbles in the liquid. This cleansing action is an effective way to clean tiny crevices that are impossible to reach with a brush. However, without an effective disinfectant solution, these devices will only sanitize implements.

Ultrasonic cleaners are a useful addition to your disinfection process, but are not required equipment. Many systems disinfect with great effectiveness without such devices. However, some feel this added cleaning benefit is well worth the extra expense. It also saves time by eliminating hand cleaning. (Fig. 3.5)

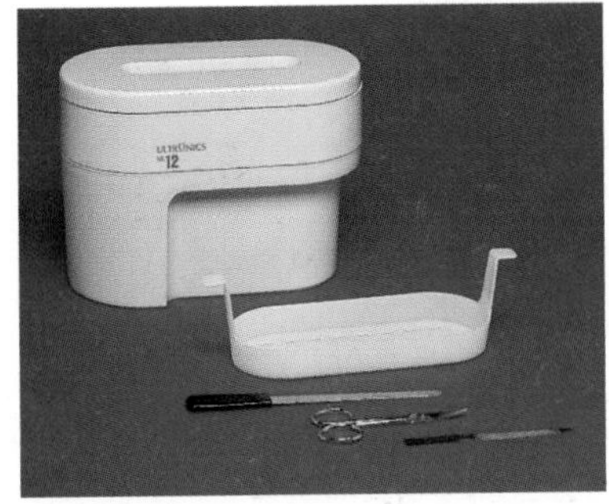

FIGURE 3.5 — Ultrasonic cleaners save time by eliminating hand-scrubbing of implements.

DISINFECTANT SAFETY

Disinfectants are powerful, professional-strength tools that may be hazardous if used incorrectly. Some disinfectants are poisonous if ingested, and some can cause serious skin and eye damage, especially in a concentrated form.

A good rule to remember is: **Use caution!** Wear gloves and safety glasses while mixing disinfectants. Always keep disinfectants away from children. (Fig. 3.6)

Use tongs or a draining basket to remove implements from disinfectants. Never pour quats, phenols, or any other disinfectant over your hands. This foolish practice can cause skin disease and increase the chance of infection. Wash your hands with an antibacterial soap and dry them thoroughly.

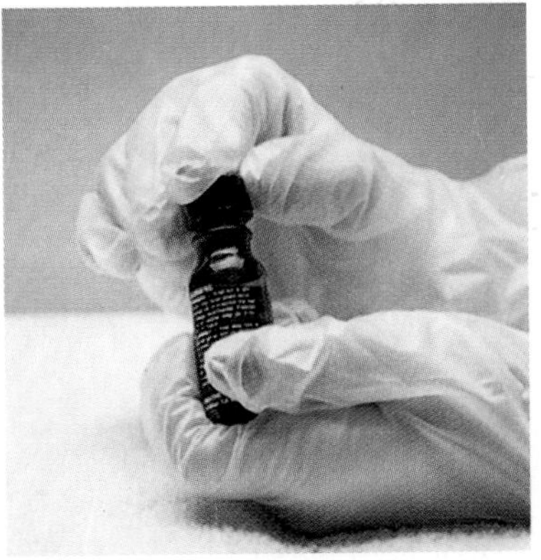

FIGURE 3.6 — Wear gloves when using strong chemicals.

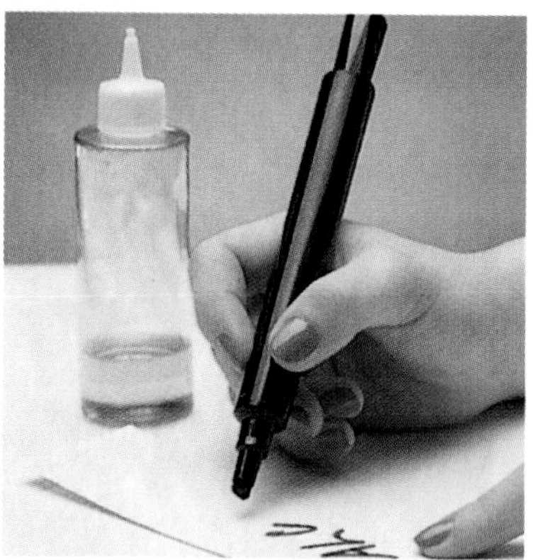

FIGURE 3.7 — Label all containers. If the container isn't labeled, don't use it.

Carefully weigh and measure all products to assure they perform at their peak efficiency. Never place any disinfectant or other product in an unmarked container. (Fig. 3.7)

CAUTION

In the past, ***formalin*** *was recommended as a disinfectant and fumigant in dry cabinet sanitizers. However,* ***formalin is not safe for salon use****.*

The gas released from formalin tablets or liquid is called ***formaldehyde*** *(for-***MAL***-de-hide). Formaldehyde is a suspected human cancer causing agent. It is poisonous to inhale and is extremely irritating to the eyes, nose, throat, and lungs. It can also cause skin allergies, irritation, dryness, and rash.*

After long-term use, formaldehyde vapors can cause symptoms similar to chronic bronchitis or asthma. These symptoms usually worsen over time with continued exposure.

Note: *Avoid using bar soaps in the salon. Bar soap can actually grow bacteria. It is much more sanitary to provide pump-type liquid antibacterial soaps.*

Other Surfaces

It is very important to properly disinfect combs, brushes, scissors, razors, nippers, electrodes, and other commonly used tools. But there are many other surfaces in the salon to consider, for example: table or counter tops, foot baths, finger bowls, tanning beds, telephone receivers, door knobs, cabinet handles, mirrors, and cash registers. Any surface can be contaminated, especially if touched by clients and staff. These items must also be sanitized regularly.

Cosmetologists also must disinfect mixing utensils, combs, clipper blades, brushes, pins, clips, curlers, hair dryers, and chairs. Dirty fans and humidifiers can spread microbes throughout the salon. These devices should be properly cleaned on a regular basis.

Look around and you will see, there is far more to keeping the salon safe and sanitary than rinsing the sinks and wiping up spills. (Fig. 3.8)

Note: *To properly disinfect a surface, first clean with suitable cleaner, apply disinfectant, and leave wet for at least ten minutes. Wipe the surface dry with a clean damp cloth or paper towel.*

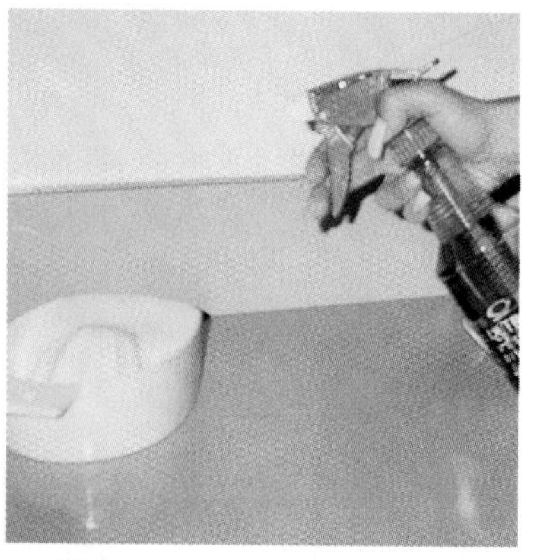

FIGURE 3.8 — All salon work surfaces, as well as implements, should be disinfected.

Proper Storage of Implements

Once tools are properly disinfected, they must be stored where they will remain free from contamination. Ultraviolet (UV) sanitizers are useful storage containers; however, they will not disinfect salon implements. Never use these devices to disinfect!

If you do not wish to use a UV cabinet, disinfected implements should be stored in a disinfected, dry and covered container.

Electric or Bead "Sterilizers"

These devices do **not** sterilize implements. They don't even properly disinfect tools; only the tip of the implement can be inserted into the hot glass beads, and the handles remain contaminated. They only give users a false sense of security. These devices are a dangerous gamble with your client's health.

To effectively sterilize an implement with dry heat, the tool must be thoroughly cleaned with soap, water, and a brush, then heated to 325°F (approximately 163°C) for at least 30 minutes. Effective disinfection can occur only if the entire implement, including the handle, is submerged in an EPA-registered disinfectant solution.

SANITATION

The lowest level of decontamination is called ***sanitation*** or ***sanitization***. These words are also frequently misused and misunderstood.

Sanitation means to "significantly reduce the number of pathogens found on a surface." Salon tools and other surfaces are sanitized by cleaning with soaps or detergents.

Sanitized surfaces may still harbor pathogens or other organisms. Removing hair from a brush and washing the brush with detergent is considered sanitation. Putting antiseptics on skin or washing your hands is another example of sanitation. Your hands may be very clean when you are finished, but they are covered with microorganisms found in the tap water and on the towel.

The Professional Image

Sanitation should be a part of everyone's normal routine. In this way, you and your co-workers can maintain a professional image. Following are some simple guidelines that will help keep the salon looking its best.

1. Floors should be swept clean after each client service.
2. Hair, cotton balls, etc. should be picked up immediately.
3. Deposit all waste materials in a waste receptacle with a self-closing lid.
4. Mop floors and vacuum carpets daily.
5. It is important to control all types of dust.
6. Windows, screens, and curtains should be clean.
7. Regularly clean fans, ventilation systems, and humidifiers.

8. All work areas must be well lighted.
9. Salons need both hot and cold running water.
10. Rest rooms must be clean and tidy.
11. Remember to clean bathroom door handles.
12. Toilet tissue, paper towels, and pump-type antibacterial liquid soap must be provided.
13. Wash hands after using the rest room and between clients.
14. Clean sinks and drinking fountains regularly.
15. Separate or disposable drinking cups must be provided.
16. The salon must be free from insects and rodents.
17. Salons should never be used for cooking or living quarters.
18. Food must never be placed in refrigerators used to store salon products.
19. Eating, drinking, and smoking are prohibited in areas where services are performed in the salon.
20. Waste receptacles must be emptied regularly throughout the day.
21. Employees must wear clean, freshly laundered clothing.
22. Always use freshly laundered towels on each client.
23. Capes or other covering should not contact client's skin.
24. Makeup, lipstick, puffs, pencils, and brushes must never be shared.
25. Clean cotton balls or sponges should be used to apply cosmetics and creams.
26. Remove products from containers with clean spatulas, not fingers.
27. All containers must be properly marked, tightly closed, and properly stored.
28. The outside of all containers should be kept clean.
29. Soiled or dirty linens are to be removed from the workplace and properly stored for cleaning in a covered container.
30. Do not place any tools, combs, rollers, or hairpins in your mouth or pockets.
31. Client gowns and headbands should be properly cleaned before being reused.
32. All tools and implements should be properly cleaned and disinfected after each use and stored in a clean, covered container.

33. Professionals should avoid touching their face, mouth, or eye area during services.
34. No pets or animals should ever be allowed in salons, except for trained Seeing Eye® dogs.

These are only a few of the things professionals must do in order to safeguard themselves and clients. Contact your local state board of cosmetology or health department for a complete list of regulations.

ANTISEPTICS

Antiseptics (an-ti-**SEP**-tiks) can kill bacteria or slow their growth, but they are not disinfectants. Antiseptics are weaker than disinfectants and are safe for application to skin. They are considered to be sanitizers and are not adequate for use on instruments and surfaces.

Completed:
Learning Objective
#4
CLEANERS, EQUIPMENT, AND DISINFECTANTS

UNIVERSAL PRECAUTIONS

In most instances, clients who are infected with Hepatitis B Virus or other blood-borne pathogens are ***asymptomatic,*** which means that they have no symptoms or signs of infection. Consequently, many individuals who have minor, nonspecific symptoms may not know that they have an infection. Exposure to blood in the salon setting presents a *risk* of exposure to various diseases, including AIDS. Therefore, the blood of all clients should be treated as if they were infected.

Because not all clients with infectious diseases can be identified, ***the same infection control practices should be used with all clients.*** This approach is known as ***universal precautions.***

Infection control procedures include handwashing, the use of personal protective equipment such as gloves and safety glasses when needed, and proper disinfection of all salon implements and surfaces to prevent the transfer of microorganisms from one person to another.

YOUR PROFESSIONAL RESPONSIBILITY

You have many responsibilities as a salon professional. You have the responsibility to protect your clients from harm. You also have a responsibility to yourself. You must protect your health and safety, as well. Don't take short cuts when it comes to sanitation and disinfection. These important measures are designed to protect you, too!

Completed: Learning Objective #5

UNIVERSAL PRECAUTIONS AND PROFESSIONAL RESPONSIBILITIES

Finally, you have a responsibility to your craft. When anyone acts unprofessionally in the salon, everyone's image is tarnished. Clients expect to see you act in a professional manner. This is how trust and respect are earned!

REVIEW QUESTIONS

DECONTAMINATION AND INFECTION CONTROL

1. What is decontamination?
2. Why is sterilization the most effective type of decontamination?
3. Define sanitation and describe how salon tools and surfaces can be sanitized.
4. What is the difference between an antiseptic and a disinfectant?
5. What is the only way to ensure that a disinfectant is both safe and effective?
6. What is an MSDS?
7. EPA-registered disinfectants are effective against what pathogens?
8. Name three types of salon disinfectants.
9. Why is it recommended to avoid bar soaps in a salon?
10. Why is formalin considered unsafe to use in the salon?
11. What are the elements of universal precautions?

CHAPTER 4

Properties of the Hair and Scalp

LEARNING OBJECTIVES

After completing this chapter, you should be able to:

1. Explain the purposes of hair.
2. Define what hair is.
3. Describe the composition of hair.
4. Define the divisions of hair.
5. Describe the process of hair growth.
6. Define basic scalp care.
7. Describe the causes of hair loss.
8. Discuss hair loss treatment options.
9. Recognize the scalp and hair disorders commonly seen in the salon and school and know which can be treated there.

NATIONAL SKILL STANDARDS

This chapter provides you with the necessary information to master these National Industry Skill Standards for Entry-Level Cosmetologists:

- Consulting with clients to determine their needs and preferences
- Using a variety of salon products while providing client services

INTRODUCTION

As a hairstylist, it is important to have a technical knowledge of hair. This knowledge will be an asset to you as a professional cosmetologist.

Hair, like people, comes in a variety of colors, shapes, and sizes. To keep hair healthy and beautiful, proper attention must be given to its care and treatment. Applying a harsh product or providing improper hair services can cause the hair structure to become weakened or damaged. Knowledge and analysis of the client's hair, tactful suggestions for its improvement, and a sincere interest in maintaining its health and beauty should be primary concerns of every hairstylist.

HAIR

Completed: Learning Objectives #1 & #2
PURPOSE AND DEFINITION OF HAIR

The study of hair, technically called ***trichology*** (treye-**KOL**-o-jee), is important because stylists deal with hair on a daily basis.

The chief purposes of hair on the head are ***adornment*** and ***protection*** of the head from heat, cold, and injury. Hair is an ***appendage,*** a slender, threadlike outgrowth of the skin and scalp. Due to the absence of nerves, there is no sense of feeling in hair.

HAIR DISTRIBUTION

Hair is distributed all over the body except on the palms of the hands, soles of the feet, lips, and eyelids. There are three types of hair on the body (Fig. 4.1):

1. ***Long hair*** protects the scalp against the sun's rays and injury, gives adornment to the head, and forms a pleasing frame for the face. Soft, long hair also grows in the armpits of both sexes and on the faces of men. Male hormones, however, make a man's facial hair coarser than a woman's.
2. ***Short*** or ***bristly hair***, such as the eyebrows and eyelashes, adds beauty and color to the face. Eyebrows divert sweat

from the eyes. The eyelashes help protect the eyes from dust particles and light glare.

3. ***Vellus hair*** (also called ***lanugo***) is the fine, soft, downy hair on the cheeks, forehead, and nearly all other areas of the body. It helps in the efficient evaporation of perspiration.

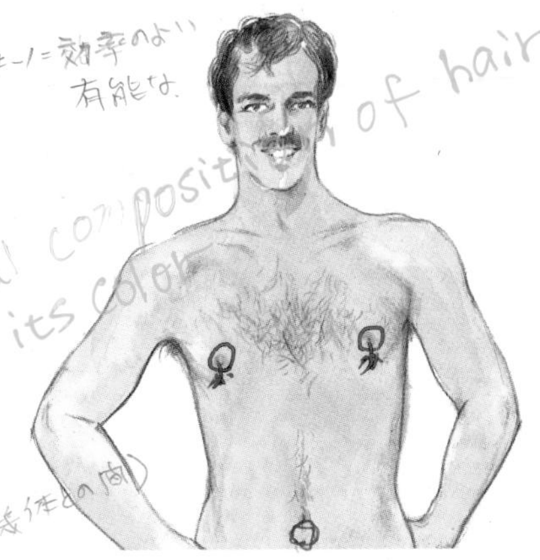

FIGURE 4.1 — Hair is distributed all over the body.

Technical Terms for Hair on the Head and Face

Barba (**BAR**-ba)—the face
Capilli (kah-**PIL**-i)—the head
Cilia (**SIL**-ee-a)—the eyelashes
Supercilia (soo-per-**SIL**-ee-a)—the eyebrows

COMPOSITION OF THE HAIR

Hair is composed chiefly of the protein ***keratin*** (**KER**-ah-tin), which is found in all horny growths including the nails and skin. (Fig. 4.2) The chemical composition of hair varies with its color. Darker hair has more carbon and less oxygen; the reverse is true for lighter hair. Average hair is composed of 50.65% carbon, 6.36% hydrogen, 17.14% nitrogen, 5.0% sulfur, and 20.85% oxygen.

Completed:
Learning Objective
#3
COMPOSITION OF HAIR

DIVISIONS OF THE HAIR

Full-grown human hair is divided into two principal parts: the root and the shaft. (Fig. 4.3)

1. The ***hair root*** is that portion of the hair structure located beneath the skin surface. This is the portion of the hair enclosed within the follicle.
2. The ***hair shaft*** is that portion of the hair structure extending above the skin surface.

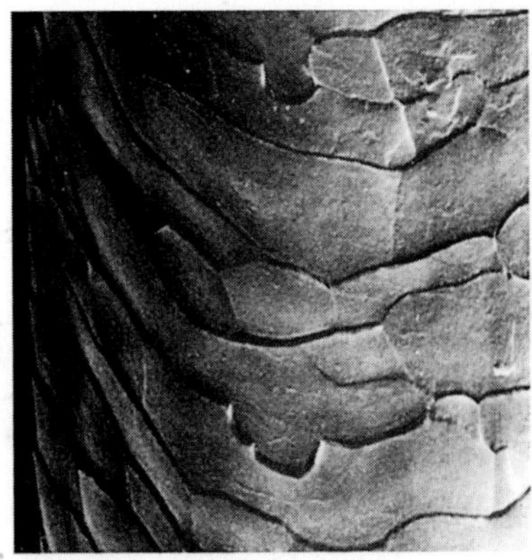

FIGURE 4.2 — Magnified view of hair cuticle, which is composed of keratin.

Structures Associated with the Hair Root

The three main structures associated with the hair root are the follicle, the bulb, and the papilla.

The ***follicle*** (**FOL**-ih-kel) is a tubelike depression, or pocket, in the skin or scalp that encases the hair root. Each hair has its own follicle, which varies in depth depending on the thickness and location of the skin. (We will talk later in this chapter about the different types of hair.) One or more oil glands are attached to each hair follicle.

The follicle does not run straight down into the skin or scalp, but is set at an angle so that the hair above the surface flows naturally to one side. (This natural flow, called the ***hair stream***, is addressed later in this chapter.)

Completed:
Learning Objective
#4
DIVISIONS OF HAIR

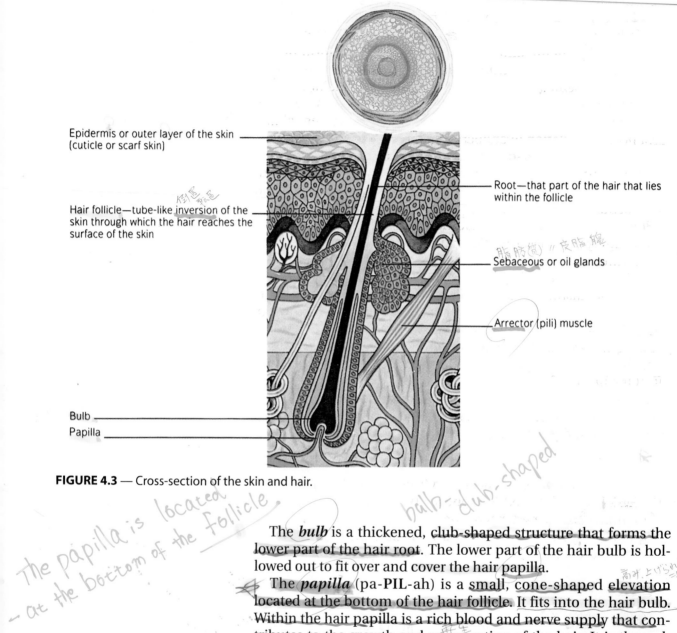

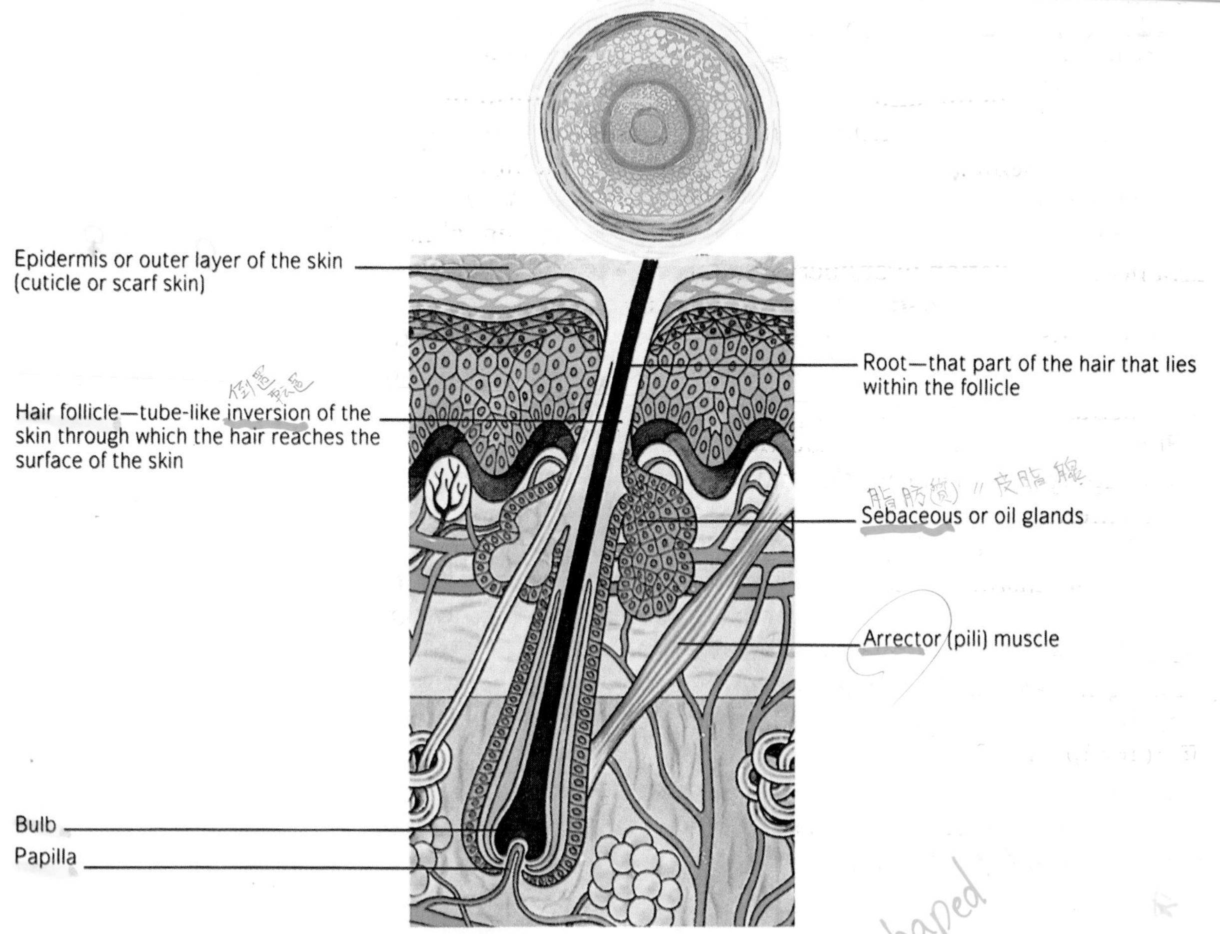

FIGURE 4.3 — Cross-section of the skin and hair.

The ***bulb*** is a thickened, club-shaped structure that forms the lower part of the hair root. The lower part of the hair bulb is hollowed out to fit over and cover the hair papilla.

The ***papilla*** (pa-**PIL**-ah) is a small, cone-shaped elevation located at the bottom of the hair follicle. It fits into the hair bulb. Within the hair papilla is a rich blood and nerve supply that contributes to the growth and regeneration of the hair. It is through the papilla that nourishment reaches the hair bulb. As long as the papilla is healthy and well nourished, it produces hair cells that enable new hair to grow.

Structures Associated with Hair Follicles

The ***arrector pili*** (a-**REK**-tohr **PEYE**-leye) is a small involuntary muscle attached to the underside of a hair follicle. Fear or cold causes it to contract, which makes the hair stand up straight, giving the skin the appearance of "gooseflesh." Eyelash and eyebrow hair do not have arrector pili muscles.

Sebaceous (si-**BAY**-shus) glands, or oil glands, consist of little sac-like structures in the dermis. Their ducts are connected to hair follicles. Sebaceous glands frequently become troublemakers by overproducing and bringing on a common form of oily dandruff. Normal secretion of an oily substance from these glands, called ***sebum*** (**SEE**-bum), gives luster and pliability to the hair and keeps the skin surface soft and supple. The production of sebum is influenced by diet, blood circulation, emotional disturbances, stimulation of endocrine glands, and drugs.

Diet. The food a person eats influences the general health of the hair. Eating too much sweet, starchy, and fatty foods can cause the sebaceous glands to become overactive and secrete too much sebum.

Blood circulation. The hair derives its nourishment from the blood supply, which in turn depends on the foods we eat for certain elements. In the absence of necessary foods, the health of the hair can be affected.

Emotional disturbances. Emotions are linked with the health of the hair through the nervous system. Unhealthy hair can be an indication of an unhealthy emotional state.

Endocrine glands. The secretions of the endocrine glands influence the health of the body. Any disturbance of these glands can affect the health of the body and, ultimately, the health of the hair.

Drugs. General anesthetics, as well as many prescription medications, can adversely affect the hair's ability to receive permanent waving and other chemical services.

Layers of the Hair Shaft

Hair is composed of cells arranged in three layers (Fig. 4.4):

1. ***Cuticle*** (**KYOO**-ti-kel). The outside horny layer is composed of transparent, overlapping, protective scalelike cells that point away from the scalp toward the hair ends. Chemicals raise these scales so that solutions such as chemical relaxers,

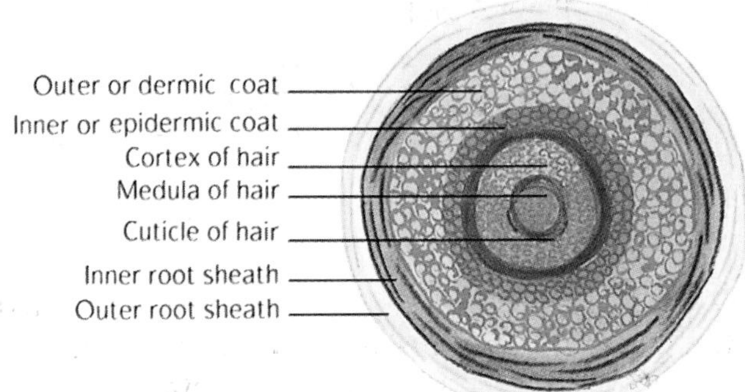

FIGURE 4.4 — Cross-section of the hair and follicle.

NORMAL HAIR CYCLE

As normal, healthy hair grows and sheds, each follicle repeatedly cycles through three stages, from active to inactive. All hair follicles have the same structure and cycle through the same three phases: ***anagen*** (AN-ah-jen, growing), ***catagen*** (CAT-ah-jen, transitional), and ***telogen*** (TELL-oh-jen, resting). (Fig. 4.6)

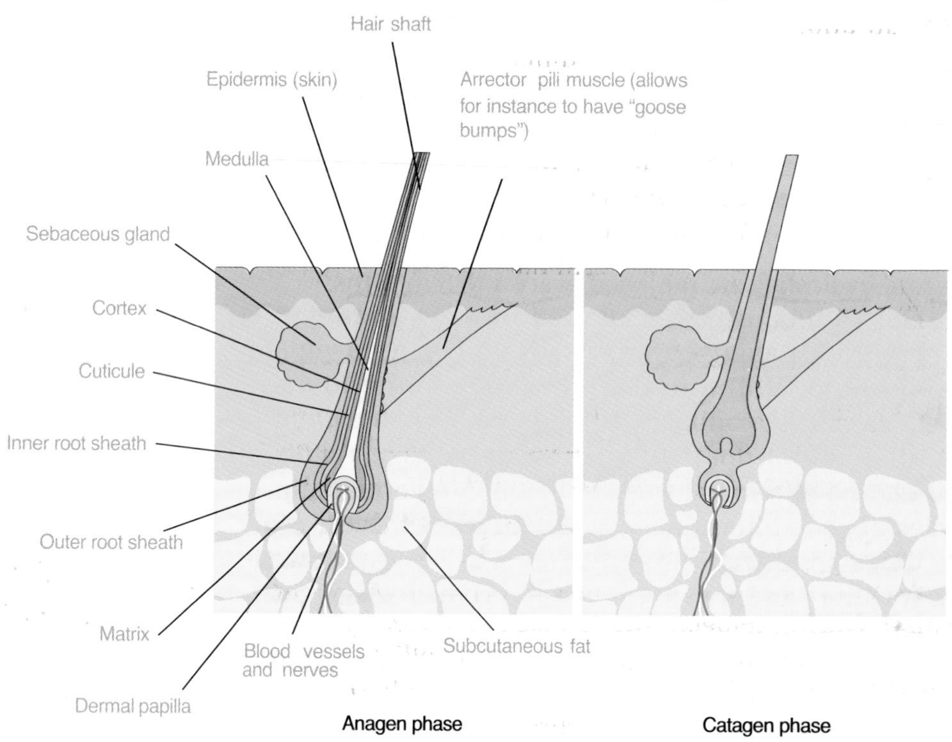

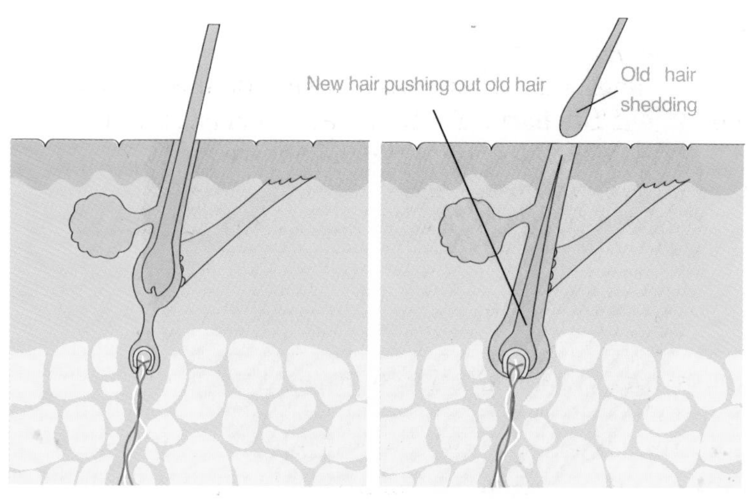

FIGURE 4.6 — Phases of the hair follicle. *(Courtesy of Pharmacia & Upjohn Company)*

Anagen: The Growing Phase

The average growth of healthy hair on the scalp is about ½" (1.25 cm) per month. At any one time, as much as 90% of the hair on our head is growing. It keeps growing for a period lasting from 2 to 6 years, during which the hair-shaft diameter increases in size and (if not cut) the hair reaches maximum length. Factors such as gender, age, type of hair, heredity, nutrition, and health have a bearing on the duration of hair life.

The rate of growth of human hair can differ on specific parts of the body, between sexes, and with age. Scalp hair grows faster on women than on men. Between the ages of 15 and 30, scalp hair grows rapidly, but slows down sharply after age 50. Hair growth also is influenced by nutrition, health, and hormones. During puberty, for example, follicles on some parts of the body increase in size, producing longer and thicker terminal hairs instead of the short, fine, vellus hairs it had before.

Catagen: The Transitional Phase

The transitional phase signals the end of the growth phase. It is very short, lasting one to two weeks. During catagen, the follicle rapidly decreases in volume and the lower part of the follicle is destroyed.

Telogen: The Resting Phase

When catagen ends, the hair follicle begins a two- to six-month phase of resting. During telogen, the follicle is shorter, approximately one half to a third of the length of an active follicle.

Only about 10% to 15% of our hair is in the resting phase at any one time. Hair follicle cycles are not synchronized; each one goes through these three phases independently.

After telogen, activity in the hair follicle begins again, returning to the anagen, or growing, phase. A new hair shaft forms and grows alongside the old hair, forcing it to fall out.

Under normal circumstances, everyone loses some hair every day—between 40 and 100 hairs. That's not as much as it sounds, since the the average head has about 100,000 individual shafts of hair. The number of hairs on the head varies with the color of the hair: blonde, 140,000; brown, 110,000; black, 108,000; red, 90,000.

DIRECTION OF HAIR GROWTH

Because the hair follicle is set at an angle, the hair above the surface of the skin slants in one direction or another. This results in hair streams, whorls, and cowlicks.

Hair stream. Hair flowing in the same direction is known as the hair stream. It is the result of the follicles sloping in the same direction. Two such streams, sloping in opposite directions, form a natural parting of the hair.

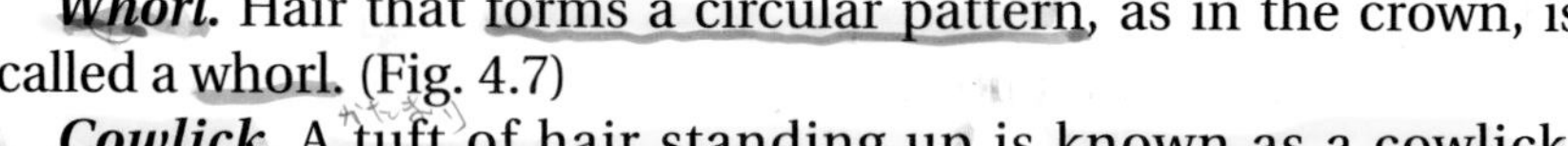

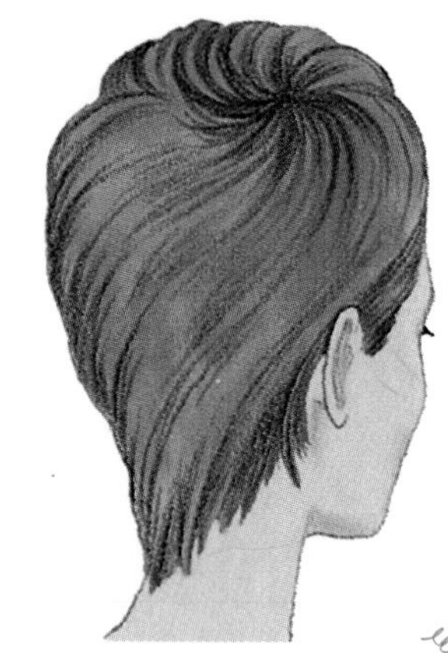

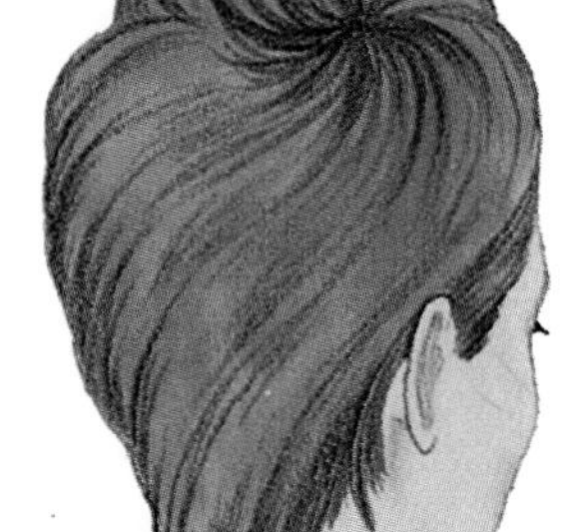

FIGURE 4.7 — Whorl.

Whorl. Hair that forms a circular pattern, as in the crown, is called a whorl. (Fig. 4.7)

Cowlick. A tuft of hair standing up is known as a cowlick. Cowlicks are more noticeable at the front hairline. However, they may be located on other parts of the scalp. When shaping or styling the hair, it is important to consider the direction of cowlicks. (Fig. 4.8)

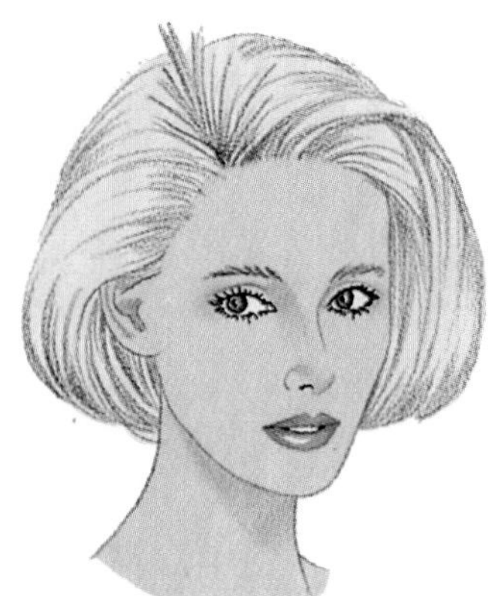

FIGURE 4.8 — Cowlick.

HAIR SHAPES

Hair usually has one of three general shapes. As it grows out, hair assumes the shape, size, and curve of the follicle. A cross-sectional view of the hair under the microscope reveals that:

1. Straight hair is usually round. (Fig. 4.9a)
2. Wavy hair is usually oval. (Fig. 4.9b)
3. Curly or kinky hair is almost flat. (Fig. 4.9c)

There is no strict rule regarding cross-sectional shapes of hair. Wavy, straight, and curly hair have been found in all shapes. A myth exists that race or nationality determines the shape of hair; this is false. Anyone can have straight, wavy, or curly hair no matter what race or nationality. The direction of a hair as it projects out of the follicle determines each person's hair shape.

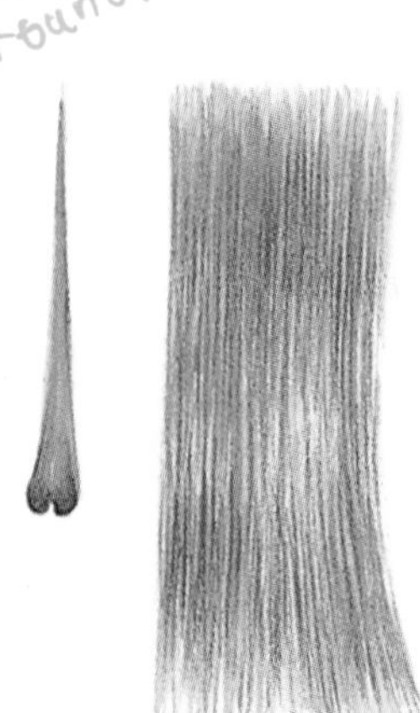

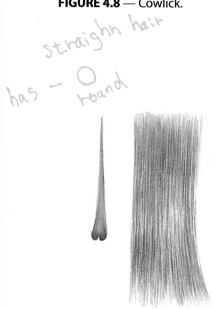

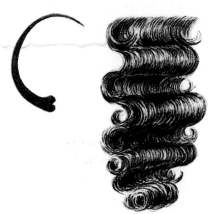

FIGURE 4.9a — Straight hair.

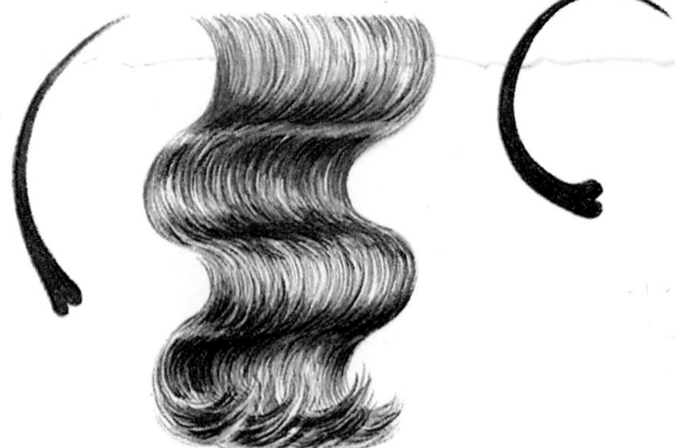

FIGURE 4.9b — Wavy hair.

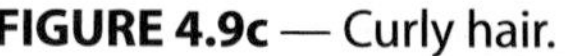

FIGURE 4.9c — Curly hair.

HAIR GROWTH MYTHS

Here are some myths about hair growth:

1. Close clipping, shaving, trimming, cutting, or singeing have an effect on the rate of hair growth. This is *not* true.
2. The application of oils increases hair growth. This is *not* true. Oils lubricate the hair shaft, but they *do not* feed the hair.
3. Hair grows after death. This is *not* true. The flesh and skin contract, thus there is the appearance of hair growth.
4. Singeing the hair seals in the natural oil. This is *not* true.

Completed:
Learning Objective
#5
DESCRIBE HAIR GROWTH

HAIR ANALYSIS

Much of the cosmetologist's time is taken up with servicing and styling clients' hair. For your hairstyling to be successful, you need to be able to recognize the type and condition of a client's hair and be able to analyze it before you begin any services.

CONDITION OF THE HAIR

Knowledge of hair and skill in determining its condition can be acquired by constant observation using the senses available to you: sight, touch, hearing, and smell.

1. ***Sight.*** Observing the hair will immediately give you some knowledge about its condition. Looking at the hair contributes approximately 15% of your analysis; touching the hair is the final determining factor.
2. ***Touch.*** Cosmetologists are guided by the touch or feel of the hair in making a professional hair analysis. When the sense of touch is fully developed, fewer mistakes will be made in judging the hair.
3. ***Hearing.*** Listen to what clients tell you about their hair, health problems, reactions to cosmetics, and medications they might be taking. You will be in a better position to analyze the condition of hair more accurately.
4. ***Smell.*** Unclean hair and certain scalp disorders create an odor. If the client generally has good health, you might suggest regular shampooing and proper rinsing.

QUALITIES OF THE HAIR

Qualities by which human hair is analyzed are texture, porosity, and elasticity.

Texture

Hair texture refers to the degree of coarseness or fineness of the hair, which may vary on different parts of the head. Variations in hair texture are due to:

1. ***Diameter of the hair,*** whether coarse, medium, fine, or very fine. Coarse hair has the greatest diameter; very fine hair has the smallest.
2. ***Feel of the hair,*** whether harsh, soft, or wiry.

Medium hair is the normal type most commonly seen in the salon or school. This type of hair does not present any special problems. ***Fine*** or ***very fine hair*** requires special care. Its microscopic structure usually reveals that only two layers, the cortex and cuticle, are present. ***Wiry hair***, whether coarse, medium, or fine, has a hard, glassy finish caused by the cuticle scales lying flat against the hair shaft. It takes longer for chemicals such as permanent wave solutions, tints, or lighteners to penetrate this type of hair.

Porosity

Hair porosity is the ability of all types of hair to absorb moisture ***(hygroscopic quality)***. Hair has good porosity when the cuticle layer is raised from the hair shaft and can absorb a fair or normal amount of moisture or chemicals. Moderate porosity (normal hair) is most often seen in the salon or school. It is less porous than hair with good porosity. Usually hair with good or moderate porosity presents no problem when receiving hair services, whether permanent waving, hair tinting, or lightening. Poor porosity (resistant hair) exists when the cuticle layer is lying close to the hair shaft and absorbs the least amount of moisture. Hair with poor porosity requires thorough analysis and strand tests before the application of hair cosmetics. Extreme porosity is seen in hair in poor condition. It may be due to tinting, lightening, or damage from continuous or faulty treatments.

Elasticity

Hair elasticity is the ability of hair to stretch and return to its original form without breaking. Hair can be classified as having good elasticity, normal elasticity, or poor elasticity. (Refer to the chapter on permanent waving for more information.) Hair with normal elasticity is springy and has a lively and lustrous appearance. Normal dry hair is capable of being stretched about one-fifth of its length; it springs back when released. Wet hair can be stretched 40% to 50% of its length. Porous hair stretches more than hair with poor porosity.

CAUTION

You should see by now that hair is complex and you must analyze each client individually. Never make a snap judgment that a client will have a particular hair type.

SCALP CARE

Two basic requisites for a healthy scalp are cleanliness and stimulation. The scalp and hair should be kept clean by frequent treatment and shampooing. A healthy, clean scalp will resist a variety of disorders.

SCALP MANIPULATIONS

Since the same manipulations are given with all scalp treatments, you should learn to give them with a continuous, even motion, which will stimulate the scalp and/or soothe the client's tension. Scalp massage is most effectively applied as a series of treatments: once a week for normal scalp and more frequently for scalp disorders, under the direction of a dermatologist.

Anatomy

Knowing the muscles, the location of blood vessels, and the nerve points of the scalp and neck will help guide you to those areas in which massage movements are to be directed for the most beneficial results. (See chapter on cells, anatomy, and physiology.)

Scalp Manipulation Technique

There are several ways in which scalp manipulations may be given. The following routines may be changed to meet your instructor's requirements.

With each massage movement, place the hands under the hair so the length of the fingers, balls of the fingertips, and cushions of the palms can stimulate the muscles, nerves, and blood vessels of the scalp area.

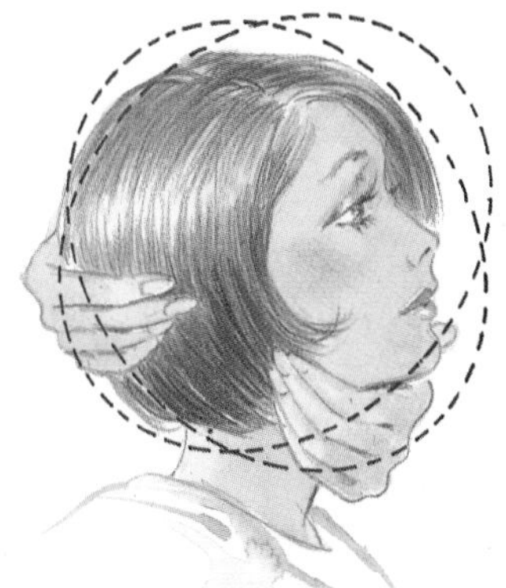

FIGURE 4.10 — Relaxing movement.

1. RELAXING MOVEMENT. Cup the client's chin in your left hand; place your right hand at the base of her skull, and rotate head gently. Reverse positions of your hands and repeat. (Fig. 4.10)
2. SLIDING MOVEMENT. Place your fingertips on each side of the client's head; slide your hands firmly upward, spreading the fingertips until they meet at the top of the head. Repeat four times. (Fig.4.11)

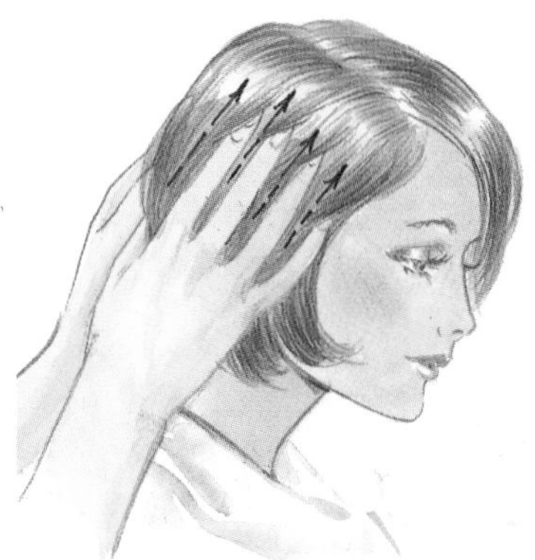

FIGURE 4.11 — Sliding movement.

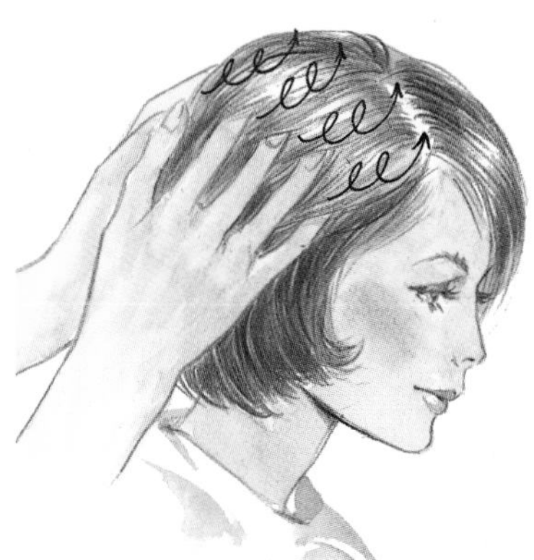

FIGURE 4.12 — Sliding and rotating movement.

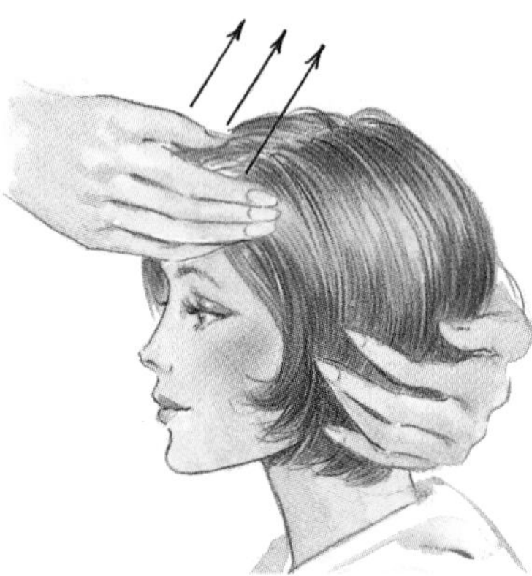

FIGURE 4.13 — Forehead movement.

3. SLIDING AND ROTATING MOVEMENT. Same as movement No. 2, except that after sliding the fingertips 1" (2.5 cm), you rotate and move the client's scalp. Repeat four times. (Fig. 4.12)
4. FOREHEAD MOVEMENT. Hold the back of the client's head with your left hand. Place stretched thumb and fingers of your right hand on the client's forehead. Move your hand slowly and firmly upward to 1" (2.5 cm) past the hairline. Repeat four times. (Fig. 4.13)
5. SCALP MOVEMENT. Place the palms of your hands firmly against the client's scalp. Lift the scalp in a rotary movement, first with your hands placed above her ears, and second with your hands placed at the front and back of her head. (Fig. 4.14)
6. HAIRLINE MOVEMENT. Place the fingers of both hands at the client's forehead. Massage around her hairline by lifting and rotating. (Fig. 4.15)
7. FRONT SCALP MOVEMENT. Dropping back 1" (2.5 cm), repeat preceding movement over entire front and top of the scalp. (Fig. 4.16)
8. BACK SCALP MOVEMENT. Place the fingers of each hand on the sides of the client's head. Starting below her ears, manipulate the scalp with your thumbs, working upward to the crown. Repeat four times. Repeat thumb manipulations, working toward the center back of the head. (Fig. 4.17)
9. EAR-TO-EAR MOVEMENT. Place your left hand on the client's forehead. Massage from the right ear to the left ear along the base of her skull with the heel of your hand, using a rotary movement. (Fig. 4.18)

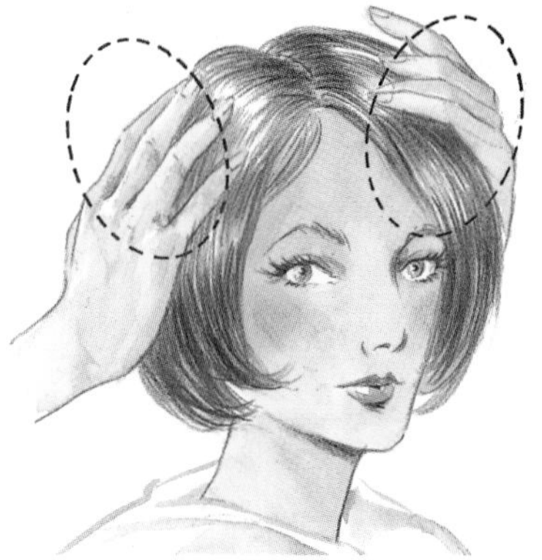

FIGURE 4.14 — Scalp movement.

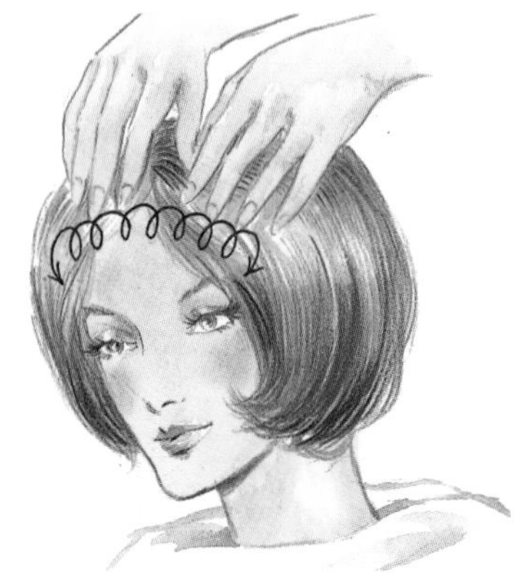

FIGURE 4.15 — Hairline movement.

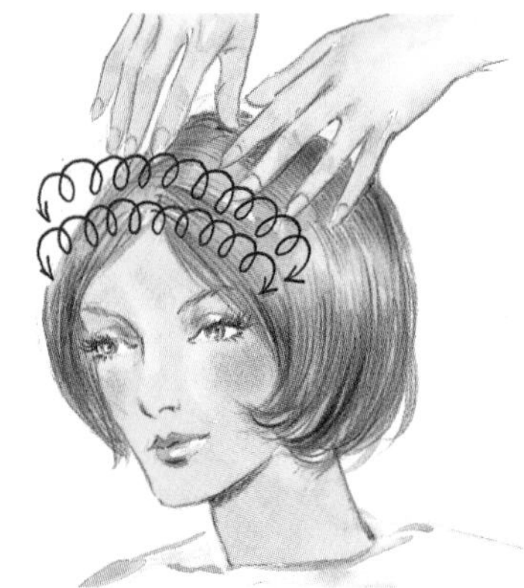

FIGURE 4.16 — Front scalp movement.

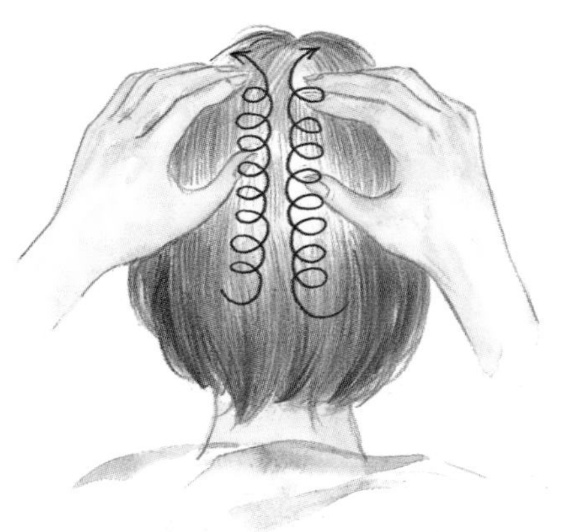

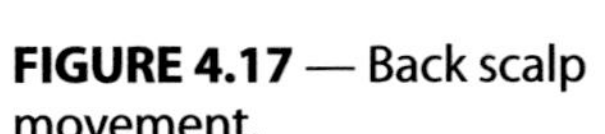

FIGURE 4.17 — Back scalp movement.

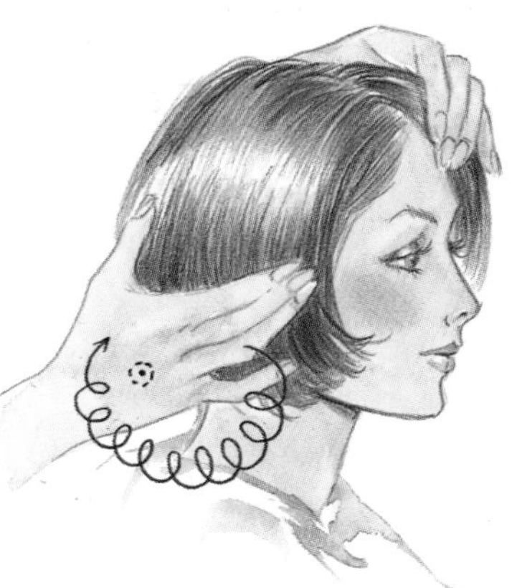

FIGURE 4.18 — Ear-to-ear movement.

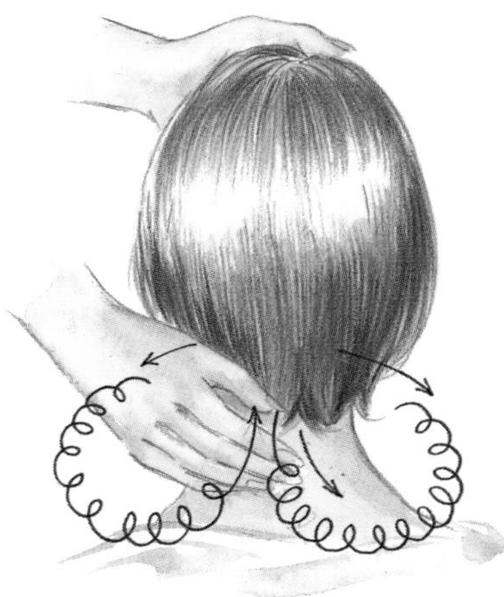

FIGURE 4.19 — Back movement.

10. BACK MOVEMENT. Place your left hand on the client's forehead and stand to the left of her. Using your right hand, rotate from the base of the client's neck, along the shoulder, and back across the shoulder blade to the spine. Slide your hand up the client's spine to the base of her neck. Repeat on the opposite side. (Fig. 4.19)
11. SHOULDER MOVEMENT. Place both your palms together at the base of the client's neck. With rotary movement, catch muscles in the palms and massage along the shoulder blades to the point of her shoulders, and then back again. Then massage from the shoulders to the spine and back again. (Fig. 4.20)
12. SPINE MOVEMENT. Massage from the base of the client's skull down the spine with a rotary movement. Using a firm finger pressure, bring your hand slowly to the base of the client's skull. (Fig. 4.21)

Completed:
Learning Objective
#6
BASIC SCALP CARE

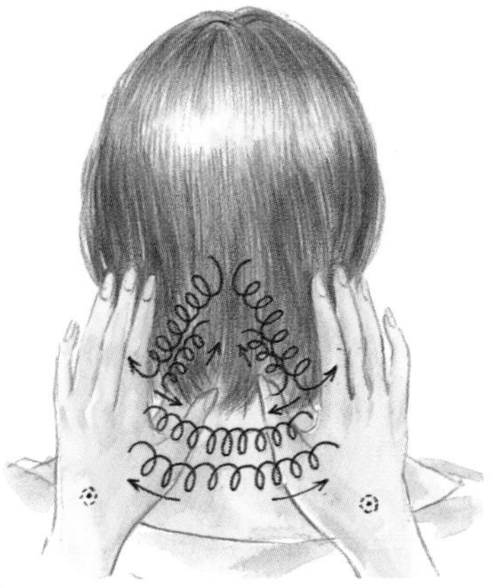

FIGURE 4.20 — Shoulder movement.

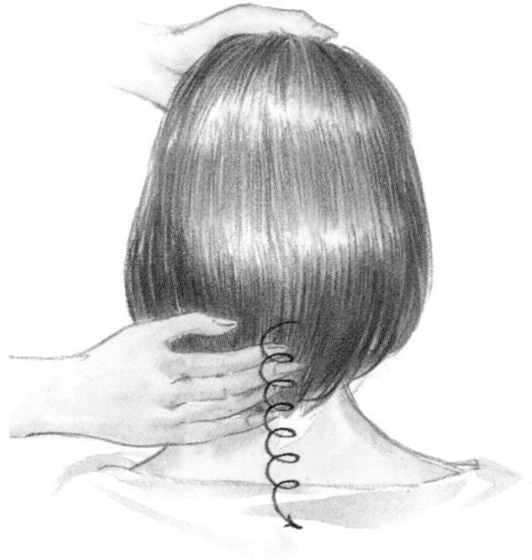

FIGURE 4.21 — Spine movement.

GENERAL HAIR AND SCALP TREATMENTS

The purpose of a general scalp treatment is to keep the scalp and hair in a clean and healthy condition. Regular scalp treatments may help slow some types of hair loss.

NORMAL HAIR AND SCALP TREATMENTS

1. Drape client.
2. Brush hair for about 5 minutes.
3. Apply scalp cream.
4. Apply infrared lamp for about 5 minutes.
5. Give scalp manipulations for 10 to 20 minutes.
6. Shampoo the hair.
7. Towel-dry the hair to remove excess moisture.
8. Apply suitable scalp lotion.
9. Set, dry, and style hair.
10. Clean up your work station.

DRY HAIR AND SCALP TREATMENTS

This treatment should be used when there is a deficiency of natural oil on the scalp and hair. Select scalp preparations containing moisturizing and emollient materials. Avoid the use of strong soaps, preparations containing a mineral oil or sulfonated oil base, greasy preparations, and lotions with a high alcohol content.

1. Drape client.
2. Brush client's hair for about 5 minutes.
3. Apply the scalp preparation for this condition.
4. Apply the scalp steamer for 7 to 10 minutes, or wrap the head in warm steam towels for 7 to 10 minutes.
5. Give a mild shampoo.
6. Towel-dry the hair and scalp thoroughly.
7. Apply moisturizing scalp cream sparingly with a rotary, frictional motion.
8. Stimulate the scalp with direct high-frequency current, using the glass rake electrode, for about 5 minutes.

9. Set, dry, and style the hair.
10. Clean up your work station.

OILY HAIR AND SCALP TREATMENTS

Excessive oiliness is caused by the over-activity of the sebaceous (oil) glands. Manipulate the scalp and knead it to increase blood circulation to the scalp. Any hardened sebum in the pores of the scalp will be removed with the correct degree of pressing or squeezing. To normalize the function of these glands, excess sebum should be flushed out with each treatment.

1. Drape client.
2. Brush client's hair for about 5 minutes.
3. Apply a medicated scalp lotion to the scalp only with a cotton pledget. (Fig. 4.22)
4. Apply infrared lamp for about 5 minutes.
5. Give scalp manipulations. (Optional: Faradic or sinusoidal current may be used.) (Figs. 4.23, 4.24)
6. Shampoo with a corrective shampoo for oily scalp.
7. Towel dry the hair.
8. Apply direct high-frequency current for 3 to 5 minutes.
9. Apply a scalp astringent.
10. Set, dry, and style the hair.
11. Clean up your work station.

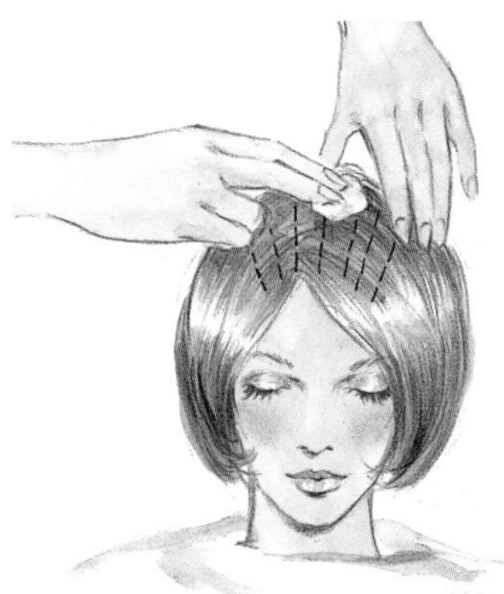

FIGURE 4.22 — Applying scalp lotion with cotton pledget.

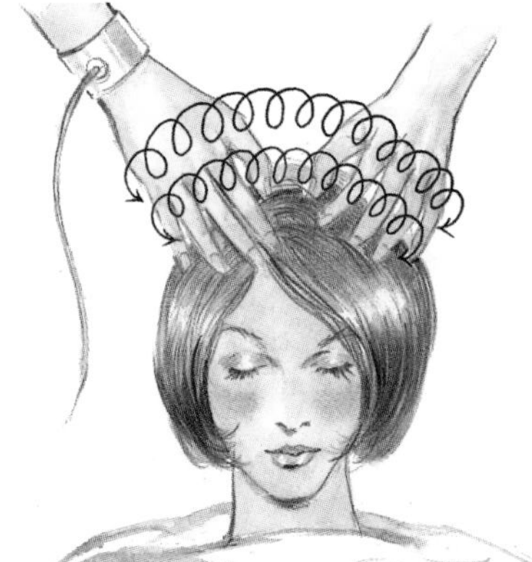

FIGURE 4.23 — Applying faradic current, cosmetologist manipulates scalp.

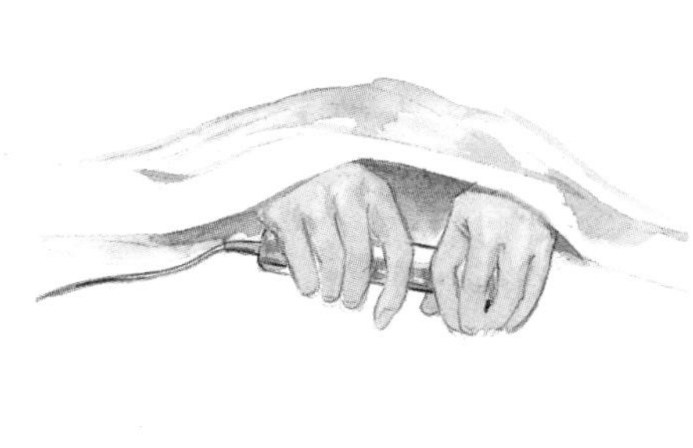

FIGURE 4.24 — While cosmetologist manipulates scalp, client holds electrode.

CAUTION

Do not use high-frequency current on hair treated with tonics or lotions that contain alcohol.

CORRECTIVE HAIR TREATMENT

A corrective hair treatment deals with the hair shaft, not the scalp. Dry and damaged hair can be greatly improved by conditioners. Hair treatments are especially beneficial and extremely important when given approximately a week or 10 days before, and a week or 10 days after, a permanent wave, tint, lightener, toner, or chemical hair straightening treatment.

Dry hair may be softened quickly with a conditioning preparation applied directly on the hair shaft. The product used for this purpose is usually an emulsion containing cholesterol and related compounds.

Some conditioners function more effectively when heat is applied to induce penetration into the cortex. The heat applied to the hair opens the cuticle's imbrications, and permits significantly more corrective agents to enter the hair shaft. This provides more conditioning benefits.

1. Drape client.
2. Brush the client's hair for about 5 minutes.
3. Apply a mild shampoo.
4. Towel-dry the hair.
5. Apply a conditioner according to the manufacturer's directions.
6. Set, dry, and style hair.
7. Clean up your work station.

HAIR LOSS

Over 63 million people in the United States suffer from hair loss. As a salon professional, you may be the first person many of these people will come to with questions about hair loss. You provide a comfortable and confidential environment for clients to discuss hair loss, and you must be informed to advise your clients and provide them with correct information. The information and services you provide will greatly affect the well-being and self-esteem of your clients.

Hair loss is a relatively new area of research. Scientists believe that approximately 95% of the hair loss seen in men and women is caused by a progressive condition called ***androgenetic alope-***

cia (an-droh-je-**NE**-tik al-oh-**PEE**-shee-ah), or common hereditary hair loss.

ANDROGENETIC ALOPECIA

The most common type of hair loss, androgenetic alopecia affects some 40 million men and 20 million women in the United States. Hair loss can begin as early as the teens and is frequently fully seen by the age of 40. By age 35, almost 40% of men and women show some degree of hair loss.

The gene for androgenetic alopecia can be inherited from either side of the family or from both sides. Affected members of the same family may have varying degrees of thinning. In men, this is known as male pattern baldness and usually progresses to the familiar horseshoe-shaped fringe of hair. In women, it turns up as a generalized thinning of the hair over the entire crown of the head. Over time, the hair on the sides may also become thinner. Women retain their frontal hair line, which may be straight or M-shaped. It is extremely rare for a woman to go bald.

Miniaturization of the Hair Follicle

In androgenetic alopecia, a combination of heredity, hormones, and age causes progressive shrinking, or miniaturization, of certain scalp follicles. This causes a shortening of the hair's growing cycle. Over time, as the active growth phase becomes shorter, the resting phase becomes longer. Eventually, there is no growth at all. The number of follicles that become miniaturized depends on the heredity of the person.

Because hair length and thickness are determined by how long the hair is allowed to grow before entering the next resting and shedding phase, the hair loss process is thus a gradual conversion of terminal hair follicles to vellus-like hair follicles. (Fig. 4.25) The net result is an increasing number of short, thin hairs that are barely visible above the scalp surface. Eventually no more hair is produced out of these follicles. In addition, more follicles are in the resting phase at the same time. Consequently, there is less scalp coverage.

Despite the dramatic change in follicle size with androgenetic alopecia, the follicle is not altered in structure and the number of follicles does not change.

OTHER TYPES OF HAIR LOSS

Alopecia Areata

There is a sudden loss of hair in round or irregular patches; the scalp is not inflamed. This type of hair loss occurs in individuals who have no obvious skin disorder or serious disease. It is often

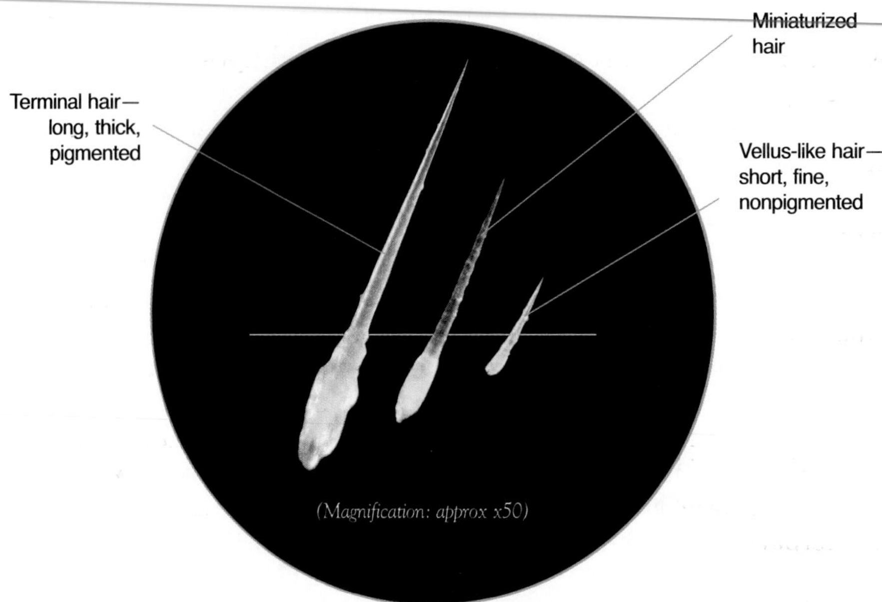

FIGURE 4.25 — Progressive miniaturization of the hair follicle.

attributed to stress. Alopecia areata is confined to a few areas and is often reversed in a few months, though recurrences may occur. The National Alopecia Areata Foundation estimates that 2.5 million men, women, and children suffer from this type of hair loss.

Telogen Effluvium

This premature shedding of hair in the resting phase (telogen) can result from various causes, such as difficult childbirth, shock, drug intake, fever, etc. Some women also experience sudden hair loss when they stop taking birth-control pills or if they follow a crash diet too low in protein. The hair loss is usually reversed once the condition is resolved.

Traction or Traumatic Alopecia

Patchy or diffuse hair loss is sometimes due to repetitive traction on the hair by pulling or twisting. This type of hair loss also occurs after excessive application of chemicals, such as permanent wave solutions, or after excessive use of hot combs. This condition is usually reversed once trauma has stopped.

Postpartum Alopecia

Women sometimes experience temporary hair loss at the conclusion of a pregnancy. While some women can lose tremendous amounts of hair in the weeks following the birth of their child, the abnormal hair loss slows as hormone levels in the body return to pre-pregnancy levels.

Completed: Learning Objective #7

CAUSES OF HAIR LOSS

THE EMOTIONAL IMPACT OF HAIR LOSS

Generally, the medical community has looked upon hair loss with complacency, stating that it was a nonmedical condition. But the mental anguish that many hair loss sufferers feel is very real, overlooked, and not fully addressed.

Psychosocial Effects of Hair Loss in Men

Thomas F. Cash, Ph.D., a professor of psychology at Old Dominion University in Norfolk, Virginia, investigated perceptions of bald or balding men in Western society.

Subjects were asked to rate photographs of balding and nonbalding men according to seven different dimensions, such as age, success, and attractiveness, but were never told that baldness was a variable.

Results showed that, when compared to nonbalding matched counterparts, balding men were perceived as follows:

- Less physically attractive (by both sexes)
- Less assertive
- Less successful
- Less personally likable
- Older (by about 5 years)

Only perceptions of intelligence seemed to be unaffected by baldness.

In another study, Dr. Cash investigated how balding men perceive themselves. Results of this study showed that greater hair loss had a more significant negative impact than did moderate hair loss. Men with more severe hair loss:

- Experience significantly more negative socioemotional effects.
- Are more preoccupied with their baldness.
- Make marginal efforts to conceal or compensate for hair loss.

Dr. Cash concluded the following:

- It is improbable for baldness not to impair overall functioning.
- Balding men are less satisfied not only about their hair, but also about their appearance in general.
- For those with a poor self-image initially, hair loss may be the focal concern.

Emotional Distress in Women

"To a woman, hair loss is devastating," states Dr. Vera H. Price, MD, clinical professor of dermatology at the University of

California in San Francisco. According to studies conducted by Dr. Price, women with hair loss often master the art of camouflage to disguise their alopecia from everyone, many times even from their physicians. When they realize that their hair is thinning, women tend to worry that their alopecia is the symptom of a serious illness.

Studies indicate that women have a greater psychosocial investment in their appearance. The vast majority of women with hair loss feel anxious, helpless, and less attractive. In a survey, many women with hair loss thought they were the only ones experiencing that problem. Several feared that friends and family would blame them for not taking good care of themselves. A few women even had suicidal thoughts. For some, the embarrassment was such that they stopped socializing and stayed at home.

It may take some time for a woman experiencing hair loss to develop the courage to discuss the situation with her physician, hairdresser, or significant other. Some investigators believe it takes about 50% hair loss before that hair loss is noticeable to someone else. A woman may notice that she is shedding more and that her hair is thinner. But if she starts out with a very thick head of hair the loss may not be that obvious to others.

RECOGNIZING HAIR LOSS

The earlier hair loss is detected, the higher the chances to successfully treat it. Cosmetologists are in a position to help detect early signs of hair loss and, where appropriate, recommend treatment.

Recognizing Androgenetic Alopecia

In general, asking questions about family history will give a good indication as to whether the hair loss is androgenetic. Ask your client if her/his parents or more distant relatives have hair loss and whether their thinning has been gradual over several years.

In the area where the scalp shows the most, look for a large number of miniaturized follicles that are producing shorter, thinner, less pigmented hairs than the long ones. Unlike hairs that have been cut short and have a flat end, miniaturized hairs have a pointy end. Hold an index card near the scalp to help you see the miniaturized hairs. (Fig. 4.26a) If you see a lot of miniaturized hairs, your client has androgenetic alopecia.

In men with balding of the vertex, the size of the bald spot has progressively increased over the years. In frontal balding, the hair line has been progressively receding.

In women, use the following techniques to determine hair loss:

1. Part the hair in the middle of the scalp and look at the width of the part. A part that shows more scalp than normal indicates hair loss. (The part on a normal head of hair is very narrow.)

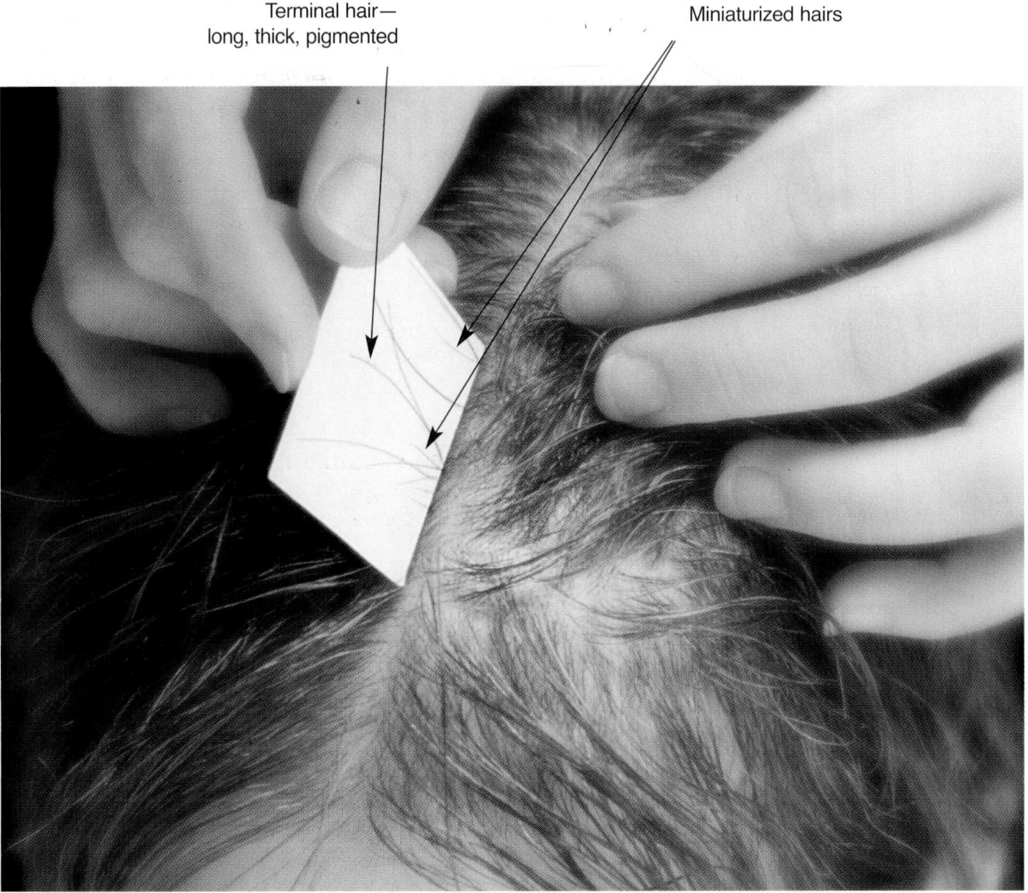

FIGURE 4.26a — Hair-loss evaluation. Note miniaturized hair. *(Courtesy of Pharmacia & Upjohn Company)*

2. Check if the size of the diameter of the ponytail has become smaller over time.

Recognizing Alopecia Areata

Ask your client if hair loss was sudden or patchy. If the hair loss was sudden or patchy, advise your client to talk to a physician. Severe stress or other health factors are causing the hair loss. (Fig. 4.26b)

Recognizing Telogen Effluvium

If your client is a woman, ask her about crash diets and oral contraceptives. Some women experience sudden hair loss when they follow a crash diet too low in protein or stop taking birth control pills. The hair loss is usually reversed when these conditions are resolved.

Another way to check for telogen effluvium is to grasp 30 to 40 hairs between thumb and forefinger at the base of the hair and gently pull to the tips. Check eight to ten different areas of the

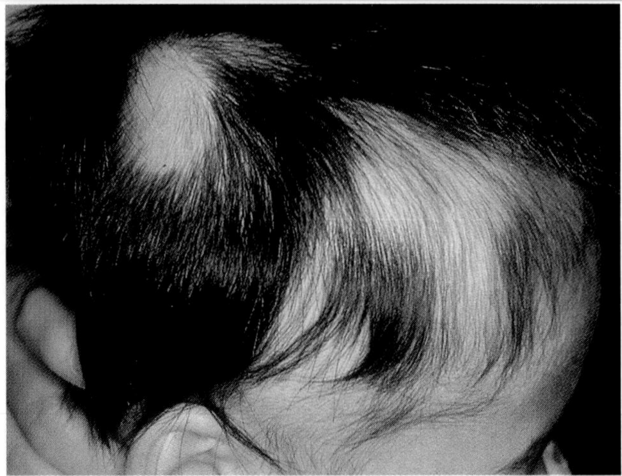

FIGURE 4.26b — Alopecia areata. *(Courtesy of Robert A. Silverman, MD, Clinical Associate Professor, Department of Pediatrics, Georgetown University)*

scalp. If more than three to five hairs come out easily, the woman has active shedding and may be going through telogen effluvium (temporary sudden hair loss). Unlike anagen hairs, telogen hairs do not have attached root sheaths so when they are pulled they do not have visible translucent tissue attached to the base.

The Savin Classification System

A universal methodology to classify and record pattern and density variations of androgenetic alopecia was developed by Dr. Ronald C. Savin, MD. The Savin scales provide you with the tools to evaluate the degree of hair loss and also the degree of response to a hair loss treatment.

Because hair grows slowly, the time lapse between evaluations should be two to four months. These scales are excellent tools to perform consistent evaluations from one visit to the other.

The degree of hair loss can be evaluated by rating pattern and density. ***Pattern*** refers to the shape and location of the area with hair loss, and ***density*** refers to how much hair is covering the scalp in the area of hair loss. In men, it is important to evaluate pattern separately from density because a man with a small pattern but a poor density may not respond to treatment as well as a man with a large area of hair loss and a fair density.

In male pattern baldness, three areas of the scalp intersect:

- The front
- The middle area
- The vertex

As balding progresses, the vertex and the mid-area appear to overlap. In advanced stages of hair loss, the vertex and the frontal areas converge.

Because of these three distinct areas of hair loss in men, it was necessary to divide the head into three areas and create three pattern scales:

- Frontal hair loss scale
- Mid-area hair loss scale
- Vertex hair loss scale

The scales allow for over 100,000 staging combinations in male-pattern baldness.

Because women experience a single pattern of hair loss (central diffuse hair loss), only density needs to be evaluated. In addition, a density scale was developed to assign a density value to each of the three pattern areas and for diffuse hair loss in women. (Fig. 4.27)

HAIR LOSS TREATMENTS

After consulting with your client, if you are confident that the hair loss is androgenetic alopecia, you can actually offer him/her a few options. If you are not sure of the cause of hair loss, recommend that your client see a doctor.

Nonmedical Cosmetology Options

Wigs, toupees, and hair weaving/hair extensions are services a trained cosmetologist can offer. Many of your clients will appreciate your knowledge and skills in fitting and styling wigs and toupees. Hair weaving/hair extensions allows you to enhance a client's natural hair, boosting their self-esteem while creating a look that meets their needs.

In addition, there are many thickening and volumizing hair products available today. It is important to note that they do not physiologically thicken hair. Nor do they put a halt to hair loss or actually grow hair. Volumizing products coat the hair, giving it more body.

Medical Treatments

Two effective treatments for hair loss are available, one a topical treatment and the other a drug.

Topical treatment. Minoxidil is a topical solution medically proven to regrow hair when applied to the scalp, usually twice a day. Since April 1996 it has been sold without a prescription and is available in two strengths. It has no adverse effects on hormones or sexual function, and is not associated with adverse effects on blood pressure, pulse rate, body weight, electrocardiograms, or laboratory assays.

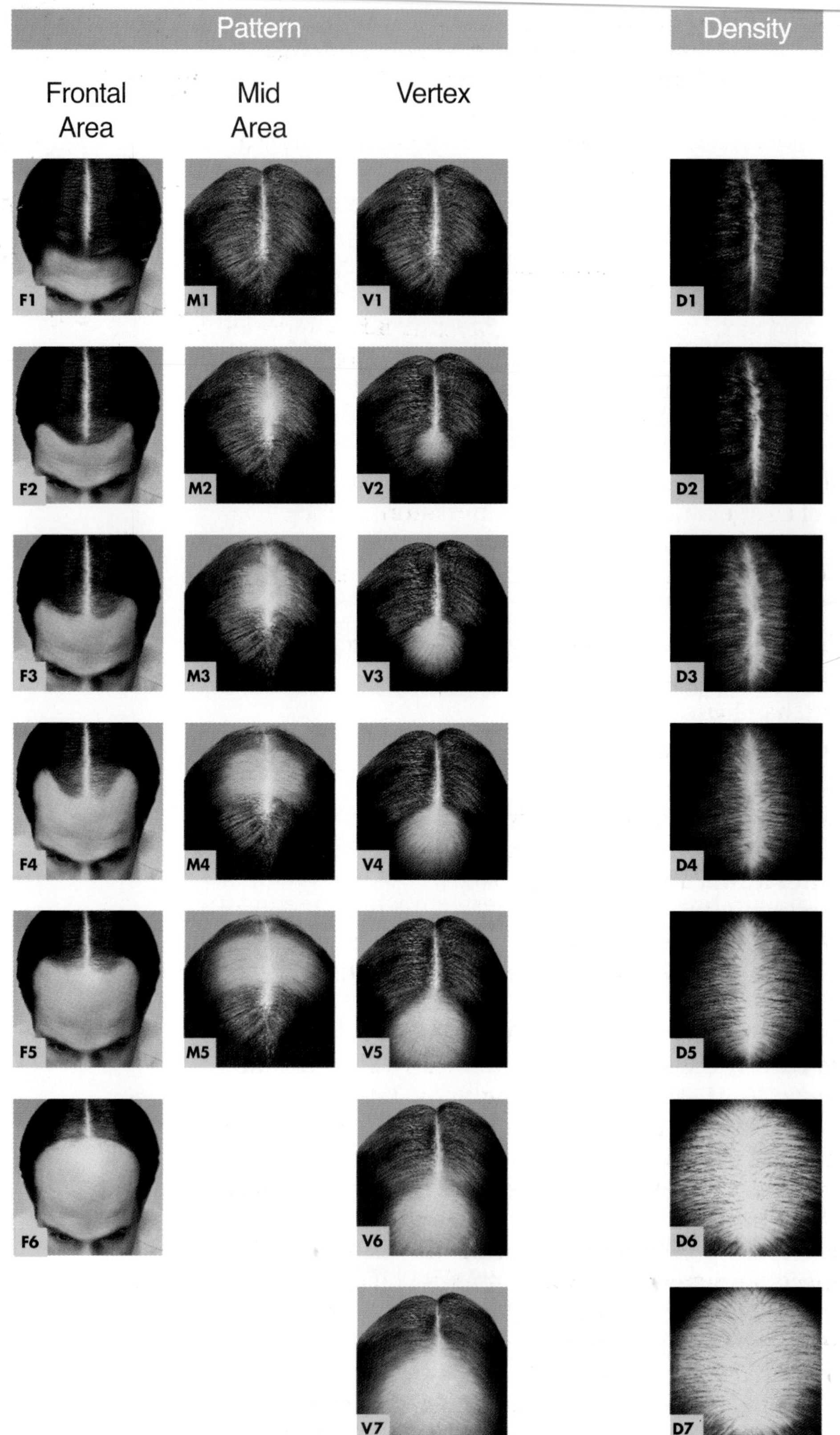

FIGURE 4.27 — Savin scales. *(Courtesty of Pharmacia & Upjohn Company)*

Minoxidil works by partially enlarging miniaturized follicles and reversing the miniaturization process. This prolongs the growth phase of the hair cycle, allowing the hair to become longer and thicker.

With more follicles in the growth phase at the same time, scalp coverage is improved. Although the growth phase may be prolonged, the follicle will continue to cycle. Better results are seen after twelve months of usage.

Best responses are seen in Savin Scales' patterns of 2, 3, 4 and densities of 2, 3, 4, 5, 6. At four months, regrowth was reported by 59% of men and at 12 months, by 84%. In women 59% reported regrowth at eight months. In a separate study, 80% of minoxidil users reported at least maintaining the amount of hair they had.

Factors favoring regrowth with minoxidil are:

- Active follicles. An important factor that favors regrowth is the presence of a large number of partially miniaturized follicles that are still producing hair 3/8 of an inch or more in length. Any area of the scalp where only vellus-like hair remains is less likely to respond to treatment.
- Age. Clinical studies suggest that people who are younger have a better response.
- More recent hair loss.
- Smaller area of hair loss.

As we discussed, it takes time for hair to grow. Follicles must go through a full cycle before they can grow hair to their maximum potential. Miniaturized follicles will need to cycle to produce new, stronger hair. New growth may first appear as soft, downy, and barely visible hairs (like peach fuzz). This is a very encouraging sign because it shows that new regrowth is actually being stimulated.

By continuing treatment, the soft, downy growth should change into hair of the same color and thickness as the other hairs on the scalp. If clients stop using the solution, the new regrowth may be lost in a few months and hair loss will begin again. Minoxidil is a *treatment* for hair loss, not a cure.

Drug treatment. In 1998 another medically proven treatment, finasteride, became available to physicians in the United States. This is a once-a-day prescription pill for the treatment of androgenetic alopecia in men only. It works through male hormones. Pregnant women or women who might possibly become pregnant are not to touch crushed tablets because of the strong potential for birth defects.

Surgical options. Surgical options are mostly available for men. Hair transplants, hair plugs, and scalp reductions are

Completed: Learning Objective #8
HAIR LOSS TREATMENT

performed by physicians. Several surgeries are necessary to achieve results. The cost of each surgery ranges from $5,000 to more than $20,000.

DISORDERS OF THE HAIR

CANITIES

Canities (ka-**NIT**-eez) is the technical term for gray (unpigmented) hair. Its immediate cause is the loss of natural pigment in the hair. There are two types:

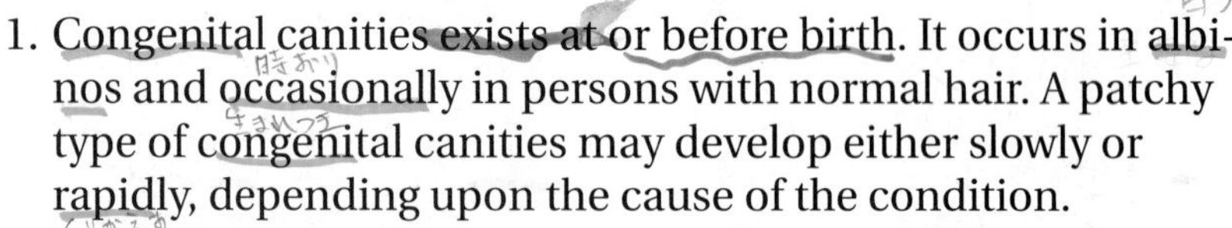

1. Congenital canities exists at or before birth. It occurs in albinos and occasionally in persons with normal hair. A patchy type of congenital canities may develop either slowly or rapidly, depending upon the cause of the condition.
2. Acquired canities may be due to old age, or onset may occur prematurely in early adult life. Causes of acquired canities may be worry, anxiety, nervous strain, prolonged illness, or heredity.

RINGED HAIR

Ringed hair is alternate bands of gray and dark hair.

HYPERTRICHOSIS

Hypertrichosis (hi-per-tri-**KOH**-sis), or ***hirsuties***, means superfluous hair, an abnormal development of hair on areas of the body normally bearing only downy hair. *Treatment:* Tweeze or remove by depilatories, electrolysis, shaving, or epilation.

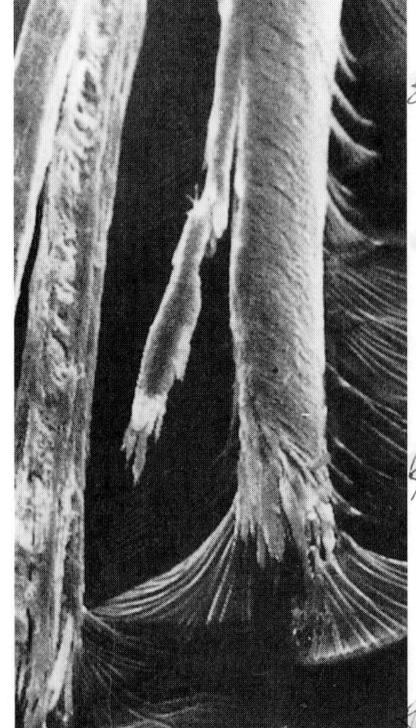

FIGURE 4.28 — Split hair ends.

TRICHOPTILOSIS

Trichoptilosis (tri-kop-ti-**LOH**-sis) is the technical term for split hair ends. (Fig. 4.28) *Treatment:* The hair should be well oiled to soften and lubricate the dry ends. The ends also may be removed by cutting.

TRICHORRHEXIS NODOSA

Trichorrhexis nodosa (**TRIK**-o-rek-sis no-**DO**-sa), or knotted hair, is a dry, brittle condition including formation of nodular swellings along the hair shaft. (Fig. 4.29) The hair breaks easily, and there is a brushlike spreading out of the fibers of the broken-

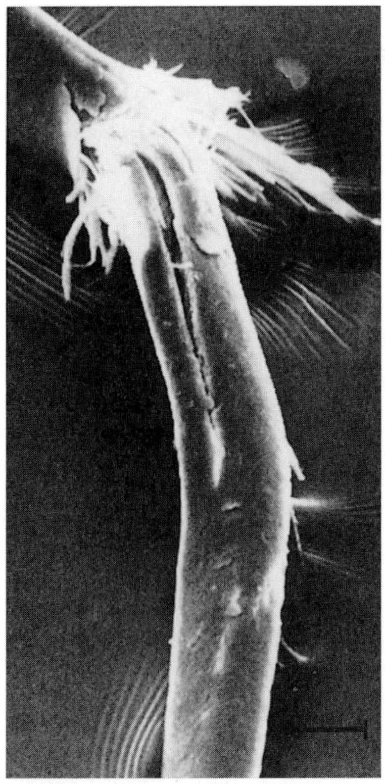

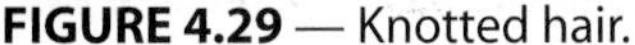

FIGURE 4.29 — Knotted hair.

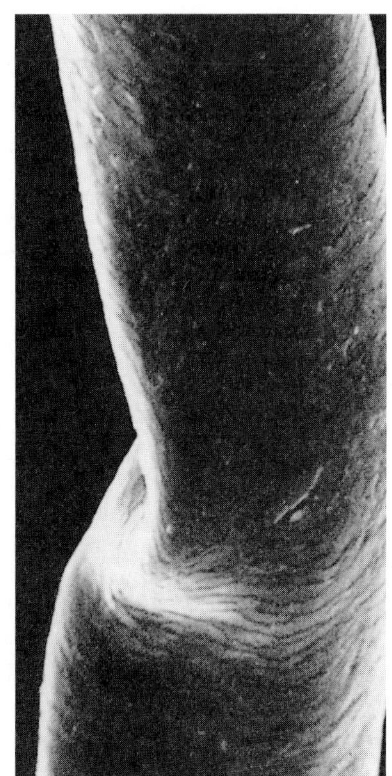

FIGURE 4.30 — Beaded hair.

off hair along the hair shaft. *Treatment:* Softening the hair with conditioners may prove beneficial.

MONILETHRIX

Monilethrix (moh-**NIL**-e-thriks) is the technical term for beaded hair. (Fig. 4.30) The hair breaks between the beads or nodes. *Treatment:* Scalp and hair treatments may improve the hair condition.

FRAGILITAS CRINIUM

Fragilitas crinium (frah-**JIL**-i-tas **KRI**-nee-um) is the technical term for brittle hair. The hairs may split at any part of their length. *Treatment:* Conditioning hair treatments may be recommended.

DISORDERS OF THE SCALP

Just as the skin is continually being shed and replaced, the uppermost layer of the scalp is also being cast off all the time. Ordinarily, these *horny scales* loosen and fall off freely. The natural shedding of these horny scales should not be mistaken for dandruff.

DANDRUFF

Dandruff consists of small, white scales that usually appear on the scalp and hair. The medical term for dandruff is ***pityriasis*** (pit-i-**REYE**-ah-sis). If neglected for long, excessive dandruff can lead to baldness. The nature of dandruff is not clearly defined by medical authorities although it is generally believed to be of infectious origin. Some authorities hold that it is due to a specific microbe.

A direct cause of dandruff is the excessive shedding of the ***epithelial,*** or surface, ***cells.*** Instead of growing to the surface and falling off, these horny scales accumulate on the scalp.

Indirect or associated causes of dandruff are a sluggish condition of the scalp, possibly due to poor circulation, infection, injury, lack of nerve stimulation, improper diet, and uncleanliness. Contributing causes are the use of strong shampoos and insufficient rinsing of the hair after a shampoo. The two principal types of dandruff are:

1. ***Pityriasis capitis simplex*** (kah-**PEYE**-tis **SIM**-pleks): dry type. (Fig. 4.31)
2. ***Pityriasis steatoides*** (ste-a-**TOY**-dez): greasy or waxy type. (Fig. 4.32)

Pityriasis capitis simplex (dry dandruff) is characterized by an itchy scalp and small white scales that are usually attached to the scalp in masses or scattered loosely in the hair. Occasionally, they are so profuse that they fall to the shoulders. Dry dandruff is often the result of a sluggish scalp caused by poor circulation, lack of nerve stimulation, improper diet, emotional and glandular disturbances, or uncleanliness. Frequent scalp treatments, use of mild shampoos, regular scalp massage, daily use of antiseptic scalp lotions, and applications of scalp ointments are all recommended for this disorder.

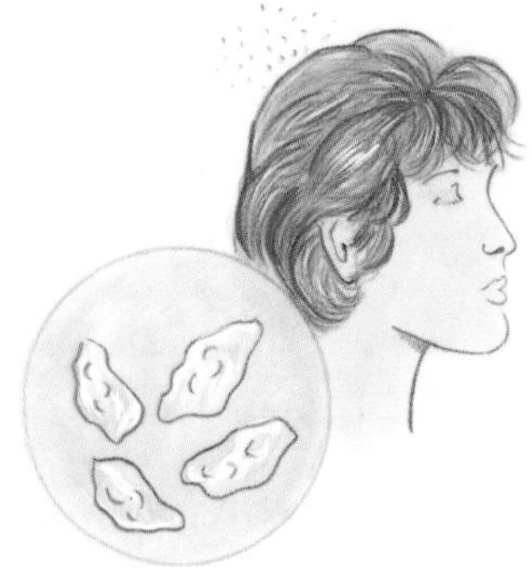

FIGURE 4.31 — Pityriasis capitis simplex.

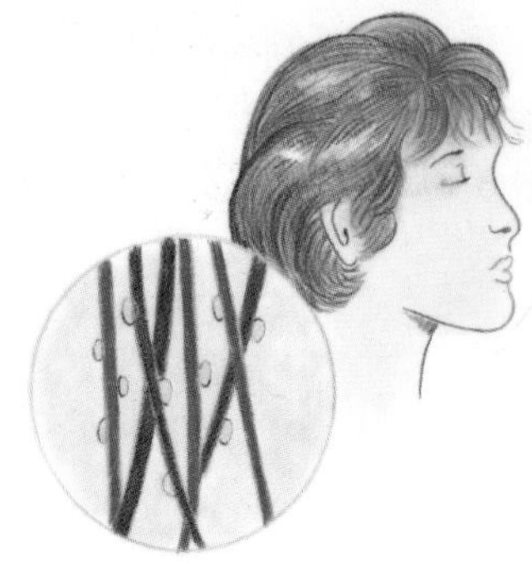

FIGURE 4.32 — Pityriasis steatoides.

Pityriasis steatoides (greasy or waxy type of dandruff) is a scaly condition of the epidermis (surface skin). The scales become mixed with sebum, causing them to stick to the scalp in patches. There may be itchiness, causing the person to scratch the scalp. If the greasy scales are torn off, bleeding or oozing of sebum may follow. Medical treatment is advisable.

Both forms of dandruff are considered to be contagious and can be spread by the common use of brushes, combs, and other articles. Therefore, the cosmetologist must take the necessary precautions to sanitize everything that comes into contact with the client.

Dandruff Treatment

A scalp with a dandruff condition may be treated by using the following procedure:

1. Drape client. (See chapter on draping.)
2. Brush the client's hair for 5 minutes.
3. Apply a scalp preparation according to the scalp's condition (dry or oily). (See sections on dry and oily hair scalp treatments on pages 62 and 63.)
4. Apply infrared lamp for about 5 minutes. (See chapter on electricity and light therapy.)
5. Give scalp manipulations, using indirect high-frequency current. (Figs. 33a, 33b) (See Chapter 24 on electricity and light therapy.)
6. Shampoo with corrective antidandruff lotion.
7. Thoroughly towel-dry the hair.

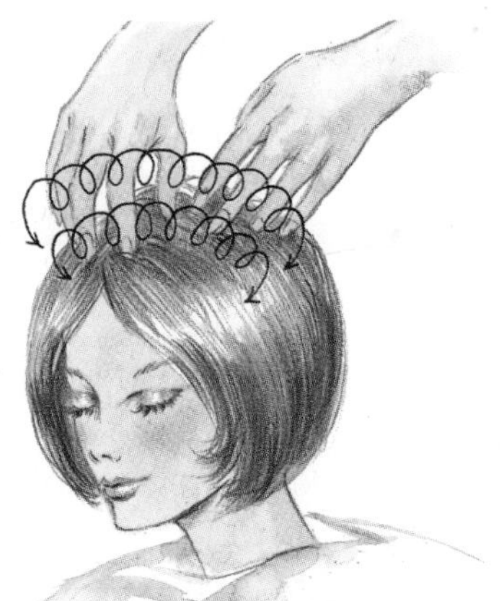

FIGURE 4.33a — Applying indirect high-frequency current, cosmetologist manipulates scalp.

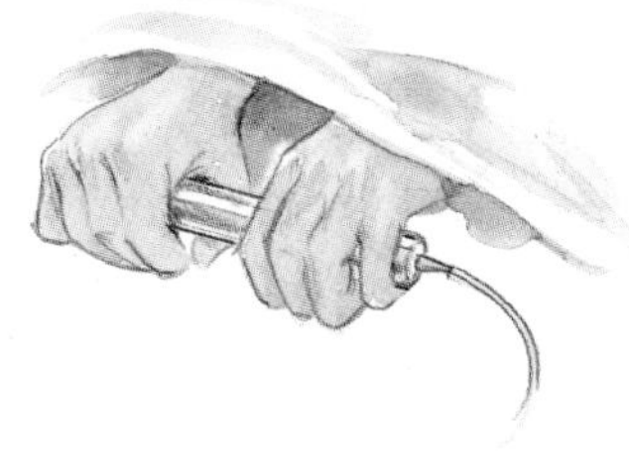

FIGURE 4.33b — While cosmetologist manipulates scalp, client holds metal electrode.

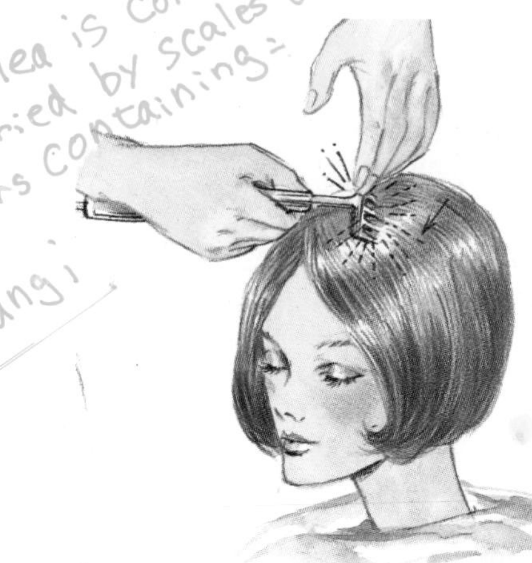

FIGURE 4.34 — Applying high-frequency current with glass rake electrode.

8. Use direct high-frequency current for 3 to 5 minutes. (Fig. 4.34) (See Chapter 24.)
9. Apply scalp preparation suitable for the condition.
10. Set, dry, and style the hair.
11. Clean up your work station.

VEGETABLE PARASITIC INFECTIONS

Tinea (TIN-ee-ah) is the medical term for ***ringworm.*** Ringworm is caused by vegetable parasites. All forms are contagious and can be transmitted from one person to another. The disease is commonly carried by scales or hairs containing fungi. Bathtubs, swimming pools, and unsanitized articles are also sources of transmission.

Ringworm starts with a small, reddened patch of little blisters. Several such patches may be present. Any ringworm condition should be referred to a physician.

Tinea capitis (kah-**PEYE**-tis), ringworm of the scalp, is characterized by red papules, or spots, at the opening of the hair follicles. (Fig. 4.35) The patches spread and the hair becomes brittle and lifeless. It breaks off, leaving a stump, or falls from the enlarged open follicles.

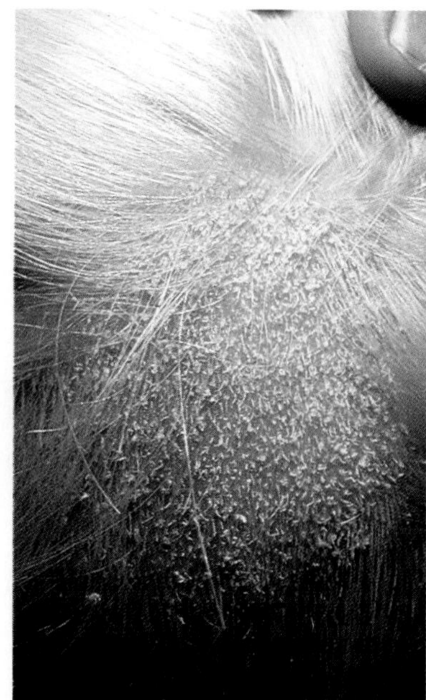

FIGURE 4.35 — Tinea capitis. *(Courtesy of Robert A. Silverman, MD, Clinical Associate Professor, Department of Pediatrics, Georgetown University)*

Tinea favosa (fa-**VO**-sah), also favus (**FAY**-vus) or ***honeycomb ringworm***, is characterized by dry, sulfur-yellow, cuplike crusts on the scalp, called ***scutula*** (**SKUT**-u-la), which have a peculiar odor. Scars from favus are bald patches that may be pink or white and shiny. It is *very contagious* and should be referred to a physician.

ANIMAL PARASITIC INFECTIONS

Scabies "itch" is a highly contagious, animal parasitic skin disease, caused by the itch mite. Vesicles and pustules can form from the irritation of the parasites or from scratching the affected areas.

Pediculosis (pe-dik-yōō-**LOH**-sis) ***capitis*** is a contagious condition caused by the head louse (animal parasite) infesting the hair of the scalp. (Figs. 4.36, 4.37) As the parasites feed on the scalp, itching occurs and the resultant scratching can cause an infection. The head louse is transmitted from one person to another by contact with infested hats, combs, brushes, or other personal articles. To kill head lice, advise the client to apply larkspur tincture, or other similar medication, to the entire head before retiring. The next morning, the client should shampoo with germicidal soap. Treatment should be repeated as necessary. Never treat a head lice condition in the salon or school.

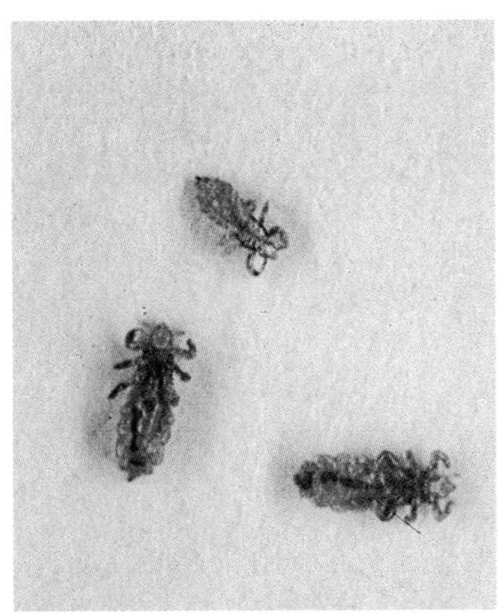

FIGURE 4.36 — Head lice do not jump or fly but run very quickly.

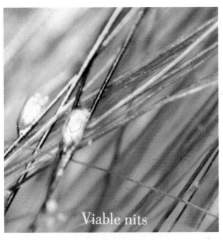

FIGURE 4.37 — Nits are the tiny, yellow-white eggs of lice. They are firmly attached to the hair and difficult to remove. *(Courtesy of Hogil Pharmaceutical Corporation)*

STAPHYLOCOCCI INFECTIONS

Furuncle (fu-**RUN**-kel), or boil, is an acute staphylococci infection of a hair follicle that produces constant pain. (Fig. 4.38) It is limited to a specific area and produces a pustule perforated by a hair.

Carbuncle (**KAHR**-bun-kul) is the result of an acute staphylococci infection and is larger than a furuncle. Refer the client to a physician.

Completed:
Learning Objective
#9
SCALP AND HAIR DISORDERS

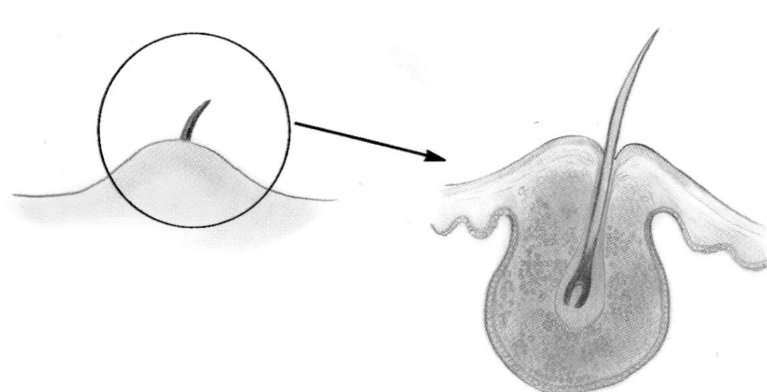

FIGURE 4.38 — Furuncle (boil).

REVIEW QUESTIONS

PROPERTIES OF THE HAIR AND SCALP

1. What are the purposes of hair?
2. What is hair?
3. What is hair composed of?
4. What are the two principal parts of hair?
5. What factors influence hair growth?
6. What are the three follicle cycles in hair growth?
7. What factors influence hair loss?
8. What are the basic requisites for a healthy scalp?

CHAPTER 5

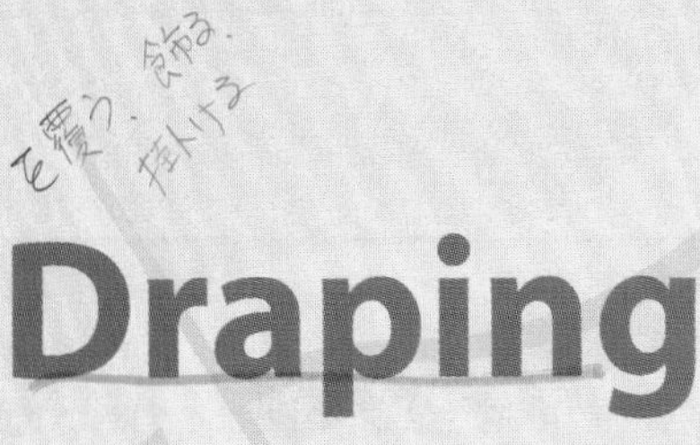

Draping

LEARNING OBJECTIVES

After completing this chapter, you should be able to:

1. List the methods of draping and preparing the client for cosmetology services.
2. Demonstrate draping for wet hair services.
3. Demonstrate draping for chemical services.
4. Demonstrate draping for dry hair services.

NATIONAL SKILL STANDARDS

This chapter provides you with the necessary information to master this National Industry Skill Standard for Entry-Level Cosmetologists:

- Conducting services in a safe environment, taking measures to prevent the spread of infectious and contagious disease

INTRODUCTION

The comfort and protection of the client must always be considered during cosmetology services. Protection of the skin and clothing assures clients that the cosmetologist is personally and professionally concerned about their comfort and safety.

Methods of draping depend on the service being performed. Several procedures are presented in this text, although those taught by your instructor are also acceptable. Consideration for the client is one of your most important responsibilities as a cosmetologist.

The following instructions are important before draping a client for any type of service:

1. Prepare materials and supplies for the service.
2. Sanitize hands.
3. Ask the client to remove all neck and hair jewelry and store it away.
4. Remove objects from the client's hair.
5. Turn the client's collar to the inside. (Fig. 5.1)
6. Proceed with the appropriate draping method.

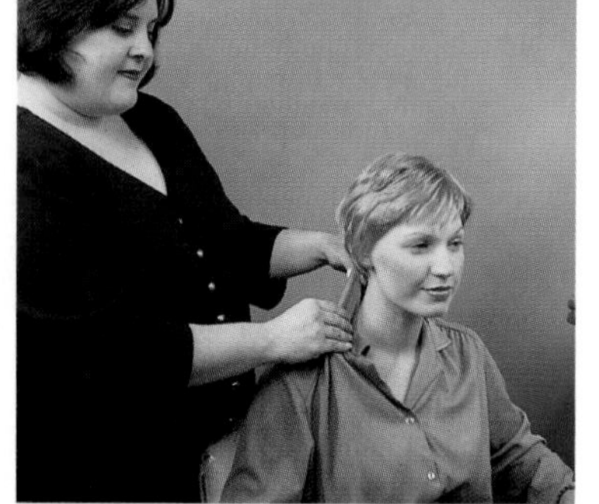

FIGURE 5.1 — Turning collar in.

In the following procedures the purpose of the towel or neck strip is for sanitary reasons, to prevent contact of the cape with the client's skin.

Completed:
Learning Objective
#1
METHODS OF DRAPING AND PREPARING THE CLIENT FOR SERVICES

DRAPING FOR WET HAIR SERVICES

Shampooing, Scalp and Hair Care, and Haircutting

1. Place a towel lengthwise across the client's shoulders, crossing the ends beneath the chin.

2. Place the cape over the towel and fasten in the back so that the cape does not touch the client's skin.
3. Place another towel over the cape and secure in front.

For haircutting, the towel should be removed after shampooing and replaced with a neck strip. This allows the hair to fall naturally without obstruction.

Completed: Learning Objective #2

DRAPING FOR WET HAIR SERVICES

DRAPING FOR CHEMICAL SERVICES

Hair Color, Perms, and Relaxers

1. Slide towel down from back of client's head and place lengthwise across the client's shoulders. (Fig. 5.2)
2. Cross the ends of the towel beneath the chin and place the cape over the towel. Fasten in the back and adjust the towel over the cape. (Figs. 5.3, 5.4)
3. Fold the towel over the top of the cape and secure in front. (Fig. 5.5)
4. It is advisable to apply a protective cream around the hairline immediately prior to the application of chemicals to the hair. This prevents possible skin irritation.

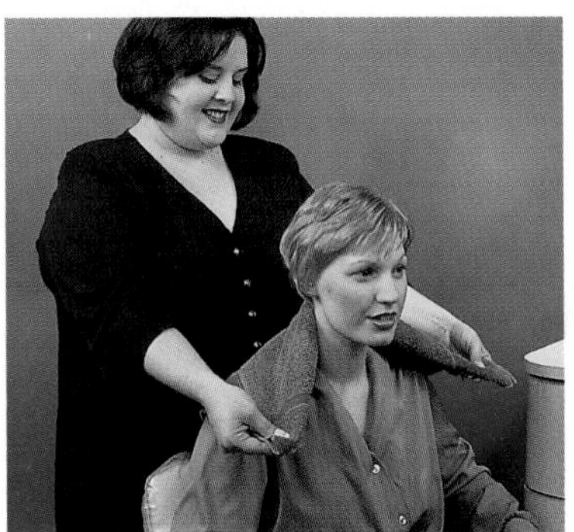

FIGURE 5.2 — Placing towel around client's neck.

DRAPING FOR DRY HAIR SERVICES

Brushing or Thermal Design

1. Secure a neck strip around the client's neck. (Fig. 5.6)
2. Place the cape over the neck strip and fasten so that the cape does not touch the client's skin. (Fig. 5.7)

Completed: Learning Objective #3

DRAPING FOR CHEMICAL SERVICES

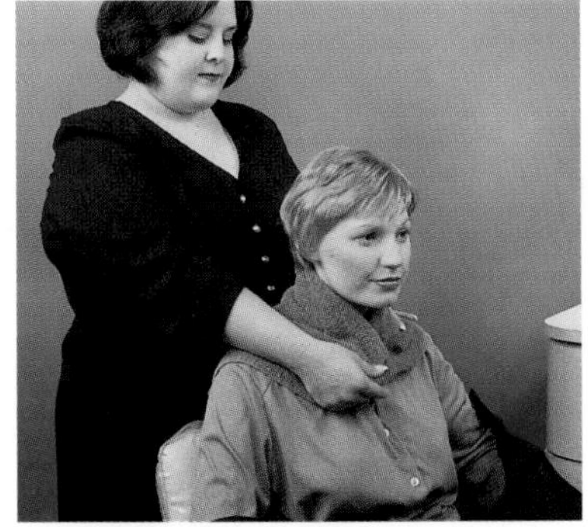

FIGURE 5.3 — Crossing ends of the towel under chin.

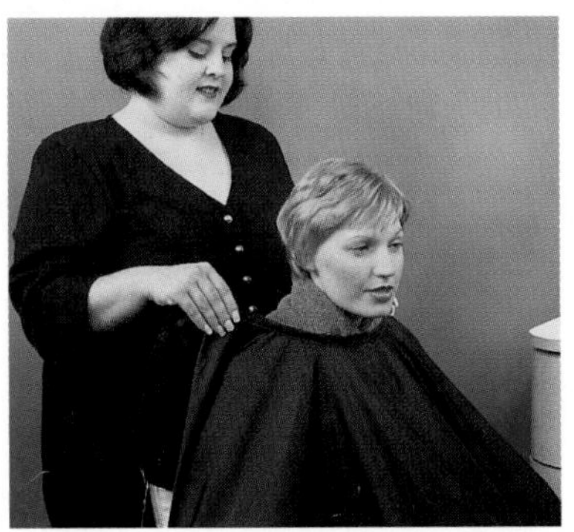

FIGURE 5.4 — Placing cape over towel.

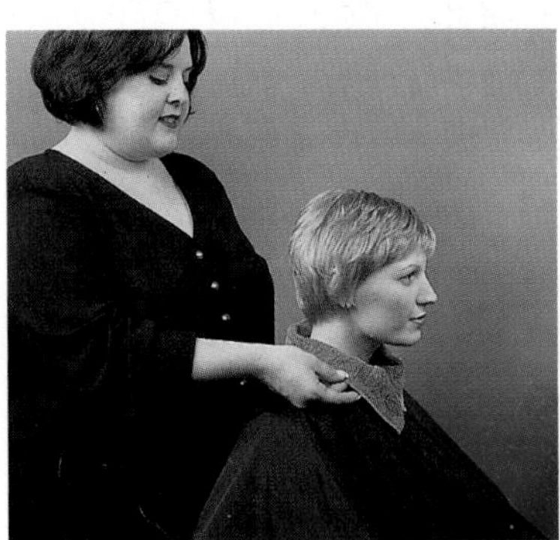

FIGURE 5.5 — Folding towel over cape.

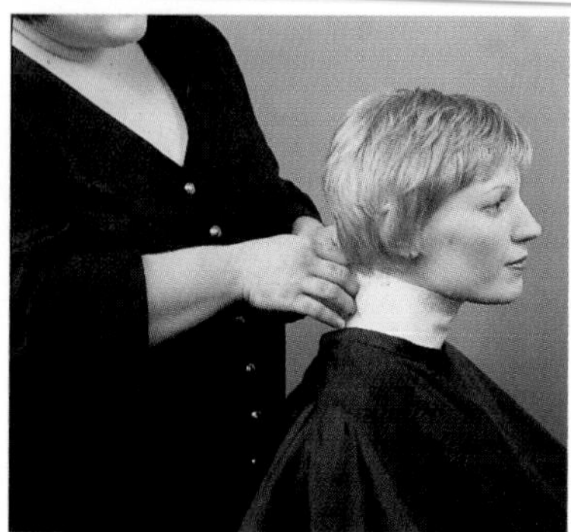

FIGURE 5.6 — Placing neck strip.

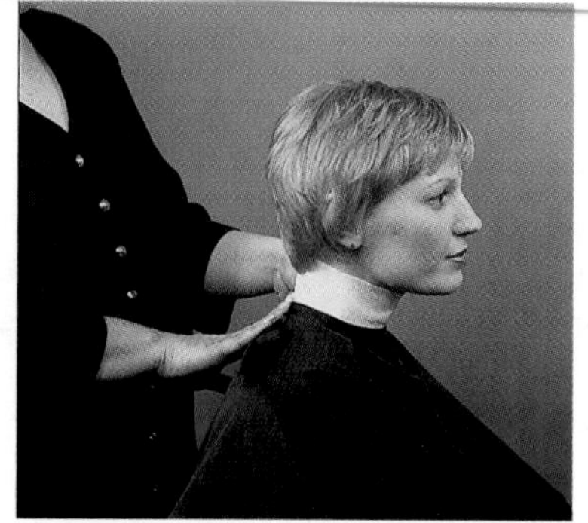

FIGURE 5.7 — Placing cape over neck strip.

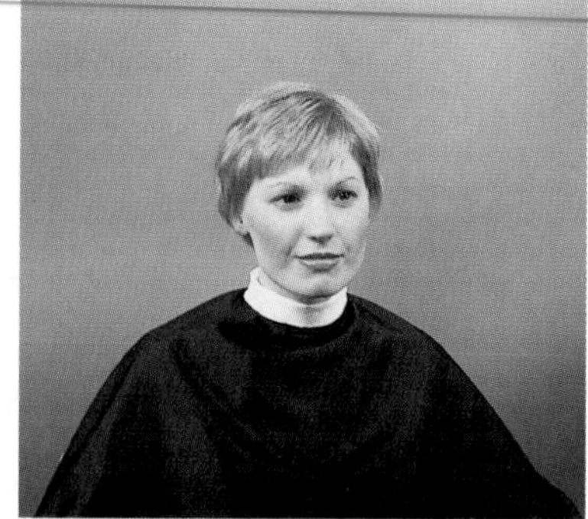

FIGURE 5.8 — Neck strip folded down over cape.

3. Fold the uncovered portion of the neck strip down over the cape. Make sure that no part of the cape touches the client's neck.

Completed: Learning Objective #4
DRAPING FOR DRY HAIR SERVICES

Comb-Out

1. Secure a neck strip around the client's neck.
2. Place the cape over the neck strip and fasten so that the cape does not touch the client's skin. (Fig. 5.8) Capes especially designed for this service can be used. ✔

REVIEW QUESTIONS

DRAPING

1. What must a cosmetologist take into consideration when performing any service?
2. What is draping?
3. Why is draping so important?
4. Why is a towel or neck strip used in draping?
5. What are the four preliminary steps before draping a client?
6. What are the differences when draping for wet hair services, dry hair services, and chemical services?

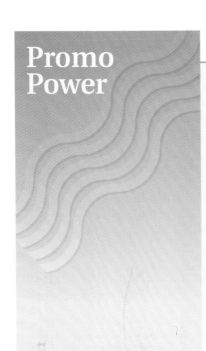

THE IN-SALON PROMO

Promotions are great business. They can cause excitement among existing clients, while bringing in new ones.

Set the rules and regulations of any contests. Plan contests at least three months ahead of time so that you are able to do everything and have everything made. Decide on all of the features and benefits of the contest to the salon. List all the pros and cons, and plan for the worst-case scenario to make sure expenses could still be covered; then have a staff meeting to inform your people what you're planning and get their input. Without their consent and participation, you could have a mess on your hands. Excite them about the idea, and reward them with something that will be exciting to them. Staff prizes could be educational classes, bonuses, time off, or something that has meaning to an individual.

The planning stages of your promo are most important. All of the preparations must be thoroughly thought out and prioritized. It's important to know that everything is ready to go at least a couple of weeks ahead of time so people are aware of what is happening. At the actual time of the promo, follow up and keep your staff updated about what is happening on a daily or weekly basis.

—*From* The Salon Biz: Tips for Success *by Geri Mataya*

CHAPTER 6

Shampooing, Rinsing, and Conditioning

LEARNING OBJECTIVES

After completing this chapter, you should be able to:

1. List the reasons for good hygienic care of the hair and scalp.
2. Identify when, why, and how to brush hair.
3. Demonstrate the procedure for shampoo manipulations.
4. Understand the meaning of pH levels in shampoos.
5. Identify the various types of shampoos.
6. Identify the various types of rinses.

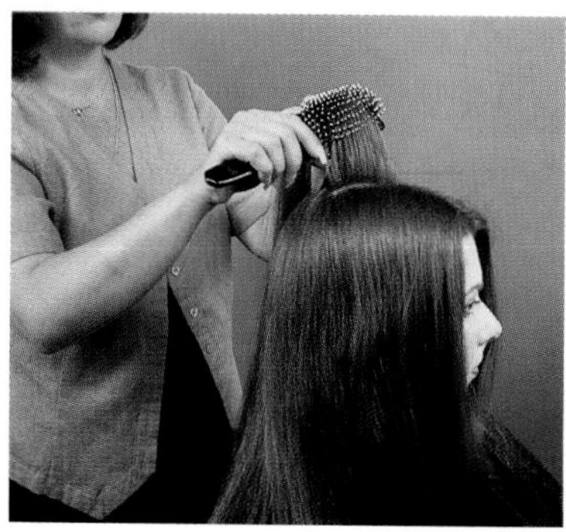

FIGURE 6.1 — Brushing the hair.

You should include a thorough hair brushing as a part of every shampoo and scalp treatment, with the following exceptions:

1. Do not brush before giving a chemical service.
2. Do not brush if the scalp is irritated.

Brushing stimulates the blood circulation to the scalp, helps remove dust, dirt, and hair spray buildup from the hair, and gives hair added sheen. (Fig. 6.1) Therefore, you should brush the hair whether the scalp and hair are in a dry or oily condition. Do not use the comb to loosen scales from the scalp.

To brush the hair, first part it through the center from front to nape. Then part a section about ½" (1.25 cm) off the center parting to the crown of the head. Holding this strand of hair in the left hand between the thumb and fingers, lay the brush (held in the right hand) with the bristles well down on the hair close to the scalp; rotate the brush by turning the wrist slightly, and sweep the bristles the full length of the hair shaft. Repeat three times. Then part the hair again ½" (1.25 cm) from the first parting and continue until the entire head has been brushed.

Completed: Learning Objective #2

BRUSHING THE HAIR

SHAMPOO PROCEDURE

Preparation

1. Seat your client comfortably at your work station.
2. Select and arrange the required materials.
3. Wash your hands.
4. Place a neck strip and shampoo cape around the client's neck. (Be sure that the client's collar lies smoothly under the garment before the neck strip is adjusted or turn collar to inside of garment.)
5. Remove all hairpins and combs from the hair.
6. Ask client to remove earrings and glasses and to put them in a safe place.
7. Examine the condition of the client's hair and scalp.
8. Brush the hair thoroughly.
9. Redrape with shampoo cape and towel.
10. Seat the client comfortably at the shampoo sink.
11. Adjust the shampoo cape over the back of the shampoo chair. (Fig. 6.2)
12. Adjust the volume and temperature of the water spray.

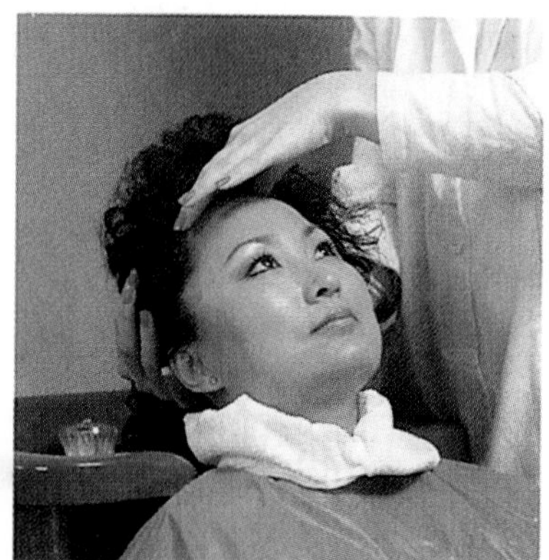

FIGURE 6.2 — Support client's head with your right hand and place the cape over the back of the chair.

Consider the client's preference in adjusting the water temperature. Turn on the cold water first and gradually add warm water until you obtain a comfortably warm temperature. Test the temperature of the water by spraying it on the inner side of your wrist. The temperature of the water must be constantly monitored by keeping one finger over the edge of the spray nozzle and in contact with the water.

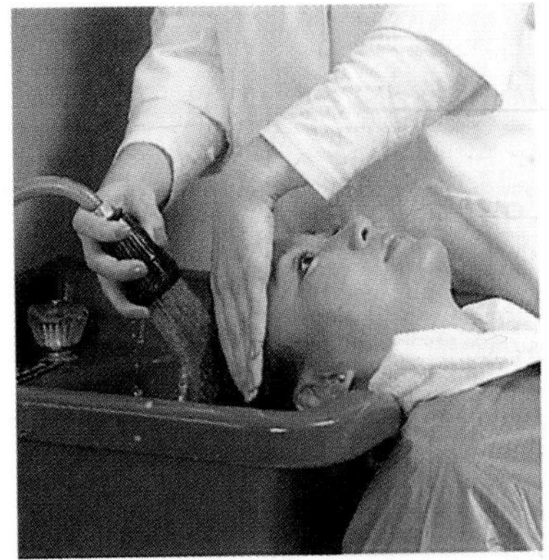

FIGURE 6.3 — Protecting the face.

Procedure

1. ***Saturate, wet hair thoroughly***, with warm water spray. Lift the hair and work it with your free hand to saturate the scalp. Shift your hand to protect the client's face, ears, and neck from the spray when working around the hairline. (Figs. 6.3–6.5)

2. ***Apply small quantities of shampoo to the hair***, beginning at the hairline and working back. Work into a lather using the pads or cushions of the fingers.

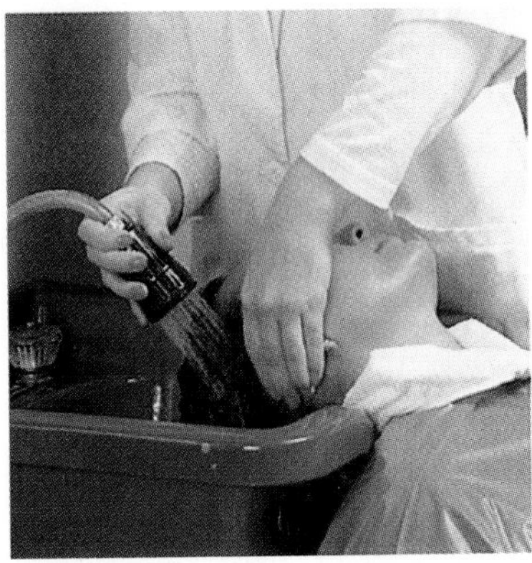

FIGURE 6.4 — Protecting the ears.

Reminders

In massaging the scalp, do not use firm pressure if:

- You will be giving the client a chemical service after the shampoo.
- The client's scalp is tender or sensitive.
- The client requests less pressure.

3. ***Manipulate scalp.***
   a) Begin at the front hairline and work in a back-and-forth movement until the top of the head is reached. (Fig. 6.6)
   b) Continue in this manner to the back of the head, shifting your fingers back 1" (2.5 cm) at a time.
   c) Lift the client's head, with your left hand controlling the movement of the head. With your right hand, start at the top of the right ear and, using the same movement, work to the back of the head. (Fig. 6.7)
   d) Drop your fingers down 1" (2.5 cm) and repeat the process until the right side of the head is covered.
   e) Beginning at the left ear, repeat steps c and d.
   f) Allow the client's head to relax and work around the hairline with your thumbs in a rotary movement.
   g) Repeat these movements until the scalp has been thoroughly massaged.
   h) Remove excess shampoo and lather by squeezing the hair.

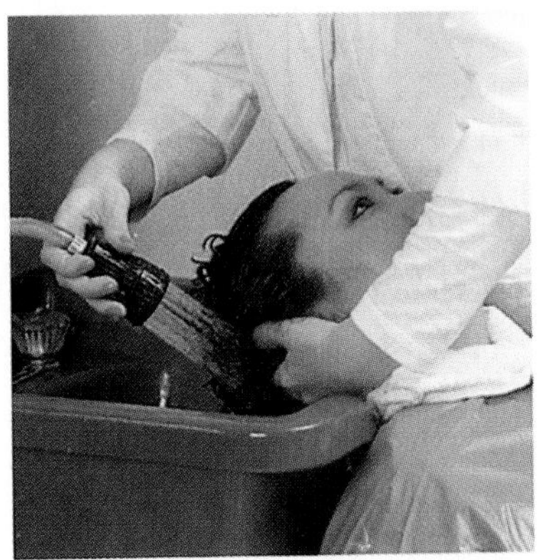

FIGURE 6.5 — Protecting the neck.

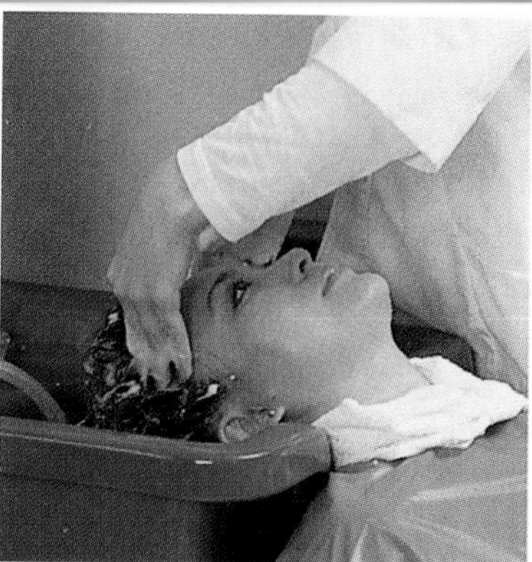
FIGURE 6.6 — Manipulating scalp.

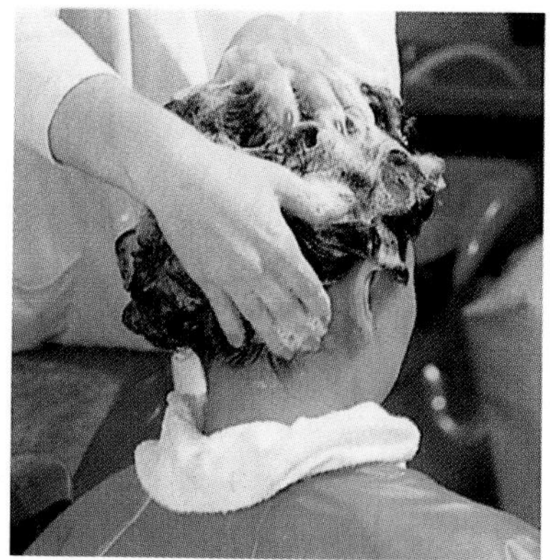
FIGURE 6.7 — Lifting client's head.

4. ***Rinse hair thoroughly*** with a strong spray.
   a) Lift the hair at the crown and back with the fingers of your left hand to permit the spray to rinse the hair thoroughly.
   b) Cup your left hand along the napeline and pat the hair, forcing the spray of water against the base scalp area.
5. ***If required, apply shampoo again.***
   a) Repeat the procedure using steps 2, 3, and 4 as outlined. You will need less shampoo because partially clean hair lathers more easily.
6. ***Partially towel-dry.***
   a) Remove excess moisture from the hair at the shampoo bowl.
   b) Wipe excess moisture from around the client's face and ears with the ends of the towel.
   c) Lift the towel over the back of the client's head and drape the head with the towel.
   d) Place your hands on top of the towel and massage until the hair is partially dry. (Fig. 6.8)

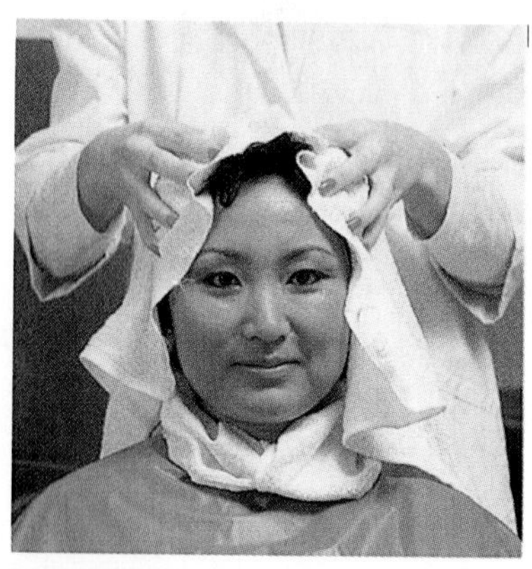
FIGURE 6.8 — Towel drying the hair.

Completion

1. Comb the hair, beginning with the ends at the nape of the client's neck.
2. Change the drape if necessary.
3. Style the hair as desired.

Cleanup

1. Discard used materials, and place unused supplies in their proper place.
2. Place used towels in the towel hamper.
3. Remove hair from combs and brushes; wash with hot, soapy water; rinse; and place in wet disinfectant for the required time.
4. Sanitize the shampoo bowl.
5. Cleanse your hands.

Completed: Learning Objective #3

PROCEDURE FOR SHAMPOO MANIPULATIONS

SHAMPOOING CHEMICALLY TREATED HAIR

Chemically treated hair tends to be drier and more fragile than non-chemically treated hair. Therefore, a mild shampoo formulated for chemically treated hair is recommended. Chemically treated hair also tends to tangle. To remove tangles, comb gently from the nape of the head and work to the frontal area. Do not force the comb through the hair. Use a conditioner if necessary. Hair that has been relaxed or straightened tends to be less tangled, but it may mat if not moisturized properly before drying.

TYPES OF SHAMPOOS

Shampoo accounts for the highest dollar expenditure in hair care products. Consumer studies show the current growth pattern in the shampoo market to be in the direction of the professional salon. You will have to be more knowledgeable and sophisticated about the products used, more proficient in using them, and capable of selling these products to your clients.

Thousands of good shampoos exist, one for every conceivable type of hair or scalp condition a client could have: dry, oily, fine, coarse, limp, lightened, permed, relaxed, or chemically untreated. There are shampoos that add highlights and others that remove them. There are shampoos that deposit a coating on the hair, and there are shampoos to strip coating off the hair.

The ingredients list is the key to determining which shampoo will leave a client's hair lustrous and manageable, treat a scalp or hair condition, or prepare hair for chemical treatment. Most shampoos have many common ingredients, and it is your responsibility as a professional cosmetologist to understand the chemical composition in order to select the best shampoo for each particular service and client.

General descriptions of different types of shampoos are listed below. The section entitled "Chemistry of Shampoos" in the chapter on chemistry has detailed information about the chemical ingredients that make up the different types of shampoos.

Explaining pH

Before discussing acid-balanced shampoos, you should know something about pH (potential hydrogen) levels in shampoo. This will help you to select the proper shampoo for your client. The amount of hydrogen in a solution is measured on a pH scale that has a range from 0 to 14. The amount of hydrogen in a solution determines whether it is more alkaline or more acid. A shampoo that is more acid can have a pH rating from 0 to 6.9; a shampoo that is more alkaline can have a pH rating from 7 to 14. The higher

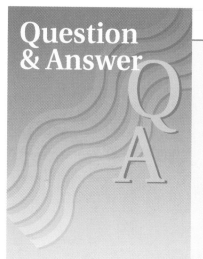

CLEANSING

During a routine shampoo service some of the shampoo accidentally went into the eye of a client. She complained of burning, and the eye turned extremely red. What should I do in such a case?

Strong synthetics in some shampoos—those containing cationics as germicides and nonionics as cleansing agents—are indeed capable of causing severe eye irritation and even permanent eye injury. Most manufacturers do not make this type of shampoo, however. Any shampoo, unless it is specifically made for use on babies and children, will cause temporary discomfort if it comes in direct contact with the eye. However, there are no documented cases of severe or lasting injury from other shampoos.

First and foremost, know your products. Purchase high-quality shampoo products that have proven effective and safe over a sufficient period of time.

Then, care in executing the cleansing service is necessary. No client wants suds and water in her face, even if it is not harmful. Scalp manipulations for shampooing purposes should be methodical but always confined to the hair portion of the head.

If shampoo accidentally gets into the client's eye, put the client in an upright position and immediately rinse the eye with clear, cold water. Allow the client to rinse her own eye to avoid rubbing beyond her personal tolerance. Blot the area dry. If the redness persists, ask the client if she would like to see her doctor; if so the salon will gladly pay for the office visit and initial treatment. Notify your insurance company at once so they can follow up if there's a problem. The law holds the manufacturer of synthetic detergent shampoo or other cosmetics solely responsible for users' safety. However, you have a co-responsibility to use it in a safe manner—only for its intended purpose.

—*From* Milady's Salon Solutions *by Louise Cotter*

the pH rating (more alkaline), the stronger and harsher the shampoo is to the hair. A high pH shampoo can leave the hair dry and brittle. (Also see pH scale in the chapter on chemistry.)

Acid-balanced Shampoos

An acid-balanced shampoo is one that falls within the 4.5 to 6.6 range, an acceptable pH range. Any shampoo can become acid balanced by the addition of citric, lactic, or phosphoric acid.

Proponents of acid-balanced shampoo state that an acid pH of 4.5 to 5.5 is essential to prevent excessive dryness and hair damage during the cleansing process, while the Consumer's Union's chemists consider the difference between a pH of 5 and a pH of 8 too small to affect the hair and scalp in the limited time of an average application. ✔

Completed: Learning Objective #4
UNDERSTANDING pH LEVELS

Conditioning Shampoos

Virtually every shampoo available on the professional market contains one or more conditioning agents designed to make the hair smooth and shiny, to avoid damage to chemically treated hair, and to improve the manageability of the hair. Protein, dimethicone, biotin, hydantoin, oleyl alcohol, and cocoamphocarboxyglycinate are just a few examples of conditioning agents that are used to assist shampoos in meeting current grooming needs.

Medicated Shampoos

Medicated shampoos contain special chemicals or drugs that are very effective in reducing excessive dandruff or other scalp conditions. These are prescribed by a physician. They generally are quite strong and will affect the color of tinted or lightened hair.

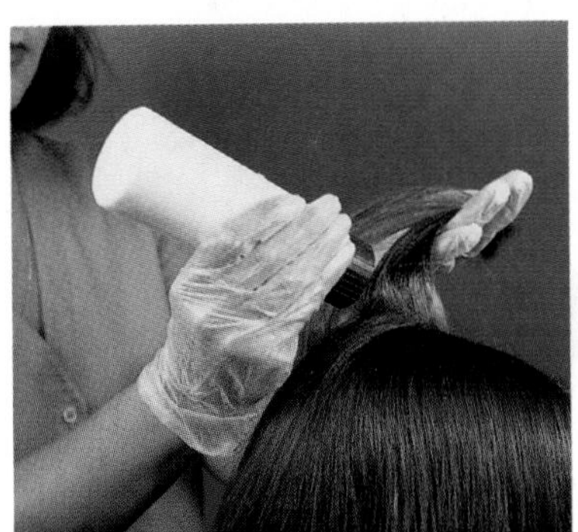

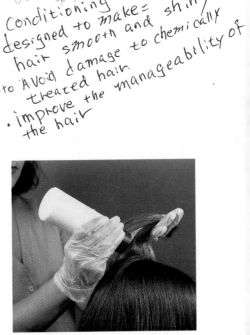

FIGURE 6.9 — Applying powder dry shampoo.

Powder Dry Shampoos

A dry shampoo is usually given when the client's health does not permit a wet shampoo. Only a few of these products are available on the market today. Follow the manufacturer's recommended directions when giving a dry shampoo. Do not give a dry shampoo before performing a chemical service. (Fig. 6.9)

Color or Highlighting Shampoos

(See chapters on hair coloring and chemistry.)

Shampoos for Hairpieces and Wigs

Prepared wig cleaning solutions are now available. (See chapter on the artistry of artificial hair.) ✔

Completed: Learning Objective #5
TYPES OF SHAMPOOS

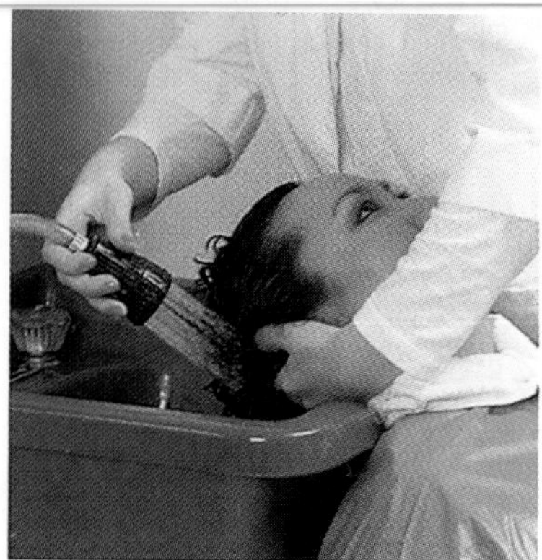

FIGURE 6.10 — Rinsing the hair after applying a hair rinse.

HAIR RINSES

A hair rinse consists of a mixture of water with a mild acid, coloring agent, or ingredients designed to serve a particular purpose. (Fig. 6.10)

Acid Rinses

Acid rinses are used to restore the pH balance to the hair and to remove soap scum. The fatty acids found in soap combine with the minerals in water to form a soap scum that cannot be completely removed from the hair with plain water. Therefore, the hair tends to become coated, dull, and difficult to comb. Because soap is not currently used in the manufacture of professional shampoos, you will not find acid rinses in many salons.

The types of acids used in prepared acid hair rinses are:

Citric acid from the juice of a lime, orange, or lemon.

Tartaric acid, which is obtained from residues in wine making.

Acetic acid, which is present in vinegar.

Lactic acid, which is derived from lactose or sugar of milk.

Conditioners and Cream Rinses

A conditioner or cream rinse is a commercial product with a creamy appearance that is used after shampooing. It is intended to soften hair, add luster, and make tangled hair easier to comb. Conditioners and cream rinses coat the hair shaft to make it slick and smooth. This temporary coating allows the comb to glide easily through the hair and often gives the false impression that the hair has been restored to its original healthy condition.

Used occasionally, conditioners and cream rinses are useful to remove tangles. However, habitual use can lead to future hair care problems. The coating ingredients can build up on the hair, making it prematurely heavy and oily. This can lead the client to shampoo more frequently, causing further damage to the hair. An endless cycle is created because conditioners and cream rinses give the illusion of curing a problem that they are actually compounding. Professional conditioning treatments are an effective solution to the problem.

Acid-balanced Rinses

Acid-balanced rinses are commercially formulated to prevent the fading of color after a tint or toner application and to give shine. This rinse is acid balanced to close the cuticle and trap within it the color molecules. This helps to prevent fading. Citric acid is probably the most commonly used ingredient in an after-rinse, but most also contain a mild moisturizer to leave the hair soft, pliable, and easy to comb.

Medicated Rinses

Medicated rinses are formulated to control minor dandruff conditions. Follow the manufacturer's instructions.

Color Rinses

Color rinses highlight or add temporary color to the hair. These rinses remain on the hair until the next shampoo. (For additional information, see the chapter on hair coloring.)

Completed:
Learning Objective
#6
TYPES OF RINSES

REVIEW QUESTIONS

SHAMPOOING, RINSING, AND CONDITIONING

1. Why is a professional shampoo important?
2. What is the purpose of a shampoo?
3. Why and how often should the hair be shampooed?
4. How do you determine the proper shampoo to use?
5. Name two types of water.
6. Why is brushing important prior to shampooing?
7. When is it not appropriate to brush before shampooing?
8. What does pH mean?
9. How is pH measured?
10. Why is pH in shampoo important?
11. What is a hair rinse?
12. What is the function of an acid rinse?
13. What type of rinse is intended to soften the hair, add luster, and remove tangles?
14. What type of rinse prevents fading of color after a tint or toner application?
15. How does an acid-balanced rinse prevent fading?
16. What is a medicated rinse?
17. What is the purpose of a color rinse?

CHAPTER 7

Haircutting

LEARNING OBJECTIVES

After completing this chapter, you should be able to:

1. Describe why professional haircutting is the foundation for hair design in the salon.
2. Conduct a scalp and hair analysis.
3. Explain the difference between a stationary guide and a traveling guide.
4. Define low elevation, high elevation, reverse elevation, and blended elevation.
5. Describe how to cut very curly hair.

NATIONAL SKILL STANDARDS

This chapter provides you with the necessary information to master these National Industry Skill Standards for Entry-Level Cosmetologists:

- Consulting with clients to determine their needs and preferences
- Providing a haircut in accordance with a client's needs or expectations

INTRODUCTION

Completed: Learning Objective
#1
HAIRCUTTING AS THE FOUNDATION FOR HAIR DESIGN

As a cosmetology student, you will learn to master the art and techniques of haircutting. Thorough instruction is required in techniques for cutting and shaping the hair using cutting shears, thinning shears, razors, and clippers. Instruction must be followed by continual practice under the guidance of an instructor.

A good haircut serves as the foundation for attractive hairstyles and other services performed in the salon. Hairstyles should accentuate the client's good points while minimizing his or her poor features. In selecting a suitable hairstyle, you should take into consideration the client's head shape, facial contour, neckline, and hair texture. However, you should also be guided by the client's wishes, personality, and lifestyle.

BASICS OF HAIRCUTTING

TERMS USED IN HAIRCUTTING

Beveled cut: Holding the shears at an angle to the hair strand other than 90 degrees.

Blunt cut: Cutting the hair straight across the strand. Lengths of hair all come to one hanging level, forming a weight line or area.

Elevation: Angle at which the hair is held away from the head for cutting.

Graduated: The graduated shape, or wedge, has a stacked area around the exterior and is cut at low to medium elevations.

Guide: Section of hair that determines the length the hair will be cut. A guide can be at the perimeter or in the interior of the cut.

Layering: Graduated effect achieved by cutting the hair with elevation or over direction. Each subsequent subsection is slightly shorter than the guide when allowed to fall naturally.

Notching or ***Pointing:*** Cutting with the points of the shears to create texture in the hair ends.

Parting (also called **subsection**)***:*** Subdivision of a section, used for control when cutting.

Sections: Divisions of the hair made before cutting.

Tension: How tightly the hair is pulled when cutting.

Undercutting: Cutting the hair with the head held in a forward position so that each parting is cut slightly longer than the previous parting to encourage the hair to curl under.

Weight line: Level at which a blunt cut falls; where the ends of the hair hang together.

GENERAL RULES OF HAIRCUTTING

- Hair must be uniformly wet, dry, or damp before cutting. Hair stretches more if it is wet than if it is dry. If the hair is cut partially wet and partially dry, the results will be uneven.
- You must use equal tension when cutting hair. If you cut one parting with light tension and the next parting with heavy tension, each parting will be a different length and will not blend.
- You must see the guide through the parting to be cut before cutting. If you cannot see the guide, reduce the size of the parting. (Fig. 7.1)
- Only cut up to your second knuckle. If you cut between the second and third knuckles, the amount of tension on the hair changes, causing an uneven haircut.
- Always comb each parting from the scalp to the guide. Comb several times to remove all tangles and distribute the hair evenly in the parting.
- Hold the shears at a consistent angle to the hair. Beginners should cut parallel to the parting.
- Partings should be uniform throughout the sections.
- Partings should be at the same angle as the cut. (Figs. 7.2, 7.3)

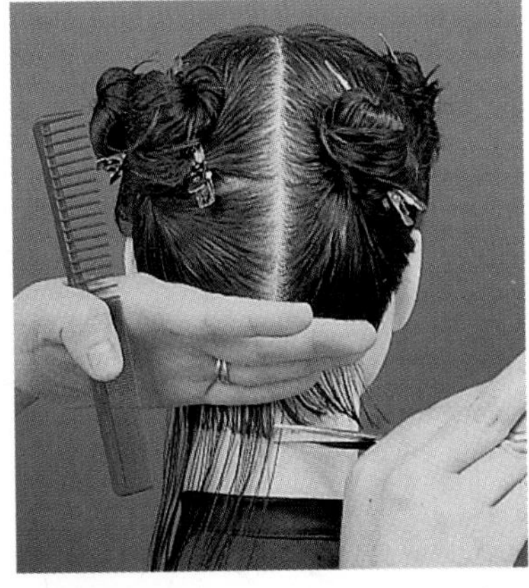

FIGURE 7.1 — Guideline should be visible through parting.

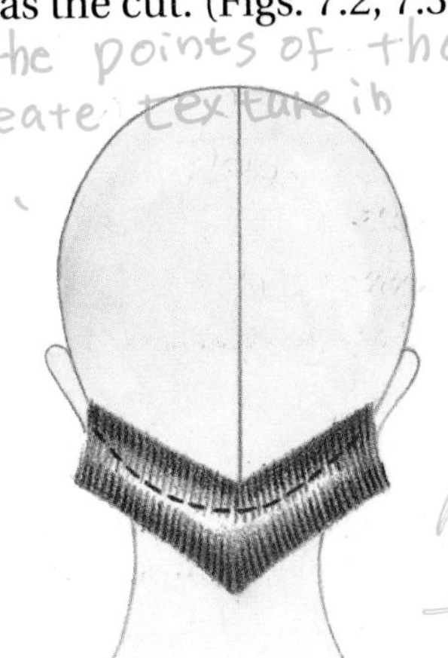

FIGURE 7.2, 7.3 — Hair parted at same angle as the cut.

- Head position should be consistent throughout a section.
- It is better to leave the hair a little long than to cut it too short. When in doubt, leave an extra ½" (1.25 cm).

UNDERSTANDING YOUR TOOLS

The quality and selection of implements is important in order to accomplish a good haircut. To do your best work, you should buy and use only superior implements from a reliable manufacturer. However, improper use will quickly destroy the efficiency of any implement, no matter how perfectly it might be made at the factory.

- ***Haircutting scissors*** or ***shears:*** Usually used to cut a blunt straight line. Can be used to thin hair by slithering (effilating). Japanese shears with razor edges can be used to slide-cut or texture the hair.
- ***Thinning shears:*** Used to remove bulk from the hair. Many different types of thinning or texturizing shears are used today. The most common are the single-notched and double-notched thinning shears. Generally the single-notched shears remove more hair. The number of teeth also determines how much hair will be removed.
- ***Straight razor*** or ***razor shaper:*** Cuts hair with a softer edge than shears. Can be used to thin the hair.
- ***Clippers:*** Used to create very short tapers quickly.

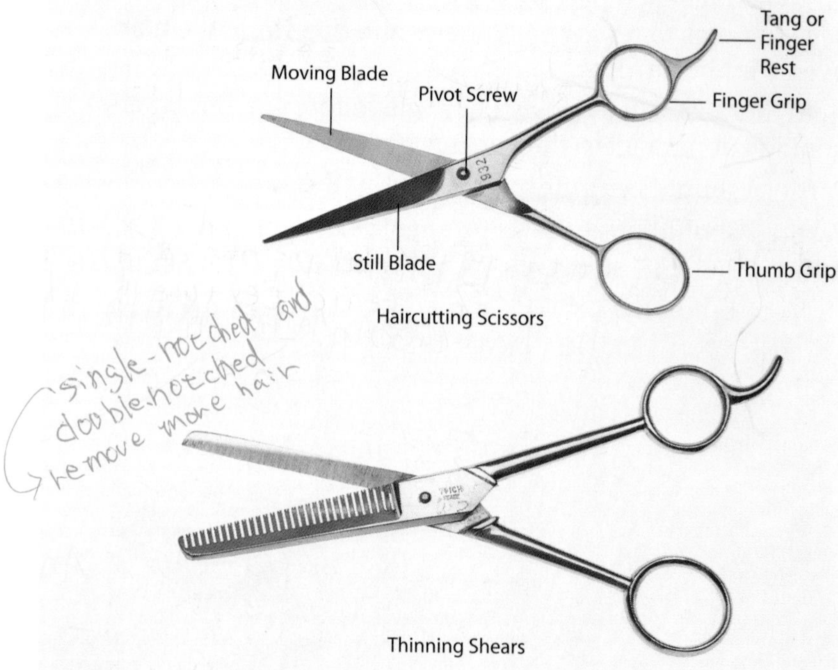

FIGURE 7.4 — Haircutting scissors and thinning shears.

- ***Edgers:*** Used to remove superfluous hair and to create clean lines around the perimeter of a short taper.
- ***Styling*** or ***all-purpose combs:*** Used for most haircutting procedures. They can be 6" to 8" (15 to 20 cm) in length and have wide teeth and close teeth.
- ***Barber comb:*** Used for close tapers in nape and sides when using the scissors-over-comb technique. The narrow end of the comb allows the shears to get very close to the head.
- ***Wide-tooth comb:*** Used to create a softer edge when cutting with shears. (Figs. 7.4, 7.5)

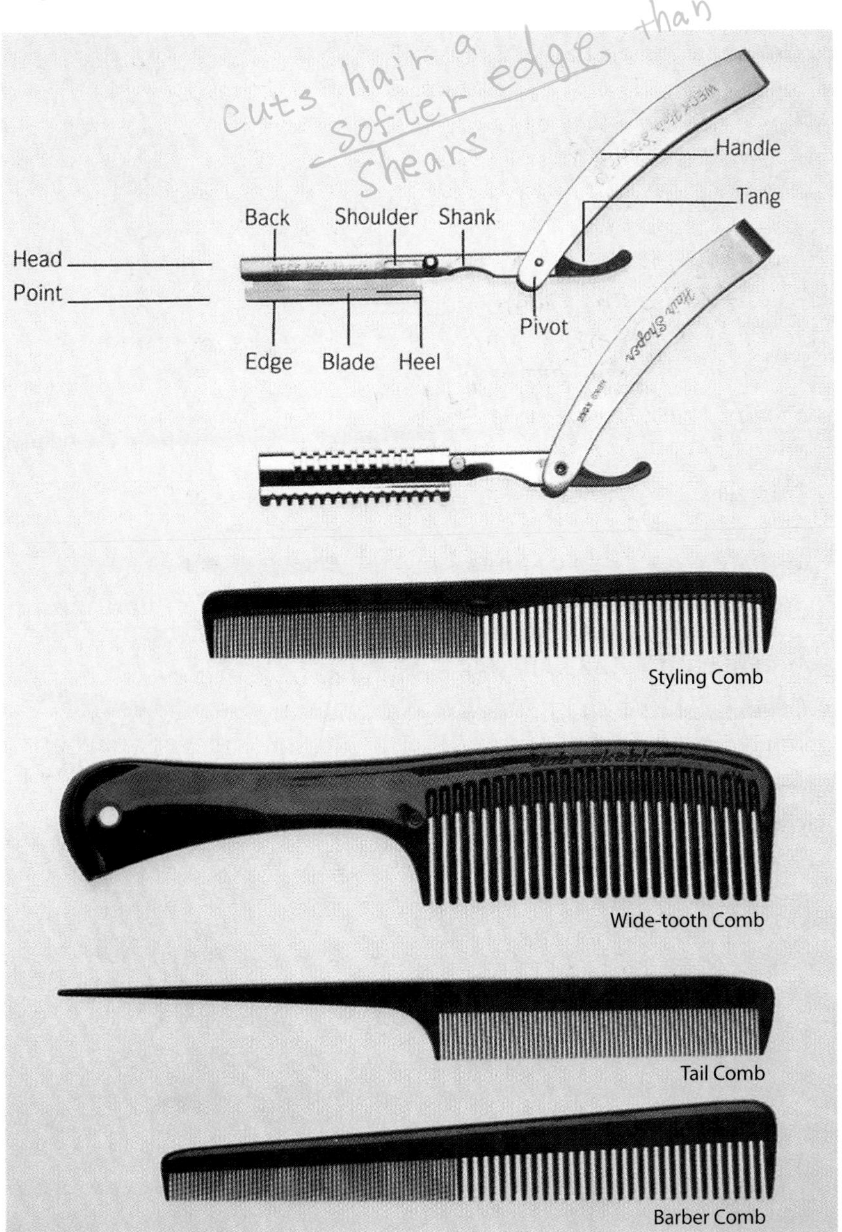

FIGURE 7.5 — Razors and combs.

GEOMETRY IN HAIRCUTTING

Geometry is used in haircutting to help insure accuracy and consistency throughout a haircut. A simple understanding of the following definitions will be beneficial in performing haircuts.

- ***Degrees:*** A way to measure circles. A complete circle measures 360 degrees from the center. The amount of elevation from the head form is measured in degrees. (Figs. 7.6, 7.7)

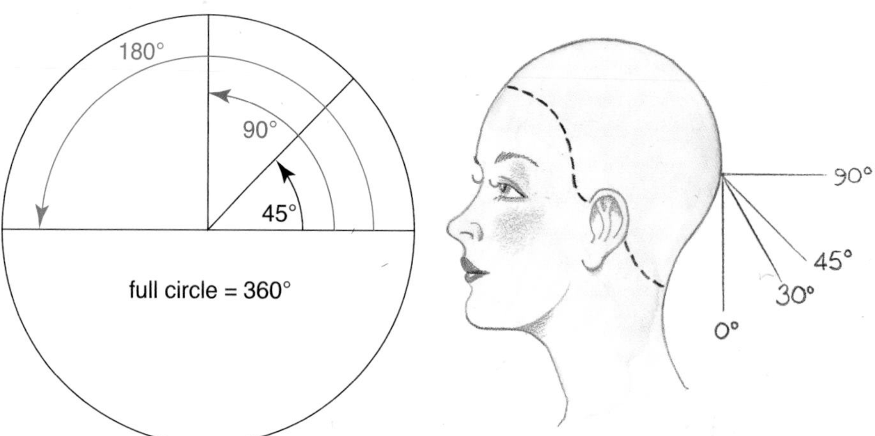

FIGURE 7.6 — Circles and angles are measured in degrees.

FIGURE 7.7 — Elevation from the head is measured in degrees.

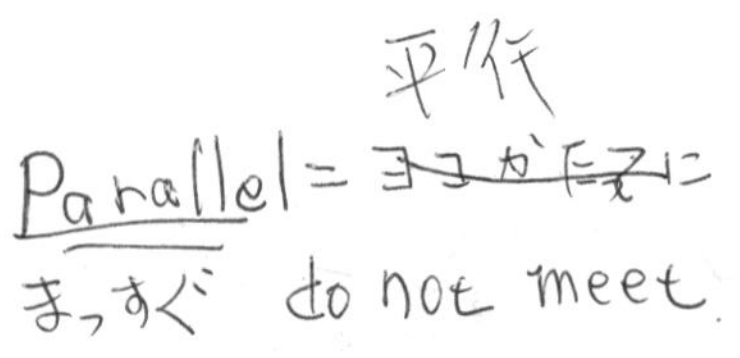

- ***Parallel lines:*** Two or more lines that do not meet in space. Parallel lines are useful to keep in mind in haircutting. Your body, hands, comb, shears, and partings must all be parallel before cutting the hair. (Fig. 7.8)
- ***Perpendicular lines:*** Two lines that intersect at a 90-degree angle. Perpendicular lines describe the hair's elevation when held at 90 degrees from the head form. Shears are held perpendicular to the parting. (Figs. 7.9, 7.10)

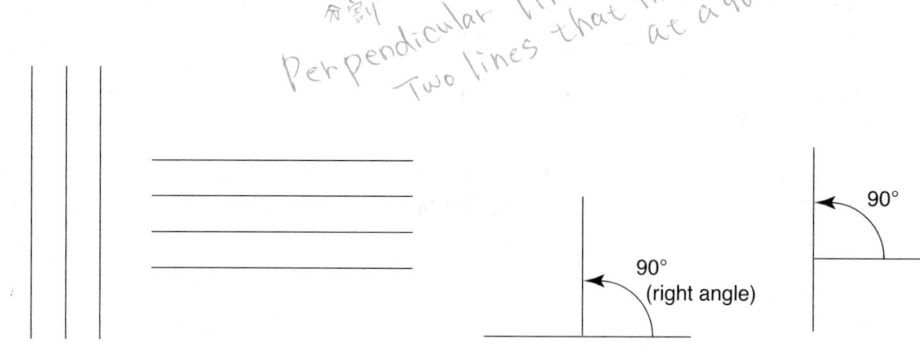

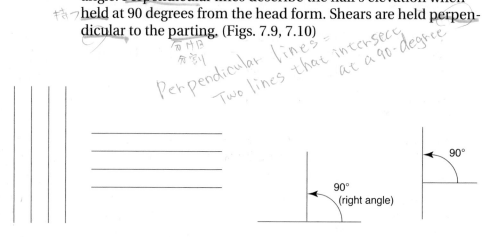

FIGURE 7.8 — Parallel lines.

FIGURE 7.9 — Perpendicular lines.

- ***Horizontal lines:*** Lines that are parallel to the floor. Horizontal lines are used in low-elevation haircuts. (Fig. 7.11)
- ***Vertical lines:*** Lines that are perpendicular to the floor. Vertical lines are used for high-elevation haircuts. (Fig. 7.12)
- ***Diagonal lines:*** Lines that are in between horizontal and vertical. Diagonal lines are used for blending and special design haircuts. (Fig. 7.13)

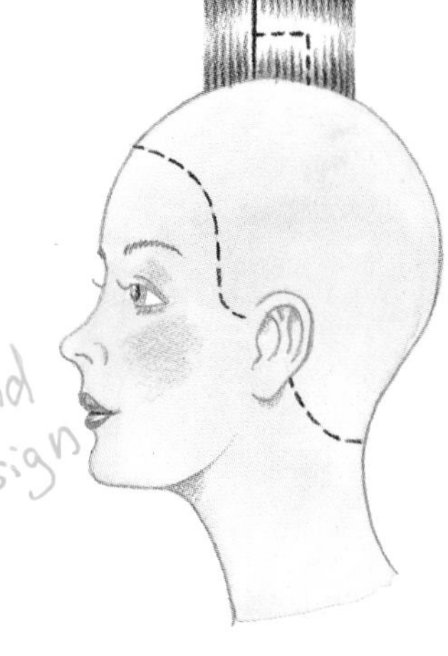

FIGURE 7.10 — 90-degree elevation from the head.

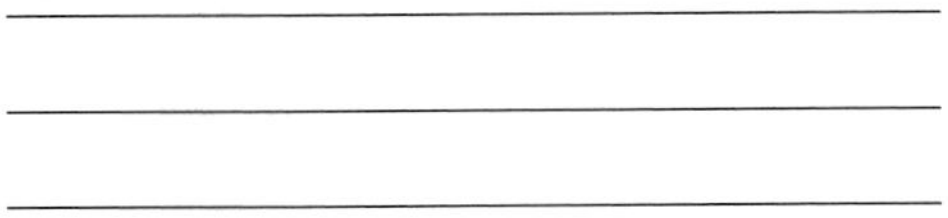

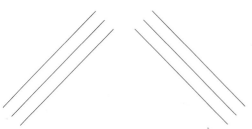

FIGURE 7.11 — Horizontal lines.

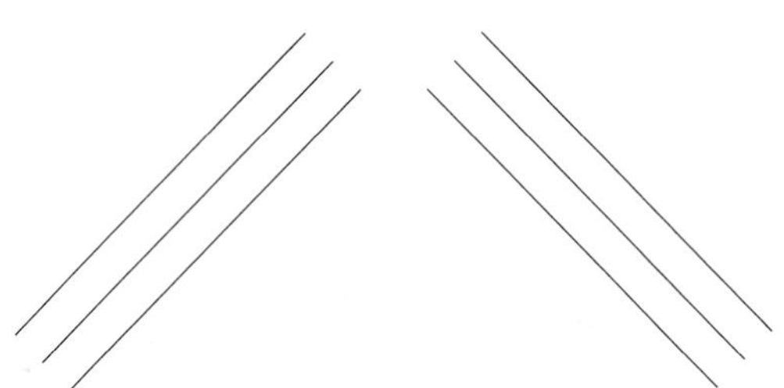

FIGURE 7.13 — Diagonal lines.

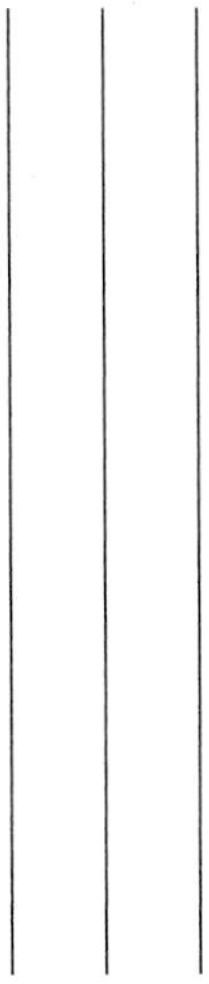

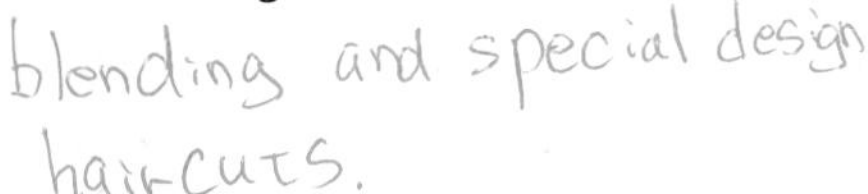

FIGURE 7.12 — Vertical lines.

CONTROLLING THE SHEARS AND COMB

During the haircutting process, you will be holding both the comb and the shears. Do not put the comb down, as this wastes time.

1. Open your right hand (left hand if you are left-handed) and place the ring finger in the finger grip of the still blade and the little finger in the finger brace (tang). (Fig. 7.14)
2. Place the thumb in the finger grip of the moving blade. (Fig. 7.15)
3. Practice opening and closing the shears, moving only your thumb while holding the comb between the thumb and index finger of the left hand. (Fig. 7.16)
4. To make partings, remove the thumb from the moving blade and transfer the comb to the right hand. Hold the comb between the thumb and the index and middle fingers of the right hand. With your ring and little fingers hold the shears

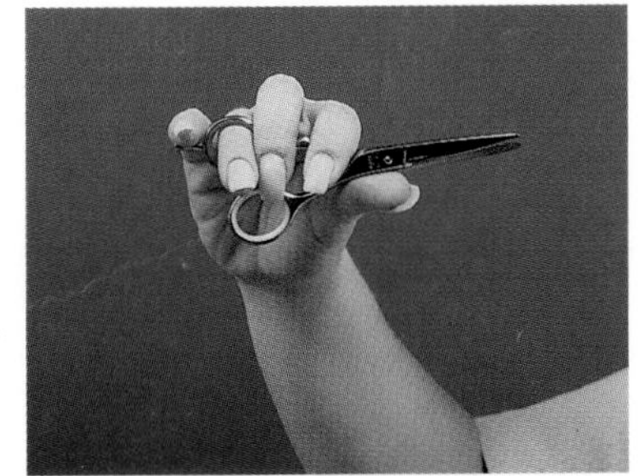

FIGURE 7.14 — Proper placement of ring finger and little finger.

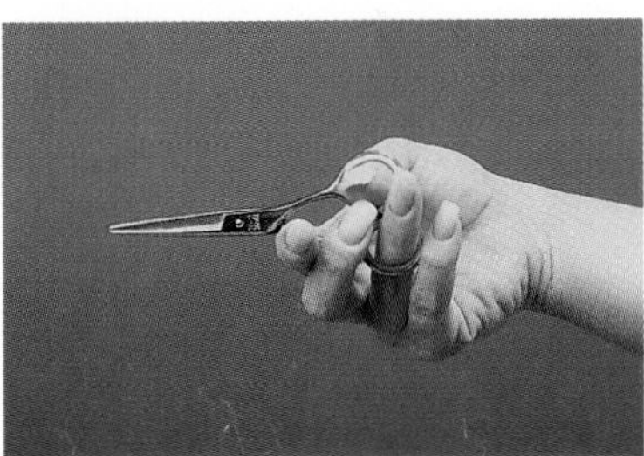

FIGURE 7.15 — Proper placement of thumb.

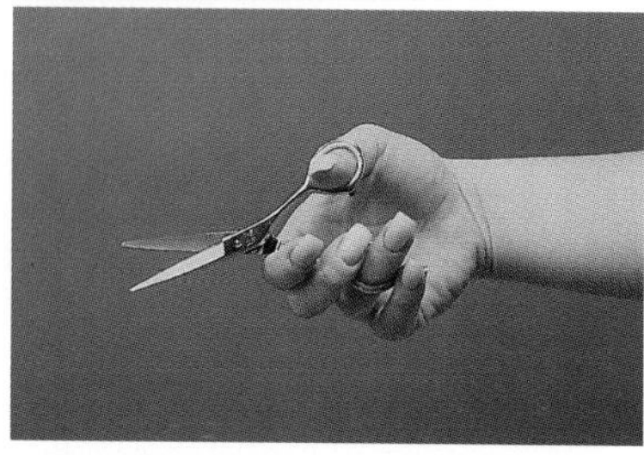

FIGURE 7.16 — Holding cutting scissors.

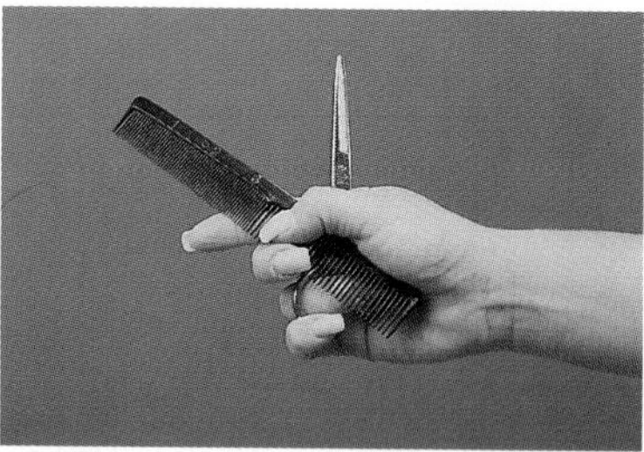

FIGURE 7.17 — Palming the comb and shears.

tightly in the palm of your hand. This is called ***palming the shears*** and is practiced for the safety of your client. (Fig. 7.17)

SAFETY IN HAIRCUTTING

1. Always palm the shears when combing the hair. This maintains control over the point of the shears while keeping your hand between the points and the client's face. Palming the shears also reduces strain on the index finger and thumb while combing the hair.
2. When cutting bangs or any area close to the skin, balance the shears by placing the tip of the index finger of the left hand (right if you cut left-handed) on the pivot screw and the knuckles of your left hand against the skin. This will prevent the client from being stabbed by the point of the shears if they suddenly move. You will be able to balance and control the shears as well.
3. Do not cut past the second knuckle when cutting on the inside of the hand. The skin is soft and fleshy past the second knuckle. It is easy to cut and takes a long time to heal.
4. Beginners should always use a guard when razor cutting.

SCALP AND HAIR ANALYSIS

Before you begin a haircut, a thorough scalp and hair analysis should be completed. Check specifically for:

1. The ***texture*** of the hair—fine, medium, or coarse. Fine hair can be cut shorter than coarse hair without sticking up or out. Coarse hair cannot be controlled when cut too short.
2. ***Cowlicks*** in the hairline and the interior of the hair. Always be careful to leave extra length to control cowlicks. (Fig. 7.18)
3. ***Whorls,*** especially in the crown. Leave extra length in the whorl area. (Fig. 7.19)

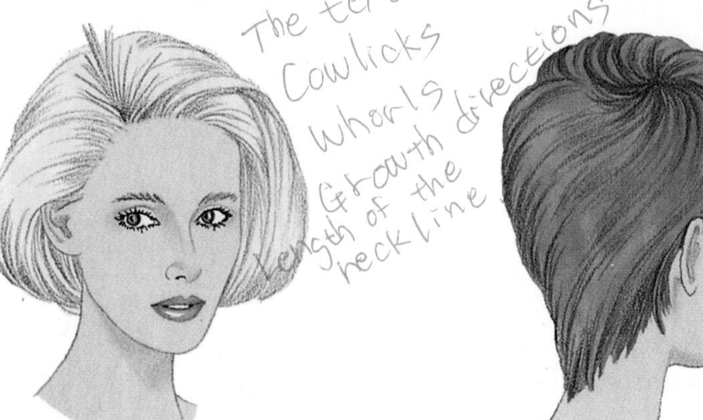

FIGURE 7.18 — Cowlick.

FIGURE 7.19 — Whorl.

4. ***Growth directions*** of the entire head, including the hairline and the top back and sides.
5. ***Length of the neckline.*** If cutting a fitted (close) neckline, check the shape the hairline forms, the growth pattern of the hairline, and if the hair in the neckline stays down or stands out from the head.

Completed: Learning Objective #2

SCALP AND HAIR ANALYSIS

SECTIONING

Dividing the head into sections helps control the hair when cutting and produces a more uniform haircut. Use four sections when cutting one-length haircuts or haircuts with low elevations and five sections when cutting high-elevation haircuts. Bang sections can be a variety of shapes, depending on the size and style. Sometimes the nape is sectioned separately when cutting a neckline. Blended sectioning is used when a high-elevation and low-elevation haircut are combined.

FOUR-SECTION PARTING

1. Part the hair from the center of the forehead to the center of the nape. (Figs. 7.20, 21)
2. Locate the top of the crown. Starting at the center part and the top of the crown, part the hair down to the point where the ear connects. (Fig. 7.22)
3. Repeat on the other side. This creates four cutting sections, two in the front and two in the back. (Figs. 7.23–7.25)

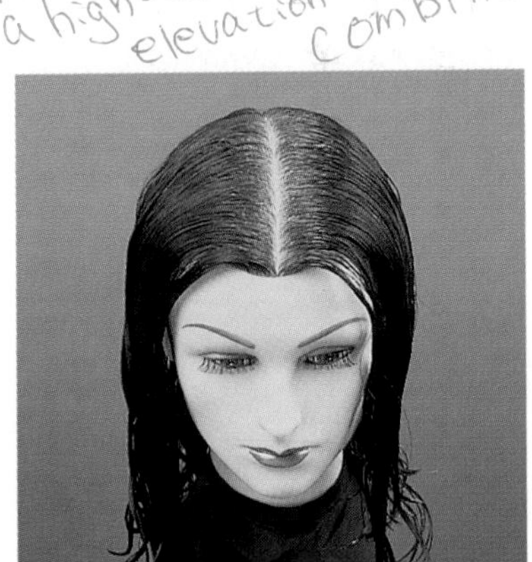

FIGURE 7.20 — Part the hair at the center of the forehead.

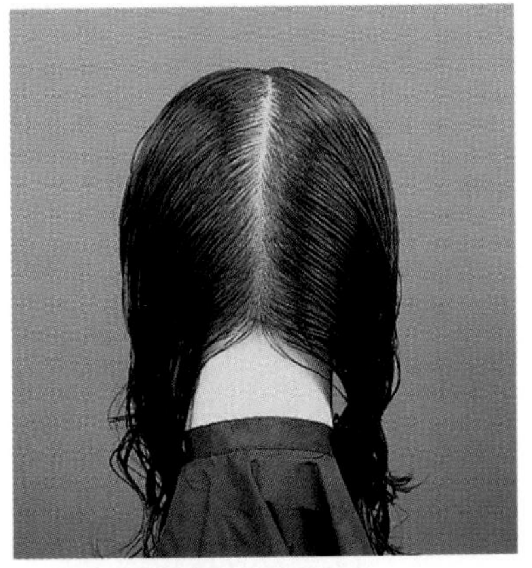

FIGURE 7.21 — Continue part down to nape.

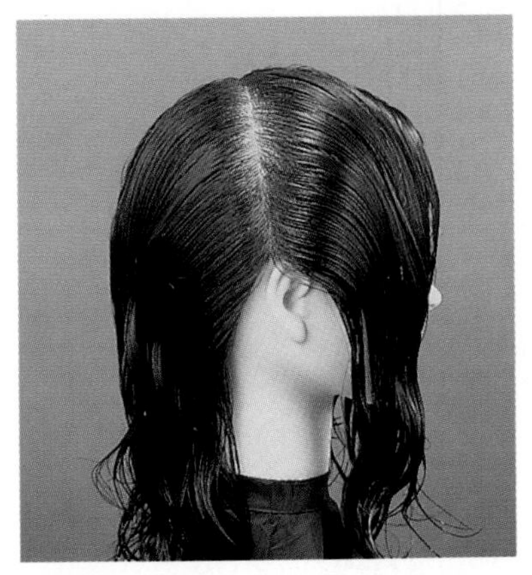

FIGURE 7.22 — Part from crown to ear.

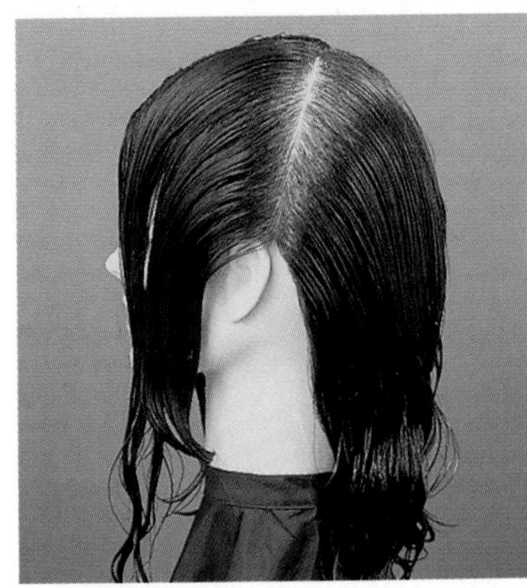

FIGURE 7.23 — Repeat on the other side.

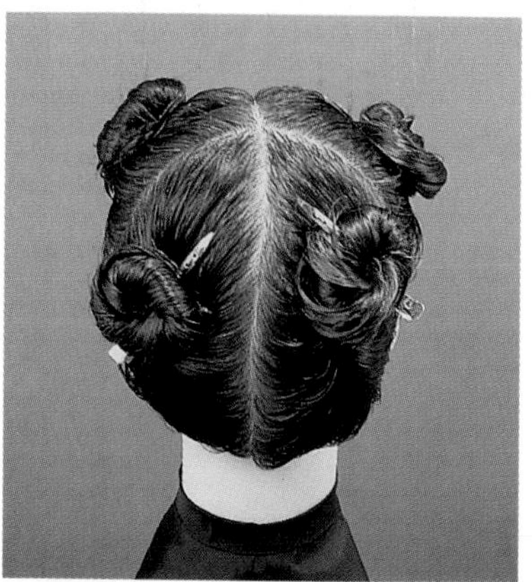
FIGURE 7.24 — Pin each section in place.

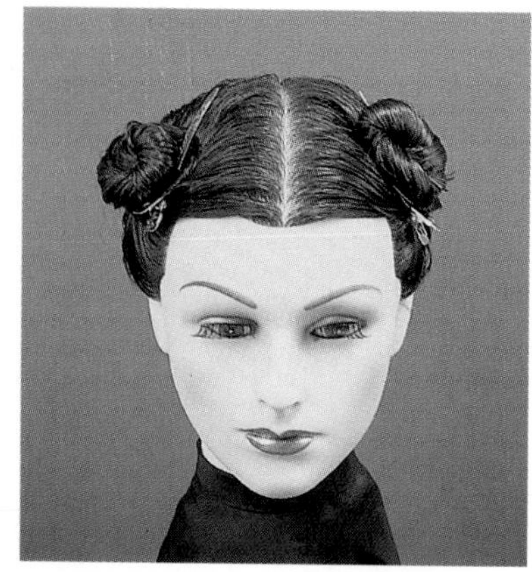
FIGURE 7.25 — Completed four-section parting.

FIVE-SECTION PARTING

1. Divide the head from the top of the crown to behind the ears. (Figs. 7.26, 7.27)
2. Divide the back in half from the center of the top of the crown to the center of the hairline in the nape. (Fig. 7.28)
3. The top front is sectioned from the center of each eye straight back to the crown, creating a square section on top and two side sections over the ears. (Figs. 7.29–7.32)
4. (optional) Section the back across from the center of one ear to the center of the other. (Fig. 7.33)

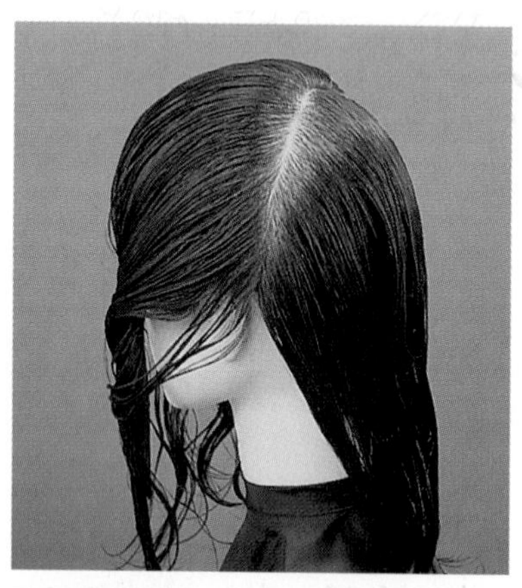
FIGURE 7.26 — Part from crown to ear.

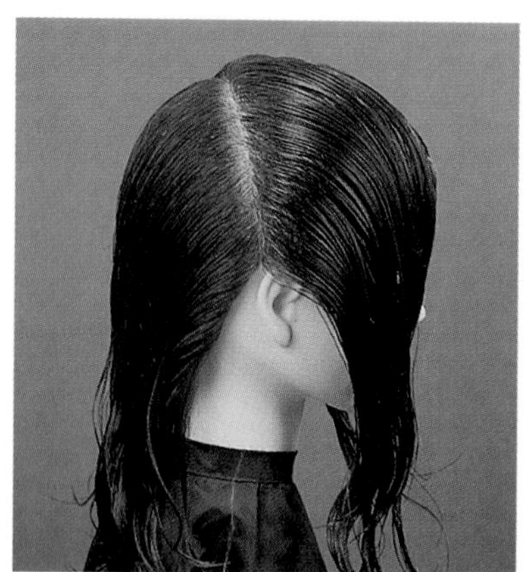
FIGURE 7.27 — Repeat on the other side.

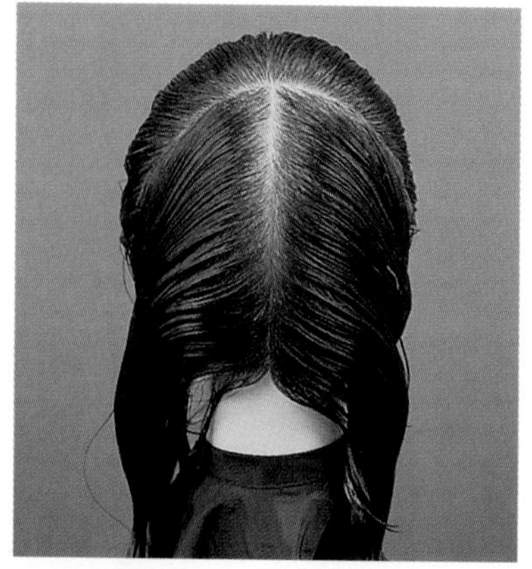
FIGURE 7.28 — Part from crown to nape.

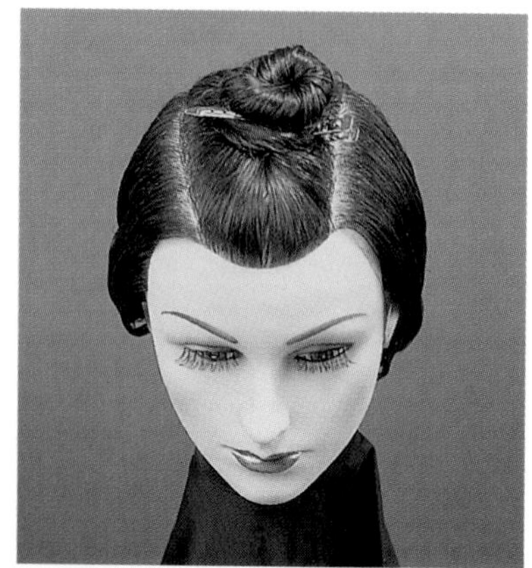
FIGURE 7.29 — Divide top front into three sections and pin top section in place.

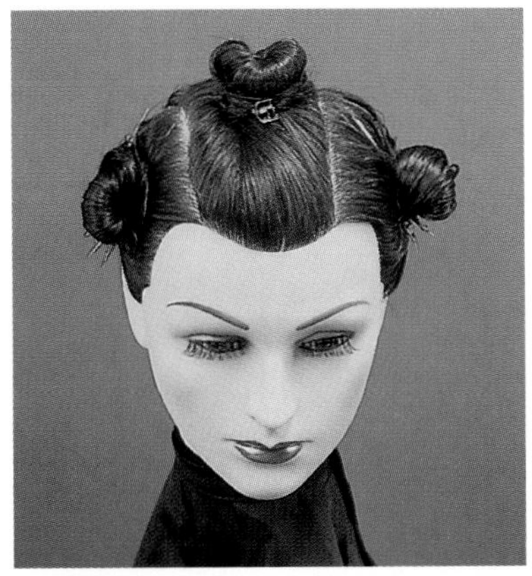
FIGURE 7.30 — Pin each side section in place.

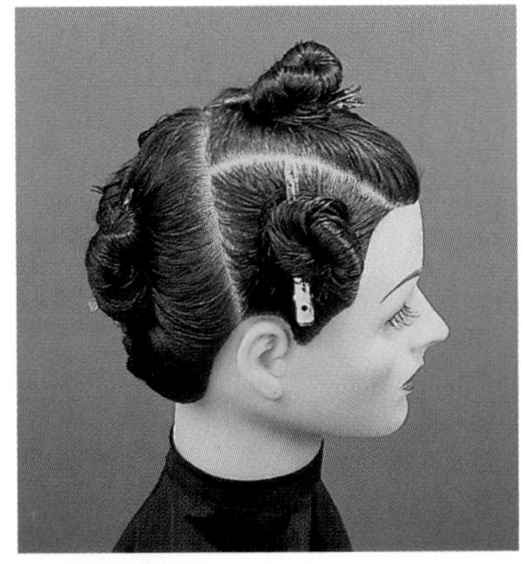
FIGURE 7.31 — Pin two back sections in place.

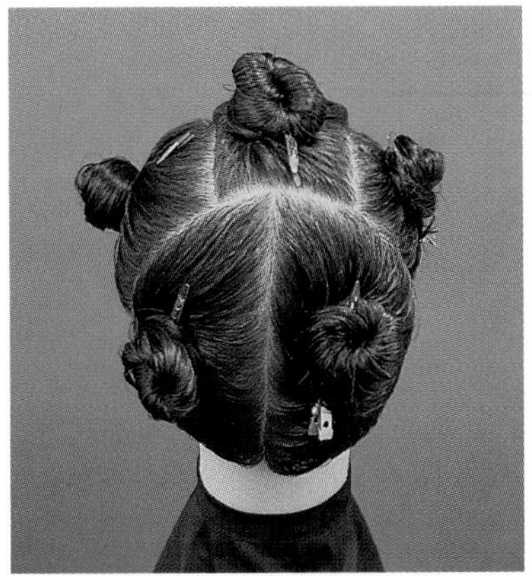
FIGURE 7.32 — Completed five-section parting.

BANGS SECTIONS

Bangs sections are used in addition to the four or five basic sections. Illustrated here are several recommended bangs sections. (Figs. 7.34–7.38)

NECKLINE SECTIONS

Neckline sections are used along the neckline when the hair is cut very short. (Figs. 7.39–7.41)

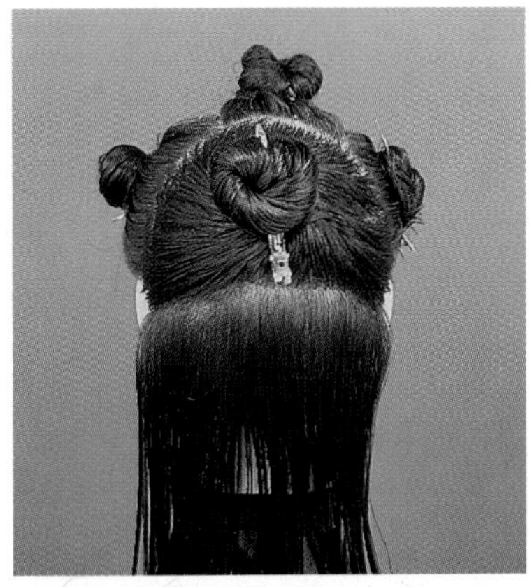
FIGURE 7.33 — Alternate five-section parting.

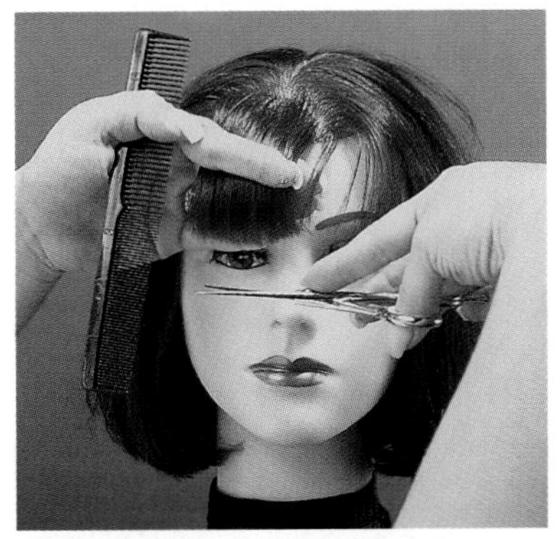
FIGURE 7.34 — When cutting bangs, keep forefinger on pivot screw.

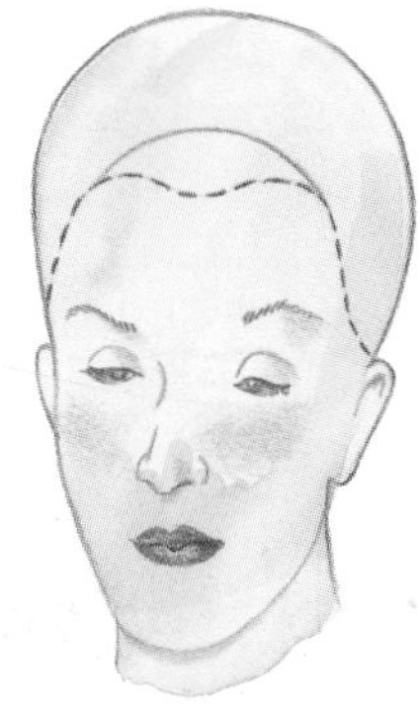
FIGURE 7.35 — Curved bangs—light.

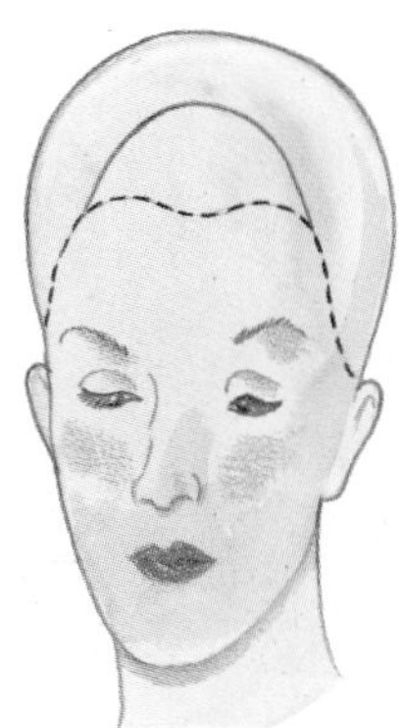
FIGURE 7.36 — Curved bangs—heavy.

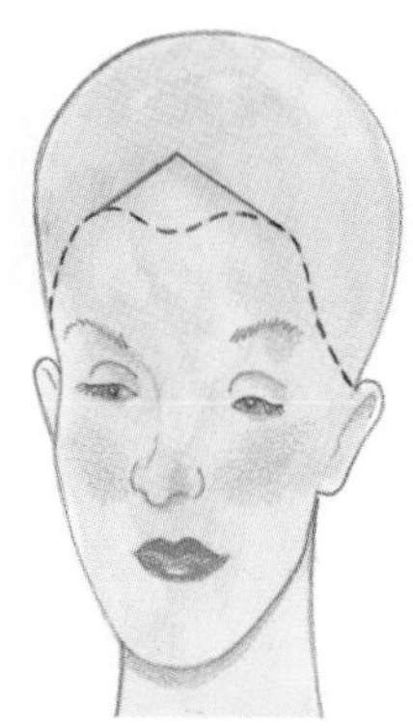

FIGURE 7.37 — Triangular bangs—light.

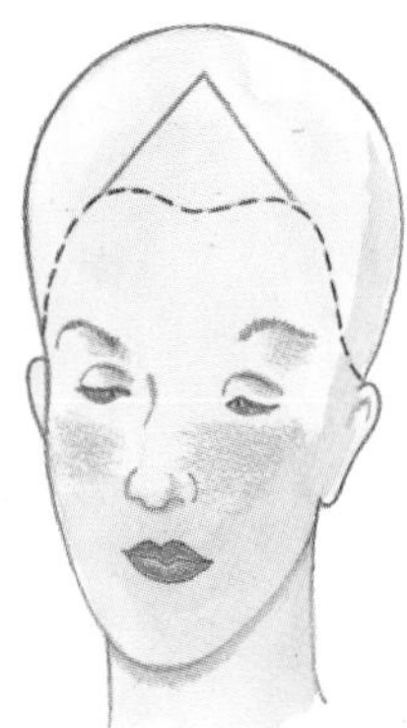

FIGURE 7.38 — Triangular bangs—heavy.

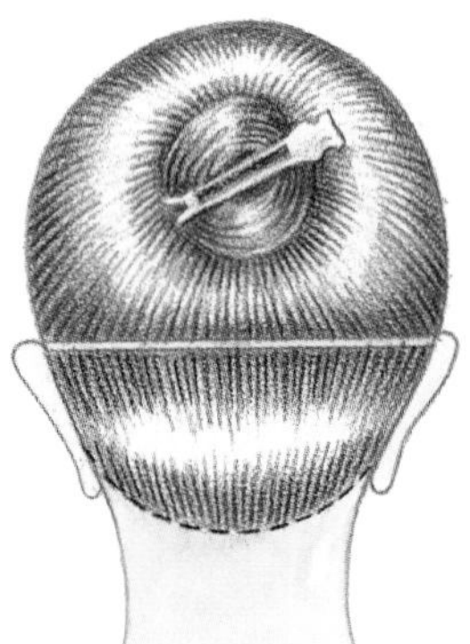

FIGURE 7.39 — Normal neckline parting.

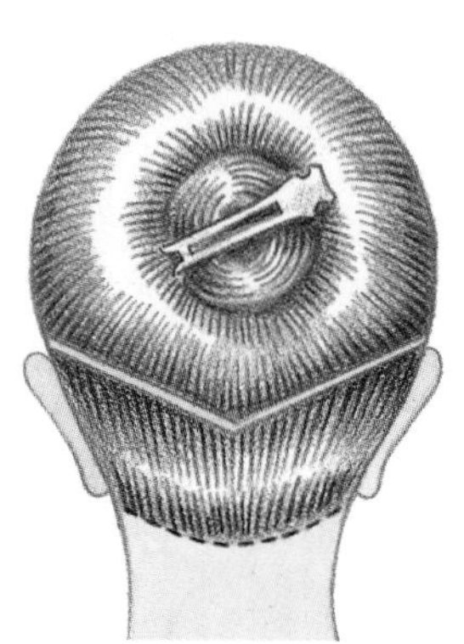

FIGURE 7.40 — Small neckline parting.

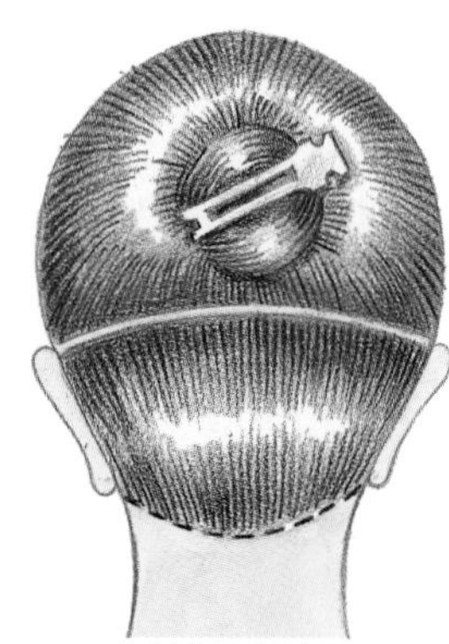

FIGURE 7.41 — Large neckline parting.

GUIDES

All haircuts have an exterior guide. This guide or design line creates the line we see around the perimeter of the haircut. Sometimes it is very definite in design—a one-length haircut, for example (Figs. 7.42, 7.43)—and sometimes it is ornamental, as in wispy bangs or sideburns.

When you layer hair at a high elevation, use an interior guide to determine the length of the hair as it is elevated. Usually a guide is a parting ½" (1.25 cm) thick. (Figs. 7.44, 7.45) A ***stationary guide*** (also called a ***stable guide***) is a guide that does not move. All the hair is directed to the guide. (Fig. 7.46) A ***moving*** or ***traveling guide*** is a guide that is directed to the next parting to be cut. (Figs. 7.47–7.49)

Completed: Learning Objective #3

STATIONARY AND TRAVELING GUIDES

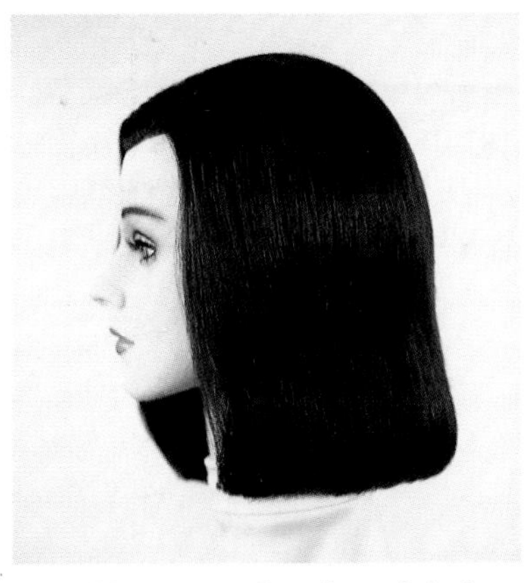

FIGURE 7.42 — One-length haircut.

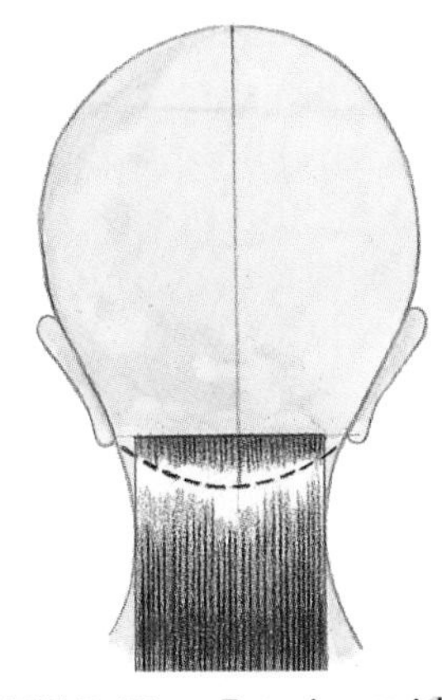

FIGURE 7.43 — Exterior guide.

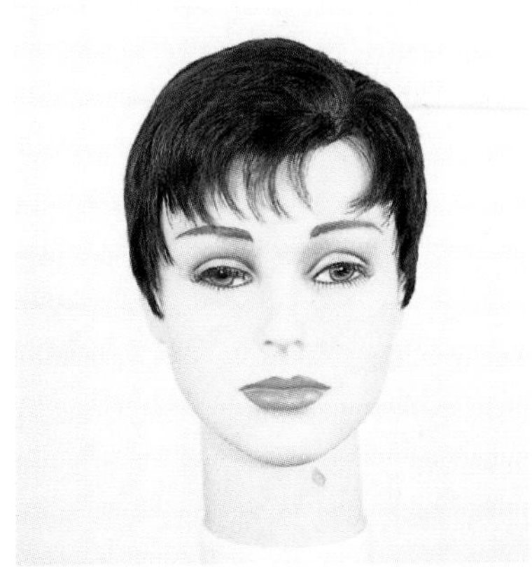

FIGURE 7.44 — Uniform layers.

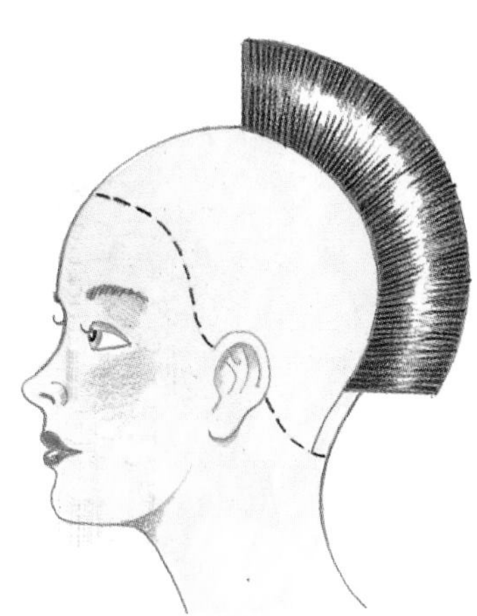

FIGURE 7.45 — Interior guide.

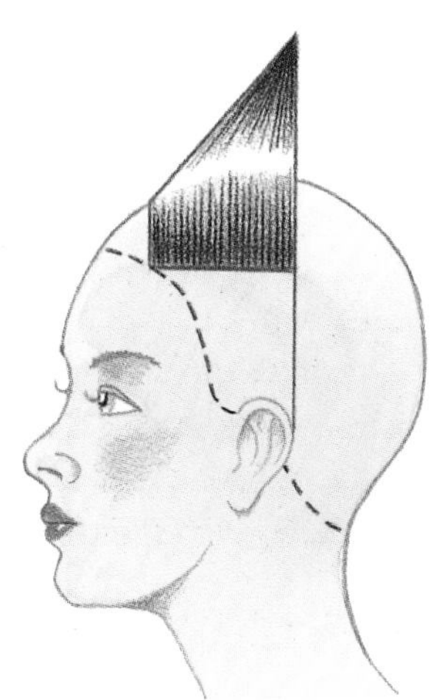

FIGURE 7.46 — Stationary guide.

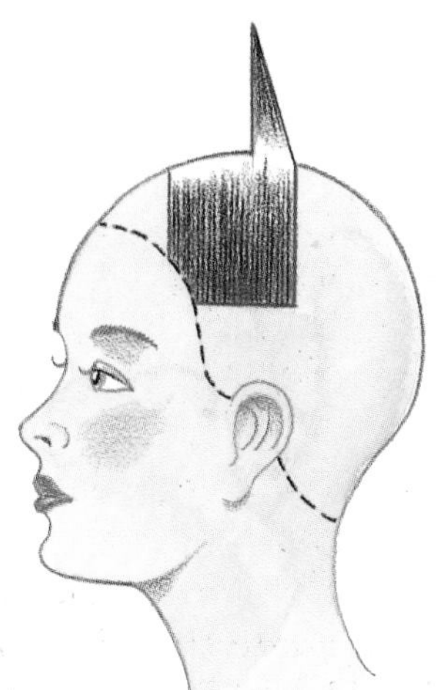

FIGURE 7.47 — Traveling guide—first parting.

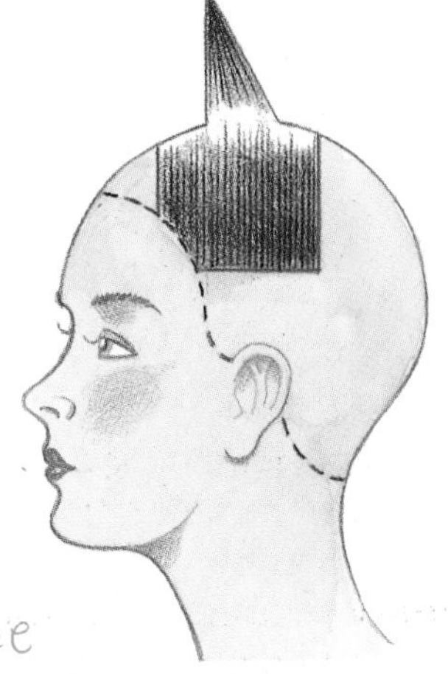

FIGURE 7.48 — Traveling guide—second parting.

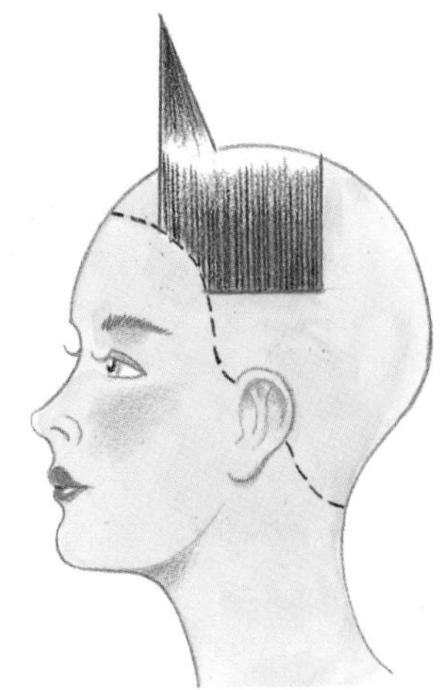

FIGURE 7.49 — Traveling guide—third parting.

EFFECTS OF HEAD POSITION

The position of the client's head has a definite impact on the finished haircut. Different positions result in a different kind of line along the perimeter. (Figs. 7.50a–7.52b) It is important that the head be held in a constant position when you are cutting the back and side sections.

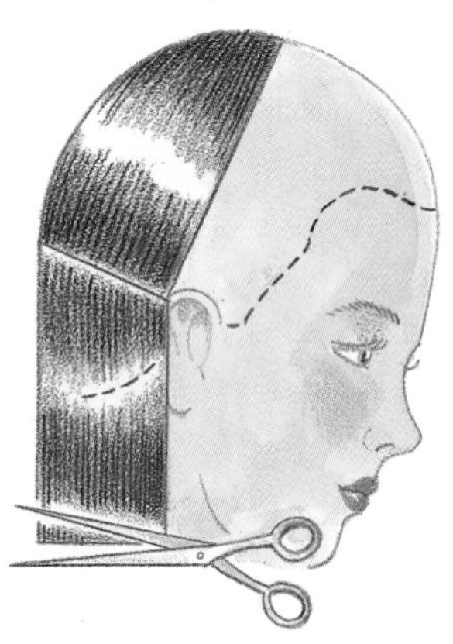

FIGURE 7.50a — Head pushed forward and down while cutting.

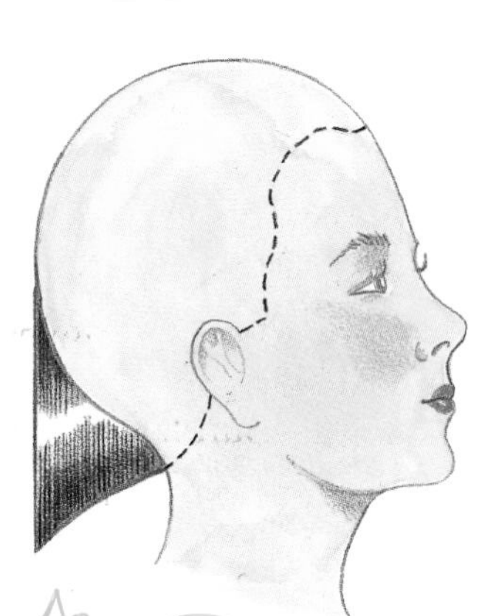

FIGURE 7.50b — Finished line: hair is undercut.

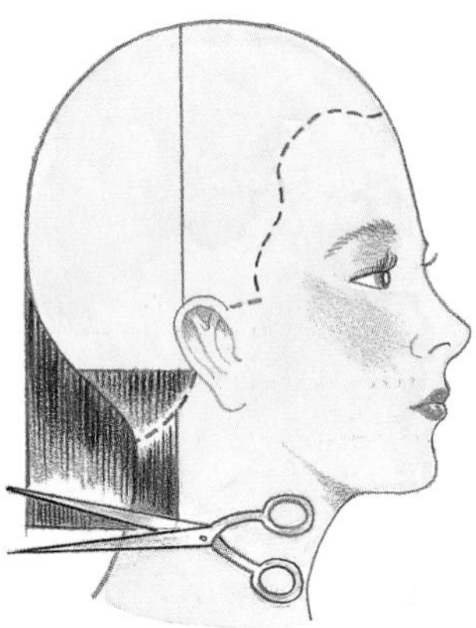

FIGURE 7.51a — Head in upright position while cutting.

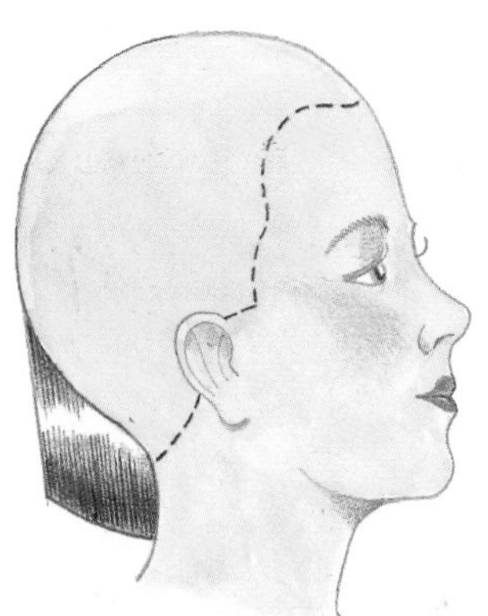

FIGURE 7.51b — Finished line: ends are graduated, slightly longer underneath.

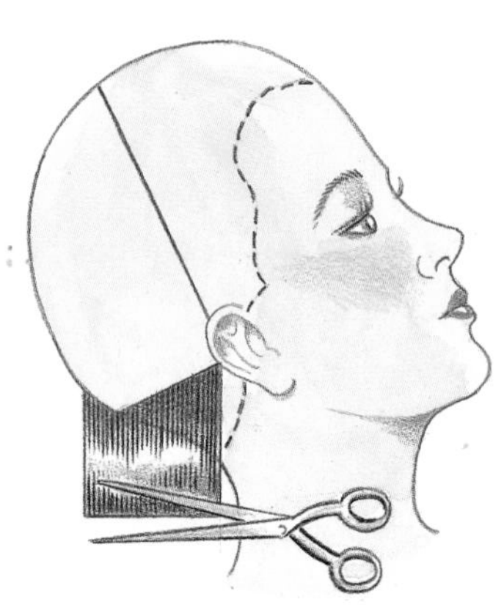

FIGURE 7.52a — Head pulled back while cutting.

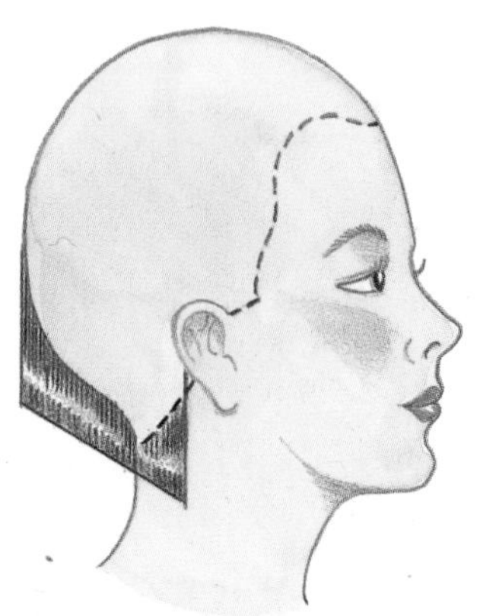

FIGURE 7.52b — Finished line: ends are graduated, longer underneath.

ELEVATIONS

There are four basic elevations used in haircutting:

1. ***Low elevation:*** also called zero-degree elevation
2. ***High elevation:*** also called 90-degree elevation
3. ***Reverse elevation:*** also called 180-degree elevation
4. ***Blended elevation:*** blending 90-degree elevation into low elevation

CUTTING THE LOW-ELEVATION, ZERO-DEGREE, OR BLUNT HAIRCUT

1. Section the hair into the four haircutting sections.
2. Start at the bottom of the nape, take a horizontal parting on the left back section (the thickness of the parting or subsection will be determined by the texture of the hair), and comb straight down. Cut the hair straight across, parallel to the floor, at the desired length. (Fig. 7.53) Repeat in the right section, matching the length to the left side. This will be the guide. (Fig. 7.54)
3. Return to the left side and make a parting (or subsection) the same thickness as your first parting. (Figs. 7.55, 7.56) Comb the hair straight down and match the length to the first cut. Repeat on the right side. (Fig. 7.57)
4. Continue working up the back of the head, alternating from the left section to the right section.

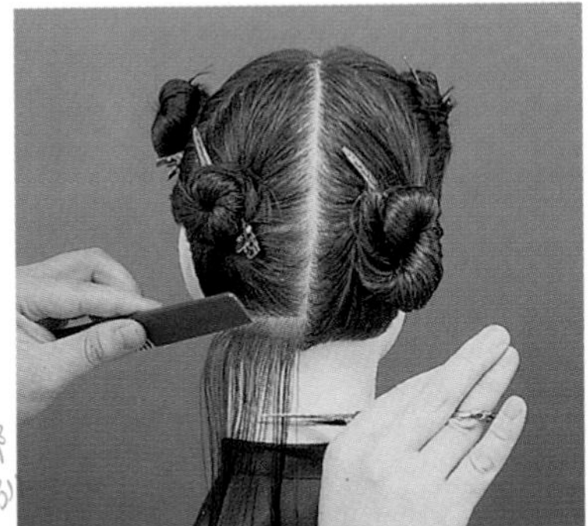

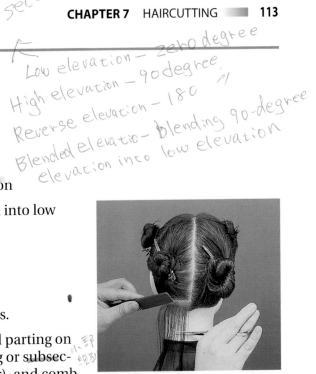

FIGURE 7.53 — First parting on left side.

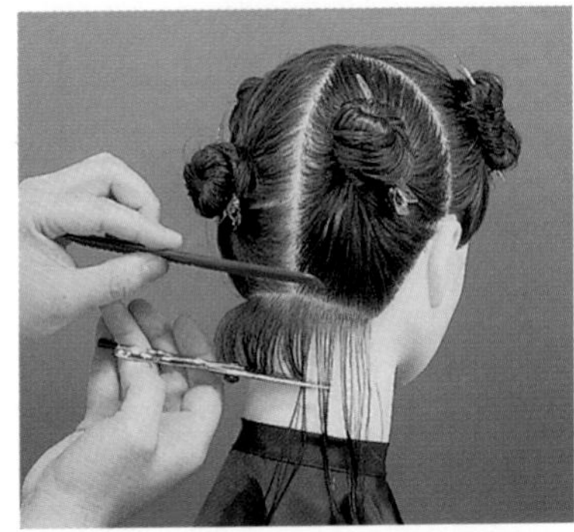

FIGURE 7.54 — Repeat on right side. This creates the guideline.

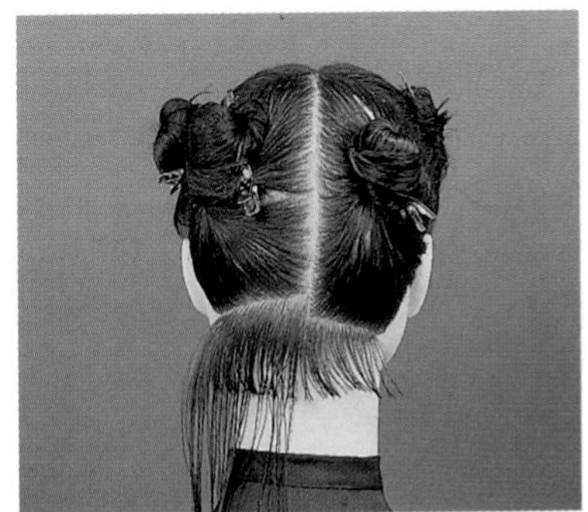

FIGURE 7.55 — Second parting, with visible guideline underneath, above the first.

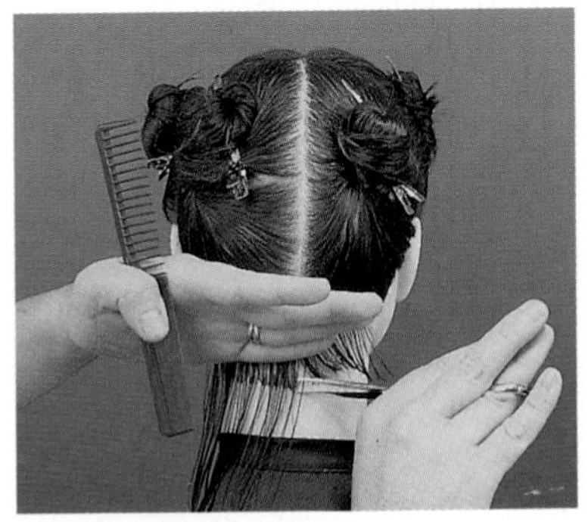

FIGURE 7.56 — Using guideline, cut across bottom.

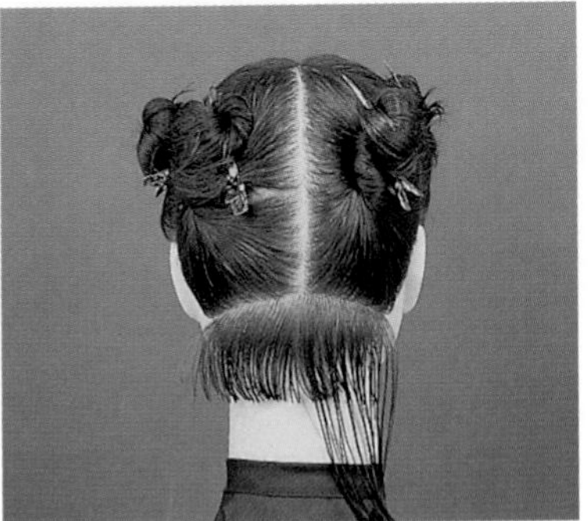

FIGURE 7.57 — Second parting on right side, above guideline.

5. Move to the left front section of the head. Starting at the bottom of the section, make a horizontal parting. Comb the hair straight down. Cut the hair parallel to the floor, matching the length in the front section with the length in the back section. (Fig. 7.58)

6. Continue working up the front section using horizontal partings until all the hair that reaches the hanging length is cut. (Fig. 7.59)

7. Repeat steps 5 and 6 on the right side. (Fig. 7.60)

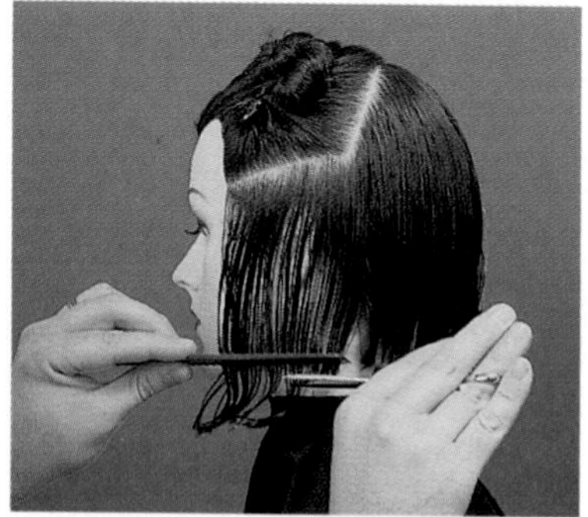

FIGURE 7.58 — Beginning on left front section.

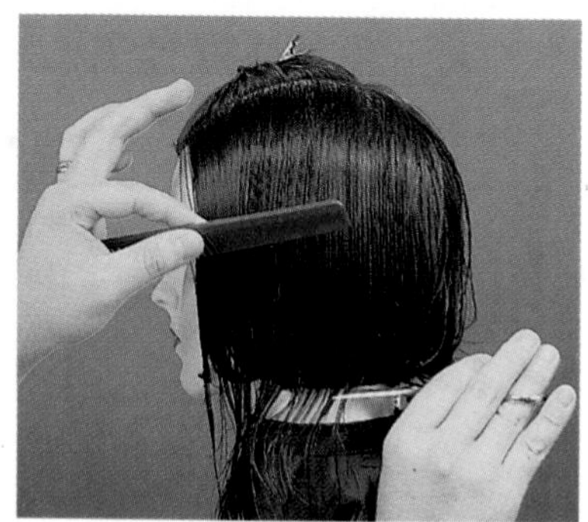

FIGURE 7.59 — Continue working up front section.

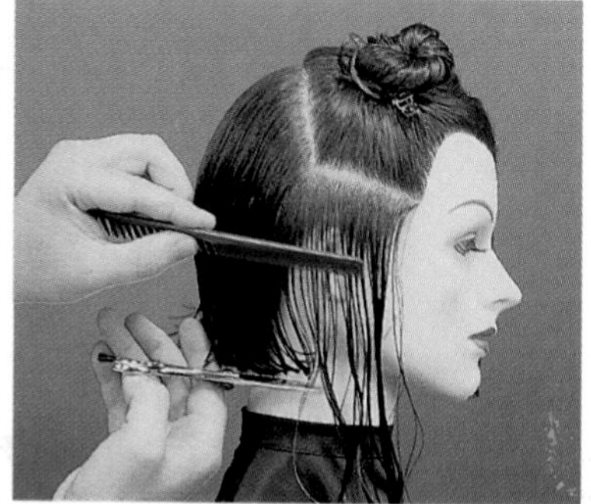

FIGURE 7.60 — Repeat on right side.

CUTTING THE HIGH-ELEVATION OR 90-DEGREE HAIRCUT

1. Part the hair into five cutting sections. Starting at the back of the top section, use ½" (1.25 cm) partings (or subsections) across the head. Hold the hair at 90 degrees from the head form and cut to the desired length. (Figs. 7.61, 7.62)

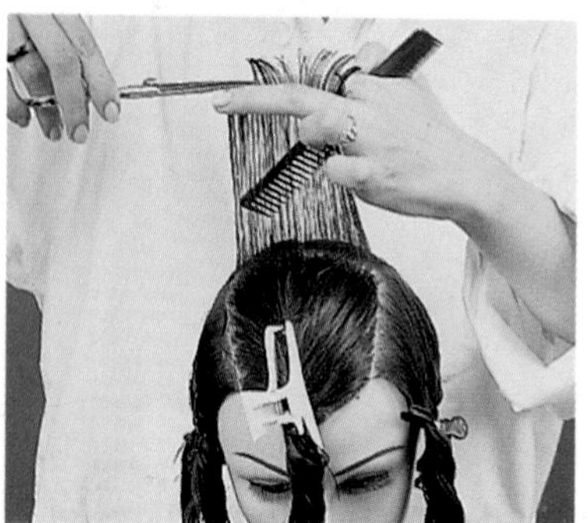

FIGURE 7.61 — First parting: creating guideline for top section.

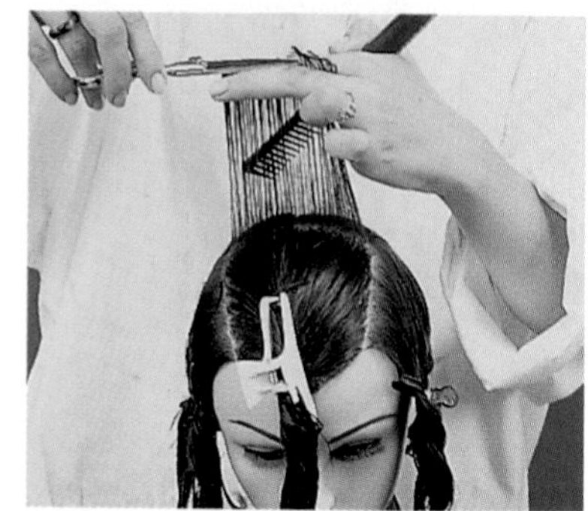

FIGURE 7.62 — Cutting first parting.

2. Make a second parting working towards the front. Direct the first parting (guide) to the second parting and cut the second parting to the same length as the guide. Continue working from back to front of the top section until all the hair has been cut to the same length. (Fig. 7.63)
3. Divide the top section in two from front to back and comb to the sides. This will be the guide for the side sections.
4. Start at the back of the right side section. Use vertical partings ½" (1.25 cm) thick. Hold the hair at a 90-degree angle from the head form. Use the previously cut hair in the top section to establish the length. Work down the section, cutting every hair the same length. This will establish a guide for the rest of the side section. (Fig. 7.64)
5. Take another ½" (1.25 cm) vertical parting. Move the previously cut parting to the parting to be cut. Use the previously cut side parting and the top section as a guide. Cut the hair from the top of the section to the bottom. (Fig. 7.65)
6. Continue using ½" (1.25 cm) vertical partings and the previously cut parting as your guide. Work forward to the front hairline. (Fig. 7.66)
7. Repeat the procedure on the left side. (Figs. 7.67, 7.68)
8. At the front of the right rear section take a ½" (1.25 cm) pie-shaped vertical parting from the center of the top of the crown to the nape. Make a second parting starting at the top section down to the bottom of the side section. This will be your guide. Direct the previously cut parting to the parting to be cut. Cut to the same length. When you get below the side parting into the nape, you will be creating a new guide for the rest of the nape area. (Fig. 7.69)

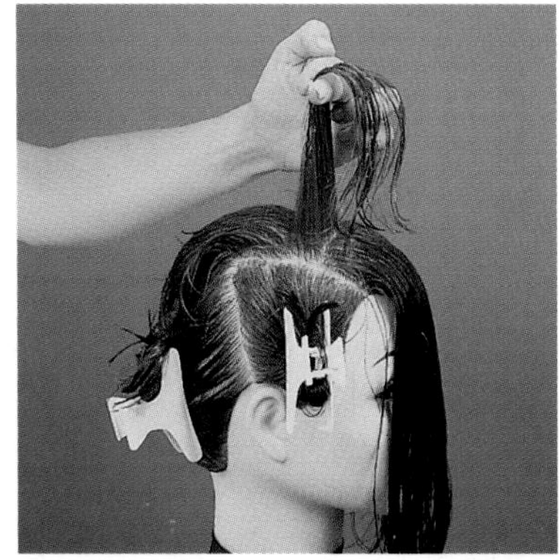

FIGURE 7.63 — Second parting in front of first.

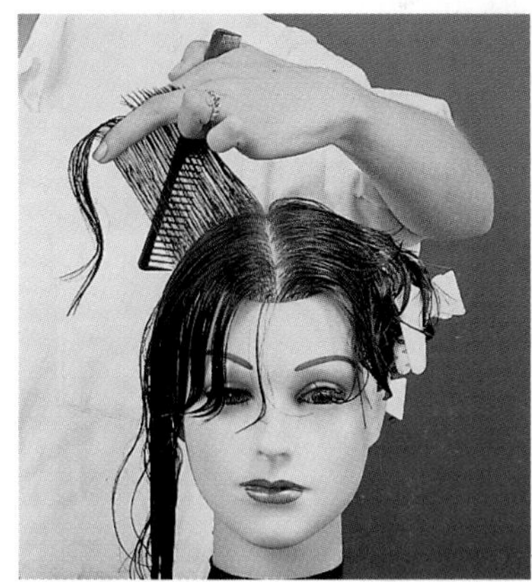

FIGURE 7.64 — First parting: creating guideline for right side section.

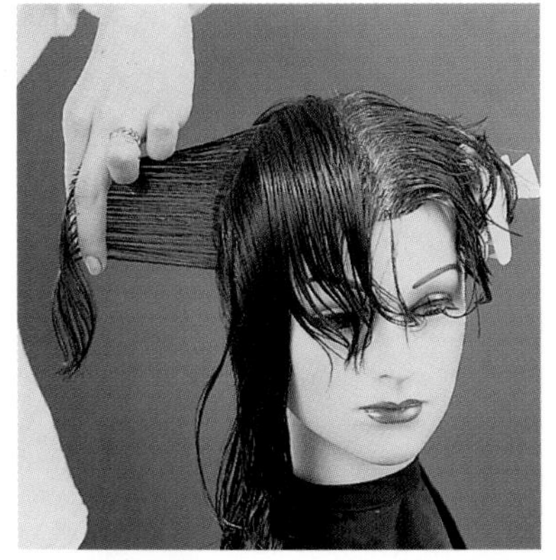

FIGURE 7.65 — Second parting in front of first.

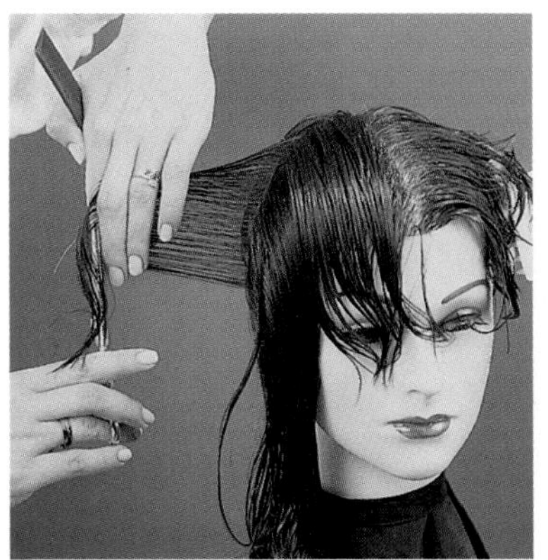

FIGURE 7.66 — Working forward with vertical partings.

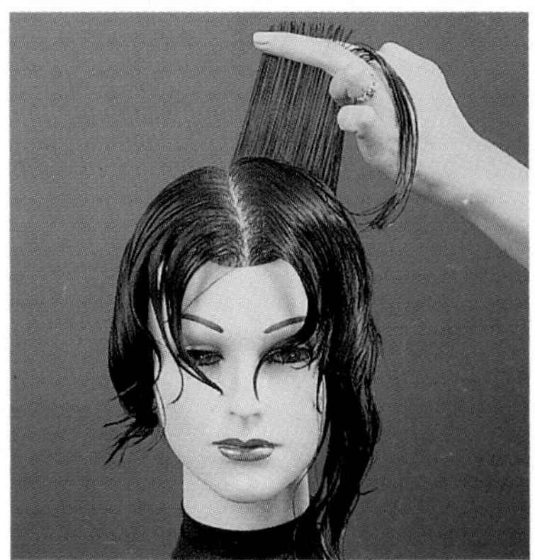

FIGURE 7.67 — Repeat on left side.

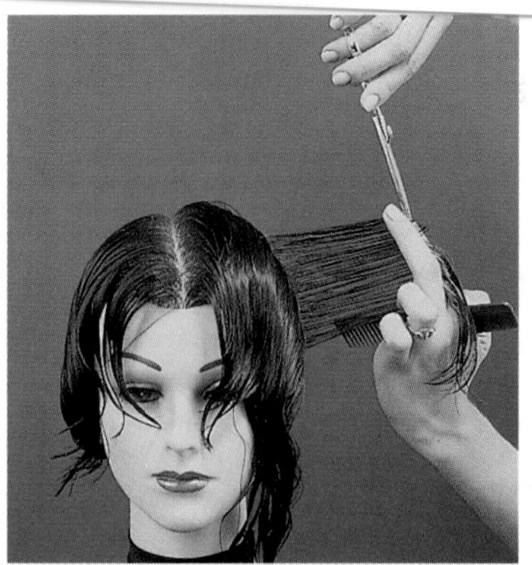

FIGURE 7.68 — Working forward with vertical partings.

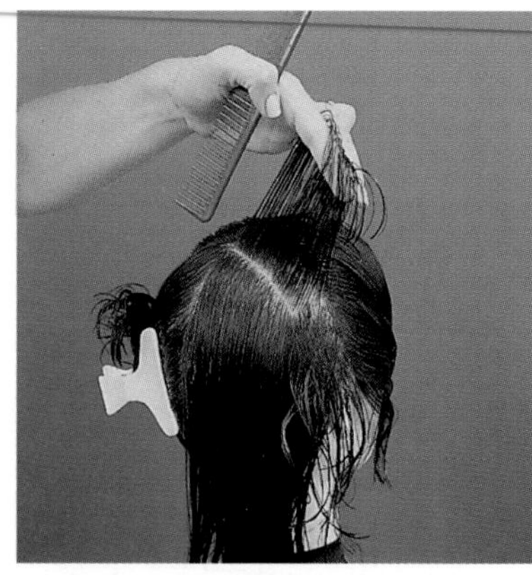

FIGURE 7.69 — Vertical pie-shaped parting.

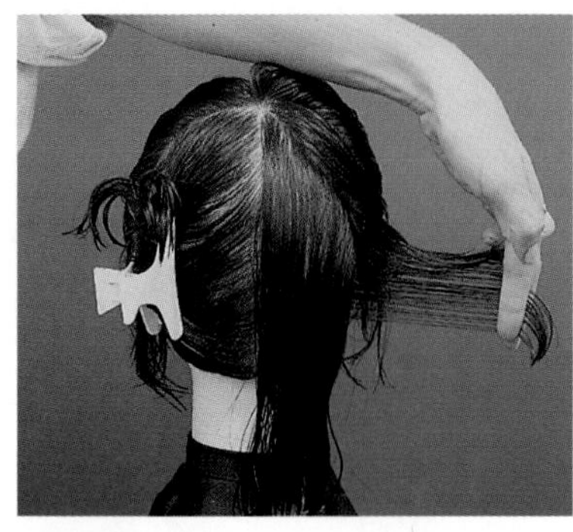

FIGURE 7.70 — Continuing with pie-shaped parting.

9. Work from right to left and continue making vertical pie-shaped partings. You should have one parting to be cut and one parting as a guide, continuing the guide down into the nape. Always move the guide to the parting to be cut. (Fig. 7.70)

10. Follow this procedure into the left rear section. When you have completed the back, the left rear section should match the left front section. (Fig. 7.71)

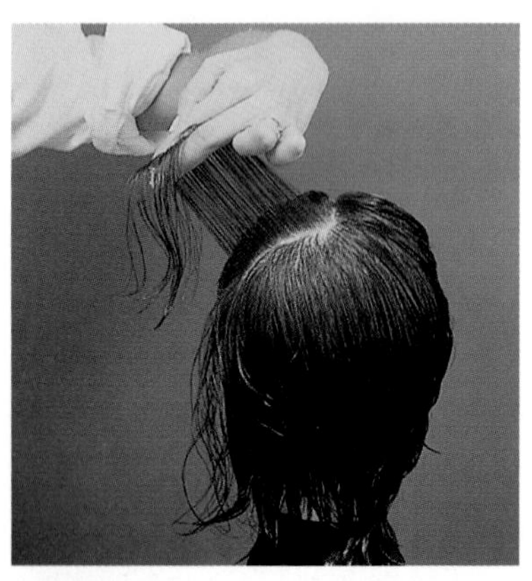

FIGURE 7.71 — Repeat on left side.

Note: *All the hair that has been cut should be the same length when measured.*

CUTTING THE REVERSE ELEVATION OR 180-DEGREE HAIRCUT

1. Part the hair into five cutting sections. Begin at the top of the crown by taking a ½" (1.25 cm) parting (or subsection) across the head. Comb straight up from the head form and cut straight across. (Fig. 7.72)

2. Work to the front of the top section by taking a second ½" (1.25 cm) parting. Direct the first parting (guide) to the second parting and cut to the same length. (Fig. 7.73)

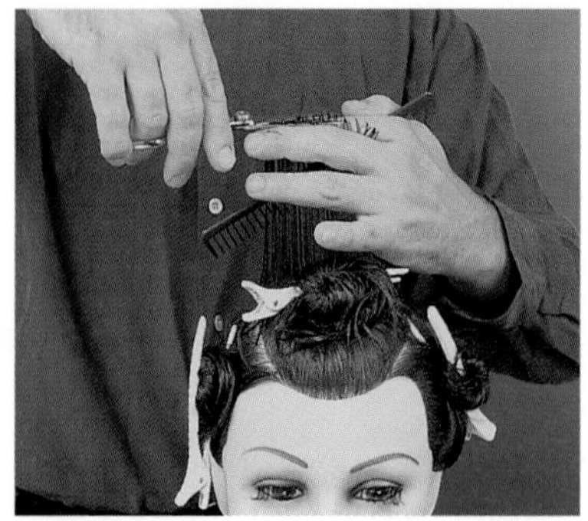

FIGURE 7.72 — Combing hair straight up for cutting.

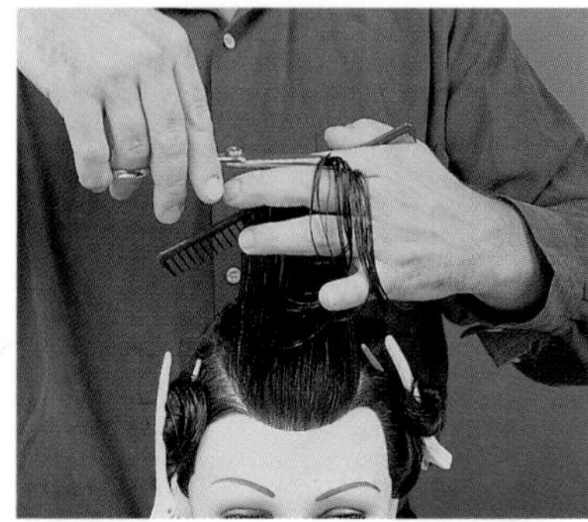

FIGURE 7.73 — Second parting cut to same length as first.

3. Continue, using the previously cut parting as your guide to cut a new ½" (1.25 cm) parting throughout the top section.
4. On the left front section, using ½" (1.25 cm) horizontal partings, comb the hair straight up, and match to the previously cut hair (guide) in the top section. Continue working down the side, using ½" (1.25 cm) partings until the hair no longer reaches the guide. (Fig. 7.74)
5. Repeat on the right side. (Fig. 7.75)
6. At the top of the left rear section, using ½" (1.25 cm) horizontal partings, comb the hair straight up from the head form, matching the length to the top section (guide), and cut straight across. (Fig. 7.76)
7. Continue, using ½" (1.25 cm) horizontal partings and working from top to bottom until the hair no longer reaches the guide.
8. Repeat on the right side. (Fig. 7.77)

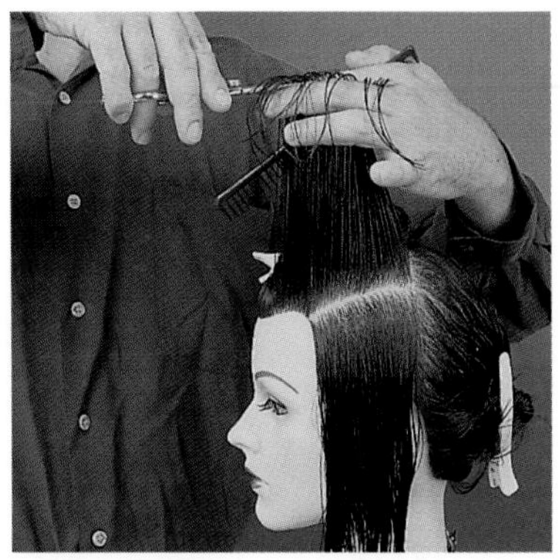

FIGURE 7.74 — Match hair to guideline on left side and cut.

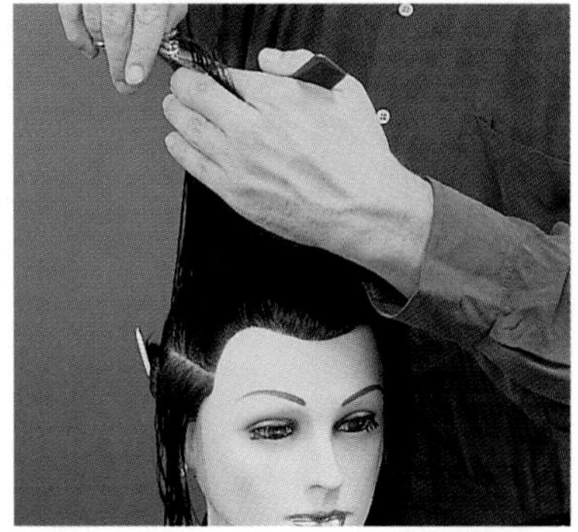

FIGURE 7.75 — Repeat on right side.

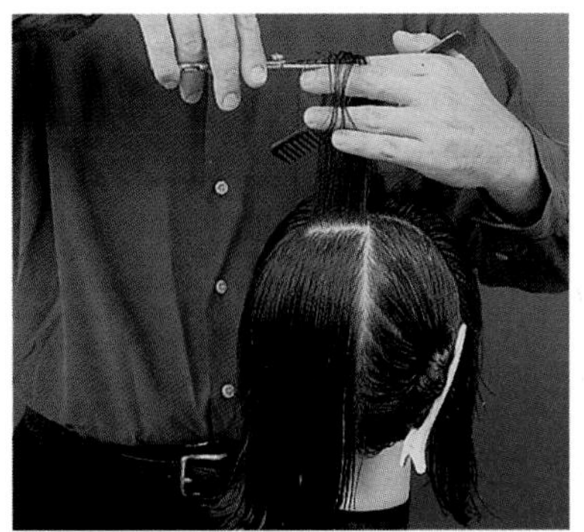

FIGURE 7.76 — Cutting left rear section.

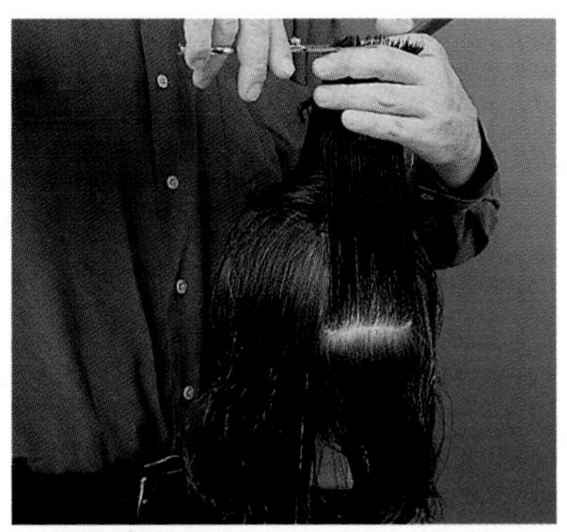

FIGURE 7.77 — Working down right rear section.

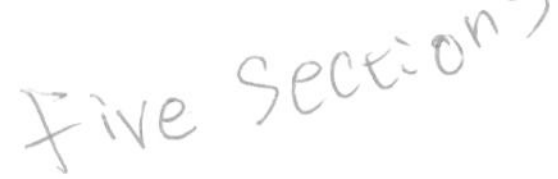

CUTTING THE BLENDED ELEVATION HAIRCUT

The blended elevation cut is short on the bottom and long on the top.

1. Section the hair into five sections, separating the crown from the nape.
2. Cut the nape at 90 degrees, holding the hair vertically to a length of 2" to 3" (5 to 7.5 cm). (Fig. 7.78)
3. Divide the crown into a left and right section. (Fig. 7.79)

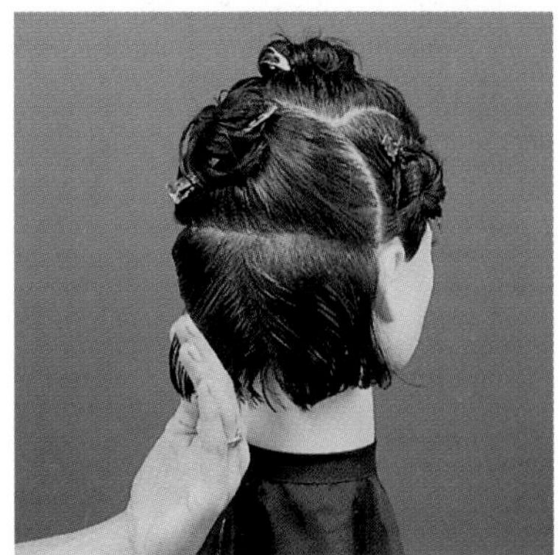

FIGURE 7.78 — Holding hair vertically at 90 degrees.

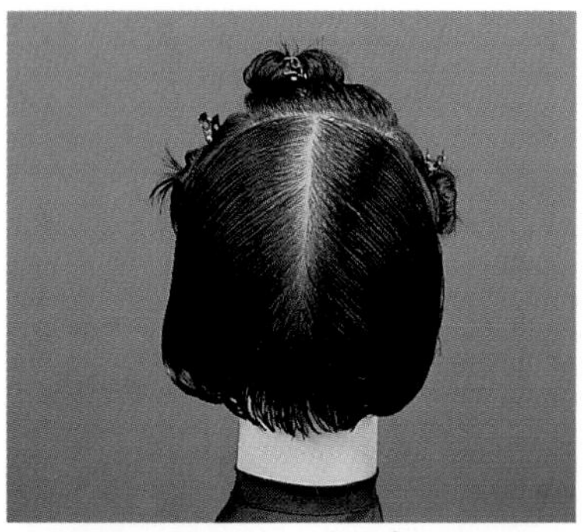

FIGURE 7.79 — Dividing crown into two sections.

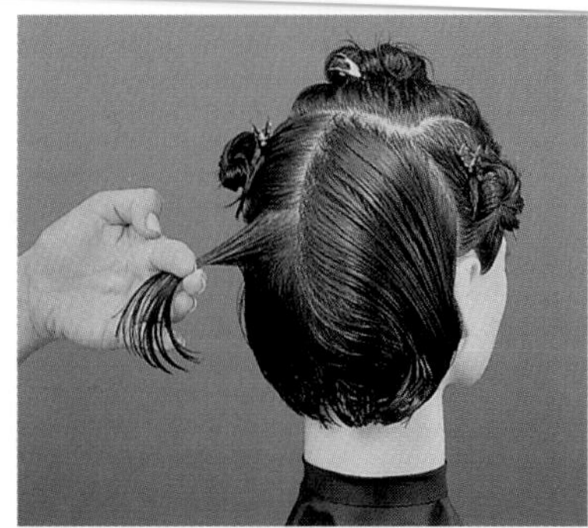

FIGURE 7.80 — Establishing guide for crown sections.

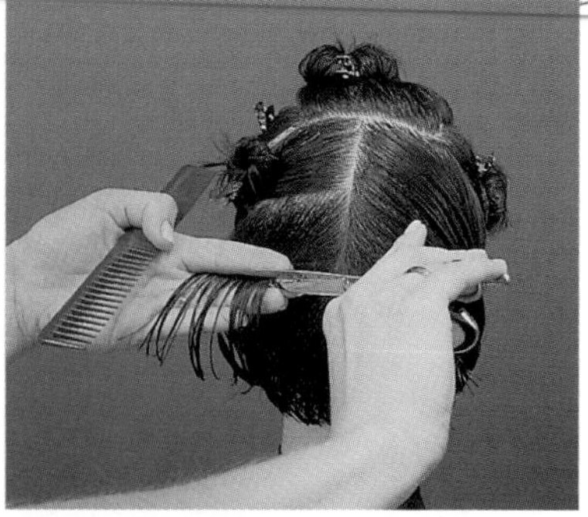

FIGURE 7.81 — Matching second parting to guide.

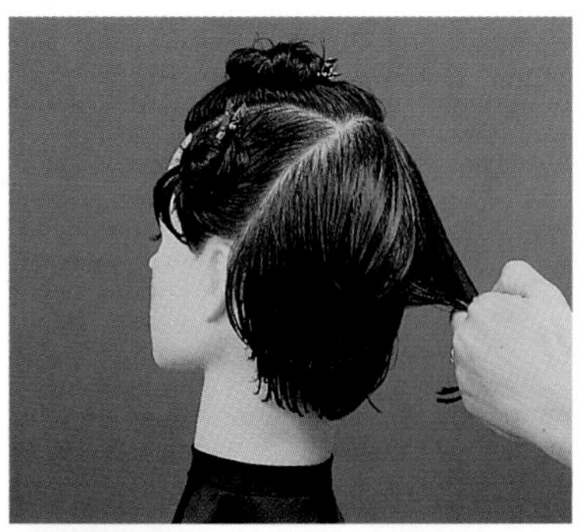

FIGURE 7.82 — Repeat on the right.

4. Take a horizontal parting (or subsection) from the nape section. This hair will be held out at 90 degrees from the head form and will be the guide for the crown sections. (Fig. 7.80)
5. Take a horizontal parting from the left crown section and direct it down to the guide from the nape. Cut the hair, matching the guide. The parting being cut will be slightly longer than the guide due to dropping the elevation. (Fig. 7.81)
6. Continue working up the left crown section, dropping the hair down to the stationary guide until the hair no longer reaches. Repeat on the right crown section. (Fig. 7.82)
7. Make a horizontal parting from the left front section into the left crown section. Hold the first parting at 90 degrees. Match the length to the left crown section and cut. Continue up the left side section, dropping each parting to the stationary guide. (Fig. 7.83)

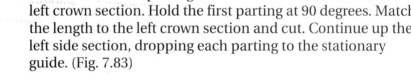

Note: *The hair should be slightly elevated on the sides as you cut.*

8. Repeat on the right side section. (Figs. 7.84, 7.85) ✔

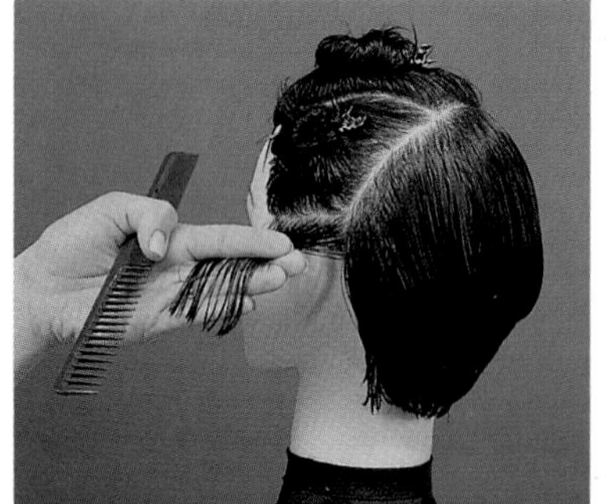

FIGURE 7.83 — Matching left front parting to left crown guideline.

Completed:
Learning Objective
#4
ELEVATIONS

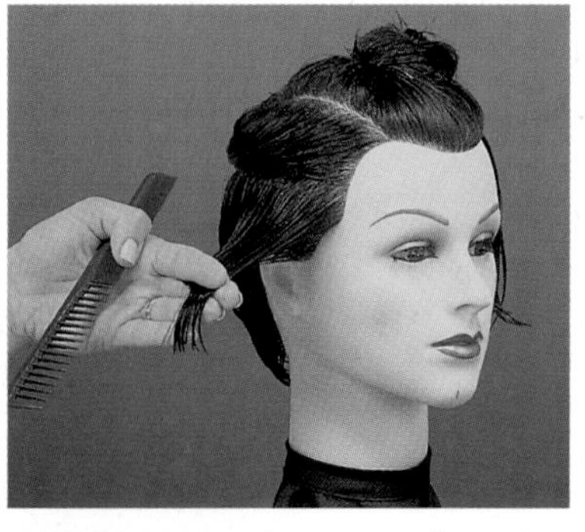

FIGURE 7.84 — Repeat on the right.

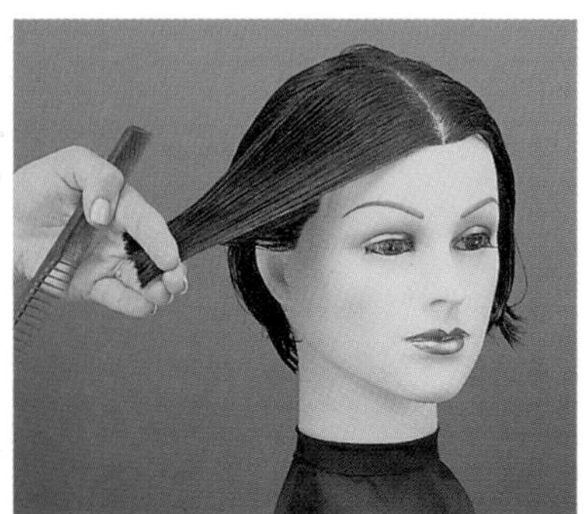

FIGURE 7.85 — Working up right side.

CHECKING A HAIRCUT

Haircuts are checked using partings opposite those used to cut the hair. If the hair is cut using vertical partings, check the cut using horizontal partings. If the hair is cut using horizontal partings, check with vertical partings. If the hair is cut across the top from ear to ear, check the cut from the front hairline back to the crown. Also be sure to check for symmetry where it is intended. (Fig. 7.86)

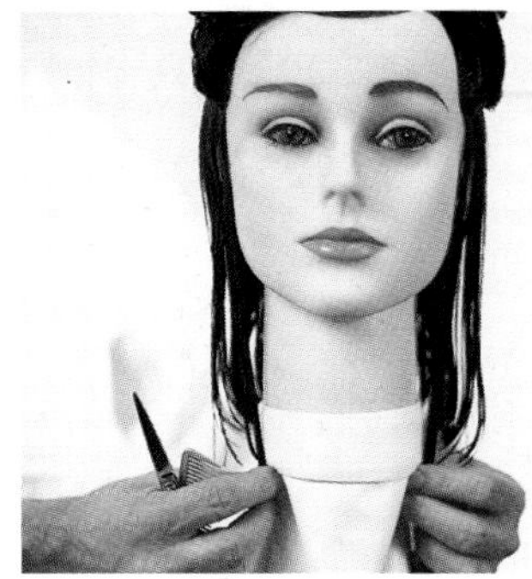

FIGURE 7.86 — Checking the haircut.

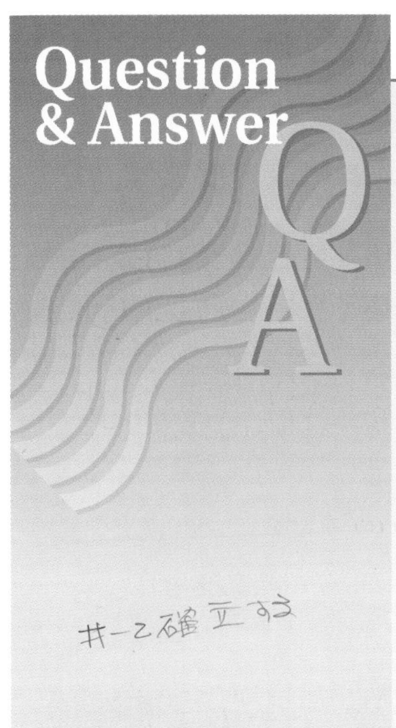

LAYERING LONG HAIR

How much layering should I put in long hair?

It's easy to be confused about "layering" the hair; the word is often misused. Layering simply means making the hair variable lengths throughout an established form.

The confusion comes from misinterpreting the various ways layering can be used to enhance a hairstyle. Most clients associate the word "layering" with shortening the hair to different lengths throughout the entire head. This is not the function of layering.

When the hair is held at 90 degrees (straight away from its natural growth) and cut to a given length throughout, it is considered an all-over layered cut.

Used to enhance long hair, perimeter layers are created by holding the hair at a slight elevation while establishing the hanging length. If you hold the hair flat against the head, no elevation equals no layering. If the hair is held at a 45-degree elevation, the perimeter will be moderately layered. This slight perimeter layering will promote softness, remove excess weight, and allow the ends to move freely.

Top and crown layering is most common, as it removes some of the length in the crown and the frontal areas so the hair will move away from the head. If the hair is left too long in the crown, the hair will lie flat to the head. If the crown hair is cut slightly shorter, the hair, with less weight and gravity pull, will stand away from the head, giving the look of volume.

—*From* Milady's Salon Solutions *by Louise Cotter*

SCISSORS-OVER-COMB TECHNIQUE

Scissors-over-comb (also called ***shear-over-comb***) is a barbering technique that has become popular with cosmetologists. In this technique, you hold the hair in place with the comb and use the tips of the scissors to remove the lengths. It is used for very short tapers and allows you to cut from an extremely short length to a longer length. A good example is a shingled neckline into a longer crown. A barber comb and longer shears (7" [17.5 cm] or more) are used in this technique.

1. Stand with your body parallel to the area of the head to be cut. The head should be at your eye level.
2. Hold the comb horizontal in the left hand and the scissors parallel to and just behind the comb. (Fig. 7.87)
3. Place the comb, teeth first, into the hairline and comb up and away from the head in a circular movement. (Fig. 7.88) The scissors should stay parallel to the comb, neither above nor below it.
4. Open and close the scissors rapidly and smoothly, cutting the hair to the desired length.
5. After completing a section, check the cut by repeating the cut diagonally. This will remove any irregularities or uneven spots. (Fig. 7.89)

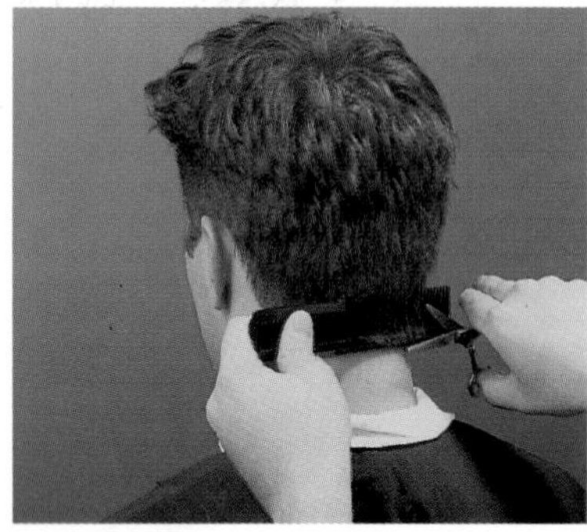

FIGURE 7.87 — Proper position for scissors-over-comb.

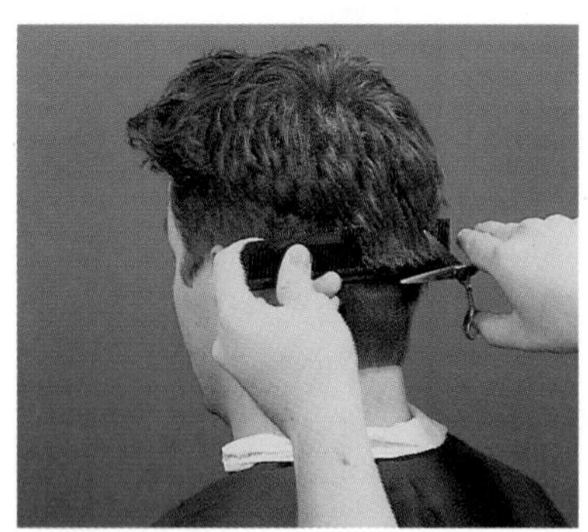

FIGURE 7.88 — Combing up and away from head.

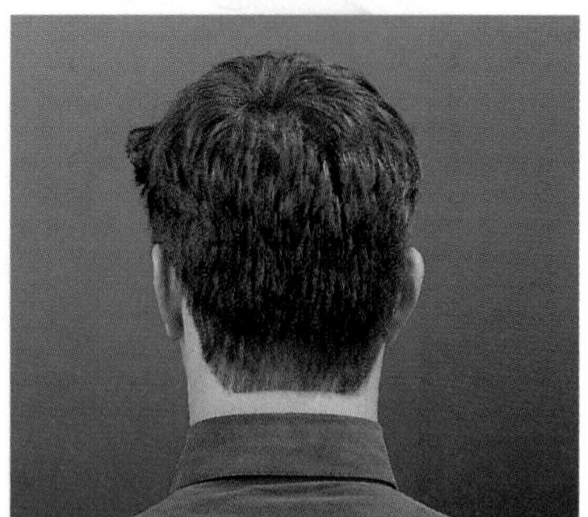

FIGURE 7.89 — Finished scissors-over-comb cut.

SPECIAL EFFECTS

BEVEL CUT

The strand is cut at an angle other than 90 degrees in a ***bevel cut.*** Beveling helps give the hair direction. (Figs. 7.90a, 7.90b)

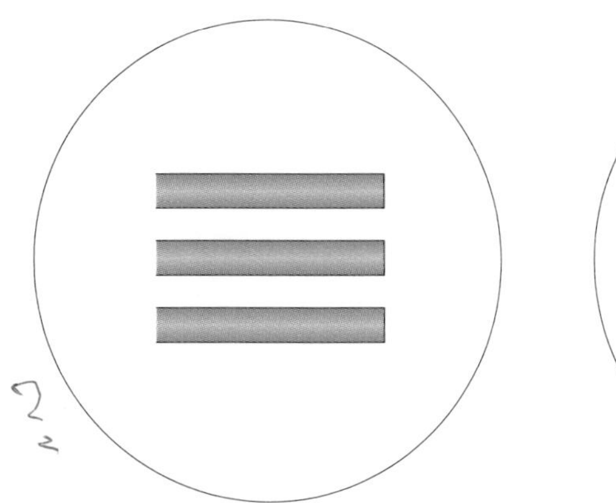

FIGURE 7.90a — Blunt-cut hair.

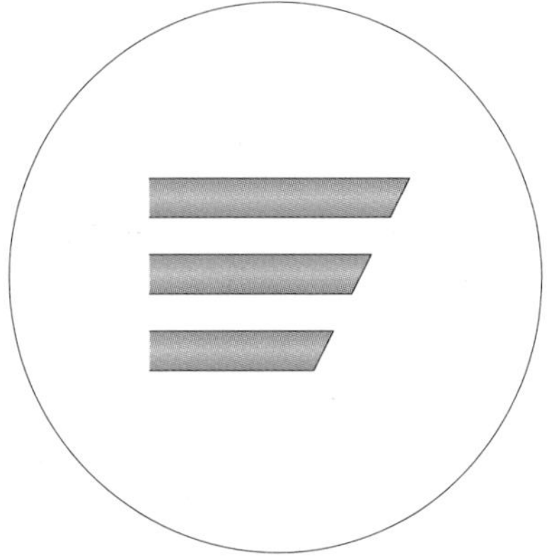

FIGURE 7.90b — Bevel-cut hair.

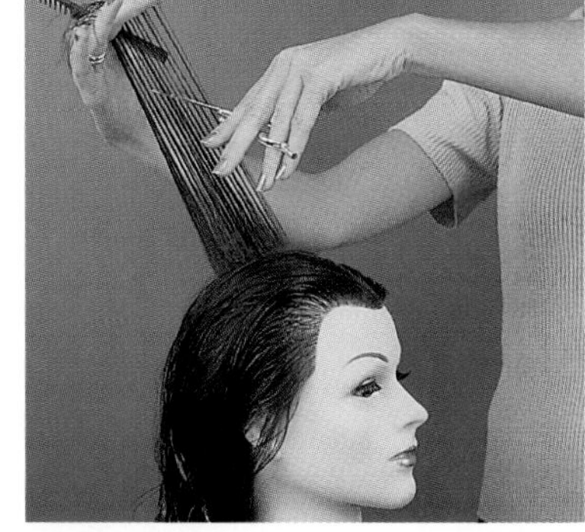

FIGURE 7.91 — Slide cutting for texturing.

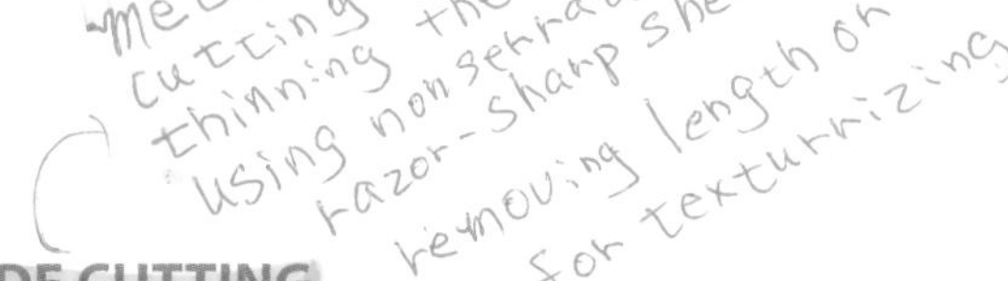

SLIDE CUTTING

Slide cutting is a method of cutting or thinning the hair using nonserrated, razor-sharp shears. Your fingers and scissors glide along the edge of the hair. The parting is placed in the open shears, starting at the shortest point of the cut. The shears, still open, "slide" through the parting to the longest length as the fingers hold the hair with slight tension. Slide cutting can be used for removing length or for texturizing. (Fig. 7.91)

NOTCHING OR POINTING

Cutting with the points of the shears to create a serrated, textured line in the hair ends is called ***notching*** or ***pointing***. (Fig. 7.92)

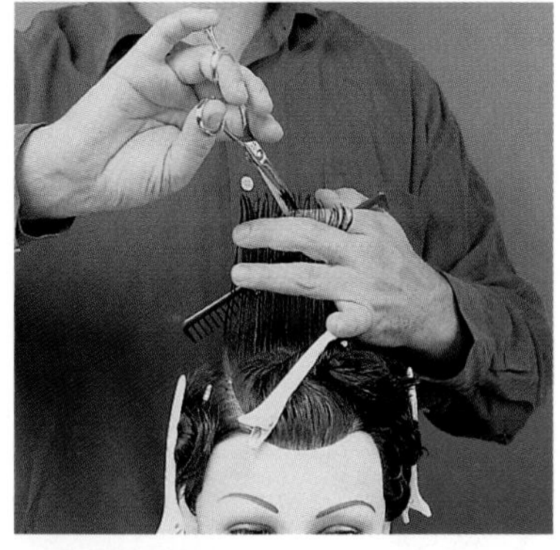

FIGURE 7.92 — Notching or pointing.

THINNING THE HAIR

The main purpose of ***thinning*** the hair is to remove bulk without shortening the length. We also thin hair to create shorter pieces of hair within the strand to aid in back-combing. Another purpose is to lighten the hair to create volume or change the texture of the hair.

GENERAL RULES FOR THINNING THE HAIR

Fine hair can be thinned closer to the scalp than coarse hair. The coarser the hair, the further from the scalp you begin texturizing. There are two places close to the scalp where it is not advisable to thin the hair: around the visible portions of the hairline and along the part. This will cause the thinned hair to stand up.

> **CAUTION**
>
> *During the thinning process, remember that you can always go back and remove more hair if necessary. However, once the hair has been cut, it is impossible to replace, and you might have difficulty achieving the desired hairstyle.*

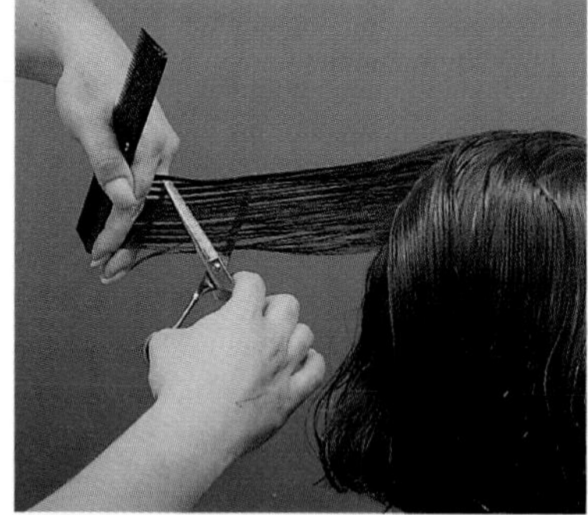

FIGURE 7.93 — Holding hair for thinning shears.

THINNING HAIR WITH THINNING SHEARS

When using thinning shears, grip the hair firmly and evenly by overlapping the middle finger slightly over the index finger. (Fig. 7.93)

1. Determine the sections of the head to be thinned.
2. Use the same partings (or subsections) you used to cut the hair.
3. Determine how much bulk you want to remove.
4. Close the thinning shears ¾ through the strand while moving out from the head form.
5. If the hair is long, step 4 can be repeated down the strand. Do not cut the same area in the strand.

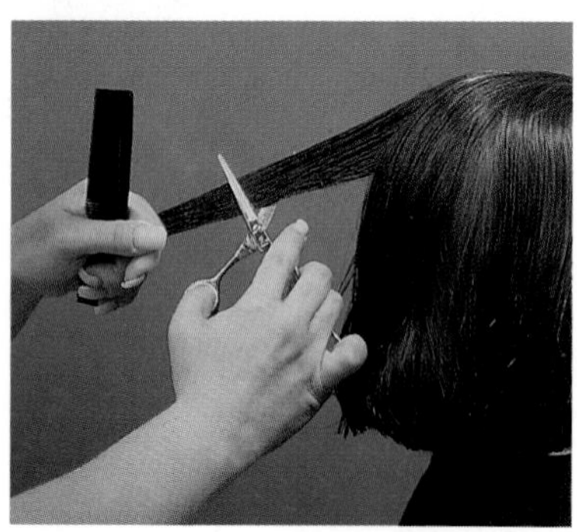

FIGURE 7.94 — Thinning with haircutting scissors.

THINNING WITH HAIRCUTTING SCISSORS

When using regular haircutting scissors or shears to thin the hair, pick up smaller sections of hair than when using thinning shears. This process of thinning with scissors is known as ***slithering*** or ***effilating*** and requires a different technique. (Fig. 7.94)

1. Hold a section of hair straight out between the middle and index fingers.
2. Place the hair in the scissors so that only the underneath hair will be cut.
3. Slide the scissors about 1" to 1-½" (2.5 cm to 3.75 cm) down the section, closing them slightly each time the scissors are moved toward the scalp.
4. Repeat this procedure twice on each section.

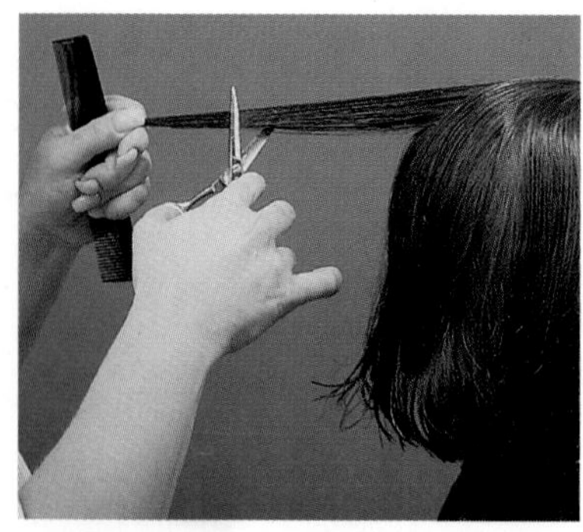

FIGURE 7.95 — Holding hair between thumb and index finger.

Alternate method: Hold the hair with the thumb and index finger. (Fig. 7.95)

THE RAZOR SHAPER

The straight razor or razor shaper is a versatile tool used to create a soft line when cutting the hair.

HOLDING THE RAZOR AND COMB

It is essential that the razor feel balanced when cutting the hair.

1. Place the thumb on the thumb grip and the index, middle, and ring fingers on the shank.
2. Place the little finger behind the pivot, either in the tang or under the handle. (Fig. 7.96)
3. Palm the razor and hold the comb between the thumb, index, and middle fingers. (Fig. 7.97)

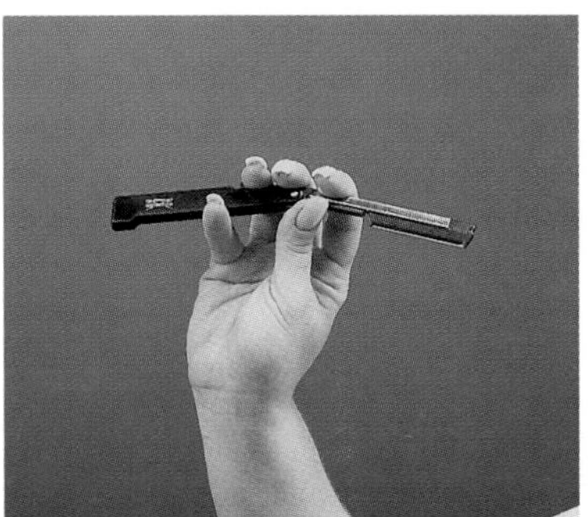

FIGURE 7.96 — Holding razor properly.

CUTTING HAIR WITH A RAZOR

Use the same procedures for cutting hair with the razor as with shears, with these exceptions:

1. Keep the hair damp to avoid pulling it and dulling the razor.
2. Hold the hair with your knuckles facing the head form.
3. Use short strokes just behind the knuckles to remove length.

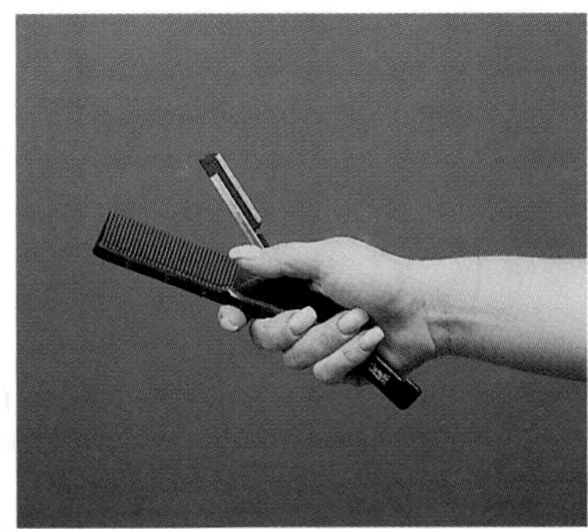

FIGURE 7.97 — Holding razor and comb.

THINNING HAIR WITH A RAZOR

Method 1

1. Hold the parting (or subsection) straight out from the head form.
2. Lay the razor flat on the parting (or subsection).
3. Take long light strokes out to the end of the parting (or subsection). (Fig. 7.98)

Method 2

Razor rotation or razor over comb is used on short hair to help give direction to the cut.

1. Comb the wet hair in the direction the hair will be moving.
2. Place the razor flat to the head above the comb.
3. Lift the comb from the hair, then follow with the razor. (Fig. 7.99)

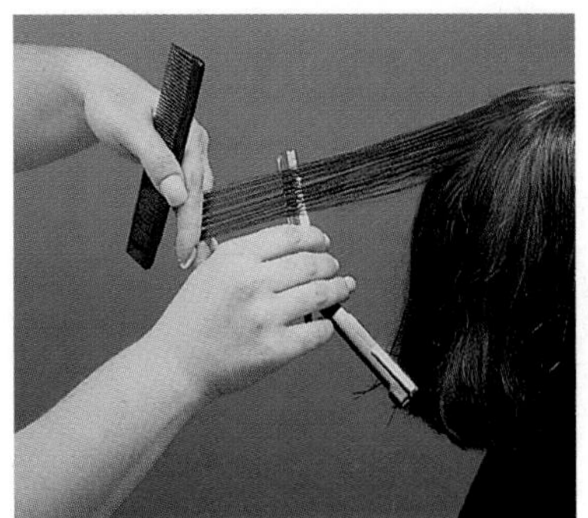

FIGURE 7.98 — Tapering ends with razor.

4. The comb and the razor follow each other in small circles with the razor only touching the hair in sections of 1" (2.5 cm). (Fig. 7.100)

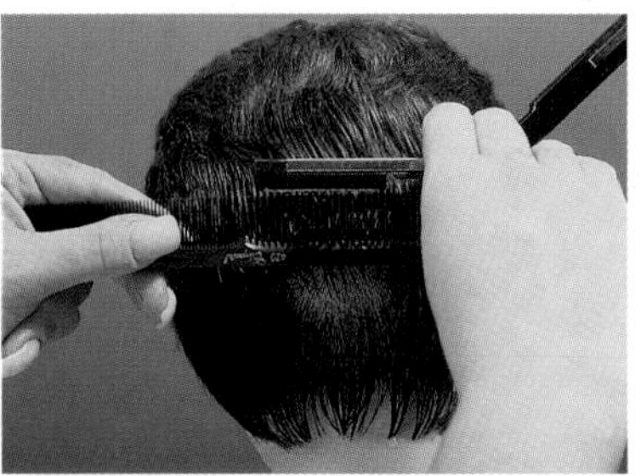

FIGURE 7.99 — Method 2.

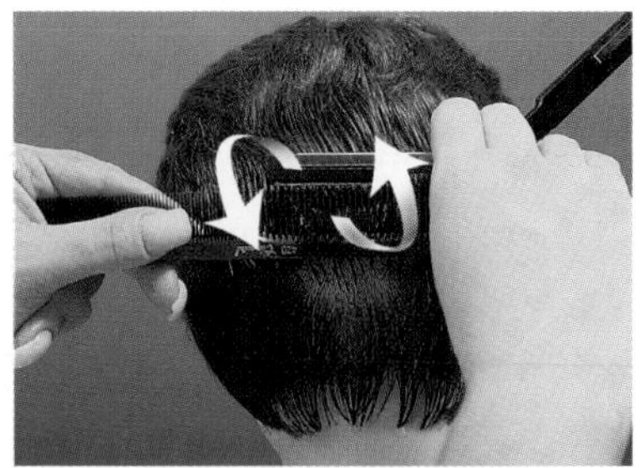

FIGURE 7.100 — Rotating with comb and razor.

CLIPPERS AND EDGERS

Clippers are used primarily for cutting short haircuts. The hair can be cut using the same method as scissors-over-comb, but substituting the clipper for the scissors. Clippers also can be used with ***clipper guards*** (sometimes called ***cheaters***). Guards are available in a variety of sizes, ranging from 1/16" to 1-½" (.15 to 3.75 cm). The most expensive clippers have different sizes of blades instead of guards.

CUTTING HAIR WITH CLIPPER GUARDS

1. Choose the length guard or guards for the haircut.
2. Begin in the nape and work up the back of the head, using the smallest guard for close-cut hair at the nape or hairline.
3. As you work up the head, use a circular motion, placing the clipper into the hair, then moving out from the head. Continue working up the head using this pattern. Increase the guard size as desired hair length increases. This will keep the clippers from jamming as well as leaving some length when increasing the size of the guard. (Fig. 7.101)
4. Cut the sides next. Start at the bottom hairline on the sides and move up to the top, using the same circular motion with the clipper.
5. Cut the top last, beginning at the center front hairline and moving into the crown. Then cut the left side of the top, working from front to back, then to the right side.

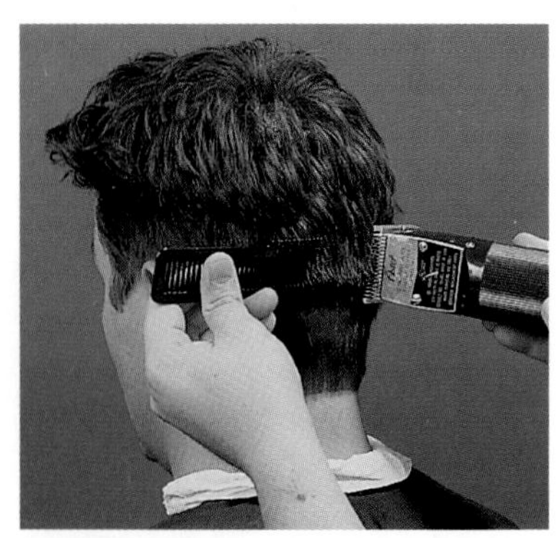

FIGURE 7.101 — Clipper over comb.

6. Blend the side and back sections into the top if there are any visible lines.
7. Clean the hairline with an edger.

CUTTING HAIR WITH TRIMMERS OR EDGERS

Trimmers or edgers are used to remove superfluous hair from the hairline. They can also be used to create straight or creative lines in short taper cuts.

1. To clean superfluous hair from the hairline, place the trimmer flat on the skin and move to the hairline. (Fig. 7.102)
2. To create a sharper line with the trimmer, point the blade toward the skin. Cut the perimeter hairline to the desired length. Then remove the hair below the line. (Fig. 7.103)

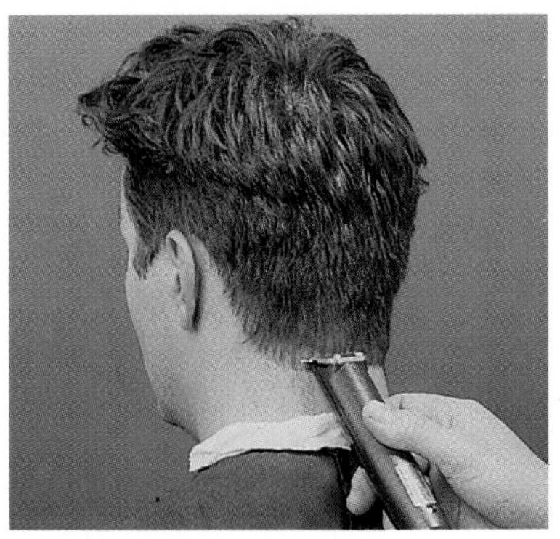

FIGURE 7.102 — Trimmer on neck.

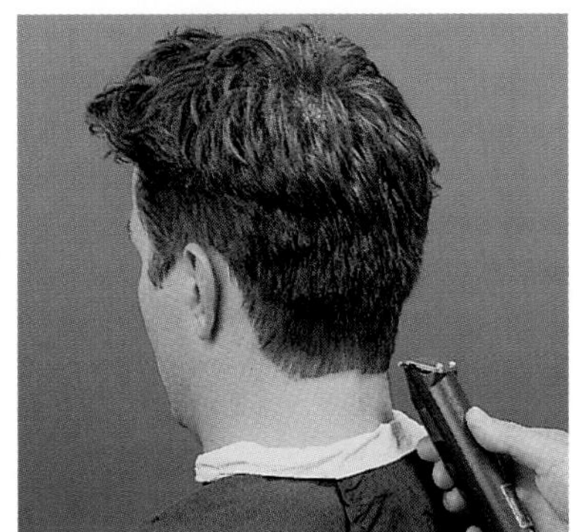

FIGURE 7.103 — Cutting a line along nape.

CUTTING CURLY HAIR

When cutting curly or overly curly hair, all the basic rules of haircutting apply, with the following additions:

1. Cut chemically relaxed hair dry. If it is wet, the hair will stretch too much to control the results.
2. Moderately wavy or curly hair is generally cut damp, with little or no tension.
3. When working with curly ethnic hair, cut it dry for very short styles. Pick the hair out, away from the scalp, then use electric clippers or shears to sculpt the desired shape. For longer styles, blow-dry it after shampooing so that it hangs straight

Completed:
Learning Objective
#5
CUTTING CURLY HAIR

for cutting. (Damp curly hair contracts as it dries, which makes it difficult to control the length as you cut.) (Figs. 7.104, 7.105)

4. Always use an electric trimmer to outline the edges of the haircut. Using a razor will cause ingrown hairs, which can get infected.

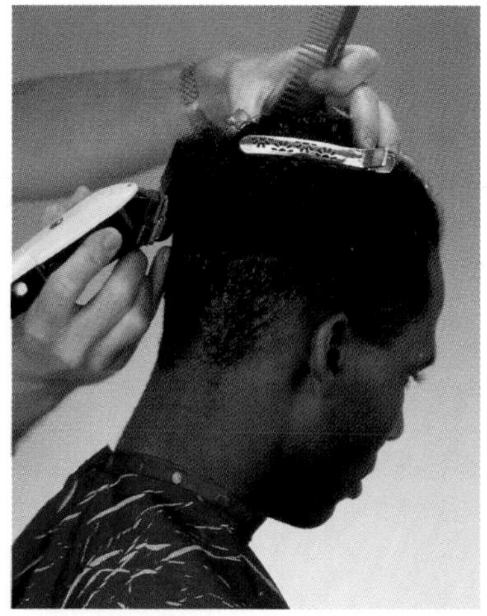

FIGURE 7.104 — Cutting curly hair with clippers.

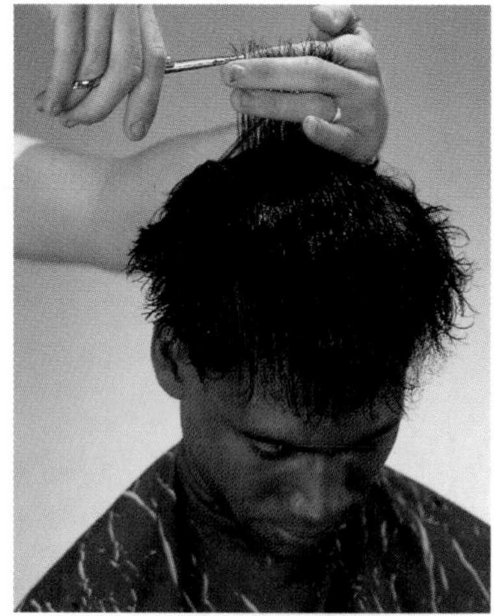

FIGURE 7.105 — Cutting curly hair with shears.

REVIEW QUESTIONS

HAIRCUTTING

1. Why is the mastery of haircutting so important to the student?
2. What four factors should be taken into consideration when choosing a hairstyle for your client?
3. What are the tools used in haircutting?
4. What is the first step in haircutting?
5. What kind of haircut do you use four sections for? Five sections?
6. What is the purpose of a guide?
7. How does the client's head position affect the haircut?
8. Name the four basic elevations.
9. What is slide cutting?
10. In which areas is it not advisable to thin the hair?
11. For what purpose is the clipper used?
12. Why is a razor used on damp hair?
13. Overly curly hair is cut wet or dry?

CHAPTER

Artistry in Hairstyling

LEARNING OBJECTIVES

After completing this chapter, you should be able to:

1. List the elements of good design.
2. List the art principles in hair design.
3. List and analyze the different facial types.
4. Demonstrate how to camouflage facial flaws with hair design.

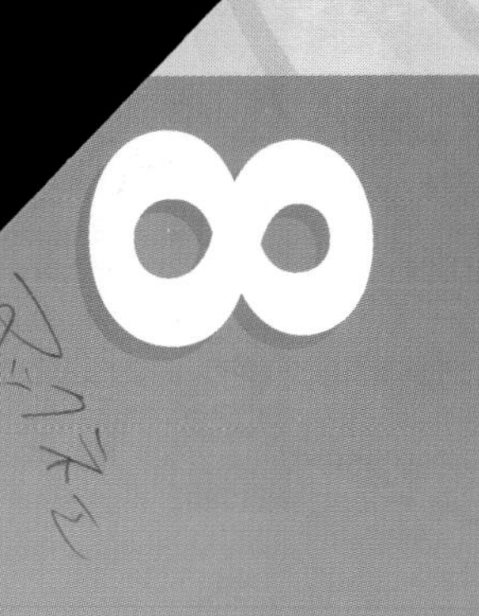

RDS

essary information
Standards for Entry-Level Cosmetologists:

their needs and preferences

iques to complete a hairstyle to the satisfaction of the client

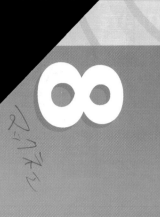

Your challenge as a professional cosmetologist will be to create a pleasing image for your client. You must be able to design a look that enhances the positive features of your client while minimizing the negative features. This is possible if you understand the elements and principles of design. Therefore, a cosmetology education is not complete until you have acquired the artistic skill and judgment necessary for successful hairstyling. A hairstyle is wearable art!

Once you have mastered the basic cutting elevations, you are ready to begin designing hairstyles. But you will need to look at more than just the client's hair. You need to analyze the entire person, keeping in mind the basic elements of design.

ELEMENTS OF DESIGN

The five elements of design are ***form, space, line, color,*** and ***texture.***

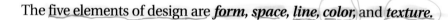

FORM

Form is the outline or silhouette of the hairstyle. It is three-dimensional and changes as it is viewed from different angles. The client will often react to the silhouette of the hairstyle first. Generally, it is best to use forms that are simple and pleasing to the eye. The hair form should be in proportion to the shape of the head and face, the length and width of the neck, and the shoulder line. (Fig. 8.1)

SPACE

Space is the area the hairstyle occupies, the area inside the form. It is also called ***volume.*** It is three-dimensional, having length, width, and depth. The space may contain curls, curves, waves, straight hair, or a combination of these. (Fig. 8.2)

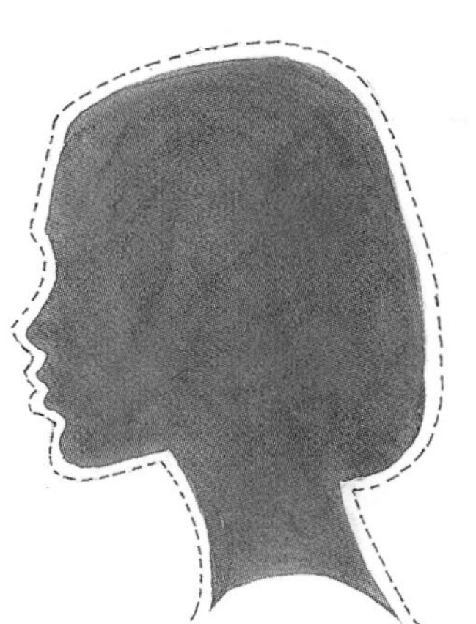
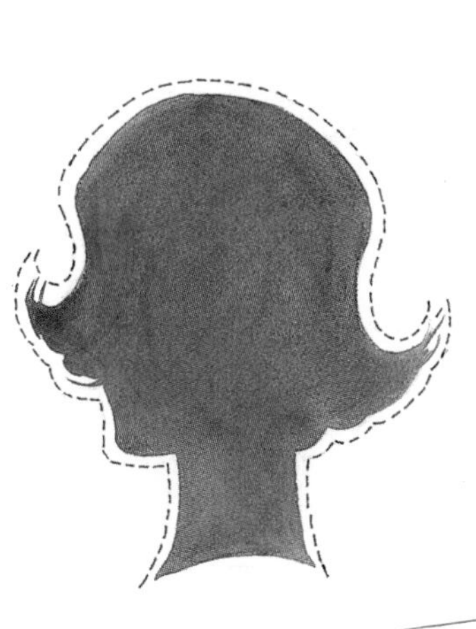

FIGURE 8.1 — The outline of the hairstyle is the form.

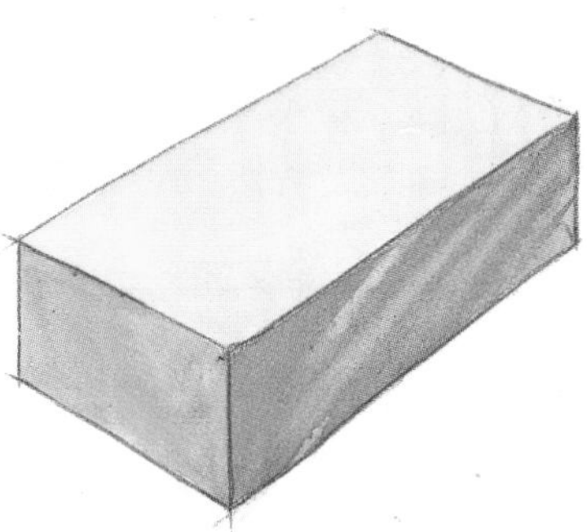
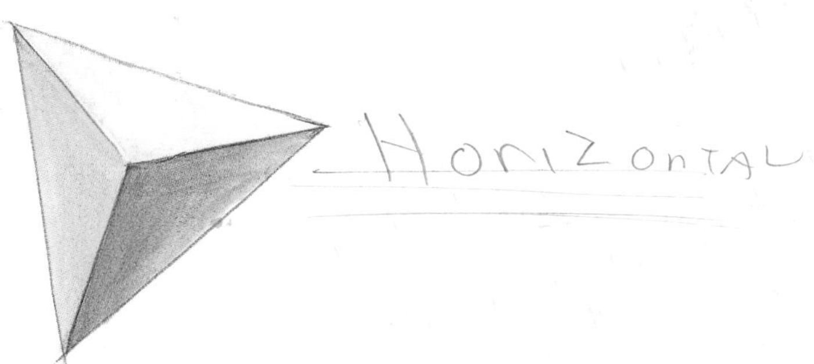

FIGURE 8.2 — Space is three-dimensional.

LINE

The eye follows the lines in a design. ***Lines*** create the form, design, and movement of a hairstyle. They can be straight or curved. There are four basic types of lines:

Horizontal lines are parallel to the floor or horizon. A horizontal line creates width in hair design because the eye follows the line from the center out to the ends. (Fig. 8.3)

Vertical lines are straight up and down. They make a hairstyle appear longer and narrower as the eye follows the lines up and down. (Fig. 8.4)

Diagonal lines are positioned between horizontal and vertical. They are often used to emphasize or minimize facial features. Diagonal lines are also used to create interest in hair design. (Fig. 8.5)

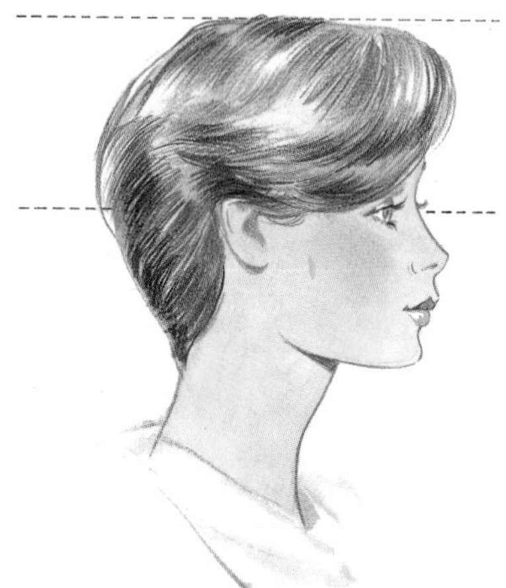

FIGURE 8.3 — Horizontal lines in a hairstyle.

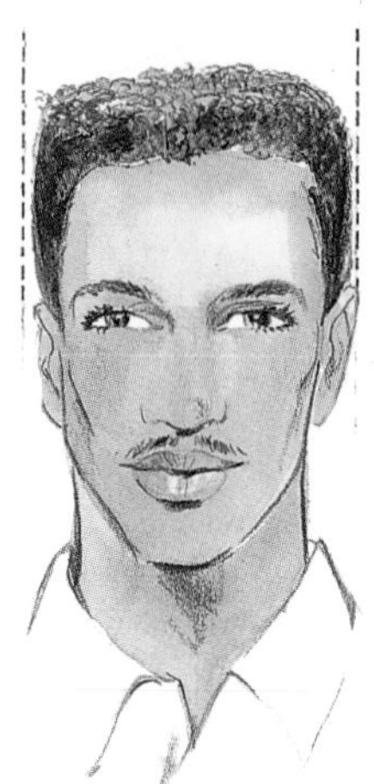

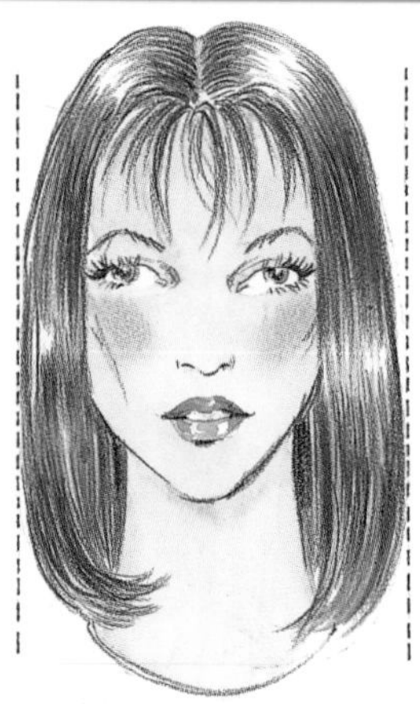

FIGURE 8.4 — Vertical lines in a hairstyle.

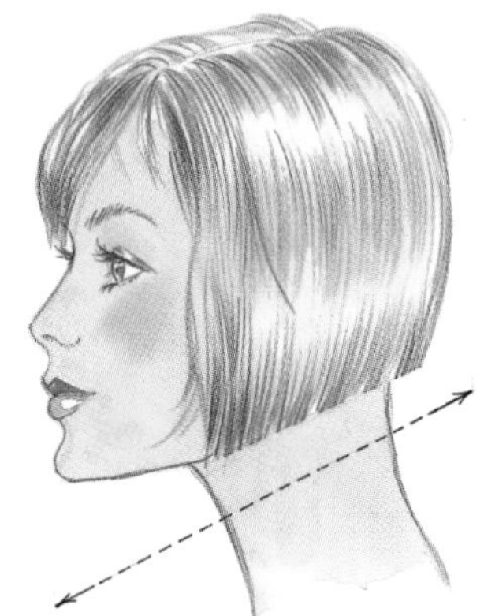

FIGURE 8.5 — Diagonal lines in a hairstyle.

Curved lines soften a design. They can be large or small, a full circle or just part of a circle. (Fig. 8.6) They can be placed horizontally, vertically, or diagonally. Curved lines repeating in opposite directions are called a ***wave.*** (Fig. 8.7)

Designing with Lines

Single line hairstyles are best on clients who require the minimum of care when styling their hair. An example of this is the one-length hairstyle. (Fig. 8.8)

Repeating lines are parallel lines in a hairstyle. They can be straight or curved. The repetition of lines creates more interest in the design. A finger wave is an example of a style using curved, repeating lines. (Fig. 8.9)

Contrasting lines are horizontal and vertical lines that meet at a 90-degree angle. These lines create a hard edge. Contrasting lines in a design are usually reserved for clients with the personality to carry off a strong look. (Fig. 8.10)

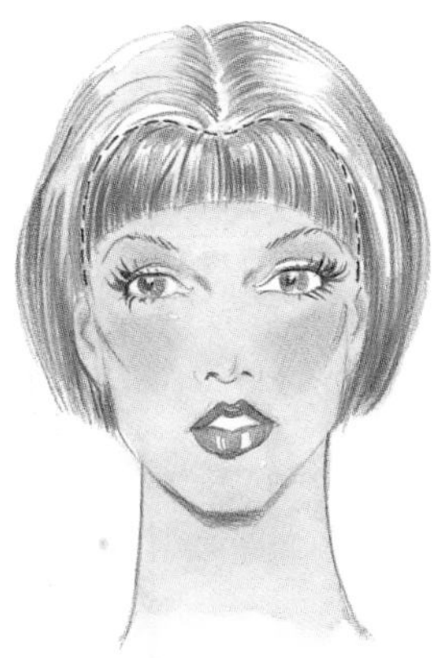

FIGURE 8.6 — Curved lines in a hairstyle.

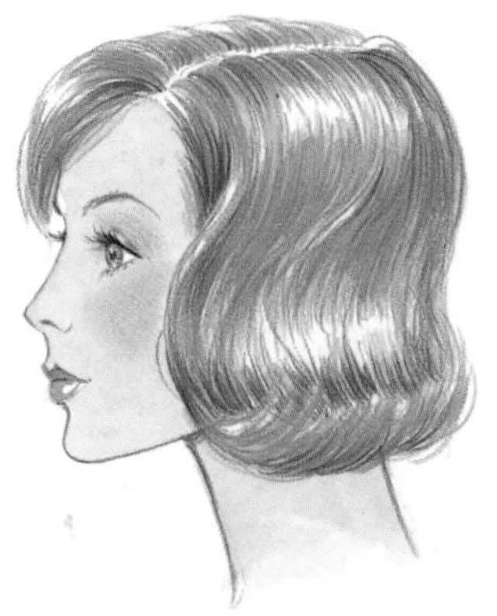

FIGURE 8.7 — Wave.

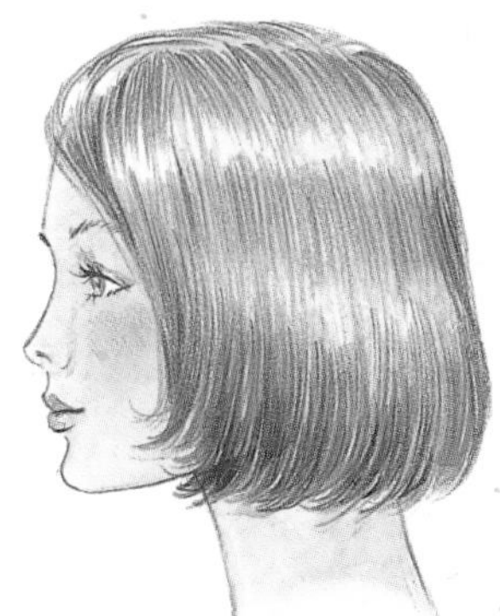

FIGURE 8.8 — Single-line hairstyle.

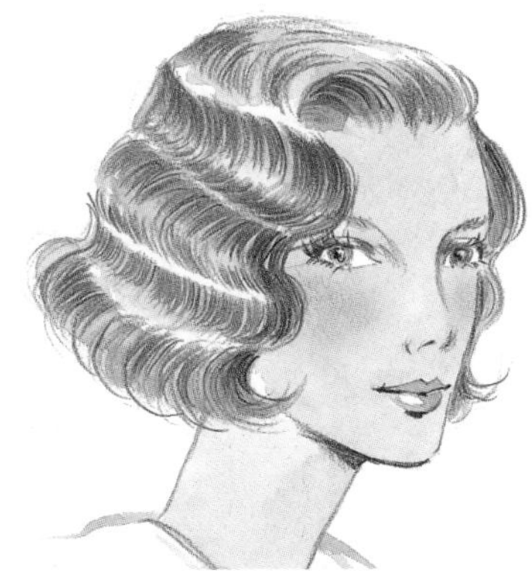

FIGURE 8.9 — Repeating lines.

Transitional lines are usually curved lines and are used to blend and soften horizontal or vertical lines. (Fig. 8.11)

COLOR

Color plays an important role in hair design, both visually and psychologically. It can also be used to make all or part of the design appear larger or smaller. Color can be used to create textures or lines; color can tie the design elements together. You will learn more about creating hair designs that include haircolor as an important element in Chapter 12, "Haircoloring."

Psychology of Color

Lighter and warmer colors are bolder and more exciting. Darker and cooler colors are demure. Darker colors tend to make people look older, and lighter colors make them look younger.

Creating Texture with Color

Light colors and warm colors recede, or move away from the head; they create the illusion of volume. Dark and cool colors move forward or toward the head, and create the illusion of less volume. When dark and light colors are used together, the light hair appears closer to the surface, while darker hair seems to recede below the surface. The illusion of texture is thus created by alternating colors that are either warm and cool or light and dark. (Figs. 8.12, 8.13)

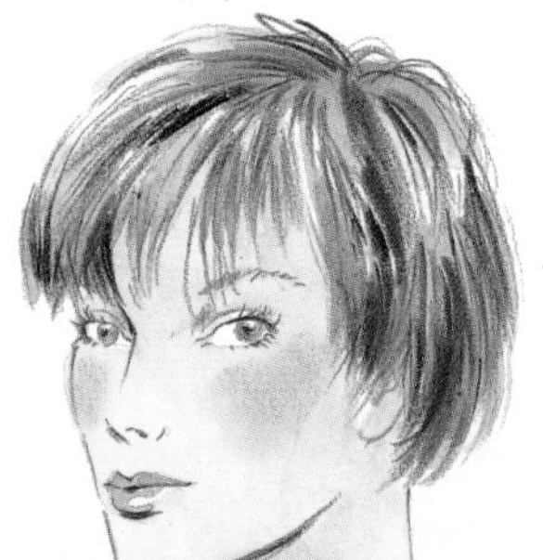

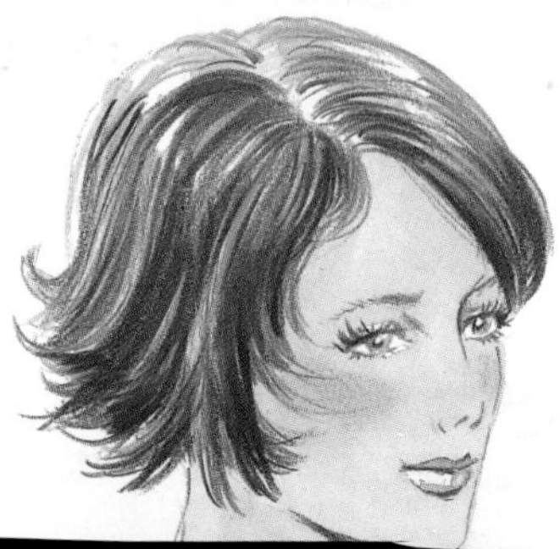

sides decrease width, while lighter or warmer colors on the sides increase width. (Figs. 8.15a, 8.15b)

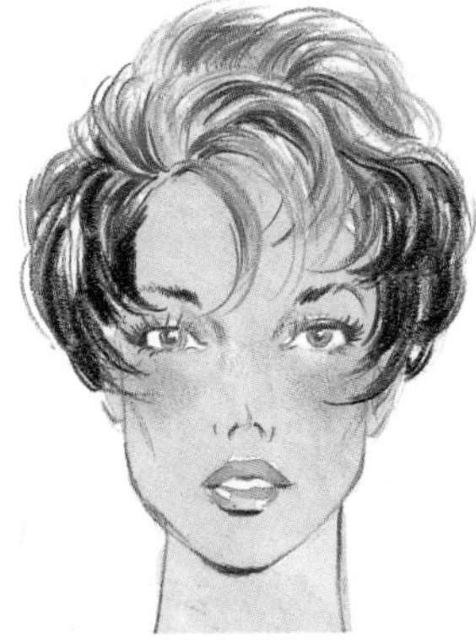

FIGURE 8.15a — Lighter color in the bangs lengthens the face.

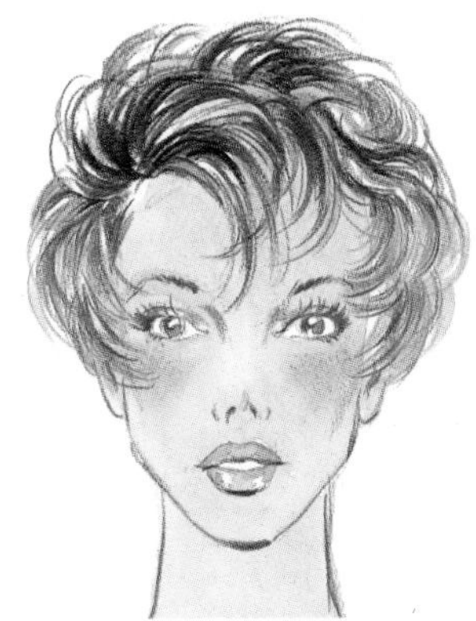

FIGURE 8.15b — Lighter color in the sides widens the face.

Color Selection

Before choosing a color, be sure that the tone is compatible with the skin tones of the client. When using two or more colors, choose colors with similar tones within two levels of each other. When using high-contrast colors, use one color sparingly. Too much contrast can create a discordant look and should be used only on the most progressive clients. (Fig. 8.16)

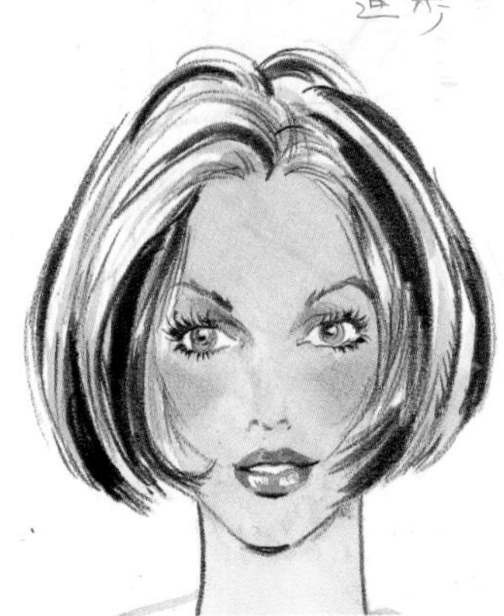

FIGURE 8.16 — Vivid color contrast.

TEXTURE

Texture is the actual surface quality of the hair. It is also what the hair looks like it might feel to the touch. Texture in hairstyling can be natural or created with styling techniques, chemical changes, or color. Textures can be used individually or combined to create a unique look for your client.

Natural Textures

Hair has a natural texture—straight, wavy, curly, or extra curly—that must be taken into consideration when designing a style for your client. Whenever possible, take advantage of the hair's natural texture. For example, since straight hair reflects light better than other textures, it is usually cut to one length so as to reflect the most light. Wavy hair can be combed into waves that create horizontal lines. Curly and overly curly hair does not reflect much light and appears coarse to the touch. It is usually layered and creates a larger form than straight or wavy hair. (Figs. 8.17–8.20)

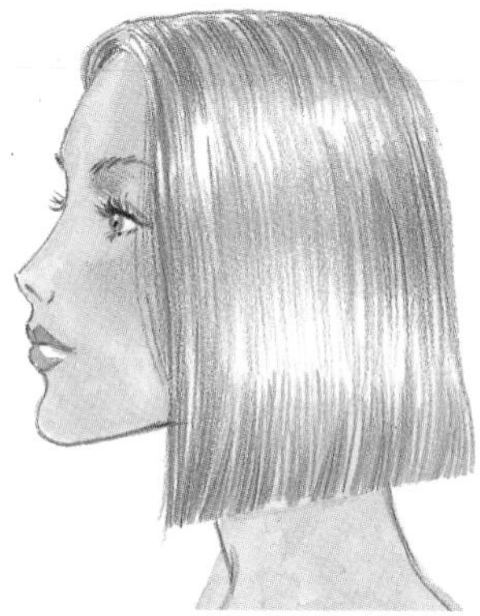

FIGURE 8.17 — Straight hair.

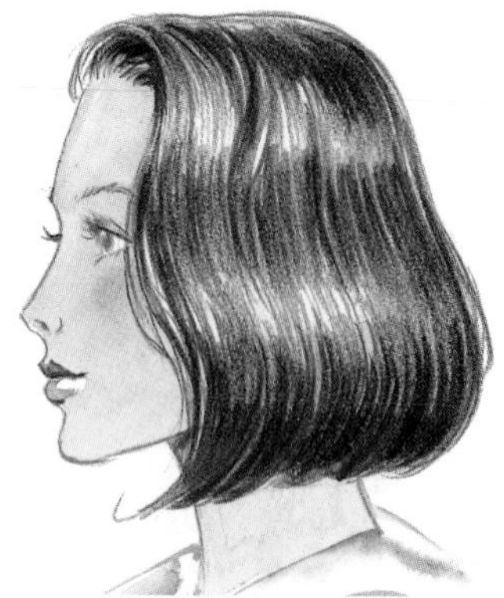

FIGURE 8.18 — Wavy hair.

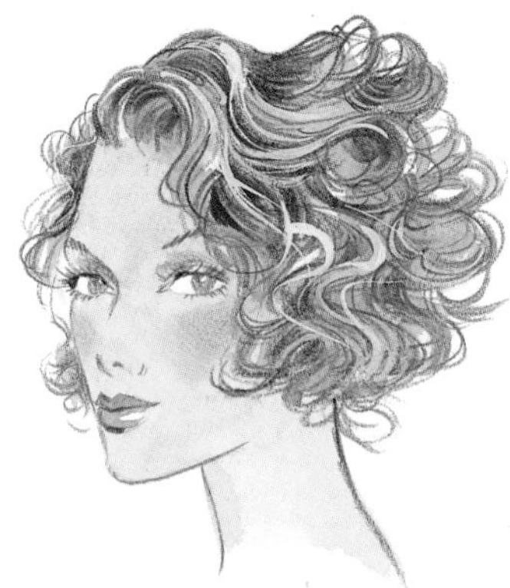

FIGURE 8.19 — Curly hair.

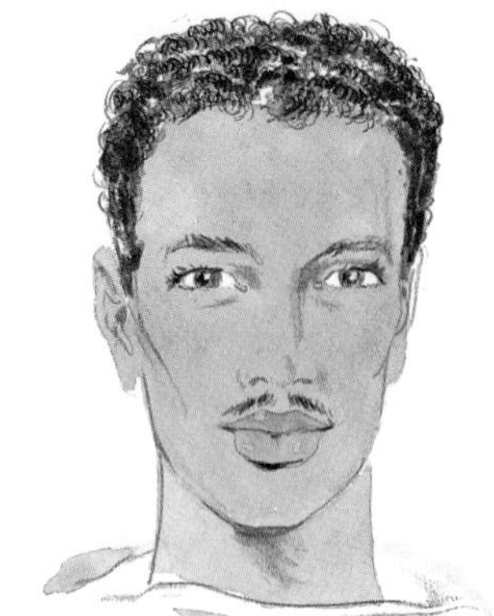

FIGURE 8.20 — Very curly hair.

Creating Texture with Styling Tools

Texture can be created temporarily with the use of heat or wet styling techniques. Curling irons or hot rollers can be used to create a wave or curly texture. Curly hair can be straightened with a blow dryer or flat iron. Crimping irons are used to create interesting, "unnatural" textures in the shape of squares or zigzags. Hair can be wet set with rollers or in pin curls to create curls and waves. Finger waves are another temporary texture change. You will learn more about styling techniques in the chapters that follow. (Figs. 8.21–8.24)

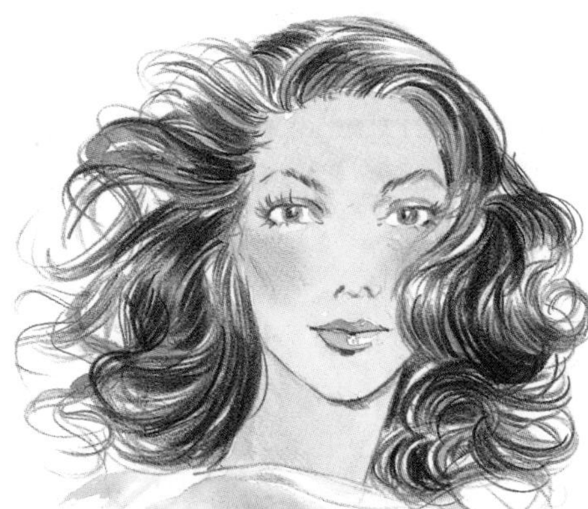

FIGURE 8.21 — Hair texture can be altered temporarily.

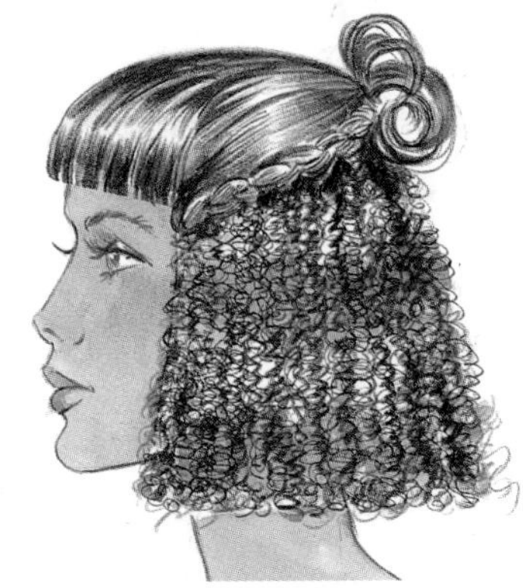

FIGURE 8.22 — Combining textures.

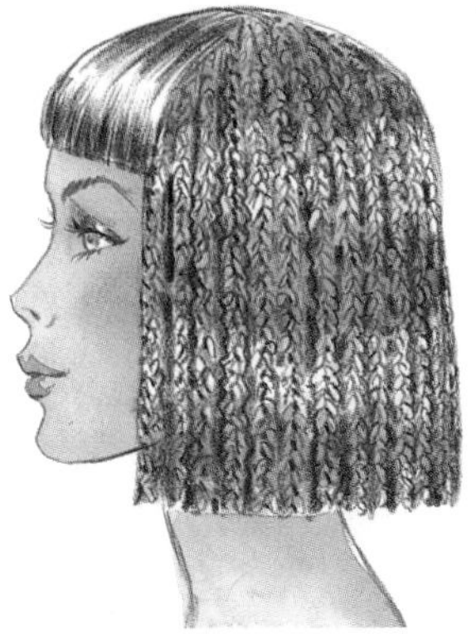

FIGURE 8.23 — Fine braids are a way to create temporary texture.

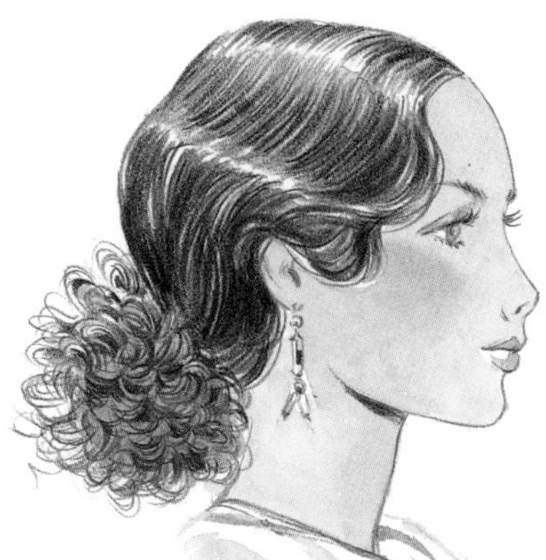

FIGURE 8.24 — Finger waves and curls.

Changing Texture with Chemicals

Chemical texture changes are considered permanent. They last until the new growth is long enough to alter the design. Curly hair can be straightened with relaxers. Straight hair can be curled with permanent waves. These techniques are covered in detail in Chapters 11 and 13. (Fig. 8.25)

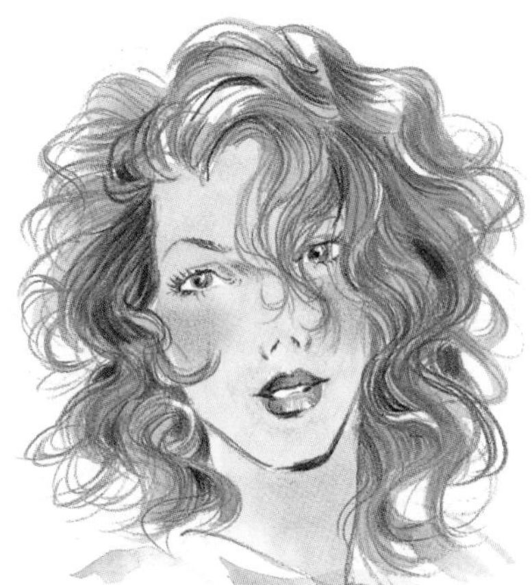

FIGURE 8.25 — Chemically altered hairstyle.

Changing Texture with Color

Alternate light and dark colors create the illusion of texture. Remember: dark colors recede or move in toward the head, while light colors move forward or away from the head. (Fig. 8.26)

Tips for Designing with Texture

- Do not use too many texture combinations together. This will create a look that is too busy. A good rule is to use a maximum of three textures.

Completed:
Learning Objective
#1
ELEMENTS OF DESIGN

- Smooth textures accent the face. Use smooth textures to narrow round head shapes. (Fig. 8.27)
- Curly textures take attention away from the face. Use curly textures to soften square or rectangular features. (Fig. 8.28)

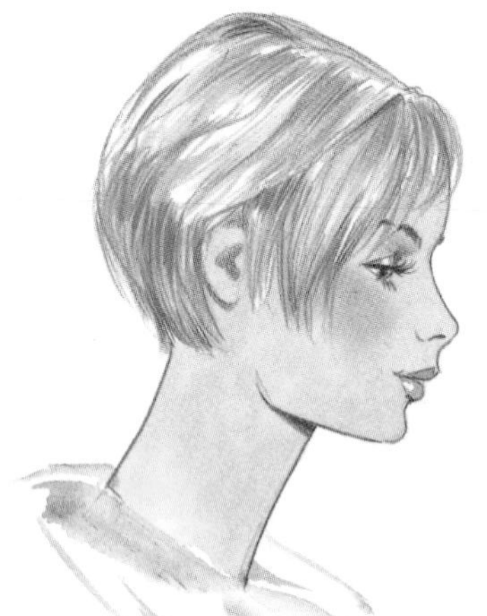

FIGURE 8.26 — Changing texture with color.

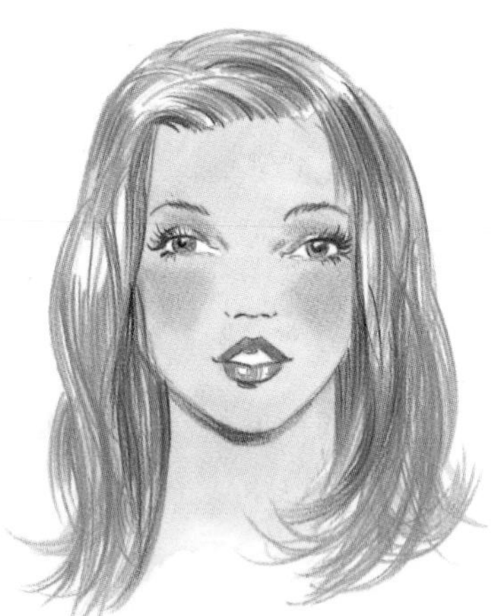

FIGURE 8.27 — Straight textures are flattering on round faces.

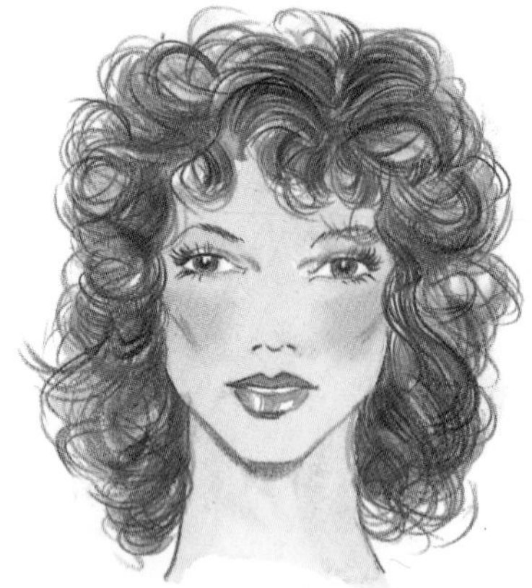

FIGURE 8.28 — Curly textures soften angular faces.

PRINCIPLES OF HAIR DESIGN

There are certain principles by which we judge the quality of a design in hairstyling. By using these principles you can be sure of creating looks that are pleasing to the eye. The five art principles important for hair design are ***proportion, balance, rhythm, emphasis,*** and ***harmony.***

PROPORTION

Proportion is the relationship between objects relative to their size. For example, a 60" television might be considered out of proportion in a very small bedroom. A 20" television would be more proportionate to the room. A person with a very small chin and a very wide forehead would be considered to have a head shape that is out of proportion. The right hairstyle would give the illusion of proper proportion. (Figs. 8.29a, 8.29b)

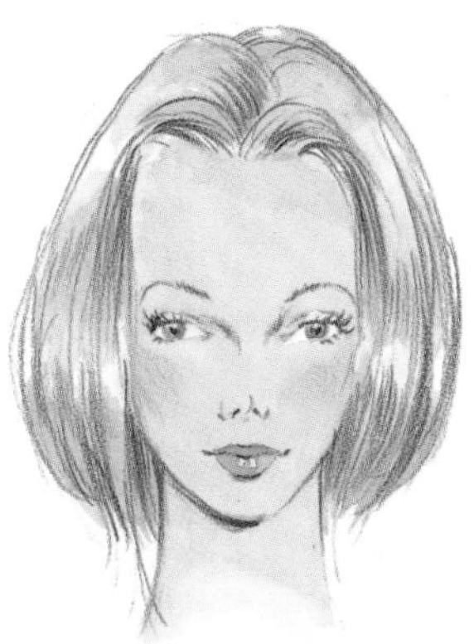

FIGURE 8.29a — Facial features out of proportion.

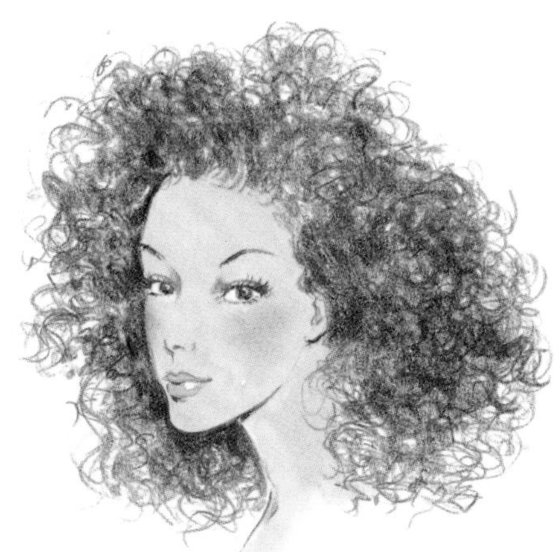

FIGURE 8.29b — Hair out of proportion to face.

Classic Proportions

The Greeks are credited with developing the ratio of 2 to 3 as the most harmonious proportions for artistic design. The same is true in hairstyle design. The ideal ratio is either 2 parts hair to 3 parts face or 3 parts hair to 2 parts face. A proportion of 2 parts face and 3 parts hair (Figs. 8.30a–8.30c) is used to minimize facial features, poor skin, or the client's reluctance to draw attention to the face. A ratio of 3 parts face and 2 parts hair (Figs. 8.31a, 8.31b) is more suitable when the client is comfortable with his or her appearance and wants attention directed to the face. When designing hairstyles, always use an odd number in your proportions.

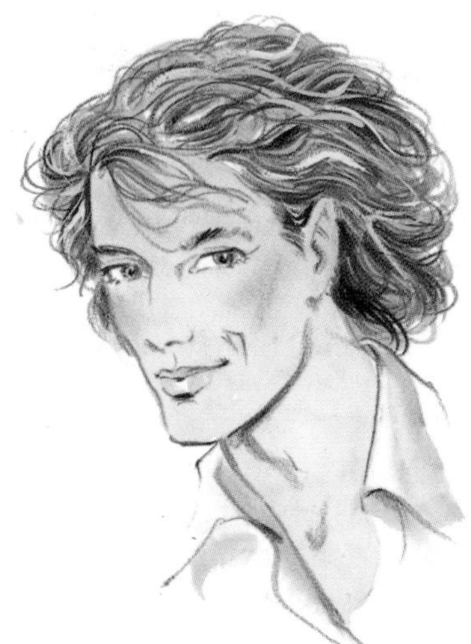

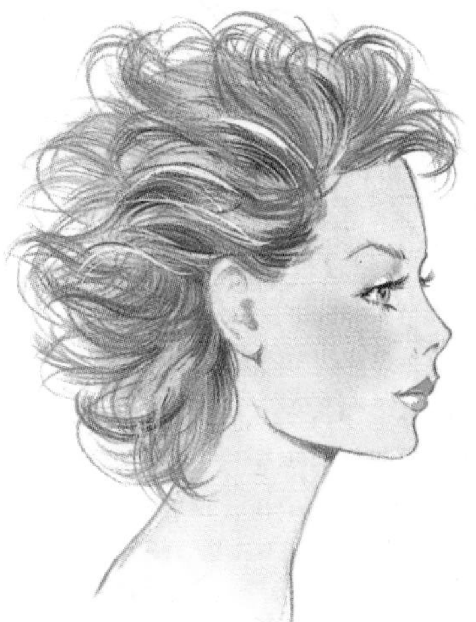

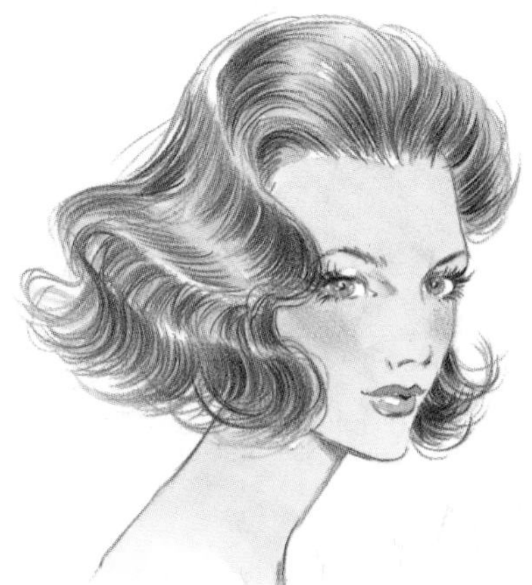

FIGURES 8.30a, b, c — Examples of the proportions 3 parts hair, 2 parts face.

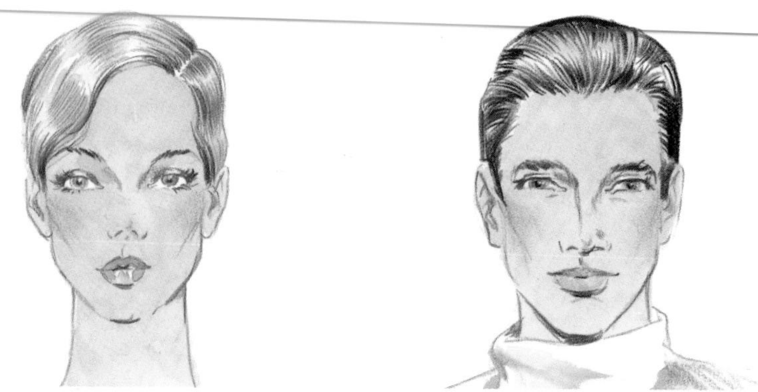

FIGURES 8.31a, b — Examples of the proportions 2 parts hair, 3 parts face.

Hair Proportion from the Profile

If you're using the ratio 2 parts face to 3 parts hair, the same ratio should apply when viewing the client's profile. If you need flexibility to correct profile problems, you can increase the proportion to 5 parts hair and 2 parts face for a more pleasing profile view. (Fig. 8.32)

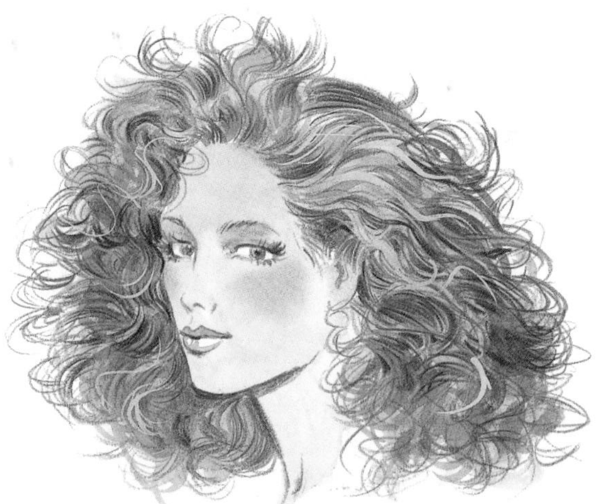

FIGURE 8.32 — 5 parts hair, 2 parts face.

Body Proportion

It is essential when designing hairstyles that you look at the client's body proportions. A body that is not in proportion will be more obvious if the hair form is too small or too large. When choosing a style for a woman with large hips or broad shoulders, for instance, you would normally create a style with a large form. (Fig. 8.33) But the same large hair form would appear out of proportion on a petite woman. When designing a hairstyle, keep in mind that the hair should not be wider than the center of the shoulders, regardless of the body structure. (Fig. 8.34)

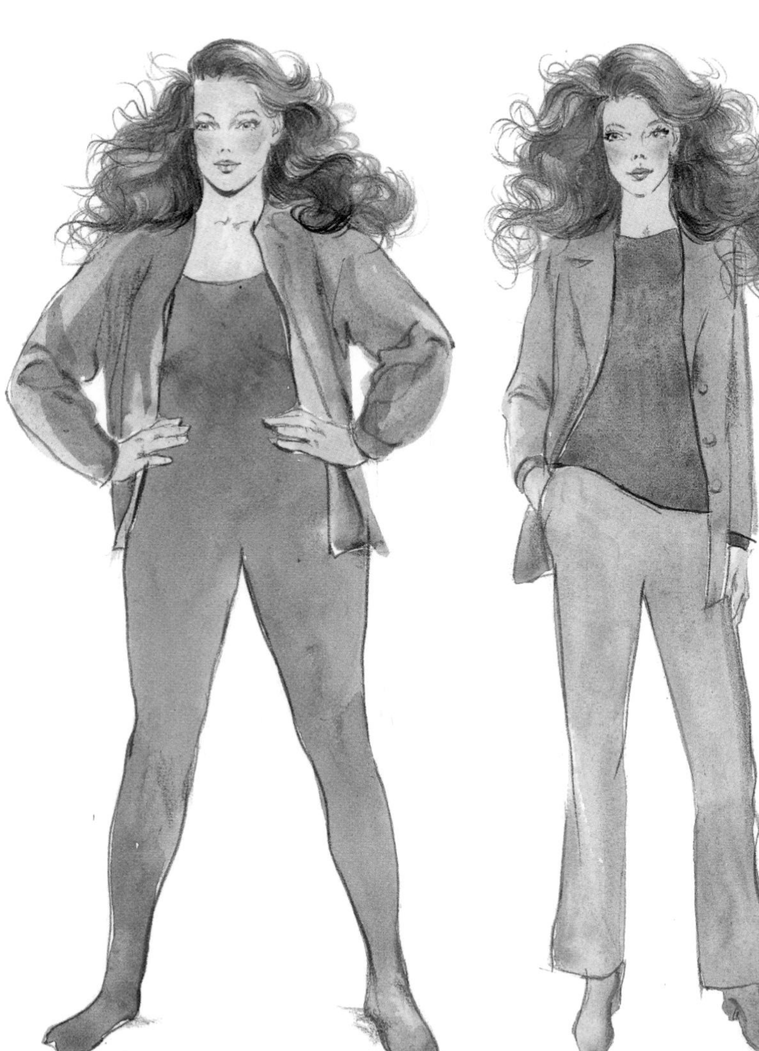

FIGURE 8.33 — Large hairstyle balances large body structure.

FIGURE 8.34 — Large hairstyle makes petite woman look smaller.

BALANCE

Balance is the harmonious arrangement of the hair. It can be symmetrical or asymmetrical. If you are dissatisfied with a finished hair design, it is often because the style is out of balance.

To measure symmetry, divide the face into four equal parts. Where the lines cross is the central axis, the reference point for judging the balance of the hair design. (Fig. 8.35)

In ***symmetrical balance,*** both sides of the hairstyle are the same distance from the center (Figs. 8.36, 8.37), the same length, and have the same volume when viewed from the front. The sides may have the same shape or a different shape but still have the same volume. (Figs. 8.38.a, 8.38b)

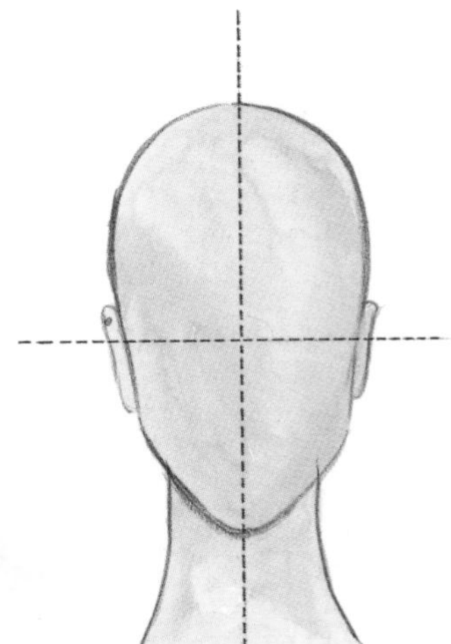

FIGURE 8.35 — Measuring symmetry of the head.

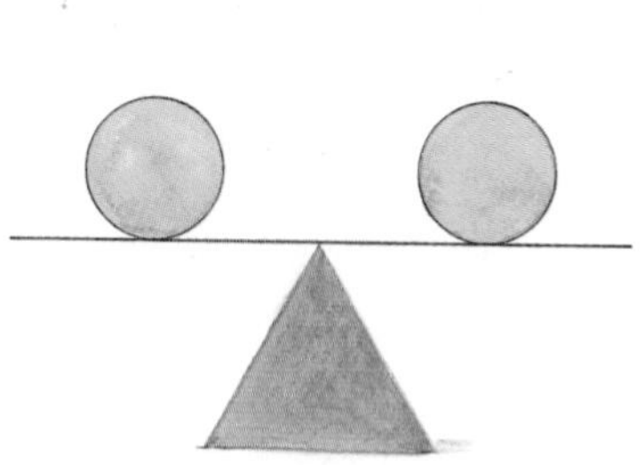

FIGURE 8.36 — Geometric symmetry.

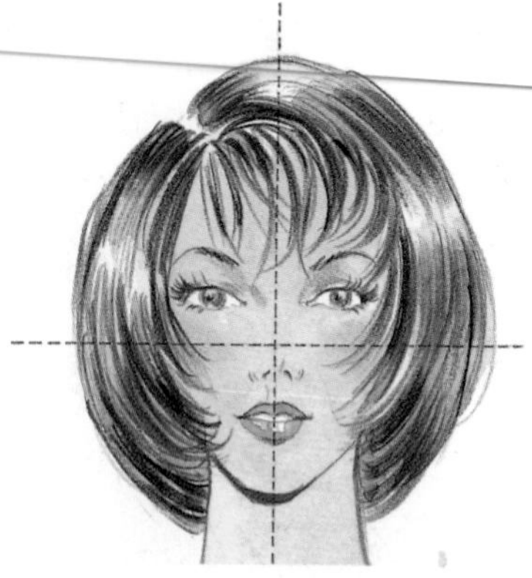

FIGURE 8.37 — Both sides equidistant from center.

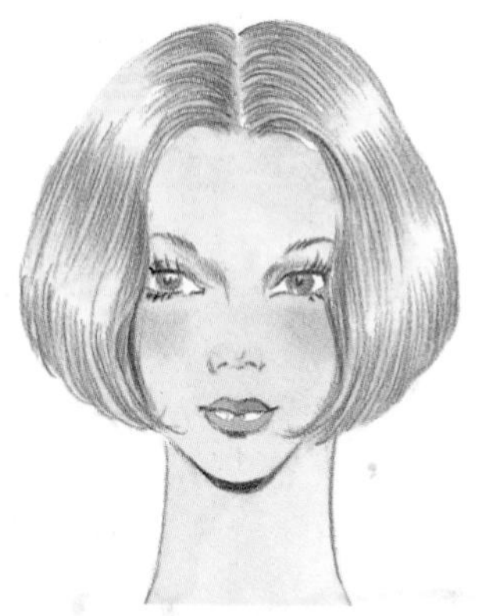

FIGURE 8.38a — Perfect symmetry.

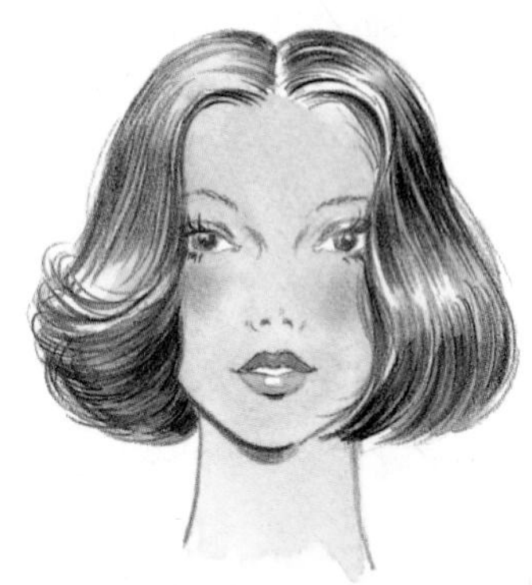

FIGURE 8.38b — Symmetry with different shapes, same volume.

In ***asymmetrical balance*** (Fig. 8.39), opposite sides of the hairstyle are a different length or have a different volume. To create balance, the larger side must be brought in closer to the center and the smaller side brought away from center. Asymmetry can be horizontal or diagonal. (Figs. 8.40, 8.41)

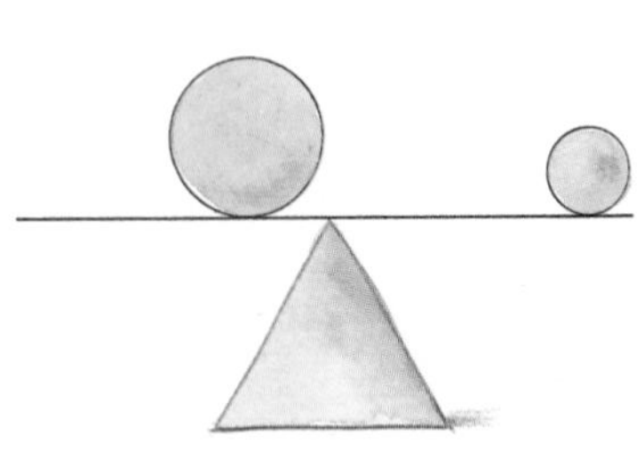

FIGURE 8.39 — Geometric asymmetry.

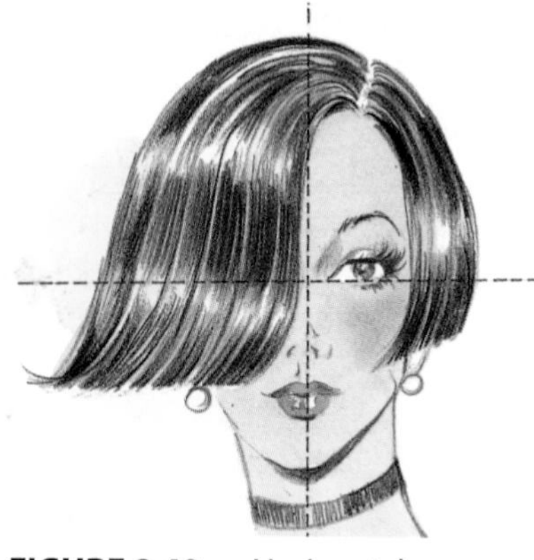

FIGURE 8.40 — Horizontal asymmetry.

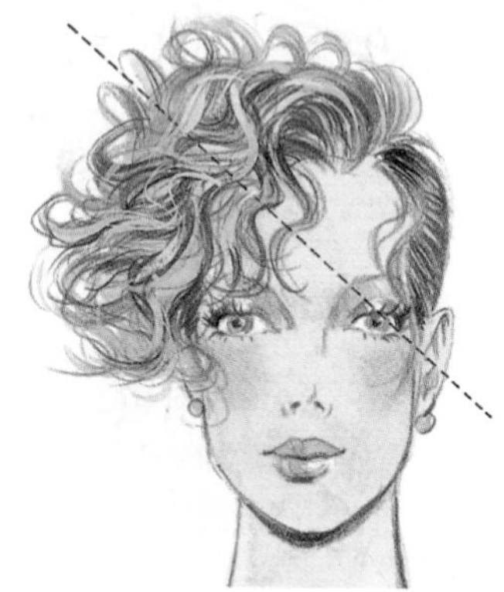

FIGURE 8.41 — Diagonal asymmetry.

When balancing hair for an updo, draw an imaginary diagonal line following the chin back to the crown. The emphasis of the hairstyle should be in the crown at the end of the line. If the emphasis is in the nape, draw an imaginary diagonal line from the eyes to the nape and place the emphasis of the design at the end of the line. (Fig. 8.42)

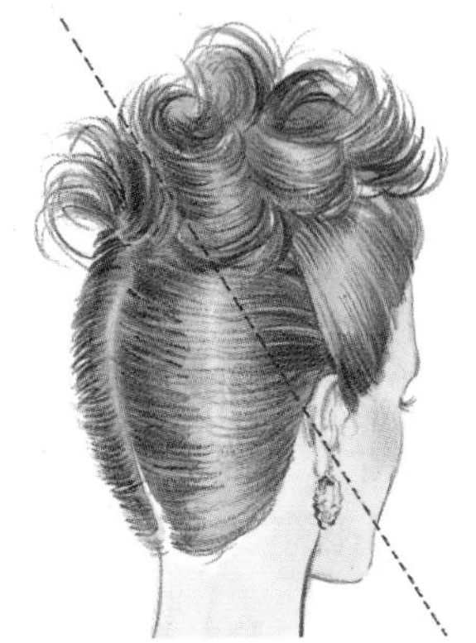

FIGURE 8.42 — Balancing with diagonal line.

RHYTHM

Rhythm is the pattern that creates movement in a hairstyle. It can be fast or slow. A fast rhythm moves quickly—tight curls are an example. A slow rhythm can be seen in larger shapings or long waves. Like music, rhythm can be simple or it can change. It is important to learn how to make varying rhythms work together to create interesting hairstyles.

In ***simple rhythm,*** the same movement is repeated throughout the hairstyle. A good example is the finger wave. (Fig. 8.43) This rhythm tends to be boring if style variations are not introduced to break the rhythm here and there.

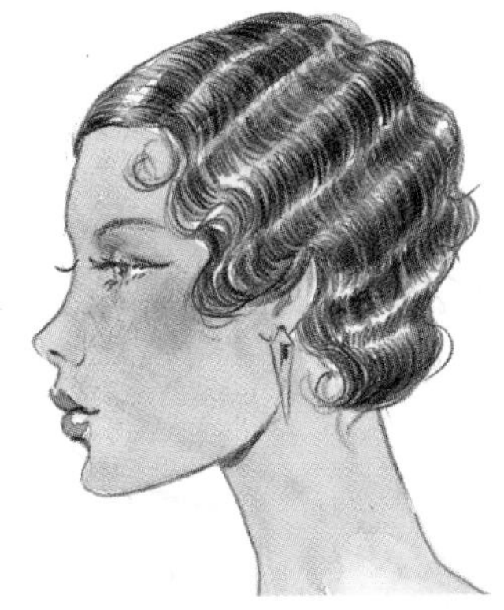

FIGURE 8.43 — Simple rhythm.

In ***increasing rhythm,*** the design patterns repeat themselves, becoming increasingly larger and creating more interest in the total design. (Fig. 8.44)

In ***decreasing rhythm,*** the design starts out with a large pattern or movement and decreases to a smaller one. (Fig. 8.45)

In ***alternating rhythm,*** the movement patterns change from small to large and back to small. This variety creates visual interest in the hairstyle. (Fig. 8.46)

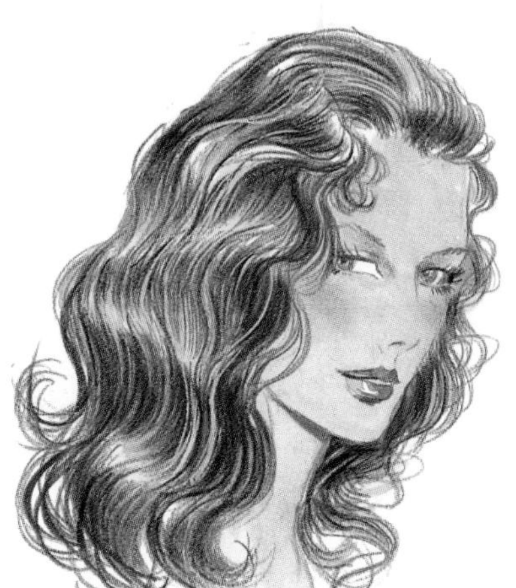

FIGURE 8.44 — Increasing rhythm.

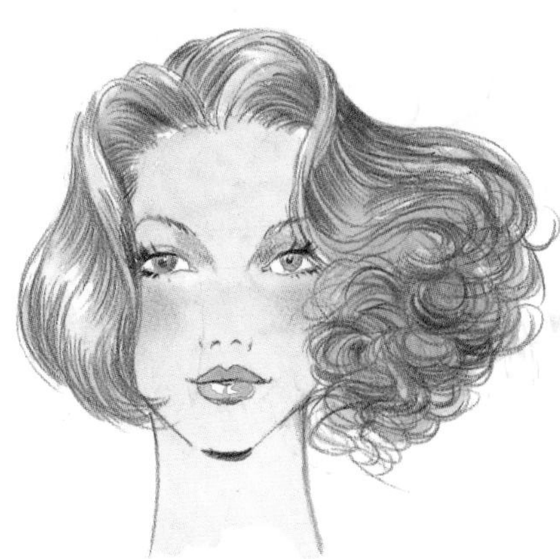

FIGURE 8.45 — Decreasing rhythm.

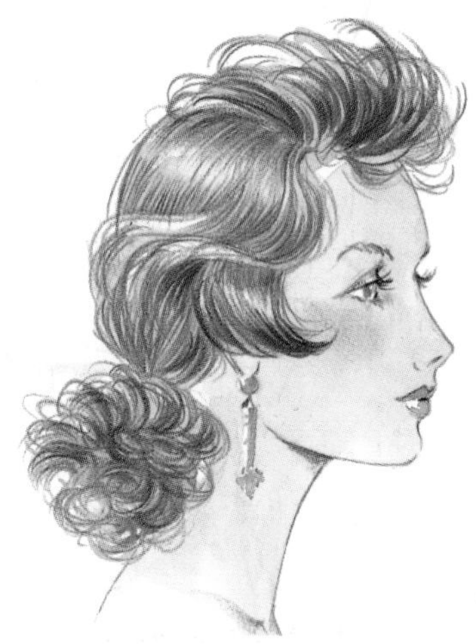

FIGURE 8.46 — Alternating rhythm.

Tips for Using Rhythm

- Generally, the rhythm should flow from small to large or large to small.
- Using only one rhythm in a design usually creates a more conservative hairstyle.
- Rhythm can be used to draw attention to the face or away from the face. (Figs. 8.47a, 8.47b)

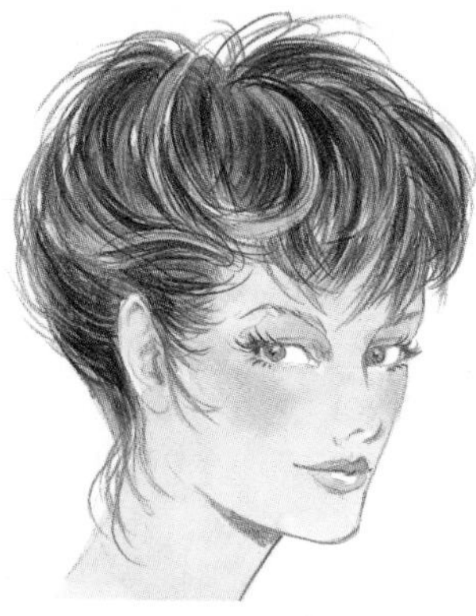

FIGURE 8.47a — Drawing attention to face.

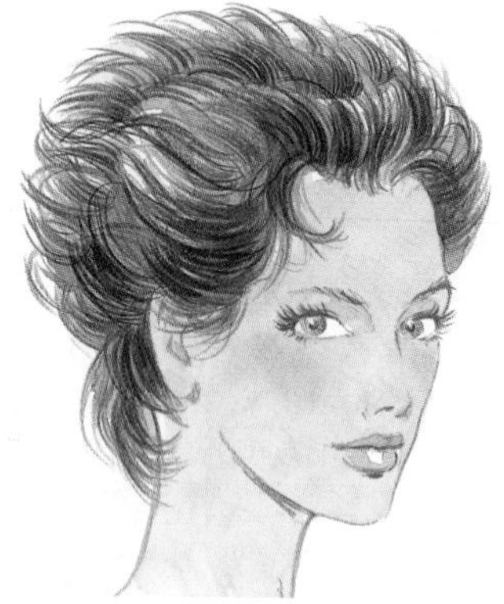

FIGURE 8.47b — Drawing interest away from face.

- Sudden changes in rhythm can be interesting. However, they should be used cautiously. If your design includes a sudden change in rhythm, use the 3-to-2 ratio: 3 parts slow to 2 parts fast. (Fig. 8.48)
- The speed of the rhythm should be carefully controlled. Moving from a soft wave (slow speed) to a very tight wave (fast speed) can create a discordant, unbalanced hairstyle. (Fig. 8.49)

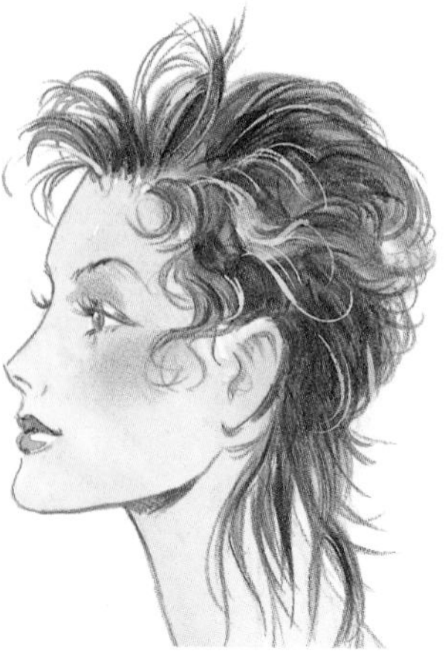

FIGURE 8.48 — Sudden change in rhythm.

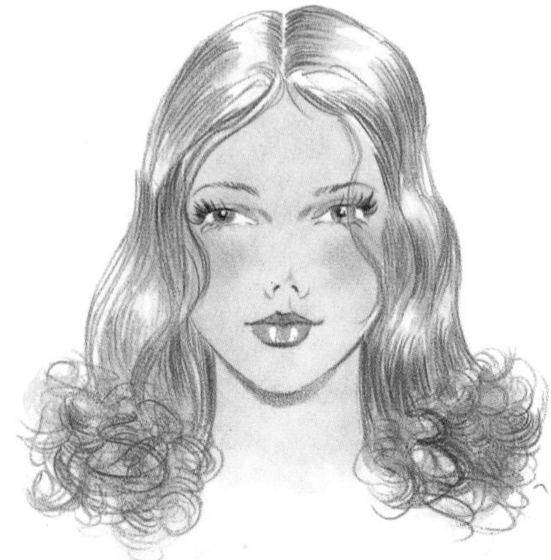

FIGURE 8.49 — Rhythm changing too rapidly.

EMPHASIS

The ***emphasis*** in a hairstyle is the place the eye sees first. The eye then travels to the rest of the design. A hairstyle may be well balanced, with good rhythm and harmony, and still lack flair. An interesting hairstyle should have an area of focus or emphasis. Emphasis can be created by using:

- texture (Fig. 8.50)
- color (Fig. 8.51)
- change in form (Fig. 8.52)
- ornamentation (Figs. 8.53a, 8.53b)

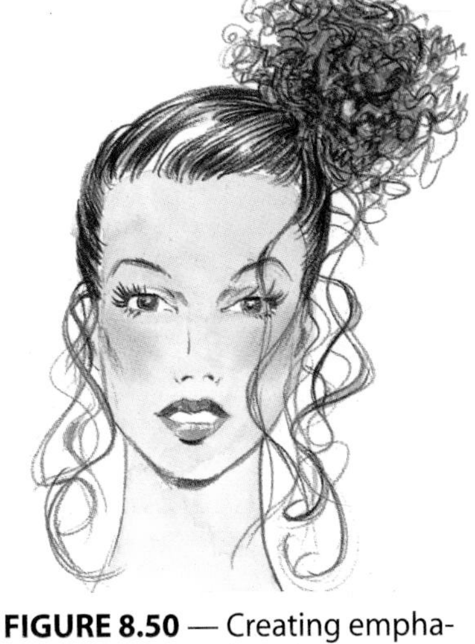

FIGURE 8.50 — Creating emphasis with texture change.

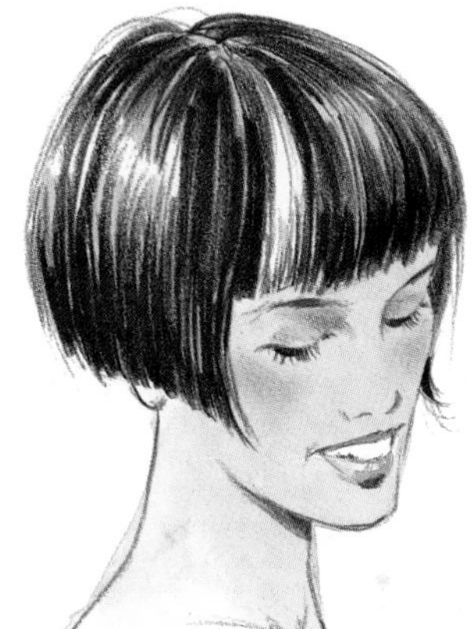

FIGURE 8.51 — Creating emphasis with color.

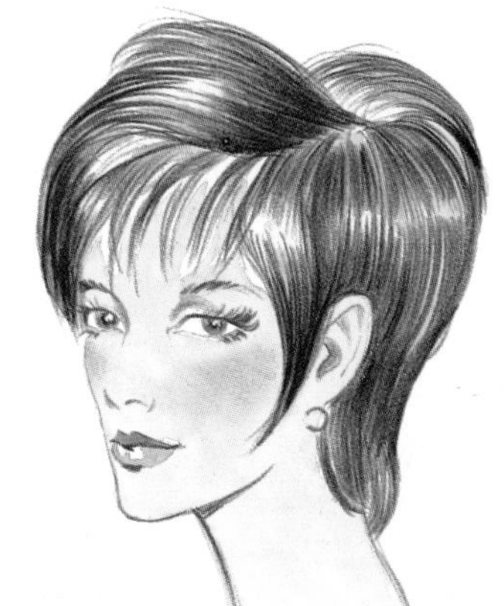

FIGURE 8.52 — Creating emphasis with form changes.

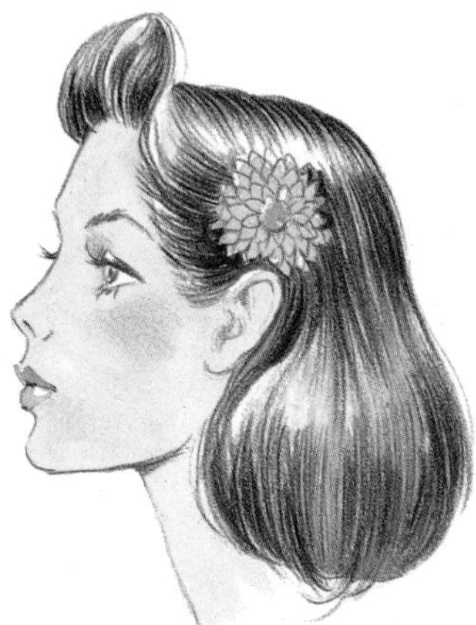

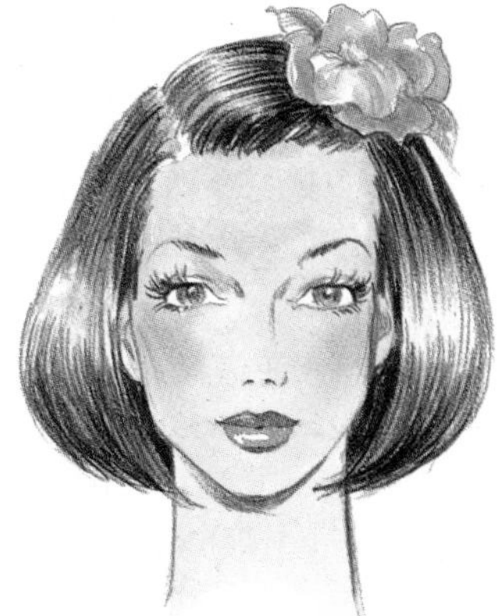

FIGURE 8.53a, b — Ornaments as focal points.

Choose the area of the head or face you want to emphasize. Keep the design simple so that it is easy for the eye to follow from the point of emphasis to the rest of the style. You can have multiple points of emphasis as long as they decrease in size and importance. Be careful not to use too many, however, as this can make the design too busy. (Fig. 8.54) Remember: less is more. When using ornaments, make sure they are appropriate to the total look of the client and do not overpower the hairstyle. (Fig. 8.55)

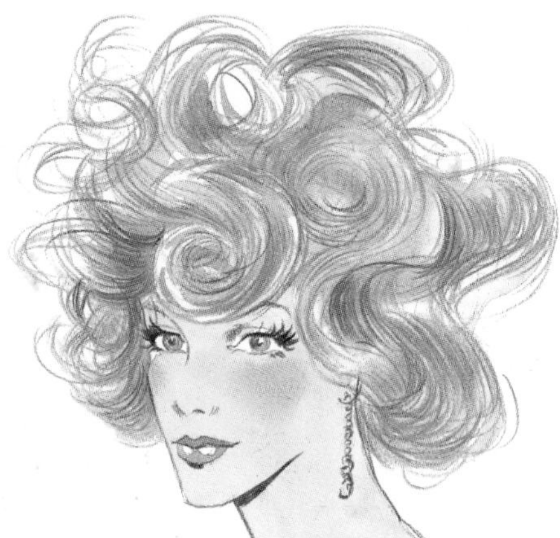

FIGURE 8.54 — Too many focal points.

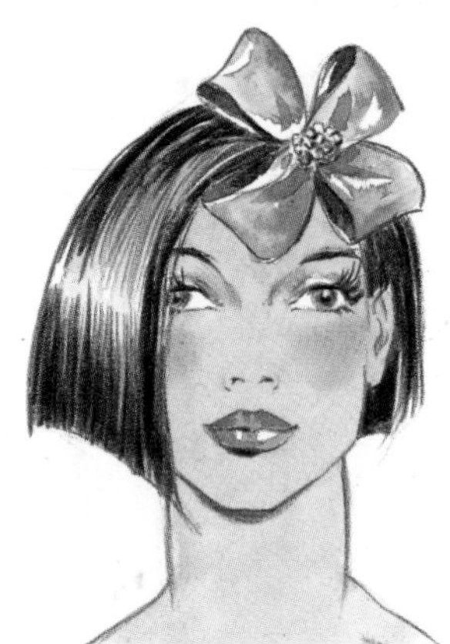

FIGURE 8.55 — Ornament dominating hairstyle.

HARMONY

Harmony is the most important of the art principles. Harmony holds all the elements of the design together. When a style is harmonious it has a pleasing form with interesting lines, a pleasing color or combination of colors, and the right texture and rhythm for the design. A harmonious style is in proportion to the client's facial and body structure and has an area of emphasis from which the eyes move to the rest of the style.

Completed: Learning Objective #2
ART PRINCIPLES OF HAIR DESIGN

CREATING HARMONY BETWEEN HAIRSTYLE AND FACIAL STRUCTURE

The principles of modern hairstyling and makeup are your guides to selecting what is most appropriate in order to achieve a beautiful appearance. The best results are obtained when each client's facial features are properly analyzed for strengths and shortcomings. Your job is to accentuate a client's best features and play down features that do not add to the person's attractiveness.

You must develop the ability to analyze hairstyles for your clients. Each client deserves a hairstyle that is properly proportioned to her body type, is correctly balanced to the head and facial features, and attractively frames the face. The essentials of an artistic and suitable hairstyle are based on the following general characteristics:

1. Shape of the head: front view (face shape), profile, and back view.
2. Characteristics of features: perfect as well as imperfect features.
3. Body structure, posture, and poise.

FACIAL TYPES

Each client's facial shape is determined by the position and prominence of the facial bones. There are seven facial shapes: oval, round, square, oblong, pear-shaped, heart-shaped, and diamond-shaped. To recognize each facial shape and to be able to give correct advice, you should be acquainted with the outstanding characteristics of each.

The face is divided into three zones: forehead to eyebrow, eyebrows to end of nose, and end of nose to bottom of chin. When you design hairstyles, you will be trying to create the illusion that each client has the ideal face shape. (Fig. 8.56)

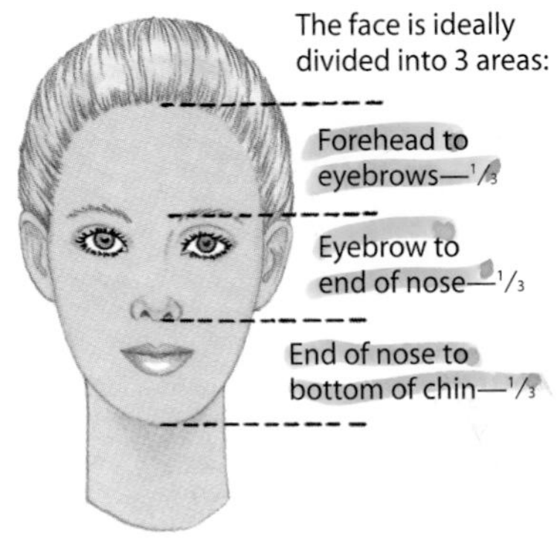
The face is ideally divided into 3 areas:
Forehead to eyebrows—1/3
Eyebrow to end of nose—1/3
End of nose to bottom of chin—1/3

FIGURE 8.56 — Ideal facial proportions.

Oval Facial Type

The oval-shaped face is generally recognized as the ideal shape. The contour and proportions of the oval face form the basis for modifying all other facial types.

Facial contour: The oval face is about 1½ times longer than its width across the brow. The forehead is slightly wider than the chin.

A person with an oval-shaped face can wear any hairstyle unless there are other considerations, such as eyeglasses, length and shape of nose, or profile. (See sections on special considerations.) (Fig. 8.57)

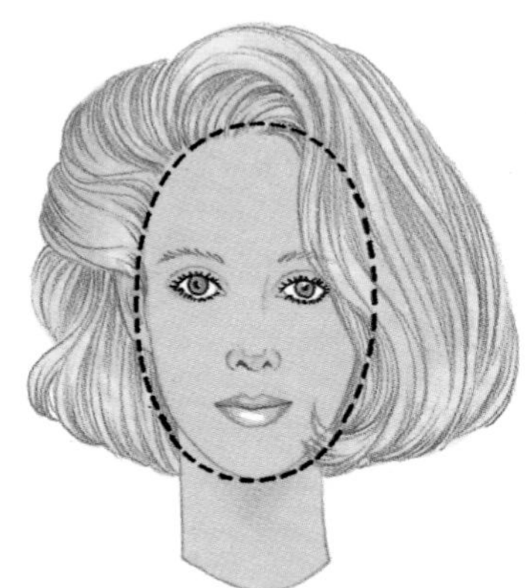

FIGURE 8.57 — Oval face.

Round Facial Type

Facial contour: Round hairline and round chin line; wide face.

Aim: To create the illusion of length to the face.

Create a hairstyle with height by arranging the hair on top of the head. You can place some hair over the ears and cheeks, but it is also appropriate to keep the hair up on one side, leaving the ears exposed. Style the bangs to one side. (Fig. 8.58)

Square Facial Type

Facial contour: Straight hairline and square jawline; wide face.

Aims: To create the illusion of length; offset the square features.

The problems of the square facial type are similar to the round facial type. The style should lift off the forehead and come forward at the temples and jaw, creating the illusion of narrowness and softness in the face. Asymmetrical hairstyles work well. (Fig. 8.59)

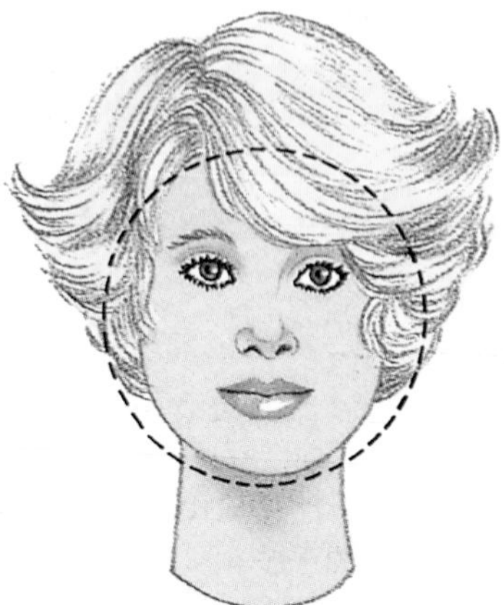

FIGURE 8.58 — Round face.

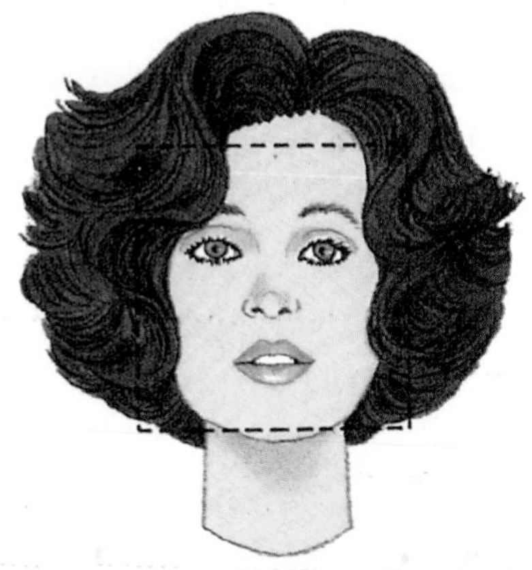

FIGURE 8.59 — Square face.

Pear-Shaped Facial Type

Facial contour: Narrow forehead, wide jaw and chin line.

Aim: To create the illusion of width in the forehead.

Build a hairstyle that is fairly full and high. Cover the forehead partially with a fringe of soft hair. The hair should be worn with a semi-curl or soft wave effect cropped over the ears. This arrangement adds apparent width to the forehead. (Fig. 8.60)

Oblong Facial Type

Facial contour: Long, narrow face with hollow cheeks.

Aim: To make the face appear shorter and wider.

The hair should be styled fairly close to the top of the head with a fringe of curls and bangs, combined with fullness to the sides. Drawing the hair out from the cheeks creates the illusion of width. (Fig. 8.61)

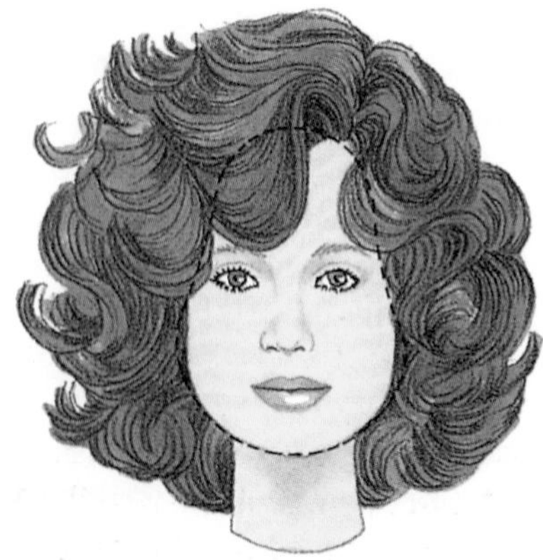

FIGURE 8.60 — Pear-shaped face.

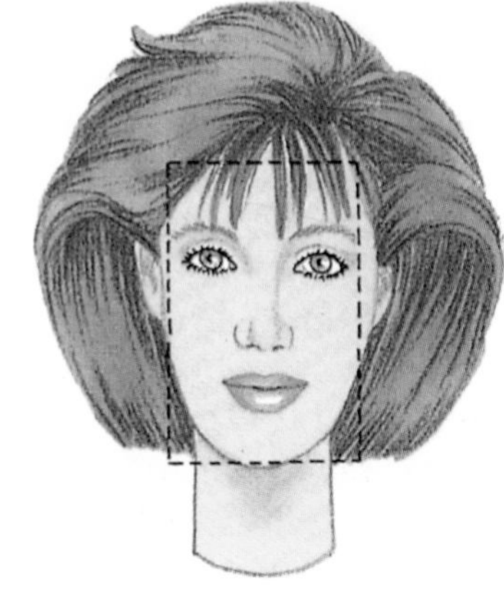

FIGURE 8.61 — Oblong face.

Diamond Facial Type

Facial contour: Narrow forehead, extreme width through the cheekbones, and narrow chin.

Aim: To reduce the width across the cheekbone line.

Increasing the fullness across the jawline and forehead while keeping the hair close to the head at the cheekbone line helps create an oval appearance. Avoid hairstyles that lift away from the cheeks or move back from the hairline. (Fig. 8.62)

Heart-Shaped Facial Type

Facial contour: Wide forehead and narrow chin line.

Aims: To decrease the width of the forehead and increase the width in the lower part of the face.

To reduce the width of the forehead, a center part with bangs flipped up or a style slanted to one side is recommended. Add width and softness at the jawline. (Fig. 8.63)

Completed: Learning Objective #3 FACIAL TYPES

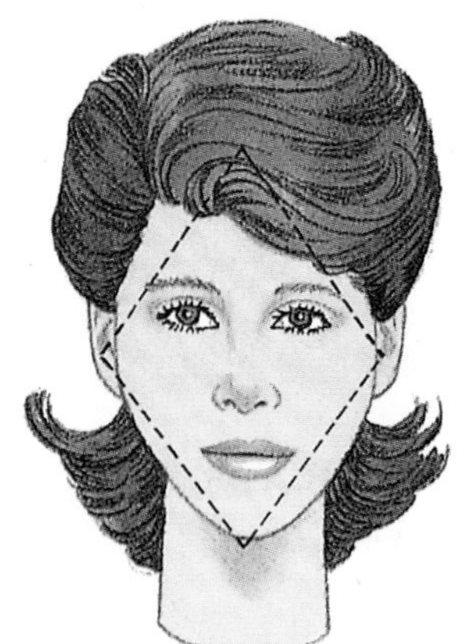

FIGURE 8.62 — Diamond face.

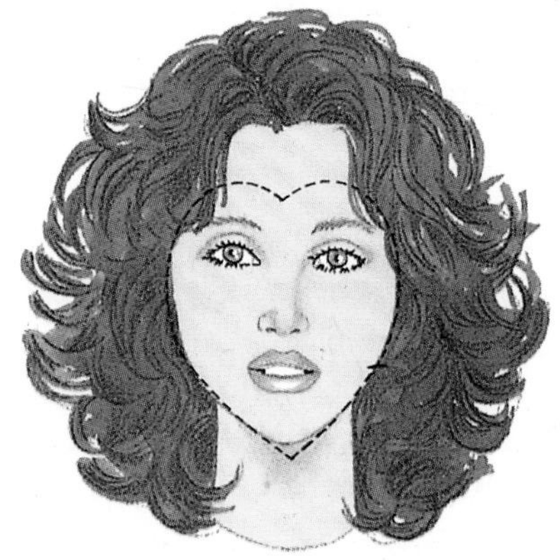

FIGURE 8.63 — Heart-shaped face.

MULTICULTURAL CLIENTS

Follow styling rules that relate to the particular face shape. If the hair has been straightened, set it on large rollers. If not, press it thermally with a large barrel iron (see chapter on thermal hairstyling). Either method will allow you to gain more control in order to style the hair according to hair art principles. (Fig. 8.64) Keep in mind that Asian hair is usually strong and may require more precise handling. (Fig. 8.65)

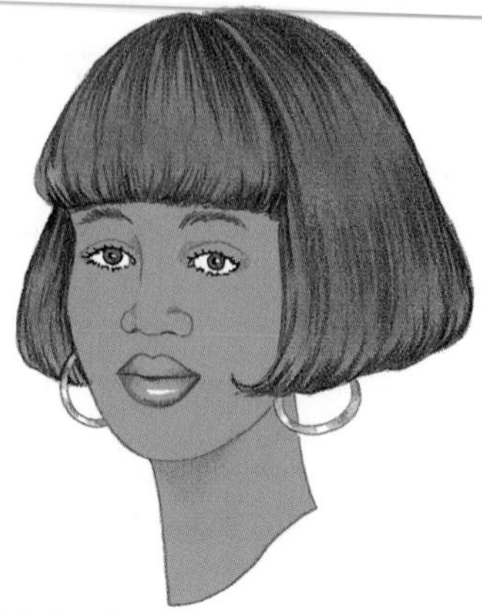

FIGURE 8.64 — African-American client.

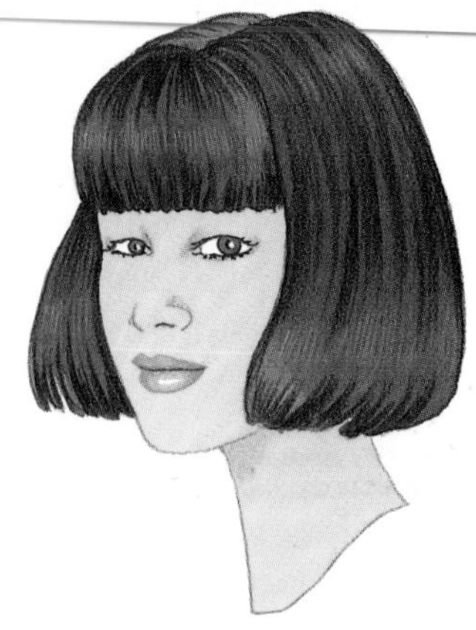

FIGURE 8.65 — Asian client.

SPECIAL CONSIDERATIONS

An understanding of facial features and proportions will make it easier for you to analyze each client's face and apply the design principles you've learned to help correct for structural problems. Dividing the face into three sections is one way to do this analysis. (Fig. 8.66)

The Top Third of the Face

Wide forehead: Direct hair forward over the sides of the forehead. (Fig. 8.67)

Narrow forehead: Direct hair away from the face at the forehead. Lighter highlights can be used at the temples to create the illusion of width. (Fig. 8.68)

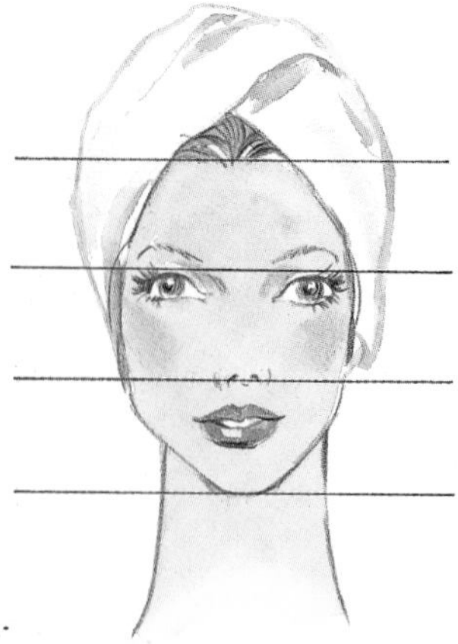

FIGURE 8.66 — Dividing face into three sections.

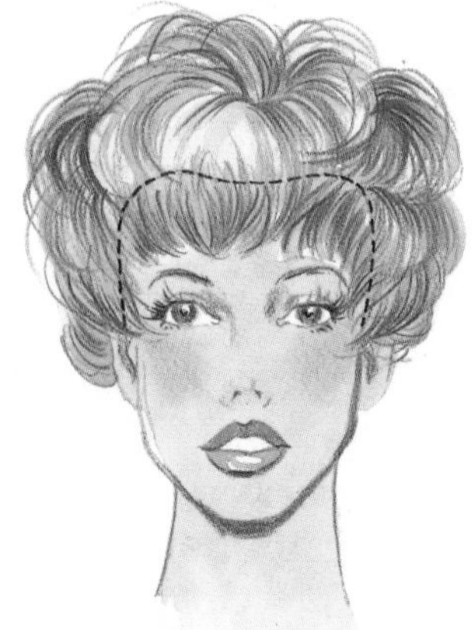

FIGURE 8.67 — Wide forehead.

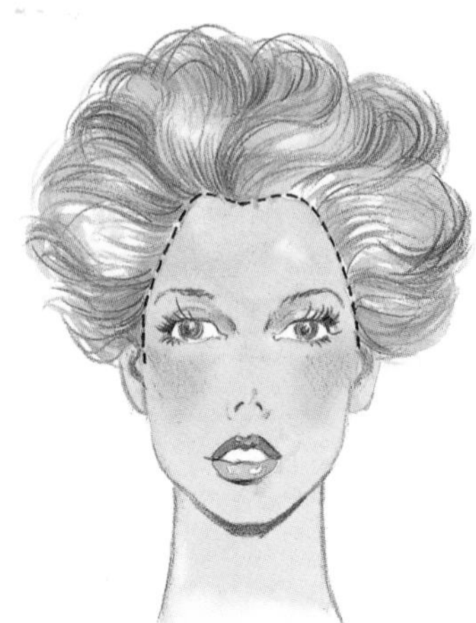

FIGURE 8.68 — Narrow forehead.

The Middle Third of the Face

Close-set eyes: Usually found on long, narrow faces. Direct hair back and away from the face at the temples. A side movement from a diagonal back part with some height is advisable. A slight lightening of the hair at the corner of the eyes will give the illusion of width. (Fig. 8.69)

Wide-set eyes: Usually found on round or square faces. Use a higher half bang to create length in the face. This will give the face the illusion of being larger and make the eyes appear more proportional. The hair should be slightly darker at the sides than the top. (Fig. 8.70)

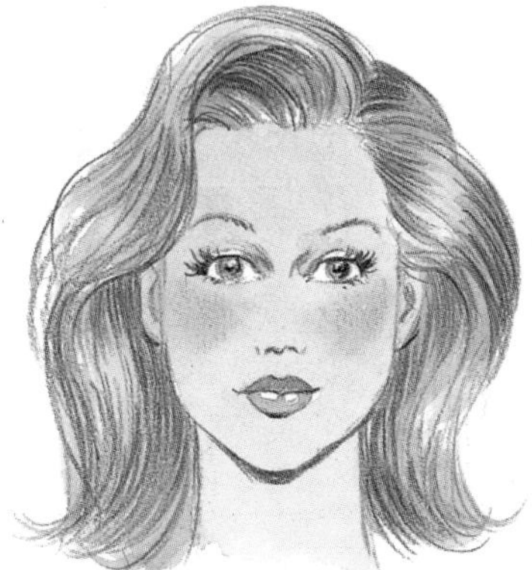

FIGURE 8.69 — Close-set eyes.

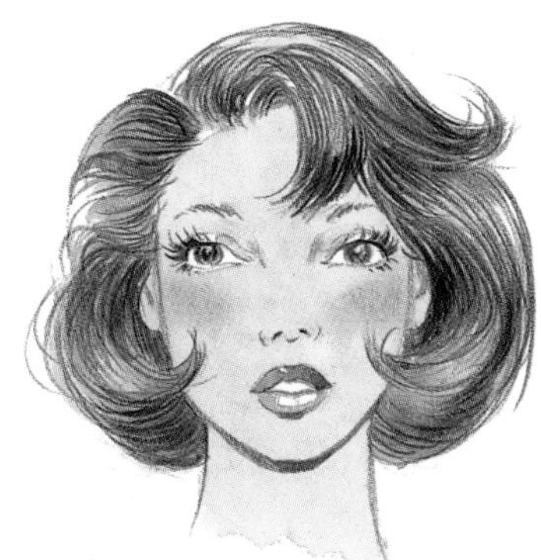

FIGURE 8.70 — Wide-set eyes.

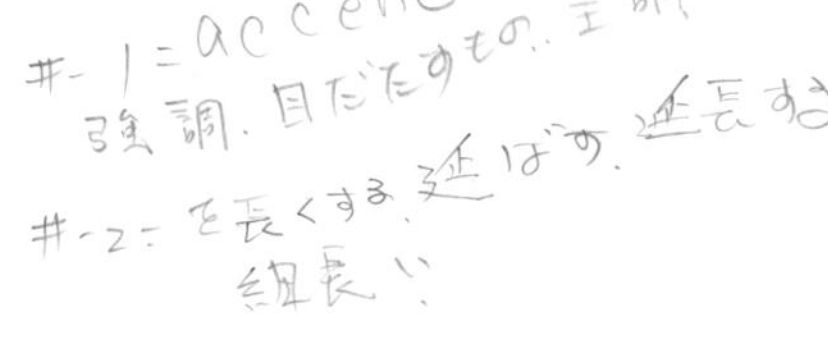

Crooked nose: Asymmetrical, off-center styles are best, as they attract the eye away from the nose. Any well-balanced style will accentuate the fact that the face is not even. (Fig. 8.71)

Wide, flat nose: Draw the hair away from the face and use a center part to help elongate and narrow the nose. (Fig. 8.72)

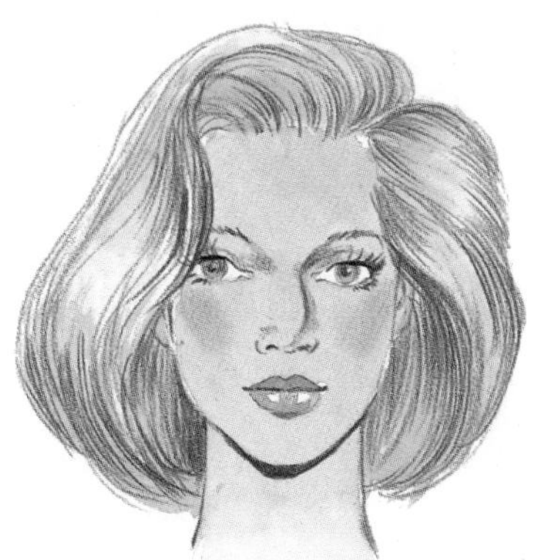

FIGURE 8.71 — Crooked nose.

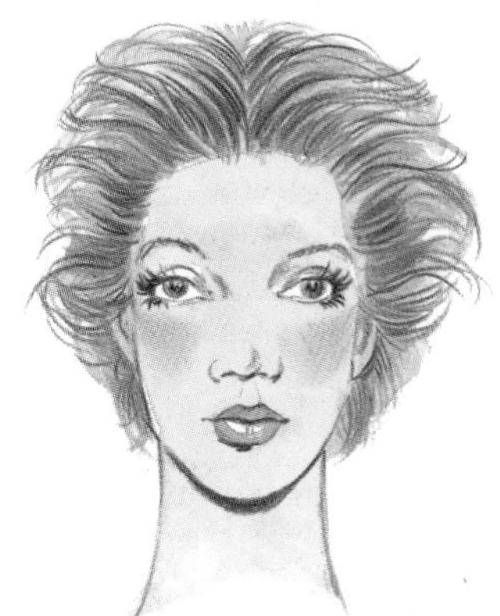

FIGURE 8.72 — Wide nose.

The Lower Third of the Face

Round jaw: Use straight lines at the jawline. (Fig. 8.73)

Square jaw: Use curved lines at the jawline. (Fig. 8.74)

Long jaw: Hair should be full and fall below the jaw to direct attention away from the jaw. (Fig. 8.75)

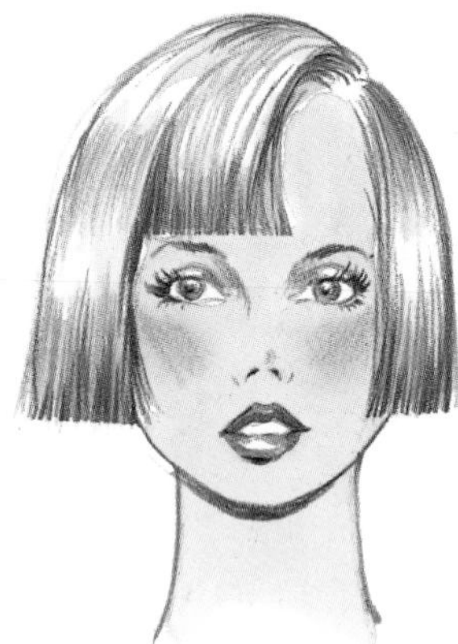

FIGURE 8.73 — Round jaw.

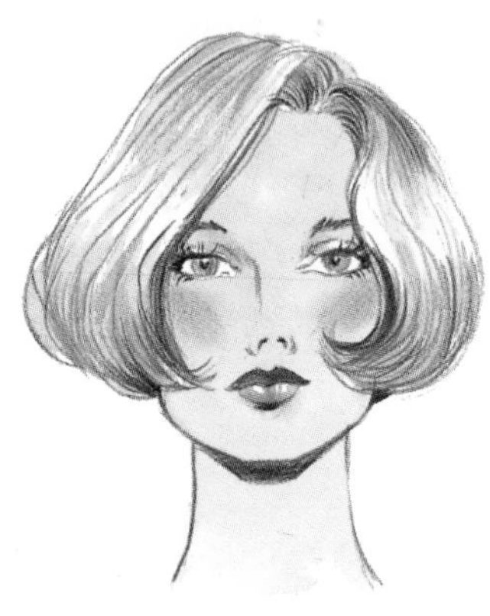

FIGURE 8.74 — Square jaw.

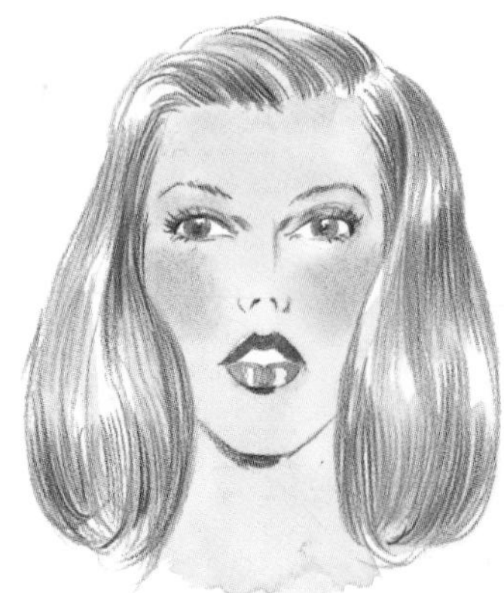

FIGURE 8.75 — Long jaw.

Profiles

When analyzing the profile, it is helpful to divide it into thirds, as you did the face. (Fig. 8.76) There are three basic profiles:

1. The ***straight profile*** is considered the ideal. It is neither concave nor convex, although it actually has a very slight curvature. Generally, all hairstyles are flattering to the straight or normal profile. (Fig. 8.77)

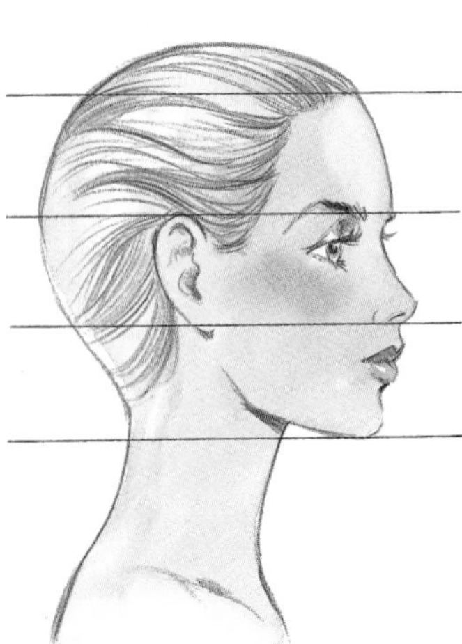

FIGURE 8.76 — Dividing profile into three sections.

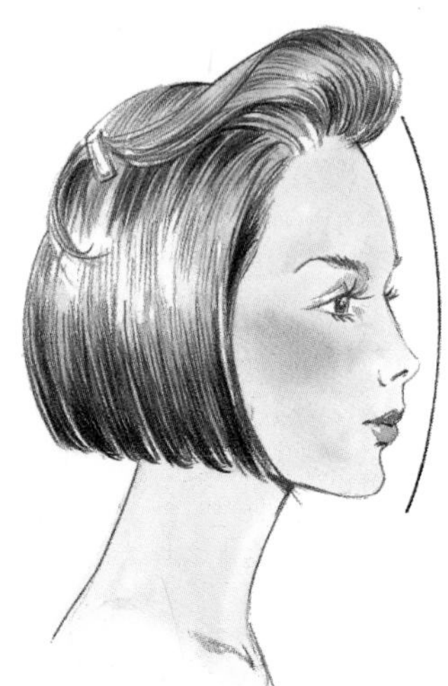

FIGURE 8.77 — Straight profile.

2. The ***convex profile*** has an exaggerated outward curvature. (Fig. 8.78) Arrange curls or bangs over the forehead. Keep the style close to the head at the nape and move hair forward in the chin area. (Fig. 8.79)

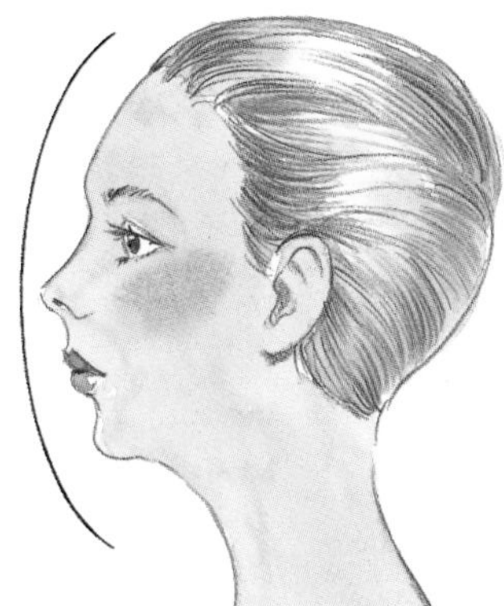

FIGURE 8.78 — Convex profile.

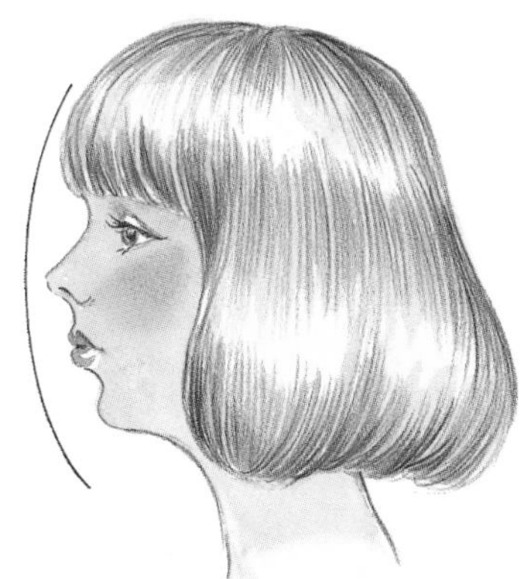

FIGURE 8.79 — Styling for convex profile.

3. The ***concave profile*** has an inward curvature. (Fig. 8.80) Hair at the nape should be styled softly, with upward movement. Do not build hair onto the forehead. (Fig. 8.81)

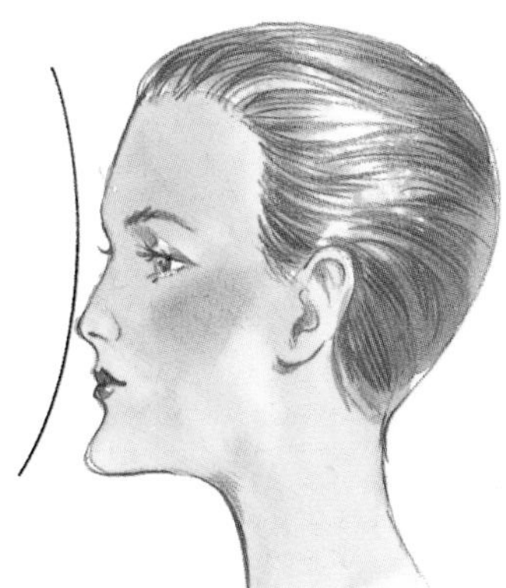

FIGURE 8.80 — Concave profile.

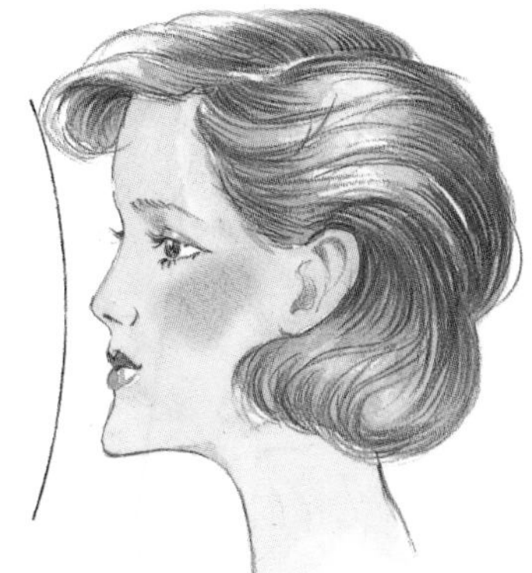

FIGURE 8.81 — Styling for concave profile.

Various hair designs can help balance other disproportionate areas of the profile, such as:

Receding forehead: Direct the bangs over the forehead with an outwardly directed volume. (Fig. 8.82)

Large Forehead: Use bangs with little or no volume to cover the forehead. (Fig. 8.83)

Small nose: A small nose is considered a childlike quality; therefore it is best to design a hairstyle that is not associated with children. Hair should be swept off the face, creating a line from nose to ear. The top hair should be moved off the forehead to give the illusion of length to the nose. (Fig. 8.84)

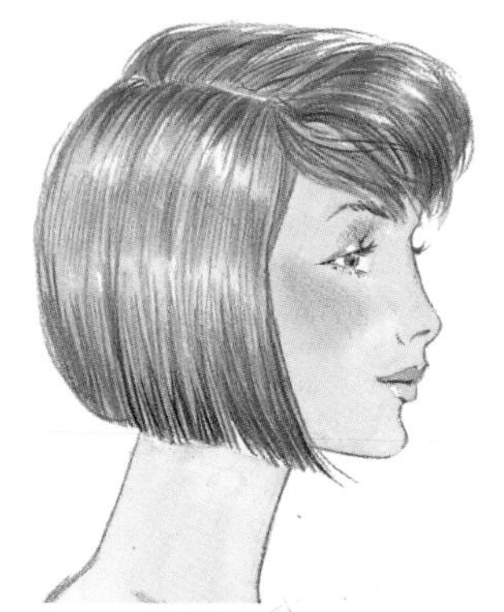
FIGURE 8.82 —Receding forehead.

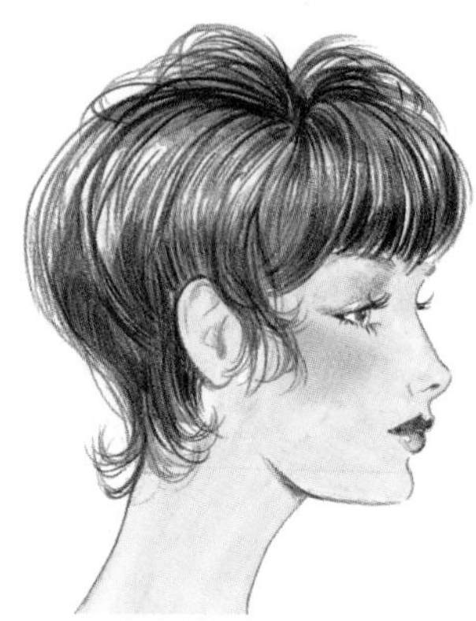
FIGURE 8.83 — Large forehead.

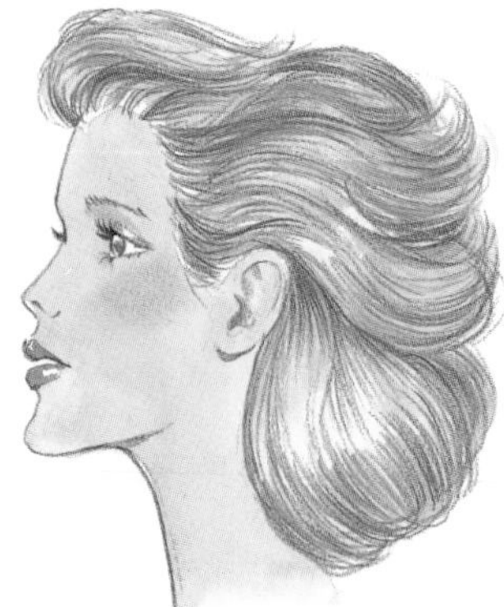
FIGURE 8.84 — Small nose.

Prominent nose: To draw attention away from the nose, bring hair forward at the forehead with softness around the face. (Fig. 8.85)

Receding chin: Hair should be directed forward in the chin area. (Fig. 8.86)

Small chin: Move the hair up and away from the face along the chin line. (Fig. 8.87)

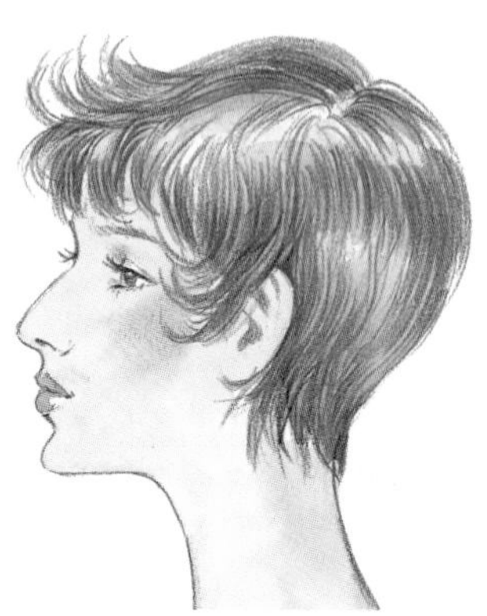
FIGURE 8.85 — Prominent nose.

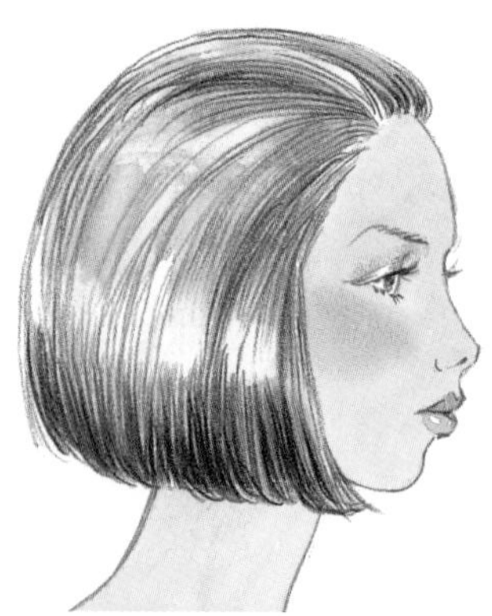
FIGURE 8.86 — Receding chin.

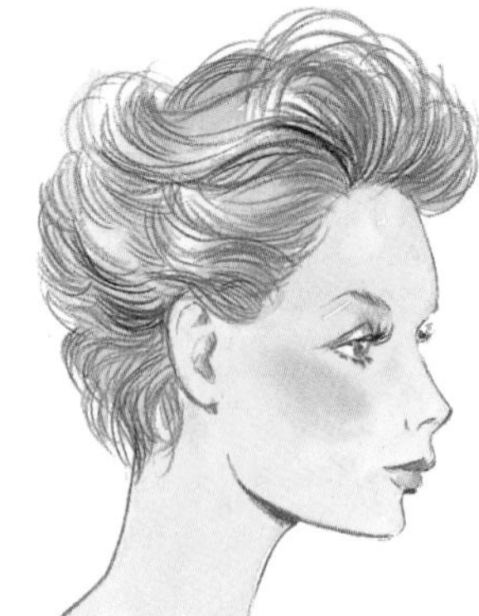
FIGURE 8.87 —Small chin.

Large chin: The hair should be either longer or shorter than the chin line so as to not draw attention to the chin. (Fig. 8.88)

The Neck

Short neck: Sweep hair up, building height on top. Avoid styles with fullness at the back of the neck, as well as styles with horizontal lines. (Fig. 8.89)

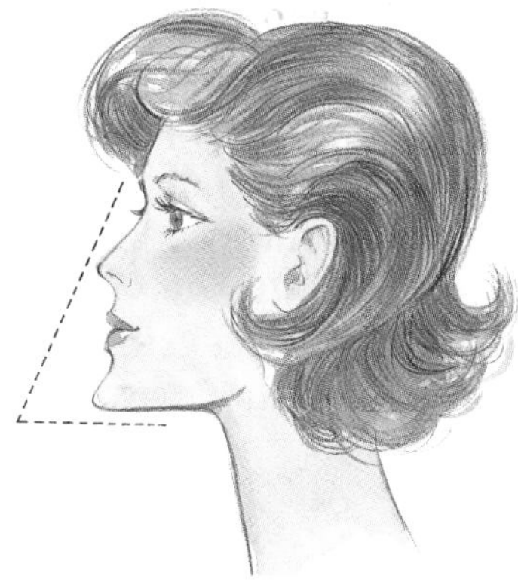

FIGURE 8.88 — Large chin.

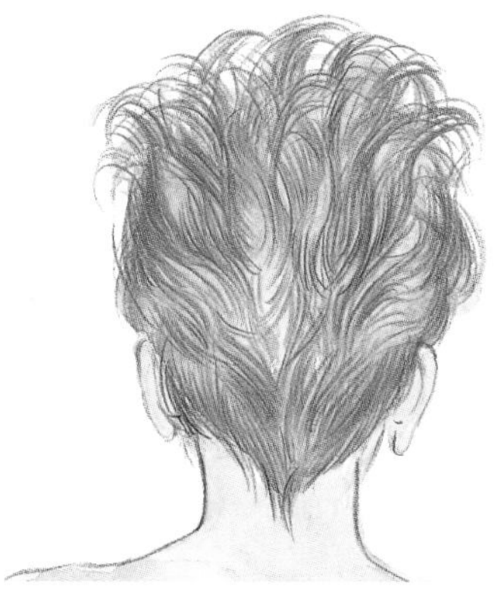

FIGURE 8.89 — Short neck.

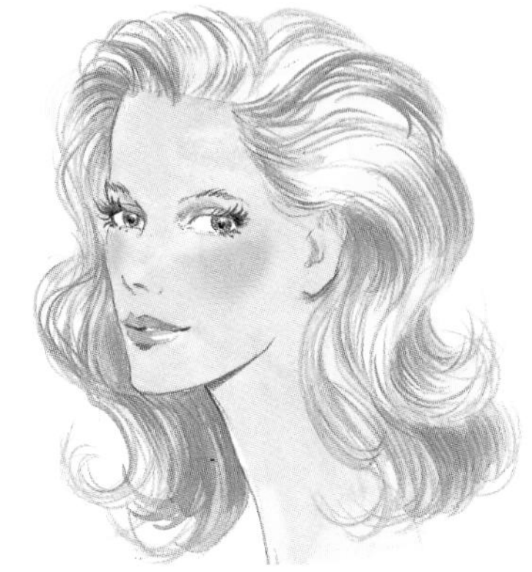

FIGURE 8.90 — Long, thin neck.

Long neck: Cover the neck with soft waves. Avoid short or sculptured necklines. Keep the hair long and full at the nape. (Fig. 8.90)

Head Shape

Not all head shapes are round. It is important to feel the head shape before deciding on a hairstyle. Design the style with volume in areas that are flat or small while reducing volume in areas that are large or prominent. (Figs. 8.91–8.96)

Completed:
Learning Objective
#4
HAIR DESIGN AND FACIAL FEATURES

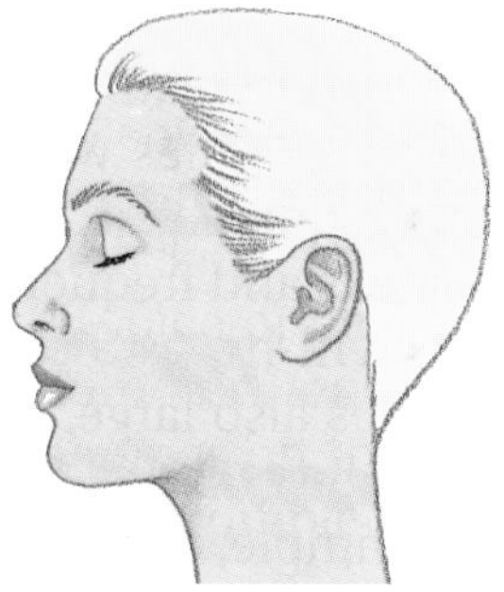

FIGURE 8.91 — Perfect oval.

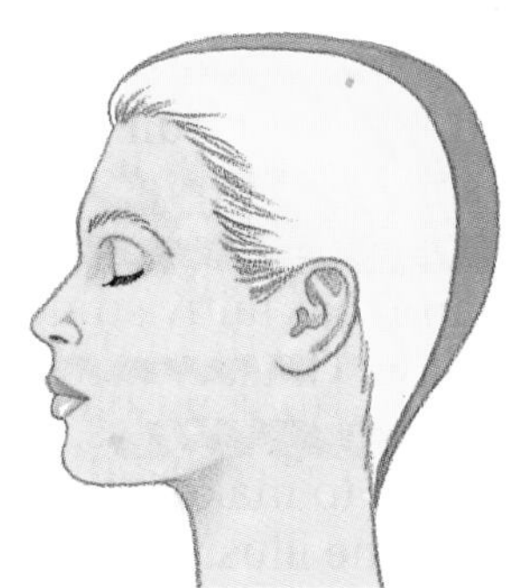

FIGURE 8.92 — Narrow head, flat back.

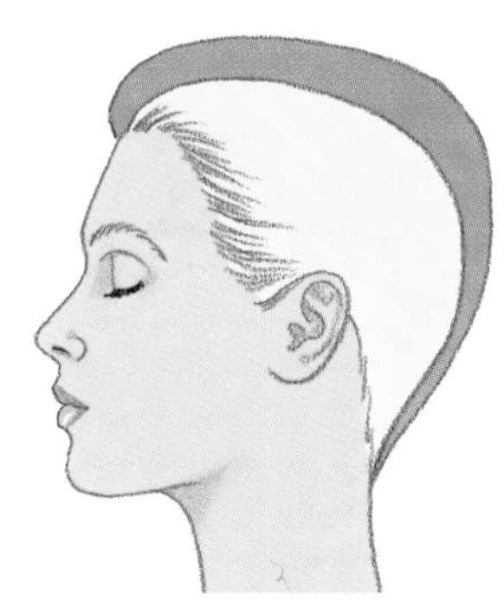

FIGURE 8.93 — Flat crown.

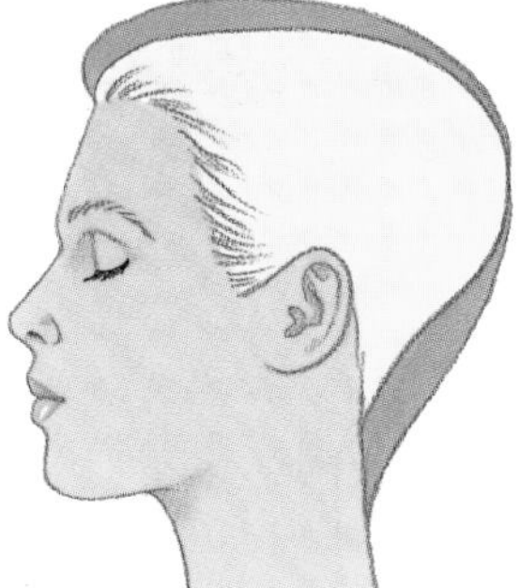

FIGURE 8.94 — Pointed head, hollow nape.

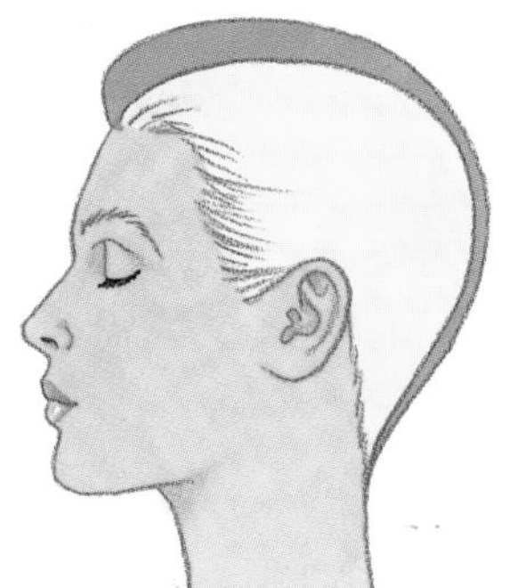

FIGURE 8.95 — Flat top.

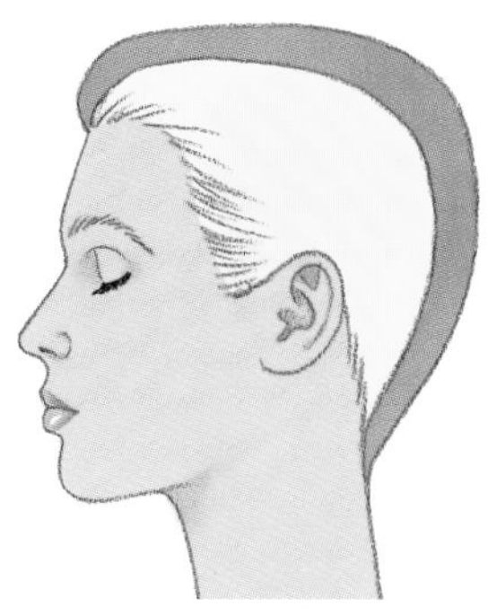

FIGURE 8.96 —Small head.

The Pear-Shaped Face

The pear-shaped or triangular face is characterized by a wide jawline and narrow cheekbones. The objective is to minimize the width of the jawline and emphasize length in the face. Larger, oval-shaped frames will soften the squareness of the jawline and emphasize the eyes. Hair should be worn up and off the face, high in the front and in the crown. Softness around the face—hair brushed forward on the lower cheeks—will reduce width and create a better balance. (Figs. 8.103, 8.104).

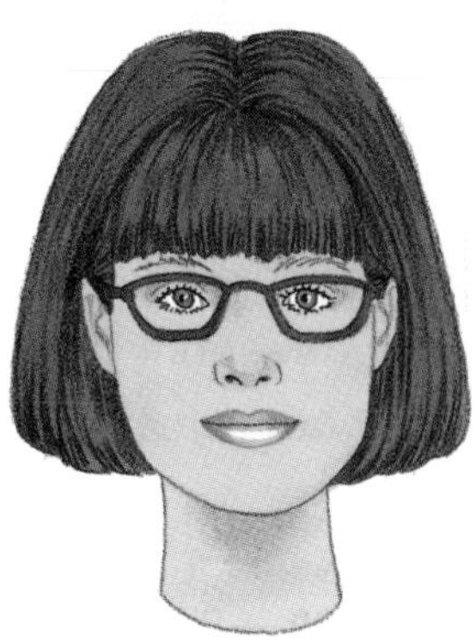

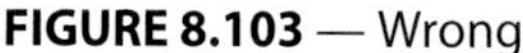

FIGURE 8.103 — Wrong.

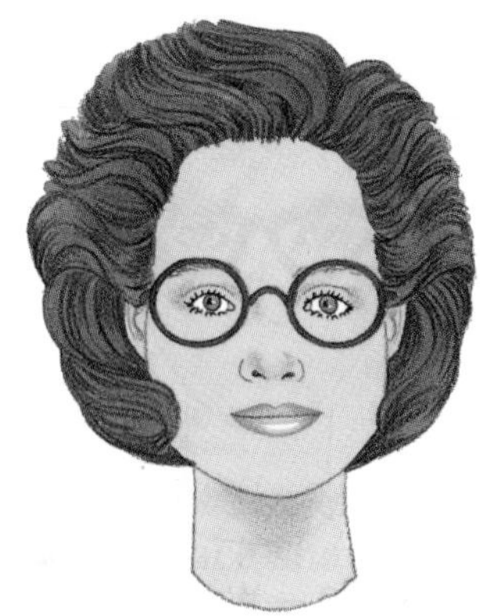

FIGURE 8.104 — Right.

Men's Eyeglasses

A man's glasses should also complement the shape of his face and facial features. The same principles of line and style apply for both men and women.

HAIR PARTS

Hair parts can be the focal point of a hairstyle. Because the eye is drawn to a part you must be careful how you use it. It must always be neat, without hairs straggling from one side or another, and it must be straight and directed positively. It is usually best to use a natural part if at all possible; however, you may want to create a part according to your client's head shape, facial features, or desired hairstyle. It is often difficult to create a lasting hairstyle when working against the natural crown part. You might be able to incorporate the natural part into the finished style.

The following are suggestions for suitable hair parts for various facial types.

Parts for Bangs

1. The ***triangular part*** is the basic parting for bang sections. (Fig. 8.105)

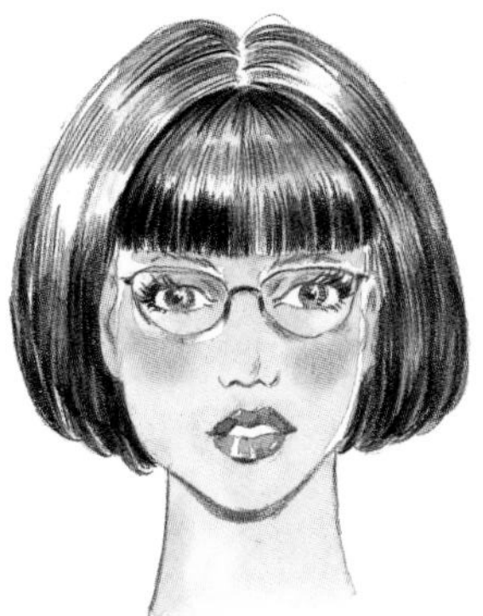

FIGURE 8.105 — Triangular part.

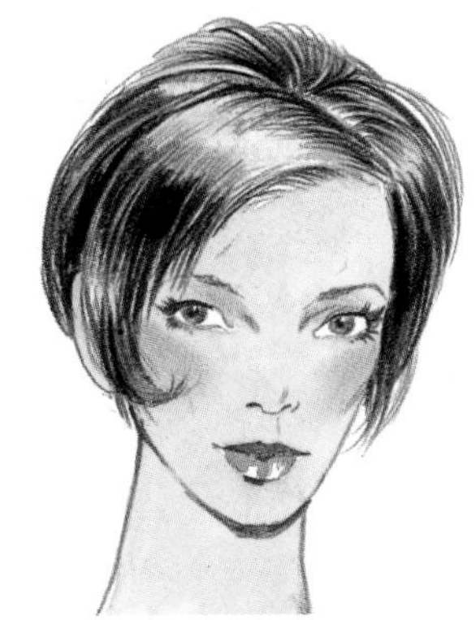

FIGURE 8.106 — Diagonal part in bangs.

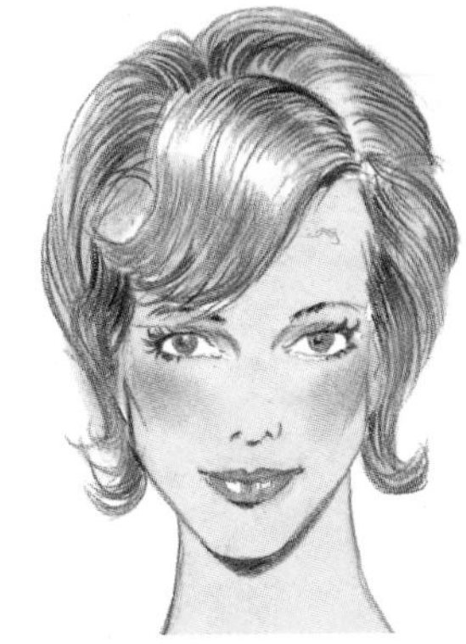

FIGURE 8.107 — Curved part.

2. The ***diagonal part*** gives height to a round or square face and width to a long, thin face. (Fig. 8.106)
3. The ***curved part*** is used for a receding hairline or high forehead. (Fig. 8.107)

Style Parts

1. ***Side parts*** are used to direct hair across the top of the head. They help develop height on top and make thin hair appear fuller. (Fig. 8.108)
2. ***Center parts*** are classical. They are usually used for an oval face, but give an oval illusion to wide and round faces. Do not use center parts on people with prominent noses. (Fig. 8.109)
3. ***Diagonal back parts*** are used to create the illusion of width or height in a hairstyle. (Fig. 8.110)
4. ***Zigzag parts*** create a dramatic effect. (Fig. 8.111)

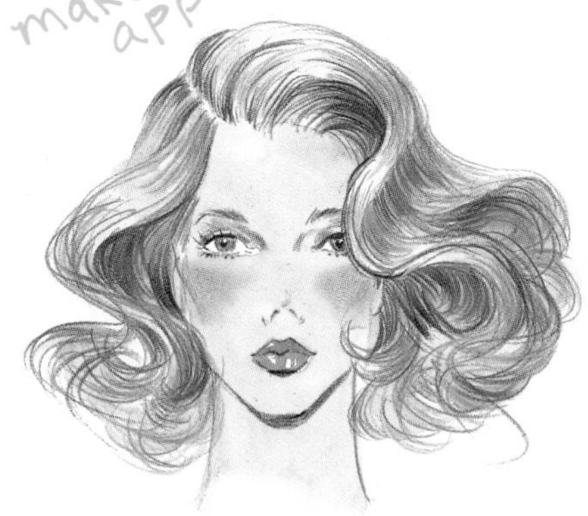

FIGURE 8.108 — Side part.

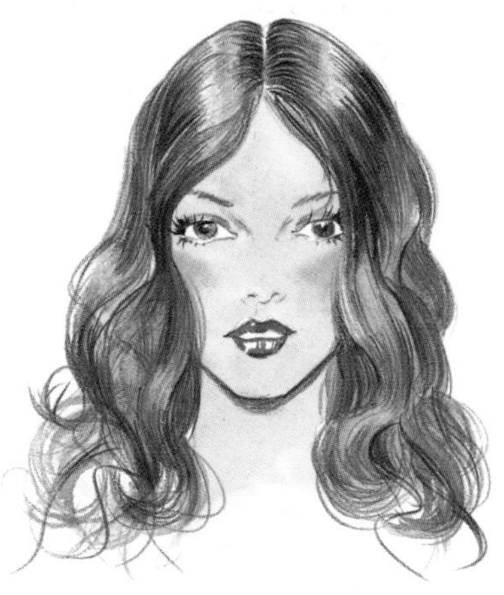

FIGURE 8.109 — Center part.

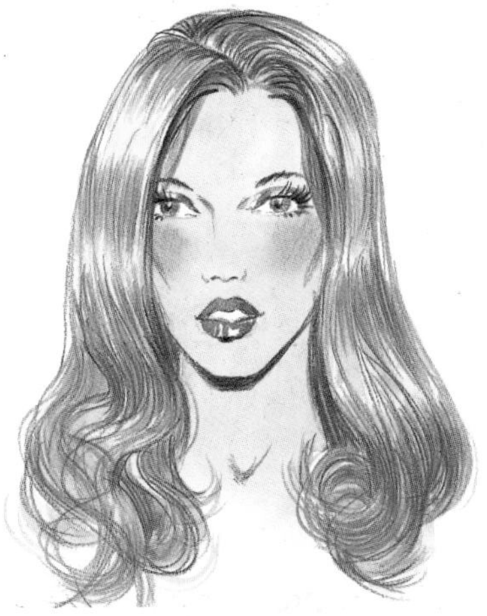

FIGURE 8.110 — Diagonal part.

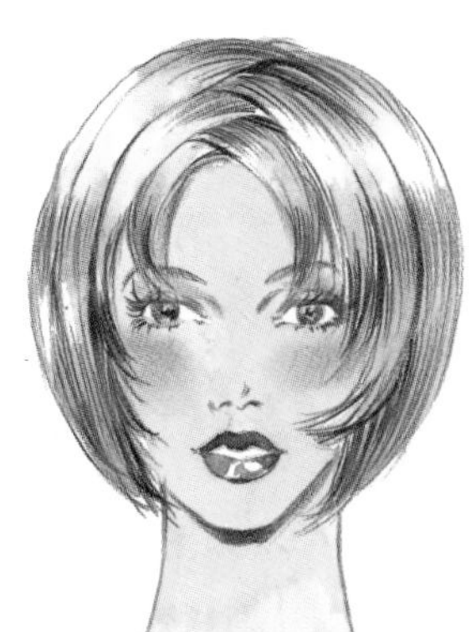

FIGURE 8.111 — Zigzag part.

REVIEW QUESTIONS

ARTISTRY IN HAIRSTYLING

1. Name the five elements of design.
2. What are the five art principles used in hair design?
3. Why must a stylist consider the entire body when designing hair?
4. What is considered the most important art principle in hair design? Why?
5. Name the seven facial shapes.
6. It is possible to correct facial flaws with the proper hairstyle. True or false?
7. Name at least three facial features that must be considered when designing a hairstyle.
8. What are the four kinds of style parts?

CHAPTER 9

Wet Hairstyling

LEARNING OBJECTIVES

After completing this chapter, you should be able to:

1. Explain the purpose of finger waving.
2. Demonstrate the various pin curl techniques.
3. Describe the differences between finger waves, pin curls, and roller setting.
4. Demonstrate proper comb-out techniques.
5. Properly execute a simple French braid style.

NATIONAL SKILL STANDARDS

This chapter provides you with the necessary information to master these National Industry Skill Standards for Entry-Level Cosmetologists:

- Consulting with clients to determine their needs and preferences
- Safely using a variety of salon products while providing client service
- Managing product supply for salon use and retail sales
- Providing styling and finishing techniques to complete a hairstyle to the satisfaction of the client

INTRODUCTION

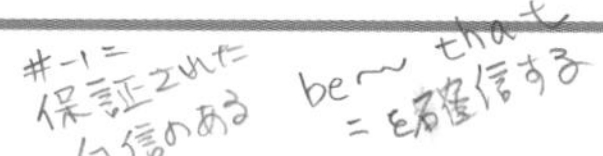

Hairstyling is creating wearable art. While roller sets, pin curls, and comb-outs may remind you of your great-grandmother's visits to the salon, be assured that these styling techniques are very much a part of hairstyling today. In fact, the stylist who is skilled and versatile in wet styling techniques as well as other cutting and styling services will always be in great demand.

HAIRSTYLING BASICS

IMPLEMENTS AND TOOLS

Rollers: short, medium, long (Fig. 9.1)

Clips: duckbill, double prong, single prong (Fig. 9.2)

Pins: bobby pins, hairpins (Fig. 9.3)

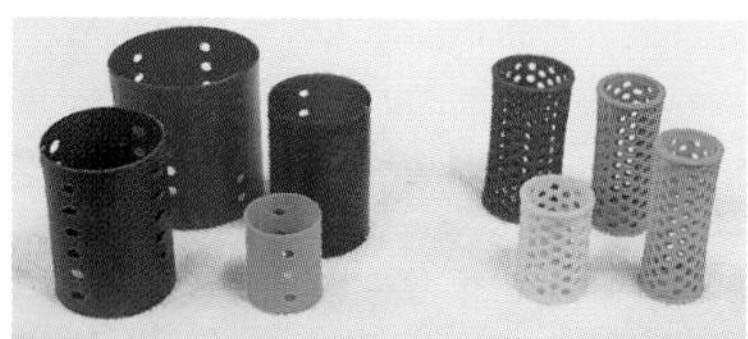

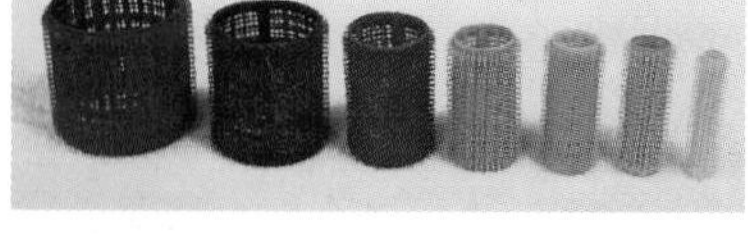

FIGURE 9.1 — Rollers are available in a variety of sizes and shapes.

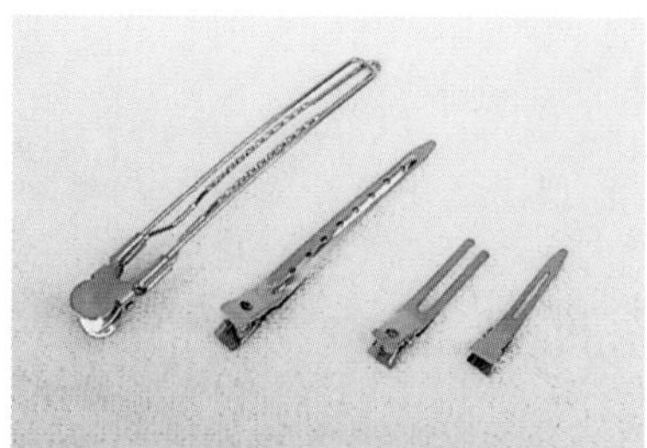

FIGURE 9.2 — Sectioning clip, duckbill clip, double-prong clip, single-prong clip.

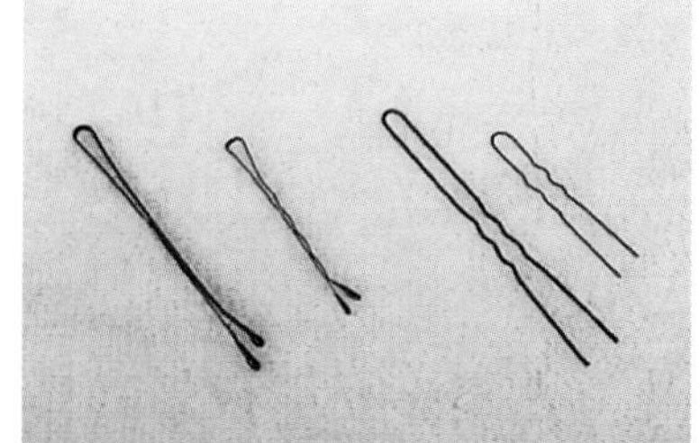

FIGURE 9.3 — Bobby pins and hairpins.

Combs: tail comb, styling comb, pick comb, wide-tooth comb (Fig. 9.4)

Brushes: boar-bristle brush, teasing brush (Fig. 9.5)

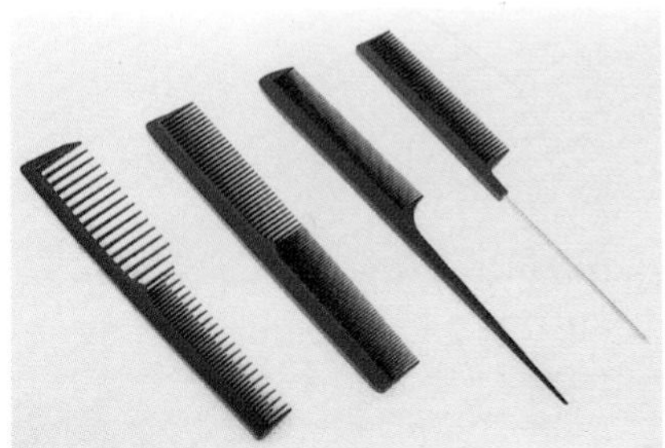

FIGURE 9.4 — Wide-tooth comb, styling comb, rat-tail combs.

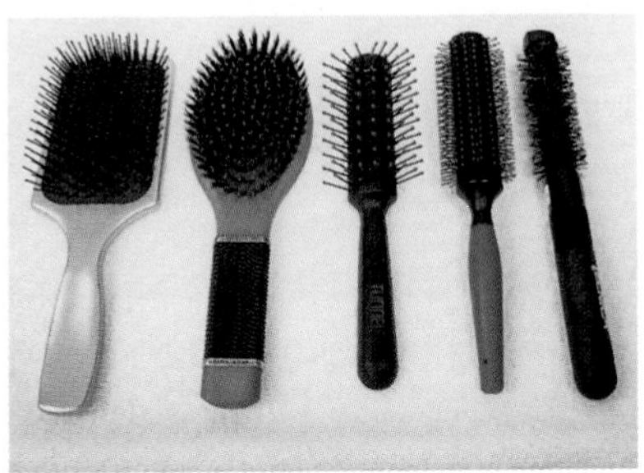

FIGURE 9.5 — Paddle brush, comb-out brush, vent brush, round brush, thermal styling brush.

PREPARING THE HAIR FOR WET STYLING

It is necessary to remove tangles or back-combing before shampooing.

1. Begin at the nape, taking a small parting.
2. Using a boar-bristle brush or wide-tooth comb, remove tangles, starting at the ends and working up to the roots. (Fig. 9.6) Work on a small area at a time, brushing or combing out to the ends.
3. Work from the bottom to the top of the back of the head. Then repeat on the sides.

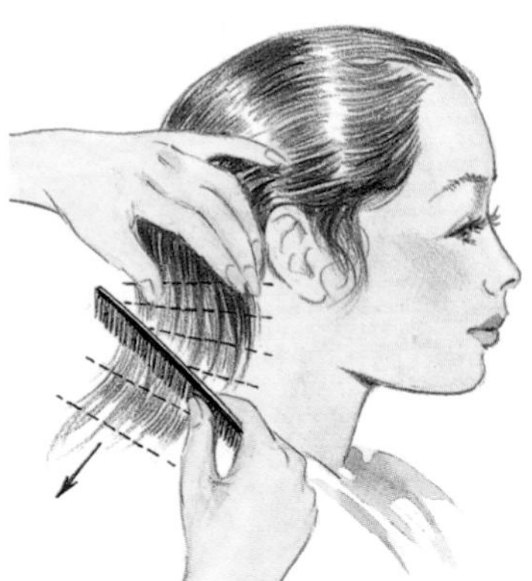

FIGURE 9.6 — Removing tangles.

Making a Part

1. Lay the wide-tooth end of a styling comb flat at the hairline.
2. Draw the comb back to the end of the desired part. (Fig. 9.7)
3. Hold the hair with the index finger on one side of the part. Pull the rest of the hair down with the comb. (Figs. 9.8, 9.9)

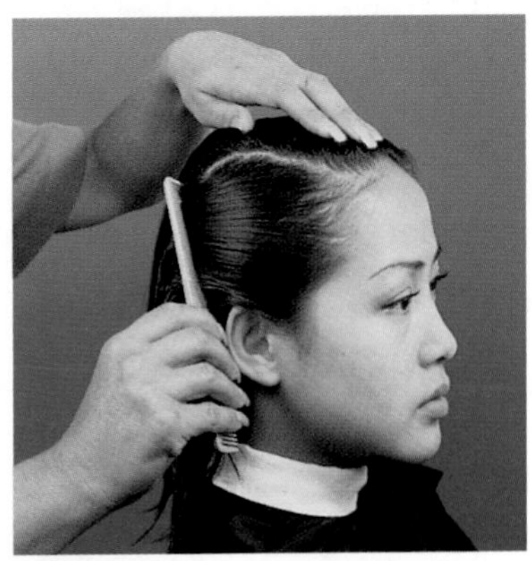

FIGURE 9.7 — Making a part.

To Find a Natural Part

1. Comb wet hair straight back from the hairline. (Fig. 9.10)
2. Push the hair gently forward with the palm of the hand. (Fig. 9.11)
3. Use your comb and other hand to separate the hair where it parts. (Fig. 9.12)

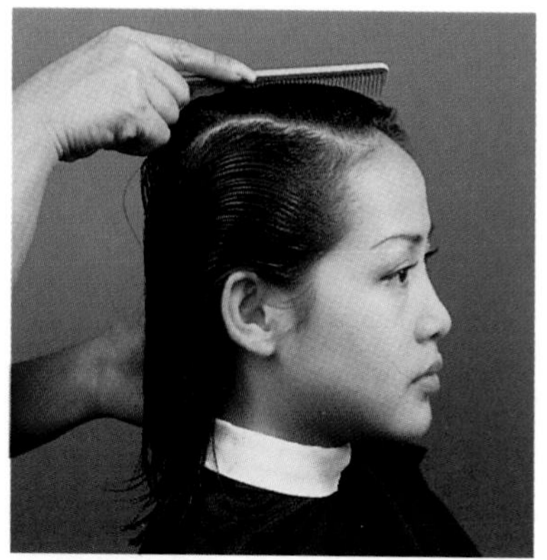

FIGURE 9.8 — Combing hair from part.

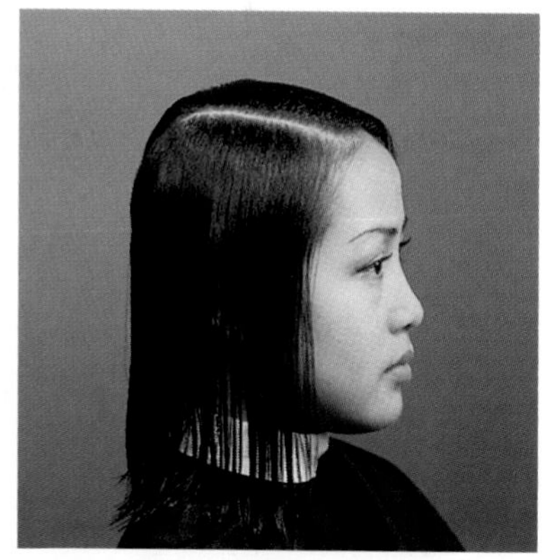

FIGURE 9.9 — Completed side part.

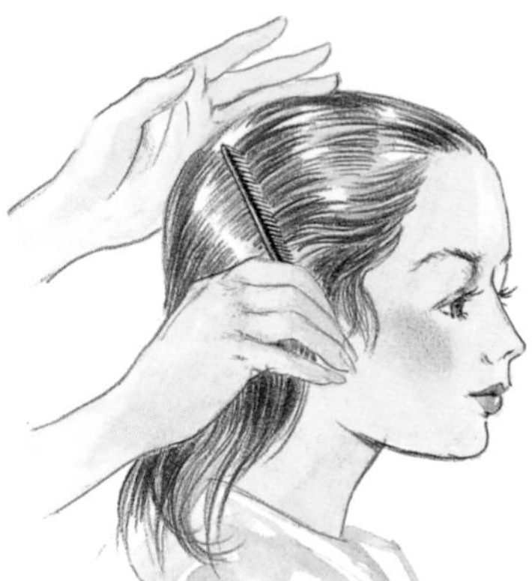

FIGURE 9.10 — Combing hair back.

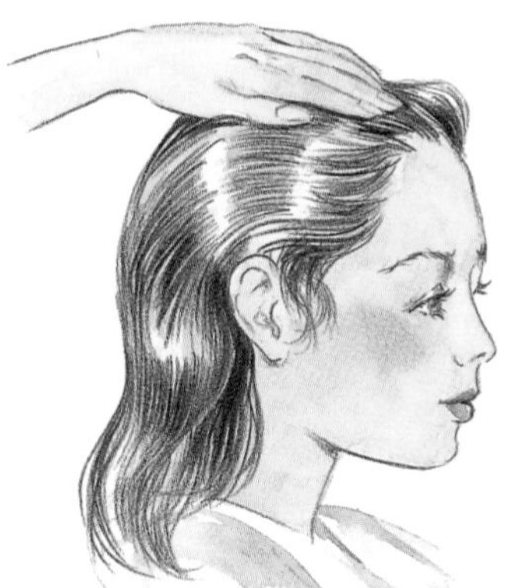

FIGURE 9.11 — Pushing hair forward.

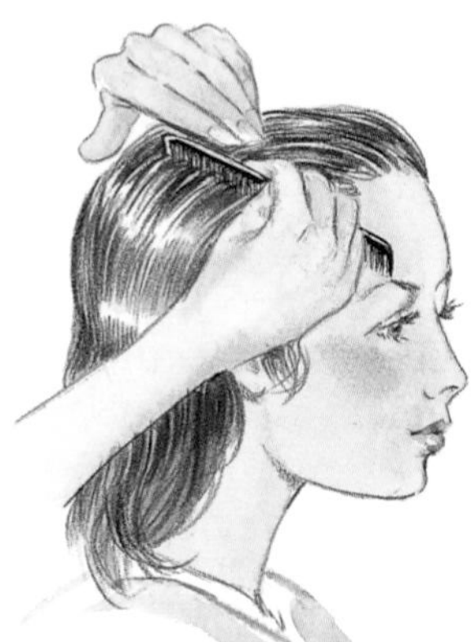

FIGURE 9.12 — Natural part.

FINGER WAVING

Finger waving is the art of shaping and directing the hair into alternate parallel waves and designs using the fingers, comb, waving lotion, and hairpins or clippies.

You may wonder why you are learning a technique that is not frequently requested by many clients anymore. Training in finger waving is important because it teaches you the technique of moving and directing hair. It also helps you develop the dexterity, coordination, and finger strength required for professional hairstyling. In addition, it provides valuable training in creating hairstyles and in molding hair to the curved surface of the head. It is an excellent introduction to hairstyling.

Completed:
Learning Objective
#1
PURPOSE OF FINGER WAVING

PREPARATION

Always wash your hands before giving your client any salon service. Make sure all necessary implements have been sanitized and towels and other supplies are clean and fresh. Prepare the client in the same manner as you would for a shampoo.

FINGER WAVING LOTION

Waving lotion makes the hair pliable and keeps it in place during the finger waving procedure.

Waving lotion is made from karaya gum, which is found in trees of Africa and India. This gum can be diluted to a thin, watery consistency, generally for use on fine hair, or its consistency can be more concentrated for use on regular or coarse hair. A good waving lotion is harmless to the hair and does not flake when it dries.

APPLICATION OF LOTION

Part the hair down to the scalp, comb smooth, and arrange it to conform to the planned style. The hair will move more easily if you use the coarse teeth of the comb. Follow the natural growth pattern when combing and parting the hair. You will find the hair easier to mold, and it will not buckle or separate in the crown area.

Apply waving lotion to the hair while it is damp. Use an applicator to apply the lotion and a comb to distribute it through the hair. Do not use an excessive amount of waving lotion.

Note: *Apply lotion to one side of the head at a time; this prevents it from drying and requiring additional applications.*

HORIZONTAL FINGER WAVING

The finger wave may be started on either side of the head. However, in this presentation, the hair is parted on the left side of the head and the wave is started on the right (heavy) side of the head.

Right Side of the Head

Using the index finger of your left hand as a guide, shape the top hair with a comb, using a circular movement. Starting at the hairline, work toward the crown in 1½" to 2" (3.7 to 5 cm) sections at a time until the crown has been reached. (Fig.9.13)

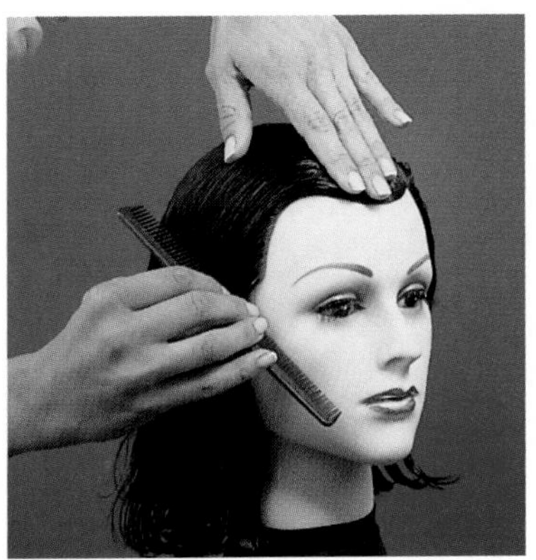

FIGURE 9.13 — Shape top area.

Forming the First Ridge

1. Place the index finger of the left hand directly above the position for the first ridge. With the teeth of the comb pointing slightly upward, insert the comb directly under the index finger. Draw the comb forward about 1" (2.5 cm) along the fingertip. (Fig. 9.14)

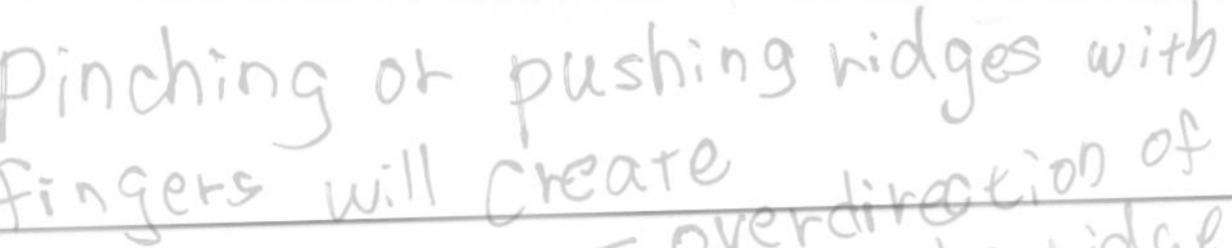
Pinching or pushing ridges with
fingers will create
= overdirection of
the ridge

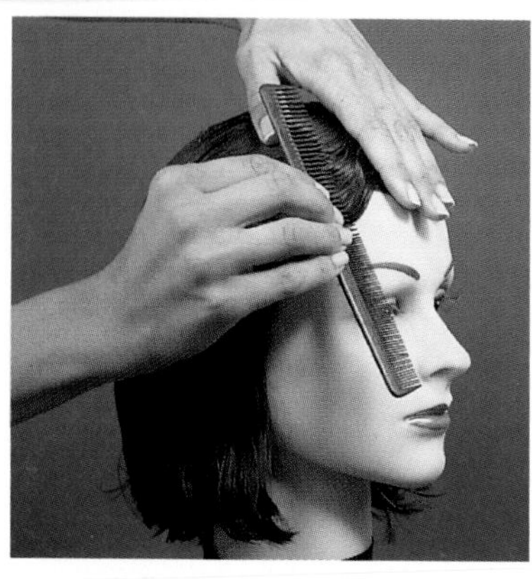

FIGURE 9.14 — Draw hair about 1″ (2.5 cm.) toward fingertip.

2. With the teeth still inserted in the ridge, flatten the comb against the head in order to hold the ridge in place. (Fig. 9.15)
3. Remove the left hand from the head and place the middle finger above the ridge and the index finger on the teeth of the comb. Emphasize the ridge by closing the two fingers and applying pressure to the head. (Fig. 9.16)

Note: Do not try to increase the height or depth of a ridge by pinching or pushing with fingers; such movements will create overdirection of the ridge.

4. Without removing the comb, turn the teeth downward, and comb the hair in a right semicircular direction to form a dip in the hollow part of the wave. (Fig. 9.17)

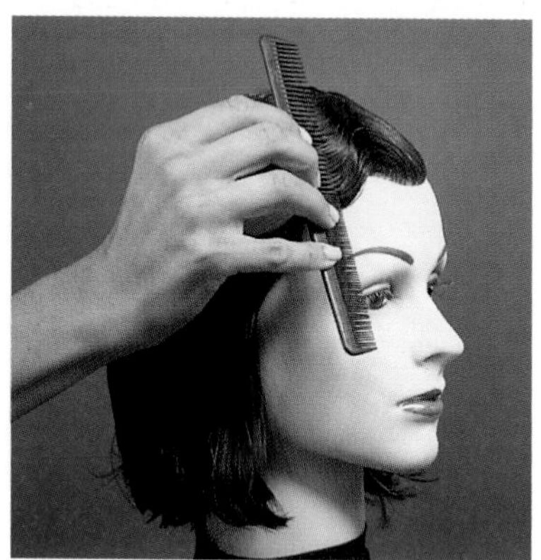

FIGURE 9.15 — Flatten comb against head.

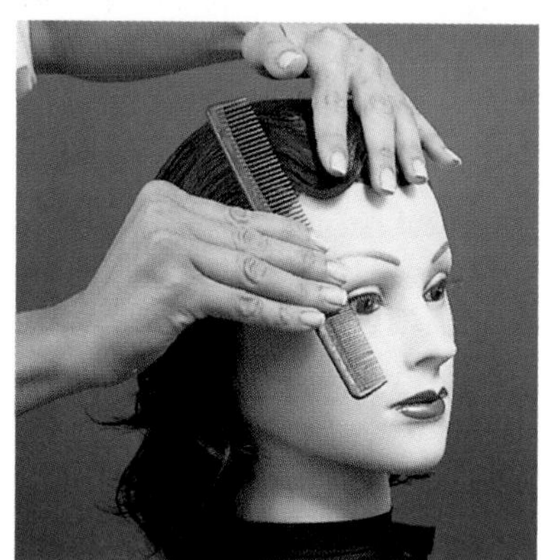

FIGURE 9.16 — Emphasize ridge.

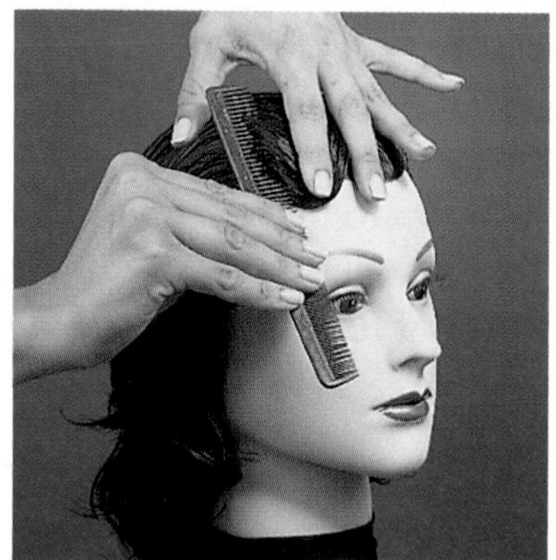

FIGURE 9.17 — Comb hair in semicircular direction.

5. Follow this procedure, section by section, until the crown has been reached, where the ridge phases out. (Fig. 9.18) The ridge and wave of each section should match evenly, without showing separations in the ridge and hollow part of the wave.

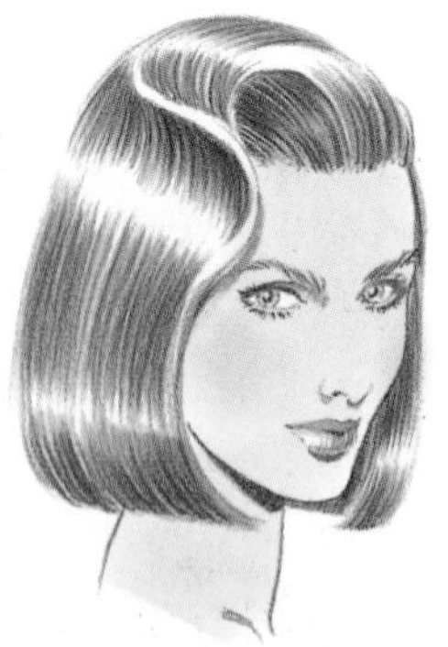

FIGURE 9.18 — Complete first ridge at the crown.

Forming the Second Ridge

Begin at the crown area. (Fig. 9.19) The movements are the reverse of those followed in forming the first ridge. The comb is drawn from the tip of the index finger toward the base of the index finger, thus directing formation of the second ridge. All movements are followed in a reverse pattern until the hairline is reached, thus completing the second ridge. (Fig. 9.20)

Forming the Third Ridge

Movements for the third ridge closely follow those used in creating the first ridge. However, the third ridge is started at the hairline and extended back toward the back of the head. (Fig. 9.21)

Continue alternating directions until the side of the head has been completed. (Fig. 9.22)

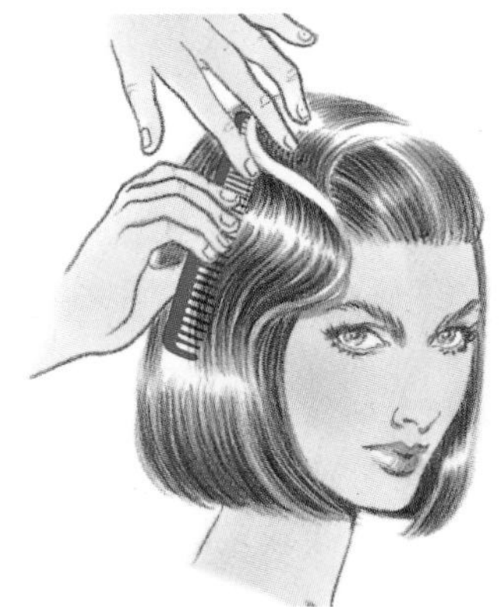

FIGURE 9.19 — Start the second ridge.

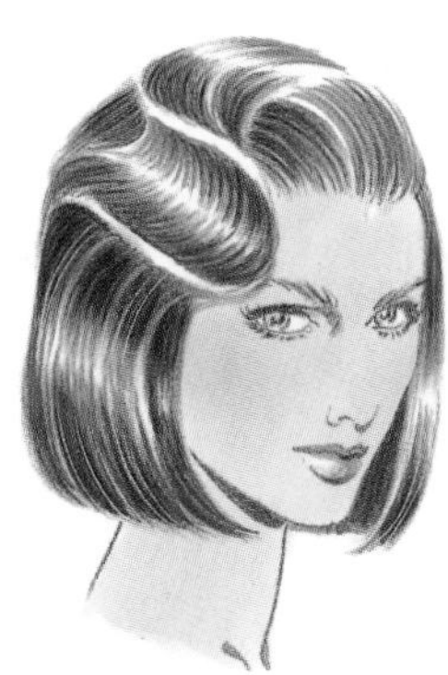

FIGURE 9.20 — Complete second ridge.

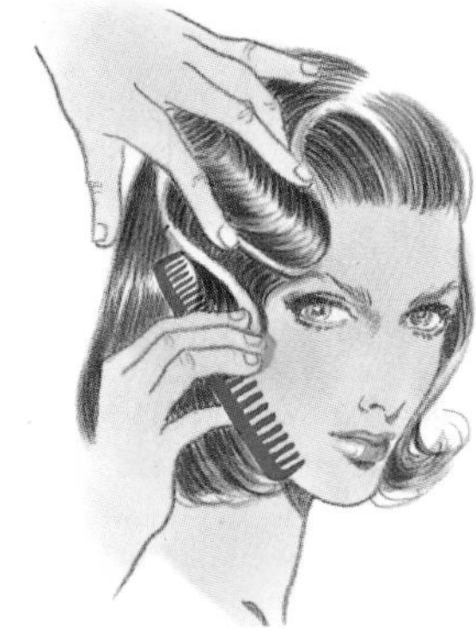

FIGURE 9.21 — Start the third ridge.

Left Side of the Head

Use the same procedure for the left (light) side of the head as you used for finger waving the right (heavy) side of the head.

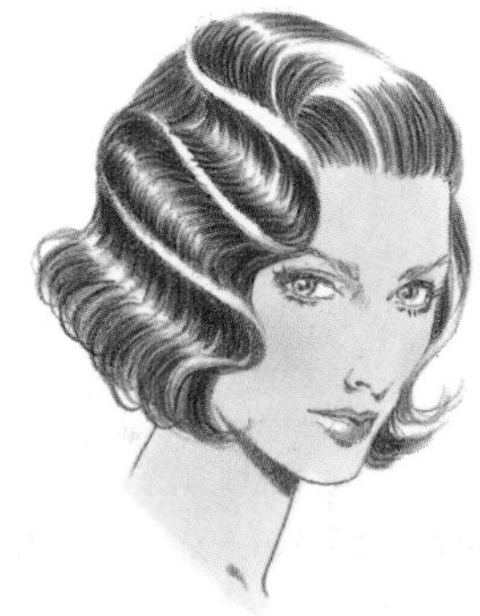

FIGURE 9.22 — Complete right side.

Procedure

1. Shape the hair. (Fig. 9.23)
2. Starting at the hairline, form the first ridge, section by section, until the second ridge of the opposite side is reached. (Fig. 9.24)
3. Both the ridge and the wave must blend without splits or breaks, with the ridge and wave on the right side of the head. (Fig. 9.25)

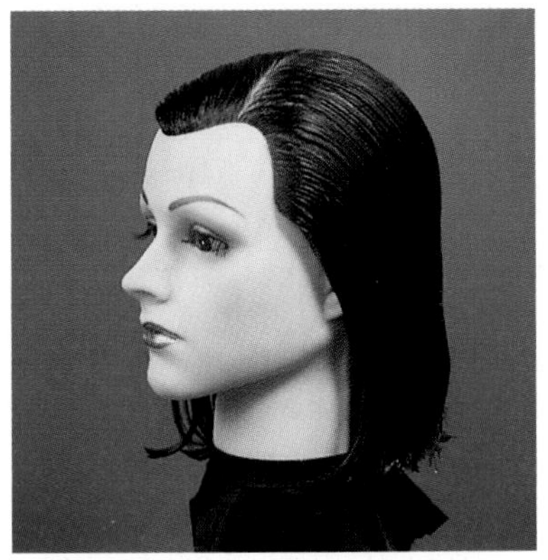

FIGURE 9.23 — Shape left side.

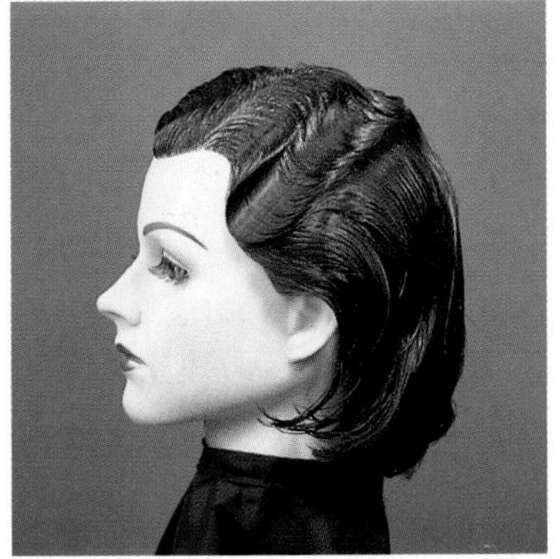

FIGURE 9.24 — First ridge starts at hairline.

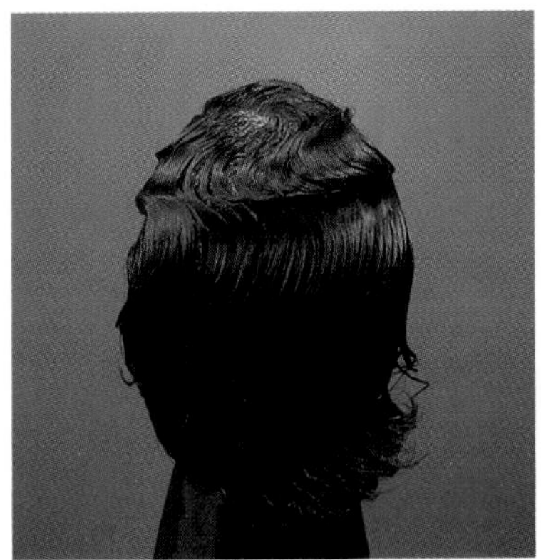

FIGURE 9.25 — Ridge and wave matched in crown area.

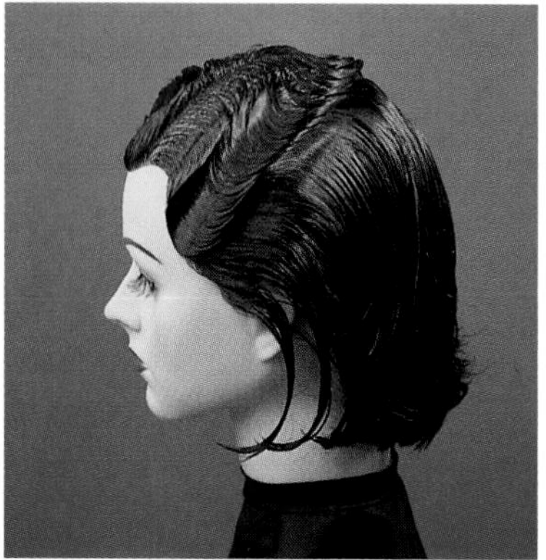

FIGURE 9.26 — Left side completed.

4. Start with the ridge and wave in the back of the head and proceed, section by section, toward the left side of the face.
5. Continue working back and forth until the entire side is completed. (Fig. 9.26)
6. Figures 9.27–9.30 illustrate the completed hairstyles.

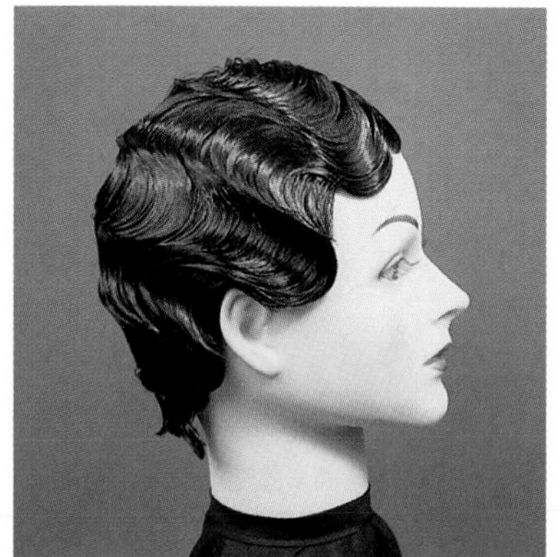

FIGURE 9.27 — Completed hairstyle, right side.

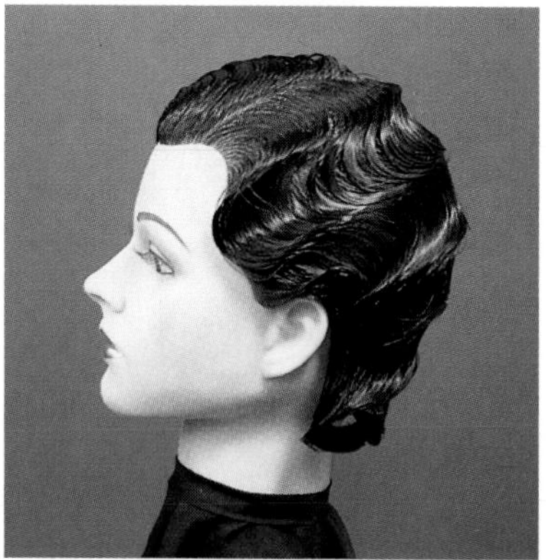

FIGURE 9.28 — Completed hairstyle, left side.

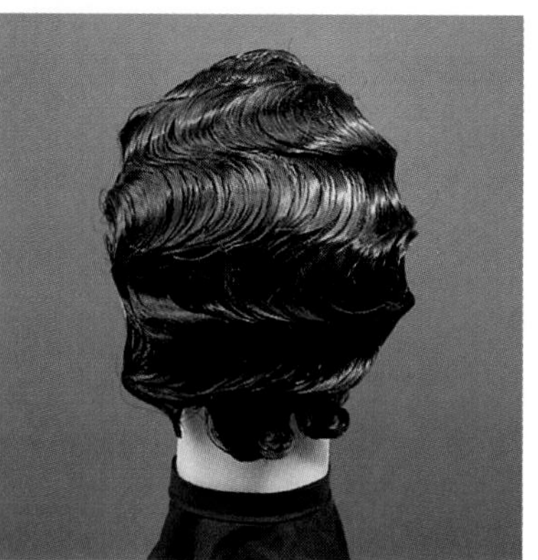

FIGURE 9.29 — Completed hairstyle, back view.

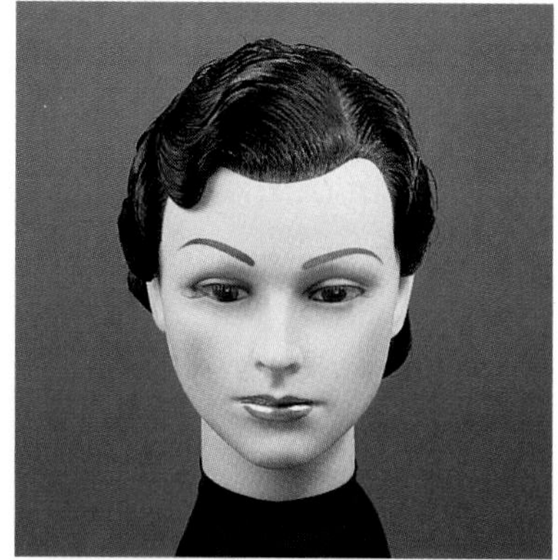

FIGURE 9.30 — Completed hairstyle, frontal view.

Completion

1. Place net over hair, secure with hairpins or clippies if needed, and safeguard the client's forehead and ears while under the dryer with cotton, gauze, or paper protectors.
2. Adjust the dryer to medium heat and allow hair to dry thoroughly.
3. Remove client from under dryer.

4. Remove clippies or pins and hairnet from hair.
5. Comb out and reset waves into a soft coiffure.
6. Sanitize combs, hairpins, clippies, and hairnet after each use.
7. Lightly spraying the hair with lacquer will hold the finger wave longer and give the hair a sheen.

ALTERNATE METHOD OF FINGER WAVING

Hair parted on left side. The following is an alternate method to perform finger waving:

1. Shape the top right (heavy) side.
2. Phase out the first ridge starting at the front ***right*** side, and working around to the crown.
3. Start a ridge on the ***left*** front side and go all around the head, finishing on the front right hairline. (Fig. 9.31)
4. Start another ridge on the front right hairline and finish on the left front side. Continue, left to right and right to left, until the entire head is completed.

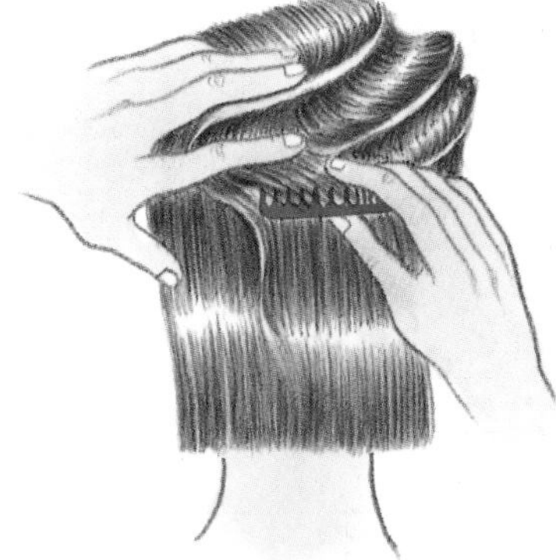

FIGURE 9.31 — Finger waving around the head.

This method eliminates the need to match ridges and waves at the back of the head. (Completion is the same as it is for the horizontal method of finger waving.)

VERTICAL FINGER WAVING

In vertical finger waving, the ridges and waves run up and down the head, while in horizontal finger waving they go parallel around the head.

The procedure for making vertical ridges and waves is the same as it is for horizontal finger waving.

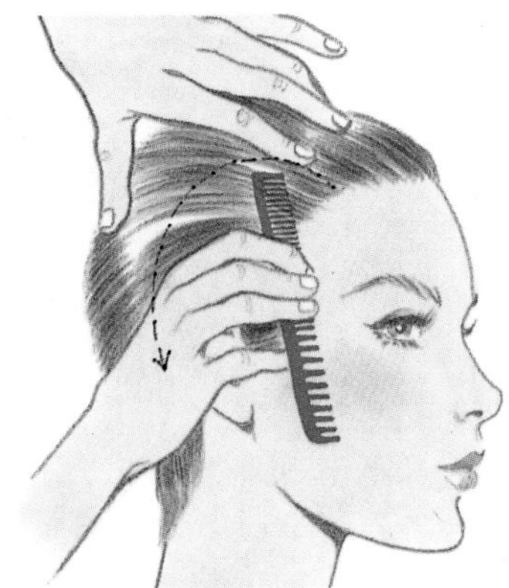

FIGURE 9.32 — Form shaping.

1. Make side part, extending from forehead to crown.
2. Form shaping in a semicircular effect. (Figs. 9.32, 9.33)
3. Make first section of ridge and wave. (See Fig. 9.34)
4. Continue with additional sections until the part is reached.

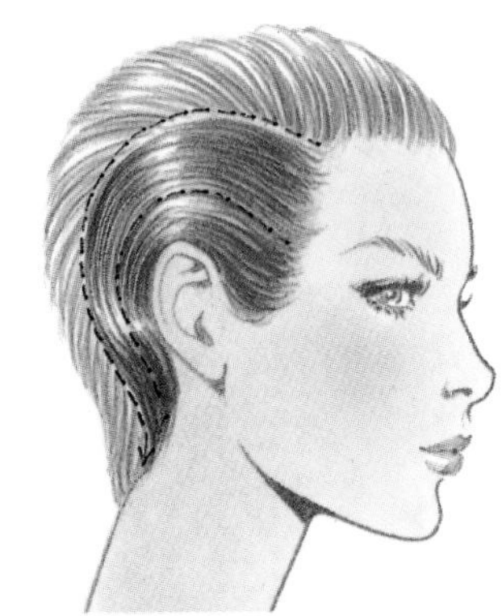

FIGURE 9.33 — First section of wave.

Start the second ridge at the hair part. Start the third ridge at the hairline. Complete side. (Fig. 9.35) (Completion is the same as it is for horizontal finger waving.)

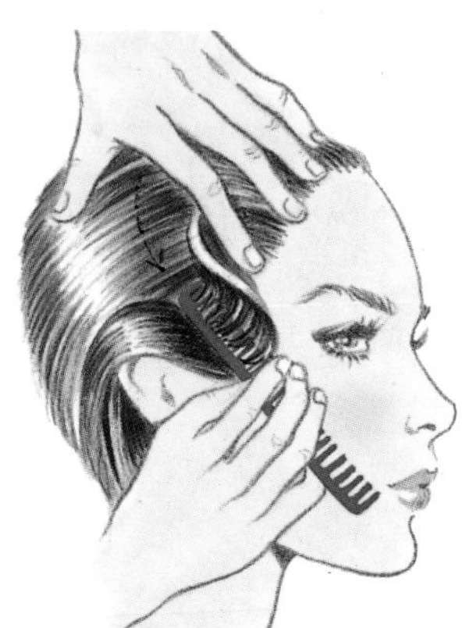

FIGURE 9.34 — Start first wave.

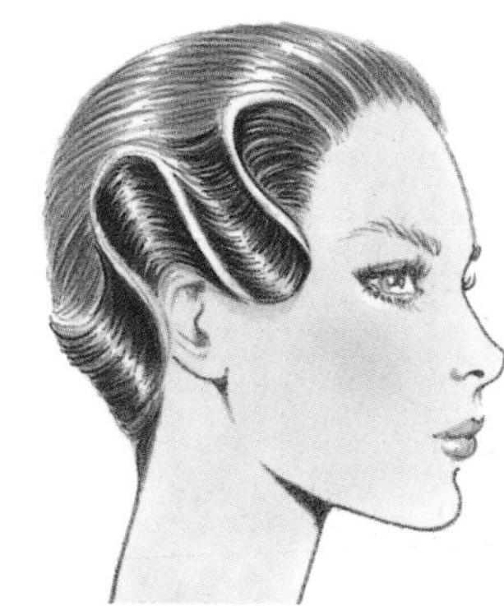

FIGURE 9.35 — Completed finger wave.

SHADOW WAVE

A shadow wave is a shallow wave with low ridges that are not very sharp. The waves are formed in the regular manner, but the comb does not penetrate to the scalp. The hair layers underneath are not waved. This type of wave is sometimes desirable for a client who wishes to dress her hair very close to the head.

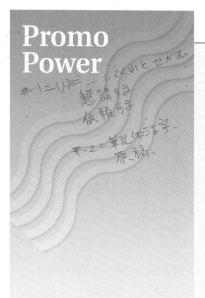

TELEMARKETING

Telemarketing can be done from within your salon anytime someone is available to spend time talking on the phone with your clients—or you can hire an outside person to do telephone soliciting for you. Either way, this kind of advertising has its advantages: It's a personal, one-on-one communication and you get instant results.

To use telemarketing effectively you must be clear about what you want to accomplish. You may want to ask a new client how the service was, how the style was, whether he or she is planning to return. This type of information can be solicited easily by a staff member.

If you're trying to mass-market your salon, you'll want to hire a telemarketing company. You must tell them what you're promoting and give them a script to use. You may want to do a survey on why customers have not returned to your salon or whether your services are satisfactory.

Telemarketing can be very beneficial, but you must have computerized telephone lists in order to do it efficiently. Keep careful records on your own clients. If you are looking for new customers, you can buy telephone lists categorized according to lifestyle, income, or geographical area. Make sure you market to people who would fit in with your type of salon.

—*From* The Salon Biz: Tips for Success *by Geri Mataya*

PIN CURLS

Pin curls provide the bases for patterns, lines, waves, curls, and rolls that you use as you create hairstyles. You can use them on straight, permanent-waved, or naturally curly hair. Pin curls work best if the hair is properly tapered and wound smoothly. This makes springy and long-lasting curls with good direction and definition. Pin curls are not usually used on overly curly hair.

PARTS OF A CURL

Pin curls are constructed of three principal parts: *base, stem,* and *circle.* (Fig. 9.36)

1. The ***base*** is the stationary, or immovable, foundation of the curl, which is attached to the scalp.
2. The ***stem*** is the section of the pin curl, between the base and first arc (turn) of the circle, which gives the circle its direction and mobility.
3. The ***circle*** is the part of the pin curl that forms a complete circle. The size of the circle governs the width of the wave and its strength.

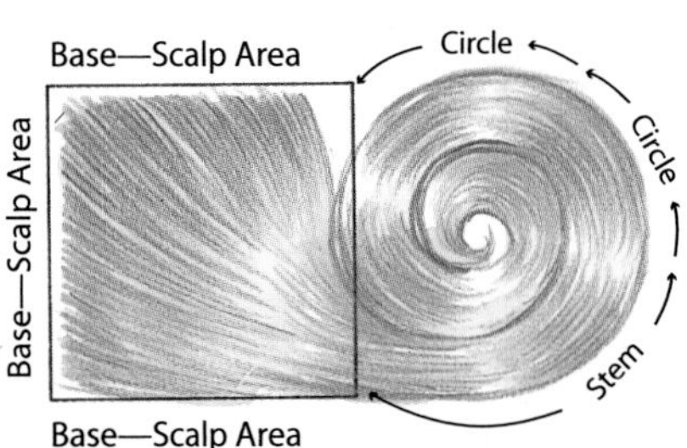

FIGURE 9.36 — Parts of a curl.

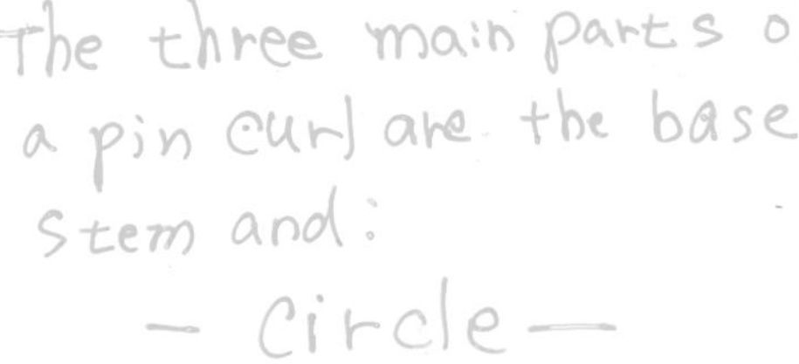

MOBILITY OF A CURL

The amount of movement (mobility) of a section of hair is determined by the *stem.* Curl mobility is classified as *no-stem, half-stem,* and *full-stem.*

1. The ***no-stem curl*** is placed directly on the base of the curl. It produces a tight, firm, long-lasting curl. (Fig. 9.37)

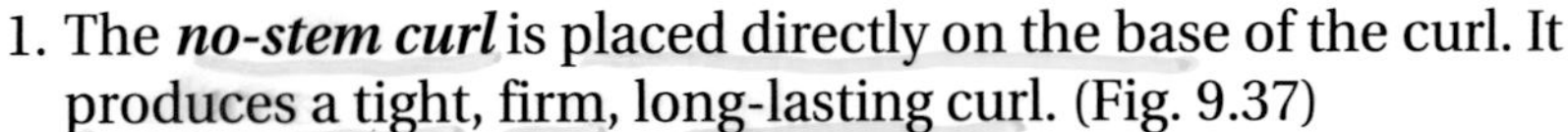

2. The ***half-stem curl*** permits more freedom, since the curl (circle) is placed one-half off the base. It gives good *control* to the hair. (Fig. 9.38)
3. The ***full-stem curl*** allows for the greatest mobility. The curl is placed completely off the base. The base may be a square, triangular, half-moon, or rectangular section depending on the area of the head in which the full-stem curls are used. It gives as much freedom as the length of the stem will permit. If it is exaggerated, the hair near the scalp will be flat and almost straight. It is used to give the hair a strong, definite direction. (Fig. 9.39)

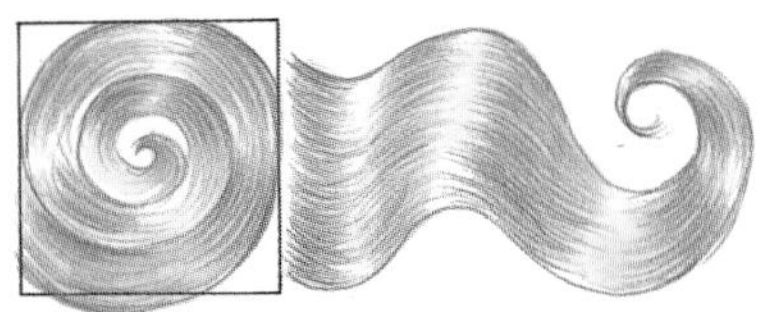

FIGURE 9.37 — No-stem curl opened out.

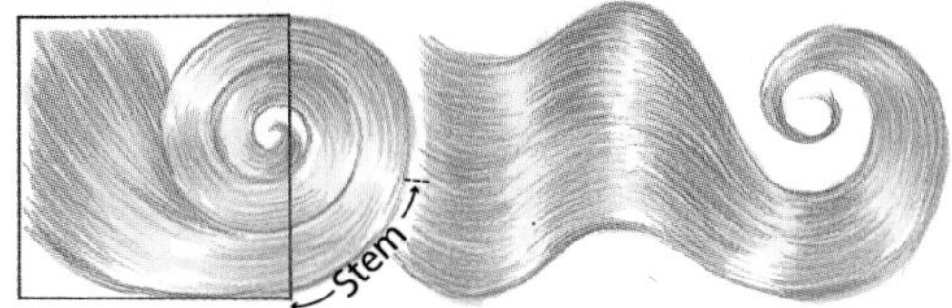

FIGURE 9.38 — Half-stem curl opened out.

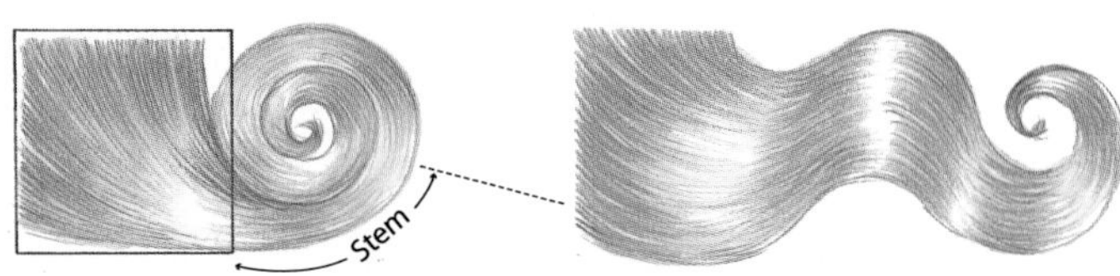

FIGURE 9.39 — Full-stem curl opened out.

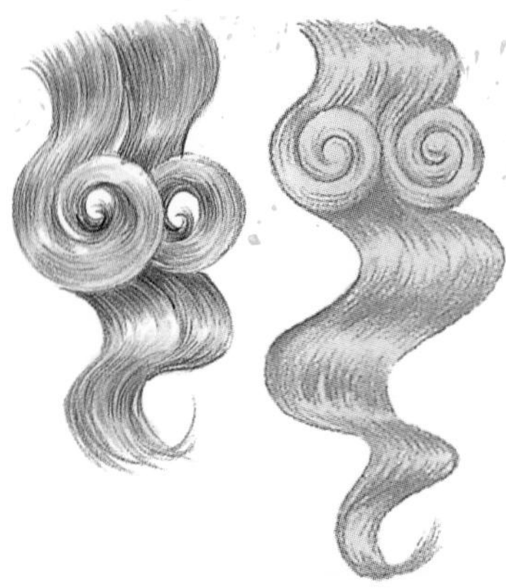

FIGURE 9.40 — Curl with open center.

FIGURE 9.41 — Curl with closed center.

OPEN AND CLOSED CENTER CURLS

Open center curls produce even, smooth waves and uniform curls. ***Closed center curls*** produce waves that decrease in size toward the end. They are good for fine hair or if a fluffy curl is desired. Notice the difference in the waves produced by pin curls with open centers and those with closed centers. The size of the curl determines the size of the wave. If you make pin curls with the ends outside the curl, the resulting wave will be narrower near the scalp and wider toward the ends. (Figs. 9.40, 9.41)

CURL AND STEM DIRECTION

Curls may be turned toward the face, away from the face, upward, downward, or diagonally. You determine what the finished result will be by the direction in which you place the stem of the curl. Curl and stem direction is referred to as:

1. ***Forward movement***—toward the face.
2. ***Reverse movement***—backward or away from the face. (Figs. 9.42–9.45)

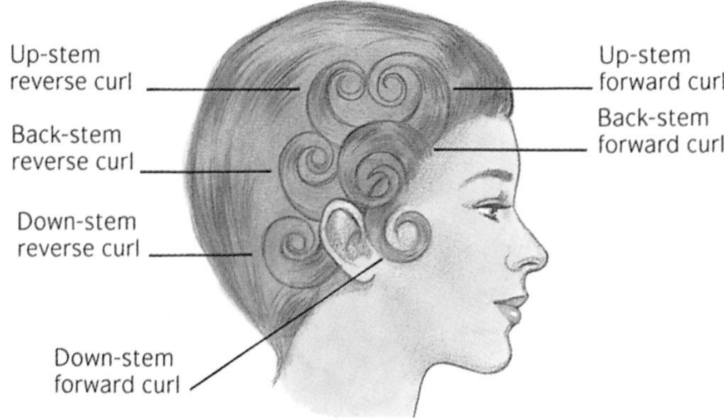

FIGURE 9.42 — Forward movement.

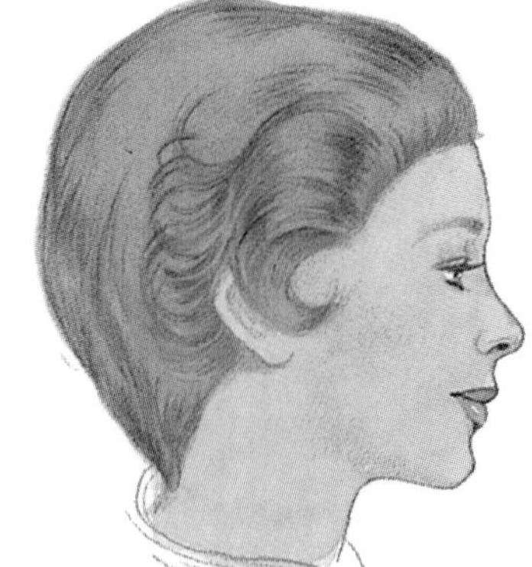

FIGURE 9.43 — Comb-out.

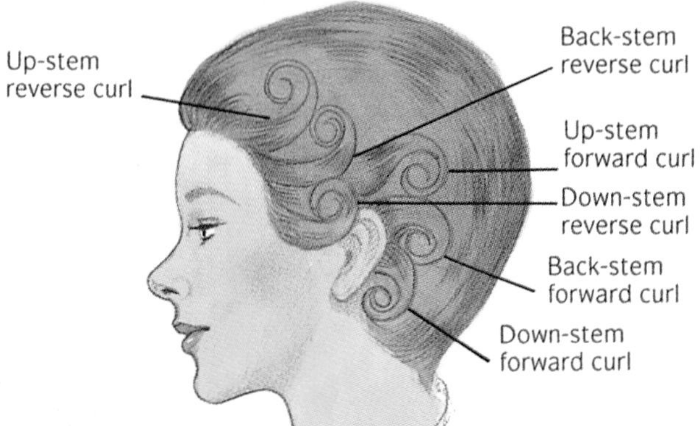

FIGURE 9.44 — Backward movement.

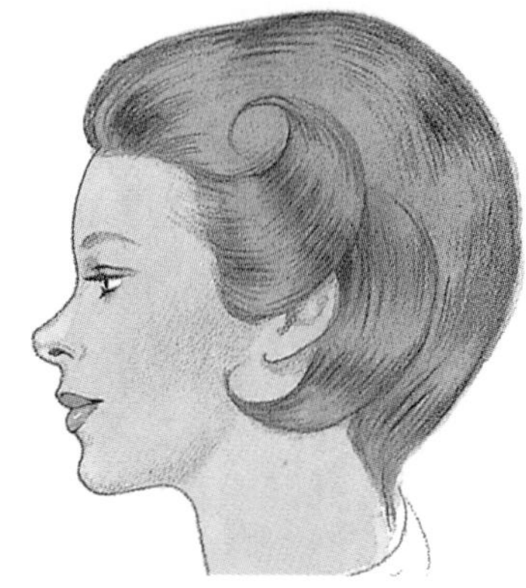

FIGURE 9.45 — Comb-out.

3. ***Upward movement***—toward the top of the head.
4. ***Downward movement***—toward the bottom of the head.

The forward or reverse movements work with up or down movements to create interesting directions in a hairstyle.

These illustrations are intended to show stem directions and curl placements and are not illustrations of pin curl patterns.

CLOCKWISE AND COUNTERCLOCKWISE CURLS

The terms ***clockwise curls*** and ***counterclockwise curls*** are used to describe the direction of pin curls. Curls formed in the same direction as the movement of the hands of a clock are known as clockwise curls. Curls formed in the opposite direction of the movement of the hands of a clock are known as counterclockwise curls. (Figs. 9.46, 9.47)

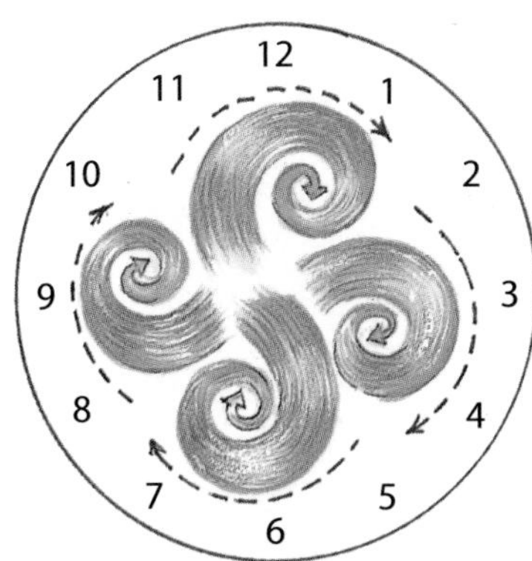

FIGURE 9.46 — Clockwise curls.

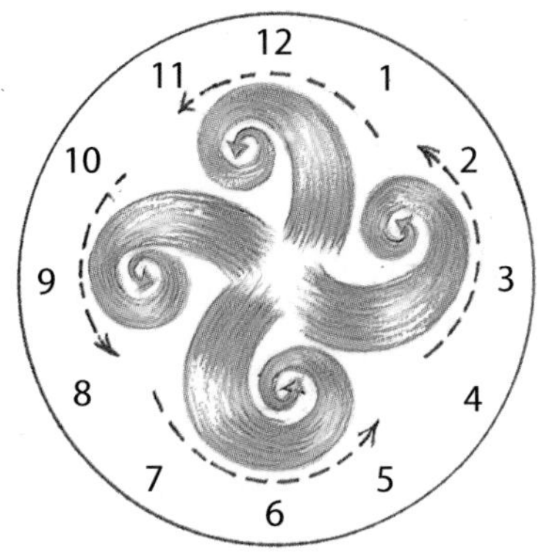

FIGURE 9.47 — Counterclockwise curls.

Sometimes the hands of the clock are used to describe the direction of the stem. In an "eight o'clock pin curl," for example, the stem would point from its base to eight o'clock. (Figs. 9.48–9.50)

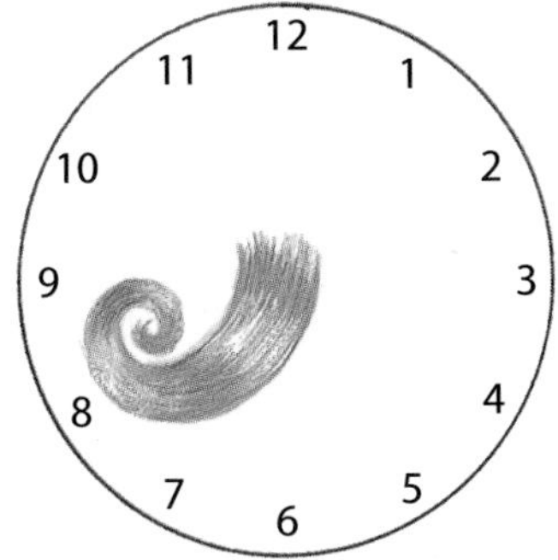

FIGURE 9.48 — 8 o'clock curl.

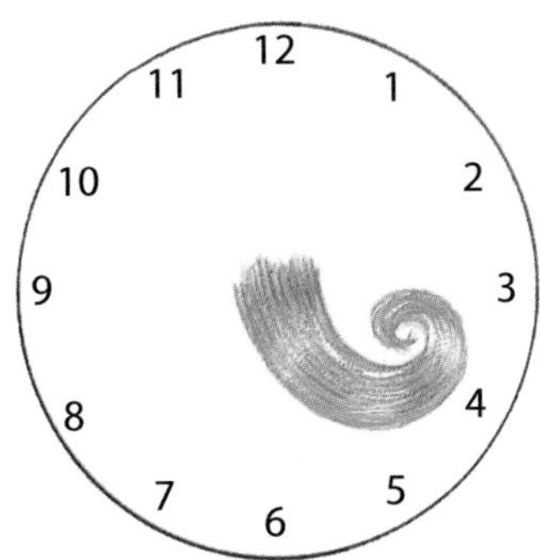

FIGURE 9.49 — 4 o'clock curl.

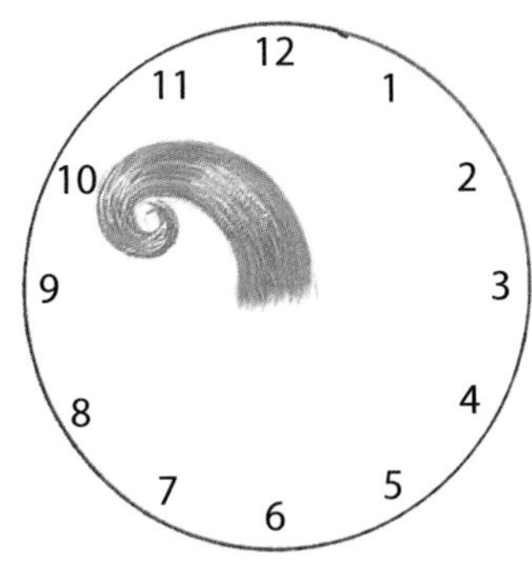

FIGURE 9.50 — 10 o'clock curl.

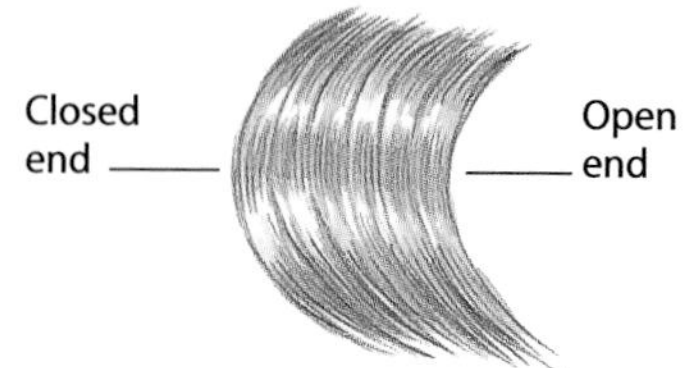

FIGURE 9.51a — Open and closed ends of curl.

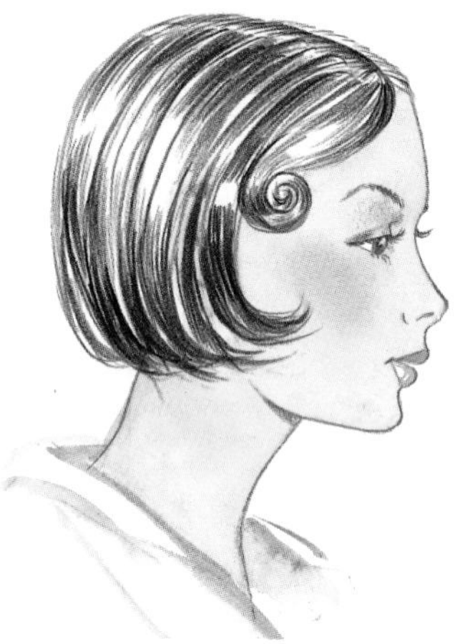

FIGURE 9.51b — Curl in the shaping.

SHAPING FOR PIN CURL PLACEMENTS

A ***shaping*** is a section of hair that you mold into a design to serve as a base for a curl or wave pattern.

Shapings are classified as forward and reverse; diagonal, vertical, or horizontal; oblong or circular.

All shapings have an open end and a closed end. Always begin a pin curl at the open end, or convex side, of a shaping. (Figs. 9.51a, 9.51b)

Circular shapings are pie-shaped with the open end smaller than the closed end. They work well as the first forward shaping in a hairstyle that moves away from the face. In a wave pattern, the forward circular shaping would be followed by a reverse circular curl.

Oblong shapings are waves that remain the same width throughout the shaping.

Forward shapings are directed toward the face. This type of shaping is *oval* (larger in size at its closed end).

Procedure

1. To make a forward, vertical shaping on the side of the head, direct the hair in a circular motion, moving back from the face, upward, then downward and toward the face. The size of the shaping determines the resulting hairstyle. (Figs. 9.52, 9.53)

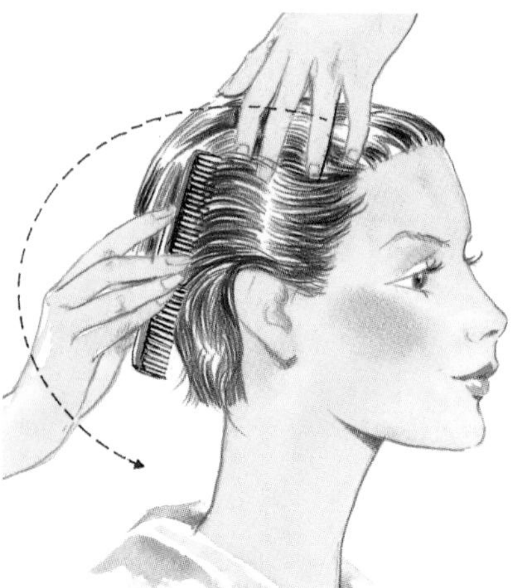

FIGURE 9.52 — Forming side forward vertical shaping.

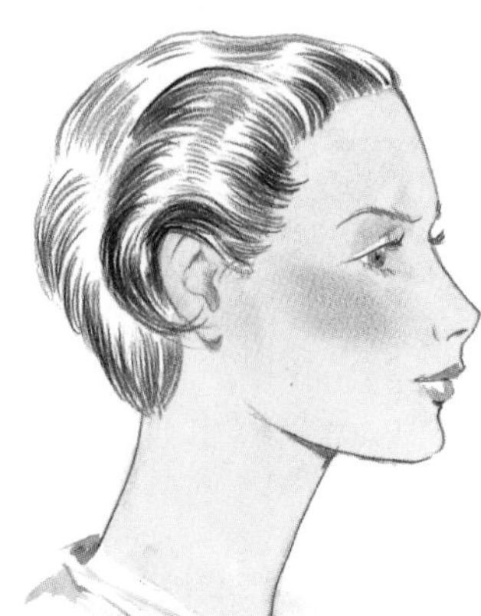

FIGURE 9.53 — Finished side forward vertical shaping.

2. To make a top forward shaping, comb-direct the hair in a circular motion, away from the forehead, pivoting the comb to create a circular effect toward the face. (Figs. 9.54, 9.55)

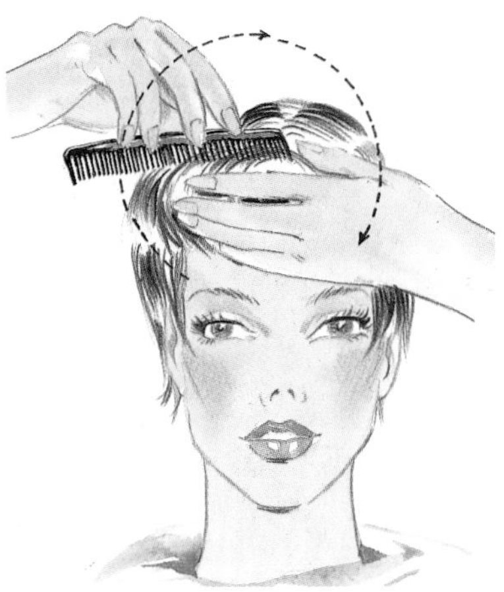

FIGURE 9.54 — Forming oval shaping for top forward movement.

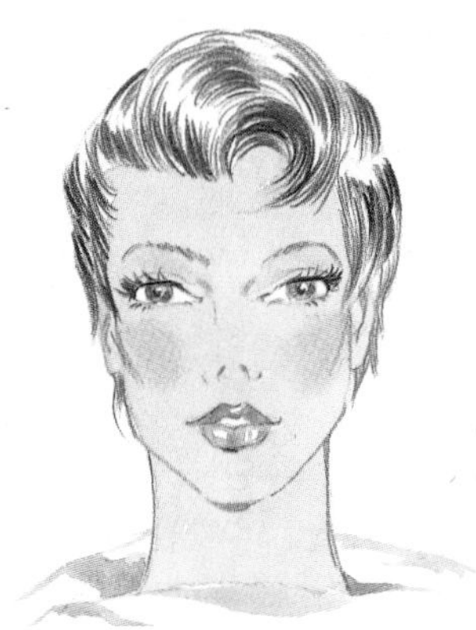

FIGURE 9.55 — Finished oval shaping for top forward movement.

Reverse shapings are comb-directed downward, then immediately upward in a circular motion, away from the face. (Figs. 9.56, 9.57)

Diagonal shapings are variations of the forward shaping with the exception that the shaping is formed diagonally to the side of the head. (Fig. 9.58)

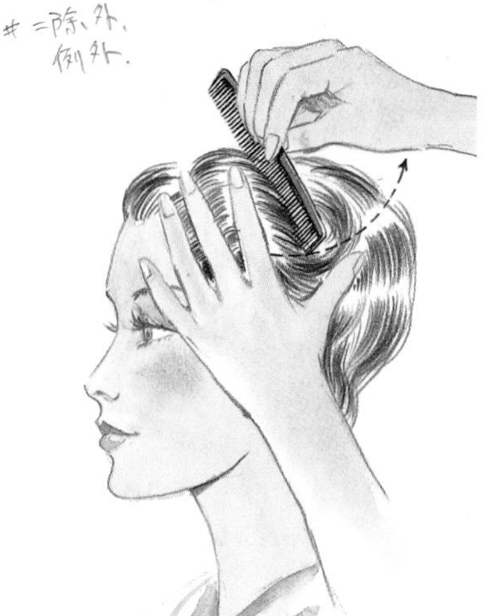

FIGURE 9.56 — Forming left side reverse vertical shaping.

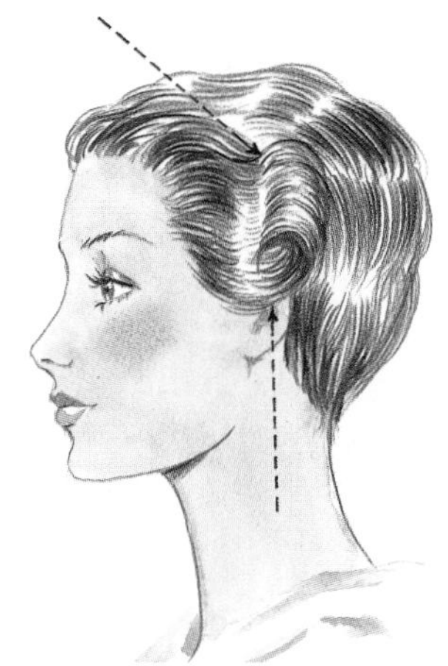

FIGURE 9.57 — Finished left side reverse vertical shaping.

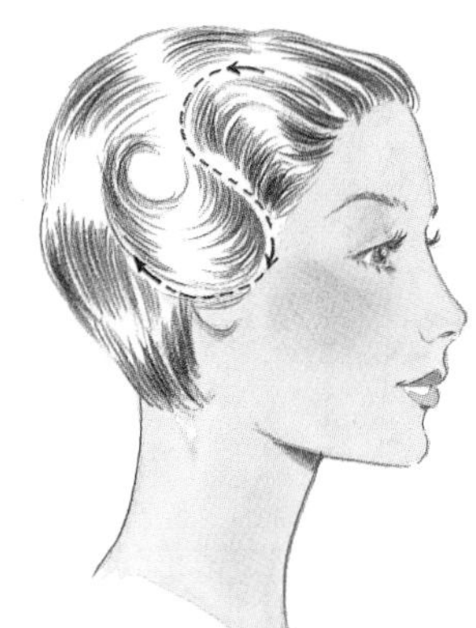

FIGURE 9.58 — Diagonal shaping.

Vertical side shapings are directed in a way that places the open and closed ends in a vertical fashion.

Horizontal shapings are comb-directed parallel with the part. They are recommended for pin curl parallel construction and where a wave design is carried completely around the head. (Figs. 9.59, 9.60)

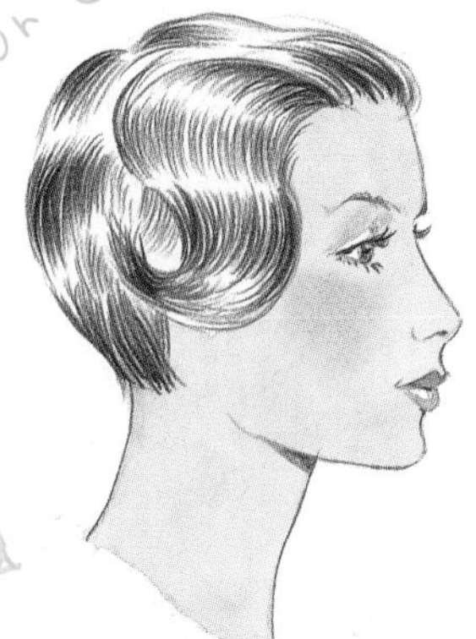

FIGURE 9.59 — Right side horizontal shaping.

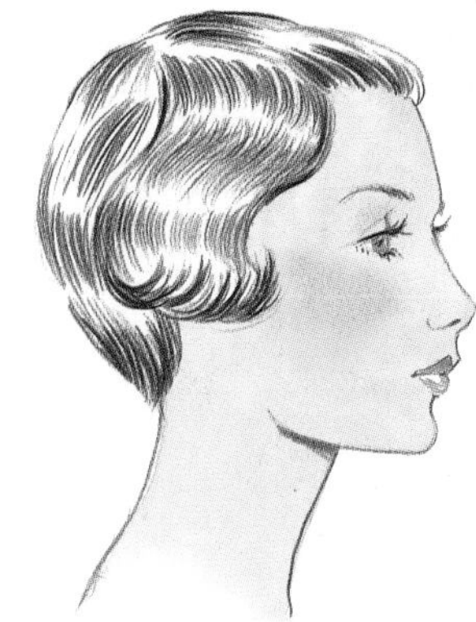

FIGURE 9.60 — Right side reverse horizontal shaping.

PIN CURL FOUNDATIONS OR BASES

Before you begin to make your pin curls, divide the hair into sections or panels. Then you are ready to subdivide the sections into the type of foundations or bases required for the various curls. The most commonly shaped bases you will use are rectangular, triangular, arc (half-moon or C-shape), and square.

To avoid splits in the finished hairstyle, you must use care when selecting and forming the curl base. Further uniformity of curl development can only be achieved if the sections of hair are as equal as possible. Each curl must lie flat and smooth on its base. If extended too far off the base you will get just direction with a loose curl away from the scalp. The finished curl, however, is not affected by the shape of the base.

Rectangular base pin curls are usually recommended at the side front hairline for a smooth upsweep effect. To avoid splits in the comb-out, the pin curls must overlap. (Fig. 9.61)

Triangular base pin curls are recommended along the front or facial hairline to prevent breaks or splits in the finished hairstyle. The triangular base allows a portion of the hair from each curl to overlap the next and comb into a uniform wave without splits. (Fig. 9.62)

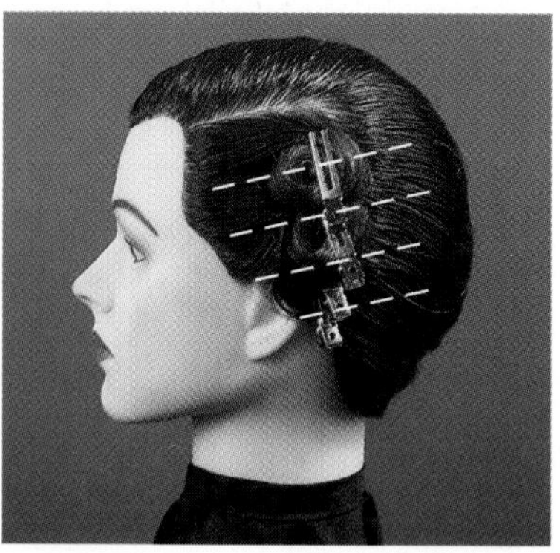

FIGURE 9.61 — Rectangular base.

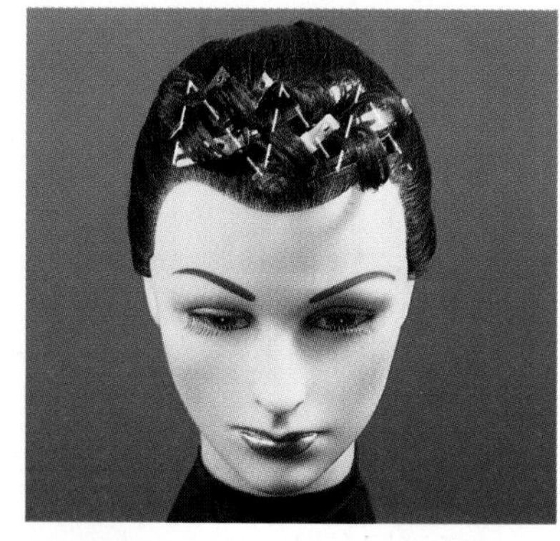

FIGURE 9.62 — Triangular base.

Arc base, also known as half-moon or C-shape base, pin curls are carved out of a shaping. Arc base pin curls give good direction and may be used at the hairline or in the nape. (Figs. 9.63a, 9.63b)

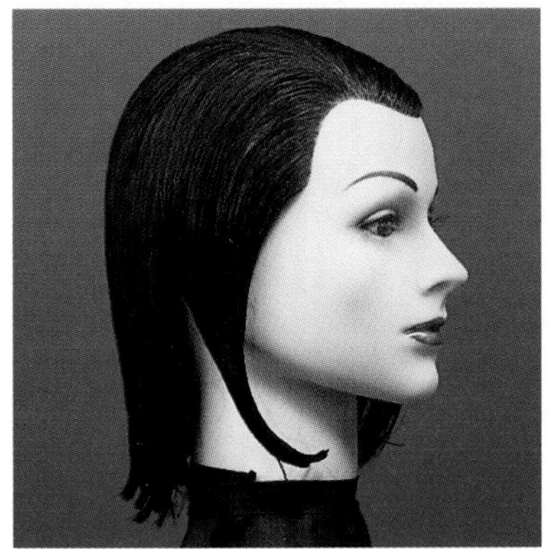

FIGURE 9.63a — Arc base, side view.

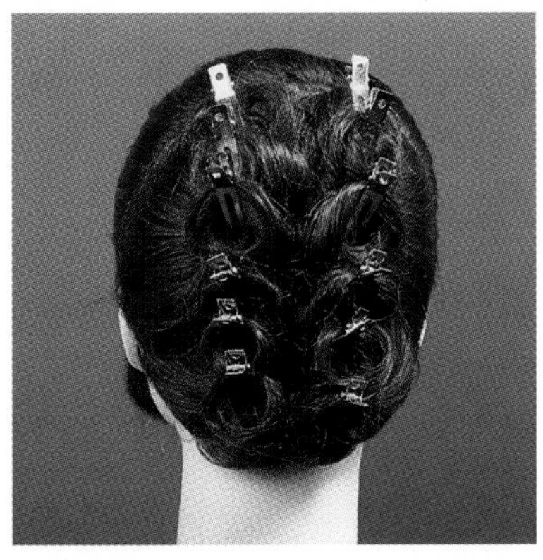

FIGURE 9.63b — Arc base, back of head.

Square base pin curls are used for even construction suitable for curly hairstyles without much volume or lift. They can be used on any part of the head and will comb out with lasting results. To avoid splits in the comb-out, stagger the sectioning as shown in the illustration (square base, brick-lay fashion). (Fig. 9.64)

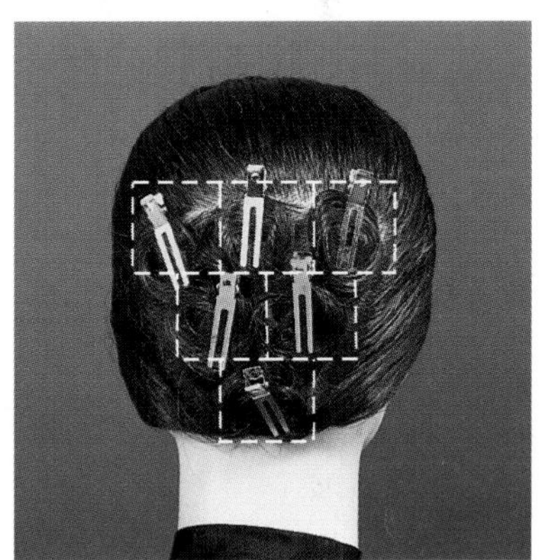

FIGURE 9.64 — Square base.

PIN CURL TECHNIQUES

You will learn to make pin curls several ways. We illustrate several methods of forming pin curls. Your instructor might demonstrate other methods that are equally correct.

Carved Curls or Sculptured Curls

Pin curls, carved out of a shaping without disturbing the shaping, are usually referred to as ***carved curls.*** You can form these curls on either the right side or the left side of the head.

Forming Pin Curls on the Right Side

1. Wet hair thoroughly with water or setting lotion.
2. Comb smoothly and form shaping. (Fig. 9.65)
3. Start making curls at the open end of the shaping.
4. Slice strand for first curl. (Fig. 9.66) Point your left index finger down and hold the strand in place.
5. ***Ribbon*** the strand by forcing it through the comb while applying pressure with the thumb on the back of comb to create tension. (Figs. 9.67, 9.68) *Or* ribbon hair by pulling the strand with pressure between your thumb and index finger out to the end.

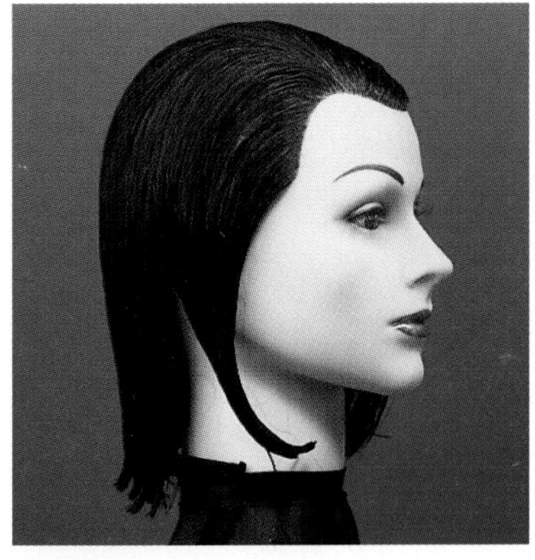

FIGURE 9.65 — Shaping.

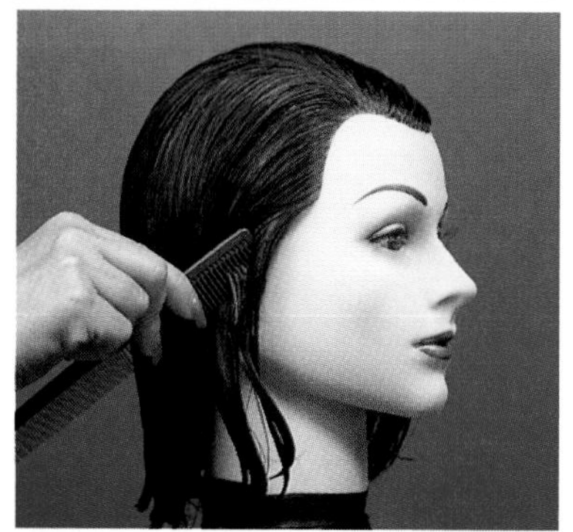

FIGURE 9.66 — Slicing.

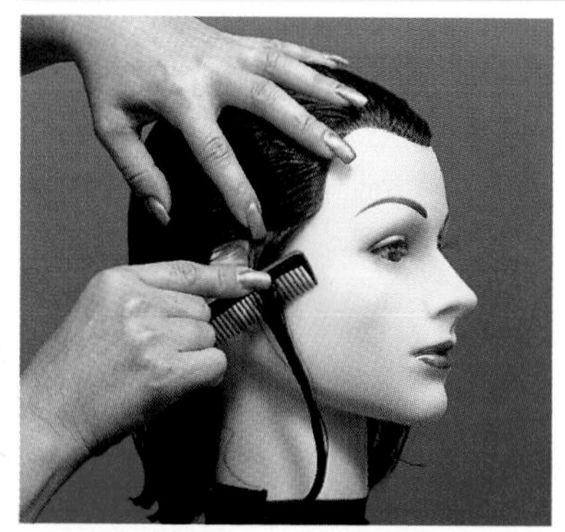

FIGURE 9.67 — Holding base with finger.

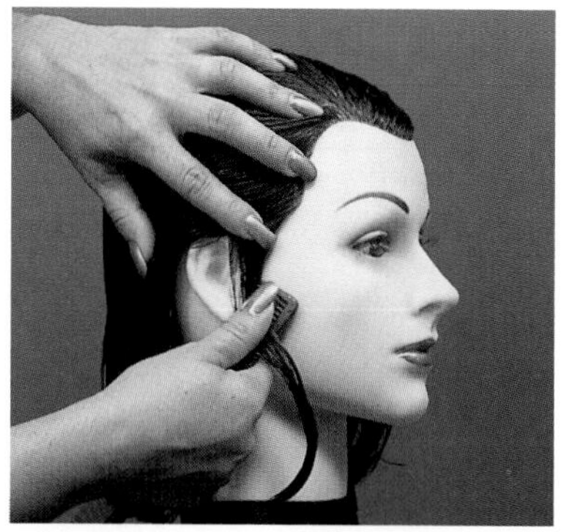

FIGURE 9.68 — Ribboning.

6. Form the curl forward. (Fig. 9.69)
7. Wind the curl around your index finger. (Fig. 9.70)
8. Slide the curl off your finger, keeping the hair ends inside the center of the curl. (Fig. 9.71)

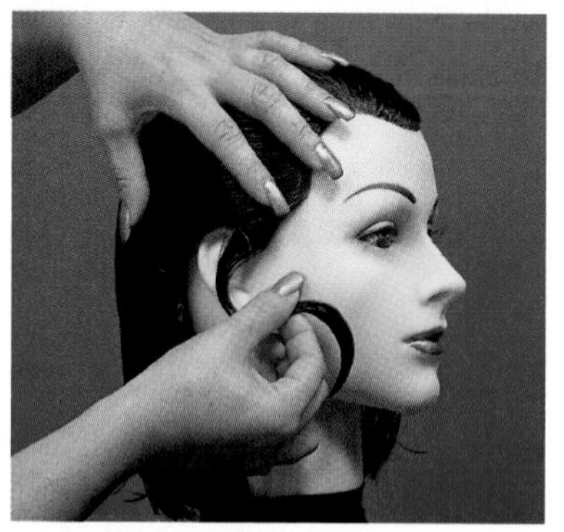

FIGURE 9.69 — Forming.

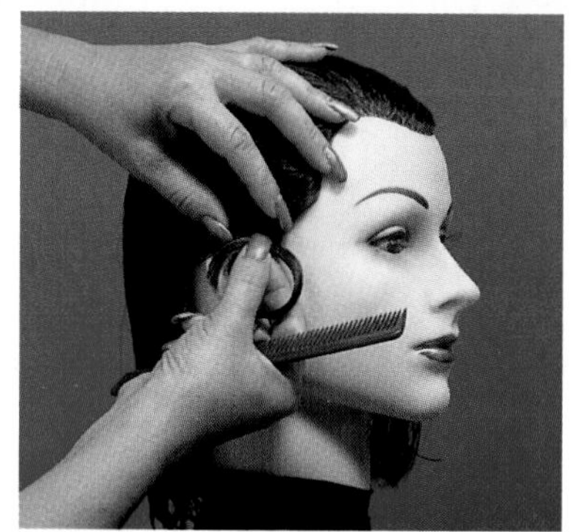

FIGURE 9.70 — Winding.

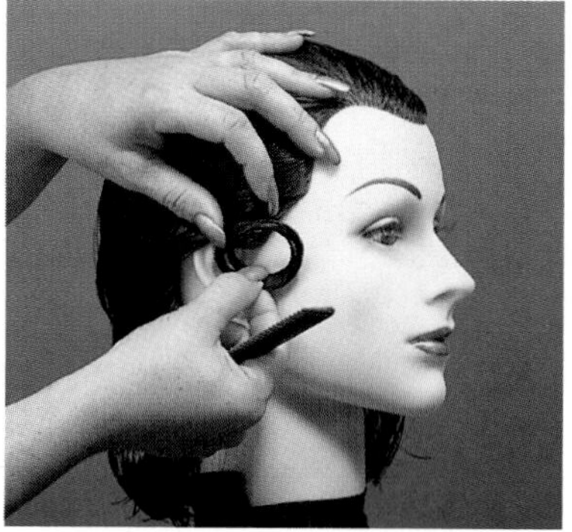

FIGURE 9.71 — Sliding off finger.

9. Mold the curl into the shaping. (Fig. 9.72)
10. Hold the curl in shaping. (Fig. 9.73)
11. Anchor the curl with clip. (Fig. 9.74)

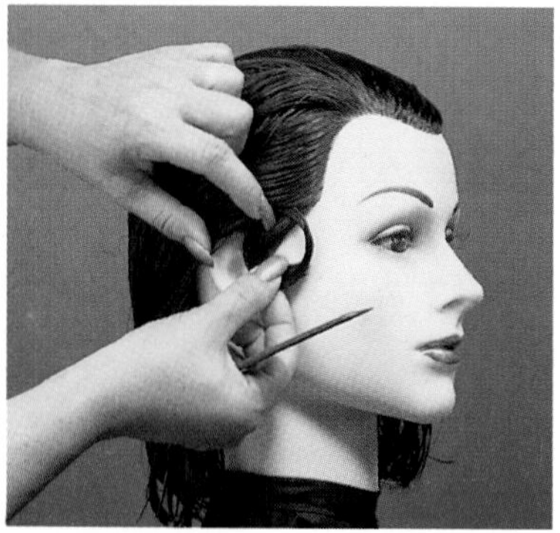

FIGURE 9.72 — Molding.

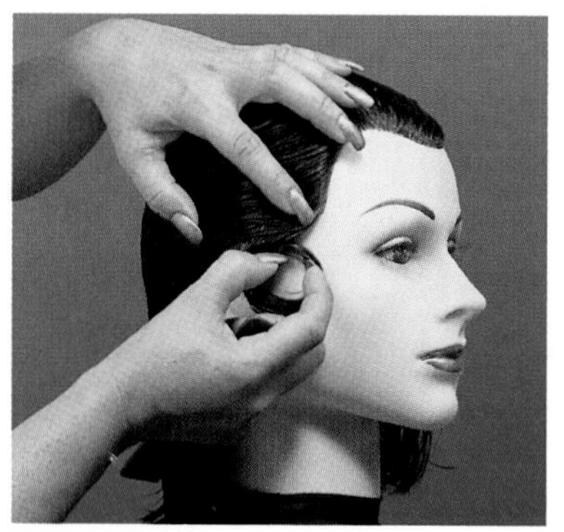

FIGURE 9.73 — Holding curl.

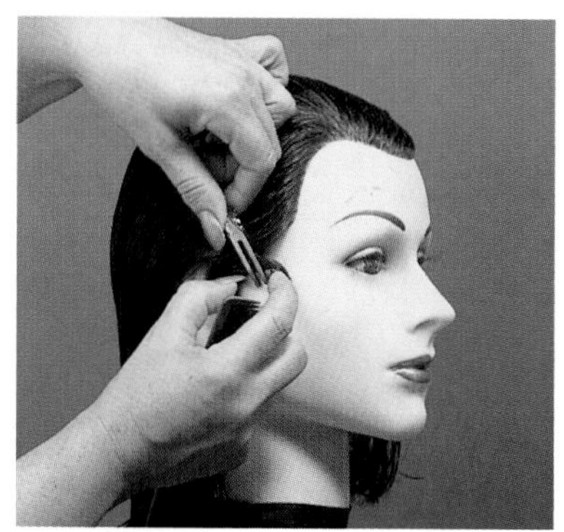

FIGURE 9.74 — Anchoring.

CAUTION

Be very careful not to destroy your shaping as you comb or pin the curl.

Whenever a longer-lasting curl movement is desired, stretch the hair strand and apply tension. You can accomplish this by ribboning and stretching the strand. Firmly comb it between the spine of the comb and the thumb in the direction of the curl movement.

Sculptured curl arrangements backed up with a second row of pin curls comb out into strong ridge waves. (Figs. 9.75–9.77)

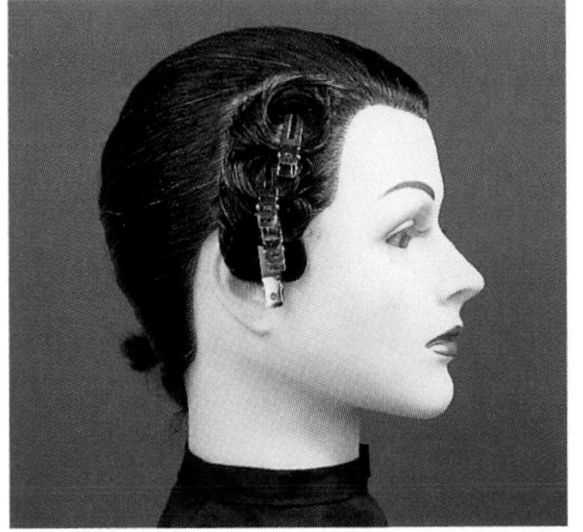

FIGURE 9.75 — Finished first row.

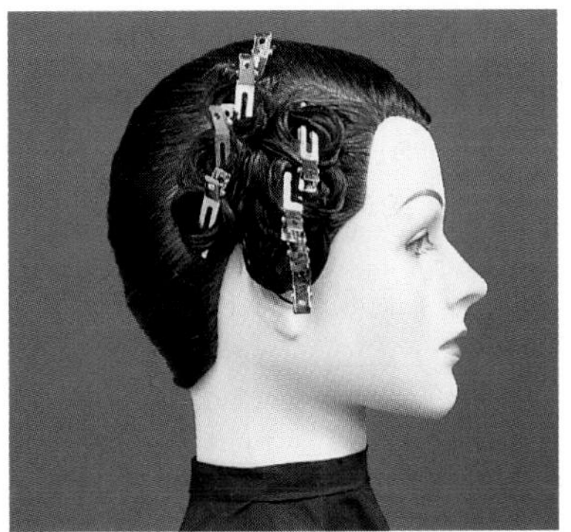

FIGURE 9.76 — Sculpture curl arrangement backed up with a second row of curls.

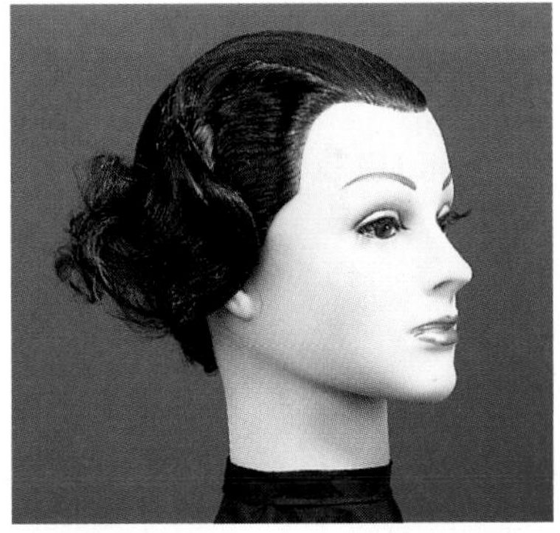

FIGURE 9.77 — Curls combined into waves with a strong ridge.

Forming Pin Curls on the Left Side

1. Wet hair thoroughly with water or setting lotion. Comb smooth and form the shaping. (Fig. 9.78) Note open and closed ends of shaping.
2. Slice a strand out of shaping and hold with your index finger. (Fig. 9.79)

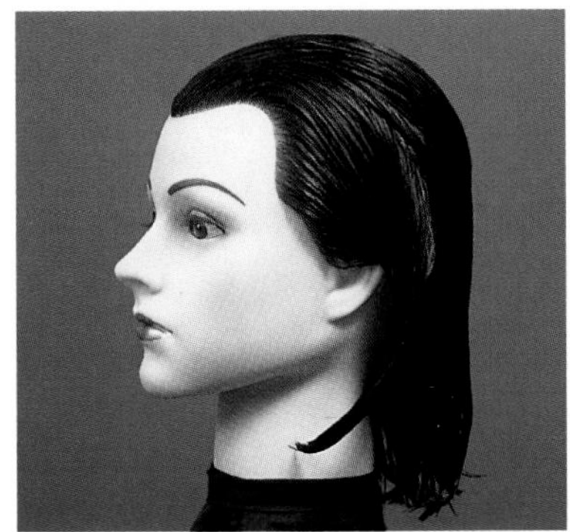

FIGURE 9.78 — Shaping.

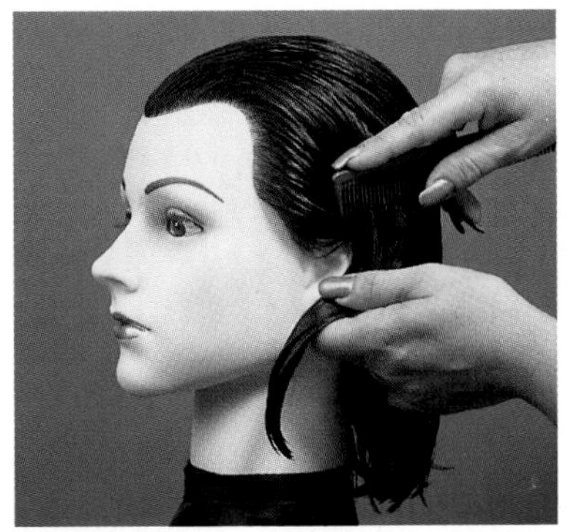

FIGURE 9.79 — Slicing.

3. Stretch a strand by ribboning it through the comb. (Figs. 9.80, 9.81)
4. Form a forward curl.

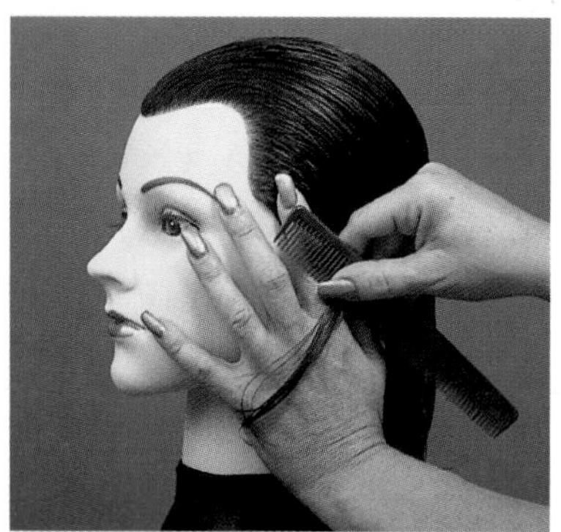
FIGURE 9.80 — Holding base with finger and stretching strand by pulling through comb.

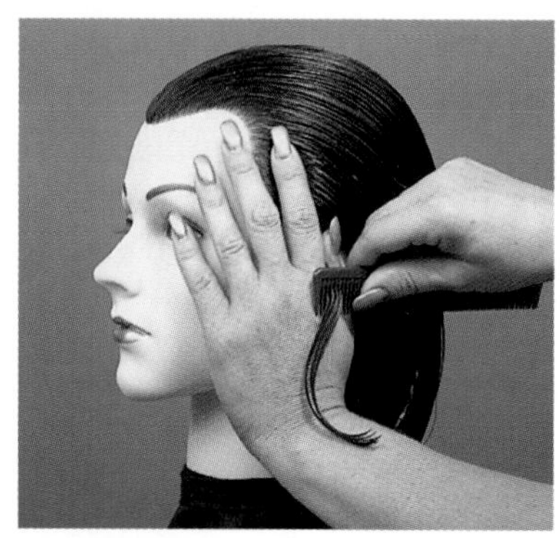
FIGURE 9.81 — Ribboning.

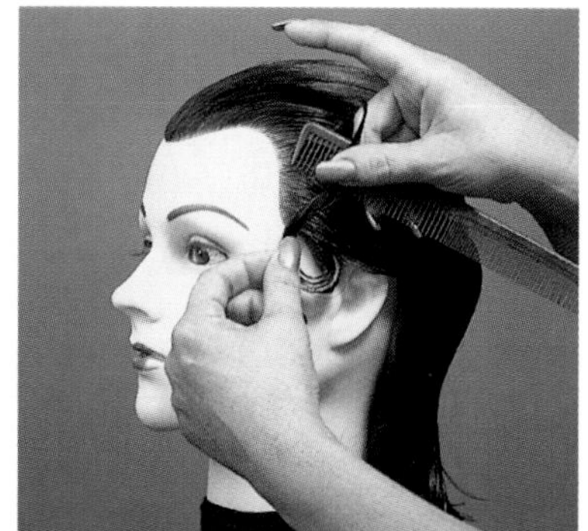
FIGURE 9.82 — Winding.

5. Wind the strand around your index finger. (Fig. 9.82)
6. Slide the curl off tip of your finger and mold into shaping. (Fig. 9.83)
7. Hold the curl in shaping. (Fig. 9.84)
8. Anchor with a clip. (Fig. 9.85) ✔

Completed: Learning Objective #2
PIN CURL TECHNIQUES

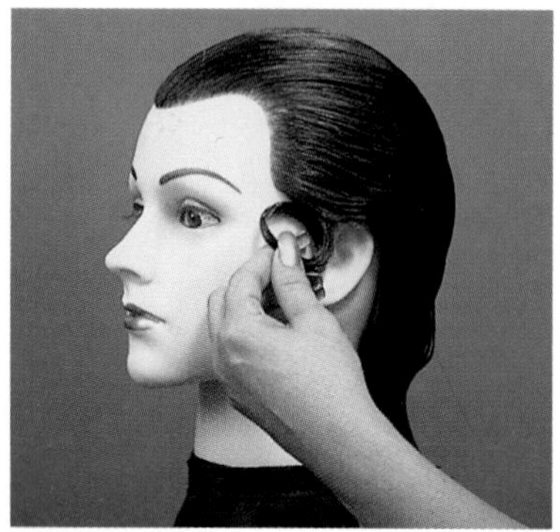
FIGURE 9.83 — Sliding off finger.

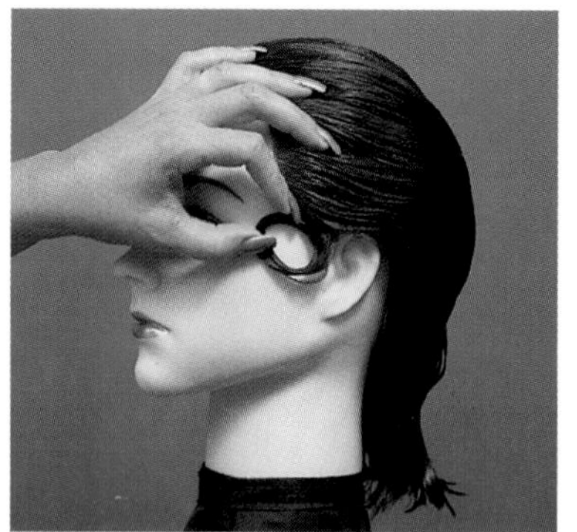
FIGURE 9.84 — Holding curl.

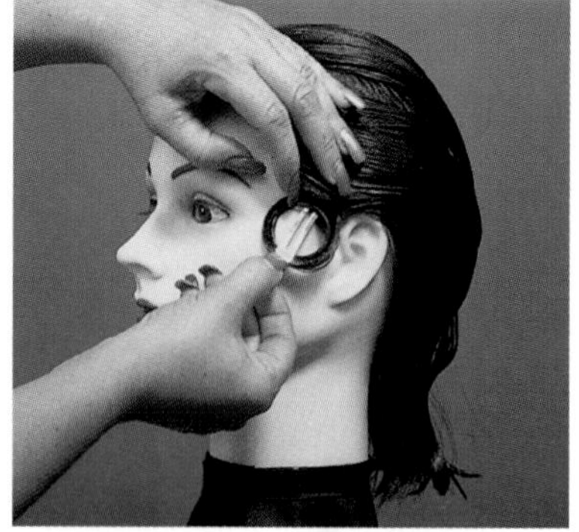
FIGURE 9.85 — Anchoring.

GENERAL RULES FOR PIN CURLING

1. Pin curls overlap in a shaping.
2. Pin curls follow the shaping.
3. To make lasting pin curls, you must ribbon the hair.
4. The size of the curl equals the size of the wave.

ANCHORING PIN CURLS

Anchor pin curls correctly to ensure that the curls hold firmly where you have placed them. This will enable you to comb the hair into the style you have planned.

1. Always anchor pin curls starting at the open end of the curl. (Fig. 9.86) This is the side opposite the stem.
2. The clip should enter the circle parallel to the stem. (Fig. 9.87)
3. Open the clip and place one prong above and one prong below one side of the circle. The upper prong should enter the hair in the center of the circle. The curl should be in the gap between the prongs. (Fig. 9.88) To avoid indentation in the curl, do not pin across the circle. (Fig. 9.89)
4. If any clips touch the skin, place cotton between the skin and the clip to keep the skin from burning.

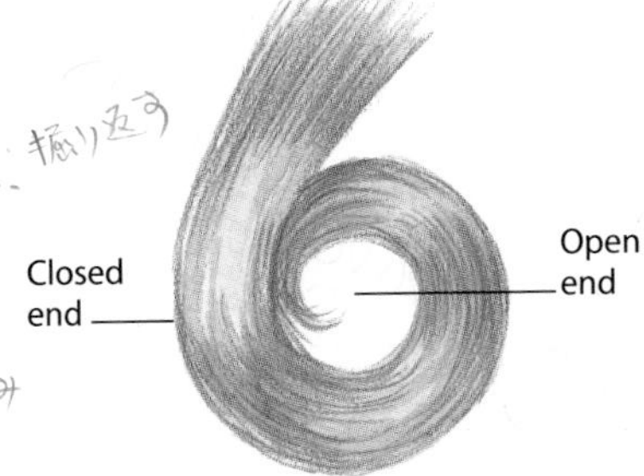

FIGURE 9.86 — Closed and open ends of curl.

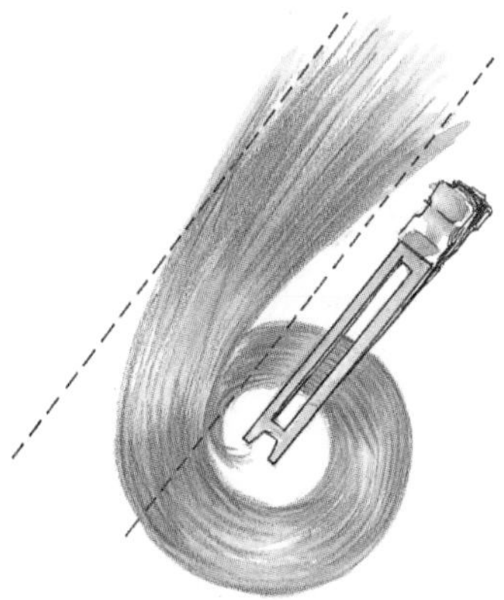

FIGURE 9.87 — Clip parallel to stem.

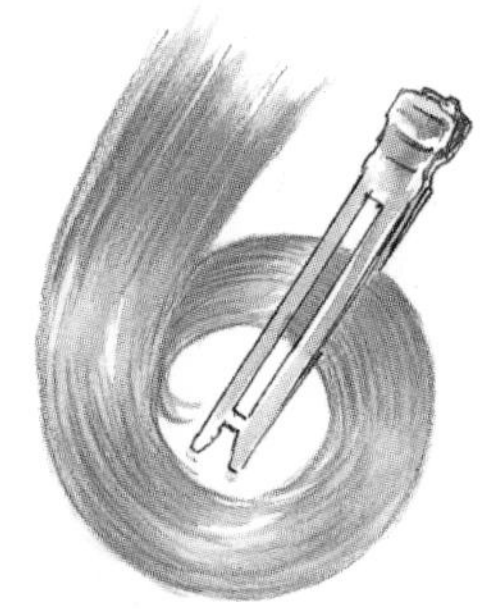

FIGURE 9.88 — Correct placing of clip.

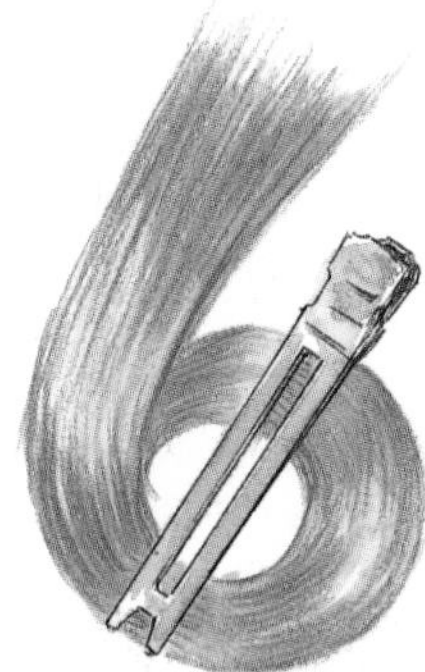

FIGURE 9.89 — Incorrect placing of clip.

DESIGNING WITH PIN CURLS

1. To create a wave, use two rows of pin curls. Set one row clockwise and the second row counterclockwise. (Figs. 9.90a, 9.90b)

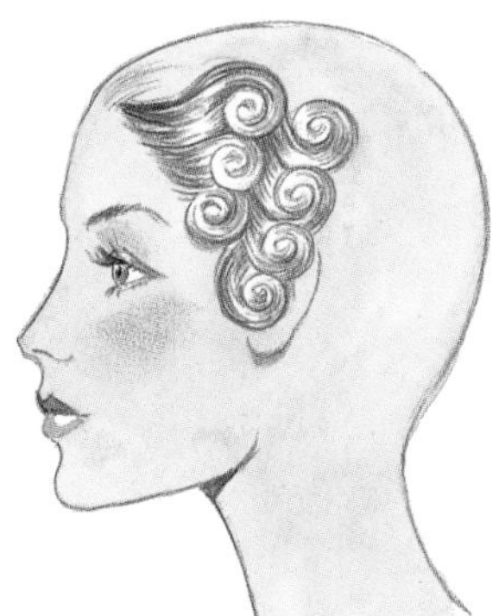

FIGURE 9.90a — Setting pattern for wave.

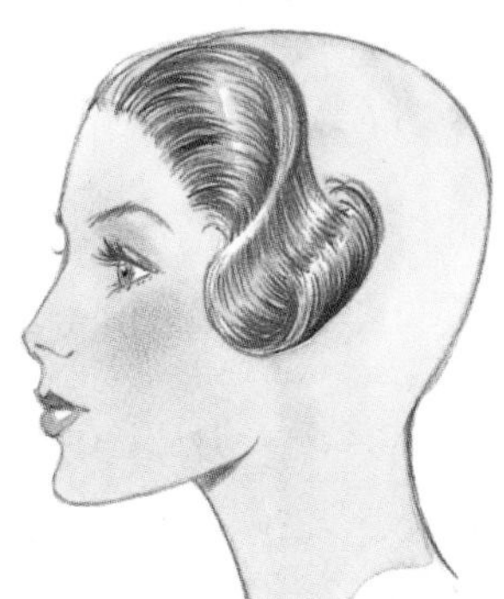

FIGURE 9.90b — Comb-out.

2. ***Brush waves*** are used to create long, soft waves. (Fig. 9.91)
3. ***Ridge curls*** are used to create a wave behind a ridge. (Fig. 9.92)
4. ***Skip waves*** are two rows of ridge curls, usually on the side of the head. They create a strong wave pattern with well-defined lines between the waves. (Figs. 9.93, 9.94)

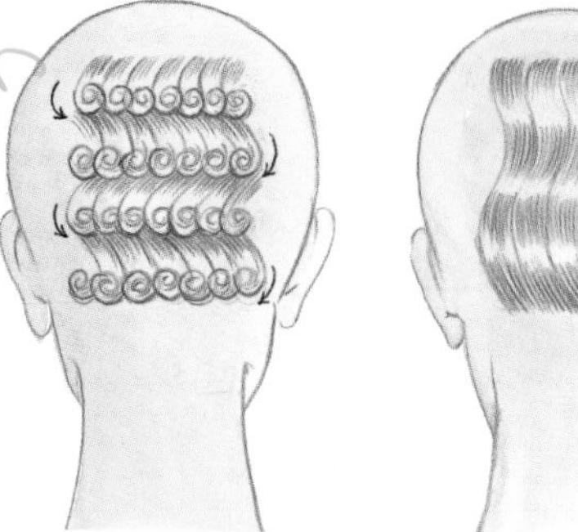

FIGURE 9.91 — Brush wave.

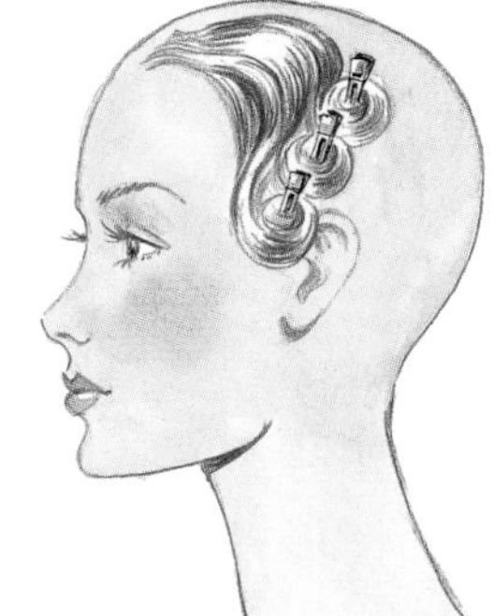

FIGURE 9.92 — Ridge curl.

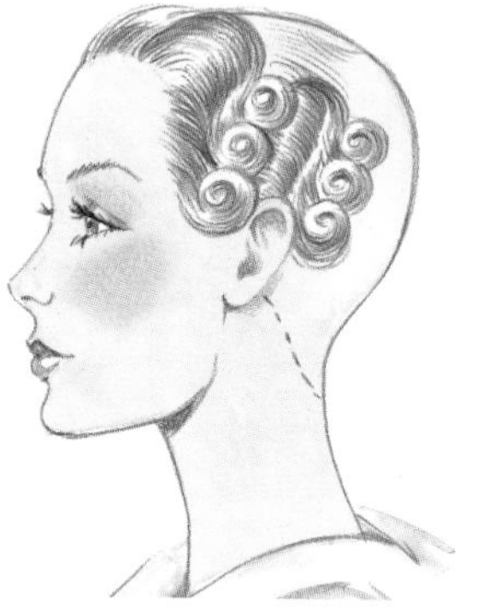

FIGURE 9.93 — Skip wave setting pattern.

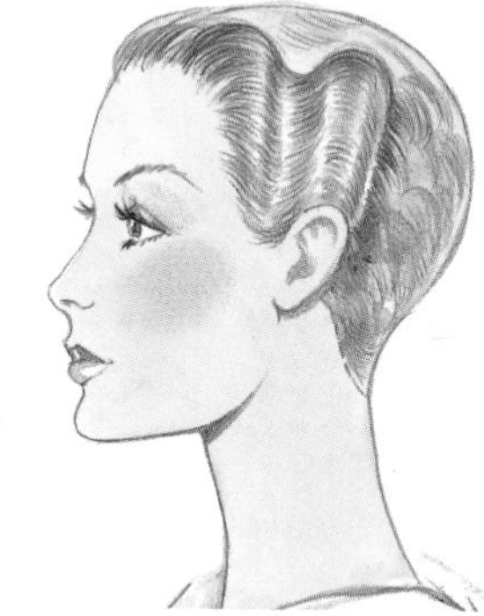

FIGURE 9.94 — Comb-out.

CREATING VOLUME WITH PIN CURLS

Cascade or ***stand-up curls*** are used to create height in the hair design. They are placed directly on the base with the circle at a 90-degree angle to the head. The size of the curl determines the amount of height in the comb-out. (Figs. 9.95–9.102)

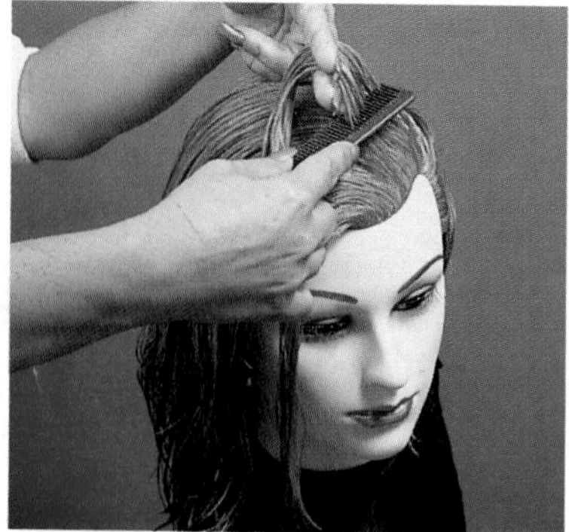

FIGURE 9.95 — Comb, divide, and smooth strand.

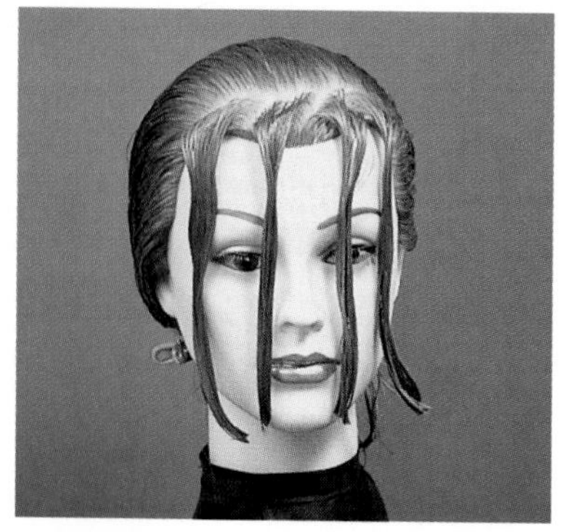

FIGURE 9.96 — Divide section into strands for individual curls.

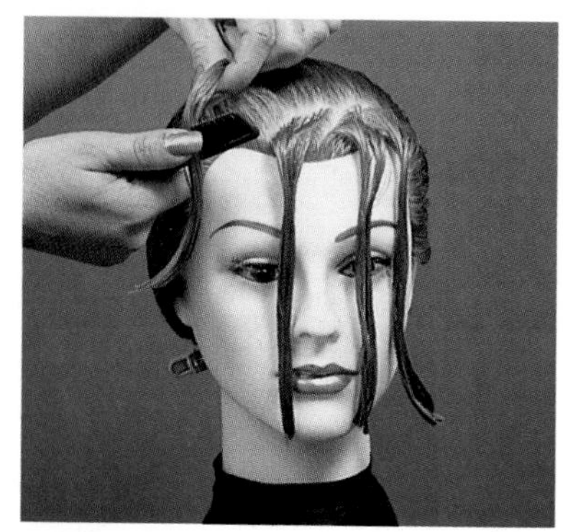

FIGURE 9.97 — Ribbon strand.

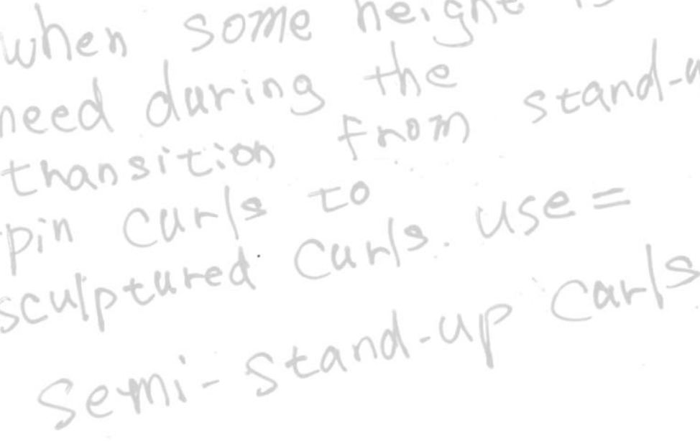

Semi-stand-up curls are used to create a transition from stand-up pin curls to sculptured pin curls. They can also be used when some height is needed, but not as much as with stand-up pin curls. (Figs. 9.103–9.106)

Barrel curls are large stand-up pin curls on a rectangular base. They have the same effect as stand-up pin curls. A barrel curl is similar to a roller but does not have the same tension as a roller when it is set.

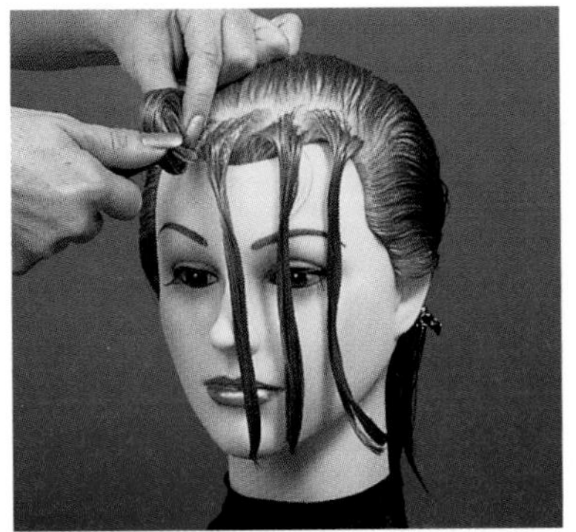

FIGURE 9.98 — Direct strand.

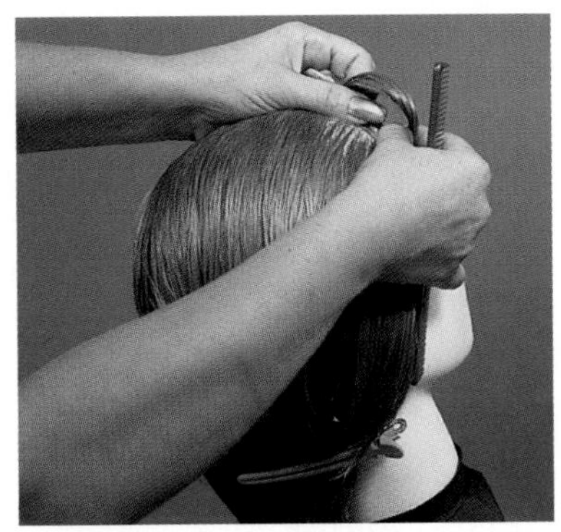

FIGURE 9.99 — Wind strand, being sure to keep curl round.

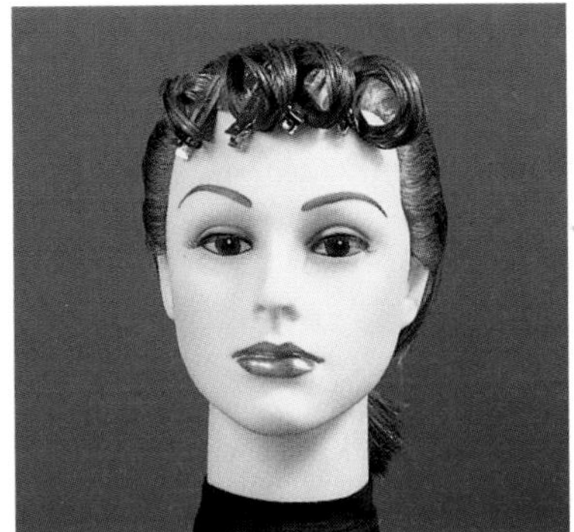

FIGURE 9.100 — Anchor curl securely at base.

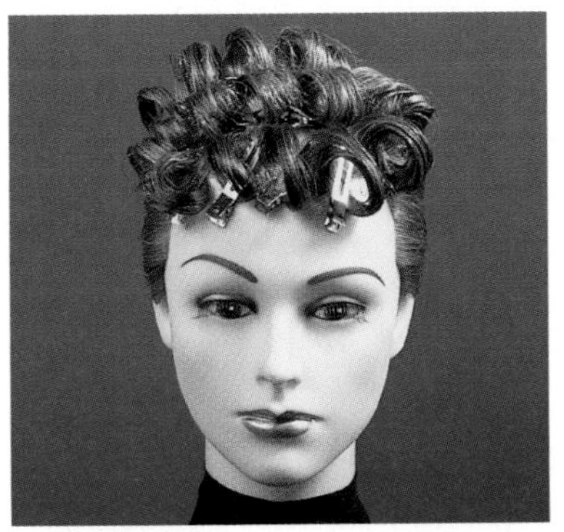

FIGURE 9.101 — Top setting.

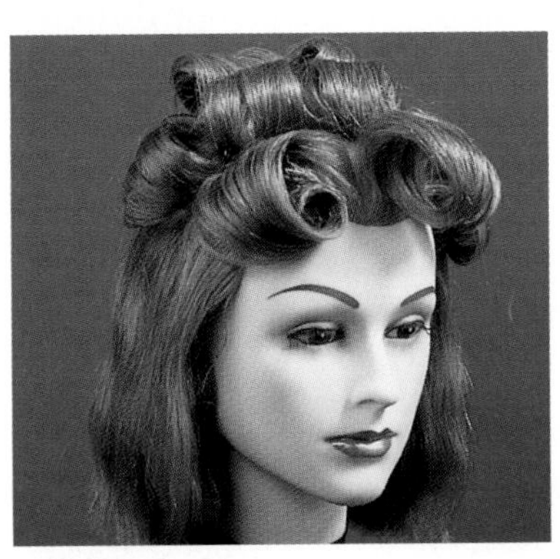

FIGURE 9.102 — Comb out as you would a roller set.

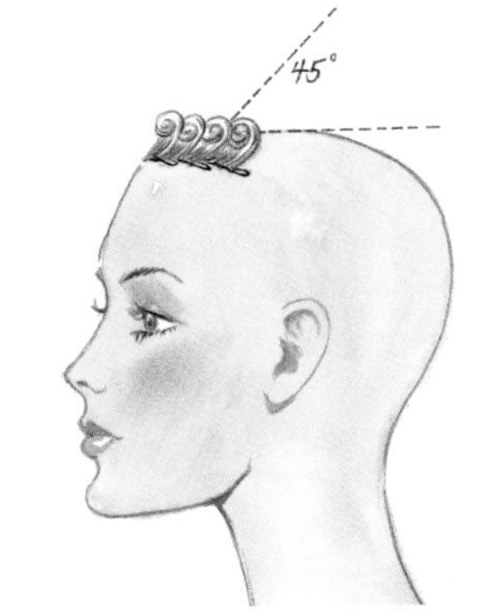

FIGURE 9.103 — Semi-stand-up curls.

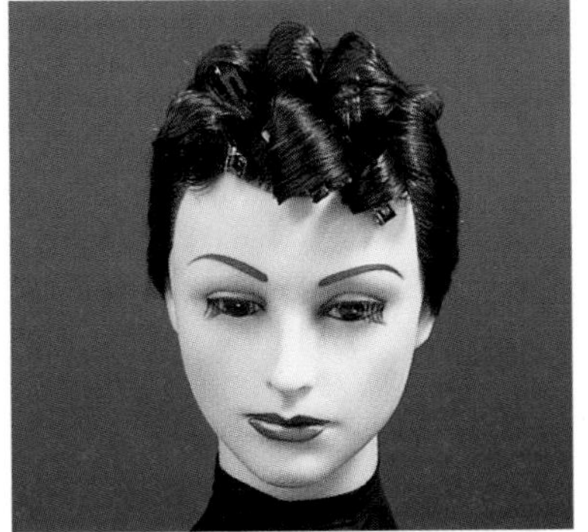

FIGURE 9.104 — Setting pattern.

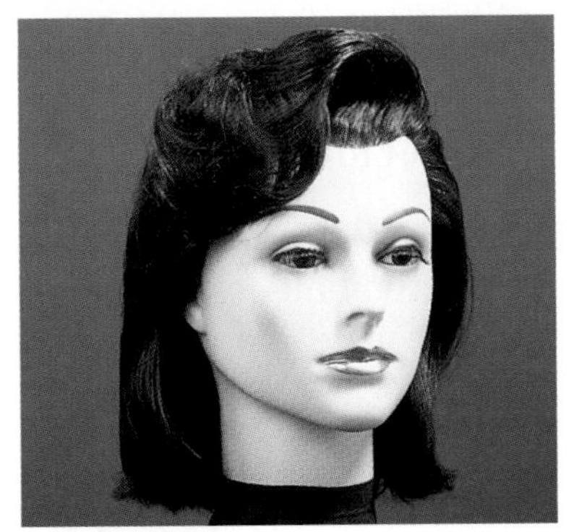

FIGURE 9.105 — Comb-out.

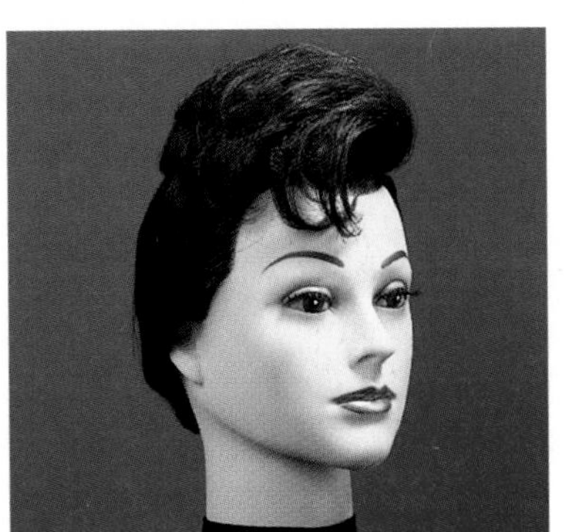

FIGURE 9.106 — Alternate comb-out.

ROLLER CURLS

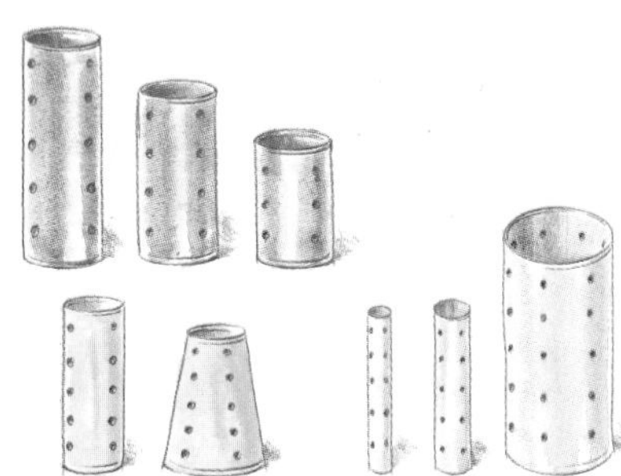

FIGURE 9.107 — Rollers.

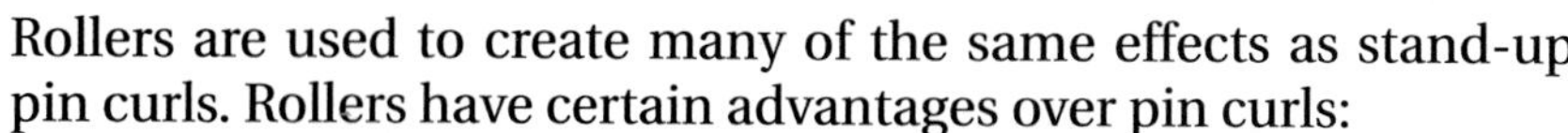

Rollers are used to create many of the same effects as stand-up pin curls. Rollers have certain advantages over pin curls:

1. Because a roller holds the equivalent of two to four stand-up curls, the roller is a much faster way to set the hair.
2. The hair is wrapped around the roller with tension, which gives a stronger and longer-lasting set.
3. Rollers come in a variety of shapes, widths, and sizes, which enhances the creative possibilities for any style. (Fig. 9.107)

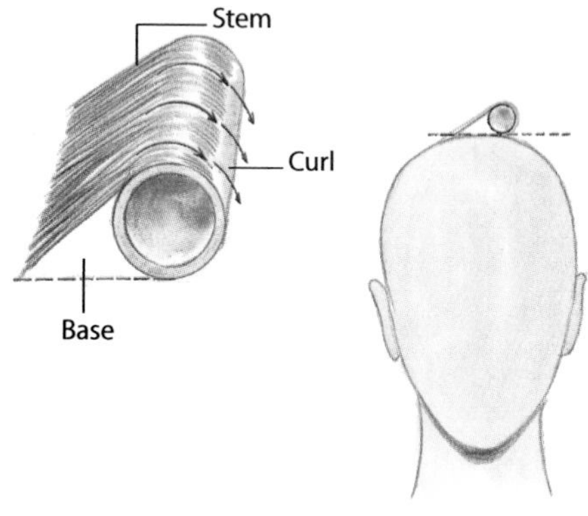

FIGURE 9.108 — Parts of a roller curl.

PARTS OF A ROLLER CURL

Base: The panel of hair the roller is placed on. The base should be the same length and width as the roller. The type of base determines the volume.

Stem: The hair between the scalp and the first turn of the roller. The stem gives the hair direction and mobility.

Curl: The hair that is wrapped around the roller. It determines the size of the wave or curl. (Fig. 9.108)

ROLLER THEORY

Roller Placement

Volume is determined by the size of the roller and how it sits on its base. The larger the roller, the greater the volume. (Fig. 9.109)

There are three kinds of bases:

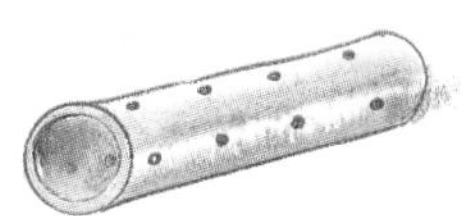

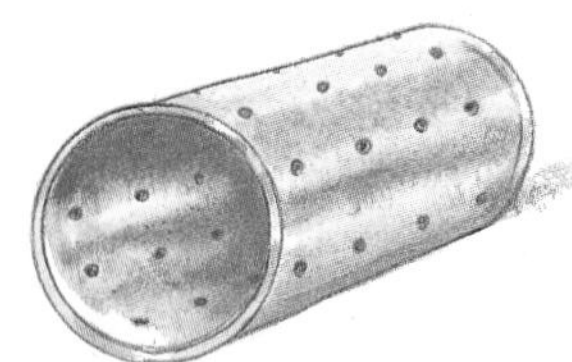

FIGURE 9.109 — Volume depends on roller size.

1. ***On base:*** For full volume, the roller sits directly on its base. Overdirect the strand 45 degrees in front of the base and roll the hair down to the base. The roller should fit on the base. (Fig. 9.110)
2. ***One-half base:*** For medium volume, the roller sits half on its base and half behind the base. Hold the strand straight up from the head and roll the hair down. (Fig. 9.111)
3. ***Off base:*** For the least volume, the roller sits behind the base. Hold the strand 45 degrees back from the base and roll the hair down. (Fig. 9.112)

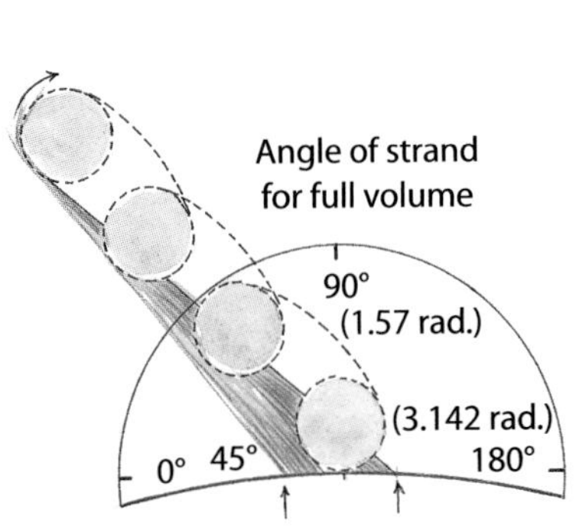

FIGURE 9.110 — On base: full volume.

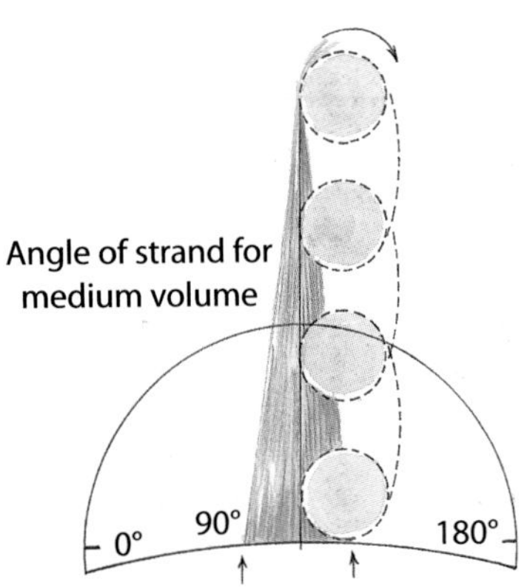

FIGURE 9.111 — One-half base: medium volume.

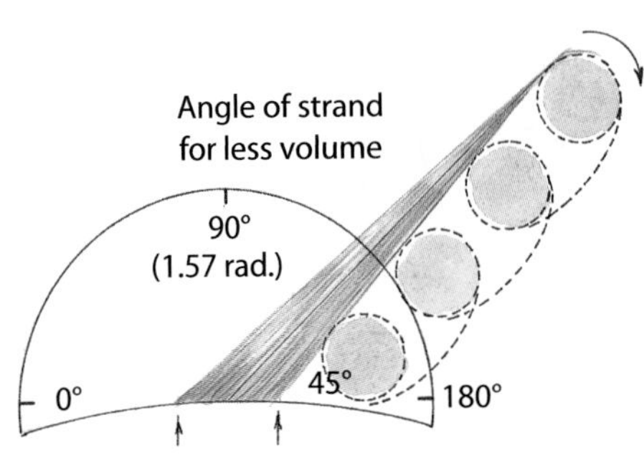

FIGURE 9.112 — Off base: less volume.

Indentation with Rollers

Rollers can be used to create an indentation in the hairstyle. An indentation roller is usually placed behind a volume roller or at the hairline.

Behind volume roller: Roll the indentation roller in the opposite direction from the volume roller. If you roll the volume roller back, roll the indentation roller forward. Comb the strand almost flat to the head form and pin it behind the base. (Figs. 9.113–9.115)

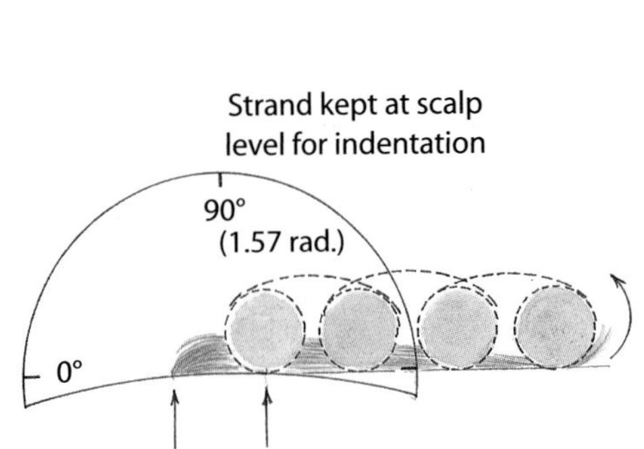

FIGURE 9.113 — Indentation.

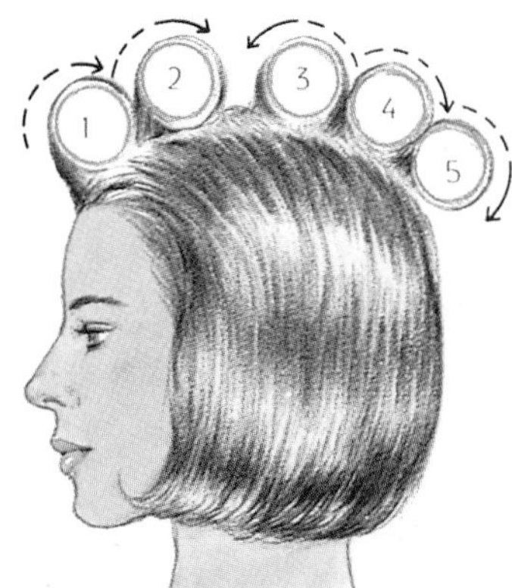

FIGURE 9.114 — Setting pattern: 1st two rollers, volume; 3rd roller, indentation; 4th and 5th rollers, volume.

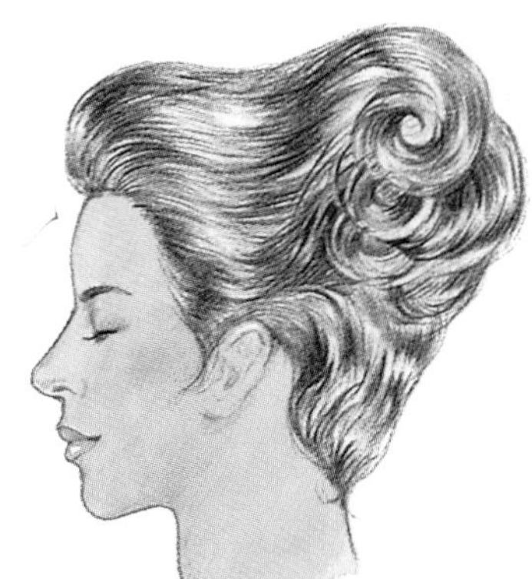

FIGURE 9.115 — Comb-out.

At the hairline: An indentation roller at the hairline creates a flat area, followed by an indentation and volume. Comb the strand flat back from the hairline. Roll the hair toward the face and pin the roller just behind the base. (Figs. 9.116, 9.117)

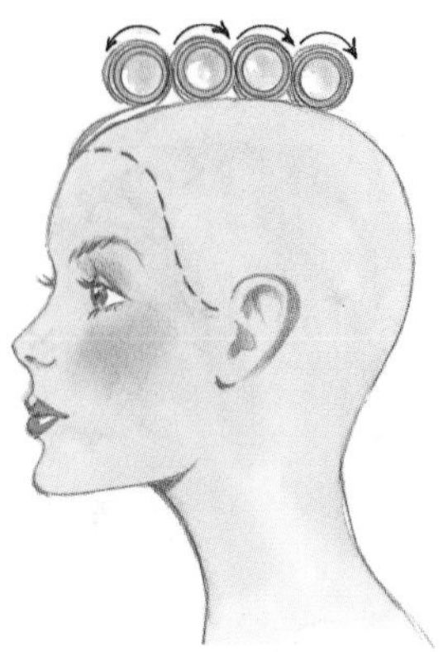

FIGURE 9.116 — Setting pattern: 1st roller, indentation; next 3 rollers, volume.

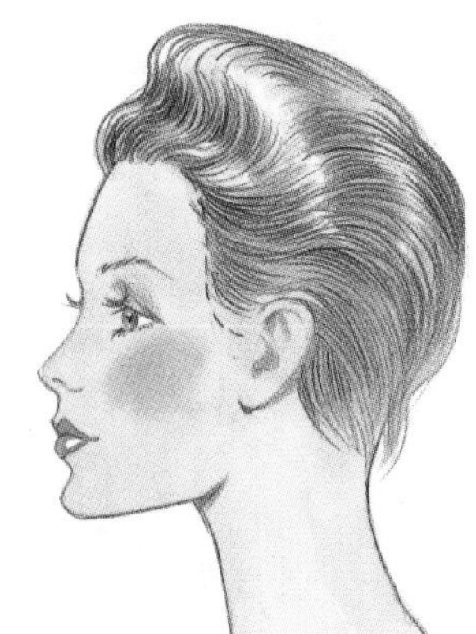

FIGURE 9.117 — Comb-out.

Choosing Roller Size

The relationship between the length of the hair and the size of the roller determines whether the result will be a C shape, a wave, or a curl.

1 complete turn around the roller will create a ***C shaped curl.*** (Fig. 9.118)

1-½ turns will create a ***wave.*** (Fig. 9.119)

2-½ turns will create an explosion of ***curl.*** (Fig. 9.120)

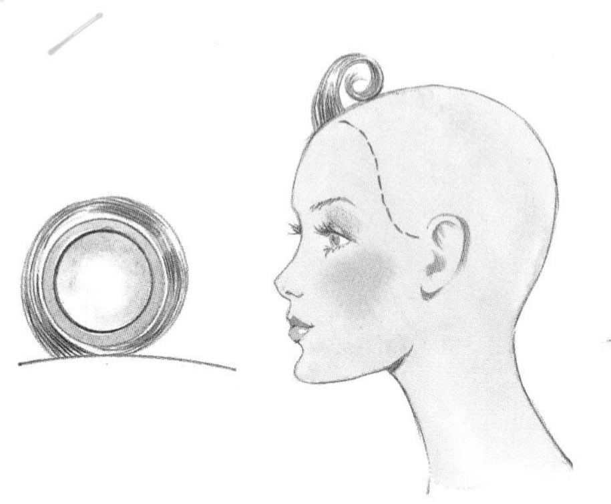

FIGURE 9.118 — C shape.

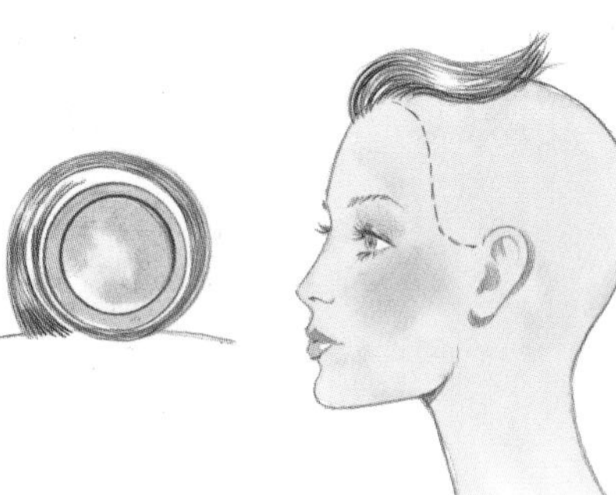

FIGURE 9.119 — Wave.

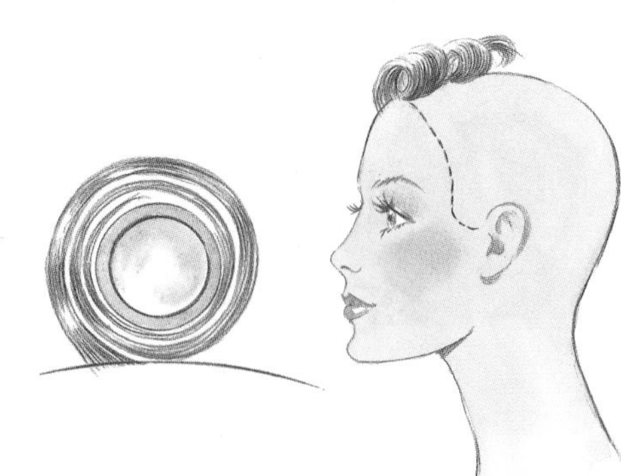

FIGURE 9.120 — Curl.

Stem Direction

The stem determines the direction and movement (mobility) of the curl. The longer the stem, the more movement in the set.

No stem = maximum volume. (Fig. 9.121)

½ ***stem*** = moderate volume. (Fig. 9.122)

Full stem = minimum volume. (Fig. 9.123)

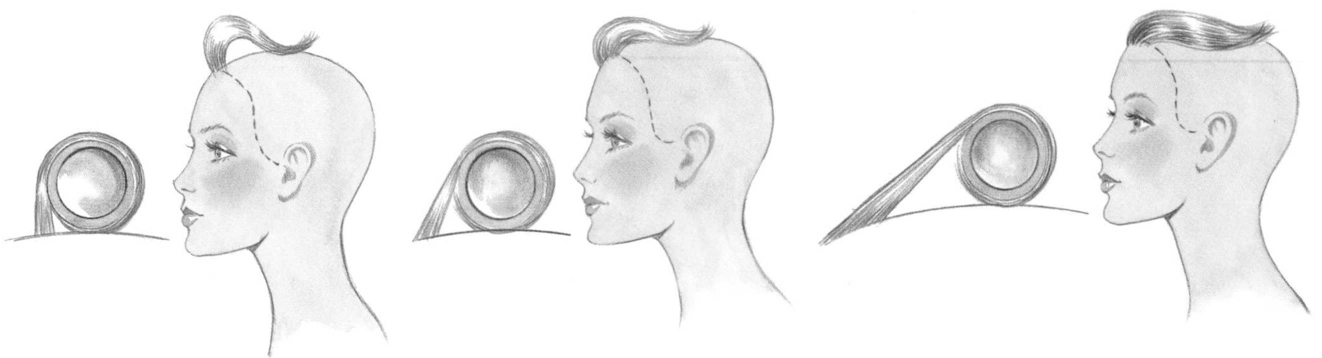

FIGURE 9.121 — No stem.

FIGURE 9.122 — One-half stem.

FIGURE 9.123 — Full stem.

ROLLER TECHNIQUE

1. Comb the wet hair in the direction of the setting pattern. Shapings may be used to accent the design.
2. Starting at the front hairline, part off a base (section) the same size as the roller. Determine the desired volume (type of base) and comb the hair out from the scalp to the ends. Repeat several times to be sure the hair is smooth.
3. Hold the hair with tension between the thumb and middle finger of the left hand. Place the roller below the thumb of the left hand. Do not converge the ends of the hair. (Figs. 9.124, 9.125) Wrap the ends of the hair smoothly around the roller until the hair catches and does not release. (Fig. 9.126)
4. Place the thumbs over the ends of the roller and roll the hair firmly to the scalp. (Fig. 9.127)
5. Clip the roller to the scalp hair. (Fig. 9.128)

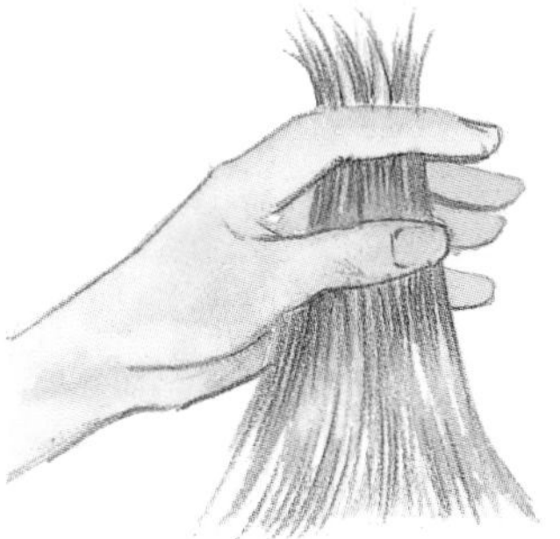

FIGURE 9.124 — Wrong way to hold hair.

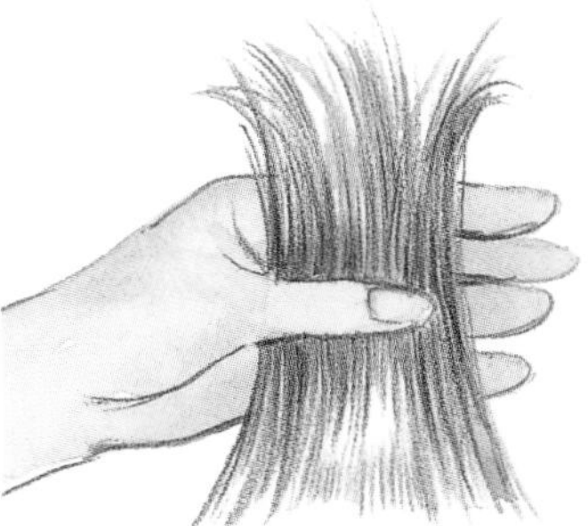

FIGURE 9.125 — Right way to hold hair.

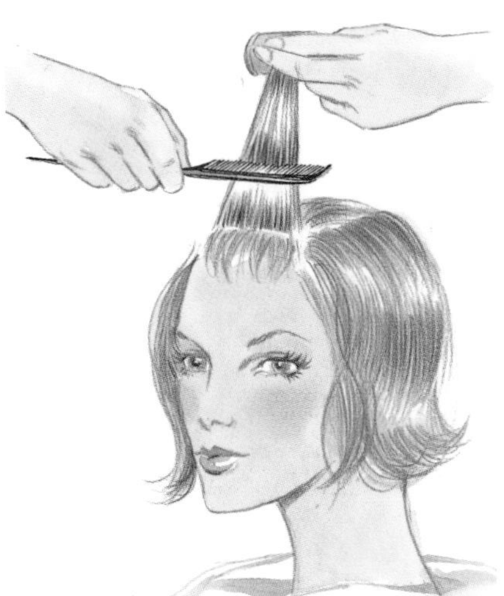

FIGURE 9.126 — Wrapping hair ends around roller.

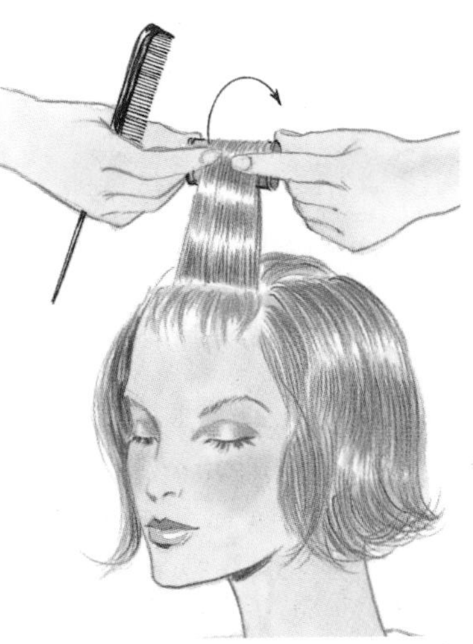

FIGURE 9.127 — Winding roller.

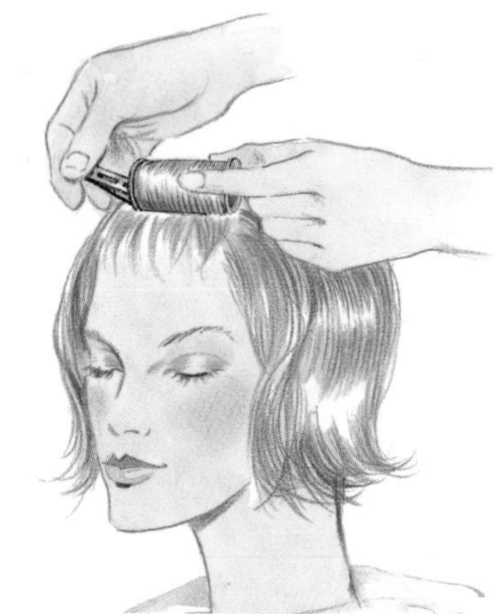

FIGURE 9.128 — Clipping roller.

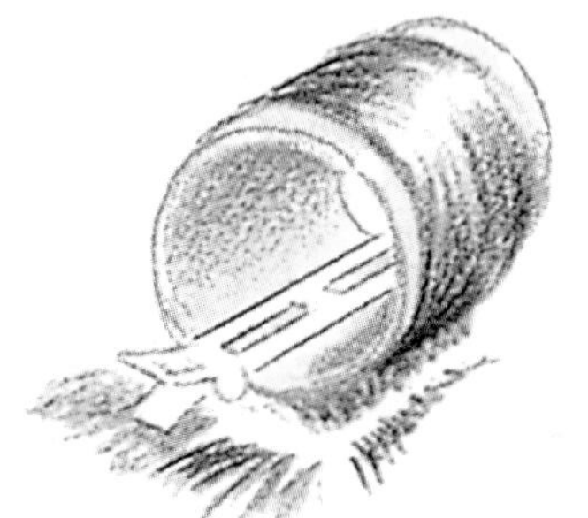

FIGURE 9.129 — Proper clipping.

When ***clipping the roller***, it is important to secure the roller properly to the head. A loose roller will lose its tension and result in a weak set. If the clip is placed at an angle against the hair, the sharp metal edge can cause the hair to break. Hold the roller against the scalp, maintaining the tension. Open the clip and slide it into the center of the roller. Place one end under the roller and one end inside the roller. (Fig. 9.129)

Cylinder Circular Roller Action

Hair that is directed in a circular fashion is referred to by various names, such as radial motion, circular movement, curvature movement, curvature roller action, rotary motion or movement, spotmatic movement, contour movement, and so on.

The spot or area from which the hair is directed to form a circular movement is also referred to by any of the following terms: balance point, swing point, terminal point, pivot point, pendulum point, radial point, fulcrum point, radiation point, rotary point, and spotmatic point.

Roller action is created by the way the hair is molded around the roller. This roller action can be varied by using different size rollers and setting patterns. (Figs. 9.130–9.143)

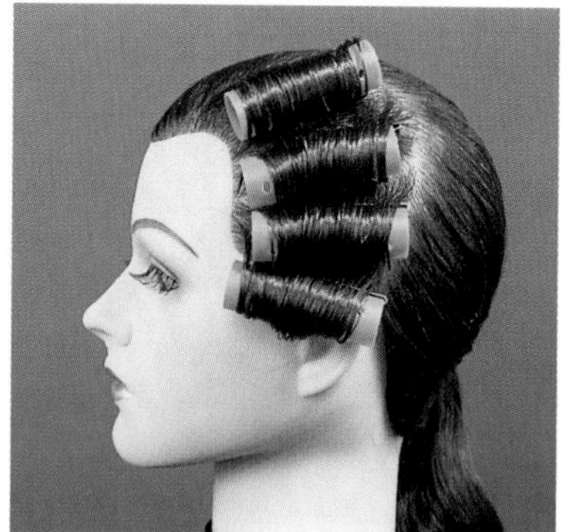

FIGURE 9.130 — Short hair (slender rollers).

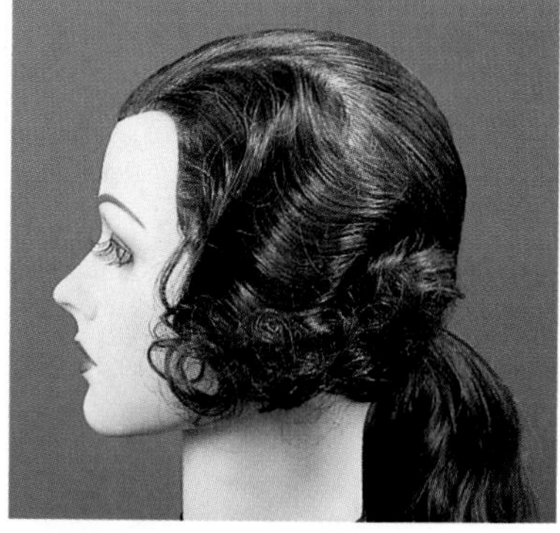

FIGURE 9.131 — Comb-out.

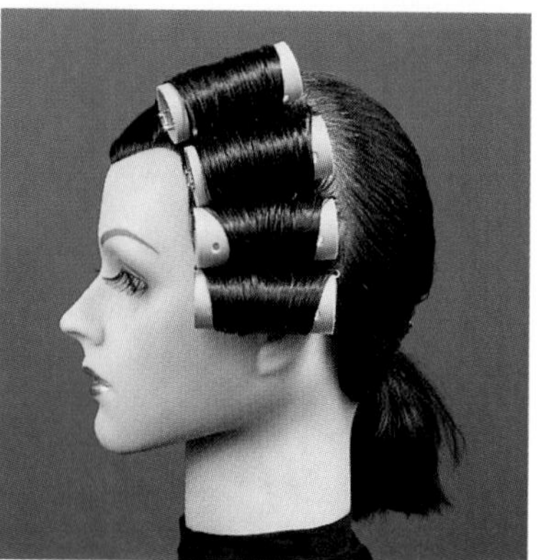

FIGURE 9.132 — Medium-length hair (medium rollers).

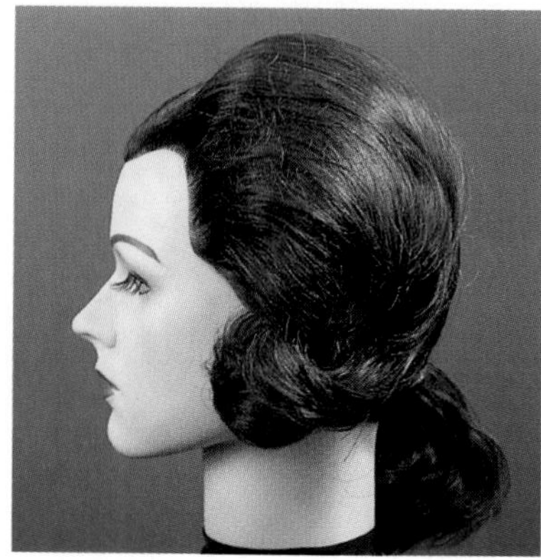

FIGURE 9.133 — Comb-out.

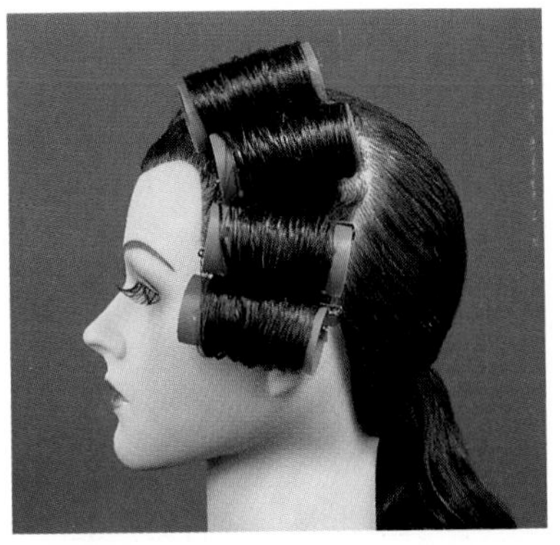

FIGURE 9.134 — Long hair (large rollers).

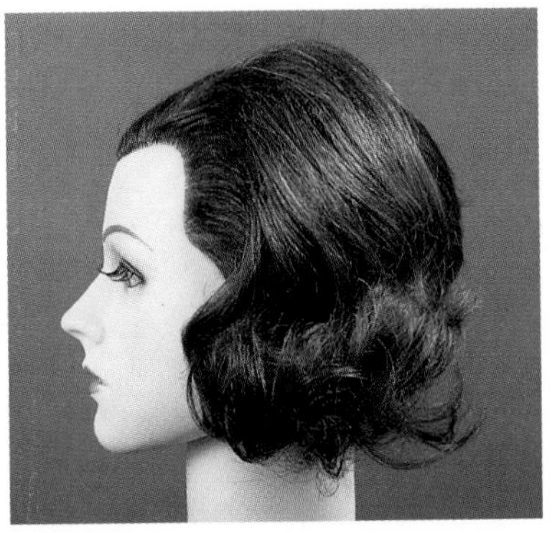

FIGURE 9.135 — Comb-out.

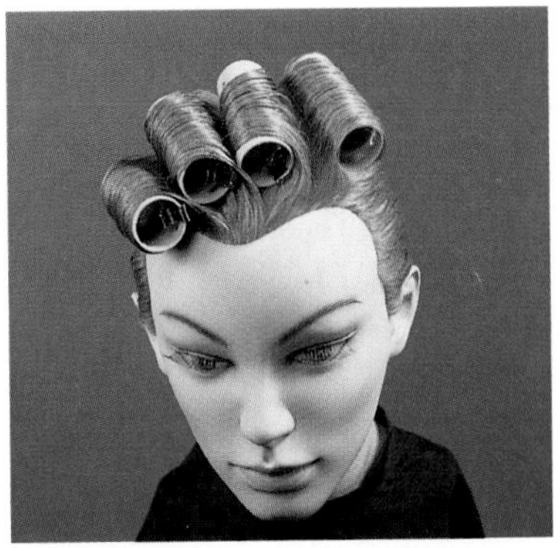

FIGURE 9.136 — Top: cylinder rollers set in wedge-shaped partings in circular manner.

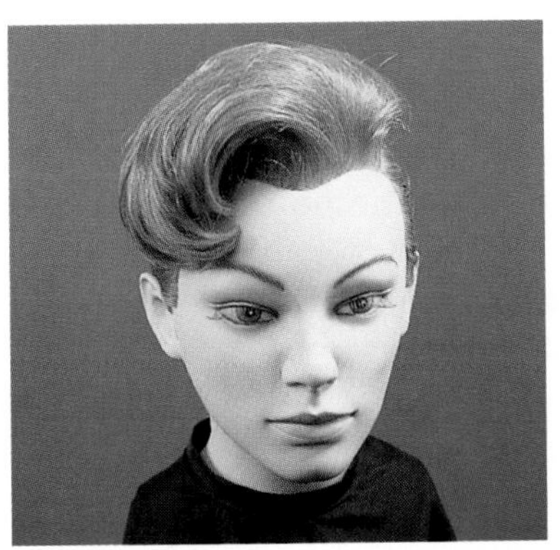

FIGURE 9.137 — Comb-out in forward shell effect with bangs.

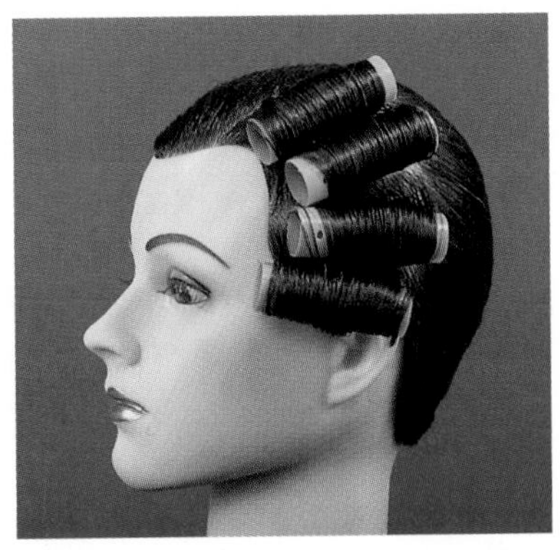

FIGURE 9.138 — Side: cylinder rollers set in wedge-shaped partings.

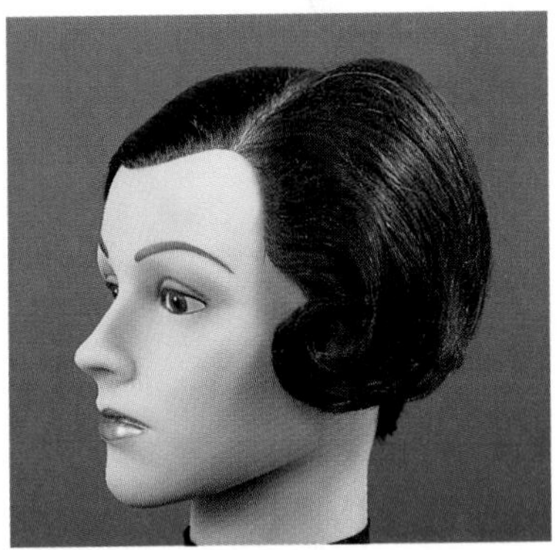

FIGURE 9.139 — Comb-out creates circular movement toward face.

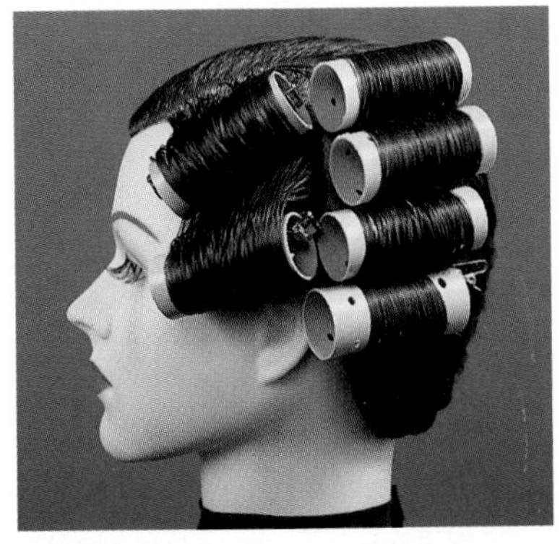

FIGURE 9.140 — Special side effects: side roller setting with sculpture curl in front of ear.

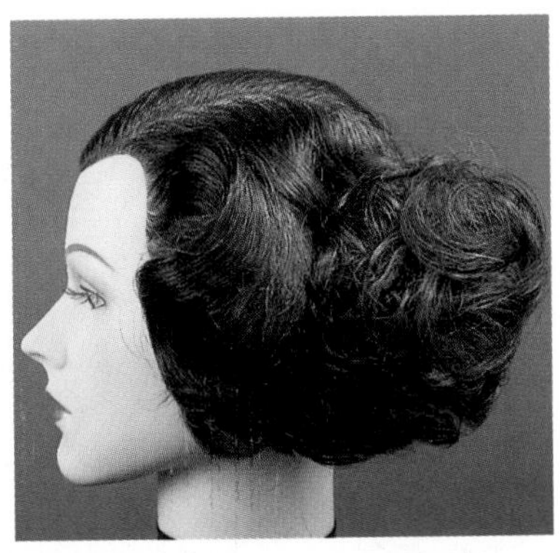

FIGURE 9.141 — Comb-out produces S-wave formation effect.

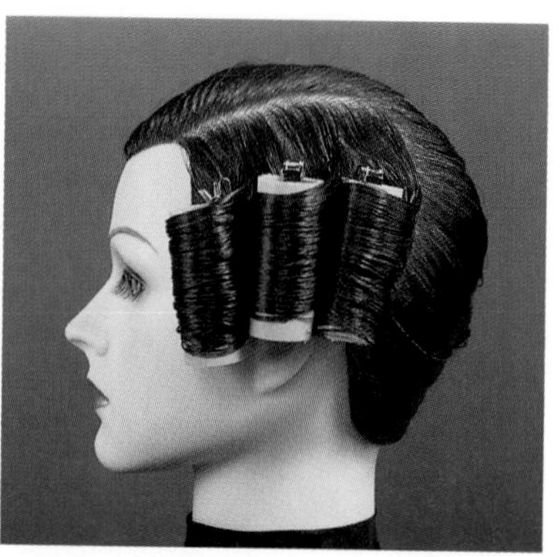

FIGURE 9.142 — To create ridge line and indentation, set hair on rollers at an angle.

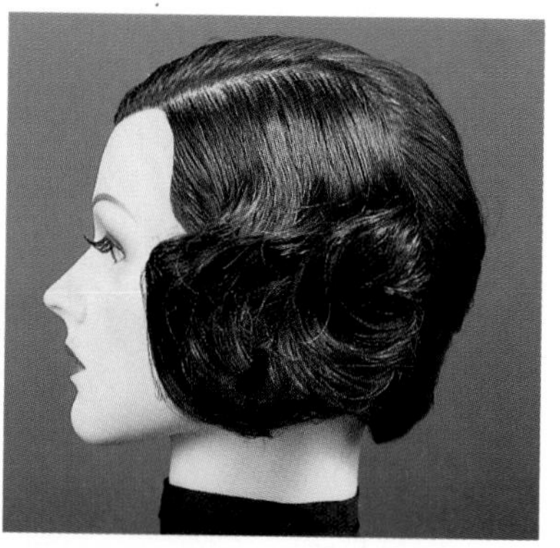

FIGURE 9.143 — Setting produces waved effect in comb-out.

Tapered Rollers

You can achieve practically the same styling results by using either cylinder or tapered rollers. However, since cylinder rollers must be placed slightly farther back from the point of distribution in a pie-shaped pattern, the movement of the hair might be weaker. The tapered roller, however, makes it possible to develop a stronger curvature movement.

Choose roller size according to the texture of your client's hair and the size of curl you desire. Fine hair requires smaller rollers; coarse hair needs larger rollers.

Completed:
Learning Objective
#3
DIFFERENT METHODS OF WET HAIRSTYLING

Effect of Tapered Rollers

Tapered rollers set along the hairline produce a shell-shaped front with bangs or curled up ends. (Figs. 9.144, 9.145)

Tapered rollers set along the side of the head comb out in a forward movement. (Figs. 9.146, 9.147)

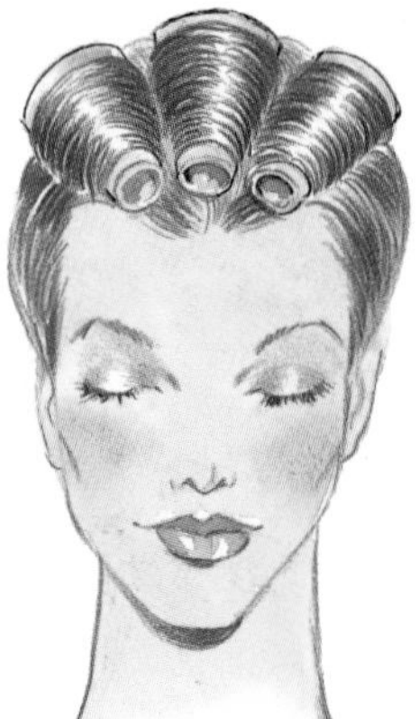

FIGURE 9.144 — Tapered roller setting.

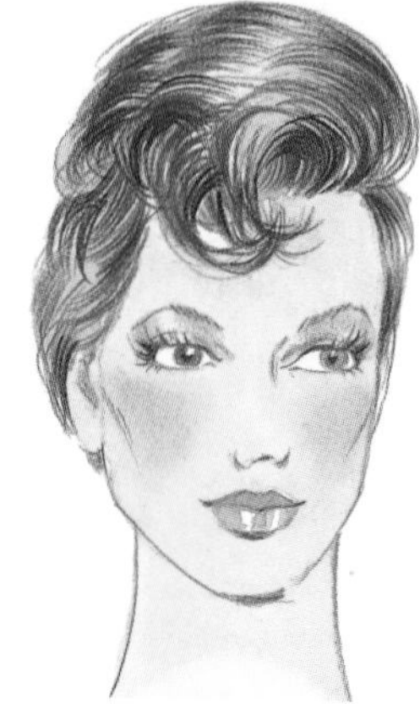

FIGURE 9.145 — Comb-out.

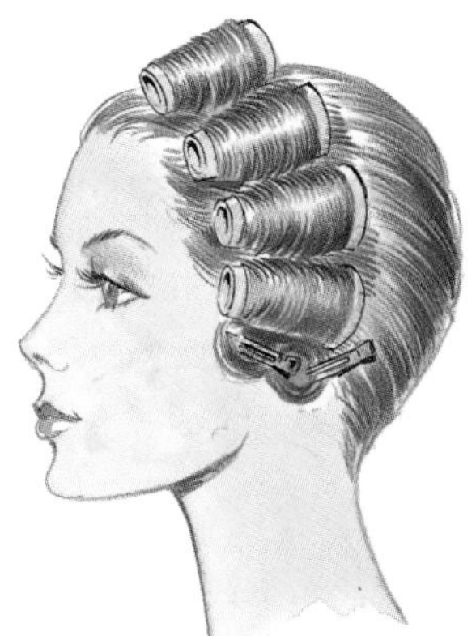

FIGURE 9.146 — Side tapered roller setting.

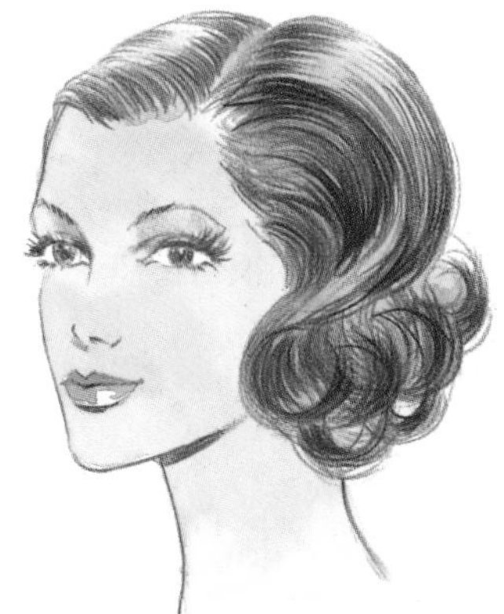

FIGURE 9.147 — Comb-out.

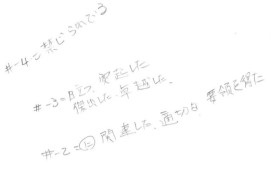

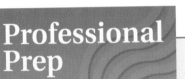

HOW TO WRITE A RESUME

You've passed your boards, and now you're ready for that first job. Everyone wants to see a resume, and in many cases it's your first chance to advertise your skills. The way you present it gives your future employer a clue as to how you do everything else.

Your resume should include your name, address, and phone number; your work history, including summer and part-time jobs; your educational background; and your skills and achievements. It should also include your employment objective (what job you want) and references from teachers, past or present employers, supervisors, or coworkers (not relatives or personal friends).

When organizing all this information, remember to place what is most relevant to the job you want in the most prominent position, so it will catch the employer's eye. Be sure to use active verbs to demonstrate your achievements—words like completed, created, designed, developed, produced, trained, won, etc.

Keep the information simple, clear, and positive; no one wants to wade through a lot of flowery language. Be sure to type your resume, and proofread it carefully—or have someone else proofread it, if grammar and spelling are your weaknesses.

Don't include personal information (age, marital status, parental status, race, religion, or physical characteristics), since it could work against you. (Employers are forbidden to ask about these things.)

Don't emphasize how much money you want (this will be discussed in the job interview) or what you need; instead, focus on how you can fill your employer's needs and wants.

—*From* Communication Skills for Cosmetologists *by Kathleen Ann Bergant*

COMB-OUT TECHNIQUES

Smooth and well-executed comb-outs result from perfect sets. To achieve success as a hairstylist, you must first master the skills of shaping and molding hair, then you must practice fast, simple, and effective methods for comb-outs.

RECOMMENDED PROCEDURE

If you follow a definite system of combing out hairstyles, you will save time, be more consistent, and build an appreciative and loyal clientele. One procedure for combing out is outlined here.

1. After removing the rollers and clips, brush the hair through to integrate roller and pin curl settings, and relax the set. A cushioned paddle brush works well. Smooth and brush the hair into a semi-flat condition that permits you to position the lines for the planned hairstyle. It is essential that this procedure is correctly executed to achieve a smooth, flowing, finished coiffure. When combing out a curly style, use a pick or pick comb to lift and separate the curls before brushing out the hair.

2. After you have thoroughly brushed the hair, direct it into the general pattern desired. This can be accomplished by placing your hand on the client's head and gently pushing the hair forward in order that waves fall into the planned design. Lines of direction should be slightly overemphasized to allow for some expected relaxation during the comb-out process.

3. Back-comb areas that require volume and back-brush sections that need to be integrated. Accentuate and develop lines and style. Take one section at a time, placing the proper lines, ridges, volume, and indentations into the hairstyle. You can create softness and evenness of flow by blending, smoothing, and combing. Exaggerations and overemphasis should be eliminated. Finished patterns should reveal rhythm, balance, and smoothness of line.

4. Final touches make hairstyles look professional; *take your time.* After completing the comb-out, you can use the tail of a comb to lift areas where the shape and form are not precise. Every touch during the final stage must be very lightly performed. When the finishing touches have been completed, check the entire set for structural balance and then *lightly* spray the hair.

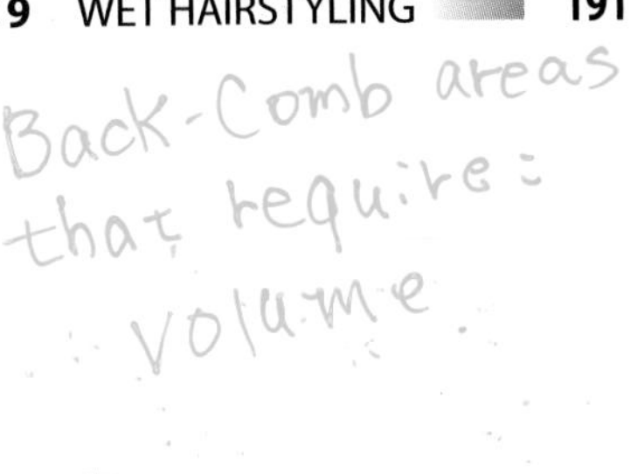

BACK-COMBING AND BACK-BRUSHING TECHNIQUES

Back-combing and back-brushing are the best means to achieve lift and increase volume. These techniques eliminate splits caused by rollers and pin curls and help the hairstyle last longer.

Back-combing is also called *teasing, ratting, matting*, or *French lacing*. This technique creates a firm cushion on which to build full-volume curls or bouffant hairstyles.

1. Starting in the front, pick up a section of hair approximately the same thickness as the teeth on your comb and 2" to 3" (5 to 7.5 cm) wide.
2. Insert the teeth of your comb about 1-½" (3.75 cm) from the scalp. (Fig. 9.148)
3. Press the comb gently down to the scalp, rotating the comb down and out of the hair. Repeat this motion two times. (Fig. 9.149)
4. If you wish to create a cushion (base), the third time you insert the comb use the same rotating motion, but firmly push the hair down to the scalp. Slide the comb out of the hair. (Fig. 9.150)

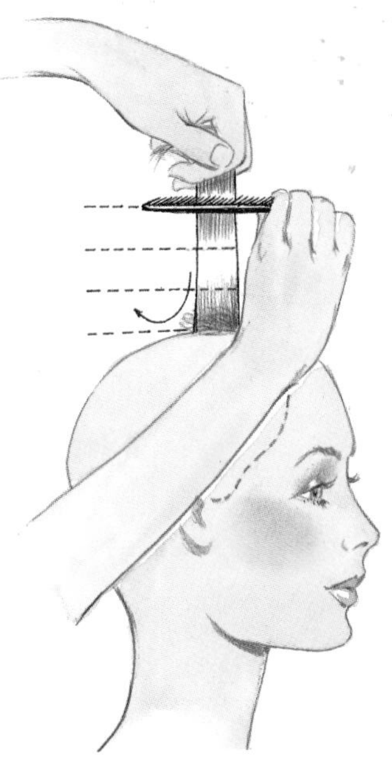

FIGURE 9.148 — Insert comb.

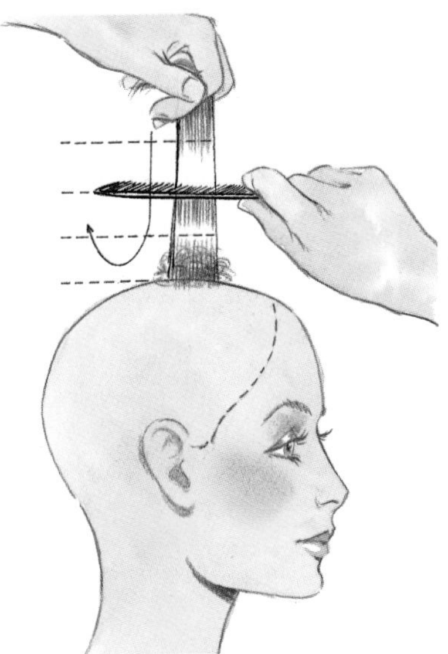

FIGURE 9.149 — Press comb down with slight circular motion.

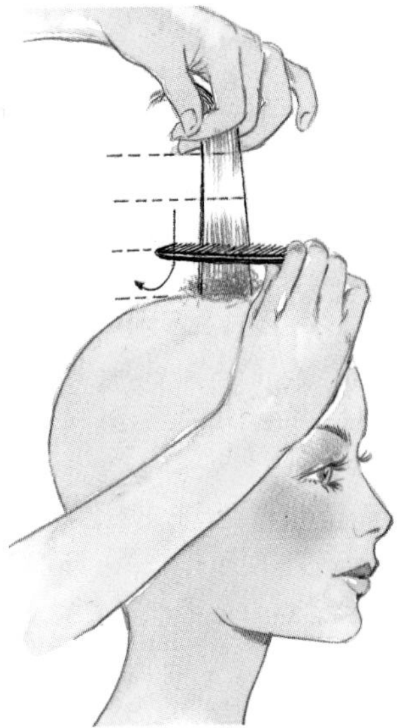

FIGURE 9.150 — Create base of back-combed hair.

5. Repeat this process, working up the strand until the desired volume is achieved.
6. To smooth hair that is back-combed, hold the teeth of the comb or the bristles of a brush at a 45-degree angle and pointed away from you. Lightly move the comb over the surface of the hair. (Figs. 9.151, 9.152)

Note: *One-length blunt-cut hair is very difficult to back-comb. Hair should be properly textured (thinned) for back-combing to be effective.*

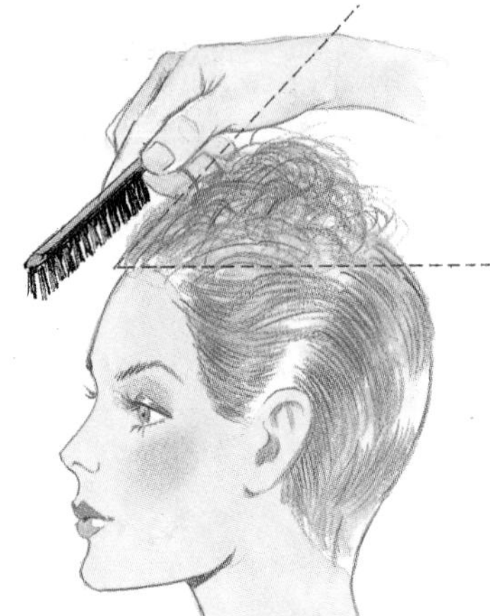

FIGURE 9.151 — Hold brush at 45 degrees to hair.

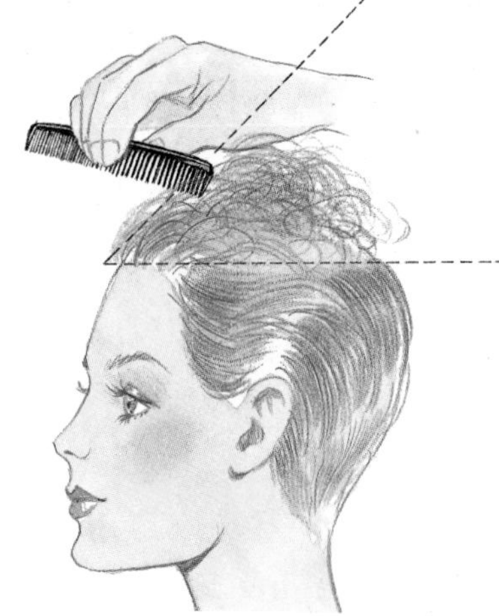

FIGURE 9.152 — Comb may also be used to smooth hair.

Back-brushing is also called ***ruffing***. It is a technique used to build a soft cushion, or to mesh two or more curl patterns together for a uniform and smooth comb-out.

1. Pick up and hold a strand straight out from the scalp.
2. With a slight amount of slack in the strand, place a narrow brush near the base of the strand. Push and roll the inner edge of the brush with the wrist until it touches the scalp. For interlocking to occur, the brush must be rolled. Then remove the brush from the hair with a turn of the wrist, peeling back a layer of hair. The shorter ends of tapered hair are interlocked to form a cushion at the scalp.
3. Repeat this procedure by moving the brush about ½" (1.25 cm) farther away from the scalp with each stroke until the desired volume has been achieved. (Fig. 9.153) ✔

Completed: Learning Objective #4

PROPER COMB-OUT TECHNIQUES

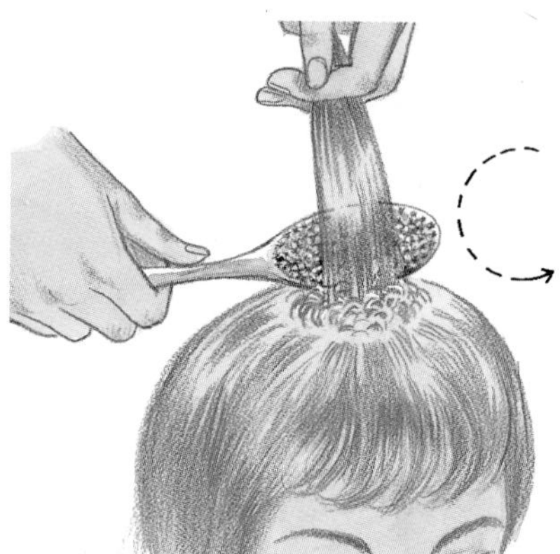

FIGURE 9.153 — Back-brushing.

BRAIDING

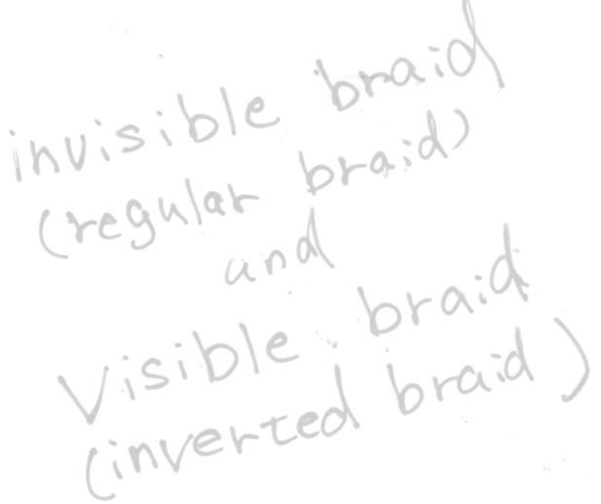

You will be asked to braid, plait, or cornrow the hair of children and adults alike. These styles must be done with a *firm* hand using even tension to all strands. It is advisable to braid on damp hair because some degree of stretch will assist in producing a long-lasting and neat style.

FRENCH BRAIDING

There are two different types of French braids: the ***invisible braid*** or regular braid and the ***visible braid*** or inverted braid.

Invisible braiding is performed by overlapping the strands on top.

1. Section the hair into two parts with a center part. (Fig. 9.154)
2. Clamp one side and divide the other side into three strands. (Fig. 9.155)
3. Start the braid by taking strand 1 (from the left) and crossing it *over* strand 2 (center strand) (strand 1 becomes the center strand). (Fig. 9.156)
4. Take strand 3 (from the right) and cross it *over* the center strand (it becomes the center strand). Hold the strands tightly. You have now completed the anchor point.
5. Pick up the strand on the left (original strand 2) and incorporate a small section (strand 2b), about ½" (1.25 cm) wide, from the scalp. Join the new section with the left strand and together draw them over the center strand. (Fig. 9.157)

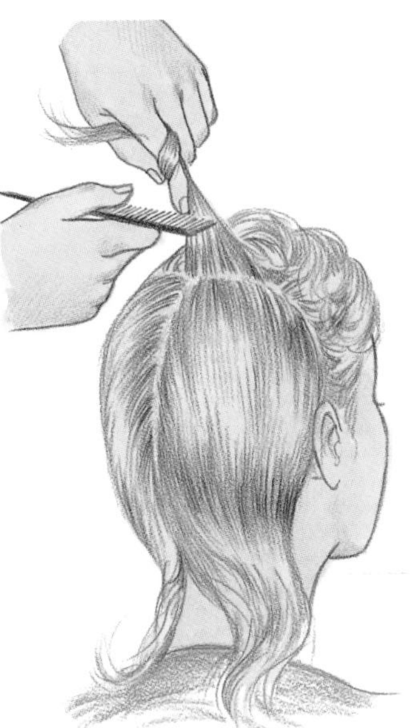

FIGURE 9.154 — Section hair.

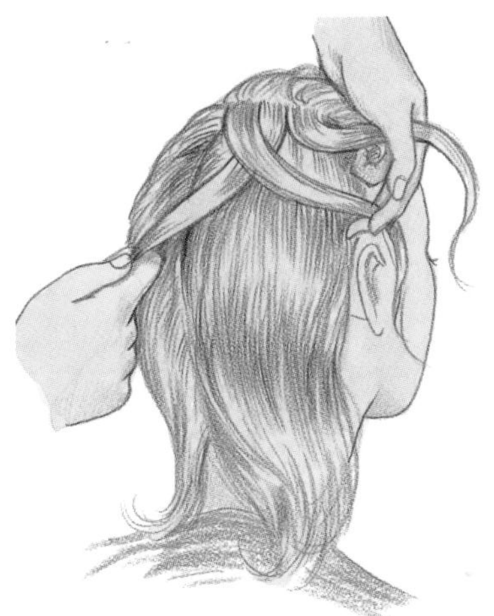

FIGURE 9.155 — Divide into three strands.

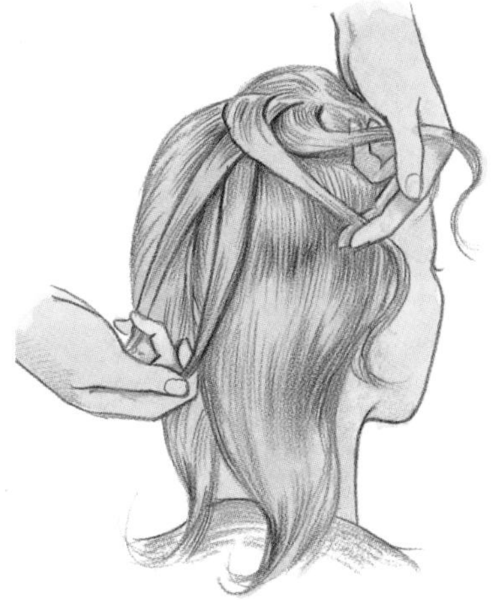

FIGURE 9.156 — Starting the braiding.

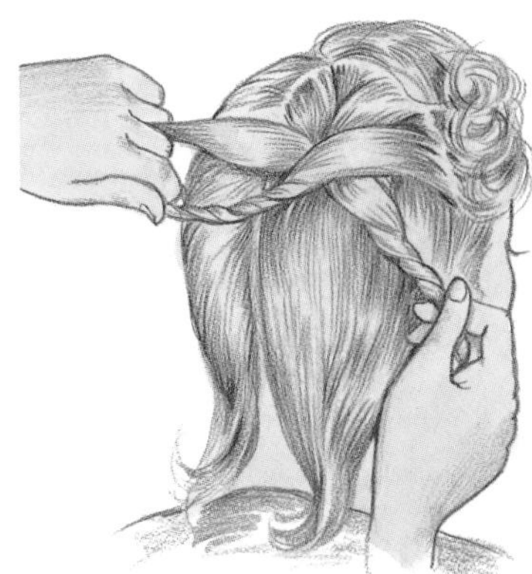

FIGURE 9.157 — Drawing over center strand.

6. Bring original strand 1 over the center hair. Bring a strand of scalp hair from the right, about ½" (1.25 cm) wide, and place it with strand 1.

7. Continue to pick up strands and braid until all the hair in the section has been taken into the braid. (Fig. 9.158)

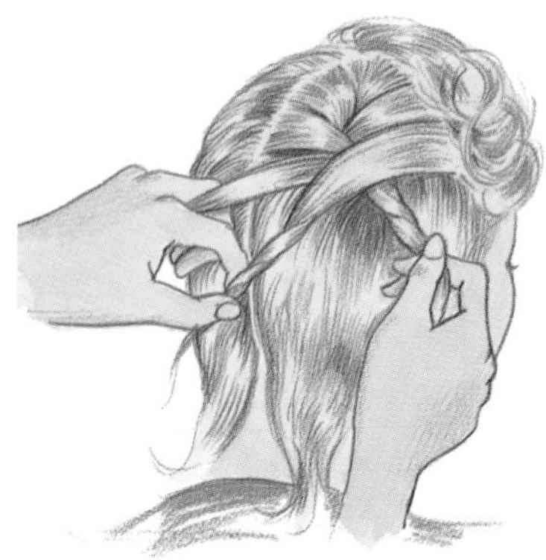

FIGURE 9.158 — Pick up strand.

Note: *To keep the braid neat with all short hair ends in place, twist each strand toward the center as you put it in place.*

8. Braid the other side in the same manner. (Fig. 9.159)

9. If the hair is long you can:

- Continue to braid through to the ends. It can then be crossed and extended up the back of the head or left to hang loose.
- Stop the braid at the hairline and tie ribbons, allowing the ends to fall into curls.

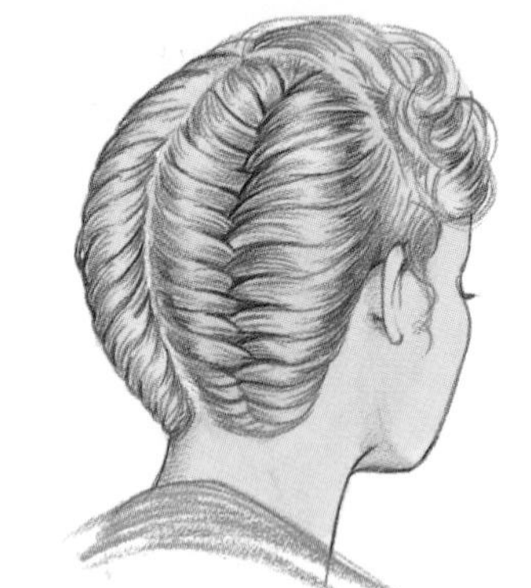

FIGURE 9.159 — Finish braiding.

If the hair is not very long you can:

- Fasten the ends with a rubber band and tuck them under and pin in place with bobby pins.
- Create design lines that travel around the head from temple to temple, or form various patterns with the braids and parting lines.
- You might want to start the French braid at the nape and work toward the face. You can tuck the ends under or finish the style with curls.

Visible French braiding (inverted braid) is done by plaiting the strands under, thus making the braid visible. It is done in the same manner as the invisible braid except that strands are placed *under* the center strand.

Part and section the hair in the same manner as for regular French braid.

1. Divide the top right section evenly into three strands. Start to braid the hair strands by placing the right side strand under the center strand and the left side strand under this one. Draw strands tightly. (Fig. 9.160)

2. Pick up ½" (1.25 cm) strand on the right side and combine with the right side strand. Place this combined strand under the center strand. Pick up ½" (1.25 cm) strand on the left side and combine with the left side strand. Place this combined strand under the center strand. (Fig. 9.161)

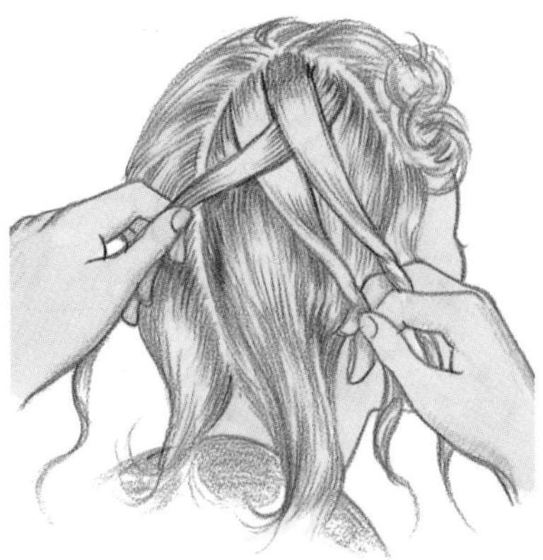

FIGURE 9.160 — Divide into three sections and begin braiding.

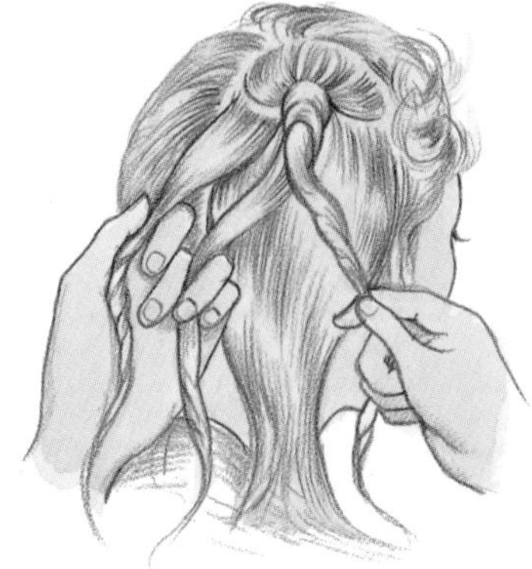

FIGURE 9.161 — Drawing under center strand.

3. Continue to pick up hair and braid as above. Finish braiding at nape, and hold in position with rubber bands. (Fig. 9.162)
4. Braid left side of the head in the same manner as right side. (Fig. 9.163)
5. The finished braids may be tucked under and held in place with hairpins or bobby pins. (Fig. 9.164) ✔

Completed:
Learning Objective
#5
SIMPLE FRENCH BRAID

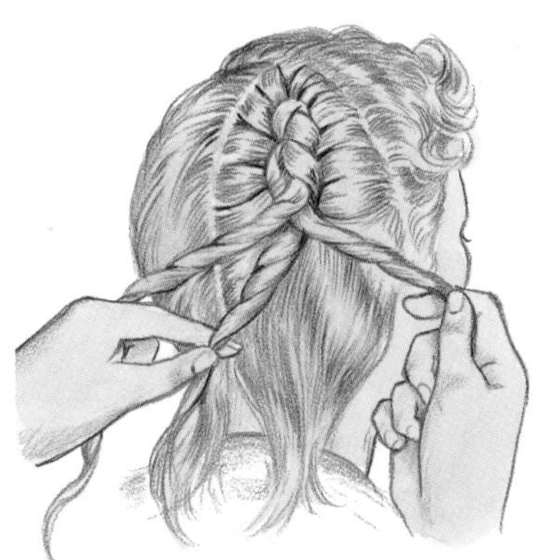

FIGURE 9.162 — Continue braiding.

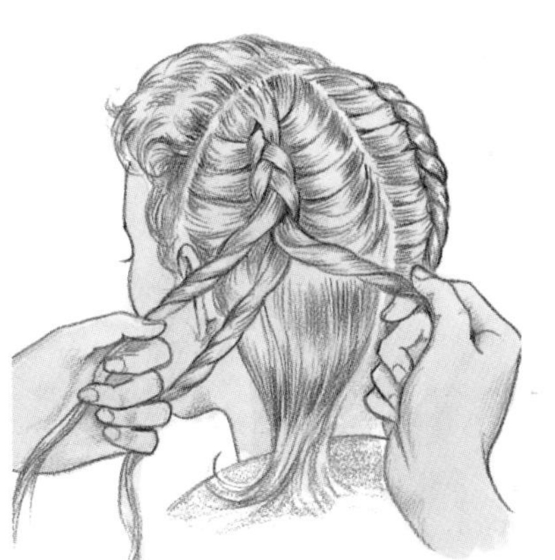

FIGURE 9.163 — Finish braiding.

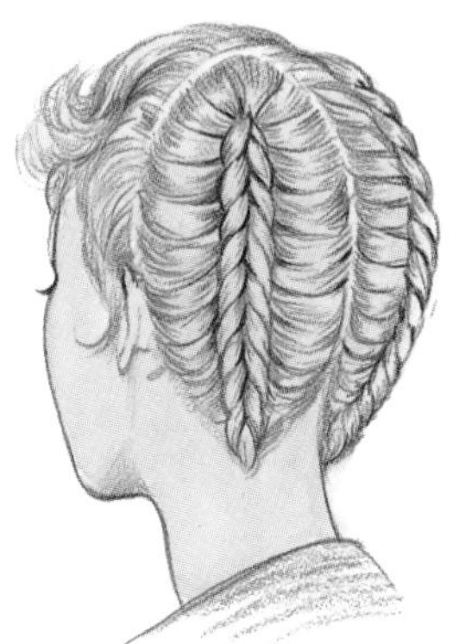

FIGURE 9.164 — Finished hairstyle.

Cornrowing is done in the same fashion as *visible French braiding* except that the sections are very narrow and form a predetermined style. It works well with overly curly hair and is popular with both children and adults. Cornrowing should last for several weeks.

PREPARATION FOR OVERLY CURLY HAIR

If your client has overly curly hair, you can prepare to cornrow as follows:

1. Shampoo in the usual way.
2. Apply conditioner and distribute it well.
3. Tie a hair net over the hair to hold it flat.
4. Place your client under a hood dryer, or blow-dry the hair.
5. Follow the visible French braid procedure using narrower sections and more tension to form the cornrow braids. (Fig. 9.165)

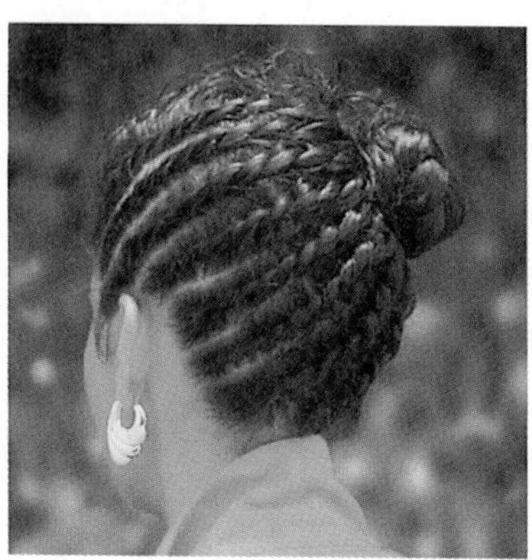

FIGURE 9.165 — A finished cornrow style.

REVIEW QUESTIONS

WET HAIRSTYLING

1. What is hairstyling?
2. List the implements used in wet hairstyling.
3. What is the purpose of finger waving?
4. What is the purpose of finger waving lotion?
5. Name the different types of finger waves.
6. List the parts of a pin curl.
7. What is a shaping for pin curl placement and how is it classified?
8. Why is stem direction important?
9. List the most commonly used bases of a pin curl.
10. List the three kinds of roller curl bases.
11. What is the purpose of back-combing?

CHAPTER 10

Thermal Hairstyling

LEARNING OBJECTIVES

After completing this chapter, you should be able to:

1. Define the purpose of thermal waving and curling.
2. Demonstrate proper thermal wave techniques and implements.
3. List safety measures used in thermal waving.
4. Define blow-dry styling.
5. Demonstrate the use of implements, techniques, and cosmetics in blow-dry styling.
6. Define air waving.
7. Demonstrate the use of implements and techniques in air waving.

NATIONAL SKILL STANDARDS

This chapter provides you with the necessary information to master these National Industry Skill Standards for Entry-Level Cosmetologists:

- Providing styling and finishing techniques to complete a hairstyle to the satisfaction of the client
- Safely using a variety of salon products while providing client services

INTRODUCTION TO THERMAL WAVING AND CURLING

Completed: Learning Objective #1

THE PURPOSE OF THERMAL WAVING AND CURLING

The art and technique of using thermal irons for waving and curling was developed in 1875 by a Frenchman, Marcel Grateau. Thermal waving is still known as ***marcel waving.***

Thermal waving and ***curling*** is the art of waving and curling straight or pressed hair (see chapter on thermal hair straightening) with thermal irons, either electrically heated or stove-heated, using special manipulative techniques. Modern implements have contributed to the continued success of these methods of waving and curling hair.

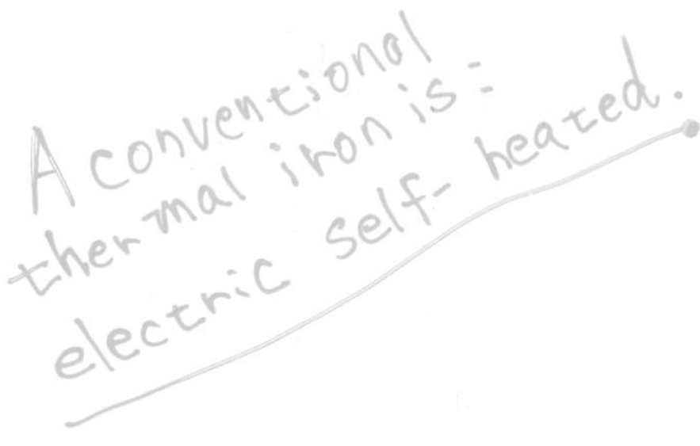
A conventional
thermal iron is =
electric self- heated.

THERMAL IRONS

Thermal irons are an important implement in hairstyling. They provide an even heat that is completely controlled by the cosmetologist. Manipulative techniques are basically the same for electric irons or stove-heated irons.

The irons must be made of the best quality steel so that they hold an even temperature during the waving and curling process. The styling portion of the irons is composed of two parts: the rod (prong) and the shell (groove or bowl).

1. The ***rod*** is a perfectly round solid steel bar.
2. The ***shell*** is perfectly round with the inside grooved so that the rod can rest in it when the irons are closed.

The edge of the shell nearest the cosmetologist is called the ***inner edge;*** the one farthest from the cosmetologist is called the ***outer edge.***

Thermal irons come in a variety of styles, sizes, and weights, from small to jumbo. They come in three different classifications:

1. Conventional (regular) stove-heated. (Fig. 10.1)
2. Electric self-heated. (Fig. 10.2)
3. Electric self-heated, vaporizing.

Note: *Do not use electric vaporizing irons on pressed hair; the moisture could cause the hair to revert to its natural overly curly state.*

There is no one correct temperature used for the irons when thermal curling and waving the hair. Temperature setting for the irons depends on the texture of the hair, whether it is fine or coarse, or whether it has been lightened or tinted. Hair that has been lightened or tinted (also white hair) should be curled and waved with lukewarm irons. Coarse and gray hair, as a rule, can tolerate more heat than fine hair.

> **CAUTION**
>
> *Do not use thermal irons on chemically straightened hair; to do so could cause breakage.*

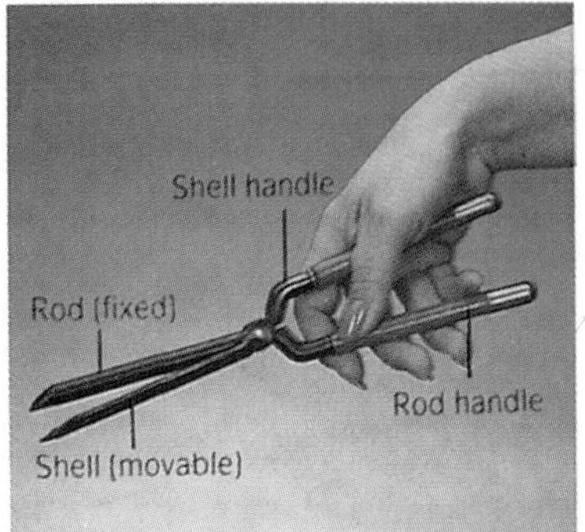

FIGURE 10.1 — Conventional thermal (marcel) irons.

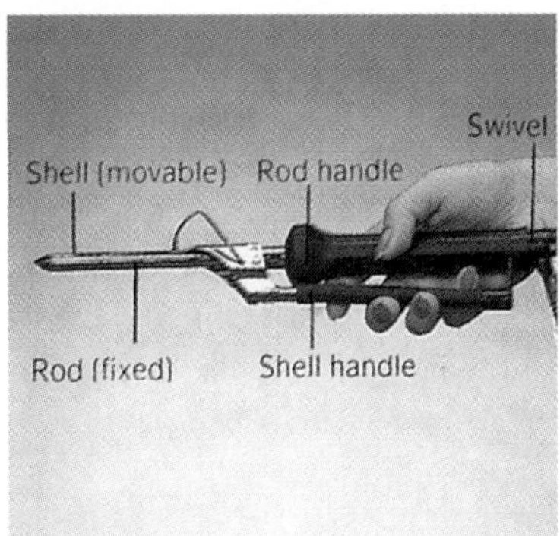

FIGURE 10.2 — Electric thermal irons.

Testing Thermal Irons

After heating the irons to the desired temperature, test them on a piece of tissue paper. Clamp the heated irons over the tissue and hold for 5 seconds. If the paper scorches or turns brown, the irons are too hot. (Fig. 10.3) Let them cool somewhat before using. Overly hot irons can burn, scorch, or damage hair, and can discolor white hair. Remember that fine, lightened, or badly damaged hair withstands less heat than normal hair.

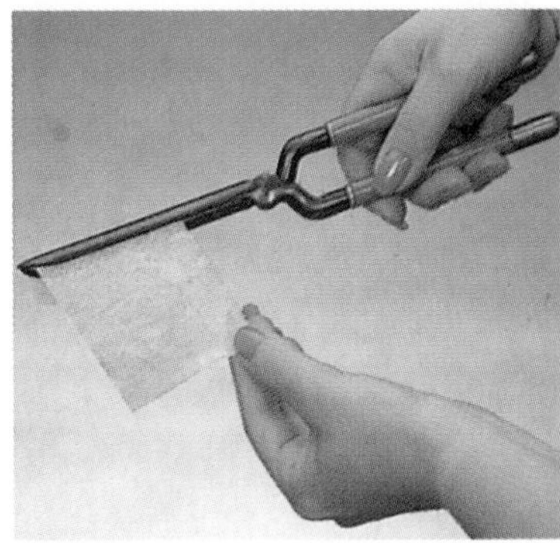
FIGURE 10.3 — Testing the heat of thermal irons.

Care of Thermal Irons

Thermal irons should be kept clean and free from rust and carbon. To remove dirt or grease, wash the irons in a soap solution containing a few drops of ammonia. This cuts the oil and grease that usually adhere to the irons. Fine sandpaper, or steel wool with a little oil, helps to remove rust and carbon. It also polishes the irons. To permit greater facility in movement, oil the joint of the irons.

New thermal irons are ***tempered*** at the factory in order to hold heat uniformly. If you overheat the irons they usually lose their temper, and, in most cases, are ruined.

Holding the Thermal Irons

Hold the irons in a comfortable position that gives you complete control. Grasp the handles of the irons in the right hand, far enough away from the joint to avoid the heat. Place the three middle fingers on the back of the lower handle, the little finger in front of the lower handle, and the thumb in front of the upper handle.

Comb Used with Thermal Irons

The comb should be about 7" (17.5 cm) long, made of hard rubber or another nonflammable substance, and should have fine teeth; fine teeth hold the hair more firmly than coarse teeth.

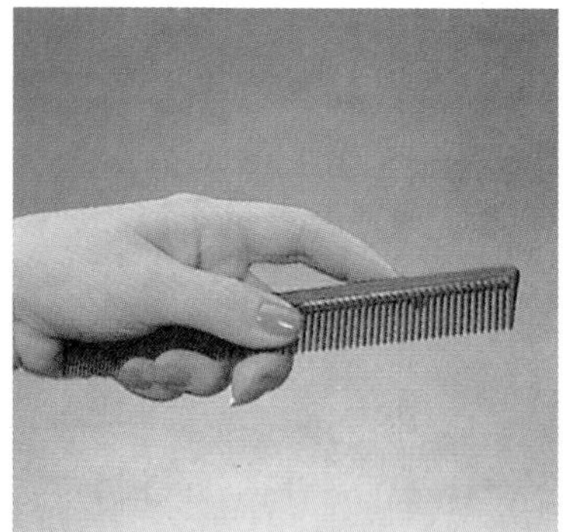

FIGURE 10.4 — Holding the comb.

Holding the Comb

Hold the comb between the thumb and all four fingers of the left hand, with the index finger resting on the backbone of the comb for better control and one end of the comb resting against the outer edge of the palm. This position assures a strong hold and a firm movement. (Fig. 10.4)

Practicing with Cold Thermal Irons

Since thermal curling and waving is a somewhat difficult operation that uses heated irons, practice with cold irons on a mannequin or hairpiece pinned to a block until you have thoroughly mastered the technique.

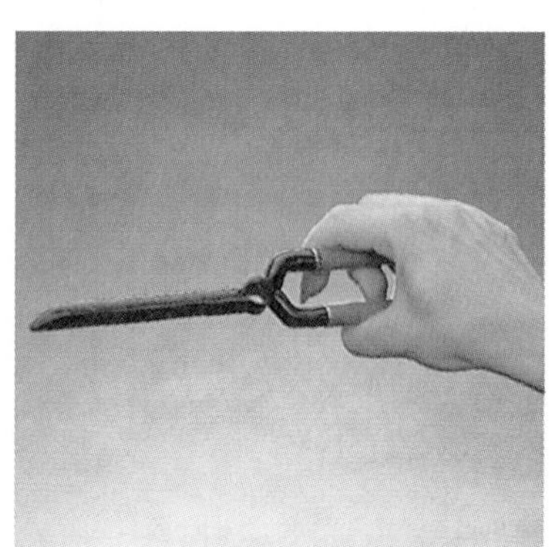

FIGURE 10.5 — Rolling the irons.

Rolling the Thermal Irons

Practice rolling the cold thermal irons in the hand, first forward, then backward. The rolling movement should be done without any sway or motion in the arm; only the fingers are used to roll the handles in either direction. (Fig. 10.5)

Exercises with Cold Thermal Irons

Exercise 1

At the starting position the rod of the thermal iron will be on top of the hair strand. (Fig. 10.6a) To make the curl, rotate the iron one-half turn (Fig. 10.6b) and then one full turn to complete. (Fig. 10.6c)

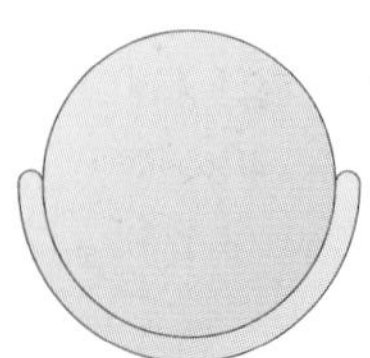

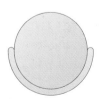

FIGURE 10.6a — Starting position.

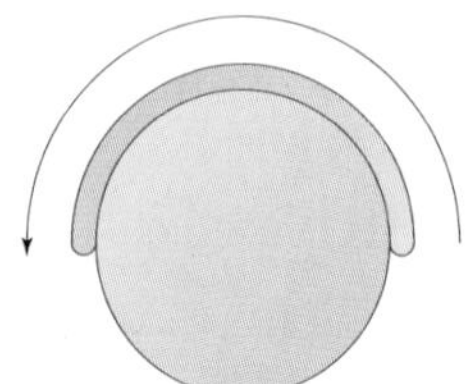

FIGURE 10.6b — One-half turn.

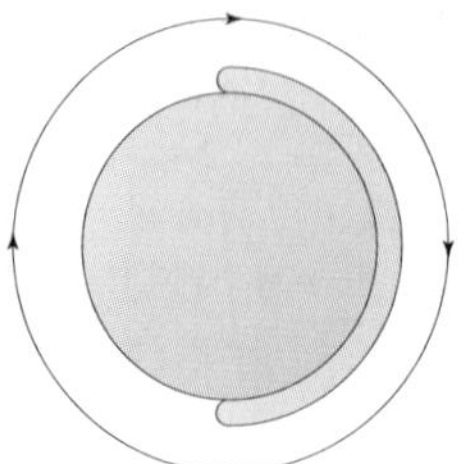

FIGURE 10.6 c — Full turn.

Exercise 2

1. Insert hair in irons with rod on top (groove facing upward).
2. Turn irons forward for one-half turn (away from you).
3. Turn irons back to starting position.
4. Open irons slightly and slide down 1" (2.5 cm), then clamp.
5. Turn irons backward for full turn (toward you).
6. Turn irons forward to starting position.
7. Release.

THERMAL WAVING WITH CONVENTIONAL THERMAL (MARCEL) IRONS

Thermal waving is the art of waving hair using conventional marcel irons. The process requires no setting creams or lotions.

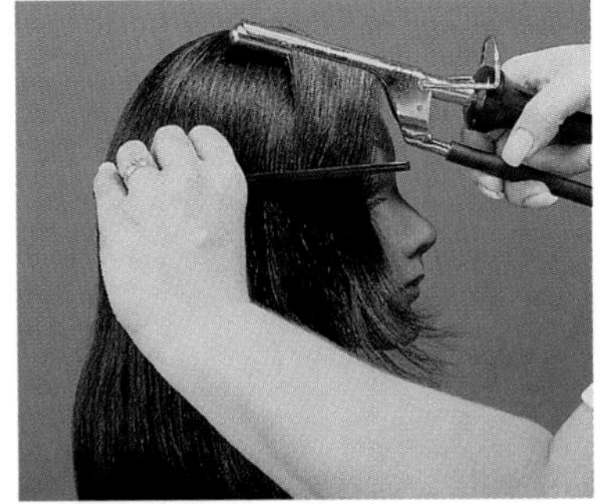

FIGURE 10.7 — Insert irons in the hair.

Procedure for Left-Going Wave

Comb the hair thoroughly, following its directional growth. The natural growth will determine whether or not the first wave to be formed will be a left-going wave or a right-going wave. The procedure given here is for a left-going wave.

Before the wave is begun, comb the hair in the general shape desired by the client.

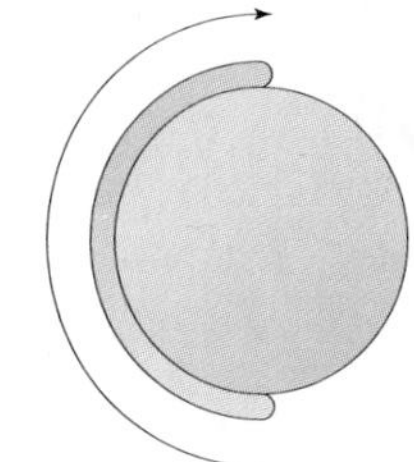

FIGURE 10.8 — One-quarter turn.

1. With the comb, pick up a strand of hair about 2" (5 cm) in width. Insert the irons in the hair with the groove facing upward. (Fig. 10.7)
2. Close irons and turn them about one-quarter turn forward (away from you). At the same time, draw the hair with the irons about ¼" (.625 cm) to the left, (Fig. 10.8) and direct the hair ¼" (.625 cm) to the right with the comb. (Fig. 10.9)
3. Roll the irons one full turn forward (away from you). (Fig. 10.10) (In doing this, keep the hair uniform with the comb. You will find that the hair has rolled on a slight slant on the prong of the irons.) Keep position No. 3 for a few seconds in order to allow the hair to become sufficiently heated throughout.
4. Reverse movement No. 3 by simply unrolling the hair from the irons, bringing them back into their first resting position. (Fig. 10.11) (When this movement is completed, you will find the comb resting somewhat away from the irons.)

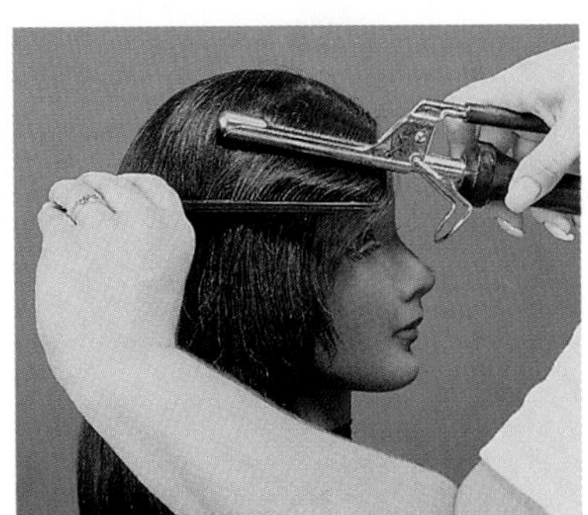

FIGURE 10.9 — Direct hair to the right with the comb.

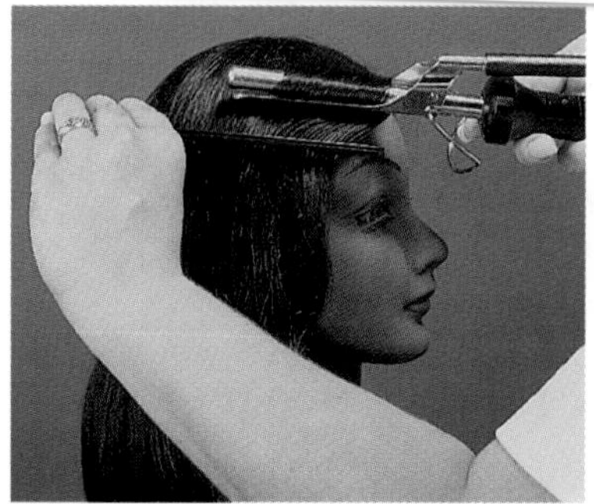

FIGURE 10.10 — Roll irons one full turn forward.

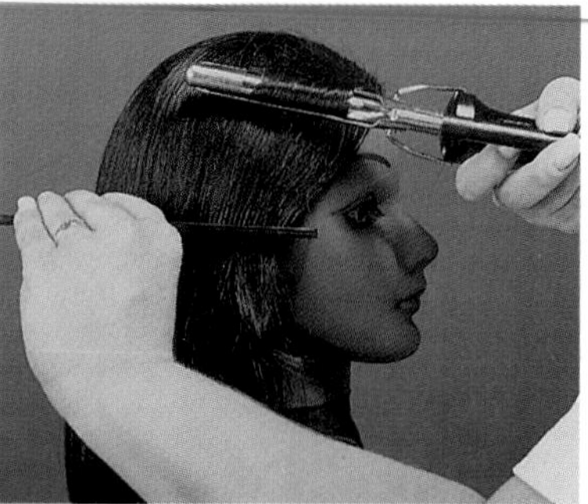

FIGURE 10.11 — Reverse movement.

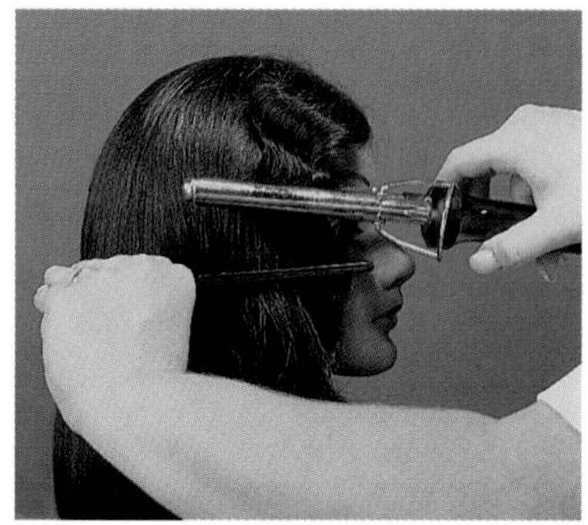

FIGURE 10.12 — Start to form the curl.

5. Open the irons with the little finger and place them just below the ridge, or crest, by swinging the rod of the irons toward you and then closing them. (Fig. 10.12) (The outer edge of the groove should be directly underneath the ridge just produced by the inner ridge.)

6. Keep the irons perfectly still and direct the hair with the comb upward about 1" (2.5 cm), thus forming the hair into a half circle. (Fig. 10.13) (You must remember that, in order to perform movement No. 6 properly, you do not move the comb from the position explained in movement No. 5.)

7. Without opening the irons, roll them one-half turn forward (from you). (Fig. 10.14) (In this movement, keep the comb perfectly still and unchanged.)

8. Slide the irons down about 1" (2.5 cm). (Fig. 10.15) (This movement is done by opening the irons slightly [loose grip] and then sliding them down the strand of hair.)

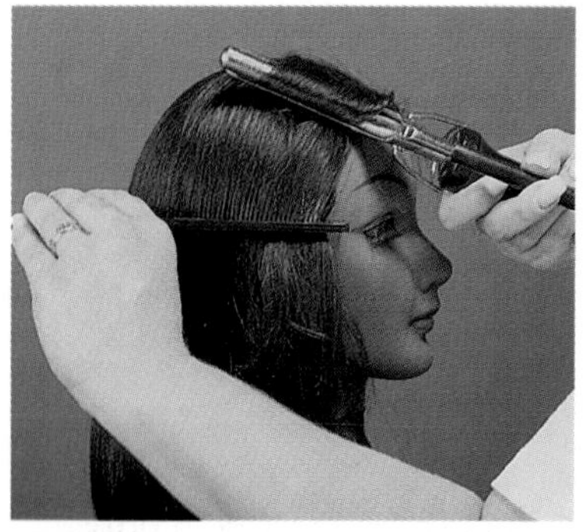

FIGURE 10.13 — Form the hair into a half circle.

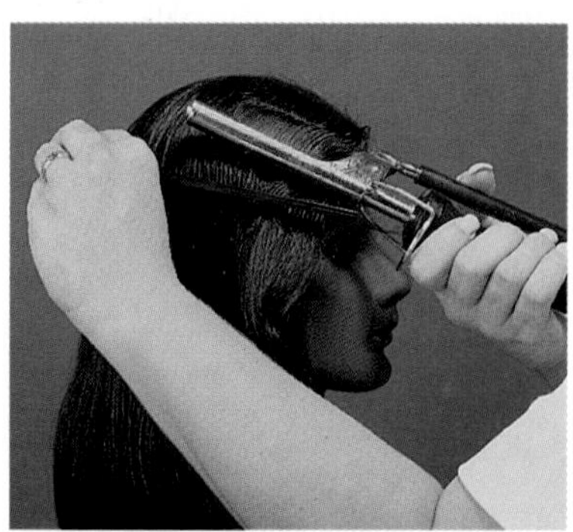

FIGURE 10.14 — Roll irons one-half turn forward.

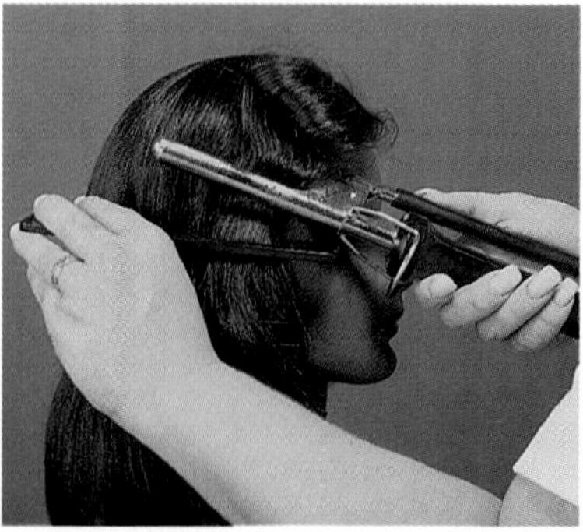

FIGURE 10.15 — Slide irons down.

Right-Going Wave

After completing movement No. 8, you will find the irons and comb in a position to make the second ridge. This is the beginning of a right-going wave. As you might expect for a right-going wave, the hair is directed opposite to that of a left-going wave.

Joining or Matching the Waves

After completely waving one strand of hair, wave the next strand to match. When picking up the unwaved hair in the comb, include a small section of the waved strand as a guide to the formation of the new wave. (Fig. 10.16)

When waving the second strand of hair, be sure that the comb and irons movements are the same as in the first strand of hair; otherwise the waves will not match.

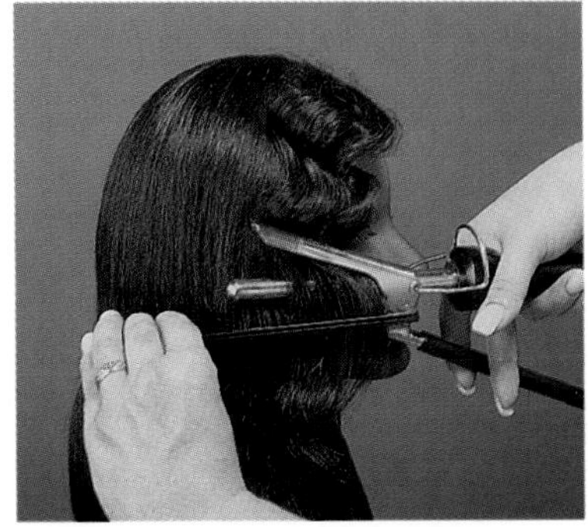

FIGURE 10.16 — Matching the wave.

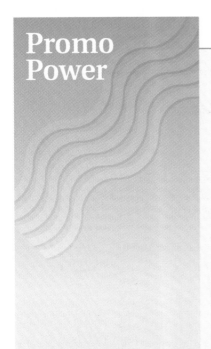

DIRECT MAILING

Direct mailing is probably the most advantageous of all types of advertising and marketing for a salon owner to do, especially if you mail to your existing clientele. They know and like you and are more likely to purchase what you are offering. And because your clients usually live nearby (within a five-mile radius is the norm), this is a relatively inexpensive way to advertise. Direct mail can entice first-time clients to return and keep regular clients coming back as well.

Design what you are presenting in a fashionable manner. If it is a special on permanent waves or color, use a photograph or sketch as part of the design. You will find that postcards cost less, but for a more formal or personal special, use envelopes.

If you plan to use direct mail frequently in your salon, you will save yourself a great deal of time and trouble if you purchase a computer, which can store all of your customer files and print out address labels. It is very important to keep track of the people who respond to mailings; your computer can help do this. If you don't know your rate of return, your mailing won't do you any good. And it's important to plan ahead, since having something typeset and printed takes time.

—*From* The Salon Biz: Tips for Success *by Geri Mataya*

THERMAL CURLING WITH ELECTRIC THERMAL IRONS

Thermal curling is the art of creating curls in the hair using modern thermal irons and a comb. Since thermal curling requires no setting creams or lotions, it may be used to great advantage for the following:

1. ***Straight hair***—permits quick styling. Thermal curling eliminates working with wet hair, use of rollers, and a long hair-drying process.
2. ***Pressed hair***—permits styling the hair without the danger of its reverting to its former overly curly condition. Thermal curling prepares the hair for any desired style. (See Chapter 14.)
3. ***Wigs*** and ***hairpieces***—presents a quick and effective method for their styling. (See Chapter 15.)

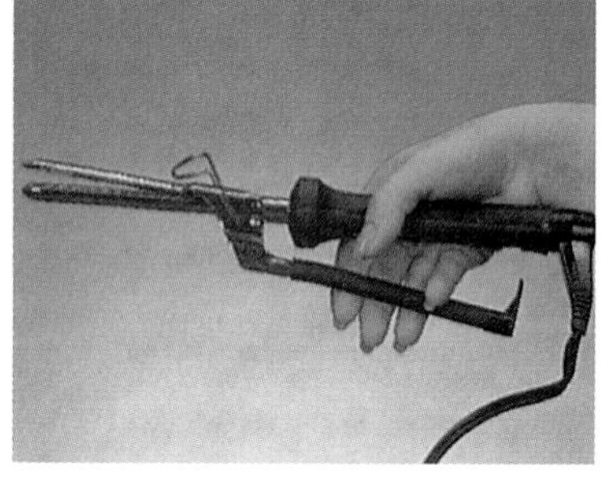

FIGURE 10.17 — Use the little finger to open the clamp.

Curling Irons Manipulations

The following is a series of basic manipulative movements for using heated curling irons. Most other curling irons movements are variations of these basic movements.

The following illustrations show a grip with only the little finger used for opening the clamp. (Figs. 10.17–10.23) Some cosmetologists prefer to use the little finger plus the ring finger for this purpose. Either method is correct.

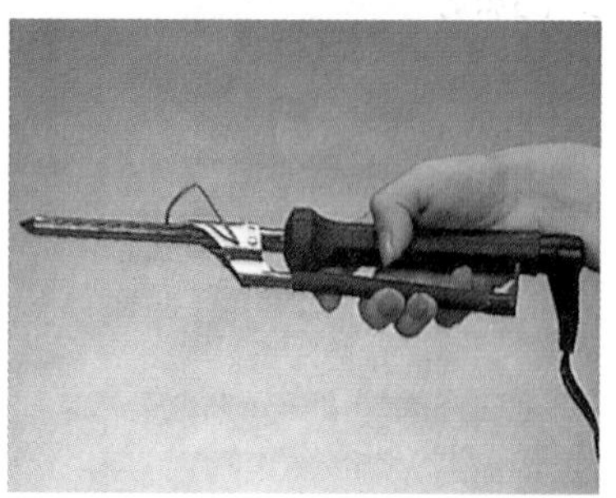

FIGURE 10.18 — Use three middle fingers to close and manipulate irons.

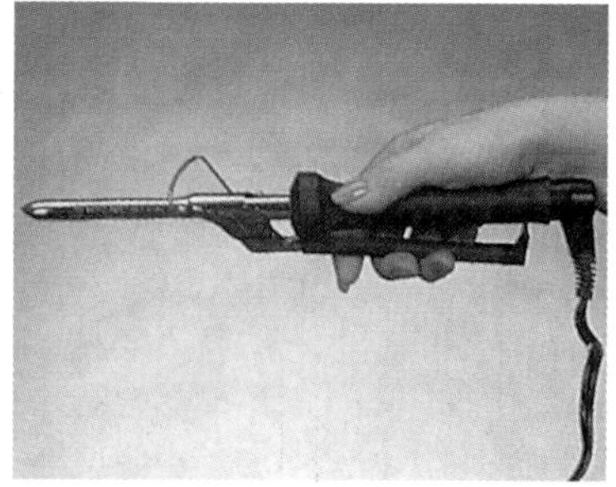

FIGURE 10.19 —Shift the thumb when manipulating the irons.

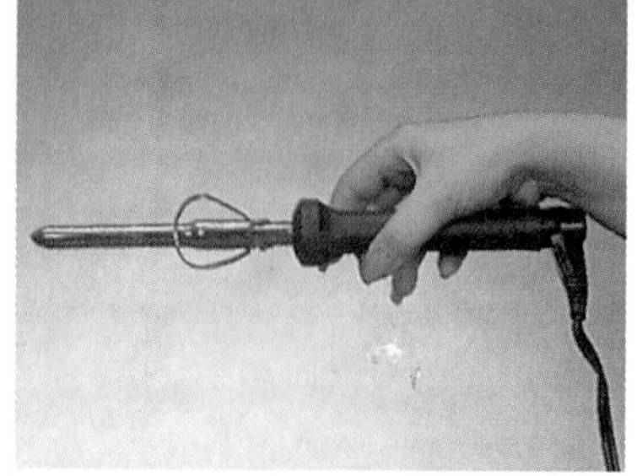

FIGURE 10.20 — Close clamp and make a one-quarter turn downward.

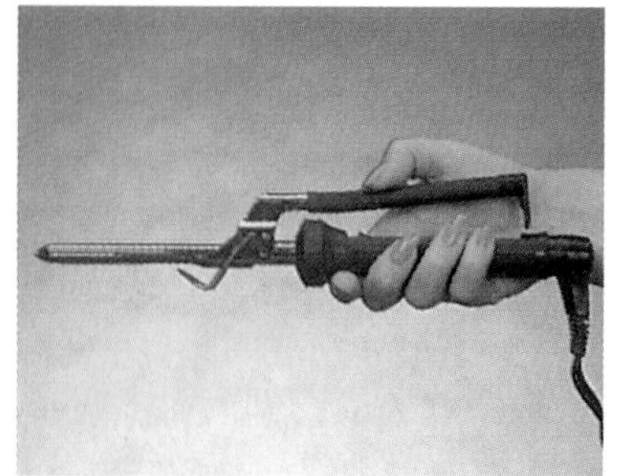

FIGURE 10.21 — Irons have made a one-half turn. Use the thumb to open clamp and relax hair tension.

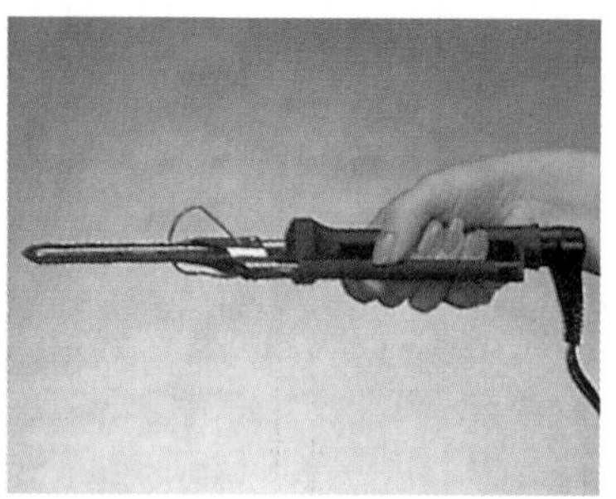

FIGURE 10.22 — Rotate irons to three-quarters of a complete turn.

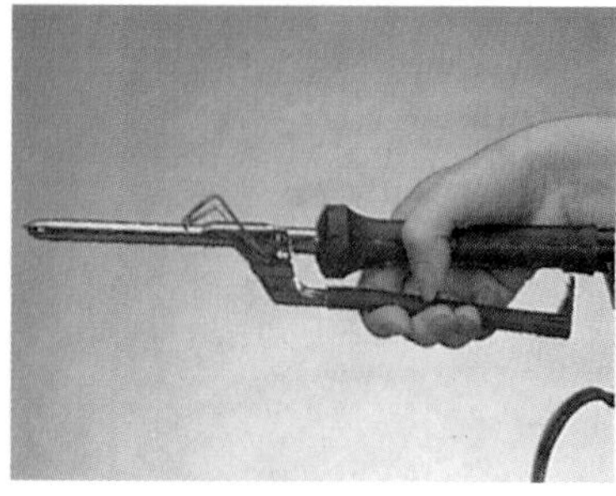

FIGURE 10.23 — Full turn.

The method of holding the irons is a matter of personal preference. The technique used should be the one that gives you the greatest ease, comfort, and facility of movement.

Practice in manipulating the curling irons is recommended to develop proficiency in their use. Remember to practice with cold irons. The following four exercises are designed to help achieve an effective use of the irons.

1. Since it is important to develop a smooth rotating movement, practice turning the irons while opening and closing them at regular intervals. Practice rotating the irons in both directions. Examples: downward (toward you) and upward (away from you). (Fig. 10.24)
2. Practice releasing the hair by opening and closing the irons in a quick, clicking movement.
3. Practice guiding the hair strand into the center of the curl as you rotate the irons. This exercise results in the end of the strand being firmly in the center of the curl. (Fig. 10.25)
4. Practice removing the curl from the irons by drawing the comb to the left and the rod to the right. (Fig. 10.26) Use the comb to protect the client's scalp from burns.

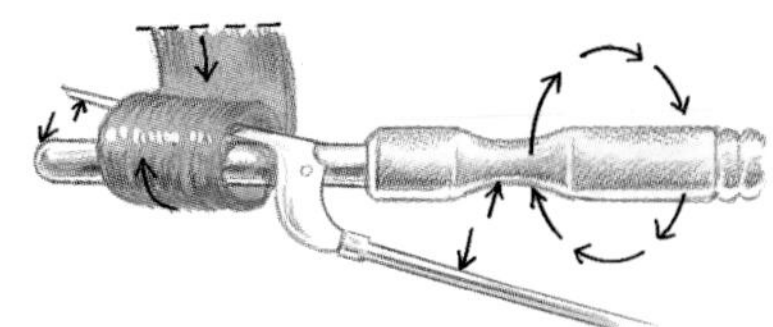

FIGURE 10.24 — Rotating movement while opening and closing the irons.

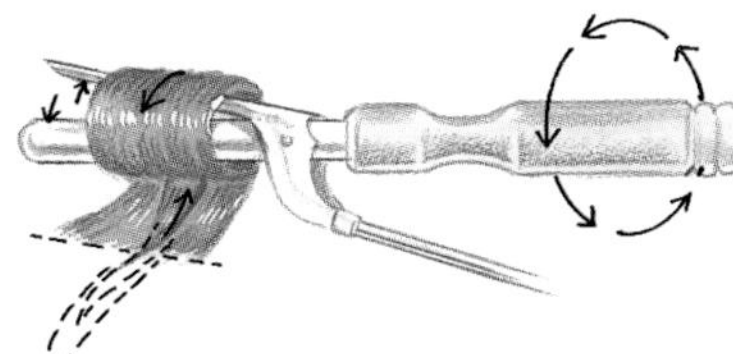

FIGURE 10.25 — Guiding the hair strand into the center of the curl while rotating the irons.

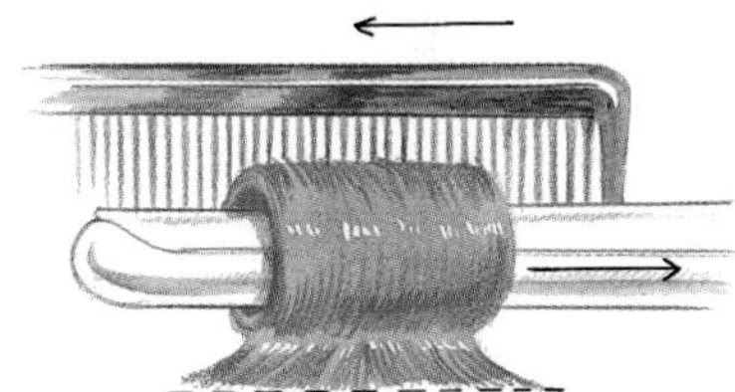

FIGURE 10.26 — Removing the curl using comb as guide.

THERMAL IRONS CURLING METHODS

Today's thermal irons curling methods have improved over the older techniques. The following methods may be changed or modified to conform with your instructor's procedures.

Preparation

1. Comb the hair thoroughly, removing all tangles.
2. Divide the head into five sections.
   a) First section, about 2½" (6.25 cm) wide, extends from center of forehead to nape of neck.
   b) Divide two side panels in half, from top parting to neck, to provide four additional sections.
3. Heat thermal irons (large or jumbo size).
4. Subdivide sections into ¾" by 2½" (1.875 by 6.25 cm) subsections. (Fig. 10.27) The same procedure is followed for electric irons and stove-heated irons.

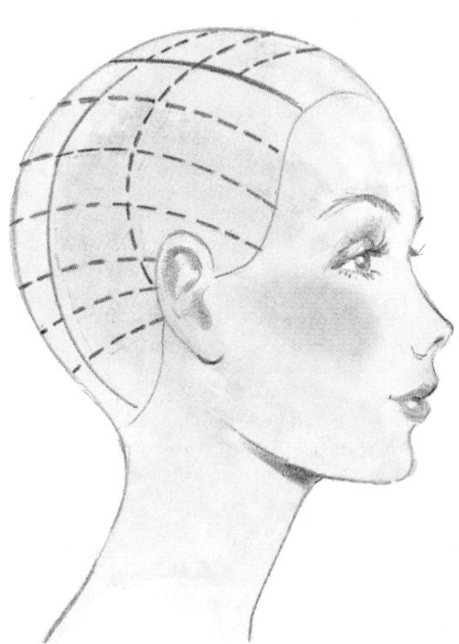

FIGURE 10.27 — Hair sectioned and subdivided.

Curling Short Hair

The base of each curl is formed by sectioning and parting to conform with the size of the curl desired. It is important to consider hair length, density, and texture. The base is usually about 1½" to 2" (3.75 cm to 5 cm) in width and approximately ½" (1.25 cm) in depth.

After sectioning off the base, comb the hair smooth and straight out from the scalp. The hair must be combed smooth in order that the heat and tension are the same for all hair in the section. Loose hairs may result in an uneven and ragged curl.

1. After the irons have been heated to the desired temperature, pick up a strand of hair and comb it up and smooth. With the groove on top, insert the irons about 1" (2.5 cm) from the scalp and hold for a few seconds to form a base. (Fig. 10.28)

2. Hold the ends of the hair strand with the thumb and two fingers of the left hand, using a medium degree of tension. Turn the irons downward (toward you) with the right hand. (Fig. 10.29)

3. Open and close the irons rapidly as you turn, to prevent binding. Guide the ends of the strand into the center of the curl as you rotate the irons. (Fig. 10.30)

4. The result of this procedure will be a smooth, finished curl, with the ends firmly fixed in the center. Remove the irons from the curl. (Fig. 10.31)

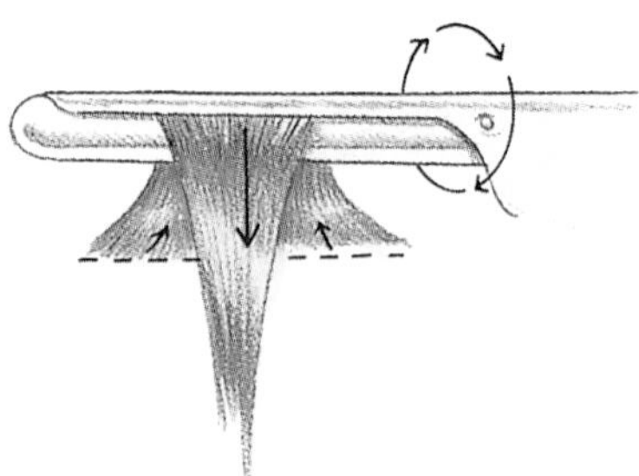

FIGURE 10.28 — Form a base.

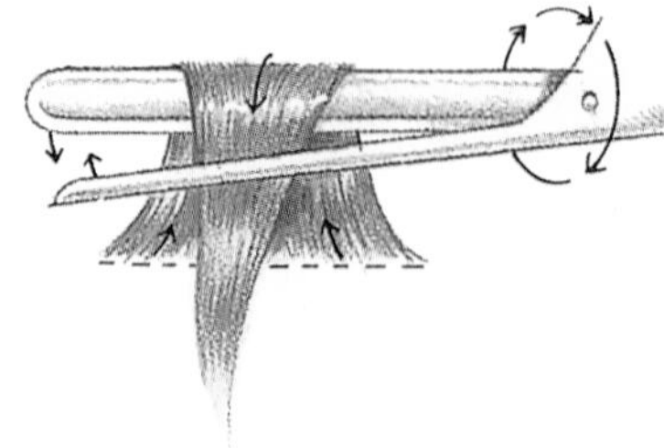

FIGURE 10.29 — Turn irons downward.

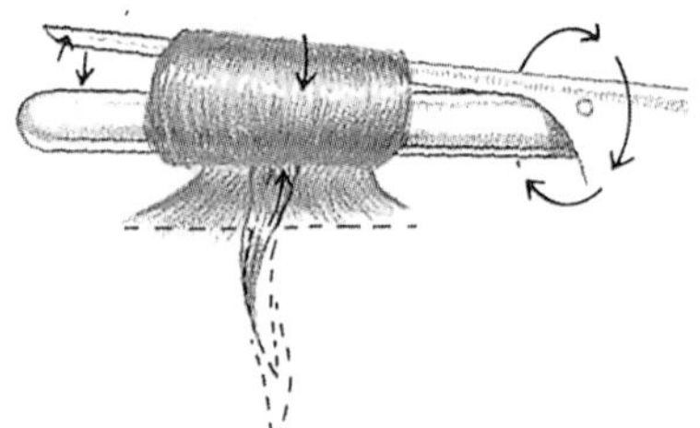

FIGURE 10.30 — Rotate irons and guide ends of strand into center.

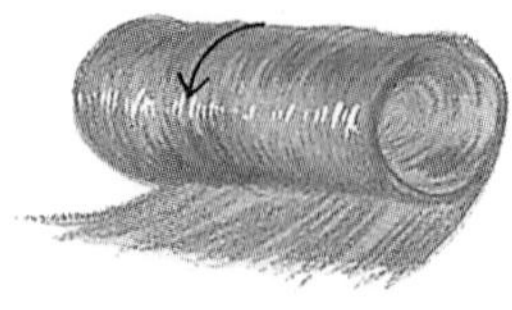

FIGURE 10.31 — Finished curl.

Curling Medium Length Hair (Using One Loop or "Figure 6")

Section and form the base of the curl as described for short hair.

1. Insert the hair into the open irons at the scalp. Pull the hair over the rod in the direction of the curl and close the shell. Hold irons in this position for about 5 seconds to heat the hair, and then slide irons up to 1" (2.5 cm) from the scalp. The shell must be on top. (Fig. 10.32)
2. Turn irons downward one-half revolution; pull the end of the strand over the rod to the left and direct the strand toward the center of the curl. (Fig. 10.33)
3. Complete the revolution of the irons, and continue directing the ends toward the center. (Fig. 10.34)
4. Make another complete revolution of the irons. The entire strand has now been curled with the exception of the ends. Enlarge the curl by opening the shell. Insert the ends of the curl into the opening created between the shell and the rod. (Fig. 10.35)
5. Close the shell and slide irons toward the handles. This technique will move the ends of the strand into the center of the curl. Rotate irons several times to even out the distribution of the hair in the curl. (Fig. 10.36)

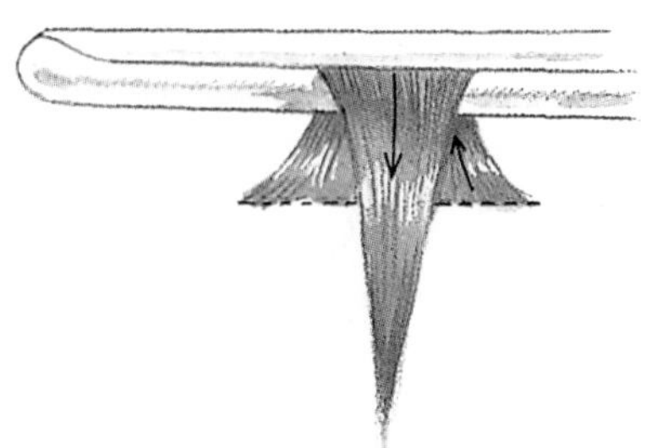

FIGURE 10.32 — Insert the hair into open irons at the scalp.

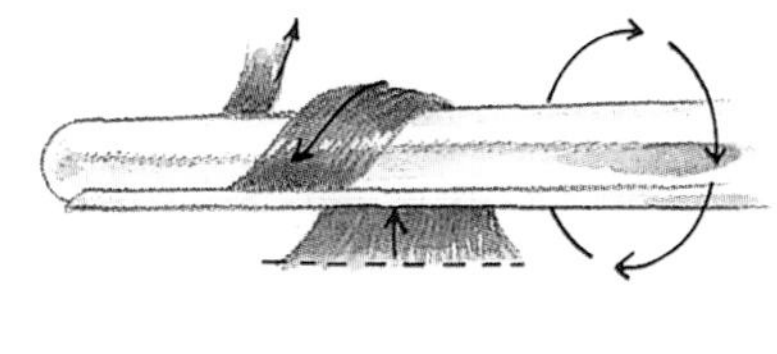

FIGURE 10.33 — Turn irons downward one-half revolution.

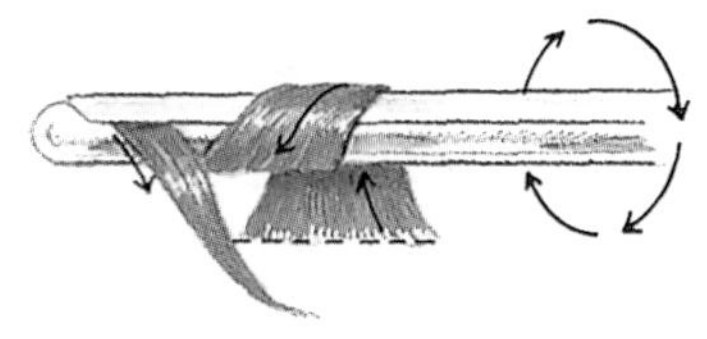

FIGURE 10.34 — Complete the revolution of the irons.

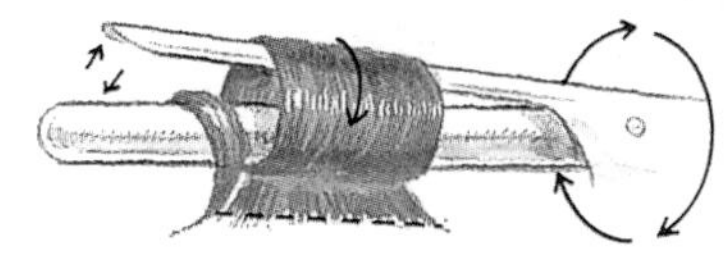

FIGURE 10.35 — Make another complete revolution.

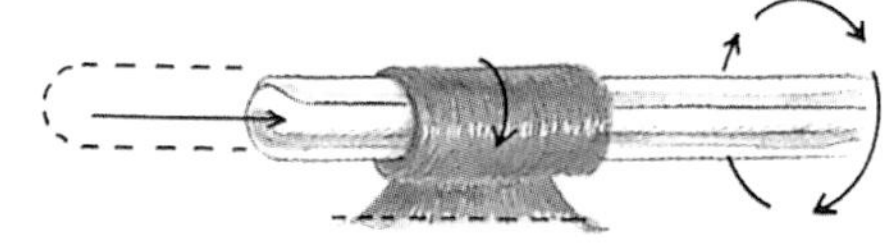

FIGURE 10.36 — Close the shell and slide irons toward the handles.

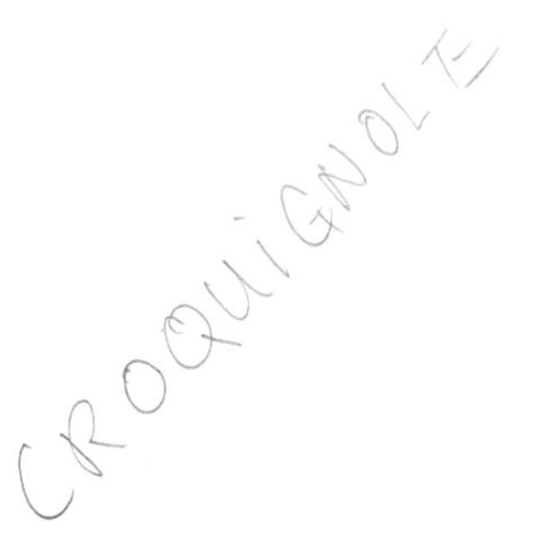

CAUTION

To protect the client during the curling process, use the comb between the scalp and irons.

When the curl is formed and the ends are freed from between the rod and the shell, make one complete revolution of the irons inside the curl. This final revolution smoothes the ends and loosens the hair away from the irons. The comb is then used to help remove the curl from the irons. The irons are drawn slowly in one direction, while the comb draws the hair in the opposite direction. In this way the curl is removed from the irons.

Curling Long Hair

(Using Two Loops or "Figure 8,")

Section and form the base of the curl as previously described.

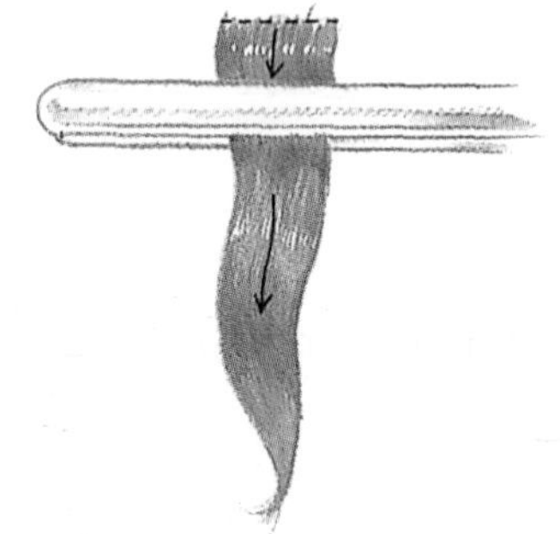

FIGURE 10.37 — Insert hair about 1" (2.5 cm) from the scalp.

1. Insert the hair into the open irons about 1" (2.5 cm) from the scalp. Pull the hair over the rod in the direction in which the curl is to move and close the shell. Hold irons in this position for about 5 seconds, in order to heat the hair. Hold the strand of hair with a medium degree of tension. (Fig. 10.37)
2. Roll irons under. Click and roll the irons until the groove is facing you. (Fig. 10.38)
3. With the left hand, pick up the ends of the hair. (Fig. 10.39)
4. Continue to roll and click the irons, keeping them the same distance from the scalp. (Fig. 10.40)
5. Draw the hair strand toward the tip of the irons. (Fig. 10.41)

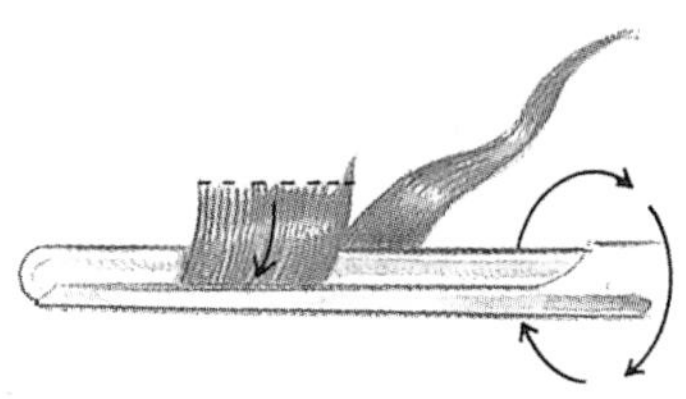

FIGURE 10.38 — Roll irons under.

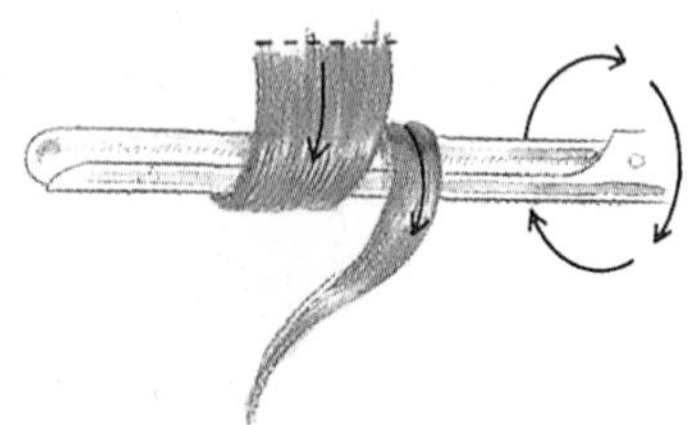

FIGURE 10.39 — Pick up the ends of the hair.

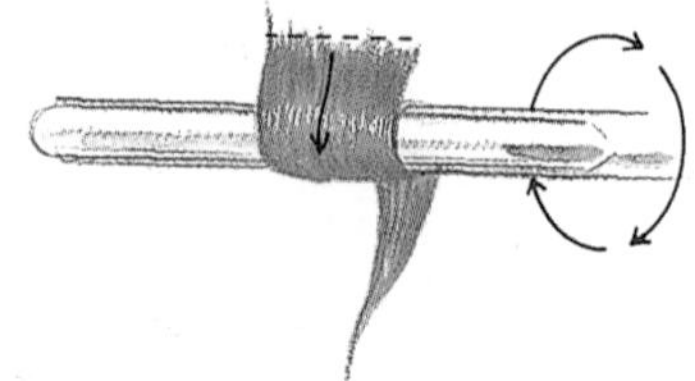

FIGURE 10.40 — Continue to roll the irons.

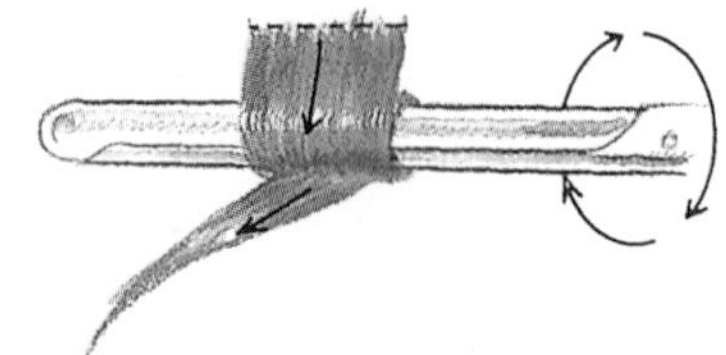

FIGURE 10.41 — Draw hair strand toward the point of the irons.

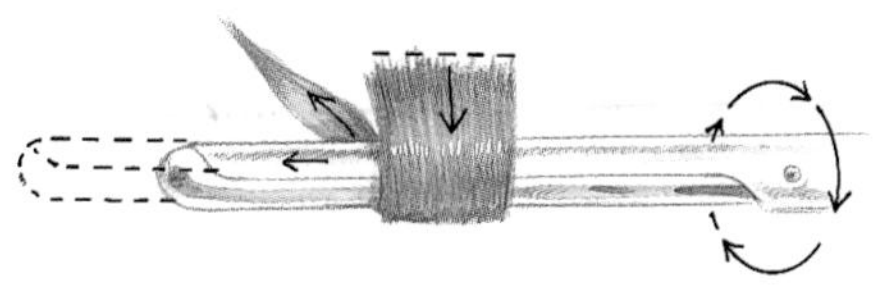

FIGURE 10.42 — Draw strand right, push irons left.

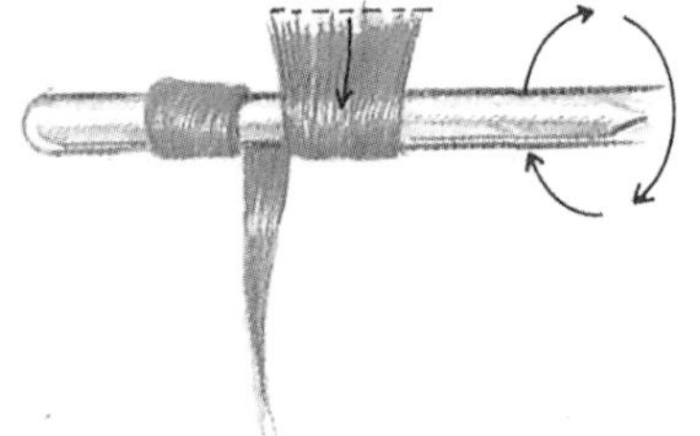

FIGURE 10.43 — Form two loops around the closed irons.

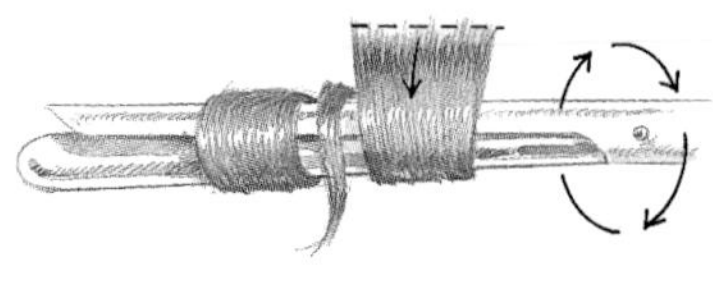

FIGURE 10.44 — Roll irons until hair ends disappear.

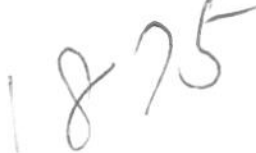

6. Draw the strand a little to the right, and, at the same time, push the irons slightly to the left. (Fig. 10.42)
7. By pushing irons forward and pushing the hair with the left hand, you form two loops around the closed irons, with the ends of the strand extending out between the loops. (Fig. 10.43)
8. Roll under and click irons until the ends of the hair disappear. (Fig. 10.44)
9. Rotate irons several times to even out the distribution of the hair in the curl and to facilitate the movement of the curl off the irons.

Other Types of Curls

Spiral curls are hanging curls that are suitable for long hairstyles.

Part the hair into as many sections as there will be curls and comb smooth. Insert the irons at an angle, with the bowl (groove) on top near the base of the strand, and rotate irons until all the hair is wound. Hold the curl in this position for 4 to 5 seconds, and remove the irons in the usual manner. (Figs. 10.45–10.48)

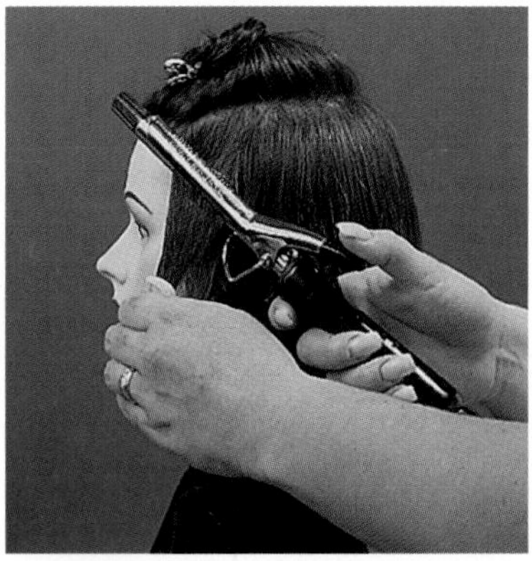

FIGURE 10.45 — Insert irons at an angle.

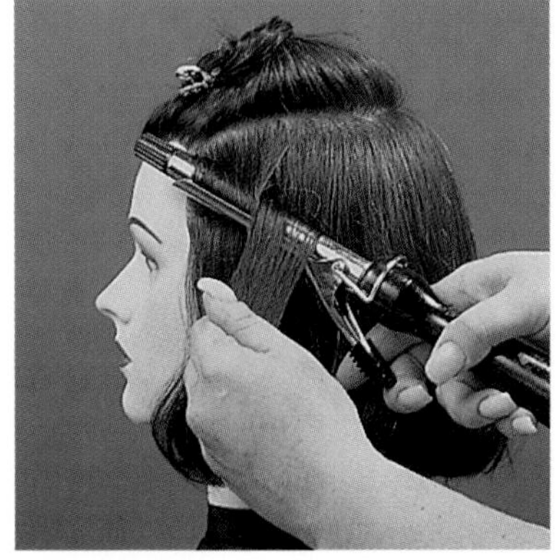

FIGURE 10.46 — Rotate irons until hair is wound.

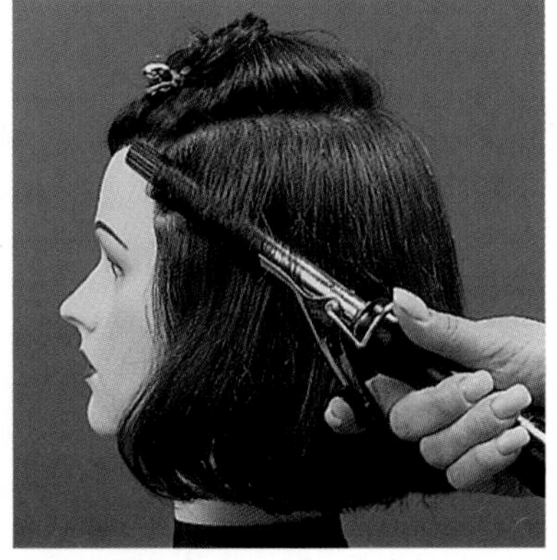

FIGURE 10.47 — Hold curl in position.

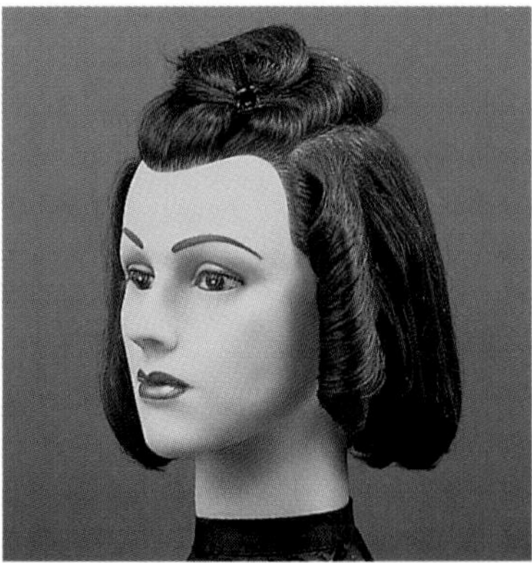

FIGURE 10.48 — Finished curl.

End curls can be used to give a finished appearance to hair ends. Long, medium length, or short hair may be styled with end curls. The hair ends can be turned under or over, as desired.

The position of the curling irons and the direction of their movements will determine whether the end curls will turn under or over. (Figs. 10.49, 10.50)

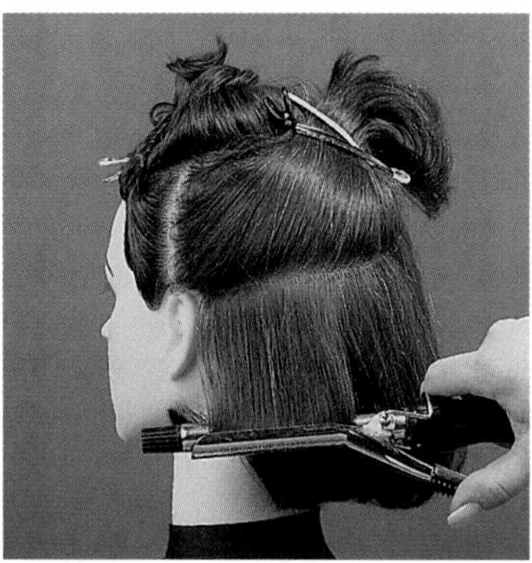

FIGURE 10.49 — Turning irons under.

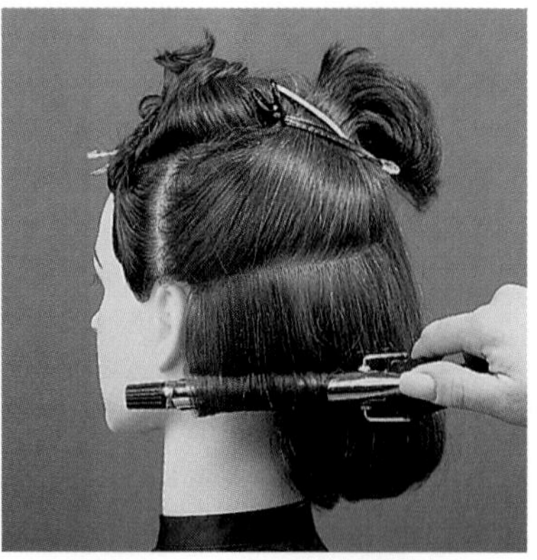

FIGURE 10.50 — Turning irons over.

VOLUME THERMAL IRON CURLS

Volume thermal iron curls are used to create volume or lift in a finished hairstyle. The degree of lift desired determines the type of volume curls to be used.

Volume-Base Curls

Volume-base curls provide maximum lift or volume, since the curl is placed very high on its base. Section off the base as described on pp. 201–202. Hold the curl strand at a 135° (2.36 rad.) angle. Slide irons over the strand about ½" (1.25 cm) from the scalp. Wrap the strand over the rod with medium tension. Maintain this position for approximately 5 seconds to heat the strand and set the base. Roll the curl in the usual manner and firmly place it forward and high on its base.

Full-Base Curls

The full-base curl provides a strong curl with full volume. Section off the base as described on pp. 201–202. Hold the hair strand at a 125° (2.18 rad.) angle. Slide irons over the hair strand about ½" (1.25 cm) from the scalp. Wrap the strand over the rod with medium tension. Maintain this position for about 5 seconds to heat the strand and set the base. Roll the curl in the usual manner, and place it firmly in the center of its base. (Fig. 10.51)

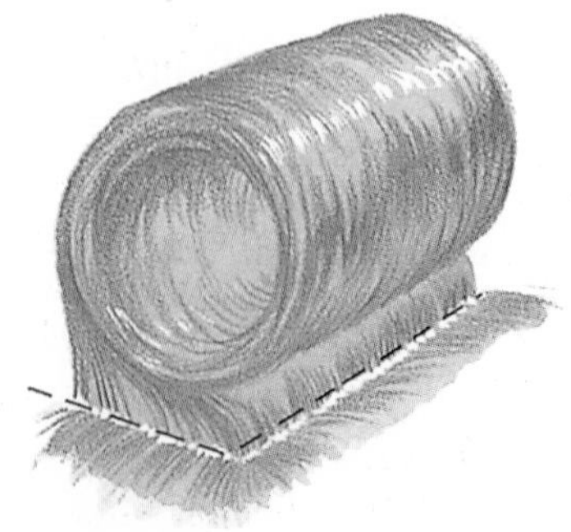

FIGURE 10.51 — Full base.

Half-Base Curls

The half-base curl provides a strong curl with moderate lift or volume. Section off the base as described on pp. 201–202. Hold the hair at a 90° (1.57 rad.) angle. Slide irons over the hair strand about ½" (1.25 cm) from the scalp. Wrap the strand over the rod with medium tension. Maintain this position for about 5 seconds to heat the strand and set the base. Roll the curl in the usual manner, and place it half off its base. (Fig. 10.52)

Off-Base Curls

The off-base curl provides a strong curl with only slight lift or volume. Section off the base as described on pp. 201–202. Hold the hair at a 70° (1.22 rad.) angle. Slide irons over the hair strand about ½" (1.25 cm) from the scalp. Wrap the strand over the rod with medium tension. Maintain this position for about 5 seconds to heat the strand and set the base. Roll the curl in the usual manner, and place it completely off its base. (Fig. 10.53)

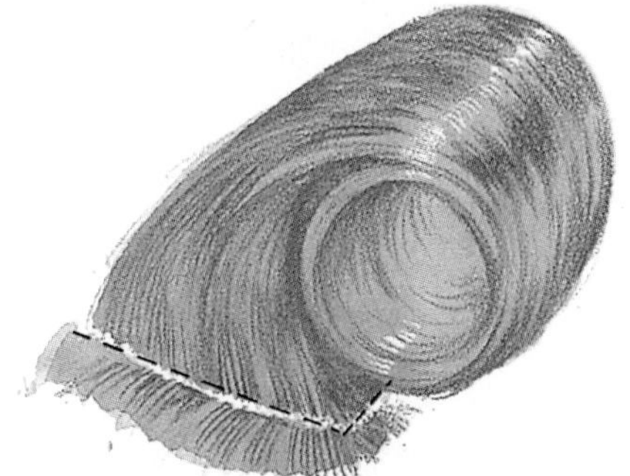

FIGURE 10.52 — One-half off base.

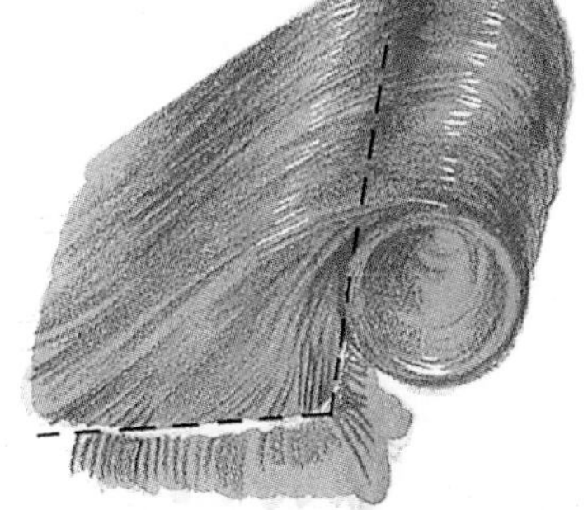

FIGURE 10.53 — Off base.

FINISHED THERMAL CURL SETTINGS

For best results when giving a thermal setting, clip each curl in place until the whole head is complete and ready for styling. (Figs. 10.54–10.56)

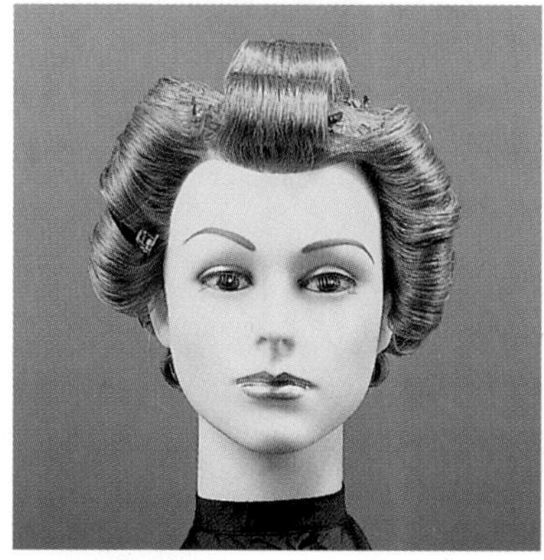

FIGURE 10.54 — Front view completely curled.

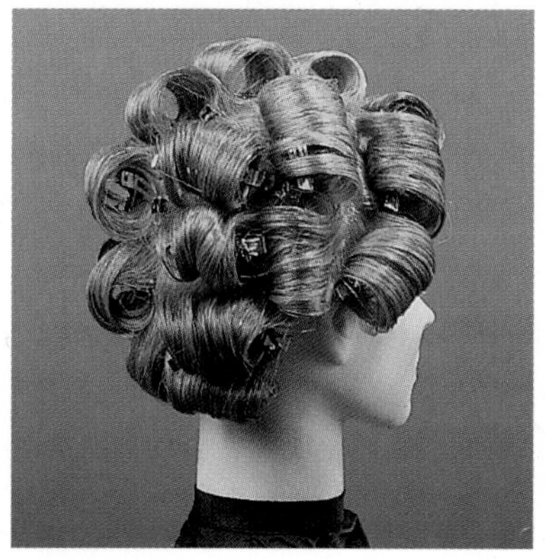

FIGURE 10.55 — Side view.

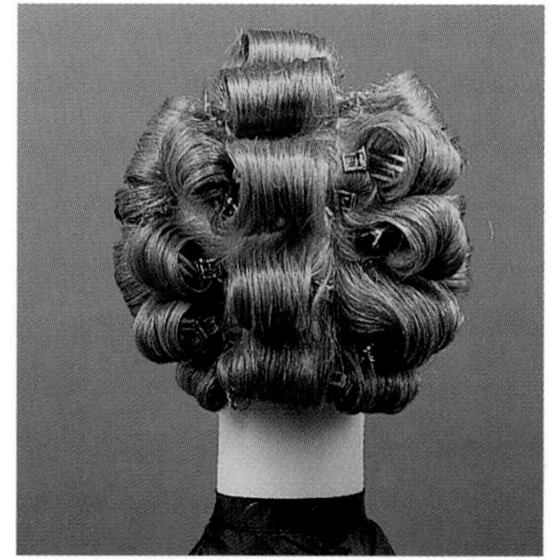

FIGURE 10.56 — Back of head completely curled.

Completed: Learning Objective #2

THERMAL WAVE TECHNIQUES AND IMPLEMENTS

STYLING THE HAIR AFTER A THERMAL CURL OR WAVE

After thermal waving or curling, style the hair according to the client's wishes. Brush the hair, working up from the neckline; push the waves and curls into place as you progress over the entire head. If the hairstyle is to be finished with curls, do the bottom curls last. (Figs. 10.57–10.60)

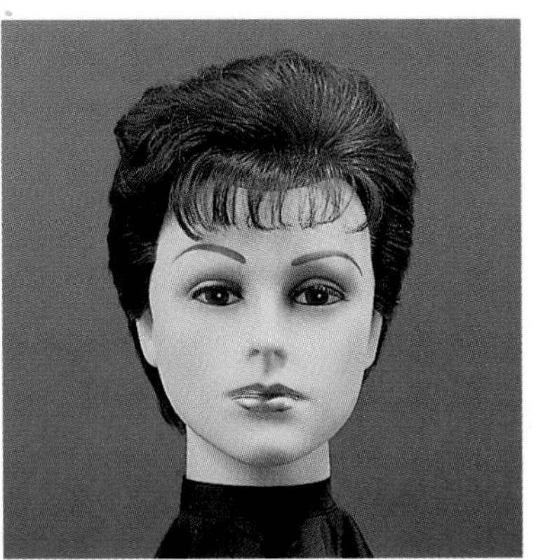

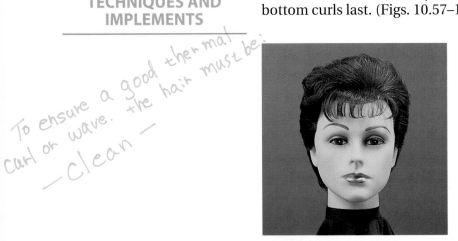

FIGURE 10.57 — Finished thermal style for short hair.

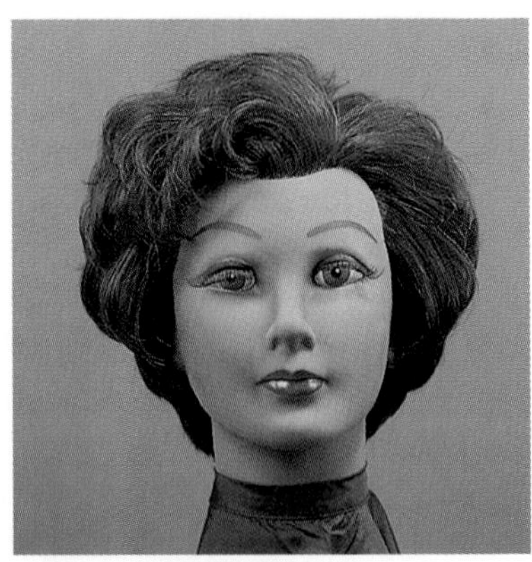

FIGURE 10.58 — Finished thermal style for short hair.

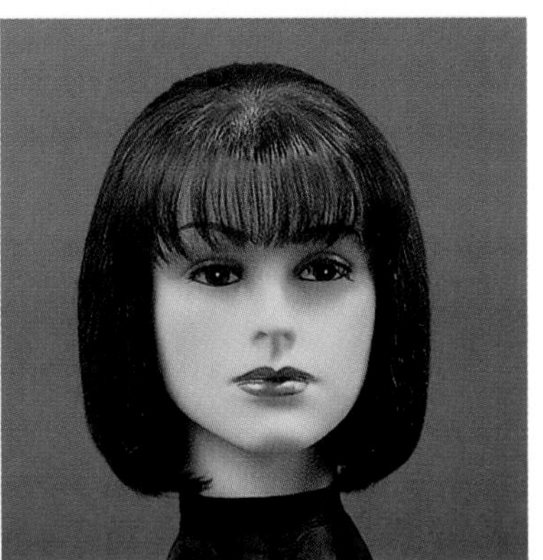

FIGURE 10.59 — Finished thermal style for medium length hair.

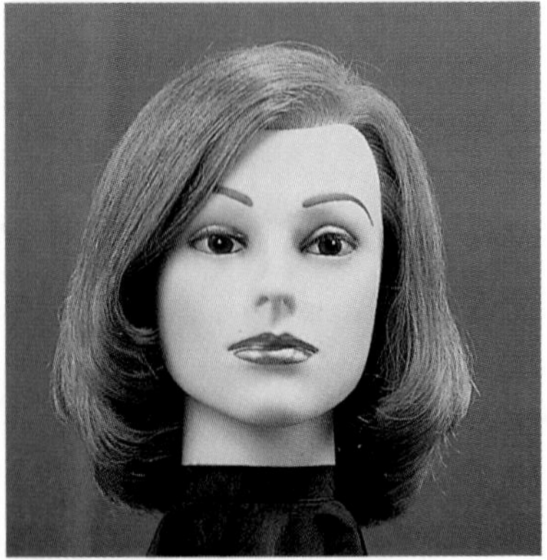

FIGURE 10.60 — Finished thermal style for long hair.

SAFETY MEASURES

1. Keep thermal irons clean and the joint oiled.
2. Use thermal irons only after receiving instruction in their use.
3. Do not overheat the irons, because this can cause the metal to lose its temper.

4. Test the temperature of the irons on tissue paper before placing them on the hair. This will prevent the hair from being burned. Do not inhale the fumes of the irons because they are injurious to the lungs.
5. Do not place the hot irons near the face to test for temperature; a burn of the face can result.
6. Handle thermal irons carefully to avoid burning yourself or the client.
7. Place hot irons in a safe place to cool. Do not leave them where someone might accidentally come in contact with them and be burned.
8. When heating the irons, do not place handles too close to the heater. Your hand might be burned when removing the irons.
9. Make sure the irons are properly balanced in the heater, or they might fall and be damaged or injure someone.
10. Use only hard rubber or nonflammable combs. Celluloid combs must not be used in thermal curling; they are flammable.
11. Do not use metal combs; they can become hot and burn the scalp.
12. Do not use combs with broken teeth. They can break or split the hair or injure the scalp.
13. Place comb between scalp and thermal irons when curling or waving hair to prevent burning the scalp.
14. The client's hair must be clean to ensure a good thermal curl or wave.
15. If the hair is thick and bulky, thin and taper it first.
16. Never use hot pressing or thermal irons on lightened or tinted hair.
17. Do not allow the hair ends to protrude over the irons; to do so will cause fishhooks (hair that is bent or folded).
18. A first aid kit must be available in case of an accident.
19. Do not use vaporizing thermal irons on pressed hair because the hair will revert to its original overly curly state.
20. Do not use thermal irons on chemically straightened hair because they might cause damage to the hair. They can be used on relaxed hair if the heat is controlled.

Completed:
Learning Objective
#3
SAFETY MEASURES FOR THERMAL WAVING

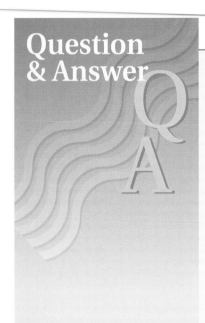

BLOW-DRYING LONG HAIR

Drying and styling hair using a blow-dryer is considered a "quick service," yet it takes me twice as long to style the hair of some of my clients who have long hair. What can I do?

Towel the hair thoroughly to remove as much moisture as possible. Use your fingers to separate the hair and further dry it.

Then start at the back and throw the hair forward. First use your fingers and hand to direct the hair as the hot air is blown from back to front. When about 50 percent of the moisture has been removed start using a vent brush to direct the hair.

Only when 90 percent of the moisture has been removed (this happens rather quickly) start bringing the hair down at the nape, drying each section thoroughly before letting down the next section. Work from the nape up the back, over the crown and toward the forehead.

Finally use a round brush to shape the ends of the hair. Spin the brush through the ends, direct the warm air onto the brush, and repeat until the ends are dry and formed. Allow the hair to cool, then while the client leans forward spray the underneath sections with styling/volumizing hair spray. Work the hair back down with your fingers while you shake the form into place. All this takes very little time if you "pre-dry" the hair as suggested.

—*From* Milady's Salon Solutions *by Louise Cotter*

BLOW-DRY STYLING

Blow-dry styling, often referred to as a "quick salon service," is the technique of drying and styling damp hair in one operation. This technique creates the basic structure of hairstyles without time-consuming setting, drying, and combing out. It helps to develop soft, natural hairstyles with free-flowing effects. These effects can also be achieved with the use of rollers and curls. (Fig. 10.61)

There are two basic techniques used in blow-dry styling:

1. Blow-dry curling with a brush.
2. Blow-dry waving with a comb.

This section covers these two basic techniques. Many other techniques can be developed with experience and advanced training. ✔

Completed: Learning Objective #4
DEFINITION OF BLOW-DRY STYLING

Note: *Take special care when blow-drying curled hair that is chemically treated or damaged. This type of hair has loss of elasticity; therefore, towel-dry the hair first to remove excess moisture.*

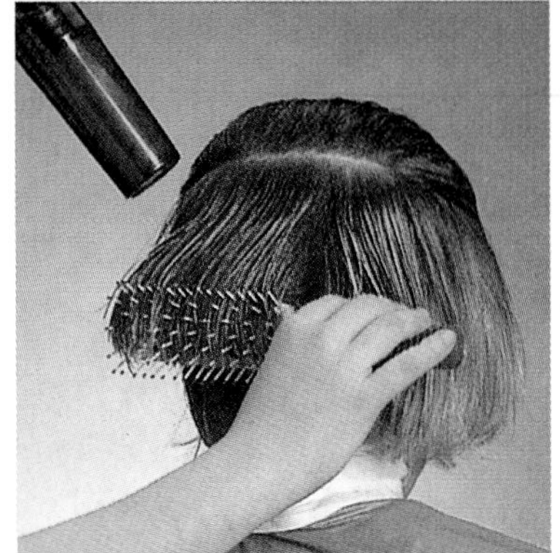

FIGURE 10.61 — Blow-dry curling with a brush.

EQUIPMENT, IMPLEMENTS, AND MATERIALS

The following equipment, implements, and materials are required for blow-dry styling:

- Blow-dryer (with or without attachments)
- Combs (hard rubber or metal)
- Shampoo
- Styling lotions, gels, mousse
- Conditioner
- Hair spray

THE BLOW-DRYER

The blow-dryer (without attachments) is an electrical device especially designed for drying and styling the hair in a single operation. Its main parts are a handle, slotted nozzle, small fan, heating element, and controls. When in operation it produces a steady stream of temperature-controlled air. The various controls permit you to make necessary heat adjustments when operating the blow-dryer. (Fig. 10.62)

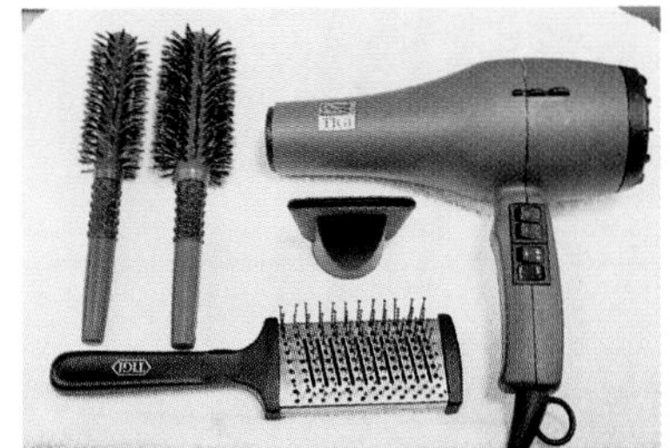

FIGURE 10.62 — Implements for blow-dryer styling—clockwise: blow-dryer; wide rounded-shoulder brush; small round brush; large round brush.

Blowdrying using a round brush creates volume or lift in a finished hairstyle. The degree of lift determines the type of volume curls to be used. Begin by sectioning off the base as described in Sectioning. For a full-base curl, hold the hair strand at a 125-degree (2.18 rad.) angle, bring the comb out to the hair ends and insert the round brush. Roll the hair down to the base with medium tension. Direct the blower very slowly through the curl in a back-and-forth movement. When the hair section is completely dry, release the brush with a rounded movement. Use clippies to secure each curl base as it is completed and to hold it in place until cool. (Fig. 10.62a) For a half-base curl, hold the hair strand at a 90-degree (1.57 rad.) angle, and for an off-base curl, hold the hair strand at a 70-degree (1.22 rad.) angle. (Fig. 10.62b and 10.62c) Follow the procedure described above.

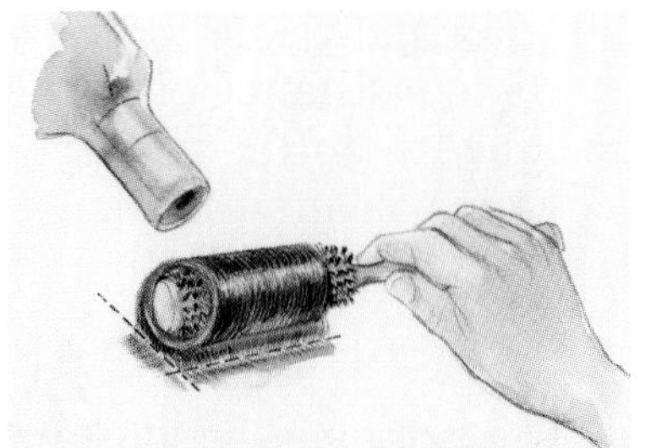

FIGURE 10.62a — Full base Curls using a Round Brush

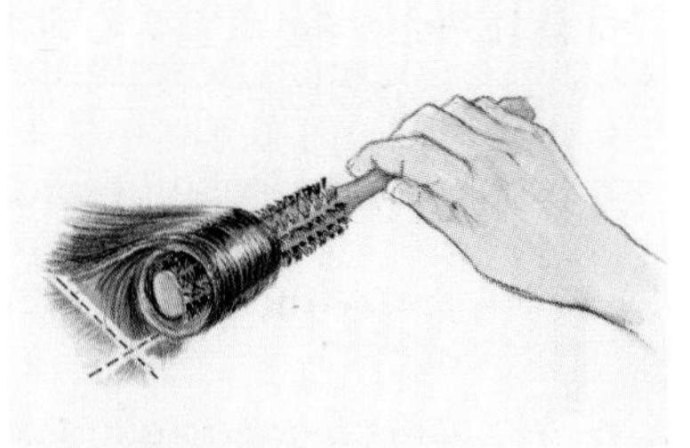

FIGURE 10.62b — Half-base Curls using a Round Brush

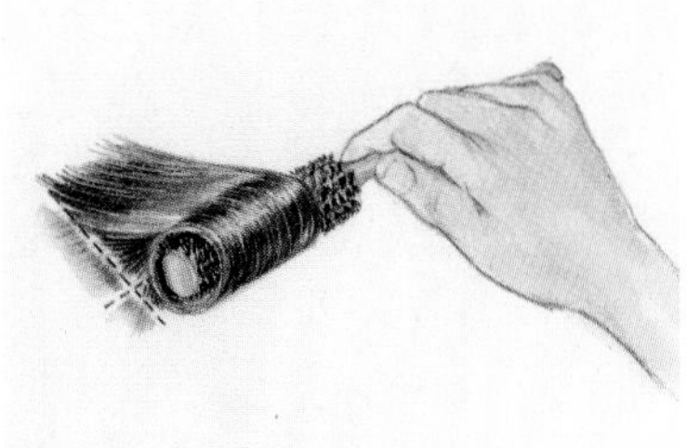

FIGURE 10.62c —Off-base Curls using a Round Brush

COMBS AND BRUSHES

Both hard rubber combs and those made of metal are used for blow waving and air waving. Some stylists prefer to use metal combs, since they retain and transmit heat better. With metal combs the hair can be re-styled in the shortest possible time. Combs are available with coarse teeth, half coarse and half fine teeth, and all fine teeth.

Special narrow synthetic bristle brushes are used in blow-dry styling. It is often easier for the stylist to brush the hair into the desired style with a narrow brush. The smaller the diameter of the brush, the tighter the curl, with better staying qualities. (Fig. 10.63)

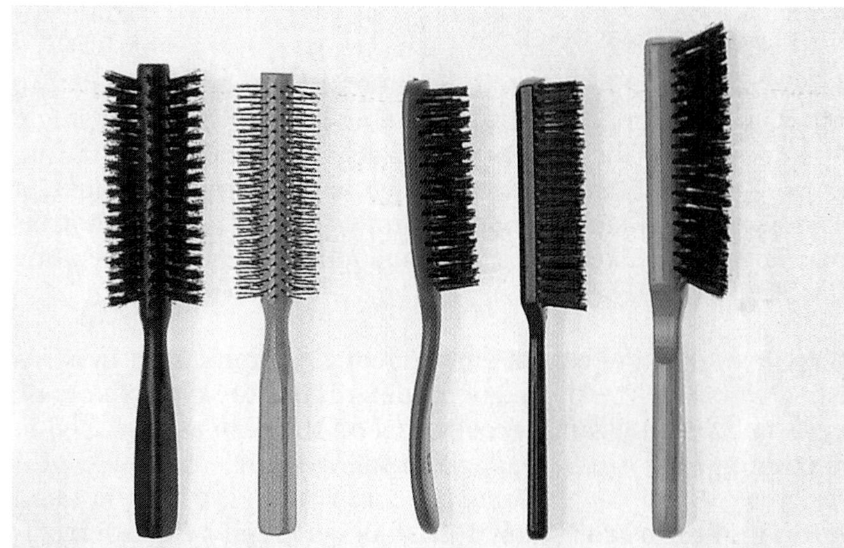

FIGURE 10.63 — Brushes used in blow-dry styling.

COSMETICS USED IN BLOW-DRY STYLING

The principal cosmetics used in blow-dry styling include styling lotions, hair and scalp conditioners, and hair sprays.

Styling Lotions

Styling lotions such as gels and mousse are applied to the hair after shampooing to make the hair more manageable for blow curling or waving. These lotions have the consistency of dense liquid and are applied with a plastic squeeze bottle or trigger (pump) action bottle. Styling lotions contain a coating substance that gives blow-dried hair more body and staying qualities.

Hair Conditioners

These are used as a corrective treatment for dry and brittle hair. They are used daily or weekly by the client or immediately prior to the blow-drying service. Excessive hairstyling by the blow-drying method can cause dryness, split ends, and loss of elasticity. Therefore, it is advisable to use hair conditioners containing a lubricant.

Hair Sprays

These are applied to the hair to keep the finished hairstyle in place.

Be guided by the manufacturer's directions or by your instructor as to the proper usage of cosmetics on the client's hair and scalp.

BLOW CURLING WITH ROUND BRUSH

Blow curling is most successful on hair that is naturally curly or has received a permanent wave. The basis for all successful blow styling is the carefully planned hair shaping. In order to properly receive a blow-curling service, hair should be shaped with tapered ends. Successful blow curling is extremely difficult on hair with blunt-cut hair ends.

The following technique is offered as one method of creating a natural-looking, easy-to-wear, informal style with a brush and blower. (Your instructor's methods are equally correct.)

Procedure

1. Shampoo and towel-dry the hair.
2. Properly shape the hair leaving tapered ends.
3. Apply styling lotion and/or conditioner.
4. Pre-plan the style. Start at the crown or top of the head, as desired. Section the hair, pick up a wide strand, and comb through. (Fig. 10.64)
5. Bring the comb out to the hair ends and insert the brush. Brush through the strand, bringing the brush out to the ends.
6. Roll the hair with the brush, making a complete downward turn, away from the face, until the brush rests on the scalp. Maintain this position and start the blower. Direct the blower very slowly through the curl in a back-and-forth movement. (Fig. 10.65) When the hair section is completely dry, release the brush with a rounded movement. Use clippies to secure each curl as it is completed and to hold it in place until it is cooled off.
7. Continue making curls in the same manner across the crown and back of the head. Clip each curl as completed.
8. Shape the neckline curls with a comb, or make pin curls on the nape for a finished, close-to-the-head look.

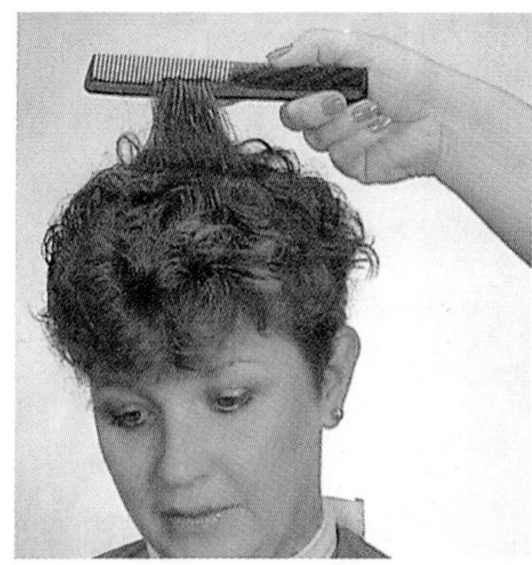

FIGURE 10.64 — Section a wide strand and comb through.

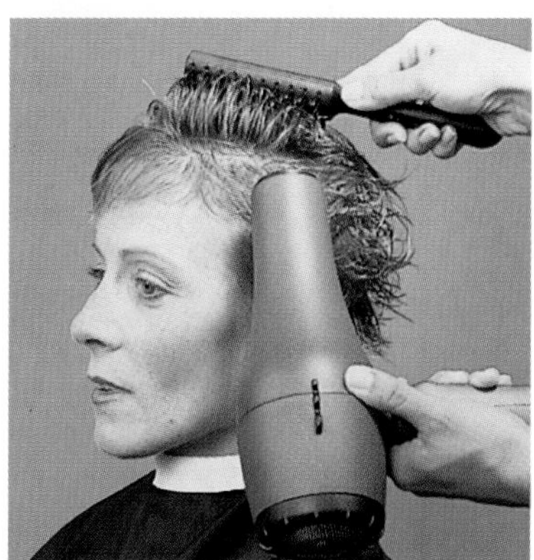

FIGURE 10.65 — Roll the hair with brush and direct blower through the curl.

REMINDERS AND HINTS ON BLOW-DRY STYLING

In order to achieve the best results from blow-dry styling, the hair should be in good condition. Permanently waved, chemically relaxed, tinted, or lightened hair should be partially towel dried before being blow curled or waved. (The hair stretches easily and could be damaged if very wet.) The hair should be shaped with tapered ends for successful blow curling or waving.

Styling lotion or mousse is important in blow waving and curling. Comb the hair thoroughly to spread the styling lotion evenly.

BLOW-DRYING THE HAIR

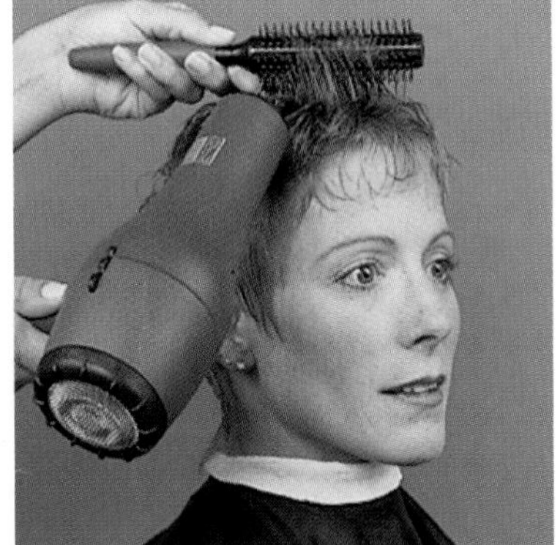

FIGURE 10.66 — Direct air from the scalp to hair ends.

Hot air is directed straight onto the head only for rough drying. For successful blow-dry styling the air should be directed from the scalp area to the hair ends. (Fig. 10.66) The flow of air is directed to the top half of the brush in a back-and-forth movement. This method acts to deflect the hot air, reduce its heat, and dry the hair nearest the scalp.

Never hold the blower too long in one place. The blower should be directed so that the hot air flows in the same direction as the hair is wound. To avoid severe scalp burns, always direct the hot air away from the client's scalp. The hair must be thoroughly cooled before it is combed out. This can be accomplished by switching the dryer to cold and cooling the hair that has been dried.

In blow styling it is essential that when the hairstyle is completed the scalp should be thoroughly dry. The hairstyle will not hold if the scalp is damp.

Complete the blow-dry styling with a light application of hair spray to give shine and holding power to the hair.

BRUSHES AND COMBS

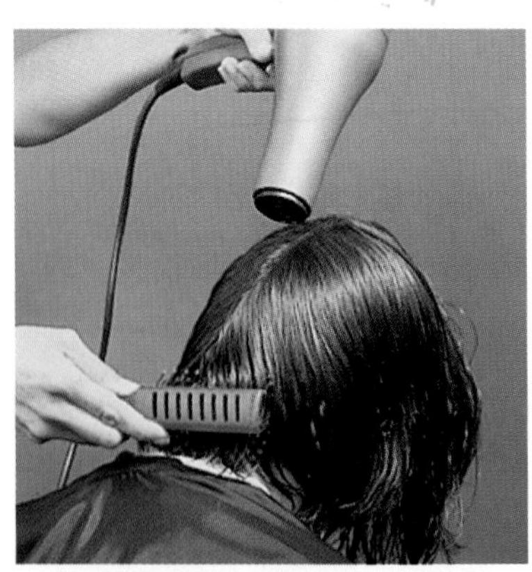

FIGURE 10.67 — Blow-drying with a vent brush.

The actual styling is performed with the brush or comb. The blow-dryer is an implement used for quickly drying the hair while the hair is being styled. The size of the styling brush used is determined by the style and length of the hair. As a general rule, short hair is styled with a small diameter or vent brush. (Fig. 10.67) For medium or longer hair, best results are achieved with large diameter or vent brushes. To avoid scalp burns, keep heated metal combs away from the scalp.

BLOW-DRYER

Make sure that the blow-dryer is perfectly clean and free of dirt, grease, hair, etc., before using. Dirt or hair can cause extreme heat and burn hair. The air intake at the back of the dryer must be kept clear at all times. If this intake is covered and air cannot pass through freely, the dryer element might burn out.

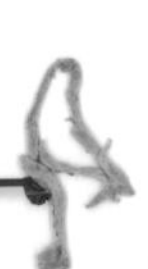

BLOW-DRYING TECHNIQUES

To give the crown hair a slight lift, a vent brush is used. This vent or open-back brush allows air from the dryer to pass through it easily. The dryer is kept on the move from side to side along the curl. Secure each curl with clippies as it is completed. (Fig. 10.68)

To create a pageboy effect, curl hair under with a brush and blow-dry. (Fig. 10.69)

To create a smooth top with flip, the hair ends are lifted by placing a brush close to the scalp. Rotate the brush. As the brush rotates, the hot air is directed to the base within the cupped area.

Completed: Learning Objective #5

BLOW-DRY STYLING IMPLEMENTS, TECHNIQUES AND COSMETICS

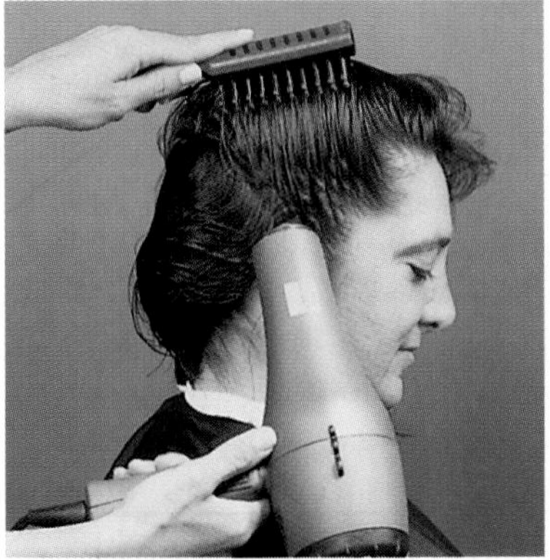

FIGURE 10.68 — Crown hair lift.

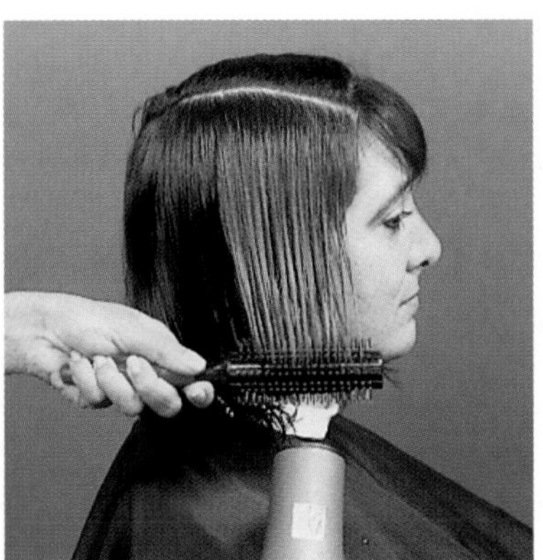

FIGURE 10.69 — Pageboy effect.

AIR WAVING

Another technique used to create attractive hairstyles without preliminary setting and drying of the hair is by the use of the electric air waver comb and styling comb. This technique is the same as finger waving, except that you use an electric air waver comb and styling comb. (Fig. 10.70)

The hair is styled after it has been shaped, shampooed, and towel dried. It is important to locate the natural wave formation in the hair. Comb the hair in the direction of the wave desired. This will help to establish the natural hair growth pattern. Comb the hair in the direction of the planned hairstyle. Comb the hair with the air waver until it is dry enough to hold a wave.

To achieve ridges and waves on various parts of the head, the hair must be slightly damp. Apply a light spray of styling lotion to assist in creating the desired hairstyle. Comb the hair in the desired direction. (Fig. 10.71)

Completed: Learning Objective #6

DEFINITION OF AIR WAVING

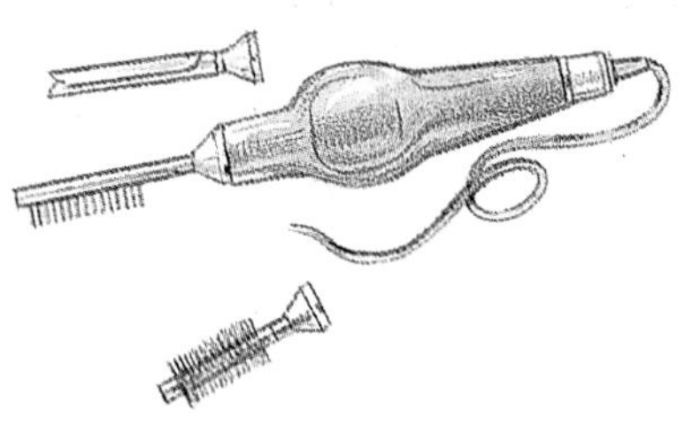

FIGURE 10.70 — Air waver with comb attachment.

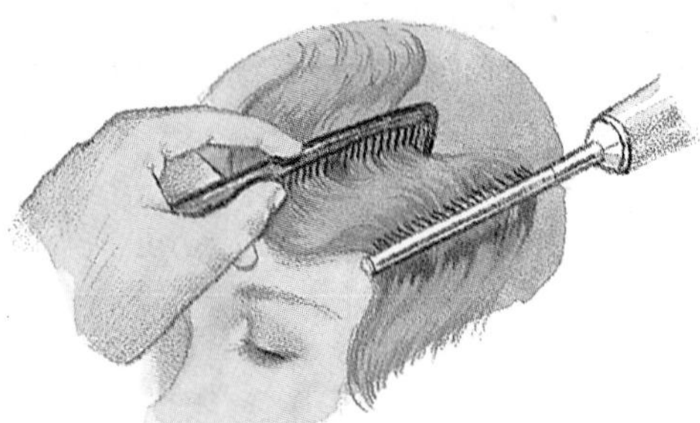

FIGURE 10.71 — Comb hair in direction of wave desired.

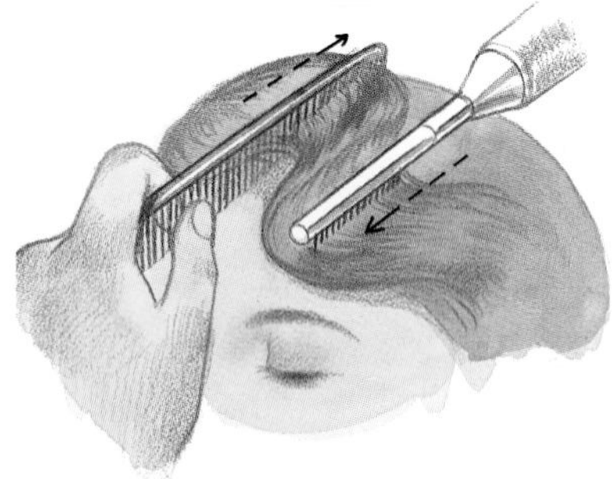

FIGURE 10.72 — Form ridge.

SHAPING HAIR WITH COMB

1. ***Left side part.*** Starting at the front section of the head, insert the styling comb into the hair about 1½" (3.75 cm) from the part. Draw the styling comb toward the back. Insert the air waver under the comb and draw the air waver comb toward the face to form a ridge. Hold both combs in this position until a firm ridge has been formed. (Fig. 10.72) Continue toward the crown until the entire length of the ridge is completed.

   Form the second ridge by starting at the crown and work toward the front. The ridge and shaping is made in reverse of the first ridge. (Fig. 10.73) Support the completed ridgeline with the styling comb while the air waver comb lifts and designs the pattern.

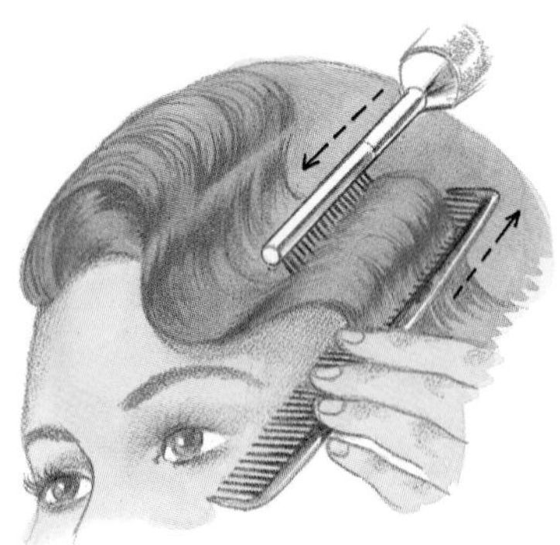

FIGURE 10.73 — Form second ridge.

2. ***Right side part.*** The procedure is exactly the same as for the left side part. The only exception is that the hand comb is held in the right hand and the air waver is controlled by the left hand. However, the waving should start at the crown and work forward toward the face.

   A finished wave is formed with the air waver comb and styling comb, taking advantage of the natural waving pattern of the hair. (Fig. 10.74)

   The air waver comb, when used in conjunction with the curling iron, presents many styling opportunities to the stylist. The number of styles and patterns that can be created with these implements working in harmony is limited only by the skill and imagination of the stylist.

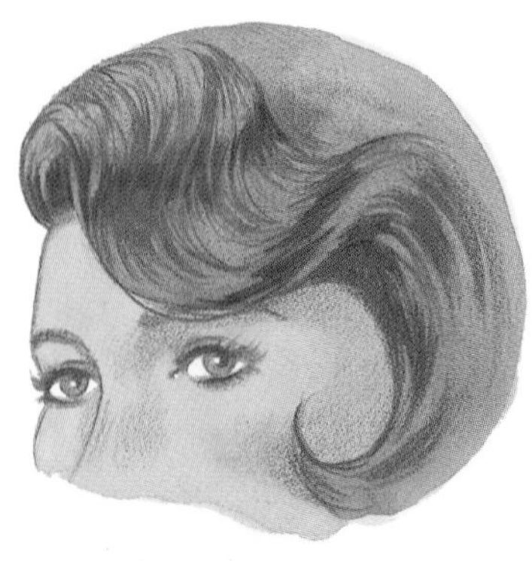

FIGURE 10.74 — Finished style.

SAFETY PRECAUTIONS

1. ***Styling dryer.*** Move moderately hot air back and forth on the hair and away from the scalp. Avoid holding the dryer too long in one place.

2. ***Metal comb.*** To avoid scalp burns, keep teeth of a heated metal comb away from the scalp.

3. ***In all blow-dry styling*** it is important that when the curling or waving is completed the scalp must be thoroughly dry. If the ends and the curls are dry but the scalp is damp, the hairstyle will not hold.

Completed: Learning Objective #7

AIR WAVING IMPLEMENTS AND TECHNIQUES

REVIEW QUESTIONS

THERMAL HAIRSTYLING

1. Define thermal waving or curling.
2. List the three types of irons used in thermal waving.
3. To avoid burning the scalp, what procedure should you follow?
4. Define blow-dry styling.
5. List the implements used in blow-dry styling.
6. What cosmetics are used in blow-dry styling?

CHAPTER 11

Permanent Waving

LEARNING OBJECTIVES

After completing this chapter, you should be able to:

1. Define permanent waving.
2. Identify the chemistry of products used in permanent waving.
3. Describe the relationship between hair structure, perm chemistry, and perming techniques.
4. Demonstrate a client consultation and hair analysis.
5. Demonstrate proper rod selection and sectioning, parting, and wrapping procedures.
6. List safety precautions required for permanent waving.
7. Demonstrate proper perming procedures.

NATIONAL SKILL STANDARDS

This chapter provides you with the necessary information to master these National Industry Skill Standards for Entry-Level Cosmetologists:

- Consulting with clients to determine their needs and preferences
- Performing hair relaxation and wave formation techniques in accordance with the manufacturer's directions

INTRODUCTION

Permanent waving (perming) is one of the most practical and lucrative techniques you will learn in cosmetology school. You'll use basic perming skills throughout your career as a salon stylist. The ability to create a beautiful perm style will bring you professional satisfaction and help build a loyal following of satisfied clients. A properly completed perm provides many valuable benefits to both the client and stylist:

1. Long-lasting style retention.
2. Easy manageability for the client when styling at home.
3. Additional volume and fullness for styling soft, fine hair textures.
4. Greater control in styling hair that is naturally coarse, wiry, and hard to manage.

HISTORY OF PERMANENT WAVING

Attempts to wave and curl straight hair date back to early civilization. Egyptian and Roman women were known to apply a mixture of soil and water to their hair, wrap it on crudely made wooden rollers, and then bake it in the sun. The results, of course, were not permanent.

THE MACHINE AGE OF PERMANENT WAVING

In 1905 Charles Nessler invented a heavily wired machine that supplied electrical current to metal rods around which hair strands were wrapped. These heavy units were heated during the perming process. They were kept from touching the scalp by a complex system of counterbalancing weights, suspended from an overhead chandelier mounted on a stand. (Fig. 11.1)

Two methods were used to wind hair strands around the metal units. Long hair was wound from the scalp to the ends, a technique called ***spiral wrapping.*** (Fig. 11.2) After World War I when many women cut their hair into the short bobbed style, the ***croquignole*** (**KROH**-ki-nohl) ***wrapping*** technique was introduced. Using this method, shorter hair was wound from the ends toward the scalp. The hair was then styled into deep waves with loose end curls. (Fig. 11.3)

The client's fear of being "tied" to an electrical contraption with the possibility of receiving a shock or burn led to the development of alternative methods of waving hair. In 1931, the ***pre-heat*** method of perming was introduced. Hair was wrapped using the croquignole method, and then clamps, pre-heated by a separate electrical unit, were placed over the wound curls.

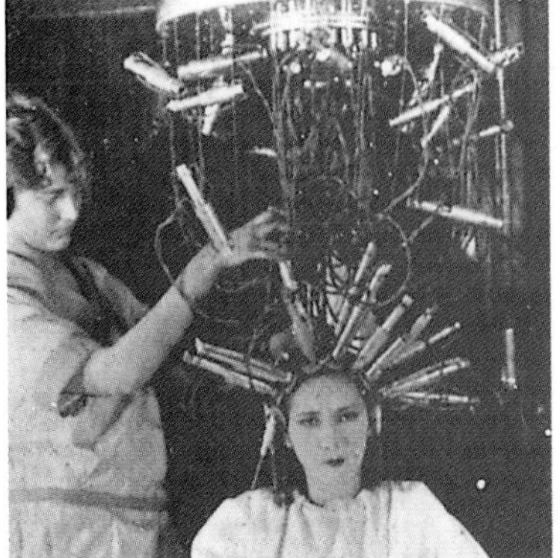

FIGURE 11.1 — Machine permanent wave.

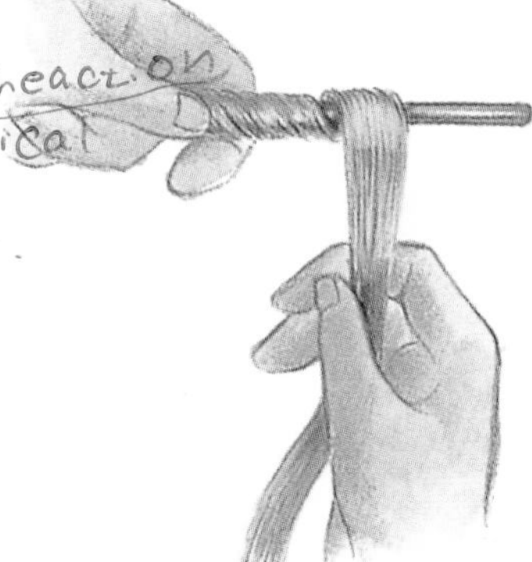

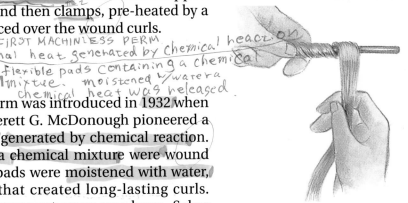

FIGURE 11.2 — Spiral flat wave.

THE FIRST MACHINELESS PERM

An alternative to the machine perm was introduced in 1932 when chemists Ralph L. Evans and Everett G. McDonough pioneered a method that used external heat generated by chemical reaction. Small, flexible pads containing a chemical mixture were wound around hair strands. When the pads were moistened with water, a chemical heat was released that created long-lasting curls. Thus, the first machineless permanent wave was born. Salon clients no longer were subjected to the dangers and discomforts of the Nessler machine.

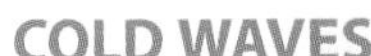

COLD WAVES

In 1941 scientists discovered another method of permanent waving. They developed the waving **lotion**, a liquid that softens and expands the hair strand. After the waving lotion has done its work, another lotion called a **neutralizer** is applied. The neutralizer hardens and shrinks that hair strand, allowing it to conform to the shape of the rod around which the hair is wrapped. It also stops the action of the waving lotion.

Because this perm does not use heat, it is called a "cold wave." Cold waves replaced virtually all predecessors and competitors, and cold waving and permanent waving became almost synonymous terms. Modern versions of cold waves, usually referred to as alkaline perms, are still very popular today.

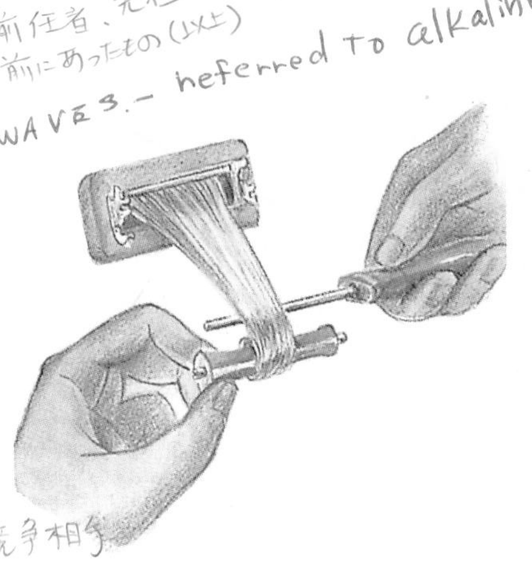

FIGURE 11.3 — Croquignole wrap.

Note: *The word "perm" is now popularly used to indicate permanent waving with either an alkaline or acid-balanced solution.*

NEUTRAL AND ACID-BALANCED PERMS

For many years, manufacturers sought to develop a permanent wave solution that would minimize hair damage and permit hair that had been damaged by lightening or tinting services to receive a perm. To achieve these goals, they developed a waving lotion that was not as highly alkaline as earlier lotions.

Neutral and acid-balanced permanent wave solutions with pH levels ranging from 4.5 to 7.9 were introduced in 1970. They did not contain strong alkalines and therefore were less damaging to the hair. Acid-balanced lotions were, however, slow to penetrate (to pass into or through; to enter by overcoming resistance) hair, and processing time was longer. To overcome this problem, the client is placed under a heated hood dryer to shorten the processing time.

Completed: Learning Objective
#1
DEFINITION OF PERMANENT WAVING

MODERN PERM CHEMISTRY

Perm chemistry is constantly being refined and improved. Perms are available today in many different formulas for a wide variety of hair types. Waving lotions and neutralizers for both acid-balanced and alkaline perms are being formulated with new conditioners, proteins, and natural ingredients that help protect and condition the hair during and after perming.

Stop action processing is incorporated in many waving lotions to ensure optimum curl development. The curling takes place within a fixed time without the risk of overprocessing or damaging the hair. Special prewrapping lotions have also been developed to compensate for hair that is not equally porous all over.

Virtually all permanent waves are achieved with a two-step chemical process:

1. Waving lotion, which softens or breaks the internal structure of the hair.
2. Neutralizer, which rehardens or rebonds the internal structure of the hair.

ALKALINE PERMS

The main active ingredient or ***reducing agent*** in alkaline perms, ***ammonium thioglycolate*** (a-**MOHN**-nee-um theye-oh-**GLEYE**-coh-layt), is a chemical compound made up of ammonia and thioglycolic acid. The pH of alkaline waving lotions generally falls within the range of 8.2 to 9.6, depending on the amount of ammonia. Because the lotion is more alkaline, the cuticle layers swell slightly and open, allowing the solution to penetrate more quickly than acid-balanced lotions. Some alkaline perms are wrapped with waving lotion, others with water. Some require a plastic cap for processing, others do not. Therefore, it is extremely important to read the perm directions carefully before beginning.

The benefits of alkaline perms are:

- Strong curl patterns (lotion wrapped alkaline perms are usually stronger than perms that are water wrapped).
- Fast processing time (varies from 5 minutes to 20 minutes).
- Room temperature processing.

Generally, alkaline perms should be used when:

- Perming resistant hair.
- A strong/tight curl is desired.
- The client has a history of early curl relaxation.

ACID-BALANCED PERMS

One of the main active ingredients in acid-balanced waving lotions is ***glyceryl monothioglycolate***, which effectively reduces the pH. This lower pH is gentler on the hair and typically gives a softer curl than alkaline cold waves. Acid-balanced perms have a pH range of approximately 4.5 to 6.5 and usually penetrate the hair more slowly. Thus, they require a longer processing time and heat for curl development. Heat is used in one of two ways:

1. The perm is activated by heat created chemically within the product. This method is called ***exothermic.***
2. The perm is activated by an outside heat source, usually a conventional hood-type hair dryer. This method is called ***endothermic.***

Recent advances in acid-balanced perm chemistry, however, have made it possible to process some acid-balanced perms at room temperature without heat. These newer acid-balanced perms usually have a slightly higher pH but still contain glyceryl monothioglycolate as the active ingredient.

All acid-balanced perms are water wrapped, require a plastic cap, and may or may not require a pre-heated hood dryer for processing. Read the manufacturer's perm directions carefully before starting the perm.

The benefits of acid-balanced perms are:

- Softer curl patterns.

- Slower, but more controllable processing time (usually 15 to 25 minutes).
- Gentler treatment for delicate hair types.

Generally, acid-balanced perms should be used when:

- Perming delicate/fragile or color-treated hair.
- Soft, natural curl or wave pattern is desired.
- Style support, rather than strong curl, is required.

THE CHEMISTRY OF NEUTRALIZERS

Neutralizers for both acid-balanced and alkaline perms have the same important function: to permanently establish the new curl shape. Neutralizing is a very important step in the perming process. If the hair is not properly neutralized, the curl will relax or straighten within one to two shampooings. Generally, today's neutralizers are composed of a relatively small percentage of hydrogen peroxide, an oxidizing agent, at an acidic pH. As with waving lotions, there are slightly different procedures recommended for individual products. To achieve the best possible results, read the directions carefully.

Completed: Learning Objective #2
THE CHEMISTRY OF PERMANENT WAVING PRODUCTS

HAIR STRUCTURE AND PERMING

Whether using an acid-balanced or alkaline formula, all perms subject the hair to two different actions:

1. Physical action—wrapping sections of hair around a perm rod.
2. Chemical action—created first by a reducing agent (waving lotion) and second by an oxidizing agent (neutralizer).

Since both of these actions work together to create a change in the internal structure of the hair, it is important to understand the composition of hair and how it is affected during perming.

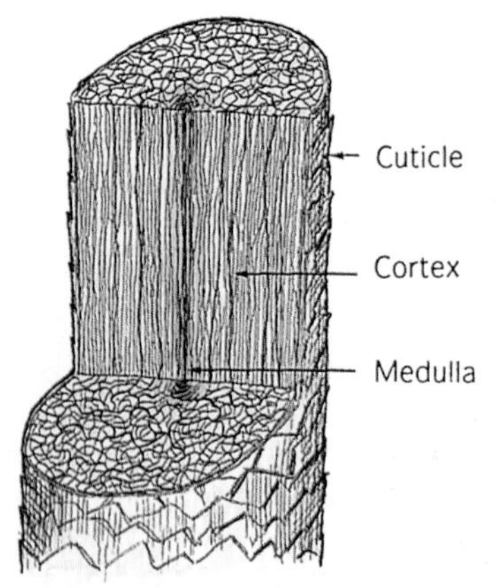

FIGURE 11.4 — Structure of a hair.

PHYSICAL STRUCTURE OF HAIR

Each strand of hair is structurally subdivided into three major components: (Fig. 11.4)

1. The ***cuticle*** or outer covering consists of seven or more overlapping layers. Although it comprises a small percentage of

the total weight of hair, the cuticle possesses unique structural properties that protect the hair. During perming, the waving lotion raises the cuticle layers and allows the active ingredients to enter the cortex.

2. The ***cortex,*** the major component of the hair structure, accounts for up to 90% of its total weight. The cortex gives hair its flexibility, elasticity, strength, resilience, and color. It is in the cortex that the physical and chemical actions take place during the perming process to restructure the hair into a new curl configuration.

3. The ***medulla*** is the innermost section of the hair structure. The function of the medulla, if any, is unknown. In fact, it is not at all unusual for an otherwise normal, healthy hair to be without a medulla.

CHEMICAL COMPOSITION OF HAIR

The chemical composition of hair consists almost entirely of a protein material called ***keratin*** (**KER**-a-tin), which is made up of approximately nineteen amino acids. When many amino acids are bonded together, they form a ***polypeptide*** (pol-ee-**PEP**-teyed) ***chain***. These chains intertwine around each other in a spiral fashion to assume a helical shape very similar to a spring. Hair contains a high concentration of the amino acid ***cysteine*** (**SIS**-teen), which is joined together crosswise with ***disulfide*** (deye-**SUL**-feyed) linkages or bonds. Disulfide bonds add strength to the keratin protein, and it is these bonds that must be broken down to allow the perming process to occur.

Processing. The chemical action of a waving lotion breaks the disulfide bonds and softens the hair. When the chemical action softens the inner structure of the hair enough, it can mold to the shape of the rod around which it is wound. (Figs. 11.5a–c)

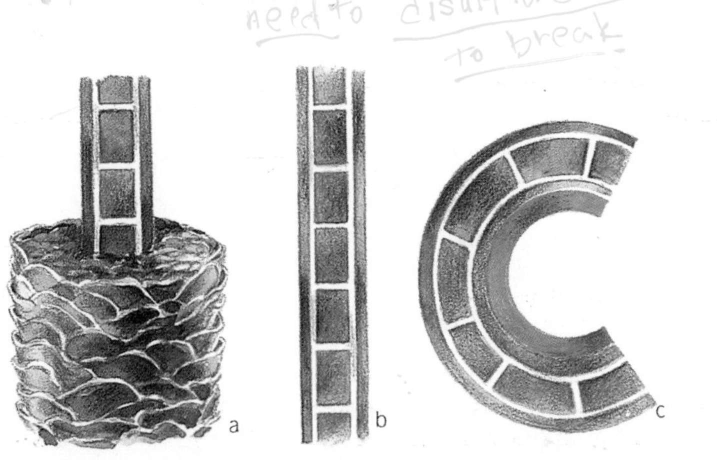

FIGURE 11.5a — Each hair strand is composed of many polypeptide chains. This series of illustrations shows the behavior of one such chain.

FIGURE 11.5b — Hair before processing. Chemical bonds (links) give hair its strength and firmness.

FIGURE 11.5c — Hair wound on rod. The hair bends to the curvature and size of the rod.

Neutralizing. When the hair has assumed the desired shape, the broken disulfide bonds must be chemically rebonded. Neutralizing rehardens the hair and fixes it into its new curl form. When the neutralizing action is completed, the hair is unwrapped from the rods, and you have a new curl formation. (Figs. 11.6a, b)

Completed:
Learning Objective
#3
HAIR STRUCTURE AND PERMING

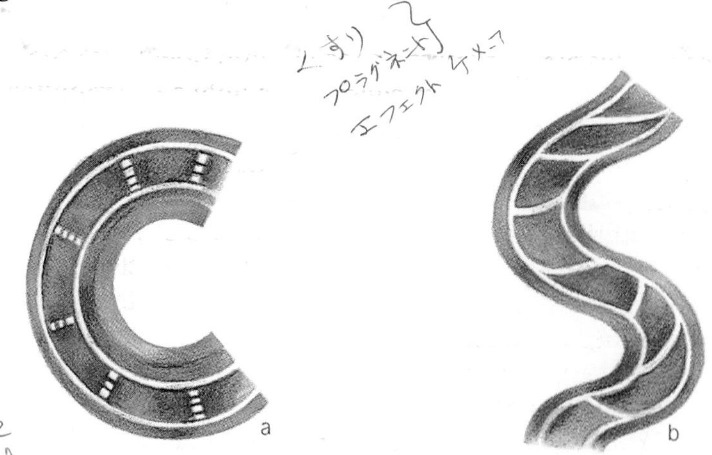

FIGURE 11.6a — During processing, waving lotion breaks the chemical cross-bonds (links), permitting the hair to adjust to the curvature of the rod while in this softened condition.

FIGURE 11.6b — The neutralizer re-forms the chemical bonds (links) to conform with the wound position of the hair, and rehardens the hair, thus creating the permanent wave.

CHOOSING THE RIGHT PERMING TECHNIQUE

How do you decide which perming technique is right for your client? You must be able to evaluate and analyze your client's hair. You must consult with your client to establish what the person expects to accomplish with a perm—a tight, curly look or a loose, wavy look. This information helps you to select the correct perm product and technique.

Basic Manual Perming Skills

Successful perming requires manual dexterity. With practice, your skills in handling and manipulating hair will improve. Before actually applying a perm, you will probably spend considerable time practicing pre-perming skills like blocking, sectioning, and wrapping. Your ability to give successful perms depends on mastering these important skills.

Client Consultation

Every perm client has a different expectation for how he or she wants the perm to look. The only way to meet your client's expectations is to determine what those expectations are. Talk to your client in a friendly but professional way. Take a few minutes to discuss:

1. What hairstyle and how much curl your client wants. Photos or magazine pictures help to make this clearly understood by both of you.

2. Your client's lifestyle. Does he or she have leisure time, or a demanding schedule that requires a low-maintenance style?
3. How your client's hairstyle relates to overall personal image. Is your client concerned about current fashion trends?
4. Your client's previous experience with perming. What did he or she like or dislike about past perm services?

Once you learn what questions to ask and how to ask them, the consultation with your perm client takes only a few minutes. It is time well-spent, however, because the consultation helps establish your credibility as a professional. It inspires your client's confidence in your technical and creative abilities, and makes the perming experience more satisfactory for both of you.

Keep the vital information you learn during the client consultation as a written permanent record, along with other important data, including the client's address, home, and business phone numbers. A release form should also be filled out by the client. It releases the school or salon owner from responsibility for accidents or damages and is required for some malpractice insurance. A sample release is shown in the hair coloring chapter. Here is an example of an organized format for maintaining client records:

PERMANENT WAVE RECORD

Name .... Tel ....

Address .... City................ State................

DESCRIPTION OF HAIR Zip.......................

Length	**Texture**	**Type**	**Porosity**	
□ short	□ coarse	□ normal	□ very porous	□ slightly porous
□ medium	□ medium	□ resistant	□ moderately porous	□ resistant
□ long	□ fine	□ tinted	□ normal	
		□ highlighted		
		□ bleached		

Condition

□ very good □ good □ fair □ poor □ dry □ oily

Tinted with ....

Previously permed with ....

TYPE OF PERM

□ alkaline □ acid □ body wave □ other.................................

No. of rods .... Lotion .... Strength................

Results

□ good □ poor □ too tight □ too loose

Date	Perm Used	Stylist	Date	Perm Used	Stylist

Other side or Record, continue with:

Date	Perm Used	Stylist	Date	Perm Used	Stylist

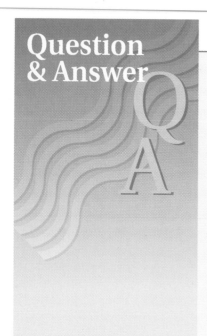

SUIT THE PERM TO THE CLIENT

The client selected the least expensive of three perms offered by the salon. Now she is dissatisfied because the perm seems dry. What should I have done?

The fault lies not with the client, but with you. It is your responsibility to advise the client what type perm she should have, based on the hair analysis

The least expensive perm imaginable is formulated with the same basic ingredients as the most expensive perm imaginable. The difference lies in the additives it contains, which influence things like moisture and gentleness.

It is far better to re-do a perm than lose a client. But you can avoid having to re-do perms by starting with a consultation. Analyze the hair and inform the client of the different perms offered (by price). Explain why each one is a different price. Tell her honestly the one you would recommend and why. Then, when she has made her choice, give her the best service you know how to give.

If you follow all the correct procedures, the perm should be a good one. The hair may need a re-conditioning treatment to restore moisture and oils that may have been reduced in the process, but it will have well-formed curl. Price is never an excuse for giving a bad perm.

—*From* Milady's Salon Solutions *by Louise Cotter*

PRE-PERM ANALYSIS

After the client consultation, you must analyze the overall condition of your client's hair and scalp. This analysis is essential for you to determine:

1. If it is safe and advisable to proceed with the perm service. The hair must be in good condition and have the necessary strength to accept a chemical alteration to achieve a successful perm.
2. Which perm product should be chosen for the best results on the particular hair type.
3. Which perm technique should be used: rod and parting sizes and wrapping pattern.

First, examine the scalp for abrasions, irritations, or open sores. If any of these conditions exist, do not give the perm. Next, judge the physical characteristics of the hair with regard to these important criteria: porosity, elasticity, density, texture, length. Finally, determine the overall condition of the hair. Observe if the hair has been previously treated with chemicals: perm, tint, bleach, highlighting (frosting, dimensionally colored). (See "Special Situations," page 257.) This will guide you in choosing the appropriate perm.

> **CAUTION**
>
> *If pre-perm analysis is not correct, poor curl development or hair damage can result.*

Determining Porosity

Porosity (po-**ROS**-i-tee) refers to the hair's capacity to absorb liquids. There is a direct relationship between the hair's porosity, the type of perm (acid-balanced or alkaline) you will use, and the strength of waving lotion you will choose.

The processing time for any perm depends more on hair porosity than on any other factor. The more porous the hair, the less processing time it takes, and a milder waving solution is required. The degree to which hair absorbs the waving lotion is related to its porosity, regardless of texture.

Hair porosity is affected by such factors as excessive exposure to sun and wind, use of harsh shampoos, tints, and lighteners, previous perms, and use of thermal styling appliances.

Porous hair might be dry—even very dry. If hair is tinted, bleached, has been exposed to sun, or was overprocessed by a previous perm, it will absorb liquids readily. Soft, fine, thin hair usually has a thin cuticle so it will absorb liquids quickly and easily. Rough, dull-looking hair and hair that tangles easily are also signs of porous hair.

While the hair is dry, check porosity in three different areas: front hairline, in front of the ear, and in the crown area. Select a single strand of hair, hold the end securely between the thumb and forefinger of one hand, and slide the thumb and forefinger of the other hand from the end to the scalp.

If the hair feels smooth and the cuticle is dense and hard, it is considered resistant and will not absorb liquids or perm lotion easily. If you can feel a slight roughness, this tells you that the cuticle is open and that the hair is porous and will absorb liquids more readily. (Fig. 11.7)

Poor porosity (resistant hair). Hair with the cuticle layer lying close to the hair shaft. This type of hair absorbs waving lotion slowly and usually requires a longer processing time and/or a strong waving lotion.

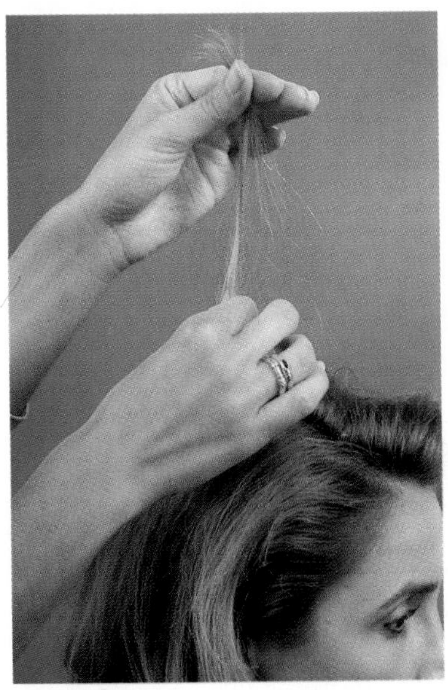

FIGURE 11.7 — Testing for hair porosity.

Good porosity (normal hair). Hair with the cuticle layer slightly raised from the hair shaft. Hair of this type can absorb moisture or chemicals in an average amount of time.

Porous (tinted, lightened, or previously chemically treated hair). Hair that has been made porous by various treatments or styling. This type of hair absorbs lotion very quickly and requires the shortest processing time. Use either an acid-balanced perm or a very mild alkaline wave.

Over-porous hair (a result of overprocessing). This type of hair is very damaged, dry, fragile, and brittle. Until the hair has been reconditioned or the damaged part has been removed by cutting, it should not be permed.

If hair is unevenly porous (usually porous or over-porous at the ends with good to poor porosity near the scalp), a pre-wrap lotion, specifically designed to even out the porosity, is recommended to achieve even curl results and help prevent overprocessing porous ends. (Figs. 11.8a–d)

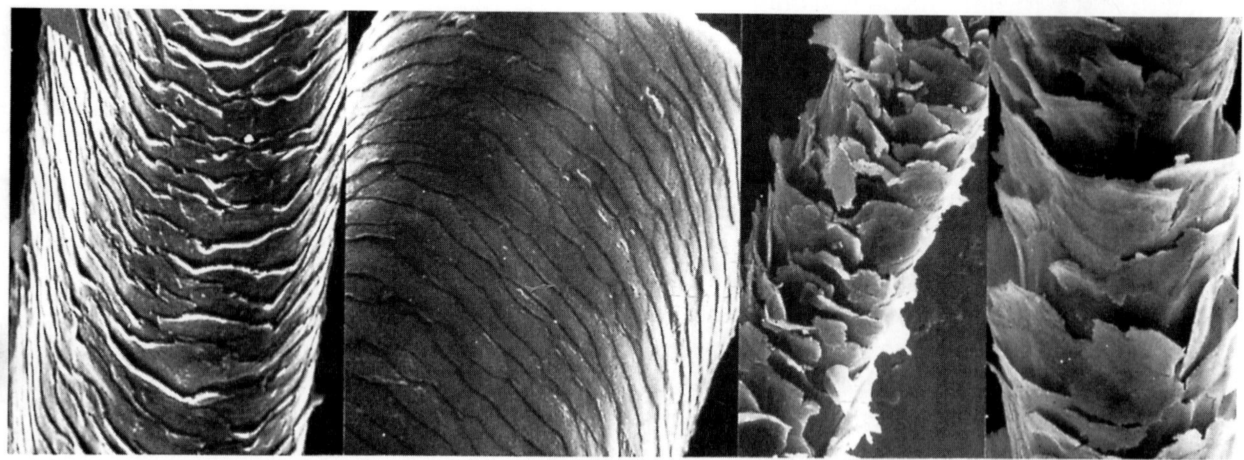

FIGURE 11.8a — Normal (moderate porosity).

FIGURE 11.8b — Resistant (poor porosity).

FIGURE 11.8c — Tinted (extreme porosity).

FIGURE 11.8d — Damaged (over-porous hair).

Determining Texture

Texture refers to how thick or thin (in diameter) each individual hair is. Fine hair has a small diameter; coarse hair has a large diameter. You can feel whether hair is fine, coarse, or medium when a single dry strand is held between the fingers.

The texture and porosity together are used to determine processing time of the waving lotion. Although porosity is the more important of the two, texture does play an important role in estimating processing time. Fine hair with a small diameter becomes saturated with waving lotion more quickly than coarse hair with a large diameter, even if both are of equal porosity. However, when coarse hair is porous, it processes faster than fine hair that is not porous.

A perm adds body to hair that appears limp, lifeless, and does not hold a style very long. For coarse, wiry hair, a perm provides greater manageability in styling. (Figs. 11.9a–c)

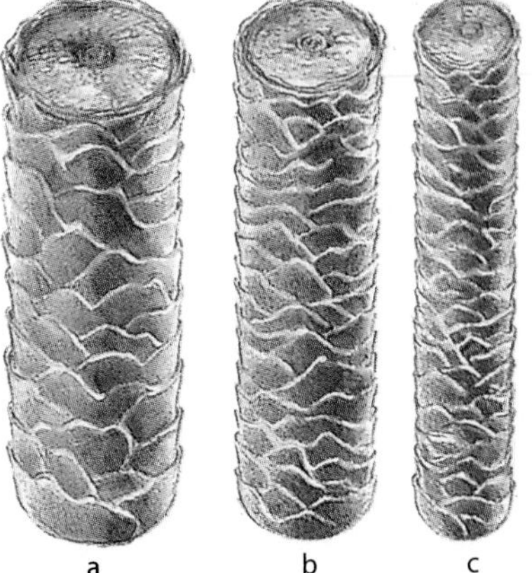

FIGURE 11.9a — Coarse.
FIGURE 11.9b — Medium.
FIGURE 11.9c — Fine.

Testing Elasticity

Elasticity is the ability of hair to stretch and contract. To test for elasticity, stretch a single dry hair. If the hair breaks under very slight strain, it has little or no elasticity. Other signs of poor elasticity include a spongy feel when hair is wet and/or hair that tangles easily. When hair is completely lacking in elasticity (for example, extremely damaged hair), it will not take a satisfactory permanent wave because it has lost the ability to contract after stretching. The greater the degree of elasticity, the longer the wave will remain in the hair, because less relaxation of the hair occurs. Hair with good elastic qualities can be stretched 20% of its length without breaking. (Fig. 11.10)

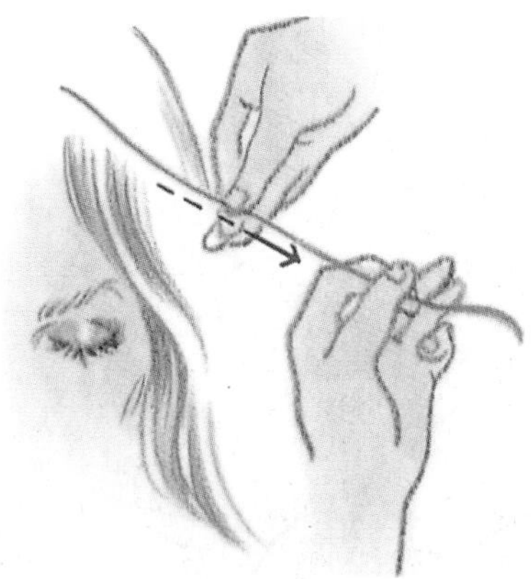

FIGURE 11.10 — Testing for elasticity.

Assessing Density

Density, or thickness, refers to the number of hairs per square inch (6.452 sq. cm) on your client's head. Density is one characteristic that determines the size of the partings you will use. Thick hair (many hairs per square inch) will require small partings on each rod. Too much hair on the rod can result in a weak curl, especially at the scalp.

If hair is thin (fewer hairs per square inch), slightly larger partings can be used, but avoid stretching or pulling the hair toward the rod because this can cause hair breakage.

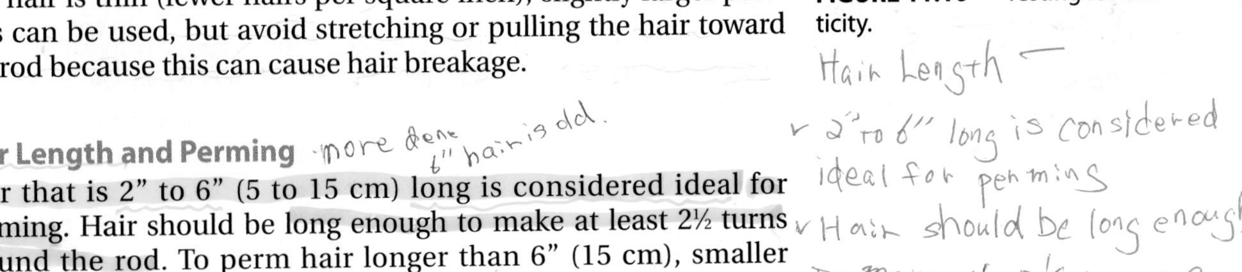

Hair Length and Perming

Hair that is 2" to 6" (5 to 15 cm) long is considered ideal for perming. Hair should be long enough to make at least 2½ turns around the rod. To perm hair longer than 6" (15 cm), smaller partings must be used to allow the waving lotion and neutralizer to penetrate more easily and thoroughly.

PERM SELECTION

The type of perm you choose depends on the total evaluation of your client's hair and wishes during the consultation and pre-perm analysis. The following is a general guide to help you decide whether to use an alkaline or an acid-balanced perm.

Hair Type	Type of Perm
Coarse, resistant	Alkaline lotion wrap or alkaline water wrap
Fine, resistant	Alkaline lotion wrap or alkaline water wrap
Normal	Alkaline water wrap or acid-balanced
Normal, porous	Alkaline water wrap or acid-balanced
Normal, delicate	Acid-balanced
Tinted, non-porous	Alkaline water wrap or acid-balanced
Tinted, porous	Acid-balanced
Highlighted/frosted/ dimensionally colored	Acid-balanced
Highlighted, tinted	Acid-balanced
Bleached	Acid-balanced

Today's perm products offer a wide selection of special features and formulas for all hair types. There are alkaline formulas for bleached hair and acid-balanced formulas for resistant hair. Each formula gives excellent results if you choose the perm carefully and follow the product directions.

PRE-PERM SHAMPOOING

Today, there are shampoos specifically formulated for pre-perm cleansing that thoroughly yet gently cleanse the hair. Use of these shampoos is recommended for optimal perm results.

When analyzing a client's hair before perming, you might notice that the hair looks and feels coated. This coating might be the buildup of shampoo or conditioners, improper rinsing, resins from styling products or hair spray, or mineral deposits from hard water. This coating can prevent penetration of the waving lotion and interfere with perm results. It is very important for the hair to be free of all coatings before beginning any perm.

CAUTION

While shampooing or doing any pre-perm preparation of a client's hair, you should avoid vigorous brushing, combing, pulling, or rubbing that can cause the scalp to become sensitive to perm solutions.

Begin the process by wetting the hair, applying the shampoo, and gently working it into a lather. If the hair is extremely coated, let the shampoo remain in the hair several minutes before rinsing. Rinse thoroughly to remove all shampoo and dissolved buildup. Towel blot excess water from hair.

PRE-PERM CUTTING OR SHAPING

If the client has chosen a hairstyle that is the same or very similar to the design he or she is currently wearing, reshape the style using either a scissors or razor. If the finished style requires texturizing or thinning of the ends, wait until after giving the perm to texturize. Tapered or thinned ends are more difficult to wrap smoothly and accurately.

If the client wants a completely new style, rough cut the hair into an approximation of the final shape. After the perm is completed, you can finish shaping the style more exactly.

Completed: Learning Objective #4

CLIENT CONSULTATION AND HAIR ANALYSIS

PERM RODS

Proper selection of perm rod size is essential for successful perm results. The size of the rod controls the size of the curl created by the waving process. Perm rods are typically made of plastic and come in varying sizes. They range in diameter (distance through the center of the rod) from small to large (⅛" to ¾" [.3125 to 1.875 cm]). Rods are color coded to identify their size. (Fig. 11.11) Typically, the color/size designations are:

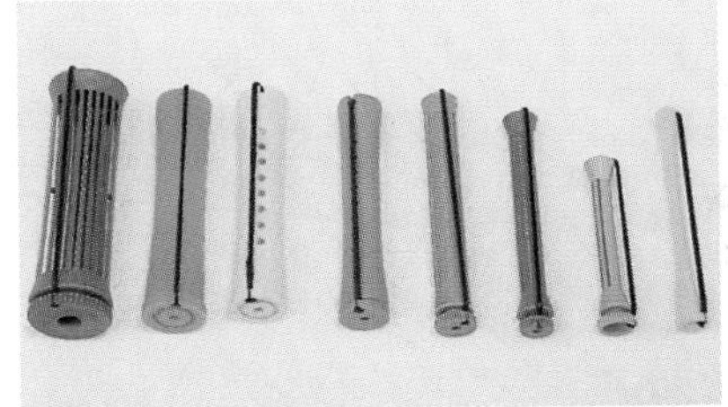

FIGURE 11.11 — Sizes of rods—left to right: extra large, large, medium, small, extra small.

Small Rods	Medium Rods	Large Rods
Yellow	Gray	Beige
Blue	Black	Purple
Pink	White	Green
		Orange

Perm rods are also available in various lengths: short, medium, and long (1¾" to 3½" [4.375 to 8.75 cm]). Rods of all diameters are available in long lengths. Medium and short lengths are not always available in all diameters. These shorter rods are used for wrapping small or awkward sections.

Types of Rods

There are two types of rods: concave and straight. Concave rods have a small diameter in the center area and gradually increase to their largest diameter at the ends, resulting in a tighter curl at the hair ends, with a looser, wider curl at the scalp. The diameter of the straight rods is the same throughout their length, creating the same size curl from end to scalp.

All rods have some means of securing the hair on the rod to prevent the curl from unwinding. Usually an elastic band, with a fastening button attached to the end, stretches across the wound hair and secures it when the button is inserted into the opposite end of the rod.

Selecting Rod Size

When selecting rod size, two things must be considered:

1. Amount of curl desired
2. Physical characteristics of the hair

Curl desired: The amount of wave, curl, or body needed is determined between you and the client during the consultation. Your success in creating a style depends primarily on the rod sizes you choose, the number of rods used, and where the rods are placed on the head.

Hair characteristics: Of the hair characteristics described earlier, three are important to rod size selection:

1. Hair length
2. Hair elasticity
3. Hair texture

Suggested Hair Parting and Rod Sizes

Although the hair length, elasticity, and texture must be considered in the choice of rods, the texture should be the determining factor.

Coarse texture, good elasticity. Requires smaller (narrower) partings and larger rods to permit better placement of rods for a definite wave pattern.

Medium texture, average elasticity. Medium or average textured hair requires average size partings and medium size rods.

Fine texture, poor elasticity. Requires smaller than average partings and small to medium size rods to prevent hair strain or breakage.

Hair in nape area. Use smaller partings and smaller rods.

Long hair. To permanently wave hair longer than 6" (15 cm), use small partings and wrap smoothly and close to the scalp. The use of smaller partings permits the waving lotion and neutralizer to penetrate more easily and thoroughly.

SECTIONING AND PARTING

Sectioning is the dividing of hair into uniform working areas at the top, front, crown, sides, back, and nape. Sectioning makes your work easier because you can pin up all sections out of your way except the section you are working with.

Parting, also known as ***blocking,*** is the overall plan for rod placement. You block so that you know where to place the rods in order to give the design the support, direction, and curl pattern it needs. It is important that the blocking is done in uniform sections. You should use the following guidelines to help you:

1. Uniformly arrange sections.
2. Equally subdivide sections (blockings).
3. Create clean and uniform partings (length and width).
4. The average parting should match the diameter (size) of the rod being used.
5. The length of the blocking should be the same as or a little shorter, but never longer, than the length of the rod. (Figs. 11.12–11.14)

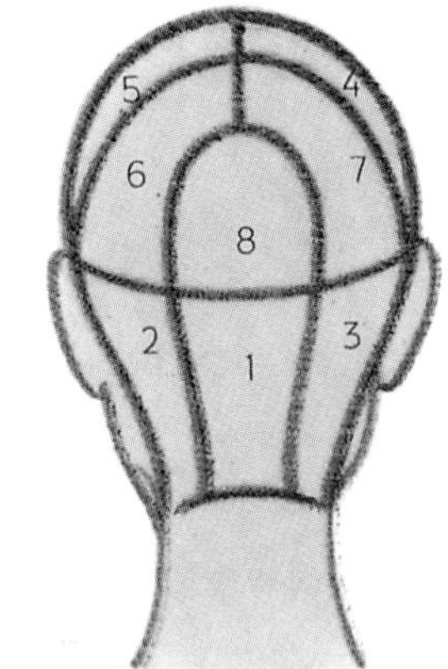

FIGURE 11.12 — Sectioning.

WRAPPING PATTERNS

Just as the rod size and parting size determine the size of the curl, the wrapping pattern determines the direction or flow of the curl.

Six popular wrapping patterns are:

1. Single halo
2. Double halo (double horseshoe)
3. Straight back
4. Dropped crown
5. Spiral wrap
6. Stack perm

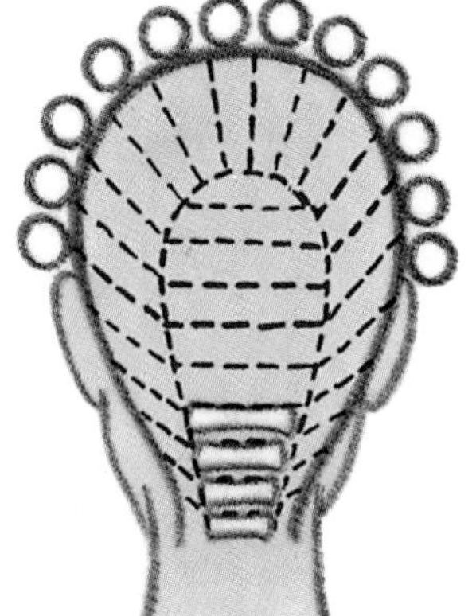
FIGURE 11.13 — Blocking (subsections).

These are known by other names in different areas of the country.

The following sections and partings are suggested for these wrapping patterns. Your instructor might suggest different sections, which are equally correct.

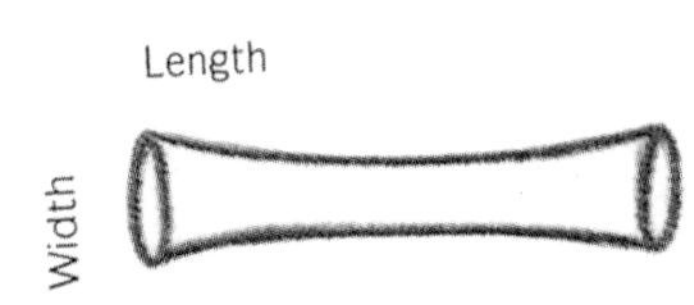

FIGURE 11.14 — Length denotes span of blocking. Width refers to the depth of the blocking. Small or large blockings usually refer to their width.

Single Halo

The single halo wrap is commonly used for average size heads to create even curls. (Figs. 11.15–11.18)

Double Halo

The double halo wrap is usually used for larger size heads. (Figs. 11.19–11.22)

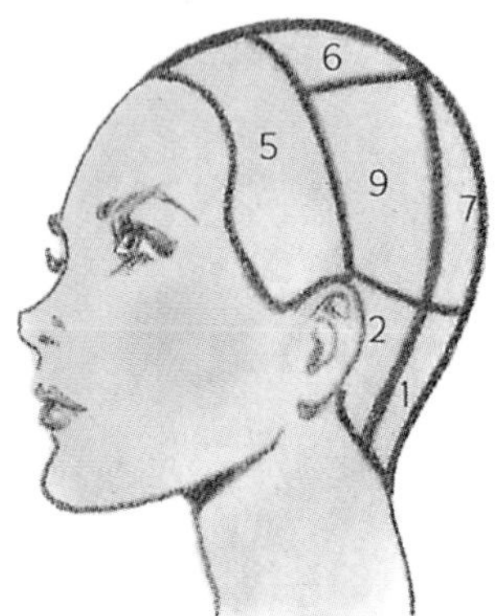

FIGURE 11.15 — Sectioning side.

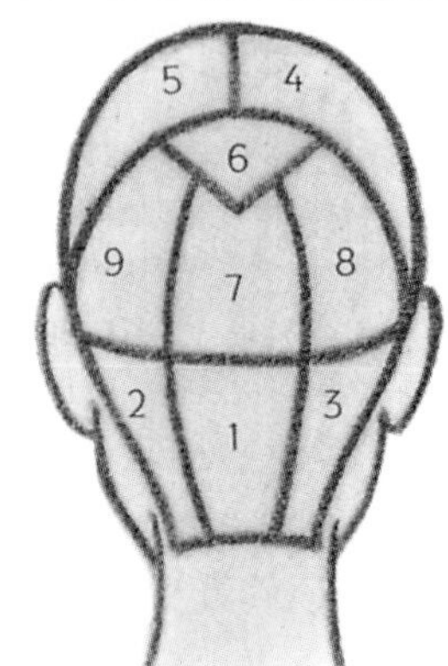

FIGURE 11.16 — Sectioning back.

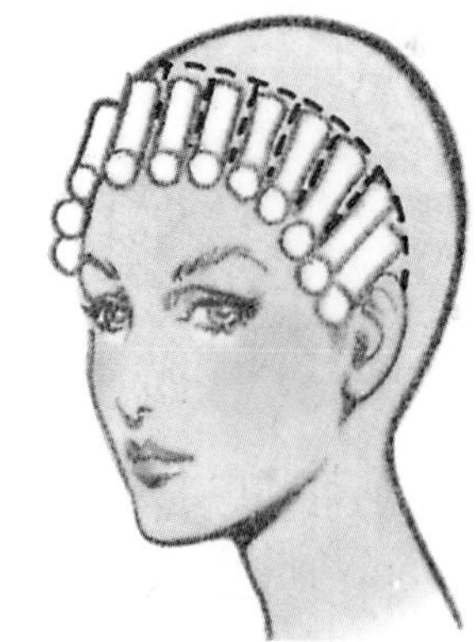

FIGURE 11.17 — Blocking side.

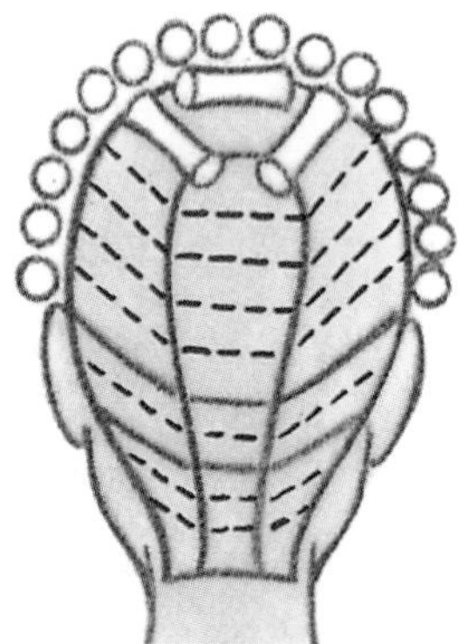

FIGURE 11.18 — Blocking back.

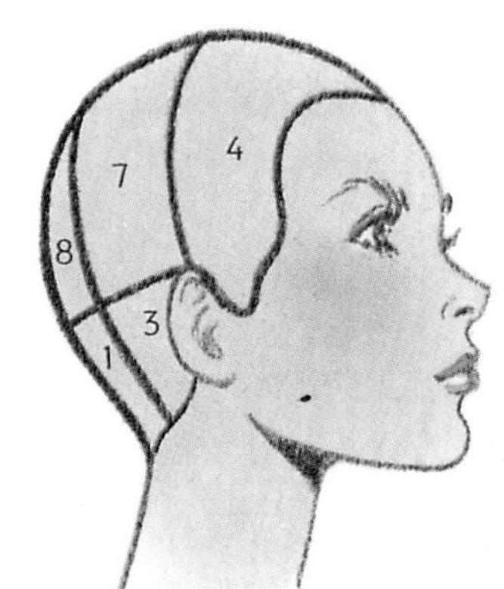

FIGURE 11.19 — Sectioning side.

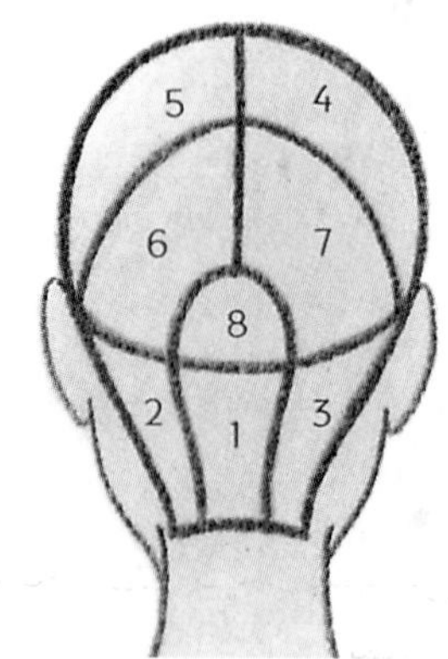

FIGURE 11.20 — Sectioning back.

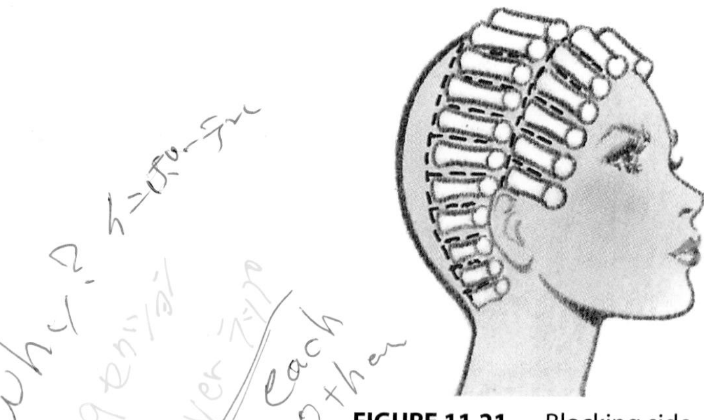

FIGURE 11.21 — Blocking side.

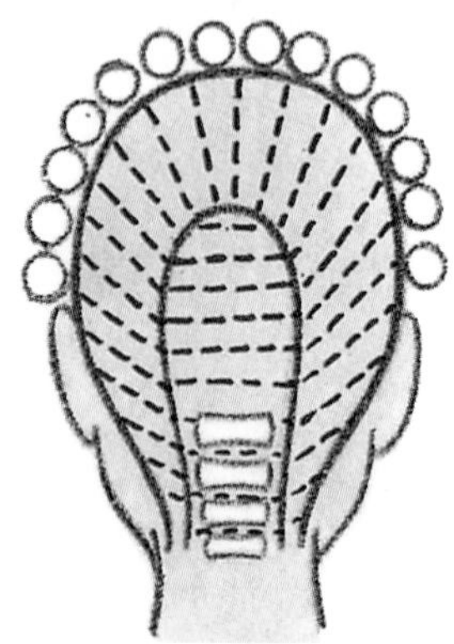

FIGURE 11.22 — Blocking back.

Straight Back

The straight back wrap is used to create a rather soft, full, and high style effect, directed off the face. (Figs. 11.23, 11.24)

To create ***bangs*** on the forehead, the first two top front curls are wrapped in a forward direction (see directional wrapping, pages 254–255). (Fig. 11.25)

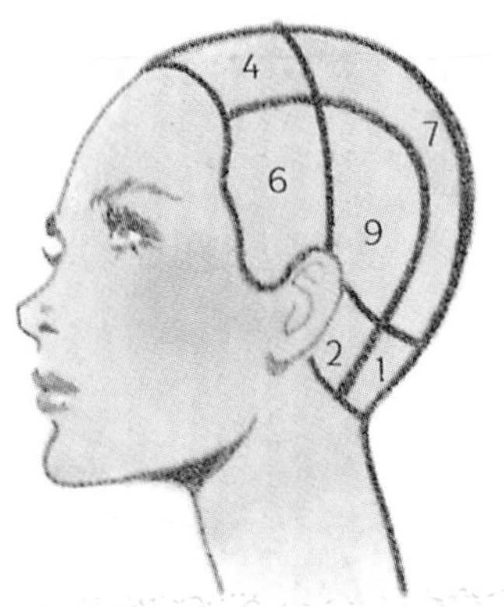

FIGURE 11.23 — Sectioning side.

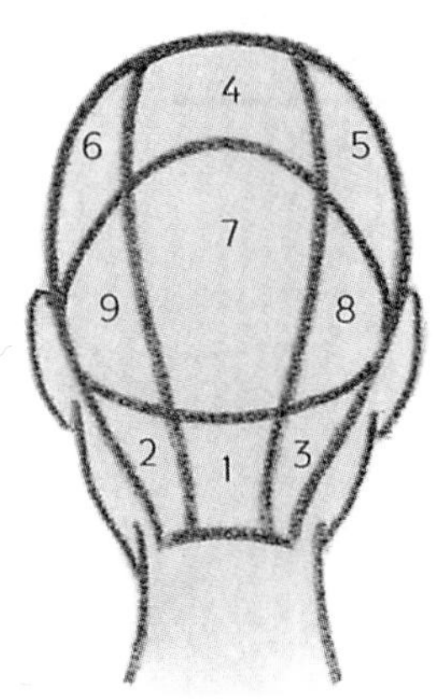

FIGURE 11.24 — Sectioning back.

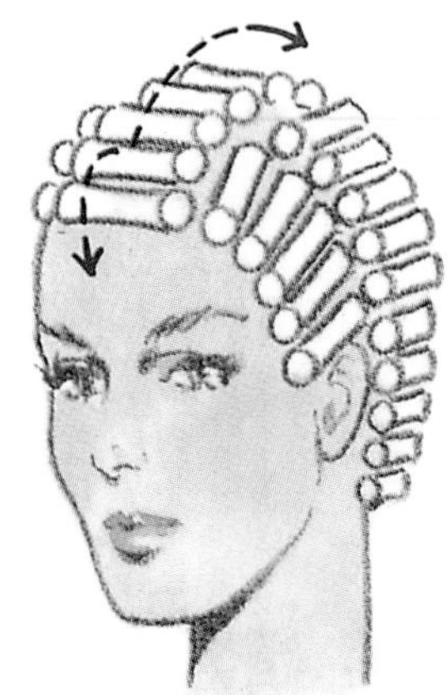

FIGURE 11.25 — Setting for bangs.

Dropped Crown

The dropped crown wrap is usually used for longer hair and for a smooth crown effect.

The hair is sectioned in the same way as for the straight back pattern. However, in the back area that is not numbered on the illustration, larger hair sections are made, depending on the amount of hair in that section. Only the hair ends are wrapped and the rods rest on the smaller rods in the nape area (sections 2, 1, 3). Be guided by your instructor. (Figs. 11.26–11.29)

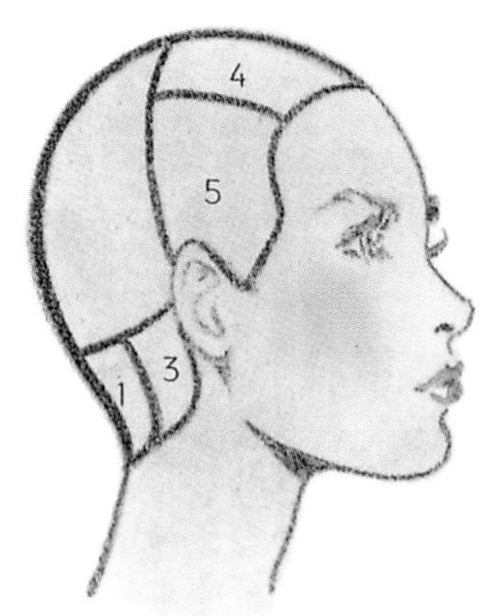

FIGURE 11.26 — Sectioning side.

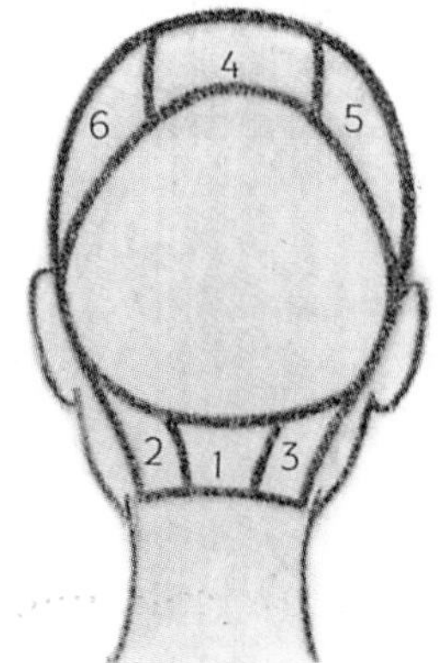

FIGURE 11.27 — Sectioning back.

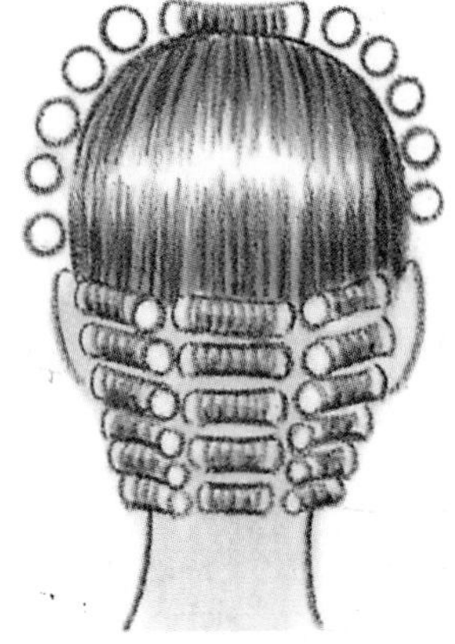

FIGURE 11.28 — Blocking (sub-sectioning) pattern.

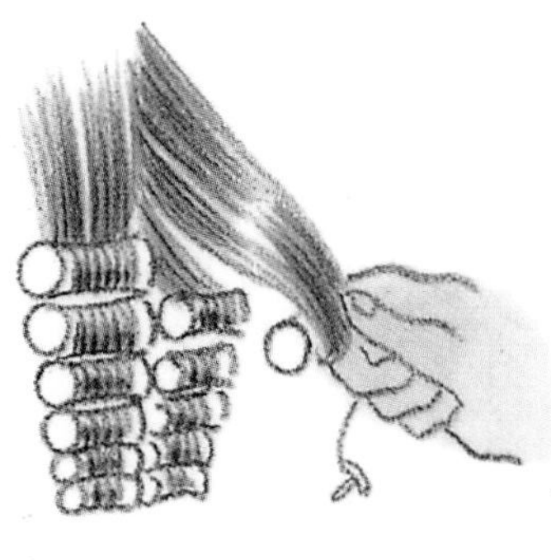

FIGURE 11.29 — Wrapping hair ends of crown area.

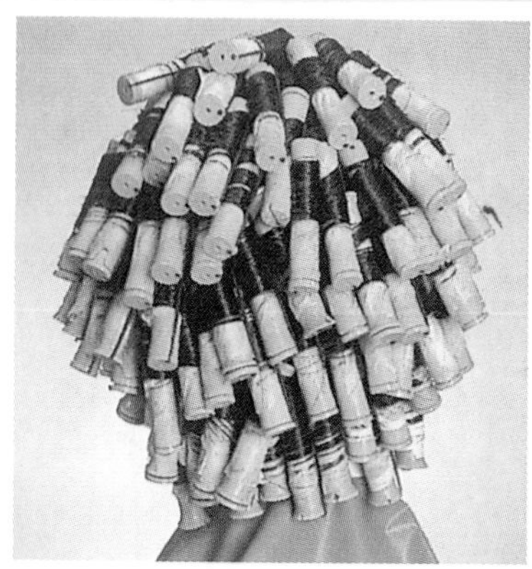

FIGURE 11.30 — Spiral wrap.

Spiral Wrap

The spiral wrap is used for long hair to create tight, springy curls. (Fig. 11.30)

Stack Perm

The stack technique is usually used for greater curl at the nape. (Fig. 11.31)

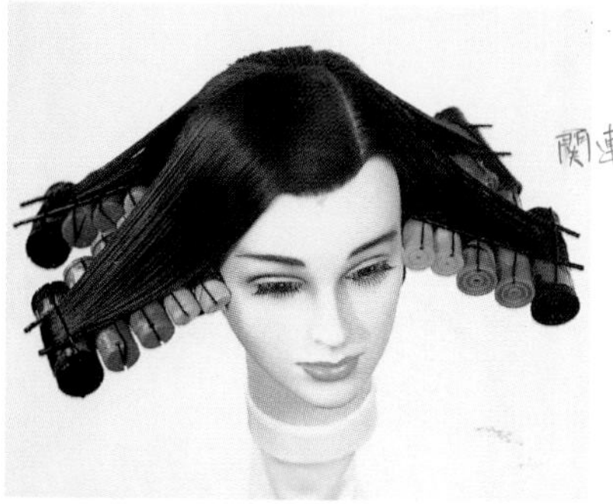

FIGURE 11.31 — Stack perm.

WRAPPING THE HAIR

To create a uniform wave or curl pattern, the hair must be wrapped smoothly and neatly on each perm rod *without stretching.* As noted earlier, the action of the waving lotion expands the hair. Hair that is tightly wrapped interferes with this action and prevents penetration of the waving lotion and neutralizer.

Hair Strand Parting in Relation to the Head

Base refers to the head or scalp and where the rod is placed in relation to the head. The rods can be wrapped on-base, off-base, or one-half off-base. Each of these rod positions creates a slightly different scalp wave direction, which will influence the overall curl pattern results.

Curl on-base. When the strand is held in an upward position and wound on the rod, the curl will rest on-base. (Fig. 11.32) Hair wound in this manner will produce curls that start close to the scalp for hairstyles that require fullness, height, and upward movement.

Curl off-base. When the strand is held in a downward position and wound on a rod, the curl will rest off-base. (Fig. 11.33) Hair wound in this manner will produce a curl that starts farther away from the scalp than hair wound on-base. Off-base winding produces close-to-the-head hairstyles that do not require fullness or height.

Curl one-half off-base. When the strand is held straight out from the head and wound on a rod, the curl will rest one-half off-base. (Fig. 11.34) Hair wound in this manner is adaptable to many hairstyles.

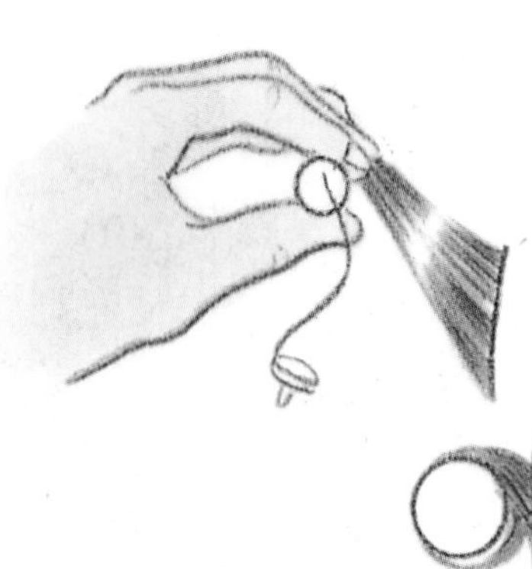

FIGURE 11.32 — Curl on-base.

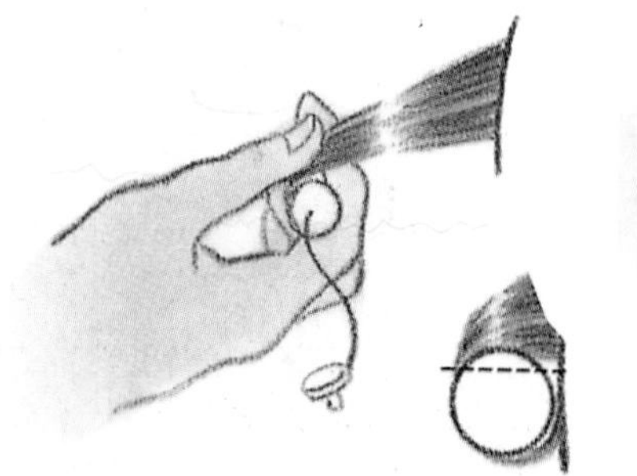

FIGURE 11.33 — Curl off-base.

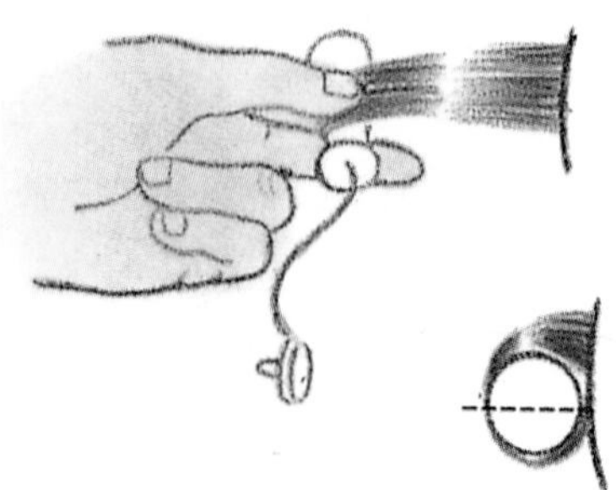

FIGURE 11.34 — Curl one-half off-base.

End Wraps

End wraps or end papers are porous papers used to cover the ends of the hair to ensure smooth, even wrapping. End wraps minimize the danger of hair breakage and help to form smooth, even curls and waves. They are especially important in helping to wrap uneven hair lengths smoothly.

There are three methods of end wrap application in general use today. Each method is equally effective, if properly used.

1. Double end paper wrap
2. Single end paper wrap
3. Book end wrap

Note: *Hair should be shampooed and left moist (not saturated) for wrapping. Section hair, then begin by making your first parting. Remember, each parting should be no longer than the length of the rod. If the parting is too long, the hair will not wave evenly. If the hair should become dry while you are wrapping, mist the hair lightly with water.*

Double End Paper Wrap

1. Part off and comb the parting up and out until all hair is smooth and evenly distributed. (Fig. 11.35)
2. Place one end wrap under the hair strand so that it extends below the ends of the hair. Place the other end wrap on top. (Fig. 11.36)
3. With your right hand, place the rod under the double end wraps, parallel with the parting at the scalp. (Fig. 11.37)

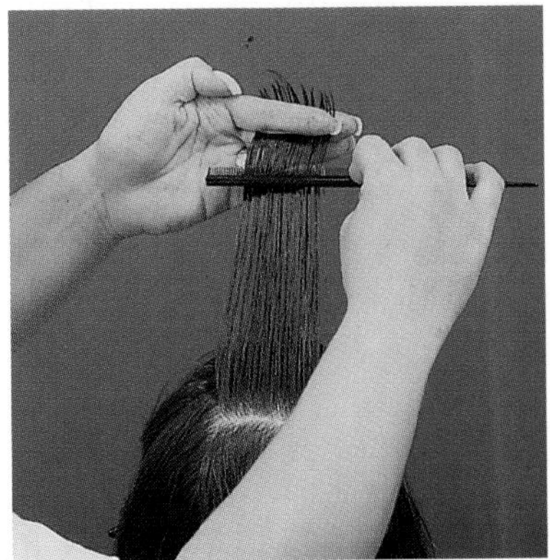

FIGURE 11.35 — Comb and distribute strand evenly.

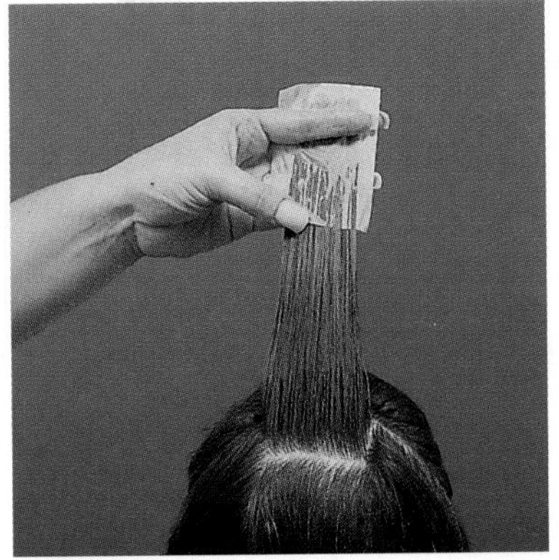

FIGURE 11.36 — Position end papers.

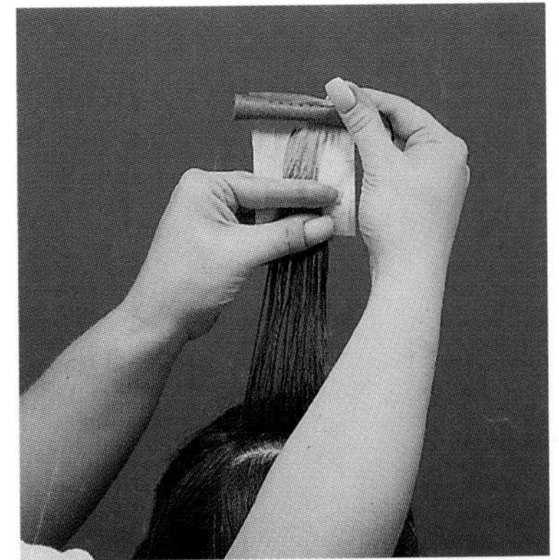

FIGURE 11.37 — Position rod.

4. Wind the strand smoothly on the rod to the scalp without tension. (Tension stretches the hair, which is in a weakened condition after lotion is applied.) (Fig. 11.38)
5. Fasten band at top of rod. (Fig. 11.39)

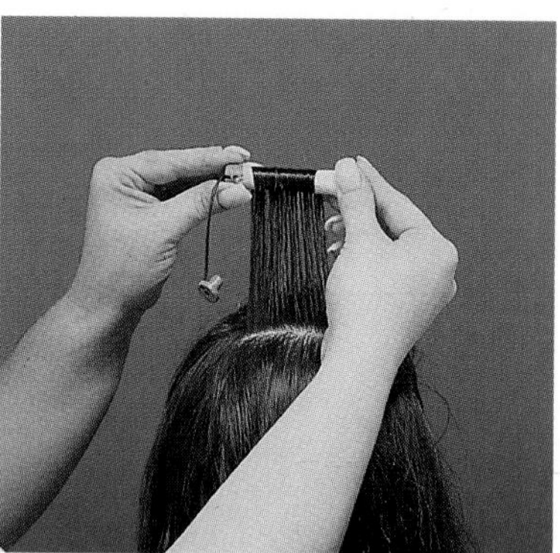

FIGURE 11.38 — Wind the strand.

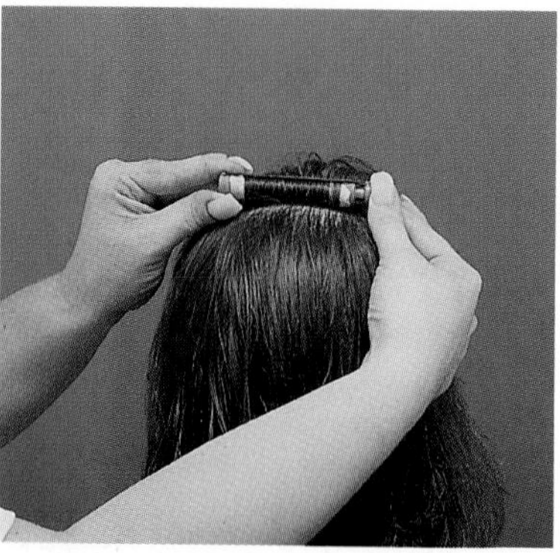

FIGURE 11.39 — Fasten band.

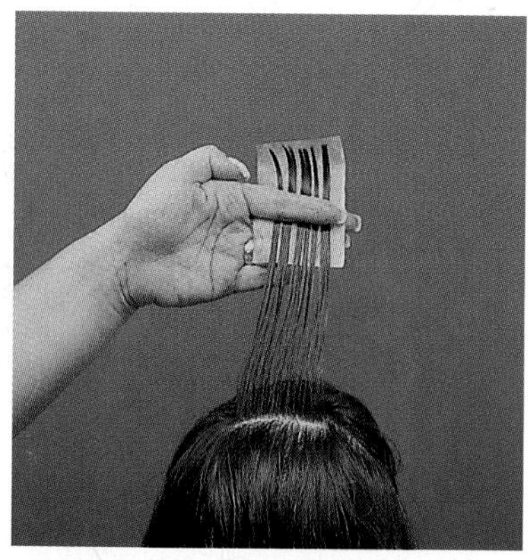

FIGURE 11.40 — Single end paper wrap.

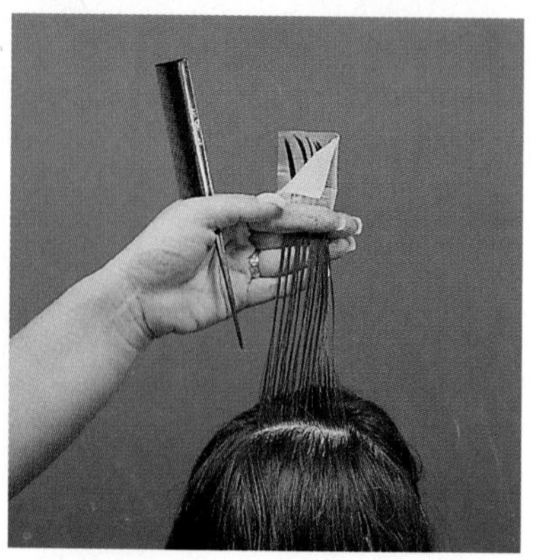

FIGURE 11.41 — Book end wrap.

CAUTION

To prevent breakage, the band should not press into the hair near the scalp or be twisted against the wound hair.

The preparation and winding of curls for the single end paper wrap and book end wrap are the same as the double end paper wrap, with the following exceptions:

Single end paper wrap. Place only one end wrap on top of the hair strand and hold it flat between the index and middle fingers to prevent bunching. (Fig. 11.40) The hair is wound in the same manner as the double end paper wrap.

Book end wrap. Hold the strand between the index and middle fingers; fold and place an end paper over the strand, forming an envelope. Wind the curl as in the double end paper wrap. (Fig. 11.41)

The Piggyback (Double Rod) Wrap

The piggyback (double rod) method of wrapping is especially suitable for extra long hair. This wrapping technique permits maximum control of the size and tightness of the curl from the scalp to the hair ends. Control of the amount of curl can be exercised by the size of the rods selected. Thus, the use of larger rods will result in a loose, wide wave; while small or medium rods will give tighter curls. The following is the procedure for wrapping in the piggyback (double rod) method:

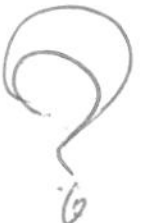

1. Section the head in the usual manner (9 sections).
2. Select the desired size rods. The rods used in the midpoint to the scalp area should be at least one size larger than those used for the hair ends.
3. About halfway up the strand, place porous end papers one on top and one underneath. (Fig. 11.42)
4. Start at the midpoint part of the strand. Place the larger rod underneath the hair strand and start wrapping. (Fig. 11.43)
5. Roll the rod toward the scalp and, at the same time, control the hair ends by holding them to the left away from the rod.
6. Secure the wrapped rod at the scalp, leaving the hair ends dangling free from the rod. (Fig. 11.44)
7. Place an end paper on the hair strand covering the ends. Using the smaller size rod, wrap the hair ends up to the above larger rod. (Fig. 11.45)

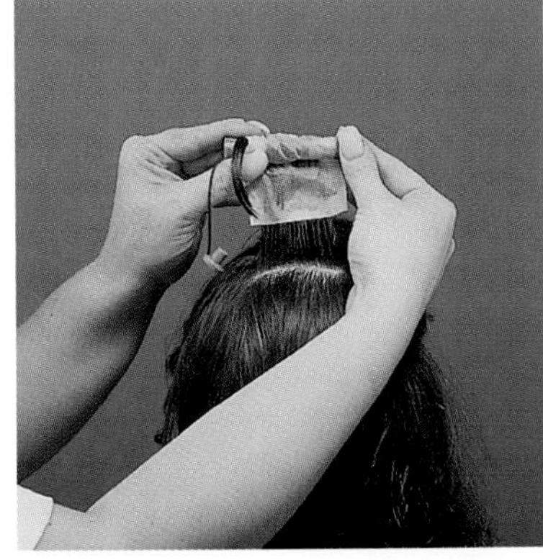

FIGURE 11.42 — Position porous end papers.

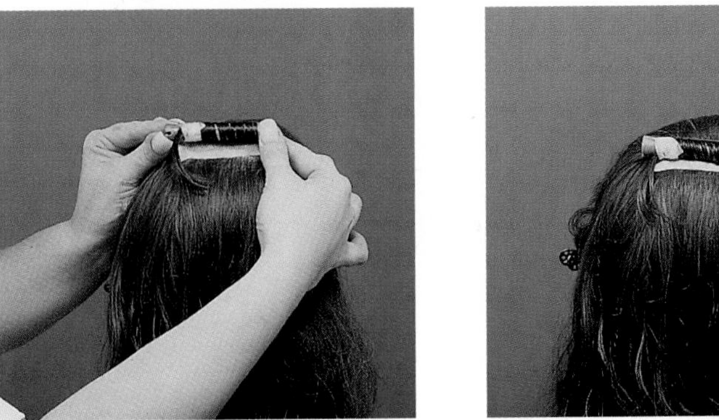

FIGURE 11.43 — Start wrapping.

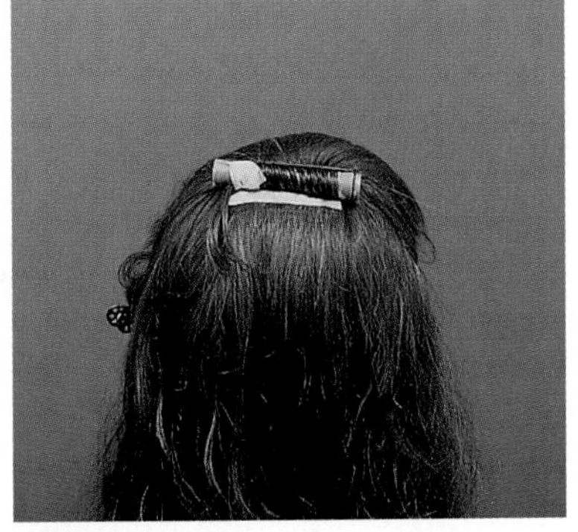

FIGURE 11.44 — Secure the wrapped rod.

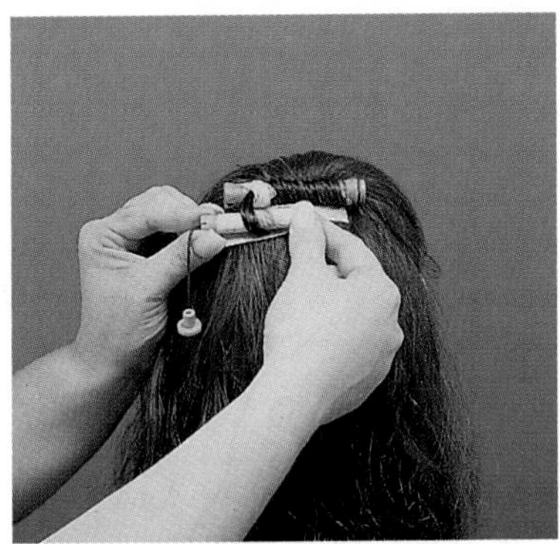

FIGURE 11.45 — Wrap the remaining hair ends.

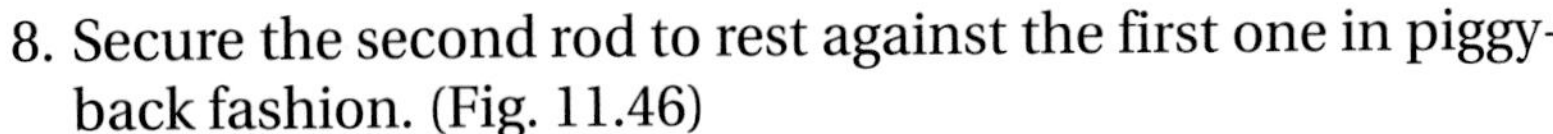

8. Secure the second rod to rest against the first one in piggy-back fashion. (Fig. 11.46)
9. To maintain better control over the wrapping and processing, it is advisable to complete the wrapping of each hair strand before proceeding to the next one.
10. Test curls should be taken from the rods closer to the scalp because the hair in this area is more resistant and might require additional processing.

Note: *When wrapping hair, always avoid bulkiness on the rod. Bulkiness prevents the formation of a good curl because the hair cannot conform to the shape of the rod, and the waving lotion and neutralizer cannot penetrate evenly and thoroughly. To ensure a smooth wave formation and avoid fishhook ends, the first turn on the rod should be the end wraps without any of the hair ends between them.*

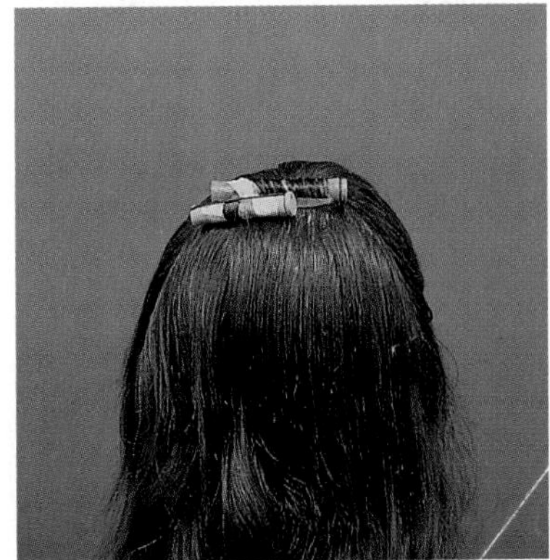

FIGURE 11.46 — Secure the second rod beneath the first rod.

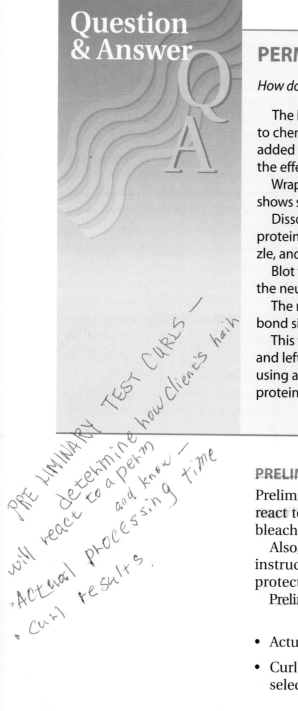

PERMING FINE HAIR

How do you deal with hair so fine and limp it will not take a perm?

The hair may not have sufficient salt bonds to respond favorably to chemical re-formation. Synthetic salt bonds can be temporarily added to the hair. They will immediately make the hair bouncier, but the effect is not permanent.

Wrap the perm, apply perm solution and process. When the test curl shows sufficient response, towel blot the solution from each perm rod.

Dissolve 1 teaspoon Epsom salts in 2 oz. of water and 2 oz. liquid protein re-conditioner. Use an applicator bottle with a very fine nozzle, and apply the solution to each rod. Leave it on for 5 minutes.

Blot the solution from the hair (do not rinse), and proceed with the neutralizing (re-bonding step).

The magnesium content in the Epsom salts creates a synthetic bond similar to salt-bonds in natural hair.

This formula may be applied to fine, limp hair after each shampoo and left on for a period of 15 minutes, as often as necessary. When using after a shampoo, omit water from the formula. Use only liquid protein and Epsom salts.

—*From* Milady's Salon Solutions *by Louise Cotter*

PRELIMINARY TEST CURLS

Preliminary test curls help determine how your client's hair will react to a perm. It is advisable to do a test on hair that is tinted, bleached, over-porous, or shows any signs of damage.

Also, before applying waving lotion, be sure to check with your instructor or state board to find out if you are required to wear protective gloves during application.

Preliminary testing gives you the following additional information:

- Actual processing time needed to achieve optimum curl results
- Curl results based on the rod size and perm product you have selected

Procedure

1. Shampoo the hair and towel dry.
2. Following the perm directions, wrap two or three rods in the most delicate areas of the hair.

3. Wrap a coil of cotton around the rod.
4. Apply waving lotion to wrapped curls, being very careful not to allow the waving lotion to come in contact with unwrapped hair.
5. Set a timer and process the hair according to the perm directions.
6. Check the hair frequently.

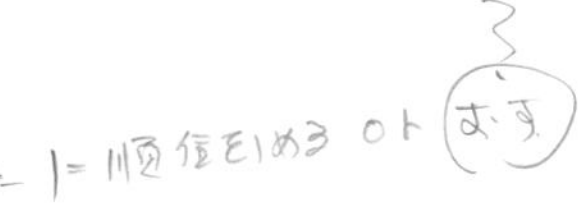

To check a test curl, unfasten a rod and carefully (remember—hair is in a softened state) unwind the curl about 1½ turns of the rod. Do not permit the hair to become loose or unwound from the rod completely. Hold the hair firmly by placing a thumb at each end of the rod. Move the rod gently toward the scalp so that the hair falls loosely into the wave pattern. Continue checking the rods until a firm and definite "S" is formed. The "S" reflects the size of the rod used. (Fig. 11.47) Be guided by the manufacturer's direction.

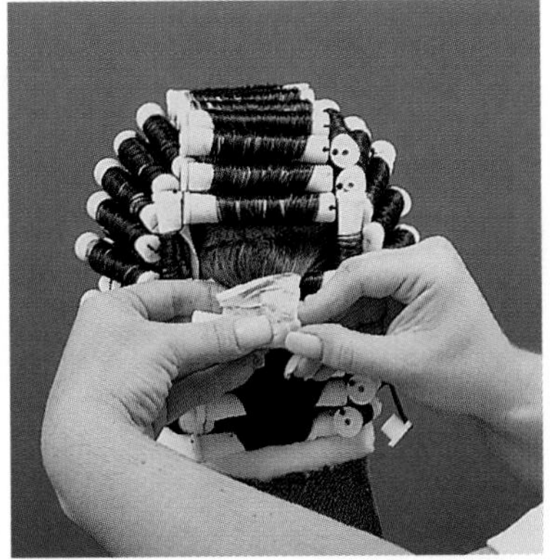

FIGURE 11.47 — Unwinding hair carefully, without pulling or pushing.

Note: *When judging test curls, different hair textures with varying degrees of elasticity will have slightly different "S" formations. Fine, thin hair is generally softer and has less bulk. The wave ridge might be less defined and more difficult to read. Coarse, thick hair has better elasticity and seems to reinforce itself, falling into the wave pattern more readily. The wave ridge will be stronger and better defined. Long hair may produce a wider scalp wave than short hair, because larger rods are used and the diameter of the wave widens toward the scalp.*

When the optimum curl has been formed, rinse the curls with warm water, blot the curls thoroughly, apply, process and rinse the neutralizer according to the perm directions and gently dry these test curls. Evaluate the curl results. If the hair is overprocessed, do not perm the rest of the hair until it is in better condition. If the test curl results are good, proceed with the perm, but ***do not re-perm these preliminary test curls.***

Overprocessing

Any lotion that can properly process the hair also can overprocess it, causing dryness, frizziness, or hair damage. Overprocessed hair is easily detected. It is very curly when wet, but frizzy when dry. It cannot be combed into a suitable wave pattern, because the elasticity of the hair has been excessively damaged, and the hair feels harsh after being dried. Reconditioning treatments should begin immediately.

Causes of overprocessing are:

1. Lotion left on too long.
2. Improperly judged pre-perm hair analysis and/or waving lotion that was too strong.
3. Test curls were not made frequently enough or were judged improperly.

Completed: Learning Objective #5

ROD SELECTION AND SECTIONING, PARTING, AND WRAPPING PROCEDURES

Underprocessing

Underprocessing is caused by insufficient processing time of the waving lotion. After perming, underprocessed hair has a limp or weak wave formation. The ridges are not well defined, and the hair retains little or no wave formation. Typically, after a few shampooings, the hair will have no curl pattern at all. (Figs. 11.48a–e)

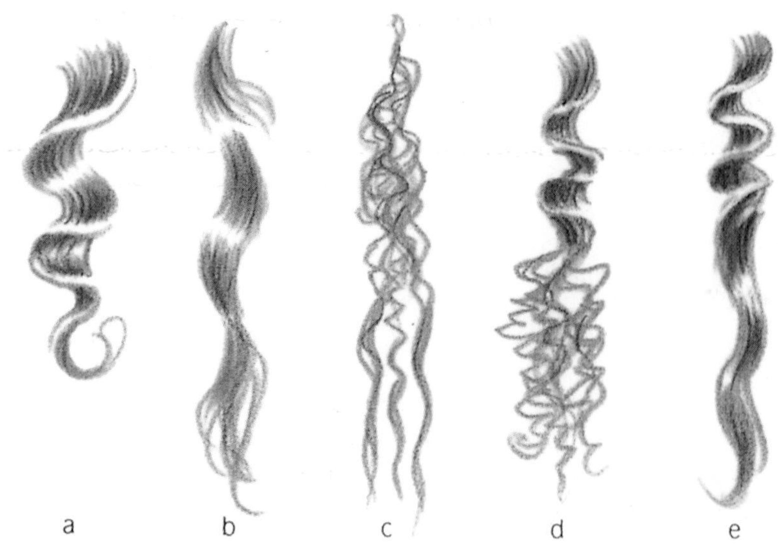

FIGURE 11.48a — Good results.
FIGURE 11.48b — Underprocessed curl.
FIGURE 11.48c — Overprocessed curl.
FIGURE 11.48d — Porous ends.
FIGURE 11.48e — Improper winding.

> **CAUTION**
>
> *Underprocessed hair, even if there is no curl, has been chemically treated. If, in your professional judgment, you decide the hair can be re-permed, condition it first, choose a milder waving lotion, and test the curls frequently.*

Important Safety Precautions

Remember that the lotions used for perming contain chemically active ingredients and therefore must be used carefully to avoid injury to you and your client. The following precautions should always be taken:

1. Protect the client's clothing with a plastic shampoo cape, or ask the client to change into a smock.
2. Ask the client to remove glasses, earrings, and necklaces to prevent damage.
3. Do not give a perm to a client who has experienced an allergic reaction to a previous perm.
4. Do not save any opened, unused waving lotion or neutralizer. These lotions can change in strength and effectiveness if not used within a few hours after opening the container.
5. Do not dilute or add anything to the waving lotion or neutralizer unless the product directions tell you to do so.
6. Keep waving lotion out of eyes and away from the skin. If waving lotion should contact these areas, rinse *thoroughly* with cool water.
7. Do not perm and apply haircolor to a client on the same day. Perm the hair first, wait one week, then apply haircolor.

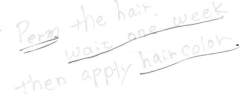

Completed:
Learning Objective
#6
SAFETY PRECAUTIONS

PERMING TECHNIQUES

Before you begin perming, make sure you have all the necessary supplies at hand. Good organization and planning will help you develop precision and speed in completing a perm. At your station, the following equipment should be laid out in an organized, easily accessible fashion:

- The perm product
- Rods (organized by size)
- End wraps
- Cotton coil
- Towels
- Plastic hair clips and pins
- Tail comb
- Protective gloves

Always Read and Follow the Product Directions Carefully. Some alkaline perm product directions call for water wrapping, some are lotion wrapped, and others require pre-wrap lotions. Some wave lotions come in two parts that must be mixed just prior to use. Some need dryer heat. (***Note:*** Dryer should be pre-heated.) Some perms require that a plastic cap be placed over the rods during the processing; others do not. (The plastic cap retains moisture and protects the hair under the dryer.) Considering all the variables, it is not a good idea to trust your memory. Make it a practice to check the printed directions that accompany every perm *each time you give a perm*.

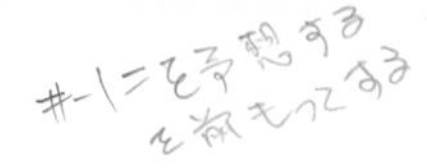

APPLYING WAVING LOTION

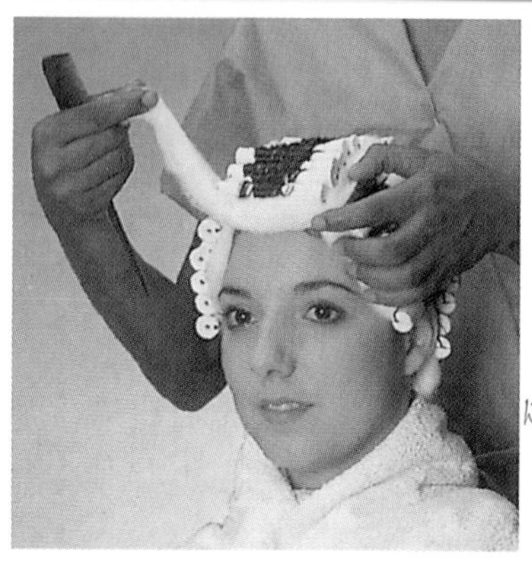

FIGURE 11.49 — Hairline protected by cotton strips or neutralizing band.

After shampooing, shaping, and wrapping the hair, place a coil or band of cotton around the entire hairline. To prevent skin irritation and for added protection, apply a barrier cream to skin around hairline before applying cotton band. This safety precaution prevents waving lotion from coming into contact with the skin and possibly causing irritation. If lotion is applied accurately there should be a minimum of dripping, but the cotton is assurance of your client's comfort and safety. After the waving lotion has been applied, remove the cotton, gently pat the skin with water-soaked cotton, and replace with dry cotton. (Fig. 11.49)

Unless otherwise specified in the product instructions, apply waving lotion liberally to the top and underside of each wound rod. Start at the crown area and progress systematically down each section. Be sure that the surface area of the wound curls is wet with lotion so penetration is even. (Fig. 11.50)

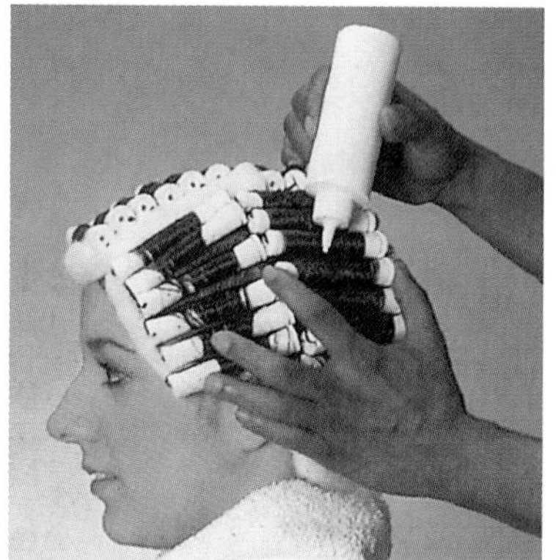

FIGURE 11.50 — Applying waving lotion.

Processing Time

Processing time is the length of time required for the hair strands to absorb the waving lotion (softening) and for the hair to re-curl (rearrangement of chemical bonds). It depends on the hair type (porosity, elasticity, length, density, texture, and overall condition) and the specific perm you are using. Again, follow the manufacturer's directions explicitly. It is usually safe to anticipate the processing time to be less than suggested by the manufacturer or a client's previous record card. Some perms have stop-action processing so that all you have to do is set a timer. (Fig. 11.51) Some perms give you a general timetable to follow and require that you do a test curl during processing. It is very important to accurately time the perm process to help prevent over- or underprocessing.

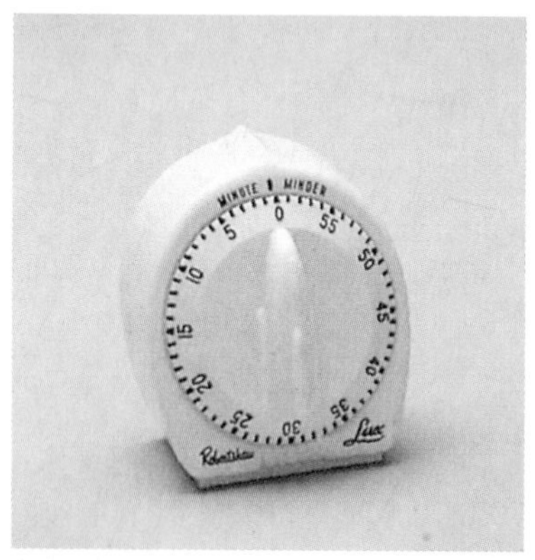

FIGURE 11.51 — Processing timer.

The ability of the hair to absorb moisture may vary from time to time in the same individual, even when the same lotions and procedures are used. A record of the previous processing time is desirable, but should be used only as a guide.

Often, it is necessary to resaturate all the rods a second time during the processing time. This might be due to:

1. Evaporation of the lotion or dryness of the hair.
2. Hair poorly saturated by the cosmetologist.
3. No wave development after the maximum time indicated by the manufacturer.
4. Improper selection of solution strength for the client's hair.
5. Failure to follow the manufacturer's directions for a specific formula.

A reapplication of the lotion will hasten processing. Watch the wave development closely. ***Negligence can result in hair damage.***

Most manufacturers provide instructions with their product. Here are some you will encounter:

1. ***Place a plastic cap over the wrapped rods.*** Be sure that the plastic cap covers all the rods and that the cap is airtight. Secure the cap with a plastic clip. The cap holds in heat and moisture and protects the hair under the dryer. If it is too loose or if all the rods are not covered, processing might take longer. (Fig. 11.52)
2. ***Pre-heated dryer.*** Turn the hood dryer to the high setting and medium airflow. Allow the dryer to warm up for approximately 5 minutes before placing your client under the dryer. (***Note:*** Dryer filters should be cleaned frequently so that optimum heat and airflow will remain constant.) (Fig. 11.53)
3. ***Process at room temperature.*** Make sure the client is not sitting in a draft or too close to an air conditioner. A room that is too cool slows the processing time.

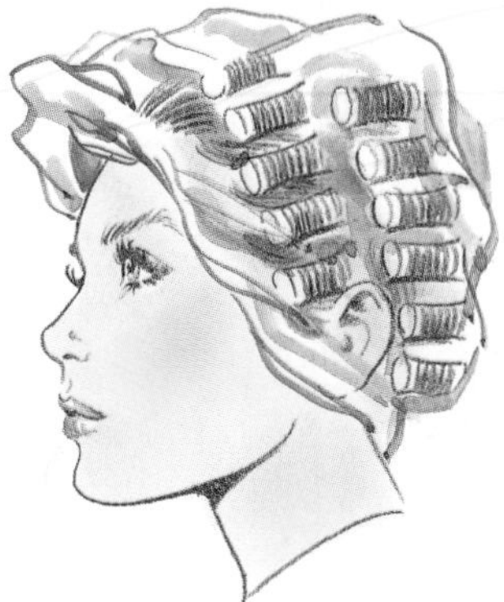

FIGURE 11.52 — Applying processing cap.

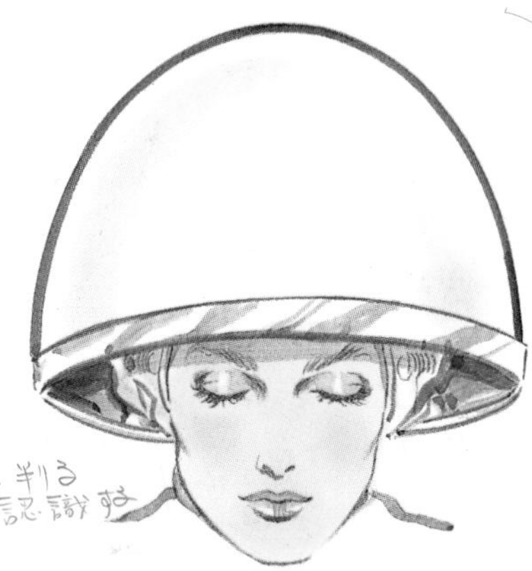

FIGURE 11.53 — Putting client under pre-heated dryer.

Testing Curls during Processing

Optimum curl development occurs only once during the processing time. The ability to read a test curl "S" formation and recognize proper wave development will help you avoid two of the most common problems in perming: overprocessing and underprocessing. Three test curls should be taken: in the crown, on top of the head, and on the side of the head. These three locations will allow you to judge the progress of curl development on the most resistant and the least resistant areas of the head. Follow the procedure for unwinding the rod and checking the "S" pattern formation described in the preliminary test curl section (pages 246–247). (Fig. 11.54)

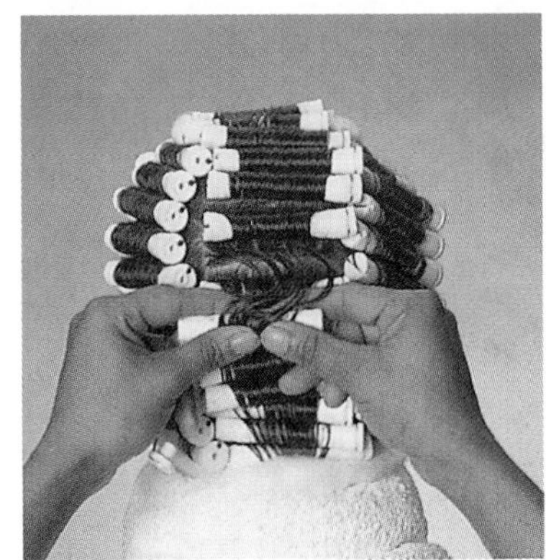

FIGURE 11.54 — Properly processed strand opens up into "S" formation.

Water Rinsing

Rinsing the waving lotion from the hair is extremely important. Any lotion left in the hair can cause poor perm results. When your test curl indicates that optimum curl has been achieved, remove the cotton from around the hairline. Rinse the hair thoroughly with a moderate force of warm water. The manufacturer's perm directions will indicate how long you should rinse—usually 3 to 5 minutes. Always set your timer for the exact time. Remember, you are rinsing the lotion *out* of the internal hair structure, not merely off the surface. Make sure that all rods are thoroughly rinsed. Pay special attention to the rods at the nape of the neck. They are a little difficult to reach, but they must be

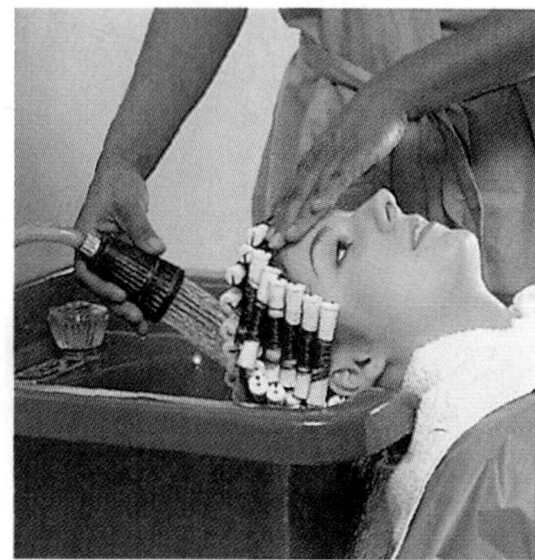

FIGURE 11.55 — Rinsing waving lotion from the hair.

rinsed as well as all the other rods. Long hair and thick hair usually require the maximum rinsing time (5 minutes) to make sure that the lotion has been removed from all the hair wrapped around the rods. (Fig. 11.55)

Undesirable effects of improper or incomplete rinsing include:

1. ***Early curl relaxation.*** Even if the perm has been processed correctly, any waving lotion left in the hair can interfere with the action of the neutralizer. If the neutralizer is not able to properly rebond the hair, the curl will be weak or will not last very long.
2. ***Lightening of hair color (natural or tint).*** Rinsing helps reduce the pH of the hair and helps to close the cuticle layer. If the hair is not rinsed properly, the hydrogen peroxide in the neutralizer can react with waving lotion left in the hair and cause the hair color to lighten. This lightening effect is usually seen on the hair ends.
3. ***Residual perm odor.*** If any waving lotion is left in the hair, it will become trapped inside the hair when the neutralizer is applied. This is especially true of acid-balanced perms. Unpleasant odors may be evident each time the hair gets wet or damp.

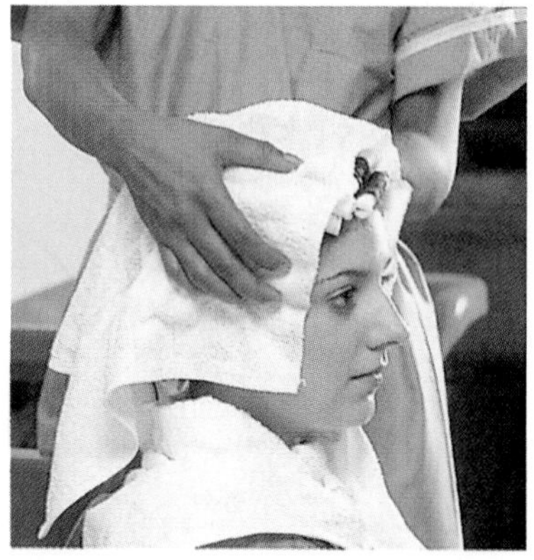

FIGURE 11.56 — Towel blotting.

Blotting after Water Rinsing

Careful blotting assures that the neutralizer will penetrate the hair immediately and completely: Do not omit this important step. To obtain the best results from towel blotting, carefully press a towel between each curl, using your fingers. Do not rock or roll the rods while blotting. When the hair is in a softened state, any such movement can cause hair breakage. Change to dry towels frequently in order to remove as much excess water as possible. Excess water left in the hair can dilute or weaken the action of the neutralizer. If this happens the curl can be either weak or relaxed. (Fig. 11.56)

After rinsing and blotting has been completed, place a fresh, clean band of cotton around the hairline before applying neutralizer.

NEUTRALIZING

Neutralizing procedures can vary according to the perm product you are using. Again, follow the manufacturer's directions explicitly. In general, the following procedure is the accepted method for neutralizing:

1. Apply neutralizer to the top and underside of all rods. Apply to the top of the rod, then gently turn the rod up and apply to

the underside of the rod in the same manner you applied the waving lotion.

2. Repeat the entire application a second time.
3. Wait 5 minutes to allow for optimum rebonding. Set a timer for accuracy. (Figs. 11.57, 11.58)
4. Remove the rods carefully and gently.
5. Work any remaining neutralizer through the hair gently with the palms of your hands.
6. Remove cotton from hairline and rinse the hair thoroughly with warm water.
7. Towel-blot the hair.

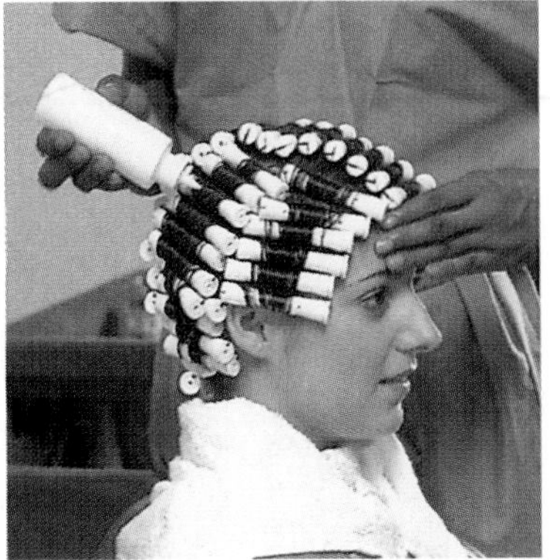

FIGURE 11.57 — Neutralizing—direct or on-the-rod method.

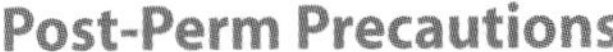

Post-Perm Precautions

After blotting, your new perm is ready for final shaping and styling. It is important to avoid shampooing, conditioning, stretching, or excessive manipulations of freshly permed hair. When styling, do not pull on the hair or use intense heat that could result in curl relaxation. Generally, hair should not be shampooed, conditioned, or treated harshly for 48 hours after perming. This special care will help ensure that the perm does not relax.

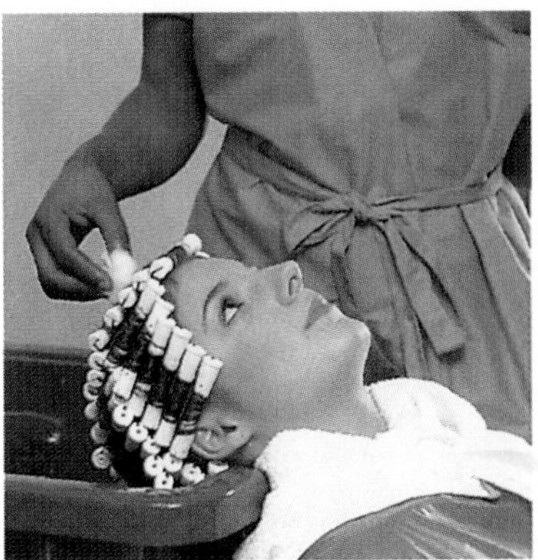

FIGURE 11.58 — Neutralizing—splash-on method.

TEN POINTERS FOR A PERFECT PERM

1. Consult with the client.
2. Analyze the hair and scalp carefully.
3. Select the correct rod size for the desired style.
4. Choose the appropriate perm product for the hair type and final design. Follow the manufacturer's directions carefully.
5. Section and make accurate partings for each rod. Wrap specifically for the style chosen.
6. Apply waving lotion to the top and underside of all wound rods. Saturate thoroughly.
7. If the perm product requires a test curl, be sure the result is a firmly formed "S" shape.
8. Water rinse for at least 3 to 5 minutes and carefully towel blot each rod.
9. Apply neutralizer to the top and underside of all rods. Saturate thoroughly.
10. Wait 5 minutes, remove the rods carefully, apply any remaining neutralizer, and gently work through the hair. Rinse with warm water.

CLEANUP

1. Discard all used supplies.
2. Clean up the work area.
3. Thoroughly clean and sanitize the rods and implements.
4. Wash and sanitize your hands.
5. Complete the client record card.

SPECIAL PERMING TECHNIQUES

DIRECTIONAL WRAPPING

Directional wrapping refers to the angle of the partings, placement of the rods, and the wrapping pattern you choose to create specific direction or movement in the final design. There are six basic directions in which hair can be wrapped. (Figs. 11.59–11.70)

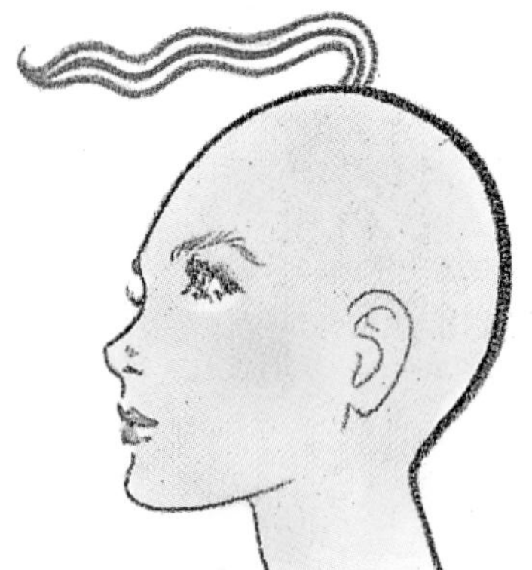

FIGURE 11.59 — Vertical direction (forward).

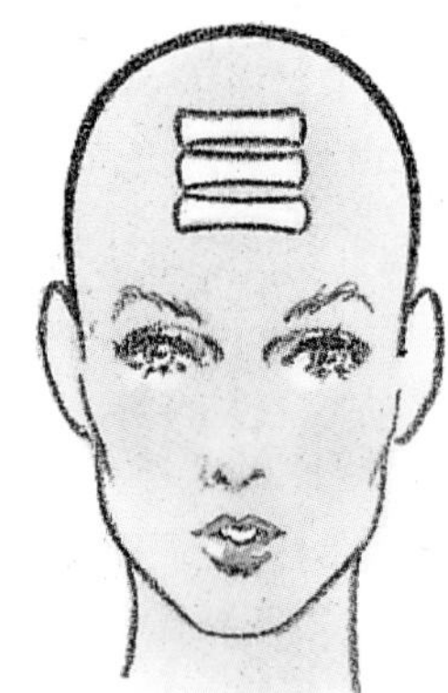

FIGURE 11.60 — Forward blocking.

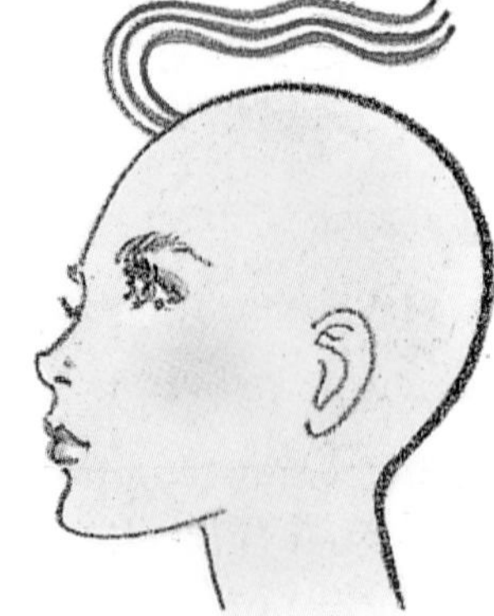

FIGURE 11.61 — Vertical direction (back).

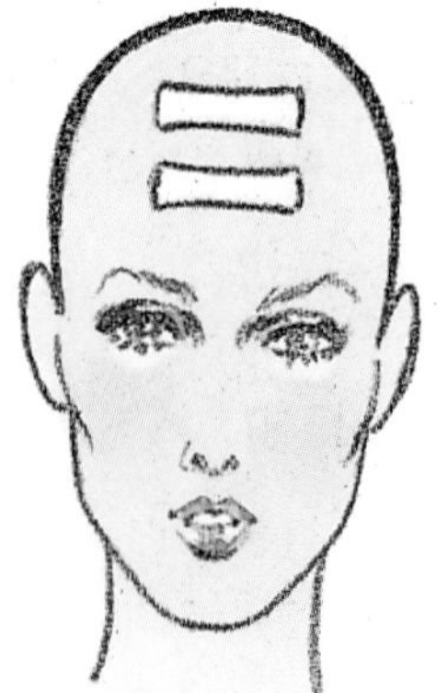

FIGURE 11.62 — Back blocking.

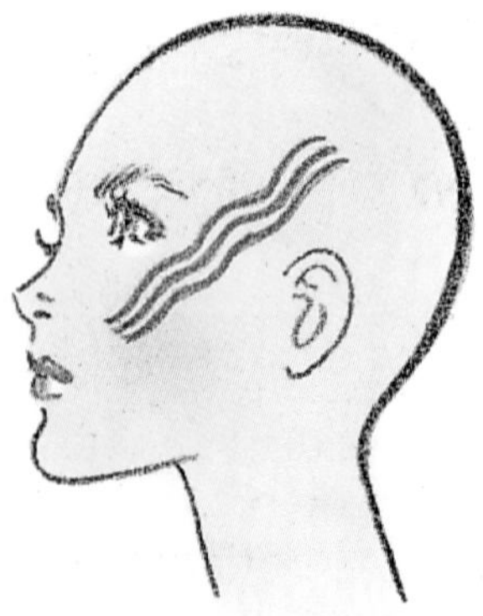

FIGURE 11.63 — Horizontal direction (forward).

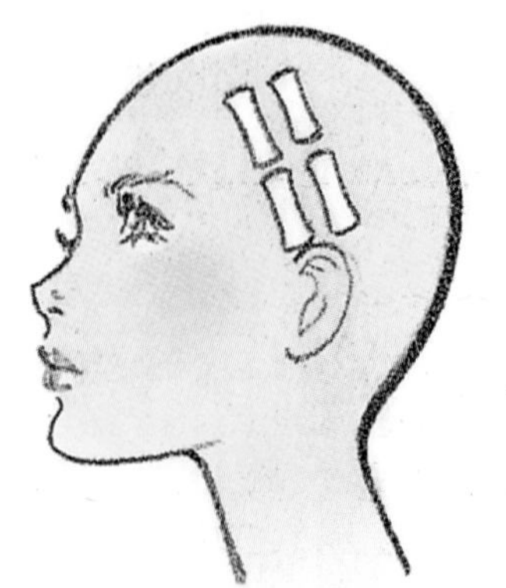

FIGURE 11.64 — Forward blocking.

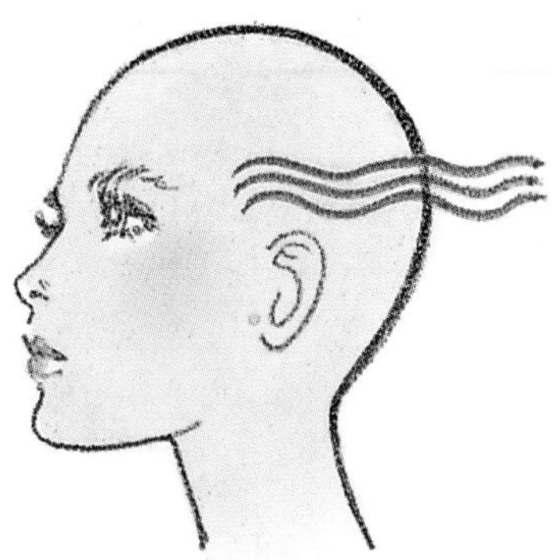

FIGURE 11.65 — Horizontal direction (back).

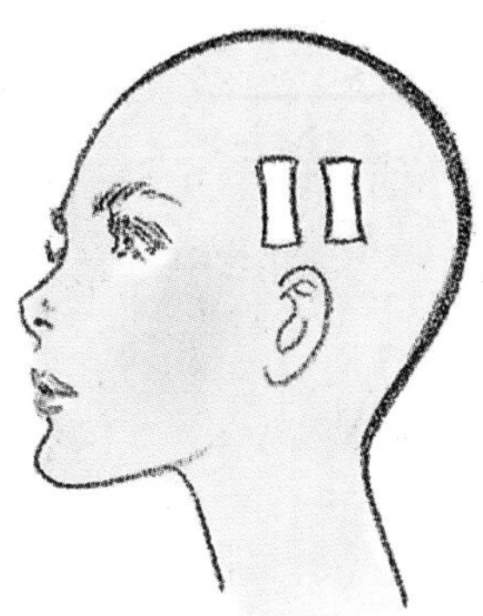

FIGURE 11.66 — Back blocking.

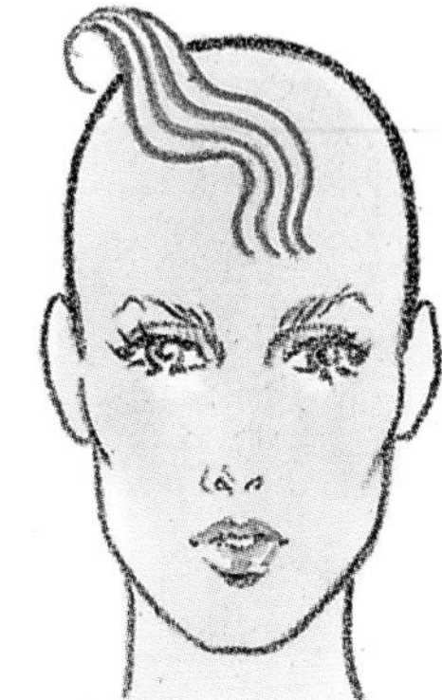

FIGURE 11.67 — Diagonal direction (down).

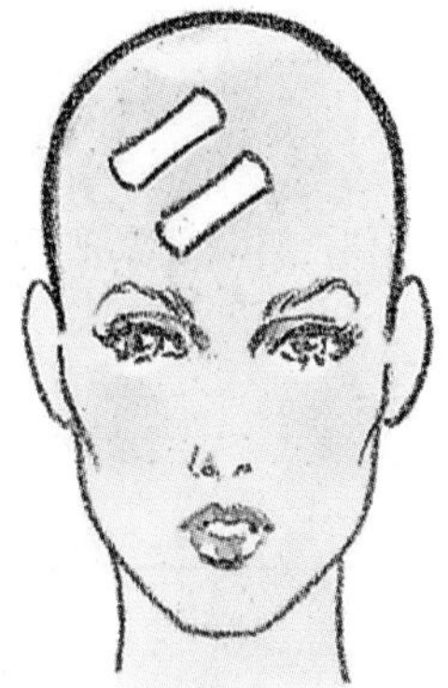

FIGURE 11.68 — Diagonal blocking (down).

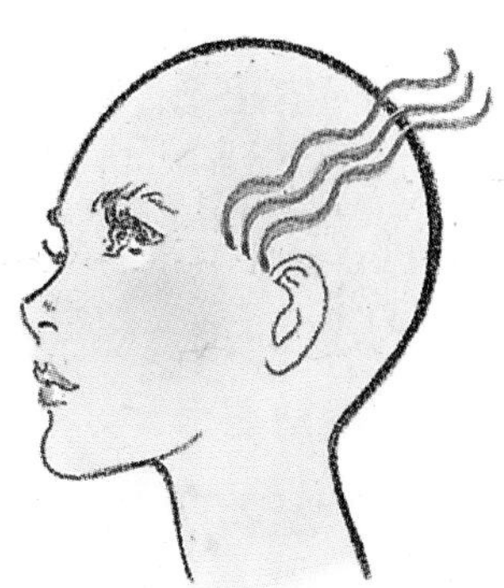

FIGURE 11.69 — Diagonal direction (up).

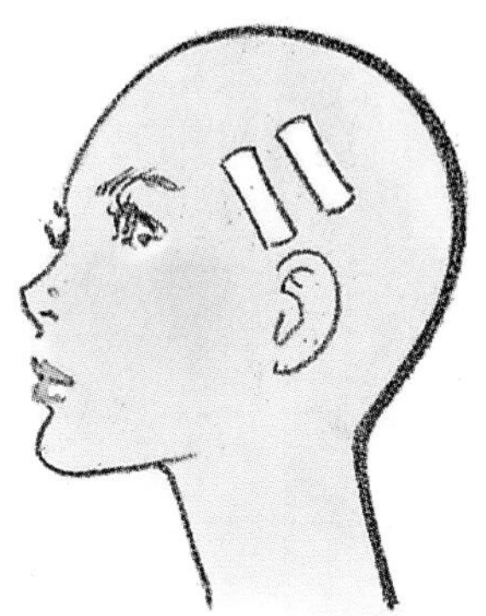

FIGURE 11.70 — Diagonal blocking (up).

By using a combination of these basic wrapping directions you will be able to create very specific designs. Directional wrapping allows for lamp or natural drying and easier styling, particularly for the client. Use the following method for directional wrapping:

1. While the hair is wet, comb it in the direction that you want in your final design, including a part if one is required.
2. Use your fingers and a comb to mold a wave pattern as if you were finger waving.
3. Wrap the hair based on the direction of the design pattern.

BODY WAVES

A body wave is a perm that gives support to a style, without definite curl. Large or extra large rods are used to give the hair softer, wider waves. Body waves are given when a softer curl or wave is desired. The wrapping patterns and techniques used for body waves are the same as those used for perming. Generally, the difference between perming and body waving is the size of rods. This affects the size of the final curl results.

The following are important considerations when giving a body wave:

1. Use large to extra large rods and make slightly larger partings. Do not take extra large partings or the waving lotion and neutralizer will not be able to penetrate all of the hair on the rod to properly form the curl/wave.
2. Follow perm directions regarding procedure, especially the processing time. Never reduce processing time to produce a softer curl/wave. Although the wave will be softer, it will be underprocessed and will not last very long.
3. Use straight rather than concave rods for body waving. The straight rods will give a more uniform wave from scalp to ends.

Note: *Body waves are softer and wider than regular perm curls because the physical force (hair wrapped around a very large rod) is not as great as in the standard perming method. The wave results from body waving will relax faster than a curl.*

PARTIAL PERMING

Perming only a section of a whole head of hair is called ***partial perming.*** Partial perming can be used on:

1. Clients (male and female) who have long hair on the top and crown and very short, tapered sides and nape.
2. Clients who need volume and lift only in certain areas.
3. Designs that require curl support in the nape area but a smooth, sleek surface.

Partial perming uses the same techniques and wrapping patterns that you have already learned. There are a few extra considerations:

1. When you are wrapping the hair and reach the area that will be left unpermed, go to the next larger rod size so that the curl pattern of the permed hair will blend into the unpermed hair.
2. After wrapping the area to be permed, place a coil of cotton around the wrapped rods as well as around the entire hairline.
3. Before applying the waving lotion, apply a heavy, creamy conditioner to the sections that *will not* be permed to protect this hair from the effects of the waving lotion (waving lotion softens and straightens unwrapped hair).

PERMS FOR MEN

Many of your male clients need the added texture and fullness that only a perm can give. A perm can also help overcome common hair problems. A perm can redirect a cowlick, help limp or unmanageable hair more easily maintain a style, and make sparse hair look fuller.

Perming techniques are basically the same for both men and women. Most often, the partial perm technique gives you and your male clients the best results.

Keep in mind that men want waves for control. (Figs. 11.71–11.73)

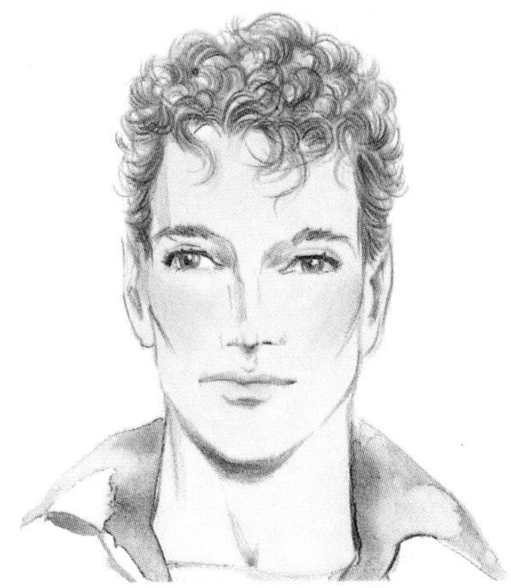

FIGURE 11.71 — Man's short, curly style.

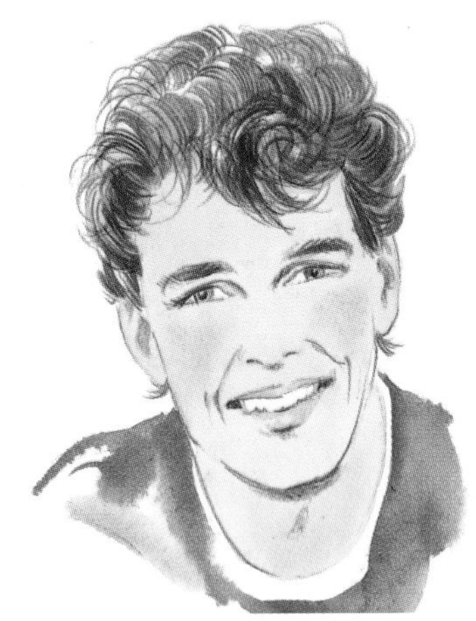

FIGURE 11.72 — Man's medium length style.

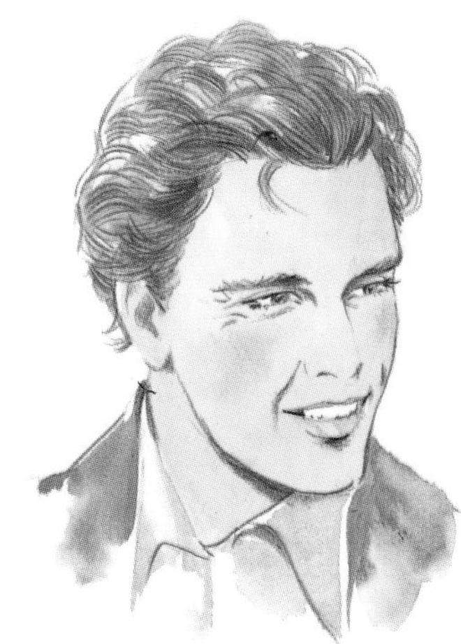

FIGURE 11.73 — Man's short, wavy style.

HEATED CLAMP METHOD

This technique of perming involves the use of heated clamps applied directly over each wound rod. After the hair is wound on rods and thoroughly saturated with the waving lotion, a preheated clamp is placed on each curl. Processing begins as soon as the heat is applied. After the hair has been processed for a predetermined period of time, the clamps are removed and the hair is rinsed and neutralized in the usual manner.

There are three special control features of the heated clamp method:

1. The temperature of the rods is strictly controlled.
2. The processing does not start until the heat is applied.
3. All curls are processed for exactly the same length of time.

SPECIAL SITUATIONS

There are certain hair types and conditions that require special attention. There also are hair types that should not be permed. If you have any doubt about perming the hair successfully, make a preliminary test curl.

1. Hair that shows signs of damage or breakage should not be permed. If the hair is excessively dry, brittle, or over-porous, it should be given reconditioning treatments until the condition improves and the damaged areas can be cut off. When you determine that the condition of the hair has improved, choose a mild perm formula and make a complete preliminary test curl before giving the perm.
2. Hair that has been previously treated with a sodium hydroxide or "no lye" relaxer (or any hair straightener that does not require a neutralizing step) should not be permed. Relaxers and perms break disulfide bonds in the hair structure. Since

the bonds are not all completely re-formed, the use of both products on the same hair can result in severe hair damage or breakage.

3. Tinted, bleached, highlighted/frosted, or previously permed hair in good condition can usually be permed successfully if the correct perm formula is chosen. Generally, these hair types vary in porosity so a product with a pre-wrap lotion to fill in porous areas is usually the best choice.

Note: *"Tinted hair" usually refers to hair that has been treated with a permanent hair color that is mixed with 20 volume peroxide. If the hair has been tinted with an ultralight shade or higher than 20 volume peroxide, it should be treated as bleached hair, which is usually more delicate and porous.*

4. Hair treated with a semi-permanent haircolor (color that is not mixed with peroxide/developer and therefore does not lighten the natural color) is frequently resistant to perming because semi-permanent color coats the surface of the hair and slows down penetration of the waving lotion. Hair treated with a semi-permanent color should be considered more resistant than tinted or color-treated (tint mixed with peroxide) hair. Perming can also cause discoloration of semi-permanent color. If you perm hair that has been treated with a semi-permanent color, it might be necessary to apply a temporary rinse after perming in order to even out the color. One week after perming you may reapply the semi-permanent color to achieve more acceptable and long-lasting color results.

5. Haircolor restorers or progressive haircolor darkeners contain metallic salts. These metallic salts form a residue on the hair, which interferes with the action of the waving lotion and can result in very uneven curls, severe discoloration, or hair damage.

To determine if hair has been treated with a haircolor restorer or darkener, a 1-20 test is recommended. In a glass bowl, mix 1 oz (30 ml) of 20 volume peroxide and 20 drops of 28% ammonia. Into this mixture immerse at least 20 strands of hair for 30 minutes.

- If there are no metallic salts present, the hair will lighten slightly. You can perm the hair.
- If hair strands lighten very rapidly, the hair contains lead. Do not perm.
- If there is no reaction after 30 minutes, the hair contains silver. Do not perm.

- If the solution begins to boil within a few minutes and a very unpleasant odor is evident, plus the hair pulls apart easily, then the hair contains copper. Do not perm.

Hair coated with metallic salts must not be permed. Do not perm until the product has been cut out of the hair. Rerun the 1-20 test to be sure that the hair is no longer coated with metallic salts before perming.

6. Unmanageable, naturally curly hair with an uneven curl pattern can be permed to form larger, more defined curls that are easier to manage. Generally, the procedure for a body wave (page 255–256) is the best approach. Keep in mind that naturally curly hair, even if it is coarse and dense, can be very porous, so choose the perm formula carefully.

7. Once the hair is permed, your client should return for another perm every 3 to 4 months depending on how quickly the hair grows, the type of curl given, and how frequently the hair is cut. Before re-perming, carefully analyze the hair again, and if necessary, use a pre-wrap lotion and/or a milder waving lotion formula. Note the product and procedure used and the results achieved on the client's record card. ✔

Completed:
Learning Objective
#7
PERMING TECHNIQUES

REVIEW QUESTIONS

PERMANENT WAVING

1. Why is permanent waving beneficial to the client?
2. What is spiral wrapping?
3. What is croquignole wrapping?
4. What is a cold wave?
5. What is the purpose of a) waving lotion, b) neutralizer?
6. Define an acid-balanced perm.
7. What is "stop-action" processing?
8. What is an alkaline perm?
9. What is the main active ingredient or "reducing agent" in an a) alkaline perm, b) acid-balanced perm?
10. Name the acid-balanced perm that is heat activated by a chemical within the product.
11. What is the main ingredient in neutralizers?
12. What are the two main actions in permanent waving?

13. Define the three major components of hair.
14. Hair is composed almost entirely of a protein material called ____________________.
15. What bonds must be broken in order for the perming process to occur?
16. How do you decide which perming technique is right for your client?
17. Why is pre-perm analysis important?
18. What is hair porosity?
19. What is a pre-wrap lotion?
20. What is hair texture?
21. What two factors determine processing time?
22. What is hair elasticity?
23. Define hair density.
24. What factor determines the size of a curl?
25. Name two types of permanent wave rods.
26. Name two factors that must be considered in choosing rod size.
27. Why is sectioning and blocking important in permanent waving?
28. Name two rules to follow when wrapping a perm rod.
29. How must the hair be wrapped on a perm rod?
30. What is the purpose of end wraps?
31. What are the three methods of end wrap application?
32. What is a test curl and how is it taken?

CHAPTER 12

Haircoloring

LEARNING OBJECTIVES

After completing this chapter, you should be able to:

1. Describe the correct procedure for a client consultation.
2. Explain the principles of color theory, and relate their importance to haircoloring.
3. List the classifications of haircolor, explain their activity on the hair, and give examples of their use.
4. Explain the activity of hydrogen peroxide in haircoloring.
5. Define single- and double-process applications.
6. Explain the types and uses of hair lighteners.
7. List preventative and corrective steps to avoid or solve haircoloring problems.
8. List the safety precautions to follow during haircolor procedures.

NATIONAL SKILL STANDARDS

This chapter provides you with the necessary information to master these National Industry Skill Standards for Entry-Level Cosmetologists:

- Consulting with clients to determine their needs and preferences
- Taking necessary steps to develop and retain clients
- Using a variety of salon products while providing client services
- Conducting services in a safe environment, taking measures to prevent the spread of infectious and contagious disease
- Managing product supply for salon use and retail sales
- Conducting a color service in accordance with a client's needs or expectations

INTRODUCTION

Cosmetology is a career that offers you the opportunity to develop your creative talents in many different ways. One of the most exciting and challenging areas of creativity in your career as a professional cosmetologist will be haircoloring and lightening.

Haircoloring is both the science and the art of changing the color of hair. Haircoloring includes the processes of:

1. Adding artificial pigment to the natural hair color.
2. Adding artificial pigment to previously colored hair.
3. Adding artificial pigment to prelightened hair.
4. Diffusing natural pigment and adding artificial pigment in one step.

(The terms *tinting* and *coloring* are used interchangeably in this text.)

Note: ***Haircolor*** *(one word) is an industry-coined term referring to artificial haircolor products and services.* ***Hair color*** *(two words) is the color of hair created by nature.*

Hair lightening, or ***decolorizing***, involves the diffusing of the natural or artificial color from the hair. Hair lightening involves the processes of:

1. Decolorizing the natural pigment to prepare the hair for the final color.
2. Decolorizing the natural or artificial pigment to the desired color.

These are profitable sources of salon income because coloring represents repeat business. The client who has tinted or lightened hair usually returns for retouching at regular intervals. Satisfactory service and trust in their colorist encourages clients to remain loyal to the same salon.

Your success as a colorist depends on the time and energy you are prepared to give to the continuous study and practice of your haircoloring skills. As you expand your skills and gain confidence you may choose to specialize in haircoloring services, just as professionals in other occupations develop one area of expertise.

Thanks to the styling revolution of the 1960s and 1970s, many stylists have mastered haircutting or perming and concentrate their energies solely on these frequently requested services. Add color to that great haircut and perfect texture, and you've got a powerful attention-getting combination. Specialist *haircolorists* are less common than cutters, and their skills are in increasingly high demand due to the renewed publicity and popularity of haircolor. Cosmetologists willing to develop their coloring skills and expertise can serve the needs of a huge and growing clientele.

REASONS CLIENTS COLOR THEIR HAIR

1. Unpigmented Hair (Graying)

- To camouflage unpigmented hair
- To keep and enhance their natural unpigmented hair

2. Self-Image Boost

- To promote a more desirable appearance

3. Experimental

- To subtly enhance their existing hair color
- To create a fashion statement or trend that expresses their personality

4. Artistic

- To accent their hairstyle design, making it look more finished
- To enhance or minimize their features, using color to create illusions

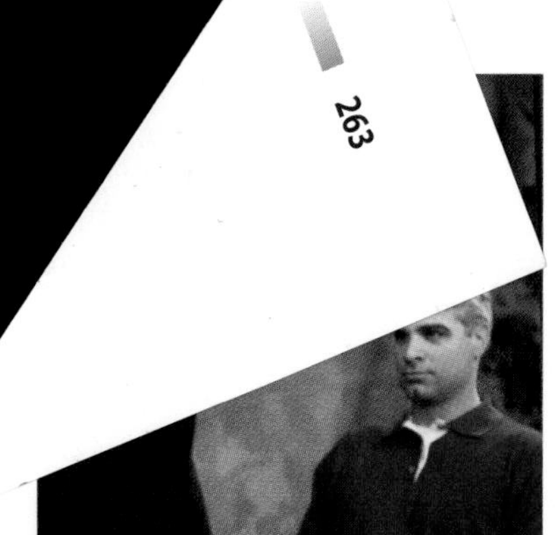

5. ***Corrective***

- To eliminate the damaged look of sun-lightened hair ends
- To remove the unsightly cast of chlorine or minerals caused by water
- To improve upon the results of previous color experimentation

Almost everyone at one time or another has considered doing something a little different with their hair. Potential clients may have already done some experimentation at home or in another salon by changing their haircut or style, their hair texture by perming, or their hair's natural color.

With the emergence and availability of nonprofessional products that your clients can buy, why should they come to you, a professional colorist, for advice and service? And who are the "typical" haircoloring clients today? (Figs. 12.1a, b)

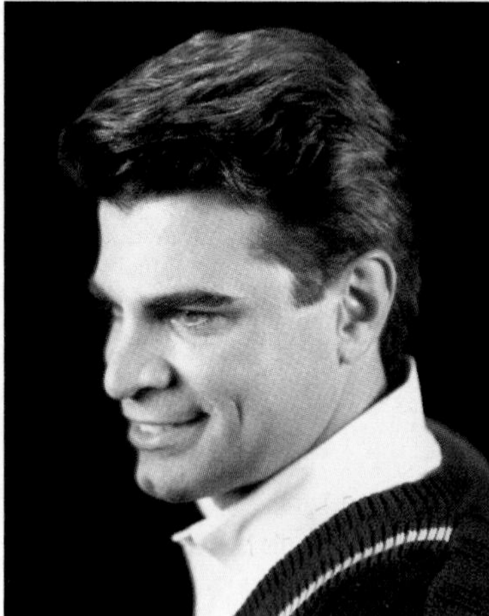

FIGURE 12.1a, b — There are many reasons clients choose to color their hair. To cover unpigmented hair is one.

TYPICAL CLIENTS

Haircoloring offers a wide variety of choices and therefore attracts the attention and interest of anyone who wants to look good and feel better. Gone are the stereotypes of the obviously tinted client: the damaged hair, the flat or unnatural appearance. Typical are those clients who want to cover or enhance their unpigmented hair; teens, women, and men who enjoy frequent fashion changes; clients currently unhappy with their natural color or who want to improve the shine and texture of their hair; and current haircoloring clients who come in for their retouch applications and a little relaxation time to themselves. Even the male clientele for haircolor is growing rapidly and is expected to be the fastest growing category of haircoloring client this decade. (Fig. 12.2)

As a trained professional haircolorist, you will have a thorough understanding of the hair structure and how haircoloring products affect it. You will have knowledge of which colors look best on your clients and which products and techniques will best achieve the desired look. You will have access to licensed-professional-only products that offer a wider range of color choices, better wearability, and greater flexibility. You will also be able to maintain the health of your clients' hair and update their appearance on a regular basis.

With continuously increasing technology and the latest advancements in haircolor education, haircolor manufacturers are moving to standardize terminology in order to simplify learning and provide greater assistance to colorists.

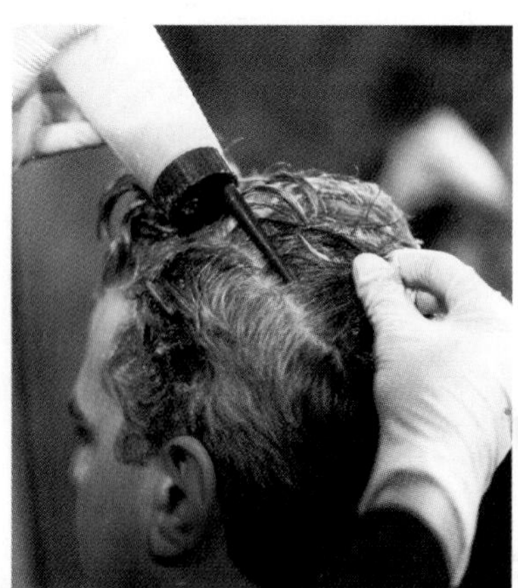

FIGURE 12.2 — Haircoloring is a popular service for male clientele today.

Note: *This chapter contains many technical terms. You should refer to the Haircoloring Glossary on pages 356–363, which was prepared by the International Haircolor Exchange to provide a standard vocabulary of haircoloring for our industry.*

NATURE'S COLOR

Natural hair color is either a dark color, a medium color, or a light color, but no two people have exactly the same hair color. Even an individual client's hair will vary from season to season and from year to year. In fact, the same head of hair will have different colors from top to bottom and front to back. That is why the same haircolor formula will produce a different result on different clients. (Fig. 12.3)

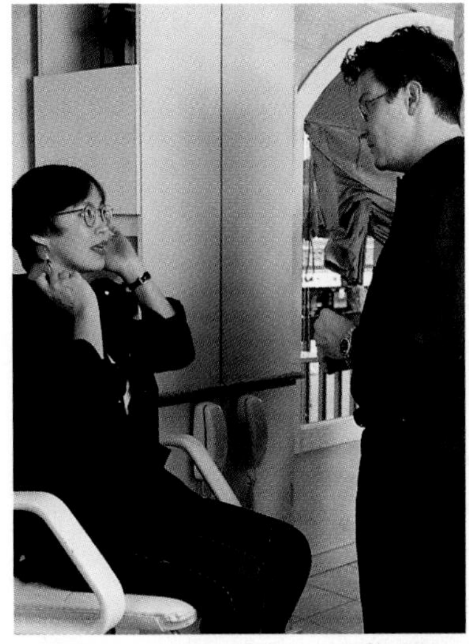

FIGURE 12.3 — It is important to analyze a client's hair before performing a haircolor service.

HOW HAIR STRUCTURE RELATES TO COLORING

Every haircolor service will affect—and be affected by—the structure of the hair. Some haircolor products cause a dramatic change in the hair's structure; others affect it very little. When a product significantly changes the hair structure, it usually creates a weaker strand of hair.

Knowing how products affect the structure will allow you to make choices. Your perceptions of what the hair can or cannot tolerate will allow you to be the best judge of what is most appropriate for each client.

As you learned in chapter 4, hair is composed of three parts: the medulla, the cortex, and the cuticle. The ***medulla*** is the innermost core of the hair shaft. The ***cortex*** is the middle layer. The natural color we see in the hair is in this layer. The cortex is made up of elongated, fibrous cells bundled together. Melanin pigment granules are scattered between the cortex cells, like the chips in a chocolate chip cookie. A healthy, intact cortex contributes to the elasticity and 80% of the overall strength of the hair. The ***cuticle*** is the outermost layer. It is made up of overlapping bands of keratinized protein that is very similar to the protein that makes up our fingernails. It is translucent, allowing diffused light to pass through. The cuticle protects the interior cortex layer. The shiny appearance of the hair depends on the cuticle layer being smooth and intact. A healthy cuticle contributes 20% of the overall strength of the hair.

Melanin

The color you see in a client's hair, skin, and eyes is the result of the body's ability to make pigment, which is called ***melanin***

(**MEL**-a-nin). The pigment molecule melanin is directly under the control of the DNA molecules of the cells. ***Pigment*** is any substance that imparts color to animal or vegetable tissues. It is the combination of pigments that determines the color you see and the underlying color as it fades or is lightened. To understand the underlying colors, let's look at the reaction from the beginning.

The chemical formation of melanin is initially formed by the reaction of naturally occurring yellow compounds called ***quinones*** (kwi-**NOHNZ**). These yellow quinones are produced from a colorless amino acid protein called ***tyrosine*** (**TYE**-ro-seen). The chemical chain of events that occurs in the transition of this colorless tyrosine into color pigment is complex but not beyond our comprehension.

First, the amino acid tyrosine is acted upon by the enzyme ***tyrosinase*** (**TYE**-ro-sin-ace), which is a copper-protein complex. Its function is to add oxygen to (oxidize) tyrosine, which yields a slightly different chemical substance called *dihydroxphenylalanine,* or *dopa.* Once dopa is formed, the enzyme tyrosinase continues oxidation and produces *dopa-quinone.* Dopa-quinone is a yellowish compound. As oxidation continues, a red, called *dopachrome,* is produced. As further oxidation occurs, a purple compound appears, called *indol-quinone.* This chemical substance proceeds through further oxidation to form larger molecules called *polymers.* Ultimately, these appear in the cell as brown and black granules, through attraction of protein in the form of particles called ***melanosomes*** (muh-**LAH**-no-sohmz).

These melanin granules are distributed by octopus-shaped cells called ***melanocytes*** (**MEL**-uh-no-sights). They are capable of dividing and producing. The color of the hair depends not so much on the number of melanocyte cells, but on the amount of melanin granules that the active melanocytes can reproduce and distribute. The more melanin granules in the melanosome, the darker the hair will appear.

Once you understand that all pigment is a series of oxidation reactions, you can apply that knowledge to the formulation of haircolor. The hardest part of haircolor and decolorization is knowing what the underlying pigment will be. Because the same process creates the coloring in the hair, skin, and eyes, you can use the eye color as an indication of the amount and tone of the underlying pigmentation of the hair. If the eye has warmth, you will usually see more red during decolorization. If the eye has a yellowish tone, there will usually be less red in the hair as it decolorizes. A cool tone in the eyes is a sign that there will be even less warmth in the hair as it lightens. Use this knowledge and the understanding of how pigment forms to assist you in anticipating the underlying tones in the hair that will appear when lightening the natural hair color.

ADDITIONAL STRUCTURAL FACTORS THAT INFLUENCE HAIR COLOR

Texture

Hair texture is described as the diameter of the individual hair strand. The terms ***coarse***, ***medium***, and ***fine*** are used to differentiate between large, medium, and small diameters. Texture has an effect on hair color because the hair's natural melanin pigment is distributed differently in the different textures. Each diameter also has a different resistance to the changes haircolor chemicals make on the hair shaft. (Fig. 12.4)

The pigment of fine-textured hair is grouped more tightly together. Because of this tighter grouping, when you deposit color, you will have a darker result on fine hair. By the same token, fine hair is less resistant to lightening, because there is less structure to resist the chemical. When lightening fine hair, a milder lightener can be used successfully.

Medium-textured hair will have average responses to haircolor products. Note any variations in texture throughout the hair. The face-line hair is usually finer in texture than the hair farther back on the head.

Coarse-textured hair has a more open grouping of hair pigment due to the larger diameter hair shaft in which the pigment is located. Because of this open grouping, you will have a slightly lighter result when depositing color. When lightening the hair, you will encounter greater resistance to the lightener, and a stronger lightening product may be needed.

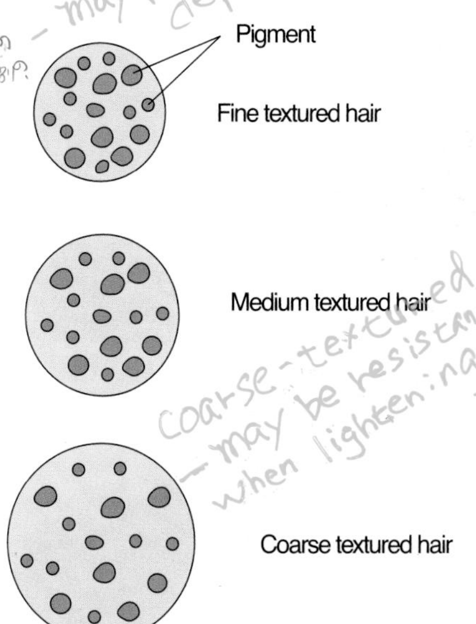

FIGURE 12.4 — The diameter of various hair strands. The fine strand appears darker because the pigment is more closely grouped together.

Porosity

Porosity is necessary for color to take properly. Each product we put on the hair requires a different degree of porosity. In simple terms, porosity is the ability of the hair to absorb moisture. Porous hair will accept liquid (haircolor, for example) more readily than nonporous hair. Uneven porosity can create problems if even color results are desired.

As hair grows longer, the ends are subject to frequent shampooing, drying, styling, and environmental influences. There will be visual and textural changes. The cuticle will be slightly abraded (worn away), and the rough hair fiber will lose some of its flexibility, body, and shine. There will also be some variation in color from strand to strand and even from the scalp area to the mid-shaft. Hair may be lighter and more faded out toward the ends.

This longer, older hair is described as ***overporous***, a condition in which hair reaches an undesirable level of porosity. This hair will respond differently to haircolor products than the newer hair closer to the scalp. Those different responses can only be determined by performing a strand test. As a general rule, overporous

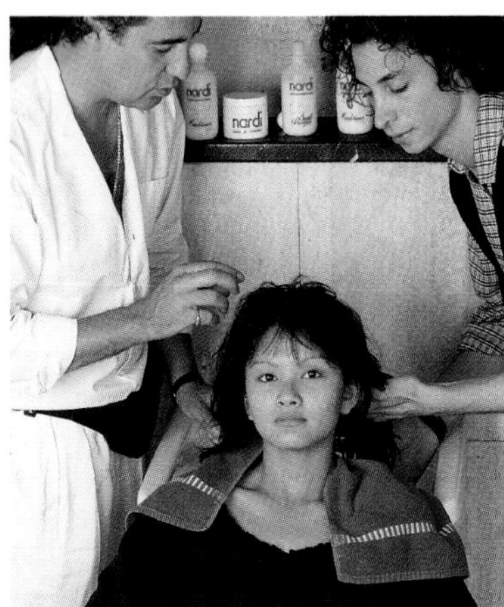

FIGURE 12.5 — Checking the porosity of hair before a coloring service is important.

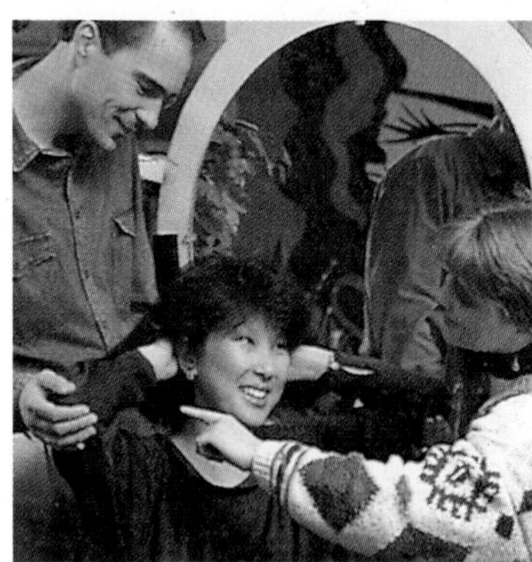

FIGURE 12.6 — Note variations in hair density prior to a haircoloring application.

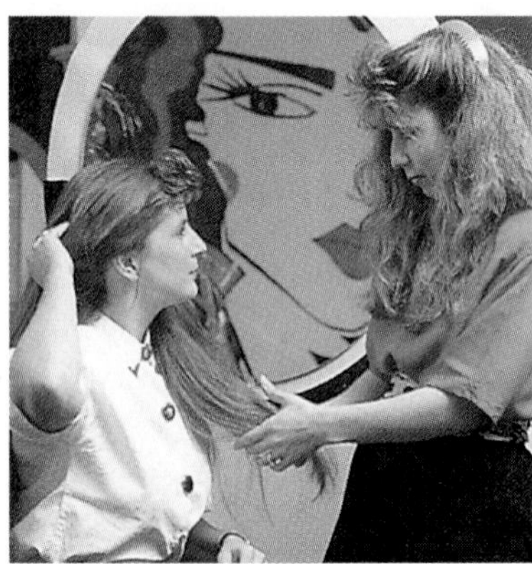

FIGURE 12.7 — Hair length will be a factor in your haircolor choice.

hair will look more dull or flat and reflect more cool tones, while the healthier hair will reflect more warm tones.

Occasionally, a client's hair has a cuticle so smooth and compact that we need to create the proper porosity for the success of our haircoloring service. This hair is considered ***resistant*** to the swelling effects of alkalies that allow haircolor to penetrate, and, if necessary, cover unpigmented hair. Presoftening of unpigmented or resistant hair will be covered later. (Fig. 12.5)

Density

Hair density is the number of hairs per square inch on the scalp. Hair can be described as sparsely, moderately, or thickly distributed on the head. It is important to notice that hair density varies, even on the same head. For some, the hair around the face line is more sparsely distributed, and the hair over the crown is more densely distributed. For others, the opposite is true.

Note the variations in density. The dense areas of your clients' hair will require more product and a more careful application. Remember, for haircolor to work effectively, each hair shaft must be surrounded by product. (Fig. 12.6)

Hair Length

Hair length will be a factor in your haircolor choice. The hair on our heads grows an average of ½" (1.25 cm) per month. This translates to 6" (15 cm) per year. If your client's hair is 12" (30 cm) long, the hair farthest away from the scalp is two years old.

Longer hair has been exposed to the elements for a longer period of time and is referred to as older hair. Older hair will vary in porosity throughout the length of the hair shaft. Unequal reactions to liquid and chemicals along the length of the hair shaft are due to variations in porosity. To observe variations in porosity, hold several strands of hair away from the scalp by their ends. Note any variations in color or surface texture. Older, more porous hair will appear lighter in color and rougher in texture.

Since the hair is of a greater length, more haircoloring product may be needed for the application. Preconditioning treatments may be necessary prior to a color application to help equalize porosity and provide the foundation for even color results. Many colorists charge for long hair accordingly, and may also prefer to use the brush-and-bowl application technique (painting the color on with a tint brush instead of using a bottle) to ensure even distribution of the haircolor product along the hair shaft. (Fig. 12.7)

Formation

The ***formation*** of the hair as it grows from the follicle is a genetic trait and is described as being straight, wavy, or curly. The smoother the hair form, the more light reflection. The curlier forms will reflect, or bounce back, light; hair colors may not reflect as strongly as on straighter hair forms. Careful color choice and application will create satisfactory color results on any hair texture. (Fig. 12.8)

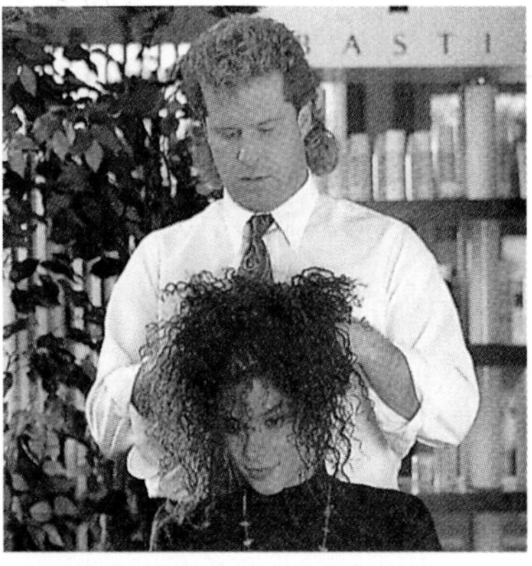

FIGURE 12.8 — Curlier hair may require a stronger tone.

IDENTIFYING THE CLIENT'S HAIR COLOR

There are three things you will need to determine about your client's natural hair color prior to formulating a haircolor to be applied. These three things will give you the information you need to anticipate the natural undertones that will appear from an oxidative haircolor service. They are: ***level***, ***tone***, and ***intensity*** of pigmentation. The level can be determined by comparing your client's existing hair color with a manufacturer's haircolor chart. The tone can be determined by looking at the skin and eye tones. The intensity of pigmentation can be identified by determining the client's natural hair color category. Each of these systems is described in detail in the following pages.

THE LEVEL SYSTEM

Whether it is natural or artificial pigment, when you are analyzing your client's color you must first identify the color level. A level is the degree of lightness or darkness of a particular color, excluding tone.

In haircoloring, cosmetologists and haircolor manufacturers use the ***Level System*** to analyze the lightness or darkness of a color. (Fig. 12.9) The materials you receive with your haircolor

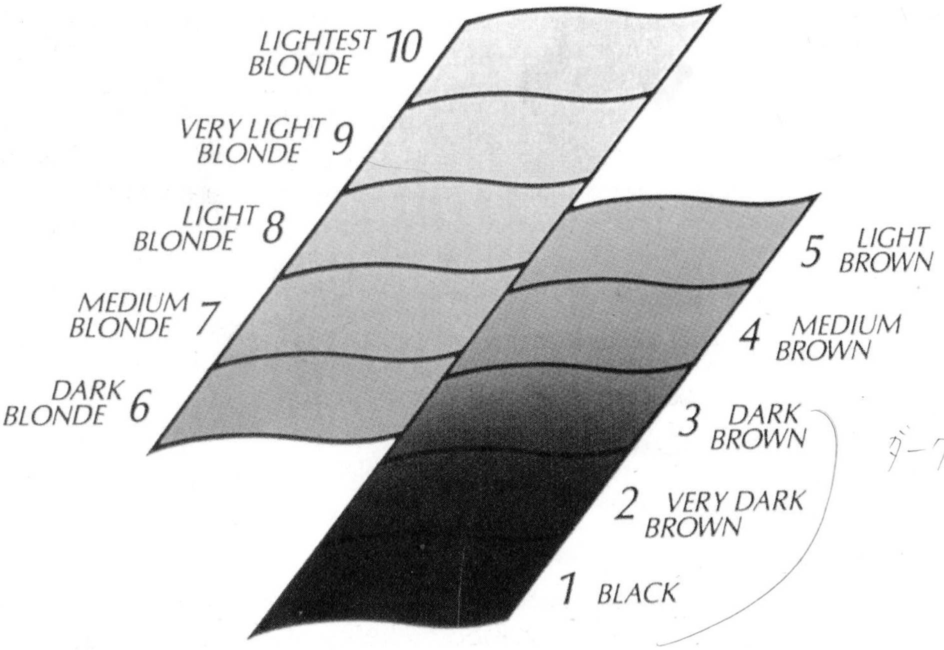

LIGHTEST BLONDE 10
VERY LIGHT BLONDE 9
LIGHT BLONDE 8
MEDIUM BLONDE 7
DARK BLONDE 6
5 LIGHT BROWN
4 MEDIUM BROWN
3 DARK BROWN
2 VERY DARK BROWN
1 BLACK

FIGURE 12.9 — Natural hair color levels.

products will describe that particular manufacturer's system. Generally, in the majority of product labeling systems, a scale of 1 to 10 is used to describe the lightness or darkness. Level 1 colors are darkest; level 10 colors are lightest. Some manufacturers use a level system starting with zero; others extend their levels up to 12. The scale works the same regardless of the starting and ending points: low numbers are darker; high numbers are lighter.

Haircolor manufacturers provide a chart depicting the colors in their product line and showing the level and tone of each. Natural hair colors can also be analyzed with this tool. By comparing the manufacturer's color chart with your client's hair, you can determine the hair color level and describe the lightness or darkness with a number from the level system.

To determine your client's natural hair color level, take a ½" (1.25 cm) square section of hair and hold it up and away from the scalp, allowing light to pass through. Take the manufacturer's level swatch and fan out the hair strands. Place it next to the hair closest to the scalp. Sometimes the hair will be a different level due to exposure to the elements or another chemical service. Be certain to identify the natural level at the base of the hair shaft, close to the scalp. Also identify the level or levels of the midshaft and ends so you can adjust your formula accordingly.

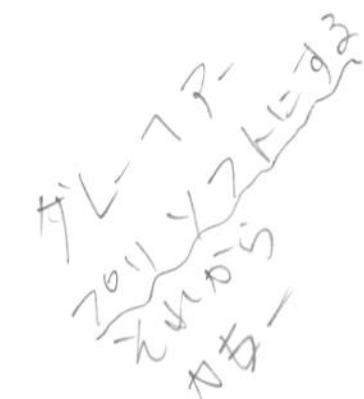

Do not part the hair and hold it flattened against the scalp; this will produce an incorrect reading, as the hair will appear darker without light. Hair that is wet or heavily soiled will also give a darker appearance.

Note: *The names for the natural hair color levels may vary from manufacturer to manufacturer. What is important is to identify the varying degrees of lightness to darkness that distinguish each level. Use the selected manufacturer's color chart as your guide in identifying your client's natural color level.*

The natural hair color levels are:

1. black
2. very dark brown
3. dark brown
4. medium brown
5. light brown
6. dark blonde
7. medium blonde
8. light blonde

9. very light blonde
10. lightest blonde

Levels 1, 2, and 3 are considered dark hair. People with dark hair comprise 75% of the population. Generally, people with dark hair want their hair to stay dark. This is usually the best choice, because their skin and eye color are also strongly pigmented. The dark hair color in combination with richly toned skin and eye color creates an intense and exotic combination.

Levels 4, 5, and 6 are the medium levels. People with medium hair comprise 15% of the population. You will note the client's pigmentation in skin and eye color is also in the medium range. There are certainly more options for someone with a medium-level hair color. Generally, you will select colors with richness or vibrancy for this client.

Levels 7 and 8 are the light levels. Again you will observe corresponding skin and eye pigmentation in this light range. People with a light color level comprise 9% of the population. Clients with light hair generally have the most options regarding their color choices. Darker or lighter hair works well.

Levels 9 and 10 are the very light levels. We don't see many of these people as clients. Their hair color is generally pleasing until it becomes unpigmented. (We will discuss unpigmented hair later in the chapter.)

TONE

The term ***tone*** is used to describe the warmth or coolness of a color. The manufacturer's color chart you used earlier to determine color level also describes hair tones.

The ***warm tones*** are red, orange, and yellow, although some haircolor labels use different names like auburn, copper, gold, or bronze. The ***cool tones*** are blue, green, and violet, often listed on labels as ash, drab, platinum, or smoky. Those words conjure up visual pictures of the properties or characteristics of the color tone.

Analyzing Eye Color

The color of clients' eyes can be a clue to what their haircolor tone could be. Eyes are rarely one color. Usually they are combinations of two or even three colors. Basically there are brown, blue, and green eyes. Look more closely. Brown eyes with olive green, reddish brown, or gold flecks are quite common. Blue eyes may have flecks of white, gold, or gray. Green eyes can range from gray-green to hazel (with brownish overtones) to yellow-green.

We can categorize eye color as warm or cool. ***Warm eye colors*** contain red, orange, yellow, or gold flecks through the iris of brown, blue, or green. Warm eye colors are:

- Brown with red, orange, yellow, or gold
- Blue with yellow or gold
- Green with reddish brown, orange, yellow, or gold

People who have warm eye colors can wear warm-toned haircolors.

Cool eye colors contain black, gray-brown, gray-green, blue, violet, gray, or white flecks through the iris of brown, blue, or green. Cool eye colors are:

- Brown with black, gray-brown, gray-green, or gray
- Blue with white, blue, gray, or violet
- Green with blue or gray

People with cool eye colors look most attractive in cool or neutral-toned haircolors.

The ***depth*** of eye color is another factor in your color choice. Lighter eyes reflect a lighter pigmentation throughout the client's coloring. A lighter-intensity color choice would be indicated. Medium eyes reflect stronger pigmentation, and more intense color options are available. Dark eyes reflect the strongest pigmentation; a deeper color choice is advisable. To choose a color that will harmonize with the client's natural pigmentation, include the depth of eye color (light, medium, or dark) in your color equation.

Note: *Many clients choose colored contact lenses to enhance their appearance. This can affect your color choice. If you are not certain of the client's natural eye color, always ask.*

Skin Tone

Skin tone can be broken down into four simple categories: olive, red, golden, and neutral. It is easiest to observe the natural skin tone by looking at the skin on the neck, close to the clavicle. Facial and arm skin is often affected by sun exposure, which masks the skin tone.

Olive skin tones have an underlying tone of gray, green, or yellow. Olive-toned clients look best in cool or neutral colors. If a warm shade is desired, it should be in a darker level.

Red skin tones have an underlying tone of red-brown, red, or blue-red. Red-toned clients look best in cool or neutral colors. Warm colors are not recommended for these clients.

Golden skin tones have an underlying tone of golden brown, gold, or peach. Golden skin tones look best in warm colors. The level chosen would be affected by the client's natural level.

Neutral skin tones are a balance of warm and cool. Neutral skin can have an underlying tone of pink and yellow in combination. You will not observe one predominant underlying skin tone. Generally, these skin tones are described as ivory, beige, or brown skin. Neutral skin tones look well in either warm or cool colors.

How does this information indicate a color choice? The chart on page [276] will help you in your selection. Remember that each person is unique, however, and consult with your instructor. Gradually, as your skill develops, you will see these items automatically. (Fig. 12.10)

INTENSITY

Intensity refers to the strength of the tonality in a color. Intensity is described as mild, medium, or strong.

Determining Natural Tone and Intensity

Each person is born with a particular combination of natural pigment. There is harmony between the hair, eye, and skin tones. At the point clients come to you for color service, their hair has changed dramatically from that original birth color. By knowing what color their hair was when they were children, you will be able to anticipate the changes the hair will undergo during treatment with an oxidative haircolor product and the intensity of pigmentation with which you will be dealing.

NATURAL HAIR COLOR CATEGORIES

One method of organizing hair colors is called ***Natural Hair Color Categories***. These categories combine intensity of tone with level to assist in reliably predicting and understanding haircolor interactions with natural color. Let us explore each natural hair color category and the changes as the hair starts to become unpigmented.

YOUR NATURAL EYE COLORS

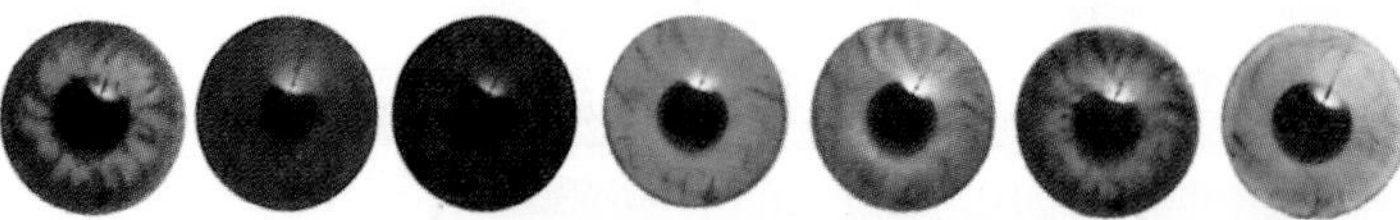

YOUR NATURAL HAIR COLORS AND MOST FLATTERING TINTS

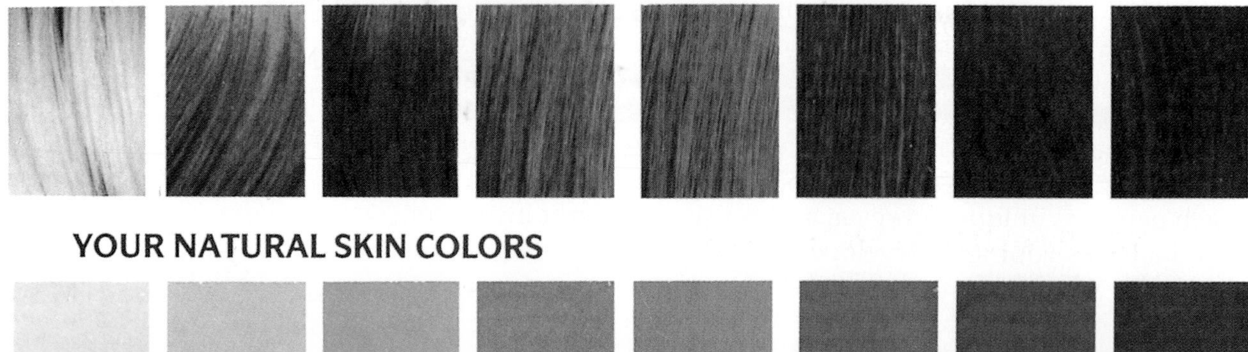

YOUR NATURAL SKIN COLORS

MAKEUP AND WARDROBE COLORS FOR PERSONS IN COLOR KEY 1

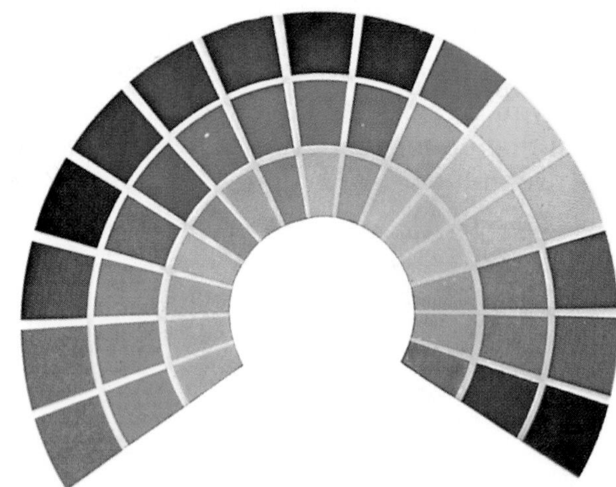

The purpose of this chart is to help you select your client's best colors for makeup, haircolor, and wardrobe; colors that will harmonize with their complexion tones. In Color Key 1, blue pigmentation predominates the undertones of the skin. When selecting a person's Color Key, the natural eye colors in the chart will be helpful in determining their correct Color Key. Light-skinned people who have a blue-pink undertone to their complexions, therefore, fall into Color Key 1. Some people in Color Key 1 have an olive undertone. Dark-skinned people in Color Key 1 may have a charcoal or occasionally an ashen gray hue to their dark complexions. If you determine that a client's personal coloring is in Color Key 1, always choose colors from the Color Key 1 selection.

FIGURE 12.10 — The Color Key System.

YOUR NATURAL EYE COLORS

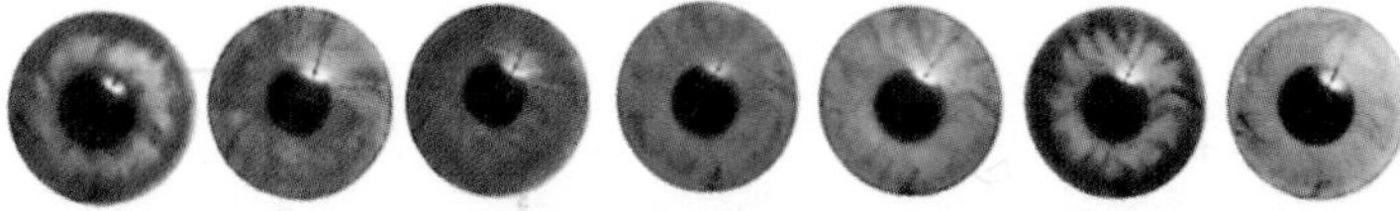

YOUR NATURAL HAIR COLORS AND MOST FLATTERING TINTS

YOUR NATURAL SKIN COLORS

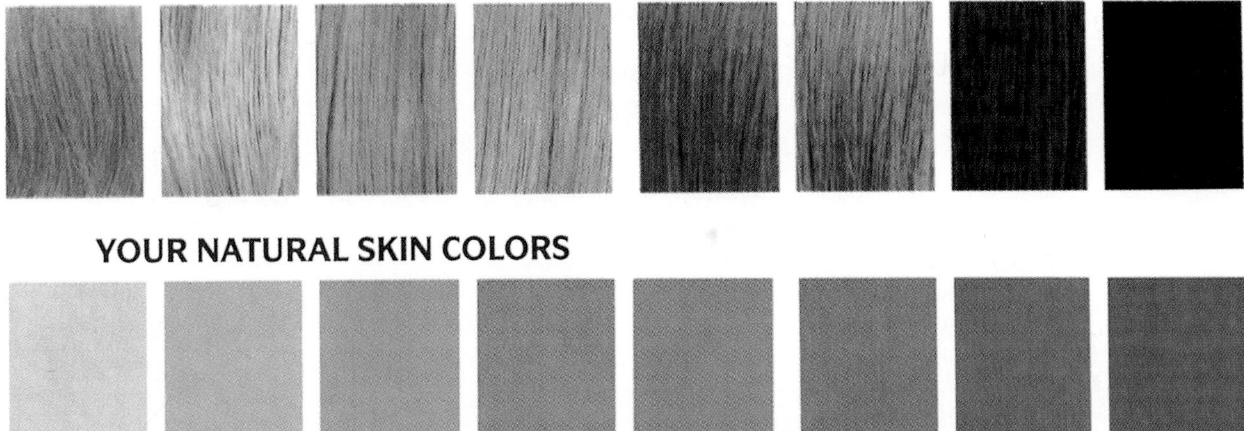

MAKEUP AND WARDROBE COLORS FOR PERSONS IN COLOR KEY 2

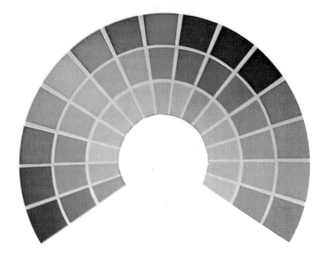

The purpose of this chart is to help you select your client's best colors for makeup, haircolor, and wardrobe; colors that will harmonize with their complexion tones. In Color Key 2, yellow pigmentation predominates. Light-skinned people with a peach-pink undertone to their complexion will, therefore, fall into Color Key 2. Dark-skinned people in Color Key 2 have a golden undertone. If you determine that a client's personal coloring is in Color Key 2, always choose colors from the Color Key 2 selection.

FIGURE 12.10 — The Color Key System (continued).

HAIRCOLOR SELECTION CHART

Natural Level	1 2 3	4 5 6	7 8	9 10
Category	"B" Dark Brown and Black	"W" Warm Brown "R" Red	"S" Light Brown	
Suggested Levels	Dark Hair	Medium Hair	Light Hair	Very Light Hair
	Recommendation: Stay close to natural level.	Recommendation: Use rich or vibrant colors.	Recommendation: A wide range of possibilities. Lighter or darker options.	Generally, you will not see as clients.
Eye Color	Cool		Warm	
	Brown with black-gray, brown-gray, green-gray. Blue with blue-gray, violet. Green with blue-gray.		Brown with red, orange, yellow-gold. Blue with yellow-gold. Green with reddish brown, orange, yellow-gold.	
Haircolor Option	Neutral Color Choice		Warm or Neutral Color Choice	
Skin Tone	Red Red-brown, red-blue, red underlying tone.	Olive Gray, green, yellow underlying tone.	Golden Golden brown, gold, peach underlying tone.	Neutral Brown, beige, ivory, pink, and yellow combined. The underlying tone is a balance of warm/cool.
Haircolor Option	Cool or Neutral	Warm or Neutral	Warm	Cool or Warm

The B Category

The B Category, black and dark brown, has strong intensity of pigmentation. People born with black or dark brown hair are in the B category. Levels 1, 2, and sometimes 3 are in this category. They may have some reddish highlights; their hair darkens with age until it turns unpigmented.

The hair is generally on the cool side, so there are no major changes in the natural hair color as the hair becomes unpigmented. The haircolorist must determine when the client can no longer color the unpigmented hair dark to match the natural hair color. At this point, the haircolorist must lighten the hair and at the same time minimize the red/orange tones that are generally unflattering to clients in this category. The red tones that this category can wear most successfully are the darker red or cool red tones.

Hair in the B category will decolorize through as many as 10 different stages. Each of the stages is warm in tone. If warm tones are desired, they exist in the hair and can be enhanced. If warm tones are not desired, caution must be exercised to avoid their appearance. An oxidative haircolor will almost always produce a warm result or fade to a warm tone. A deposit-only or semi-permanent product would be a better choice. A light, cool result would require double-process lightening followed by a cool-toned tint or toner.

The W Category

The **W Category, warm brown,** has medium intensity of pigmentation. People born with blonde hair that gradually darkens before adolescence are in the W category. Even before the hair begins to become unpigmented, the natural hair color loses its warmth and starts to appear dull. It is important to be aware that the undertones that were present prior to the hair becoming unpigmented are still there. These clients can generally wear red tones very well and often will request them. These clients also wear highlights very well.

An oxidative haircolor would lighten the hair nicely, but it would always retain some warm tones. To achieve a cool color result, you would have to use a double-process lightening product.

The S Category

The **S Category, light brown,** has mild intensity of pigmentation. People born with blonde hair that remains blonde through adolescence are in the S category. Their hair gradually darkens later in their teens to a soft brown color.

The light brown category is usually level 5 or 6. The natural hair is light and does not make for an attractive contrast when the hair color begins to become unpigmented. The color usually takes on a drab, dreary look. This category does not have the red/orange undertones that the B and W categories do. Remember, these clients were blonde when in high school, so they would generally not be averse to once again being blonde.

Clients in the S category generally can achieve attractive blonde colors with the light blonde shades of oxidative tints. Pale cool colors would probably require prelightening.

The R Category

The **R Category, red,** has medium intensity of pigmentation and usually falls in the levels 5, 6, and 7. People born with red hair that remains red throughout adolescence are in the R category. Their hair gradually darkens or loses warmth with age. The red category sometimes does not become unpigmented gracefully; once-vibrant red hair can become a muddy red color. Many times the changes happen so gradually that clients may not realize that their hair is losing its glow.

Knowing the Natural Color Category in addition to identifying the level will assist you in recommending the proper haircolor

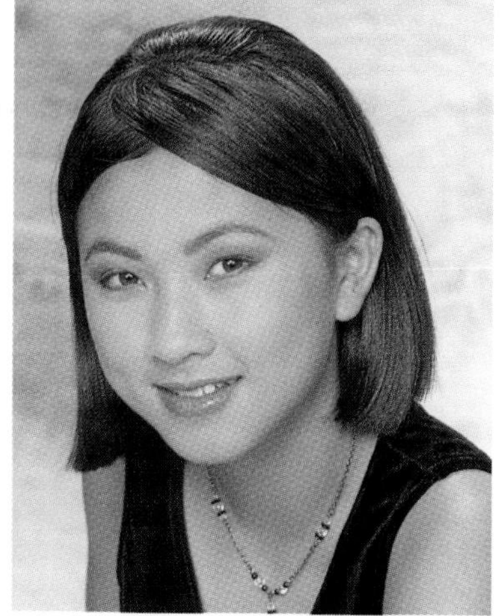

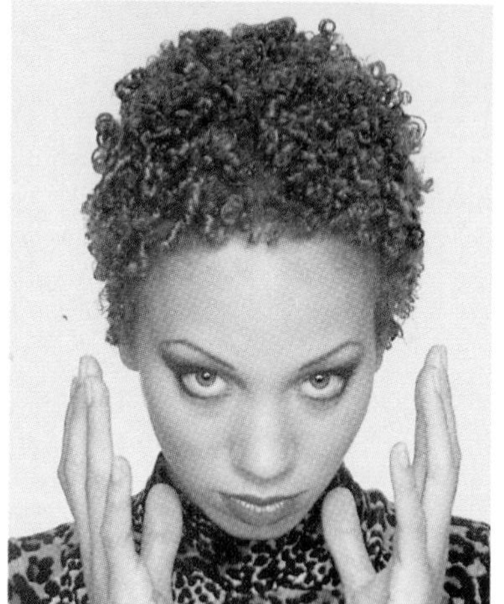

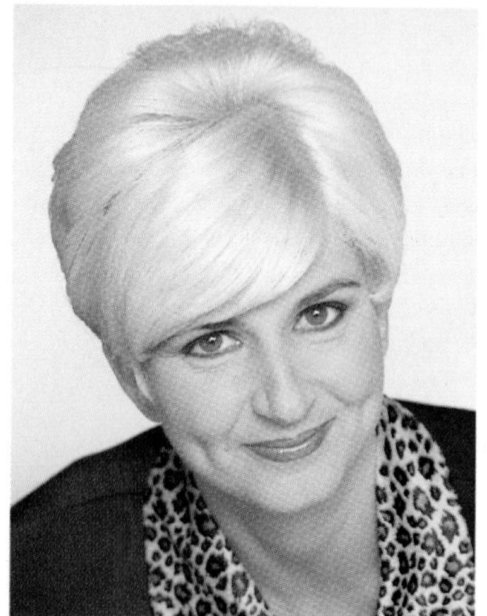

FIGURE 12.11a, b, c — Achieving natural haircolors with the Level System. *(Courtesy of Fantastic Sams, Brian and Sandra Smith, and Saverio for Julian Hans Salon)*

service to accomplish the desired end result, and the haircolor formula that is best suited for your client. (Figs. 12.11a–c)

ENHANCING THE CLIENT'S NATURAL COLORING

The key to maintaining harmony is creating a balanced relationship which is a pleasing visual blend between hair, skin, and eye colors. Natural harmony can be achieved by recreating the relationship between hair, skin, and eye colors that nature created, although the colors may be lighter than the original.

Consider how tones change with maturity. Many clients initially want to return to the color of their youth. They do not realize that the pigment of their skin is aging in a process similar to that of the hair. To tint the hair back to the natural color of their youth creates a severe contrast that can be harsh. Generally, a color of a similar tone but lighter level will be more flattering.

There will always be clients who break these rules. Many do so with great success. Attractiveness is a quality that incorporates esthetics and the laws of art and balance, along with the client's personality and self-expression.

CREATING NATURAL HAIR COLORS USING ARTIFICIAL PIGMENTS

Most hair colors represent a balance of colors, which means that they generally contain a balance of each of the primary colors. However, colors will have a predominant base and a level of lightness or darkness that must be identified before formulating a tint for the hair.

Oxidation tints are identified by the predominant base tone and the level of color formulated by the manufacturer. Most manufacturers provide literature that identifies the level and base tone for you. You may identify the level and base tone of the client's hair by comparing it to the manufacturer's color identification chart (as a guide, not an absolute). Determining the tone in the eyes and skin will help you identify your client's natural base tone. The Natural Category will indicate the intensity of pigmentation.

All colors—warm, cool, or neutral—can be formulated in tones that range from the lightest blonde to the darkest black, using the basic theory related to the Law of Color.

USING LEVEL, TONE, AND INTENSITY IN SELECTING A COLOR

When you have decided on the haircoloring products to use, you will next find the correct level, tone, and intensity to achieve your desired result. In many manufacturer's product lines, you will find more than one color tone at each level. Each of these shades will create a different tonality. Choose the one closest to what you need to achieve the desired result. To give the new haircolor the exact tonality and intensity desired, the basic shade can be adjusted or modified by adding a small quantity (¼ to ½ ounce) of a cooler or warmer shade on the same level, or by using an accent additive (usually added drop by drop) to enrich or drab the final formula.

THE FOUR RULES FOR NATURAL-LOOKING HAIRCOLOR

In order to more easily mimic the characteristics of virgin hair color, consider the following in determining your choice of color and application technique:

1. The hair should be lighter on the ends than at the base of the hair shaft.
2. The hair should be lighter on the surface than underneath.
3. Face-line hair should be lighter than the hair behind it (crown and nape).
4. The darker hair should always be the dominant color; for example, in reverse highlighting, always have more dark hair than light on the head.

PERCENTAGE AND DISTRIBUTION OF UNPIGMENTED HAIR

The changeover from natural to unpigmented hair is a gradual one. ***Unpigmented hair*** is primarily associated with aging and heredity. Even though the loss of pigment progresses in most people throughout their lives, few become completely white. Most retain a certain percentage of pigmented hair. It can be solid or blended throughout the head, as in salt-and-pepper hair. This blending creates different shades of unpigmented hair, depending on the ratio of pigmented to nonpigmented hair. Both unpigmented and white hair contain little melanin within the cortex.

Unpigmented hair can be a curse or a blessing. It is certainly most often the catalyst that convinces clients to color their hair, which is a blessing to colorists. On the other hand, unpigmented hair can also complicate the haircolor service because it does not respond to haircoloring the same as the naturally pigmented hair. Unpigmented hair tends to be coarser, less elastic, and occasionally curlier than the other hair on the head. It also becomes more resistant to chemical services, and thus requires special consideration in haircoloring practice.

Another consideration when formulating for unpigmented hair is recognizing the natural hair color that has not yet become unpigmented. Most people retain some dark hair as their hair becomes unpigmented. The pigmented hair must be analyzed for level and tone.

Be careful not to allow the reflection of the unpigmented hair next to the pigmented hair to affect your judgment. In many instances, this will cause even the most experienced colorist to identify the naturally pigmented hair as lighter than it really is. By misjudging the depth of the natural level, you may not compensate adequately for the undertones present in the hair, which will create a warmer-than-expected end result when you begin to lift the natural hair color. Using the Natural Hair Color Categories will assist you in properly identifying the pigmented hair.

It is first necessary to determine the amount of unpigmented hair (the actual percentage) on the head. Then you must determine the distribution of those unpigmented hairs (where they are located on the head). A person who is 50% unpigmented could have their unpigmented hair sprinkled equally throughout the head or located only in the front portion of the head. Each of these requires a different approach to formulating. Therefore, we must identify and note these factors regarding unpigmented hair on the client's record card.

DETERMINING THE PERCENTAGE OF UNPIGMENTED HAIR

Percentage of Unpigmented Hair	Characteristics
10%-30%	Mostly pigmented; difficult to see; generally most heavily located in temples and sides with some blending of colors throughout the head.
30%-50%	More pigmented than unpigmented; easy to see in dark colors but may blend in with lighter natural hair.
50%-70%	More unpigmented than pigmented; unnecessary to study hair to see unpigmented hair.
70%-90%	Mostly unpigmented hair; generally, majority of remaining pigmented hair is located in back with rest blended over head.
90%-100%	Virtually no pigmented hair; tends to look white.

THE COLORIST'S ROLE IN CLIENT COMMUNICATION

The ***consultation*** is of primary importance in the haircoloring service. Your consultation creates the foundation for the service that follows. But first there are other important elements to consider that will allow you to "set the stage" for your consultation success.

SETTING THE STAGE: THE PROPER ENVIRONMENT

Adequate Lighting

Light, and how it plays with haircolor, is of prime importance to the haircolorist. Bright natural light makes haircolor appear different than does dim light. Electric lights of varying intensities and hues also alter the eye's perception of color.

Perform the consultation in a well-lighted room, preferably with natural lighting. If this is not possible, arrange lighting so that there is incandescent in front of clients (around the mirror) and fluorescent behind the colorist (ceiling fixtures).

Incandescent lighting alone will make the hair and skin tones appear warmer than they truly are; fluorescent lighting alone has a cool cast and will give the skin and hair a pale, unnatural, cool appearance. Always remember to consider the lighting in which your clients will most often see themselves; a beautifully subtle highlight in natural sunlight may disappear under office lighting. Conversely, a strong, attractive color in your salon lighting could become neon looking in the sunlight.

For the best mix of lighting for haircoloring, use full-spectrum white fluorescent tubes or consider adding track lighting spotlights (incandescent) to the existing fluorescent lighting found in most buildings.

Consultation Area

Privacy and good lighting are important. Ideally, a separate room (or area) in the salon should be reserved specifically for consultations. If possible, the walls should be white or neutral, and neutral draping should be used to conceal the clients' street clothes, especially if they are strong colors that may influence your perception of the clients' hair and skin tonality. This would also be an excellent time for clients to put on chemical smocks to protect their clothes from stains.

GATHERING AND UTILIZING COLOR CONSULTATION TOOLS

In your consultation room or area, you will keep all of your professional haircoloring consultation tools—items that will make communication with your clients go smoothly. Keep a haircolor portfolio of your work or magazines and picture books with different haircolor levels, tones, intensities, and application techniques, so clients can show you the general hair color they have in mind. Photographs or paper reproductions do not exactly match haircolors but can be used as a guide.

Manufacturers' paper color charts and haircolor swatches, although showing color on white paper or on white hair, will at least give you an idea of clients' wishes. After all, your idea of red and a client's idea of red may be different—as different as strawberry blonde and burgundy. Manufacturers also make available to colorists their natural level haircolor swatches, in order to help you judge the natural hair color depth or level based on their color product's system. (Fig. 12.12)

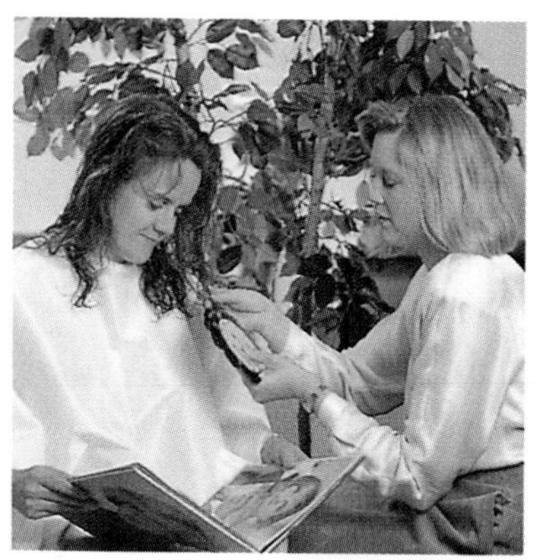

FIGURE 12.12 — Use style books and color charts and swatches when consulting with a client on a haircolor service.

A CONSULTATION, STEP BY STEP

Observe

Simple observation and listening give you a chance to use your training and analyze clients' needs. Your eyes and ears are your primary information-gathering tools. The following is a list of factors about hair that influence color choice. With time and practice, you will notice certain physical characteristics relevant to haircolor selection immediately upon seeing a client for the first time. These are items you will need to note when observing clients prior to a haircoloring service:

- Color level (natural category)
- Color tone
- Eye color
- Skin tone
- Length
- Porosity
- Density
- Texture
- Form
- Percentage of unpigmented hair

The consultation is a time when your greeting and appearance are most important. The greeting establishes your credibility and trustworthiness. Your professional appearance, confident mannerisms, and use of professional industry terminology will establish you as an authority in a client's eyes.

You have only one chance to make a first impression on your clients so make it a good one. You, and you alone, are responsible for the image you project. Make sure your clients and potential clients see you as you want them to. Establish and maintain eye contact, make clients comfortable, and listen.

Listen

Listening allows you to find out how clients view their needs. An important skill to practice is ***reflective listening***. This technique is accomplished by listening to your client and repeating back to him/her what he or she has said. For example: Mrs. Jones describes a hair color in the following manner: "I would like my hair to be lighter." You respond, "Lighter?" She says, "Yes, you know, with little golden streaks around my face." To which you reply, "Oh, you would like a few golden highlights around your face." She then replies, "Yes, a few highlights."

Her first direction was to make her hair lighter. That could have been a number of services: double- or single-process application or, as it turned out, a few highlights. If you proceed without clarification, you may not know what your client needs or wants. The reflective listening technique will support thorough communication. Practice this technique with your classmates in consultation role playing until you feel comfortable and reflective listening becomes a natural part of your behavior.

All clients expect to be treated with courtesy and attention. Reflective listening will show the client you are listening and wish to fully understand their wishes. This respect, courtesy, and attention will win their confidence. And, when a cosmetologist sincerely recommends a haircolor service, after a through consultation, clients are likely to listen carefully and seriously consider the recommendation.

Discuss Client's Expectations and Hair Limitations

Does your client want a temporary change or a more permanent one? Does your client want something close to the current color or a dramatic color change? Based on your thorough analysis, you can choose the proper product and technique that will fulfill the client's expectations, but also respect the hair's limitations.

Be realistic in discussing color selection with your client. It is best to select a general range of color lightness and tone, rather than to promise an exact shade. Some clients will be able to change their color in one process, creating the right level and tone at the same time. Other clients will need two separate products and processes to create the same effect. Be sure to consider carefully all the factors that will influence your client's decisions.

Consider the Client's Lifestyle

A few key questions will assist you in guiding your client toward a color service that will be pleasing and practical.

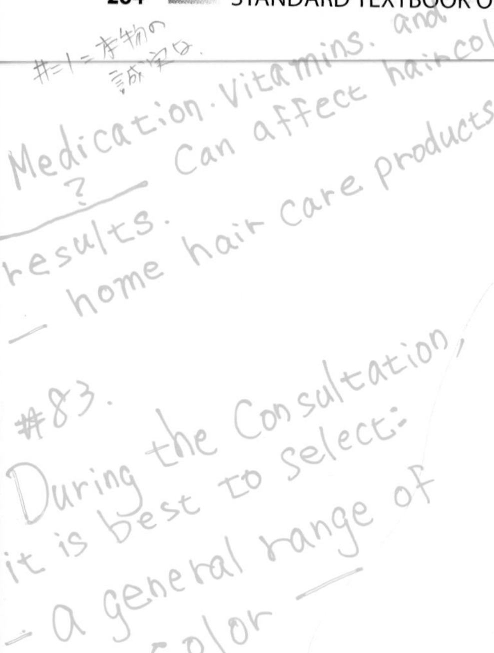

- Do you see yourself as conservative or dramatic?
- Do you work in a professional arena?
- What is your personal grooming budget?
- How much time are you willing to allow for haircolor maintenance?
- Is there someone in your life who will affect your decision-making process?

The answers to these questions will assist you in advising your client on a haircolor choice that will be practical to maintain considering the factors of his/her life.

Medicines can affect haircolor results. Sulfur-based drugs can add warmth to light blonde colors. High doses of vitamins and minerals can darken the natural hair color level. Always ask your clients and note any medications they are taking on the record card.

Home care products are of great importance for haircolor clients. A shampoo for controlling dandruff or psoriasis will change your color result. Rapid fading can occur because of highly alkaline, nonprofessional products. Some mousses, conditioners, and hair sprays can build up and coat the hair shaft. This will alter the porosity of hair, causing uneven color results. Always ask your clients about the products they use at home.

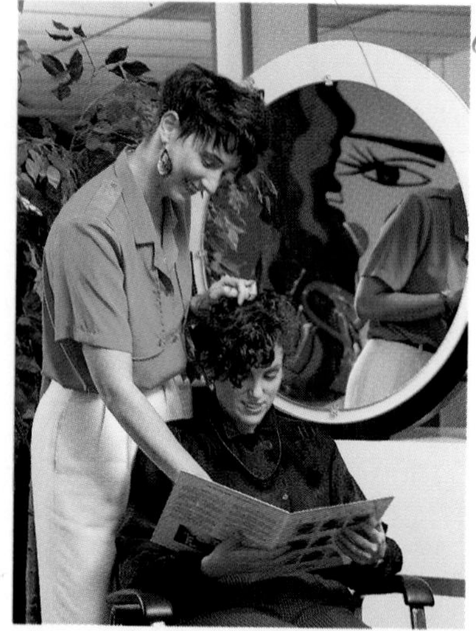

FIGURE 12.13 — Good communication is essential when discussing haircoloring service with a client.

Make Suggestions

To recommend a haircolor service with sincerity means to suggest a color only when you honestly believe that your clients would be happier and more attractive with the color service. You must be attentive to your clients' needs by listening closely, by being genuinely interested, and by treating every client as you would like to be treated yourself in the same situation. In doing so, you can be confident that your choice will reflect and meet your clients' needs, improve your clients' appearance, and enhance your reputation as a colorist. (Fig. 12.13)

Basic Rules for Color Selection

1. Make sure the client's hair is clean and dry.
2. Determine the Natural Category by asking what color the client's hair was as a child.
3. Analyze the level present in the hair. Lift a section of hair up, away from the scalp to see the level clearly.
4. Note the texture, density, and condition of the hair, especially its porosity. Check the condition of the scalp.
5. Determine with the client the desired end result. What highlights does the client want? Select the classification of haircolor product that will supply the desired effect.
6. Know the propertie s of the product you are using. Consult the manufacturer's information on each color and how it reacts on different hair color levels (light, medium, or dark hair).

7. If the client wishes to camouflage her/his gray, you may choose a deposit-only haircolor. If the client wishes a greater change and all other factors permit, a permanent oxidative haircolor may be chosen.

The directions for each manufacturer's color product will indicate the formulation for adequate lift and/or deposit. They will also indicate what haircolor classification and volume of developer (if any) is required to achieve the desired results, based on your thorough analysis of your client's hair and needs.

Examining the Scalp

Carefully examine the scalp to determine the presence of any factors that would make it inadvisable to use a haircoloring product. An oxidative tint solution should not be used if the following conditions exist:

- Positive skin test (predisposition or patch test)
- Scalp abrasions, irritations, or eruptions
- Contagious scalp disorders

Examining the Hair

Examine the hair to determine what, if any, pretreatment may be necessary prior to your haircolor service. Elements to consider are:

- Evidence of prior chemical treatments
- Different degrees of porosity over the length of the hair shaft
- Variations in texture

In some cases it may be advisable to postpone the haircolor service due to excessive damage or the presence of noncompatible chemicals in the hair.

All information about the condition of the client's hair should be recorded on the client's record card.

Explain Time and Monetary Investment Involved

At the completion of your consultation, you should have an agreement with your client as to what is needed, how long it will take, and how much it will cost.

The time and money involved in committing to a color service should be carefully explained in advance. Your conversation should be something like: "This color (show a picture or swatch) can be achieved by (indicate the type of color service—weaving, single-process color, etc.). The cost of your service today will be ($00.00). To maintain this color, it is important that you have this service every (number of weeks), and the cost each time will be ($00.00). Does that work for you?"

This is a time to make direct eye contact with your client and wait for the answer. If the time or cost is objectionable, alter your suggestion. Continue this conversation until you and your client agree to the maintenance schedule you have presented. At this point, you will have an agreement with your client and can begin your service.

A client record card (see page 287) will be necessary for transferring your hair analysis and testing and consultation information into a permanent file along with the client's release statement. You will also want to gather together your materials for strand and predisposition tests, which should be performed prior to each service in this chapter.

FULFILLING THE CLIENT'S NEEDS

Haircolor is a wonderful service that can make a tremendous difference for your client. Whether you choose a subtle change or something quite dramatic, the opportunity to create is greatly enhanced by being able to offer a haircolor service.

Haircoloring is an art, something to be learned over time and not simply by reading books. The people who walk into your salon to become your clients bring not only their hair, but their likes and dislikes, their hopes and dreams—a whole wealth of experiences in which you can share. Take your time, look carefully, listen well, and offer the gift of your art.

SELECTING THE APPROPRIATE APPLICATION TECHNIQUE

After a thorough discussion with your client, you must then select the technique that will achieve the desired effect. Sometimes a combination of application techniques is necessary to first cover the unpigmented hair, then add carefully placed highlights in order to make the transition from the lightness of unpigmented hair to the contrasting darkness of a solid color. Another example would be the use of a double-process blonding technique for clients with dark natural coloring who choose to be a pastel color with a cool tone.

Whatever you select, make sure the client understands each step of the procedure and the technique necessary to achieve your objective. This will avoid startled looks from clients when they see unexplained things happening to their hair during a procedure.

CLIENT RECORD CARD

Always record the consultation in the client's record card. It is important to keep an accurate record so that successful services can be repeated and any difficulties encountered in one service can be avoided in the next. A complete record should be kept, containing all analysis notes, strand test and whole head results, timing, and suggestions for the next service.

HAIRCOLOR RECORD

Name ______________________ Tel. ______________________

Address ______________________ City ______________________

Patch Test: ☐ Negative ☐ Positive Date ______________________

Eye Color ______________________ Skin Tone ______________________

DESCRIPTION OF HAIR

Form	Length	Texture	Density	Porosity	
☐ straight	☐ short	☐ coarse	☐ sparse	☐ very porous	☐ resistant
☐ wavy	☐ medium	☐ medium	☐ moderate	☐ porous	☐ very resistant
☐ curly	☐ long	☐ fine	☐ thick	☐ normal	☐ perm. waved

Natural hair color ______________________

Level (1-10)	Tone (Warm, Cool, etc.)	Intensity (Mild, Medium, Strong)	Category (B, W, S, R)

Scalp Condition
☐ normal ☐ dry ☐ oily ☐ sensitive

Condition
☐ normal ☐ dry ☐ oily ☐ faded ☐ streaked (uneven)

% unpigmented __________ Distribution of unpigmented ______________________

Previously lightened with ______________________ for ____________ (time)

Previously tinted with ______________________ for ____________ (time)

☐ original hair sample enclosed ☐ original hair sample not enclosed

Desired hair color ______________________

Level (1-10)	Tone (Warm, Cool, etc.)	Intensity (Mild, Medium, Strong)

CORRECTIVE TREATMENTS

Color filler used ______________________ Conditioning treatments with ____________

HAIR TINTING PROCESS

whole head ____________ retouch inches (cm) ________ shade desired ____________

formula: (color/lightener) ____________ application technique ______________________

Results: ☐ good ☐ poor ☐ too light ☐ too dark ☐ streaked

Comments: ______________________

____

____

____

____

Date	Operator	Price	Date	Operator	Price

RELEASE STATEMENT

A release statement is used for chemical services. It is designed to release the school or salon owner from responsibility for accidents or damages and is required for some malpractice insurance. A release statement is not a legally binding contract, however, and will not absolve the cosmetologist of responsibility for what has occurred to the client's hair.

A release statement is now used primarily to explain fully to clients whose hair is in questionable condition that their hair may not withstand the requested chemical treatment. It also encourages clients to be more truthful about any prior chemical experimentation that may affect your color selection and end result.

RELEASE FORM

I, the undersigned, ______________________________.

(name)

residing at ______________________________.

(street, address)

______________________________.

(city, state and zip)

about to receive services in the Clinical Department of

______________________________.

and having been advised that the services shall be performed by either students, graduate students, and/or instructors of the school, in consideration of the nominal charge for such services, hereby release the school, its students, graduate students, instructors, agents, representatives, and/or employees, from any and all claims arising out of and in any way connected with the performance of these services.

The Proprietor Is Not Responsible for Personal Property

Signed ______________________________.

Date ______________________________.

Witnessed ______________________________.

THIS RELEASE FORM MUST BE SIGNED BY THE PARENT OR GUARDIAN IF THE CLIENT BEING SERVED IS UNDER 18 YEARS OF AGE.

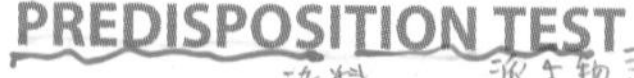

PREDISPOSITION TEST

Allergy to aniline derivative tints is unpredictable. Some clients may be sensitive, while others may suddenly develop a sensitivity after years of use. To identify an allergic client, the U.S. Federal Food, Drug, and Cosmetic Act prescribes that a patch or predisposition test be given 48 hours prior to each application of an aniline tint or toner. The tint used for the patch test must be the same type as will be used for the haircolor service.

Predisposition Test Procedure

1. Select a test area—behind one ear extending into the hairline or at the inside bend of the elbow. (Figs. 12.14a–c)

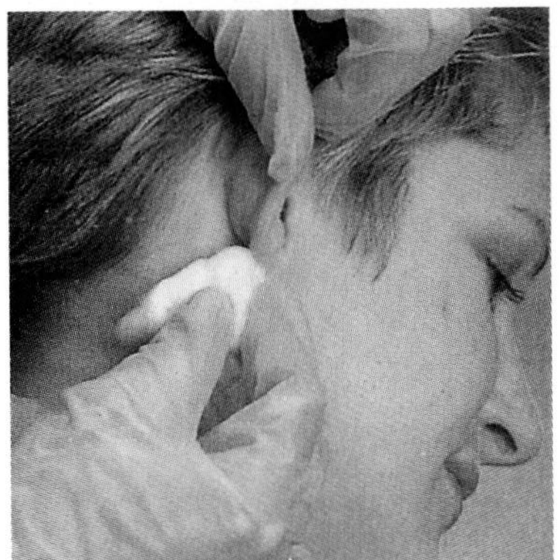

FIGURE 12.14a — Clean patch test area.

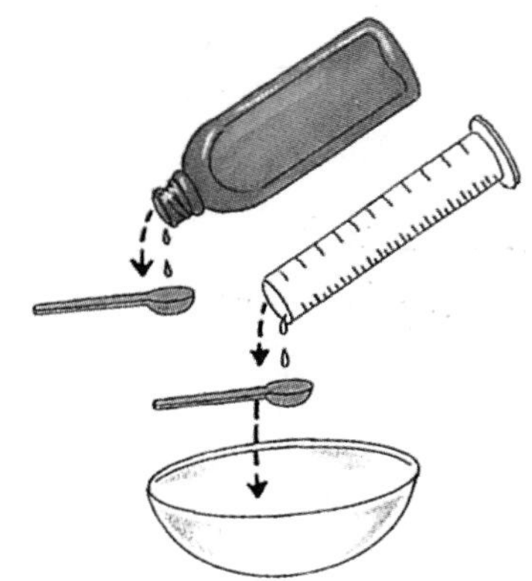

FIGURE 12.14b — Mix tint and peroxide.

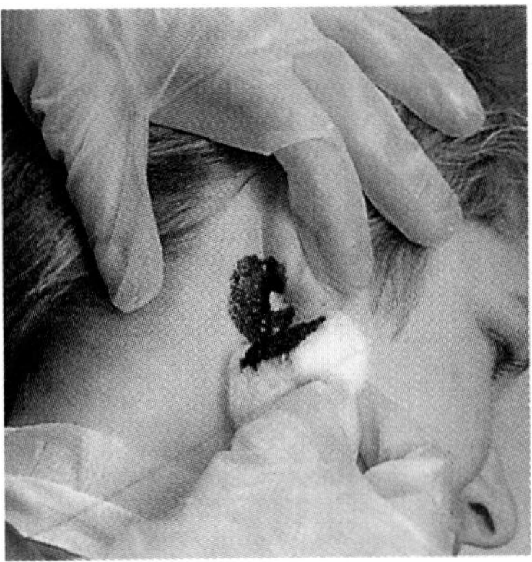

FIGURE 12.14c — Apply tint mixture.

2. Using mild soap, cleanse an area about the size of a quarter.
3. Dry the area.
4. Prepare the test solution according to the manufacturer's directions.
5. Apply to the test area with a sterile cotton swab.
6. Leave the area undisturbed for 48 hours.
7. Examine the test area.
8. Note the results on the client's record card.

In reality, most clients will not make the trip to the salon two days prior to their haircolor service to have their patch test done. As an alternative, you can make up patch test kits. Fill one small glass bottle with haircolor and another with developer. Write instructions on how to administer the patch test and give them to your clients when they book their appointment. Then just check their arm for the stain and no sign of irritation. (Fig. 12.14d)

A negative skin test will show no sign of inflammation and color may be safely applied. If the test is positive, you will see redness and a slight rash or welt. In extreme reactions, blisters and swelling

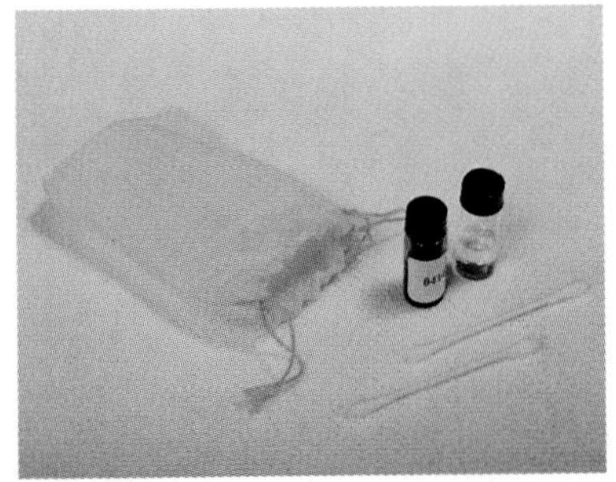

FIGURE 12.14d — Patch test kit.

will be noticeable. A client with these symptoms is allergic, and under no circumstances should receive a haircolor service.

Completed:
Learning Objective
#1
CLIENT CONSULTATION

CAUTION

Aniline derivative tints must never be used on the eyelashes or eyebrows. To do so may cause blindness.

COLOR THEORY

It is important that you understand the theory of color pigment before you begin applying haircoloring products to clients' hair. It is only through knowledge of color theory that you can think your way through color problems to the correct color formulation for each situation.

THE LAW OF COLOR

The ***Law of Color*** is a system for understanding the relationships of color. When combining colors, you will always get the same result from the same combination. Equal amounts of red and blue mixed together will always make violet. Equal amounts of yellow and blue will always make green. Equal amounts of red and yellow will always make orange. This system is called the Law of Color because these relationships have been tested over and over and have proven to be true.

This information will assist you when you wish to refine an unwanted tone in the hair. It will also facilitate your choosing appropriate toners for hair that has been decolorized.

Primary Colors

Primary colors are pure or fundamental pigments (colors that cannot be created by mixing colors together). The primary colors are, in order of their dominance, blue, red, and yellow. (Fig. 12.15) Understanding the order is essential to understanding color theory. All colors are created from these three primaries. Colors with a predominance of blue are cool-toned colors. Colors with a predominance of red or yellow are warm-toned colors.

Any natural hair color will visually include a combination of blue, red, and yellow. The physical characteristics of the colors are made up of various enzymes and chemical reactions. However, combinations of primary colors will create various visual results.

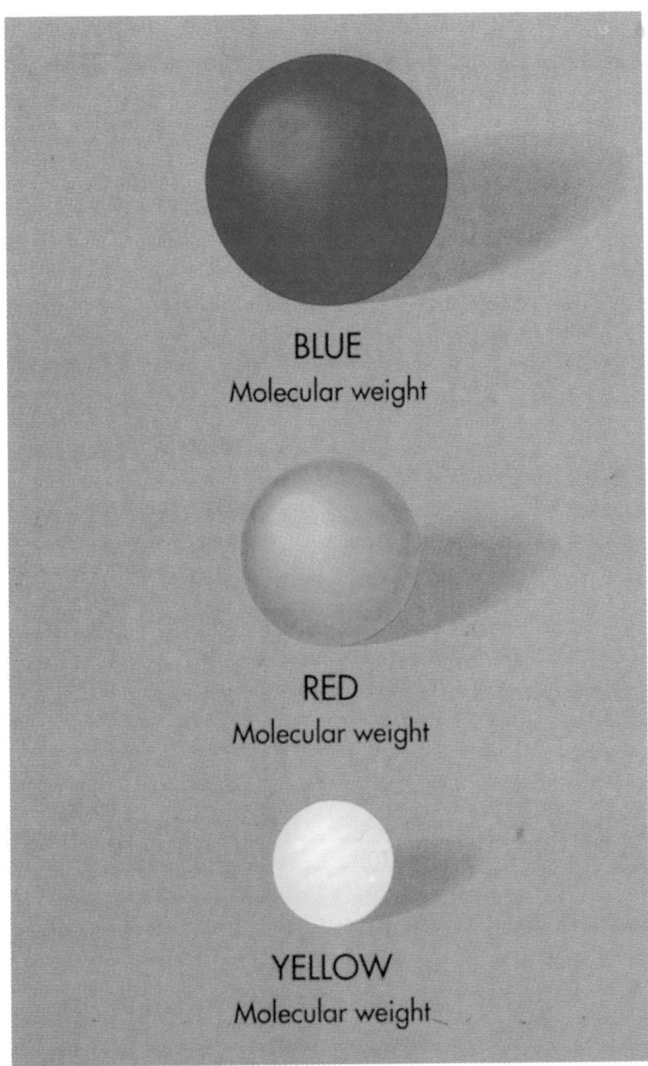

FIGURE 12.15 — Primary colors arranged by molecular size or pigment weight.

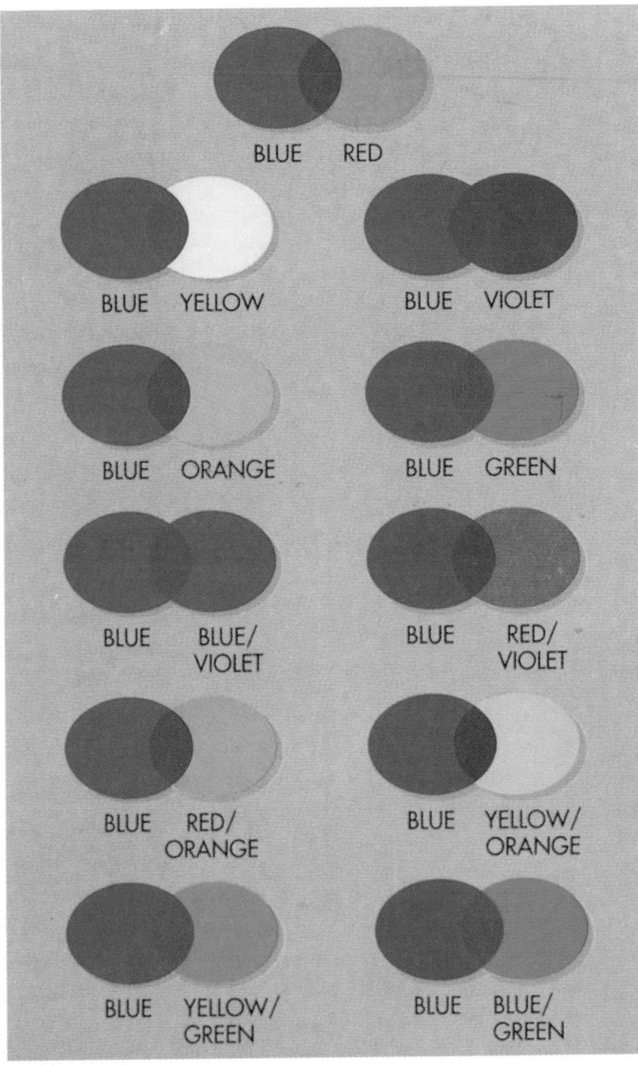

FIGURE 12.16 — Blue in combination with any secondary or tertiary color creates a cool shade.

Blue is the darkest of the primary colors. When you add blue to your mixture, you will make a color darker and cooler in appearance. Blue is the only cool primary, and when it is added to any primary, secondary, or tertiary color, it is dominant. The resulting new color will also be cool. (Fig. 12.16) In addition to a cool tone, blue also adds depth or darkness to any color to which it is added.

Red is the medium primary color. When you add red to your mixture, the resulting color will be warmer and richer. Red added to blue based colors will cause them to appear lighter. Red added to yellow toned colors will cause them to become darker.

Yellow is the lightest of the primary colors. When you add yellow to your mixture, you will make a color lighter and brighter in appearance.

When all three primary colors are present in equal proportions, the resulting color is black in its highest concentration, with shades of gray to white in its lightest level and intensity. Unequal proportions of the three primaries will produce a neutral brown or blonde, depending on the amount of pigment present. For example, unequal proportions of red, yellow, and blue with a majority of red will produce a reddish brown. A predominance of yellow would create a golden brown, and more blue than red or yellow becomes a dark or drab brown.

It is helpful to think of hair colors in terms of their proportions of the three primary colors. Neutral Brown for example, has the three primaries in the following proportions: One blue, two reds, and three yellows, or B-R-R-Y-Y-Y.

As the hair decolorizes, one of each of the primaries is eliminated, so one blue, one red, and one yellow are visually gone from the hair. You are left with one red and two yellows, which appears to our eyes as orange. As the hair continues to decolorize, one red and one yellow are eliminated. You are then left with one yellow, which will continue to appear lighter and lighter as the decolorization process continues.

Secondary Colors

Secondary colors are green, orange, and violet. They are created by combining two, and only two, primary colors in equal proportions. Green is a combination of blue and yellow. Orange is a combination of red and yellow. Violet is a combination of blue and red. Green and violet both have blue in them, so they are cool tones. Orange has red and yellow, so it is a warm tone. (Fig. 12.17)

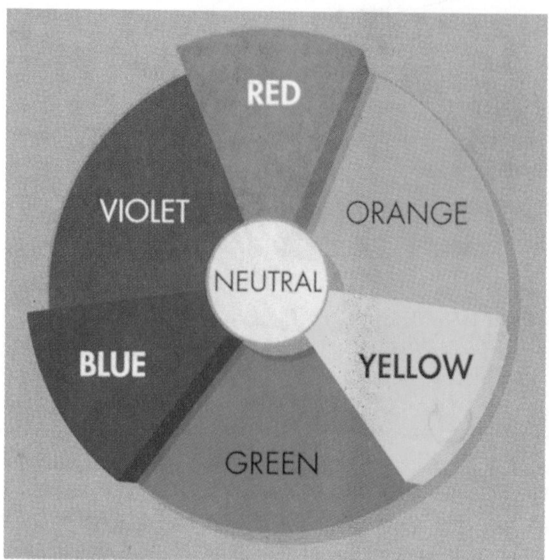

FIGURE 12.17 — Secondary colors are created from equal parts of two primaries.

Tertiary Colors

Tertiary colors are blue-green, blue-violet, red-violet, red-orange, yellow-orange, and yellow-green. When relating this basic information to haircolor, you will notice that haircolor is never one primary color. Natural-looking haircolor is made up of a combination of primary and secondary colors.

Tertiary colors are created by mixing a primary color with the adjacent secondary color on the color wheel. Blue-green and blue-violet are cool tones. Red-violet is also cool, but not as cool as the other two because of the predominance of red. Red-orange and yellow-orange are warm tones. Yellow-green is a warm tone, but not as warm as the other two because of the presence of blue. (Fig. 12.18)

Complementary Colors

The term complementary comes from the word *complement*, which means to make complete or to mutually make up what is lacking. ***Complementary colors*** are a primary and secondary color positioned opposite each other on the color wheel. Combinations are blue and orange, red and green, and yellow and violet.

These colors neutralize each other. When formulating, you are often attempting to neutralize or refine unwanted warmth in your end result. Knowing the complementary relationships can direct you in choosing the appropriate tone to color. For example, when mixed in equal amounts, red and green neutralize each other. Orange and blue neutralize each other, and yellow and violet neutralize each other. (Fig. 12.19)

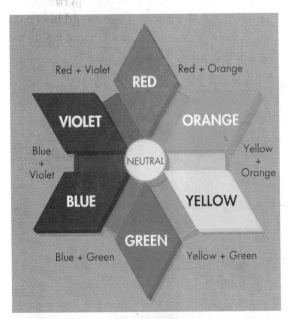

FIGURE 12.18 — The combination of primary and secondary colors creates tertiary colors.

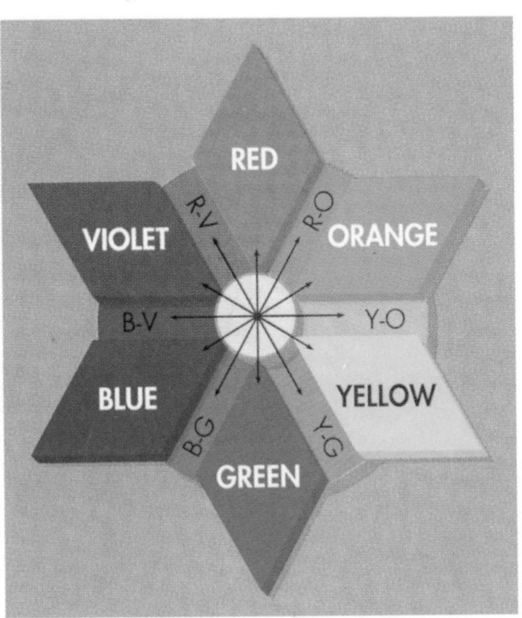

FIGURE 12.19 — Complete color wheel with arrows to indicate which colors neutralize others.

When formulating haircolor, you always work with a combination of colors. That combination may be your client's natural pigment and one haircolor product. Or it may be several colors blended together. Your client's own natural pigment contributes warm tones to the end result. Knowing how much warmth will be contributed takes practice and experimentation with each color level.

You have learned that the warm tones are red, orange, and yellow. When these warm tones are unwanted, you can refine your result by using the complementary tone, opposite on the color wheel.

Red pigment is not really a factor in hair color. The unwanted tone clients comment on most often is orange. Clients may call this unwanted tone "brassy" or "red." It will be up to your educated eye to determine whether the actual tone is orange. The complementary color to orange is blue. A blue-based haircolor product will help to neutralize orange highlights in the hair. Another unwanted tone you may need to correct is yellow. In this case, the complementary color is violet. A violet-toned haircolor product will refine yellow.

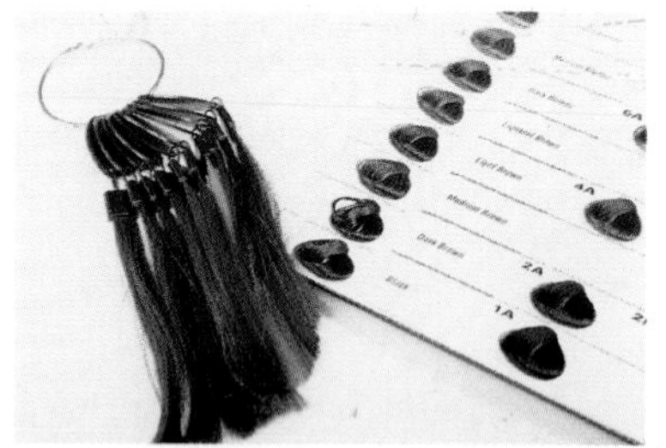

FIGURE 12.20 — A manufacturer's color guide is a useful tool for creating natural-looking haircolor.

Referring to the Color Wheel to Predict Results

The ***color wheel*** is a professional tool colorists use to create custom formulas. It is based upon the universal method of creating different colors by combining the primary, secondary, and tertiary colors. This tool, together with the colorist's knowledge of artificial coloring products, will enable the colorist to enhance or subdue tones present in the hair during the coloring process. Manufacturers' materials may provide other visual tools to clarify this information, along with recommendations for color formulation. (Fig. 12.20)

Completed: Learning Objective #2 COLOR THEORY

TYPES OF HAIRCOLOR

Haircoloring falls into five main categories: temporary, semi-permanent, oxidative deposit-only (demi), non-oxidative permanent, and oxidative/lift-deposit (permanent). The organization of haircolor products by their chemistry, action on the hair, and lasting ability created the need for a new fifth category. Previously, the permanent haircolor category was comprised of both non-oxidative permanent and oxidative/lift-deposit color products. To clarify the great differences in these products, they are separated into two different categories.

TEMPORARY HAIRCOLOR

Temporary colors utilize the largest pigments of all four classifications of haircolor. The large size of this color molecule prevents penetration of the cuticle layer of the hair shaft and allows only a coating action on the outside of the strand. The chemical composition of a temporary color makes only a physical change rather than a chemical change in the hair shaft. (Fig. 12.21)

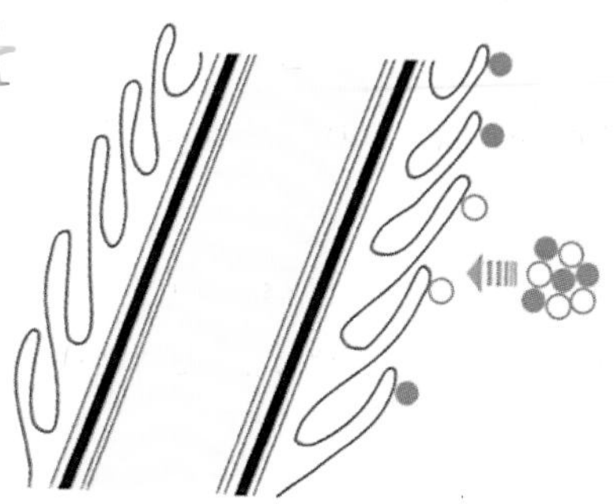

FIGURE 12.21 — Action of temporary haircolors.

Action of Temporary Color on the Hair

Since the color remains on the cuticle and does not penetrate into the cortex, it lasts only from shampoo to shampoo. However, excessive porosity can allow temporary color to penetrate, making it last much longer. Temporary colors usually contain certified colors—colors that have been approved by the Food and Drug Administration (FDA) for use in cosmetics.

Uses for Temporary Color:

1. To temporarily restore faded hair to its natural color.
2. To neutralize the yellowish tinge in white or unpigmented hair.
3. To tone down overlightened hair without creating further chemical damage.
4. To temporarily add color to the hair without changing its condition.

Disadvantages of Temporary Haircolor:

1. Color is short in duration; it must be applied after every shampoo.
2. Coating is thin and may not cover hair evenly.
3. Color may rub off on pillows or collars and may run with perspiration or other moisture.
4. They can only add color; they cannot lift.
5. Staining may result if the hair is porous or if a dark color is used on very light hair.

Temporary colors come in a wide array of shades from light to dark, warm to cool. They are easy to apply and are valuable as an introduction to haircoloring or as a "quick fix" in corrective coloring situations when the hair may not tolerate a stronger chemical.

A patch test is usually not necessary for this type of haircolor, although the recent introduction of noncertified direct dyes does not always make this claim a certainty. Consult the manufacturer's directions for recommendations.

Types of Temporary Haircolor

A wide variety of products are available within this classification: coloring crayons and mascara; coloring mousses, gels, and creams; coloring sprays; color-enhancing shampoos; color rinses; and coloring powders.

Coloring Crayons and Mascara

Hair crayons and ***mascara*** are a relatively new innovation in the temporary haircoloring category. They are available in a tube with an applicator similar to the type used with makeup mascara. They come in a wide variety of shades—from natural golden and reddish tones, to add temporary highlights, to bright blue, violet, and red to create fashion effects. The advantage of this type of color is that it can be added to the hair design to accent the exact area desired and is easily removed by shampoo. Use of this product is a good way to introduce a color-shy client to a little variety in his or her haircolor.

Coloring Mousses, Gels, and Creams

Coloring mousses are one of the most contemporary ways to temporarily color the hair. They offer a wide array of colors that are fast and easy to apply. Color mousses serve many of the same purposes as temporary color rinses. They can brighten hair, tone unpigmented hair, disguise regrowth lines, and blend uneven color as well as create dramatic effects.

Color mousses stay put on the hair shaft. They do not drip, run, or blow off the hair when blow-drying. This characteristic, and the fact that they do not appear to be a traditional haircolor, makes them popular with men. They also give the hair body and volume. Some mousses have detangling and conditioning abilities.

Coloring gels and creams are available in a variety of shades, some natural, others wild and vibrant. These colors are designed to shampoo completely out, but because they tend to be tones of great intensity, they may stain porous, bleached, or very dry hair. (Fig. 12.22)

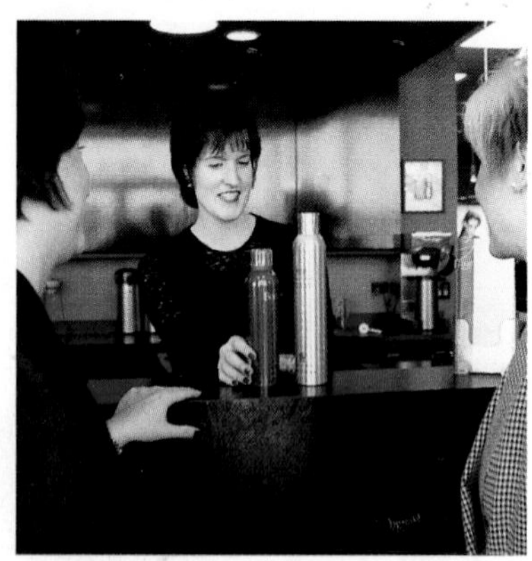

FIGURE 12.22 — A variety of color mousses and gels are available.

Coloring Sprays

Spray-on haircoloring is applied to dry hair from aerosol containers. These are generally used for special or party effects. Temporary color sprays can be sprayed over the entire head of hair to create an even tone, such as brown or auburn, but they are more popular for creating special and exotic effects.

The metallic salts in color sprays can build up after repeated use and cause an adverse reaction with future chemical services. These products are also extremely flammable, so they cannot be used around clients who are smoking.

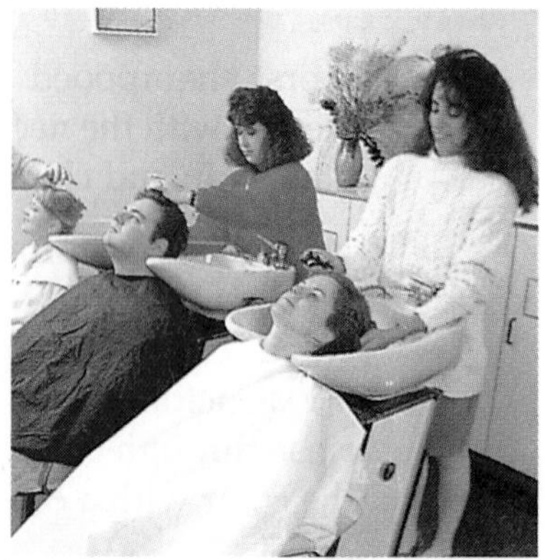

FIGURE 12.23 — Color-enhancing shampoos combine the action of a color rinse with that of a shampoo.

Color-Enhancing Shampoos

Color-enhancing shampoos are also known as highlighting shampoos. They are a combination of rinse and shampoo. They are similar to temporary color rinses in that they give only slight color changes that are removed with plain shampooing. Color shampoos are used to brighten, impart slight color, and eliminate unwanted tones. (Fig. 12.23)

Temporary Color Rinses

Temporary color rinses are prepared rinses used to add color to the hair. These rinses contain certified colors and remain on the hair until the next shampoo. Temporary rinses are also known as water rinses, since they are a simple aqueous-alcoholic solution combined with various dyes.

TRADITIONAL SEMI-PERMANENT HAIRCOLOR

Semi-permanent color offers a form of haircoloring suitable for the client who is reluctant to have a permanent color change. The semi-permanent color is formulated to be more lasting than temporary but milder than permanent color.

Semi-permanent color may be excellent for clients who feel that their hair is dull, drab, or showing unpigmented areas but who are not ready to begin permanent haircoloring. Semi-permanent color can blend unpigmented hair and deepen color tones without altering the natural color, since there is no lightening action on the hair.

Semi-permanent color is available in a wide range of shades. It can be purchased as a gel, cream, liquid, or mousse. Semi-permanent color is often chosen by younger clients as fashion trends change. It can deposit a dramatic color or even be used for special effect streaks in bright colors. Providing the hair's porosity is normal, the color will naturally fade without a regrowth, so the client can change the color at any time or discontinue the effect.

Semi-permanent haircolor is formulated to last approximately four to six shampoos. No developer is required. The color molecules penetrate the cuticle somewhat so that the color gradually fades with each shampoo. Due to this gradual fading of color tone from the hair, regrowth may be less noticeable (depending upon the color applied) and retouching may not be required as frequently. If the hair is extremely porous or if heat is used, as with some types of semi-permanent color, the results can be more permanent. Results depend on the hair's original color and porosity, processing time, and technique. (Fig. 12.24)

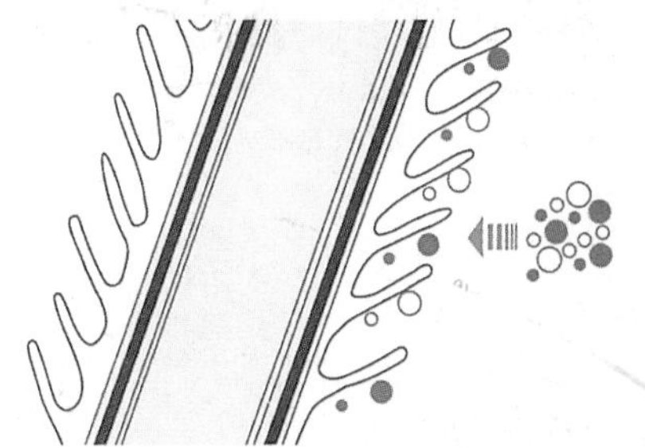

FIGURE 12.24 — Action of semi-permanent haircolor.

Advantages of Semi-Permanent Haircolor:

1. The color is self-penetrating.
2. The color is applied the same way each time.
3. Retouching is not necessary.
4. Color does not rub off on a pillow or clothing.
5. Hair returns to its natural color after approximately 4 to 6 shampoos.

Note: *Semi-permanent tints containing aniline derivatives require a patch test. Follow the manufacturer's directions carefully.*

Types of Semi-Permanent Haircolor

1. Semi-permanent tints that blend or cover unpigmented hair completely, but do not affect the remaining pigmented hair.
2. Semi-permanent tints that enhance unpigmented hair without changing the natural pigment.
3. Semi-permanent tints that add color and shine to hair that is not unpigmented.
4. Translucent tints that add gloss, tone, and sometimes special effects to the hair. These colors vary in their effect according to porosity, heat application, and timing. Consult your instructor and manufacturer's information for assistance with these products.

Uses for Semi-Permanent Haircolor

1. To enhance hair's natural color. Semi-permanent colors can be used to add golden or red highlights, and to deepen the color of the hair. This type of color is especially effective on ethnic clients and clients whose natural hair color is too light or too drab to set off their complexions.
2. To tone prelightened hair. Semi-permanent colors can serve as a nonperoxide toner for prelightened hair. Prelightened hair is porous and the toner will penetrate.
3. To refresh faded tints. Semi-permanent colors are excellent for between permanent color services and for corrective work, when a nonperoxide alternative is desired.
4. To add color to unpigmented/white hair. Most semi-permanent colors are designed to cover hair that is 25% or less unpigmented or to create a blending effect on higher percentages. They are also recommended for clients who want to keep and enhance their unpigmented or white hair.

Action on Hair

- Traditional semi-permanent colors are formulated with pigment molecules that are smaller than those of the temporary colors but larger than those of the permanent tints. They have a mild penetrating action that results in a gentle addition of color in the cortex, as well as some coating of the cuticle.
- The chemical composition of semi-permanent colors falls within the approximate pH range of 8.0-9.0, thus causing an alkaline reaction on the hair. The alkali swells the cuticle,

opening imbrications and allowing the molecules to enter the cortex. However, this solution is mildly alkaline, which causes limited swelling and opening. Only a small number of these medium-sized molecules enter and remain in the cortex.

- The pigment molecules are trapped within the cortical layer of the shaft as the hair shrinks back toward normal during the rinsing step of the service. A neutral or slightly acid after-rinse helps to close the imbrications and hold the pigment molecules within the cortex. However, even the mild swelling that occurs with shampooing allows some of the color to fade.
- Traditional semi-permanent colors have several distinct differences from temporary and permanent colors. They last longer than temporary colors and do not rub off. They are also easy to use, requiring no retouch application. Because semi-permanent colors make no significant permanent changes in the structure of the hair, they are less damaging. Some brands even give a conditioning effect. They are excellent for toning bleached hair that is too weak or porous to accept another peroxide treatment and for use on hair that is exceptionally fine or damaged from permanent wave or relaxer services.

Polymer Semi-Permanent Haircolor

The polymer colors are classified as semi-permanent colors because they use direct, disperse application and include certified dyes that require no oxidation process or the addition of an oxidizer for color development. However, they are distinctly different from traditional semi-permanent colors in color results, color fastness (holding ability), and chemical composition.

A ***polymer*** is a substance or product containing long chain-like structures. This structure actually inhibits its penetration of the cuticle and its ability to adhere to the keratin of the hair shaft. However, the dyes in polymer colors are extremely concentrated so that regardless of the long-chain structure, the color becomes well fixed to the hair. The polymers are designed to coat and penetrate the hair shaft, creating translucent shine and accent hues rather than complete coverage of the natural color.

The color fastness or staying power of the polymer colors differs from traditional semi-permanent colors. The polymer colors are advertised as colors that are removed gradually by shampooing. However, in many cases colorists have found this not to be true. The higher the heat and the longer the processing time, the deeper the color penetration and the greater the color fastness. Polymer colors have been known to become so well attached to the structure of the hair that even bleaches or dye solvents prepared with hydrogen peroxide will not remove them. Regardless of the experience of the colorist, performing a strand test is the most professional method of color selection.

The natural melanin within the hair shaft will not be changed by this type of coloring. The color achieved will be the direct result of the addition of the polymer pigment to the natural pigment of the shaft. After perming or relaxing services, the softened state of the shaft allows for more color to be deposited than can be achieved on nonchemically treated hair.

Polymer semi-permanent colors were originally available in only highly intense primary and secondary colors that added a high-fashion accent to natural hair color. They are currently also available in more natural shades, including a neutral or clear color designed to fill in the cuticle and give hair a shinier, healthier appearance.

OXIDATIVE DEPOSIT-ONLY HAIRCOLOR

When semi-permanent colors were first introduced years ago, clients shampooed their hair weekly, allowing the semi-permanent color of the time to last a satisfactory four to six weeks. Today, however, with more clients shampooing daily, a color that lasts four to six shampoos may be unsatisfactory. For a color that will act similarly in nature to the semi-permanent colors but will produce a longer-lasting effect, manufacturers have introduced a new category of haircolors called ***oxidative deposit-only*** or ***demi-permanent colors***.

Composition and Action

The effect of an oxidative deposit-only haircolor lies somewhere between those of the semi-permanent and permanent color classifications. Deposit-only colors use a form of catalyst, such as low volume peroxide developers, along with non-ammonia alkali materials, such as amino methyl propanol (AMP) or monoethanolamine (MEA). This combination of chemicals gently swells and opens the cuticle layer and drives the color precursor molecules into the cortex, enabling the color molecules to form. The use of low volume peroxide and low levels of non-ammonia alkali does not promote the destruction and solubilization of melanin. Therefore there is no lightening or bleaching of the natural pigment. Deposit-only colors produce a diffused line of demarcation. (Fig. 12.25)

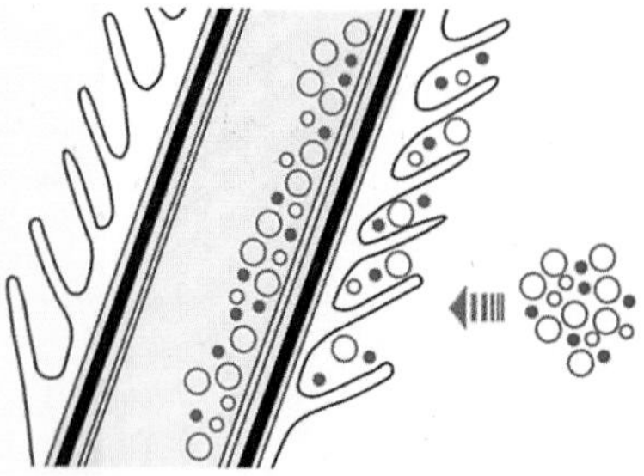

FIGURE 12.25 — Action of deposit-only haircolor.

NON-OXIDATIVE PERMANENT HAIRCOLOR

Non-oxidative permanent haircolors are prepared from a variety of materials: vegetables, flowers, herbs, salts of heavy metals, and organic and synthetic chemicals. All of these permanent colors fall into one of four classifications: vegetable tints, metallic dyes, compound dyes, or oxidative tints.

Vegetable Tints

In the past, before technology brought us the beauty industry as we now know it, many vegetable materials such as chamomile and henna were used as haircoloring ingredients.

Chamomile flowers can be ground into a powder and used as a paste that is applied in a manner similar to a henna pack, with a processing time that ranges from 15 to 60 minutes. It gives a lighter, brighter effect to the hair. Shampoos and rinses containing powdered flowers are intended to add a bright yellow color in the hair. However, chamomile's effectiveness is limited to a minimal color change.

Henna is the most noteworthy and popular of the vegetable colors and comes from plants grown in moist climates throughout Africa, Arabia, Iran, and the East Indies. The henna leaves are removed before the flowering cycle, dried, and ground into a fine powder. Hot water is added to create a paste. Henna is a natural product that esthetically appeals to the young client and the type of consumer that prefers organic products and avoids synthetics. Its "natural" qualities appeal to many.

Current technology has made available hennas in black, chestnut, and auburn, plus a lightener. These hennas are made of concentrated herbal extracts that have both a cumulative and a semi-permanent effect. The dye coats the hair and is partially removed by shampooing. The coating action of henna creates a hair strand that becomes thicker, and thus helps to give body to fine, limp hair. Because it makes no structural changes in the hair, it can be used on weak hair without damaging it. Henna fills in a roughened cuticle and holds together a split end to provide a slick, light-reflective surface. This, coupled with the additional warmth henna provides, creates hair that shines.

However, it is important to remember that excessive application will build up on the outside of the shaft and can create an unnatural brassiness. If overused, the build-up can become so heavy that conditioners cannot penetrate to the hair shaft and the hair becomes dry and coarse.

Metallic Hair Dyes

Metallic haircolors can be recognized by the descriptive terms used by manufacturers in their packaging even before reading the ingredients list. ***Metallic dyes*** are known as "progressive haircolors" and "color restorers." They are referred to as progressive because the hair progressively turns darker and darker upon each subsequent application. The term color restorer is used because the natural hair color appears to be gradually restored. When the desired color is reached, the consumer is to reduce the frequency of application to maintain the color.

Metallic hair dyes comprise a minor portion of the home haircoloring market and currently are never used professionally. Nevertheless, it is crucial for the professional colorist to be informed of the chemical composition, characteristics, and methods of removal, because metals react adversely with oxidation results.

Clients occasionally request chemical services without knowing the incompatibility of metallic color with professional products. Consumers generally do not even realize that they used a product containing metal. The colorist must be able to analyze and prescribe safe, professional treatments to avoid hair damage and discoloration.

The metallic salts react with the sulfur of the hair keratin, eventually turning the protein brown. In this reaction, the quality of the keratin is lowered from the use of this chemical. The physical result is a colored film coating the hair shaft, which gives the hair a characteristic dull metallic appearance. The metallic coating also builds up on the surface of the hair shaft. Repeated treatments leave the hair brittle and conflict with future chemical services that include in their formulation hydrogen peroxide, thioglycolate, ammonia, and/or most other oxidizers. Resulting damage can include discoloration, breakage, poor permanent waving results, and even destruction to the point of a melted hair shaft due to the heat created in this adverse chemical reaction.

Compound Dyes

Compound dyes are a combination of metallic or mineral dyes with a vegetable tint. The metallic salts are added to give the product more staying power and to create different colors. Like metallic dyes, compound dyes are not used professionally.

OXIDATIVE/LIFT-DEPOSIT HAIRCOLOR

On a professional level, permanent hair dyes are based almost entirely on the use of oxidative tints. ***Oxidative/lift-deposit (permanent) haircolors*** can lighten and deposit color in one application, a feat performed by no other color classification. This ability to create an infinite array of levels, tones, and intensities has made oxidative/lift-deposit (permanent) colors irreplaceable in the industry. These tints penetrate the cuticle of the hair and enter the cortical layer. Here, they are oxidized by the peroxide added into color pigments. These pigments are distributed throughout the hair shaft much like natural pigment. (Figs. 12.26, 12.27)

Toners also fall into the category of permanent color. Toners are aniline derivative products of pale, delicate shades designed for use on prelightened hair. (They will be covered more thoroughly later in the chapter.)

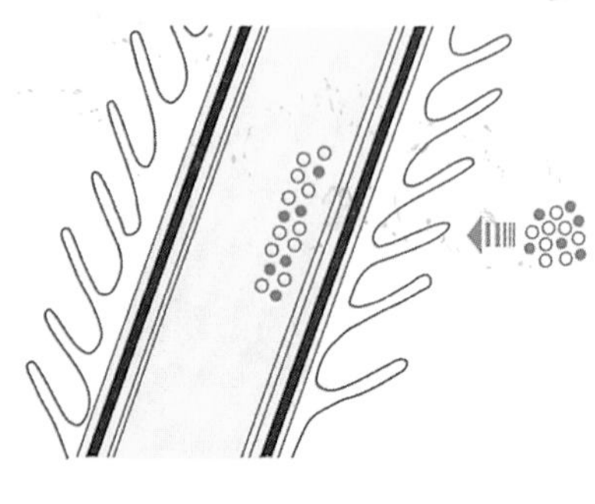

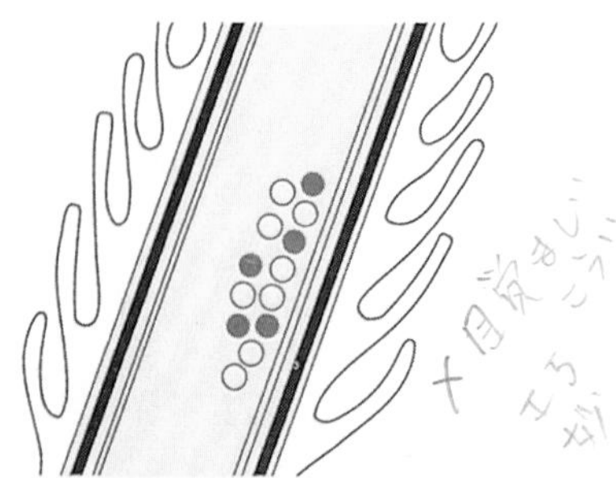

FIGURE 12.26, 12.27 — Action of permanent haircolor.

Composition of Oxidative/Lift-Deposit Haircolor

Commercially, oxidative/lift-deposit (permanent) dyes are known by a variety of names: para-dyes, aniline derivative tints, permanent tints, synthetic-organic tints, penetrating tints, cream tints, and tube colors, as well as oxidative tints.

The term ***para-dye*** refers to the colorless substances, either paraphenylenediamine or paratoluenediamine, that transform into a colored material in and on the hair shaft when mixed with an oxidizer such as hydrogen peroxide. Even though some oxidation tints no longer contain either of these derivatives, *para-dye* has become a term that refers to all oxidation tints regardless of chemical composition.

Many permanent haircolors include a type of ammonia in the formulation to activate the coloring process. Ammonia, as formulated into oxidative colors, is in selected proportions to achieve the desired amount of lift. Also, ammonia or some alternate alkalizing agent creates the proper pH for the oxidative dyes to develop.

The industry has taken strides toward manufacturing tint products that either replace or partially replace ammonia. However, the permanent tints containing no ammonia do not have the lifting power of those formulated with it.

Most oxidative tints contain aniline derivatives and require a ***predisposition test*** before the service.

Action of Oxidative Tints

Oxidative tints are sold in bottles, canisters, and tubes in either a semi-liquid or cream form. The colorist adds the oxidizing agent, hydrogen peroxide, that activates the chemical reaction known as oxidation. This reaction, which occurs at an alkaline pH, is created to a great extent by the ammonia in the tint, and begins as soon as the two compounds are combined. For this reason, the mixed tint must be used immediately. Any leftover tint must be discarded, since it deteriorates quickly.

Application of this oxidizing tint in an alkaline state causes the hair shaft to swell and the cuticle to open. The molecules of the tint base, before mixing with the oxidizer, are very small and can pass easily through the cuticle and into the cortex of the hair shaft. As the oxidation process begins, the coupling together of these small colorless tint-base molecules changes them into large chains of colored, relatively stable pigment.

These molecules become trapped beneath the cuticle as they are now too large to be shampooed out. They form acid bonds with the keratin chains in the cortex and become part of the hair structure.

Timing the application of the tint depends upon the product and the volume of peroxide selected. The general rule is: the higher the working volume of hydrogen peroxide used in your formula, the longer the color has to process. Consult the manufacturer's directions and your instructor for assistance. A test strand should always be taken to ensure satisfactory results.

Single-process tints have the ability to both lighten and deposit pigment at one time to achieve the desired color. Prelightening or presoftening is not required. Single-process tints usually contain a lightening agent, a shampoo, an aniline derivative tint, and an alkalizing agent. The alkalizing agent acts with the peroxide that is added to the formula, oxidizing the melanin and creating an alkaline environment in which the dyes can develop. Most color is formulated to be used with 20 volume peroxide. Color results are altered when other volumes are used.

The advantages of single-process tints are that they:

1. Can produce shades from the deepest black to the lightest blonde.
2. Can color the hair lighter or darker than the client's original shade.
3. Can blend white or unpigmented hair to a natural hair shade.
4. Can correct streaks, off-shades, discolorations, and faded ends.
5. Are available as creams, liquids, and gels.

Types of Permanent Tints

The cosmetic chemicals that make oxidative haircoloring possible are available to salon colorists in several forms: liquids, creams, and gels. Each of these haircoloring bases has its loyal professional users, and the choice of one form or the other is a matter of individual preference.

As the name implies, the viscosity of ***liquid haircolor*** is generally thinner, and may be applied with a bottle technique to better control the placement of the color formula. Liquid haircolor products are generally more economically priced and have excellent penetrating ability.

Cream haircolor products may come in tube or canister form from the manufacturer, and have conditioners and thickening agents. They can sometimes be too viscous (thick) to be applied from an applicator bottle, and are generally mixed with cream developer when applied by the brush-and-bowl technique.

The consistency of a ***gel haircolor*** falls between that of a liquid and a cream. It can be applied using the bottle or brush technique.

Completed:
Learning Objective
#3
CLASSIFICATIONS OF HAIRCOLOR

HYDROGEN PEROXIDE DEVELOPERS

Although other oxidizers are available, hydrogen peroxide is the oxidizing agent most commonly used in haircoloring. An ***oxidizer*** is a substance that causes oxygen to combine with another substance, such as melanin. As the oxygen and melanin combine, the peroxide solution begins to diffuse (break apart and spread out) and lighten the melanin within the hair shaft. This new smaller structure and spread-out distribution of the melanin gives hair its light appearance.

Hydrogen peroxide decomposes at a pH greater than 5.5. This higher pH exists in the haircolor product because of the alkalizing agent in the formula. The diffused melanin is in a soluble form and is partially removed from the hair.

Forms of Hydrogen Peroxide

Hydrogen peroxide (H_2O_2) is distributed for cosmetology use under a variety of names such as *oxidizer, generator, developer,* or *catalyst.* (Some manufacturers also use the word *catalyst* to mean protinator, an additive to lightening or bleach mixtures used to increase product strength.) Regardless of which name is used, hydrogen peroxide comes in three forms: dry, cream, and liquid.

Dry peroxide, in either tablet or powder form, is dissolved in liquid hydrogen peroxide to boost the volume. The availability of liquid peroxides in a variety of volumes has made this product somewhat obsolete.

Cream peroxide contains additives such as thickeners, drabbers, conditioners, and an acid for stabilization. The thickeners help to create a product that is easy to control. This extra control helps to prevent dripping during the use of brush-and-bowl method of application. This thicker formula is also advantageous when used in foil-weave wrapping, hair painting, or highlighting, because the bleach mixture is less likely to "bleed" onto places where it is not wanted. The creamy formula also tends to stay moist on the hair longer than liquid peroxide, which prevents the hair lightening or coloring mixture from drying out and stopping the product action before full development is complete. However, the thickening additives in cream peroxides may dilute the strength of the formula, making it undesirable to use when full product strength is needed, such as in tinting to cover unpigmented hair.

Liquid peroxide contains no additives, only a stabilizing acid that brings the pH to 3.5-4.0. Liquid peroxide is convenient because it can be used in almost every bleach and tint formula on the market today. Another plus is that the formula for liquid peroxide is basically the same from one manufacturer to another rather than varied as with the cream peroxide. This offers the colorist consistent results regardless of the brand used. The lack of additives in liquid hydrogen peroxide creates a color formula that generally covers unpigmented hair effectively.

The disadvantages to be considered in choosing liquid peroxide over cream are that haircoloring and lightening products tend to dry out faster, and the conditioning agents are not present. However, one peroxide is not superior to the other; they are just different. It is the responsibility of the colorist to read the manufacturer's recommended directions and select the best product for the job.

Strengths of Hydrogen Peroxide

Completed: Learning Objective #4
EXPLAIN ROLE OF HYDROGEN PEROXIDE

A variety of strengths of both liquid and cream peroxide are available. Consult your manufacturer's directions for the recommended strength. Although scientists identify the different strengths of hydrogen peroxide by percentages, cosmetologists identify the various strengths by volume, as it is the freeing of a certain volume of gases that creates the desired chemical reaction in haircoloring. Thus, 20 volume and 6% hydrogen peroxide are the same strength. ✔

COLOR APPLICATION TECHNIQUES

For successful haircoloring services, the technician must follow a definite procedure. A system makes for the greatest efficiency and the most satisfactory results. Without such a plan, the work will take longer, results will be uneven, and mistakes will be made.

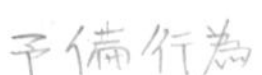

PRELIMINARY STRAND TEST

Once you have created a color formula for your client, you should try it out on a small strand of hair. This ***preliminary strand test*** will let you know how the hair will react to the formula and how long the formula should be left on the hair. The strand test is performed after the hair is completely prepared for the coloring service.

Implements and Materials

- Plastic clips
- Spray water bottle
- Towels
- Protective gloves
- Client record card
- Tint brush or bottle
- Glass or plastic mixing bowl
- Shampoo
- Mixing spoons
- Aluminum foil or plastic wrap
- Selected tint
- Developer

Procedure

1. Assemble materials.
2. Put on protective gloves.
3. Mix a small amount of formula according to manufacturer's directions.
4. Part off a ½" (1.25 cm) square strand of hair in the lower crown. Use plastic clips, as necessary, to fasten other hair out of the way.
5. Mix ½ teaspoon of the selected color formula with the amount of hydrogen peroxide recommended by the manufacturer.
6. Place the strand over the foil or plastic wrap and apply the mixture. Follow the application method for the color procedure you will be using.
7. Check the development at 5-minute intervals until the desired color has been achieved. Note the timing on the record card.
8. When satisfactory color has been developed, remove the protective foil or plastic wrap. Place a towel under the strand, mist it thoroughly with water, add shampoo, and massage through. Rinse by spraying with water. Dry the strand with the towel and observe results.
9. Adjust the formula, the timing, or the application method as necessary and proceed to color the entire head.

CAUTION

A predisposition test must be given before coloring the hair with an aniline derivative product. The client should be draped to protect clothing. Operator dermatitis, although rare, involves the same types of negative reactions to chemicals as the client can experience. Since a colorist's hands are in water and contact chemical solutions repeatedly throughout an average day, it is important to take proper precautions. You should protect yourself from allergic reactions by wearing gloves until the product is completely removed from the client's hair.

APPLICATION OF TEMPORARY RINSES

There are many methods of application, depending upon the product used. Your instructor will help you interpret the manufacturer's directions.

The pigment molecules are designed to attach to hard keratin. Skin and hair are composed of similar types of keratin; the soft keratin of the skin and scalp are even more reactive than the hard keratin of the hair. This allows rinses to stain the scalp as well as the skin. Therefore it is advisable to wear gloves to protect your hands even though the solution itself is relatively harmless.

Implements and Materials

Neck strip	Towels
Protective gloves	Shampoo cape
Comb	Applicator bottle (optional)
Temporary color	Shampoo
Record card	

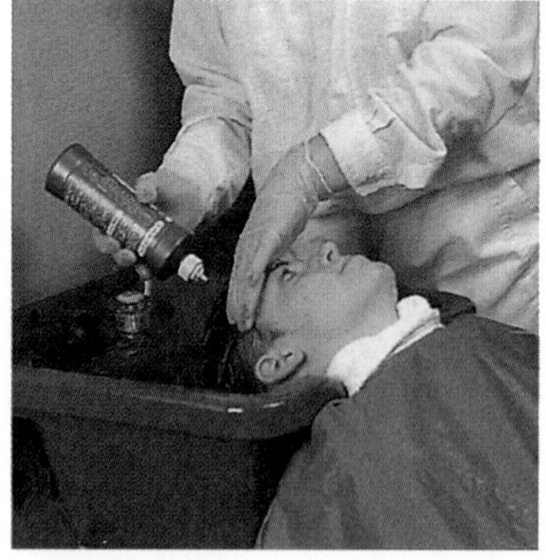

FIGURE 12.28 — Apply temporary rinse.

Procedure

1. The hair is first shampooed and towel-dried. Make sure that the client is protected with the neck strip and cape as temporary coloring can easily stain skin and clothing.
2. The client should be comfortably reclined at the shampoo bowl.
3. Shake product thoroughly to blend any pigments that may have settled. Apply color. Use an applicator bottle as directed by your instructor. (Fig. 12.28)
4. Blend rinse through entire hair shaft. (Fig. 12.29)
5. Blend the color with a comb, applying more color as necessary.
6. Do not rinse hair.
7. Proceed with styling as desired.

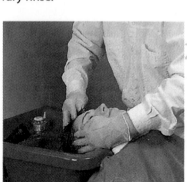

FIGURE 12.29 — Blend rinse through hair.

Cleanup

1. Discard all disposable supplies and materials.
2. Close containers, wipe them off, and store in proper place.
3. Clean and sanitize implements.
4. Organize and sanitize work area.

5. Wash and sanitize hands.
6. Record results and file record card.

Alternate Application Methods

Temporary color is also available in the form of gels, mousses, foams, and sprays. To apply, return the client to your work area and apply color as directed by the manufacturer.

APPLICATION OF SEMI-PERMANENT HAIRCOLORS

Color Selection

The following steps, used in conjunction with the manufacturer's color chart, offer a guide to selecting the correct color with which to perform a strand test:

Note: *Semi-permanent tints containing aniline derivatives require a patch test. Follow the manufacturer's directions carefully.*

1. On solid hair (no unpigmented hair) select a level of semi-permanent color that is two levels lighter than the desired shade. (For unpigmented coverage, see chart on page 341.)
2. Due to the absorption of light, the use of an ash or cool shade will create a color that the eye interprets as darker than if a warm shade is applied.
3. Due to the reflection of light, the warm colors will appear shinier.

The addition of artificial color molecules to the natural pigment of the hair shaft will create a color that is darker than the sample on the color chart. Most color charts show the approximate color that will be achieved on white hair. This color is to be used as a guide to estimate the color results when it is applied to natural hair.

The natural hair color must be considered as half the formula. Think of it as half artificial color and half natural color. Semi-permanent colors lack the strong oxidizers necessary to lift; therefore they deposit color and do no substantial lifting. Think back to laws of intensity and remember that color applied on top of color makes a darker color.

Since these products "take" based on the hair's porosity, be cautious to avoid creating ends that are darker than the base of the hair. Semi-permanent colors, due to their depositing nature, may also build up on the hair's ends with subsequent applications. A strand test will determine your formula and timing before each service.

Many semi-permanent colors are used just as they pour from the bottle. However, others require the mixing of an activator prior to application. This activator is an oxidant that helps to swell the cortex and open the cuticle for color penetration. This mild oxidizer also develops the color pigments within the formula.

Some semi-permanent colors include a color balancer in the packaging. This crystal need be added only if the semi-permanent color is to be applied immediately following the removal of a lightening or bleaching product. It stops the residual oxidation that occurs on the hair shaft until the normal pH is completely restored.

Some semi-permanent colors come packaged with an after-rinse. This rinse is acid balanced to close the cuticle and trap the color molecules within it. This helps prevent fading to a lighter color as well as fading off-tone. The chemical composition of the after-rinse is designed to leave the hair soft, pliable, and easy to comb. Whether or not the product you select is packaged in this way, it is always a good idea to finish your service with a mild conditioning rinse.

Implements and Materials

Neck strip	Applicator bottle or brush
Finishing rinse	Towels
Plastic cap (optional)	Plastic clips
Tint cape	Cotton
Protective cream	Protective gloves
Mild shampoo	Record card
Comb	Selected color
Color chart	Timer

Preliminary Steps

1. Give preliminary patch test if required. Proceed only if test is negative.
2. Thoroughly analyze hair and scalp. Record results on client's record card.
3. Assemble all necessary supplies.
4. Prepare client. Protect clothing with a towel and tint cape. Ask client to remove jewelry and put safely away.
5. Apply protective cream around hairline and over ears.
6. Put on protective gloves.

7. Perform a strand test.
8. Record results on client's card.

Procedure

1. Give a mild shampoo, if required.
2. Towel dry hair.
3. Put on protective gloves.
4. Apply semi-permanent tint to entire hair shaft (Fig. 12.30), starting near the scalp and gently working color through ends. (Fig. 12.31) Apply with bottle or brush according to the consistency of the color selected and your instructor's directions. (Fig. 12.32)

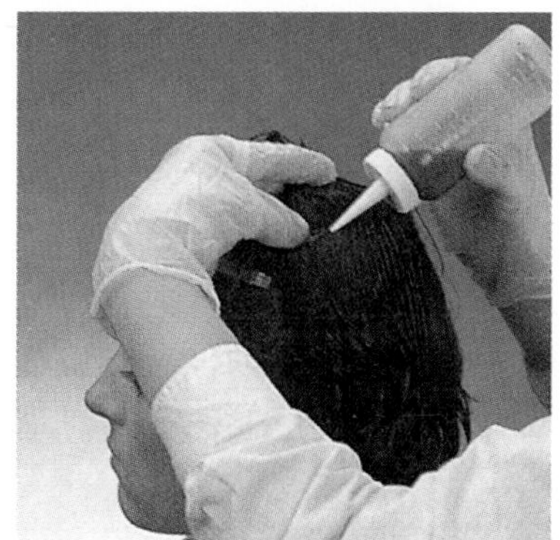

FIGURE 12.30 — Apply semi-permanent color.

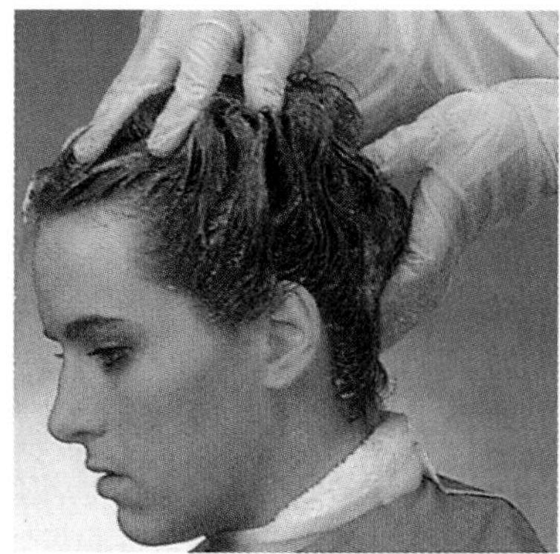

FIGURE 12.31 — Gently work color through.

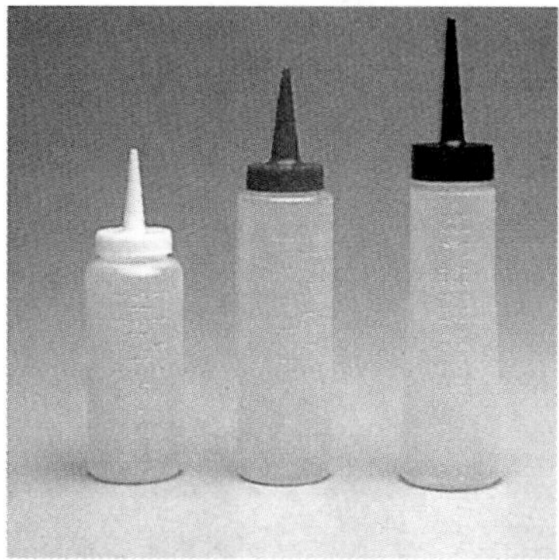

FIGURE 12.32 — Tint applicator bottles.

5. Pile hair loosely on top of head.
6. Follow the manufacturer's directions about using a plastic cap or heat. (Fig. 12.33)
7. Process according to strand test results.
8. According to the timing instructions provided by the manufacturer, when color has developed, wet hair with warm water and lather.
9. Rinse, then shampoo, if the manufacturer recommends it, then rinse again with warm water until water is clear. (Fig. 12.34)

10. Use a finishing rinse to close the cuticle and set color. (Fig. 12.35)
11. Rinse and towel blot hair. Style as desired.
12. Complete record card and file.

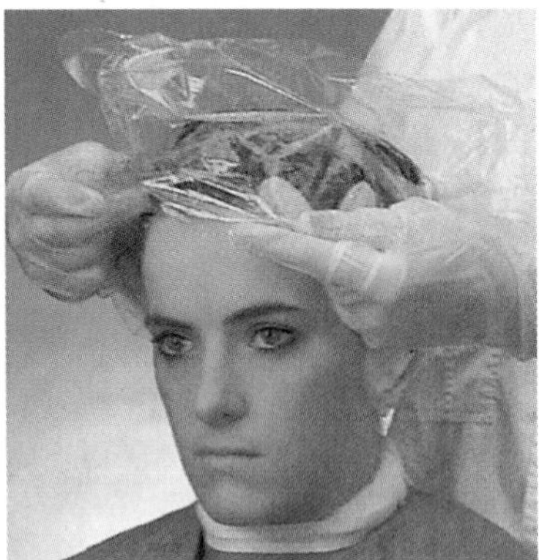

FIGURE 12.33 — Use plastic cover if required.

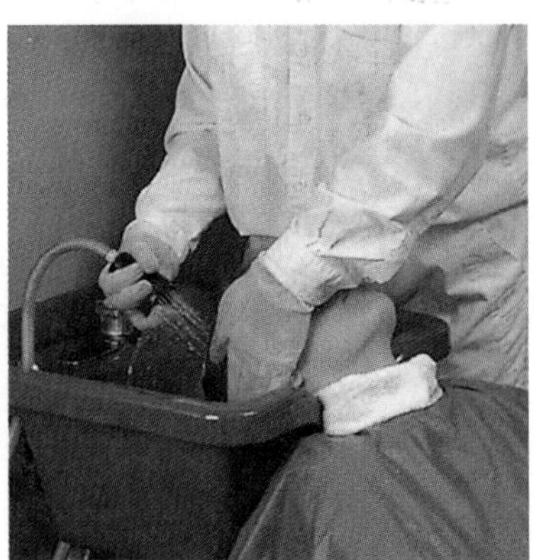

FIGURE 12.34 — Rinse hair with warm water until water is clear.

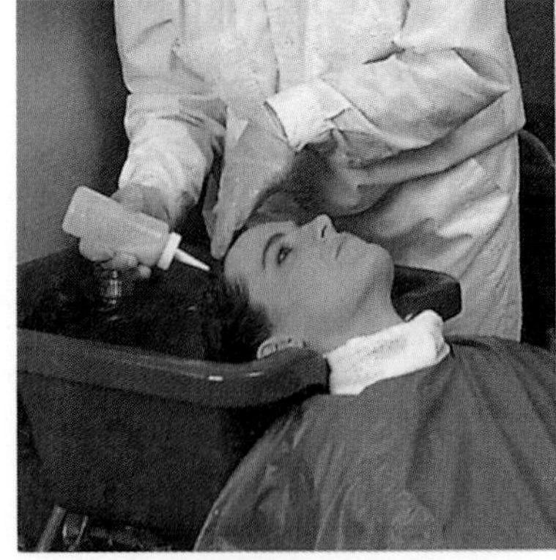

FIGURE 12.35 — Give a finishing rinse.

Cleanup

1. Discard all disposable supplies and materials.
2. Close containers, wipe them off, and store safely.
3. Clean and sanitize implements, tint cape, work area, and hands.

APPLICATION OF DEPOSIT-ONLY HAIRCOLORS

Color Selection

Deposit-only haircolors are ideal for unpigmented coverage, to refresh faded permanent tints, for corrective coloring and reverse highlighting, and for depositing tonal changes without lift.

By its very nature, a deposit-only haircolor will darken the natural hair color when applied. Remember when formulating that half of your formula will be the client's natural hair color and half will be the depositing color you have selected. Since color on top of color always appears darker, select a deposit-only color lighter than the client's natural level if your intent is to keep the same amount of depth but add tone.

Since unpigmented hair is absent of pigment and appears lighter, it is important to consider the unpigmented hair in your formulation of a deposit-only haircolor. As there is no lift, the resulting depth of color when covering unpigmented hair may appear too extreme unless you allow for some brightness in your formulation. It is often inadvisable to make unpigmented hair one even shade when coloring with any product, since natural hair color has different depths and tonalities that give the hair the added life that unpigmented hair is lacking. (Since there is no lifting ability with deposit-only haircolors, use the chart for semi-permanent colors on page 341 when selecting color.)

When taking a client from lighter to darker, it is always better to err on the side of lightness. A darker tone can easily be used to deepen the color if necessary. A too-dark result, on the other hand, will involve corrective procedures to lighten or remove the artificial pigment before reapplying to achieve the desired color.

Hair previously treated with another color service will have a greater degree of porosity, which must be considered carefully when formulating and applying a deposit-only haircolor.

Procedure

The application procedure for a deposit-only haircolor is similar to that of a semi-permanent color, since both colors do not alter the hair's natural melanin or produce lift. Follow the manufacturer's application and timing guidelines for the product that you have selected.

WORKING WITH PERMANENT COLORS

The formulation for lift and deposit of a permanent oxidative haircolor is based on the product you select. Always follow manufacturers' guidelines to obtain the precise amount of lifting of natural pigment (in order to create the proper degree of contributing pigment), as well as the correct amount of depositing pigment (in order to enhance or conceal the newly created undertone), to produce your final desired result.

The colorist adds the oxidizing agent, hydrogen peroxide, that activates the chemical reaction known as oxidation. This reaction, which occurs at an alkaline pH, is created to a great extent by the ammonia in the tint and begins as soon as the two compounds are combined. For this reason, the mixed tint must be used immediately. Any leftover tint must be discarded since it deteriorates quickly.

Timing the application of the tint depends upon the product and the volume of peroxide selected. The general rule is the higher the working volume of hydrogen peroxide used in your formula, the longer the color has to process. Consult the manufacturer's directions and your instructor for assistance. A test strand should always be taken to ensure satisfactory results.

Most oxidative tints contain aniline derivatives and require a predisposition test before the service. As long as the hair is of normal strength and kept in good condition, oxidative tints are compatible with other professional chemical services.

Uses of Hydrogen Peroxide in Haircoloring

The majority of permanent coloring products use 20 volume hydrogen peroxide for proper color development. Those that recommend the use of 40 volume are designed to achieve a greater breakdown of melanin, resulting in a lighter color than may be achieved with a standard lightening tint formula.

Formulas recommending the use of less than 20 volume are designed to allow more deposit than lift. Such formulas may be used when there is no need for breakdown of melanin to achieve the desired color.

> **CAUTION**
>
> *Increasing the strength or volume used in a formula beyond the manufacturer's recommended directions may cause excessive damage to the hair and chemical burns to the skin and scalp.*

It is especially risky to mix the higher levels of hydrogen peroxide with bleach formulated for use with 20 volume because the ingredients in the product itself, such as boosters, activators, or protinators, also work to increase the strength of the formula. However, a volume lower than 20 will not release enough oxygen to lighten the hair properly.

As the volumes of oxygen gas in any strength of hydrogen peroxide are set free, it reverts to water (H_2O). This is considered an advantage, because no dangerous residue is formed and left behind to damage the hair.

Most hydrogen peroxide solutions are packaged in opaque bottles because light causes them to break down. Heat has the same effect. Therefore, the manufacturers recommend storage in a cool, dry place. If stored safely, a stabilized, uncontaminated bottle, either partially or completely full, is expected to retain its quality for up to three years (always check your manufacturer's recommendations).

A ***hydrometer*** can be used to measure the volume of liquid peroxide for the purpose of adjusting its strength or simply confirming that the product is still potent. Occasionally a cap is left off or a product gets pushed to the back of a shelf, and it is best not to assume it is still potent. The hydrometer can also be a money-saving device. It is more economical to purchase the higher volume and dilute it in the salon than to buy an equivalent of prepackaged lower volumes. The hydrometer looks much like a thermometer and must be handled delicately and stored carefully to prevent breakage.

130 Volume Hydrogen Peroxide Chart

For 16 oz. Total Quantity

12½ oz. of H_2O_2 + 3½ oz. of H_2O (water) = 16 oz. of 100 volume H_2O_2

7½ oz. of H_2O_2 + 8½ oz. of H_2O (water) = 16 oz. of 60 volume H_2O_2

6½ oz. of H_2O_2 + 9½ oz. of H_2O (water) = 16 oz. of 50 volume H_2O_2

5 oz. of H_2O_2 + 11 oz. of H_2O (water) = 16 oz. of 40 volume H_2O_2

3½ oz. of H_2O_2 + 12½ oz. of H_2O (water) = 16 oz. of 30 volume H_2O_2

2½ oz. of H_2O_2 + 13½ oz. of H_2O (water) = 16 oz. of 20 volume H_2O_2

1¼ oz. of H_2O_2 + 14¾ oz. of H_2O (water) = 16 oz. of 10 volume H_2O_2

100 Volume Hydrogen Peroxide Dilution Chart

For 10 oz. Total Quantity

6 oz. of H_2O_2 + 4 oz. of H_2O (water) = 10 oz. of 60 volume H_2O_2

5 oz. of H_2O_2 + 5 oz. of H_2O (water) = 10 oz. of 50 volume H_2O_2

4 oz. of H_2O_2 + 6 oz. of H_2O (water) = 10 oz. of 40 volume H_2O_2

3 oz. of H_2O_2 + 7 oz. of H_2O (water) = 10 oz. of 30 volume H_2O_2

2 oz. of H_2O_2 + 8 oz. of H_2O (water) = 10 oz. of 20 volume H_2O_2

1 oz. of H_2O_2 + 9 oz. of H_2O (water) = 10 oz. of 10 volume H_2O_2

It is important to use clean implements in measuring, using, and storing hydrogen peroxide. Even a small amount of dirt or impurity can cause peroxide to deteriorate, and can cause inconsistent color results. Once hydrogen peroxide is poured from its original container, it should not be returned to the original or another stock bottle. Never measure the needed amount of hydrogen peroxide by pouring it into the lid of another product. The residue will cause the container to oxidize as it sits on the shelf, thus making it unusable. Product frothing, a popping or hissing sound when opening the bottle, or a bulging or rounded bottle, signals peroxide that has begun to break down or deteriorate.

Contact with any metal (whether from metallic haircoloring products, a metal clip, or mixing bowl) has an adverse reaction on hydrogen peroxide and should be avoided. Metal speeds up the release of the oxygen molecules, and can cause hydrogen peroxide to oxidize the product. It will then lose strength before it can penetrate the cuticle and cortical layers, reach the melanin, and allow for proper color development.

Action of Oxidative Tints

Application of an oxidizing tint in an alkaline state causes the hair shaft to swell and the cuticle to open. The molecules of the tint base, before mixing with the oxidizer, are very small and can pass easily through the cuticle and into the cortex of the hair shaft. As the oxidation process begins, the coupling together of these small colorless tint-base molecules changes them into large chains of colored, relatively stable pigment. These molecules become trapped beneath the cuticle as they are now too large to be shampooed out. They form acid bonds with the keratin chains in the cortex and become part of the hair structure.

Application Classifications

Permanent haircolor applications are classified as either *single-process coloring* or *double-process coloring.*

Single-process tints have the ability to both lighten and deposit pigment at one time to achieve the desired color. Lightening of the hair's natural pigment and depositing of the artificial pigment in the cortex is done simultaneously as the haircoloring product processes. Some examples of single-process coloring are virgin tint applications and tint retouch applications. Prelightening or presoftening is not required.

Single-process tints usually contain a lightening agent, a shampoo, an aniline derivative tint, and an alkalizing agent to activate the peroxide that is added. Most color is formulated to be used with 20 volume peroxide. Color results are altered when other volumes are used.

The advantages of single-process tints are that they:

1. Can produce shades from the deepest black to the lightest blonde.
2. Can color the hair lighter or darker than the client's original shade.
3. Can blend white or unpigmented hair to a natural hair shade.
4. Can correct streaks, off-shades, discolorations, and faded ends.
5. Are available as creams, liquids, and gels.

Completed: Learning Objective #5

SINGLE- AND DOUBLE-PROCESS APPLICATIONS

Double-process coloring achieves the desired color upon completion of two separate product applications. It is also known as double-application tinting and two-step coloring. Two examples are bleaching followed by a toner application and presoftening followed by a tint application. Because the lightening action and the color deposit are independently controlled, a wider range of haircolor possibilities is opened up for each client.

Selecting the Color

Manufacturers currently offer liquid haircoloring products that use an American "Shades System," and also cream or gel colors that are based on the European "Level System." If the client wants to go darker, simply select the desired level of oxidative tint (the tonal value may have to be adjusted, depending upon the client's current hair color), mixed with 10 or 20 volume developer (based on your test strand results), and proceed with the service.

If your client wants to go lighter, you will select the correct level of color for ***lift*** and ***deposit*** based upon which manufacturer's system you will be using (Shade or Level System). Remember that tint does not lift tint. A color remover product must first be used to lighten the tinted hair before applying the final color formula.

For the ***American Shades of Lift System,*** you would subtract the present level from the desired level. For example, if your client's natural color is a level 6 dark blonde, and the shade desired is a level 8 light blonde, you would use an oxidative tint that is 2 levels lighter (8-6=2) than the desired color to achieve the desired lift. (Remember to formulate for the contributing warmth into your depositing tone.) Always refer to the manufacturer's color selection chart accompanying your product for help in formulating properly.

In the ***European Level System***, the color level you choose is the color you will use (but not necessarily the same tone). The lift is determined by the choice of developer. For example, 10 volume developer is for deposit with minimal (up to 1 level) lift; 20 volume is the most recommended strength for adequate deposit and up to 2 levels of lift; 30 volume is for approximately 3 levels of lift; and 40 volume is for 4 levels of lift. Some manufacturers offer haircoloring additives to "boost" the color an extra level. In doing so they create lift but lose depositing pigment, which may result in inadequate refinement of the natural underlying (contributing) pigment. This could produce considerably more warmth than desired. If a client wishes to be a color more than 2 levels lighter, the end tonal result will be warm. Beyond 4 to 5 levels from the natural hair color, most manufacturers recommend a double-process lightening product to achieve the correct balance of lift and deposit.

The more lifting ability a haircolor has, the less depositing ability of the base color. Always remember to formulate with both lift and deposit in mind, to achieve the proper balance for the desired end result. A higher lifting formula than necessary may not have enough depositing tonality to subdue the warmth of a client's natural contributing pigment. Lift and deposit can further be influenced by varying the volume of hydrogen peroxide mixed with the haircolor product. (Fig. 12.36)

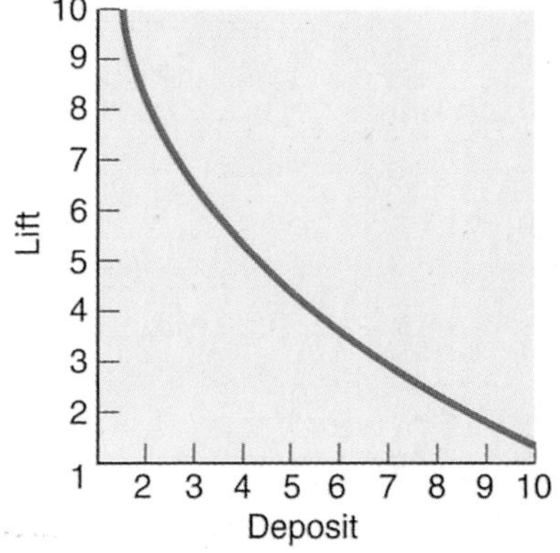

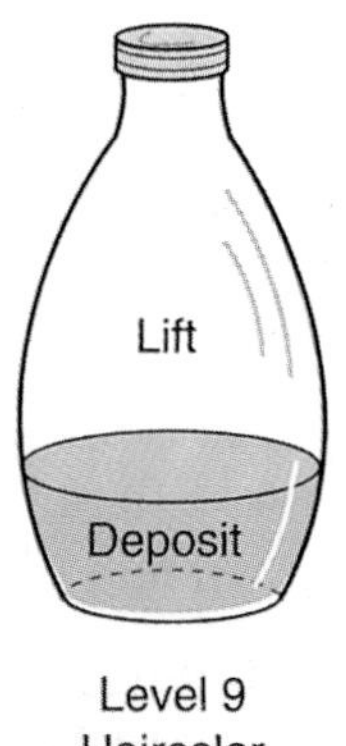

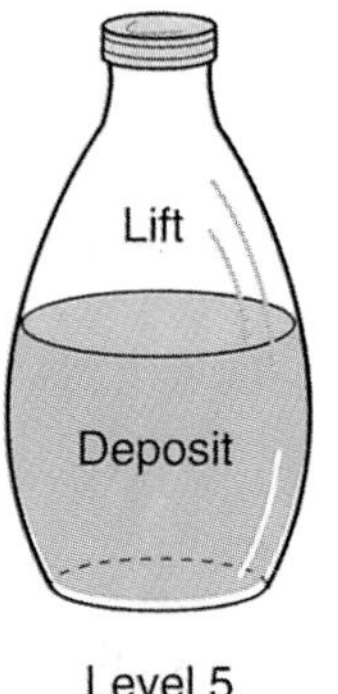

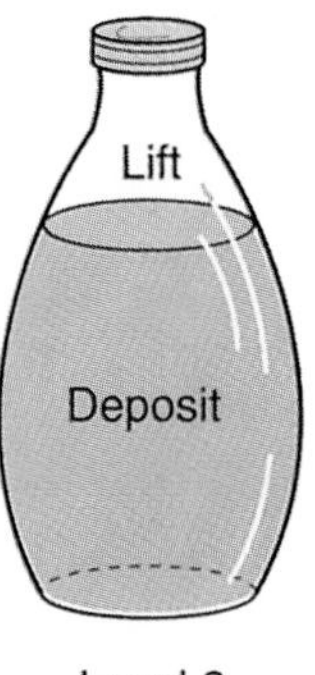

FIGURE 12.36 — Lift and deposit ratios.

Mixing Permanent Colors

Permanent color is usually applied in one of two ways: by use of an applicator bottle or by the bowl-and-brush method. Each has its own mixing procedure.

Applicator bottle: Measure into a clear applicator bottle (markings for ounces or milliliters are generally provided on the side by the manufacturer) an amount of color product sufficient to saturate hair in the areas of the head to be colored. Add the appropriate volume and consistency of developer. Be sure to select an applicator bottle large enough to accommodate both the color product and developer, with enough "air" space to shake the bottle until the mixture is thoroughly blended.

Brush-and-bowl: Using a nonmetallic mixing receptacle (glass or plastic bowl will do), add the color or colors selected by your test strand in the appropriate proportions to create the lift and tonal deposit desired. Measure and slowly add the developer (generally cream consistency for added thickness and control during application). Stir into mixture using a tint applicator brush until thoroughly blended.

Single-Process Haircolor Application

Virgin hair is hair that has had no chemical services and has not been damaged by natural factors such as wind and sun. The procedure that follows is a basic single-process color procedure for virgin hair. Your instructor may have another technique just as correct for the particular color used.

Implements and Materials

Towels	Tint cape
Protective gloves	Comb
Applicator bottle or brush	Plastic or glass bowl
Timer	Mild shampoo
Selected tint	Cotton
Color chart	Finishing rinse
Record card	Hydrogen peroxide
Protective cream	

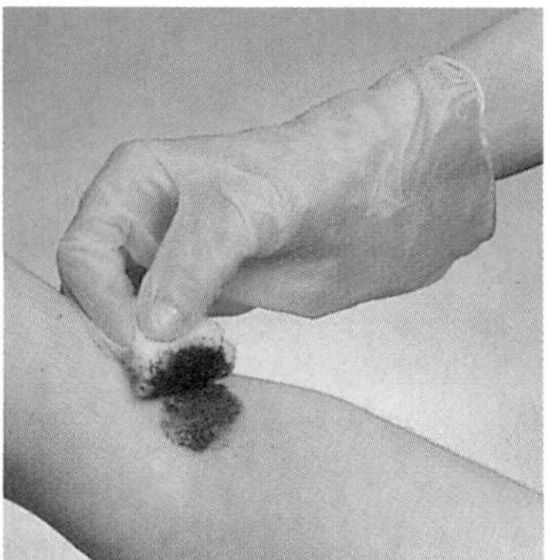

FIGURE 12.37 — Give patch test.

Preliminary Steps

1. Give patch test 48 hours before the service. (Fig. 12.37) Proceed only if test is negative. (Fig. 12.38)
2. Thoroughly analyze scalp and hair. Perform any necessary preconditioning treatments, and record results on client's record card.

3. Assemble all necessary supplies.
4. Prepare client. Protect clothing with a towel and tint cape. Ask client to remove all jewelry and place safely away.
5. Apply protective cream around hairline and over ears.
6. Put on protective gloves.
7. Perform a strand test.
8. Record results on record card.

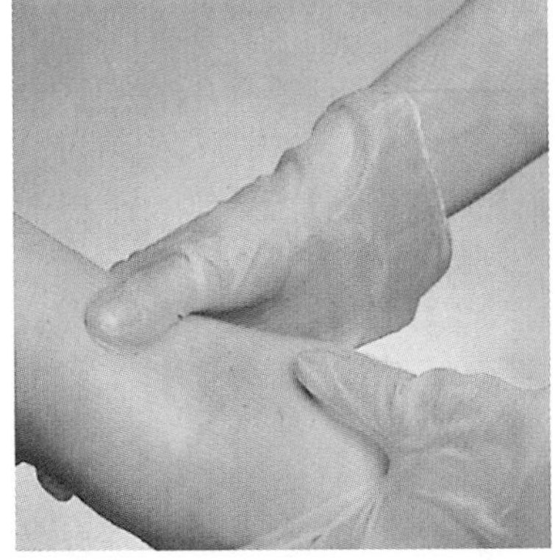

FIGURE 12.38 — Proceed if test is negative.

Procedure

1. Section the hair into four quarters. (Fig. 12.39)
2. Prepare tint formula for either bottle or brush application. (Fig. 12.40)
3. Begin in section where color change will be greatest or hair is most resistant. (Fig. 12.41)
4. Part off ¼" (.6 cm) subsection with applicator.
5. Lift subsection and apply tint to hair ½" (1.25 cm) from scalp up to, but not through, the porous ends. (Fig. 12.42)

Note: *The hair at the scalp will process faster due to body heat and incomplete keratinization. For this reason the tint is applied in the scalp area after being applied to the shaft. Your strand test will determine the application procedure and timing for even color development.*

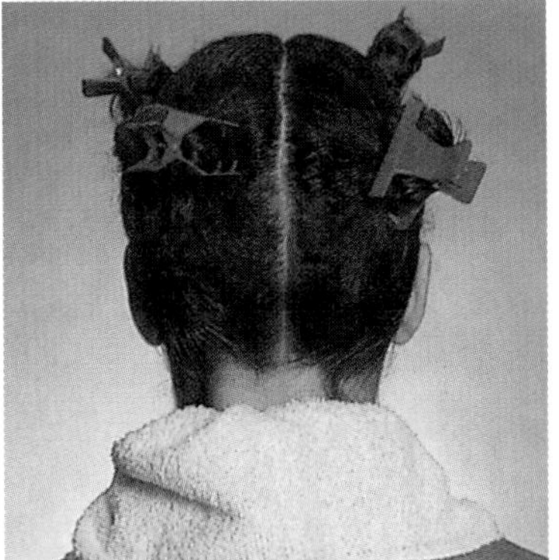

FIGURE 12.39 — Section hair into four quarters.

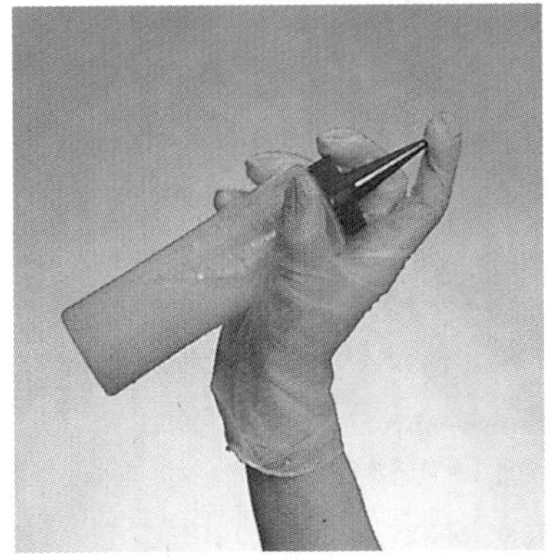

FIGURE 12.40 — Prepare and mix tint formula.

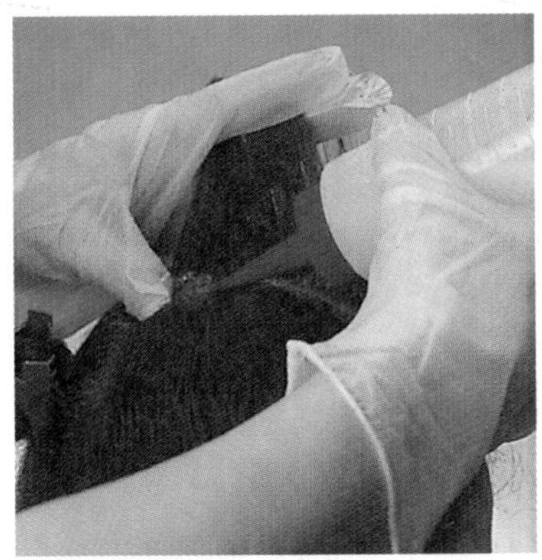

FIGURE 12.41 — Begin applying color.

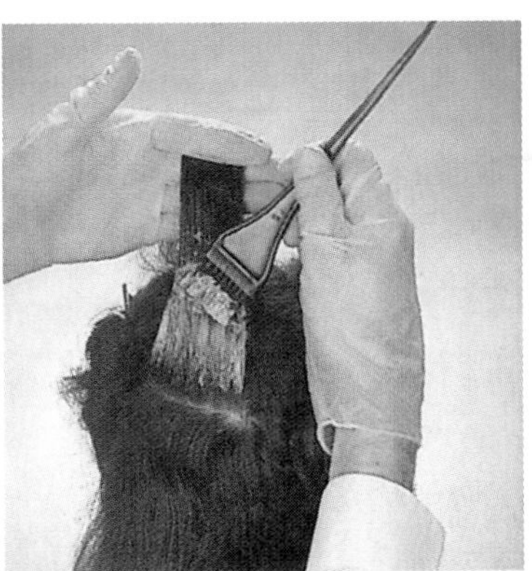

FIGURE 12.42 — Apply tint to the hair ends.

6. Process according to strand test results. Check for color development by removing color as described in the strand test procedure.
7. Apply tint mixture to hair at scalp.
8. Blend tint to hair ends. (Fig. 12.43)
9. Lightly rinse with lukewarm water. Massage color to lather and rinse thoroughly.
10. Remove any stains around hairline with remaining tint mixture, shampoo, or stain remover. Use cotton or terry towel to gently remove stains.
11. Shampoo hair thoroughly with a mild (acid-balanced) shampoo.
12. Apply an acid or a finishing rinse to close the cuticle, restore pH, and prevent fading.
13. Style hair.
14. Complete record card and file.

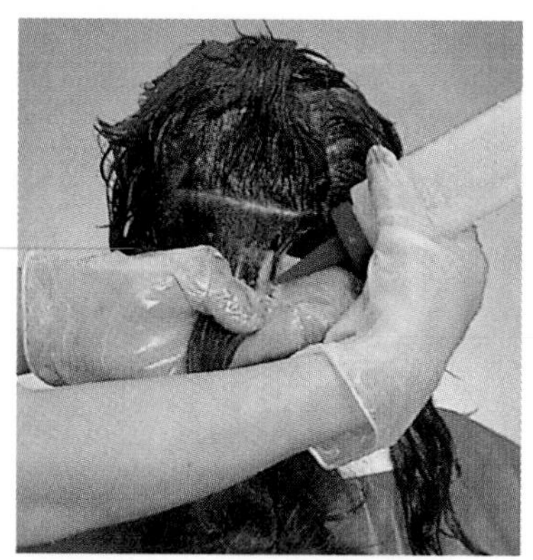

FIGURE 12.43 — Blend tint to hair ends.

Cleanup

1. Discard all disposable supplies and materials.
2. Close containers tightly, wipe them off, and put them in their proper places.
3. Clean and sanitize implements.
4. Sanitize tint cape.
5. Sanitize work area.
6. Wash and sanitize hands.

Coloring Darker

When tinting close to or darker than natural hair color, follow the same preparation and procedure as for a lighter shade. Then proceed as follows:

Procedure

1. Select appropriate color.
2. Application begins where the hair is the most resistant. (If unpigmented hair is present, application most likely will begin in the front. If no unpigmented hair is evident, then begin in the back.)

3. Apply tint from scalp to the porous ends using ¼" (.6 cm) subpartings.
4. Process according to strand test results.
5. When color has developed to desired degree, distribute the tint through the ends with a large-toothed comb to ensure complete coverage.
6. Continue processing according to strand test results.
7. Shampoo color off and complete styling and cleanup in usual manner.

Long Hair Application

The same preparation and procedure are used for long hair as for short hair. Condition the ends according to your analysis. You will probably need more color material than you used for short hair.

Single-Process Tint Retouch Application

As the hair grows, you will need to do a retouch so the hair looks attractive and not two-toned. After you assemble the materials and implements as for a virgin tint, follow the procedure below.

Preliminary Steps

1. Give a patch test 48 hours before the service. Proceed only if test is negative.
2. Assemble all necessary supplies.
3. Prepare client. Protect clothing with a towel and tint cape. Ask client to remove all jewelry and put safely away.
4. Take out client 's record card. Consult with client to see if she or he liked the original color. Carefully analyze hair and condition previously tinted hair as needed.
5. Apply protective cream around hairline and over ears.
6. Perform a strand test.
7. Record all results on record card.

Procedure

1. Section the hair into four quarters.
2. Prepare tint formula.
3. Begin in section where color was begun in the virgin application.

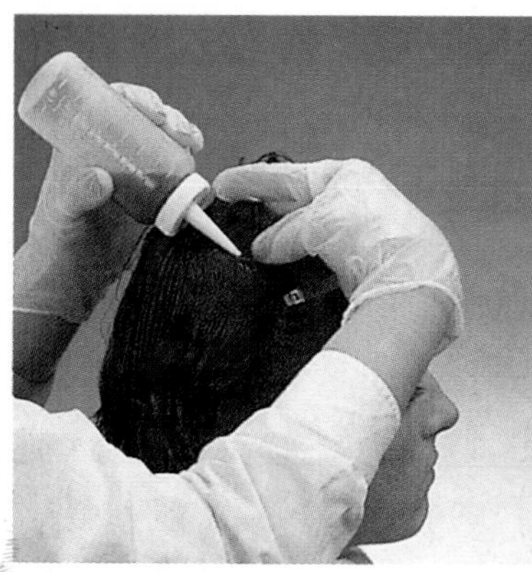

FIGURE 12.44 — Apply tint up to new growth only.

4. Part off ¼" (.6 cm) subsection with applicator.
5. Apply tint to new growth only. (Fig. 12.44) Do not overlap. Overlapping of color can cause breakage and create lines of demarcation.
6. Confirm color development by strand testing.
7. Apply diluted color formula to ends according to your analysis and strand test results. Dilute the remaining tint mixture with distilled water, shampoo, or conditioner. (This step is done only if color is faded.)
8. Lightly rinse with lukewarm water. Massage color to lather and rinse thoroughly.
9. Remove any stains around hairline with remaining tint mixture, shampoo, or stain remover. Use cotton to gently remove stains.
10. Shampoo hair thoroughly with a mild (acid-balanced) shampoo.
11. Apply an acid or a finishing rinse to close the cuticle, restore pH, and prevent fading.
12. Style hair.
13. Complete record card and file.
14. Clean up in the usual manner.

Double-Process Tint

If the client desires a drastically lighter color, the hair should first be prelightened. It is sometimes much more efficient to use a double-process application to achieve pale or cool colors. This avoids the warm undertones the hair contributes from the lightening process, which a single-process tint may not be able to overcome. Remember, the higher the amount of lift in the tint, the less pigment deposit. By decolorizing the hair with a lightener and using a separate product to add the desired tonality, you have more control over the coloring process.

It is also possible to have the hair's contributing pigment work for you in a double-process coloring application. By prelightening the hair to the desired degree of decolorization, you can create a perfect foundation for longer lasting red colors that stay true to tone, without muddiness.

The prelightener is applied in the same manner as for a regular hair lightening treatment. After the prelightening has reached the desired shade, the hair is lightly shampooed, acidified, and towel dried. The color is then applied in the usual manner after a strand test has been taken.

HAIR LIGHTENING

Hair lightening, removing pigment from the hair, is always a popular salon service. Changing styles determine if the entire head is lightened, or just one area, or if a special effect is created. Lighter strands draw attention to the individual. (Fig. 12.45)

Lighteners may be used for two purposes:

1. As a color treatment, to lighten the hair to the final shade.
2. As a preliminary treatment, to prepare the hair for the application of a toner or tint (double-process application).
   a) Toner: A lightener is always necessary before applying delicate toner shades.
   b) Tint: If the client desires a shade much lighter than the natural shade, a lightener can be used to remove some color before the tint is applied.

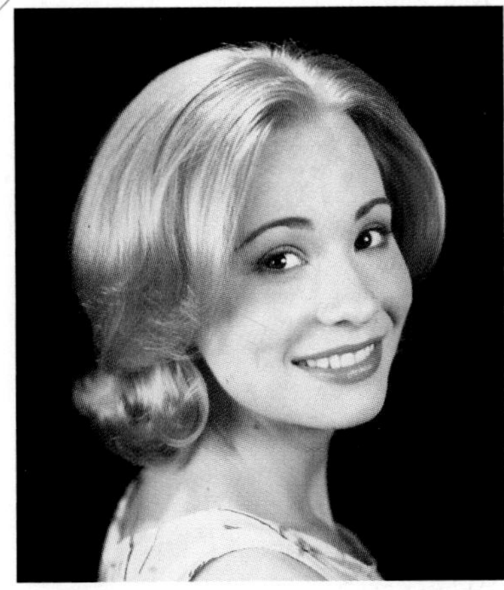

FIGURE 12.45 — Special-effects hair lightening.

Lightening creates a desired color foundation. This new color foundation may be the finished result, or it may be the first step of a double-process application. Before beginning the lightening process, it is important to understand that achieving the desired shade requires that you consider the virgin hair color, how long the product should be left on to achieve the desired stage of lightening, the resulting porosity of the hair shaft, and the selection of the appropriate product that will achieve the desired color foundation.

The hair becomes more porous during the lightening treatment, a condition necessary to permit penetration of a toner. Even naturally light hair or unpigmented hair may need a pre-lightening process in order to achieve the necessary degree of porosity for the acceptance of a toner or tint.

Hair lighteners, used according to the manufacturer's directions, can:

1. Lighten the entire head of hair for toner application.
2. Lighten hair to a particular shade.
3. Brighten and lighten existing shade.
4. Lighten only certain parts of the hair.
5. Lighten hair that has already been tinted.
6. Remove undesirable casts and off-shades.
7. Correct dark streaks or spots in lightened or tinted hair.

> **CAUTION**
>
> *Clients with dark hair may not be able to be lightened to a very pale blonde color without extreme damage to their hair.*

TYPES OF LIGHTENERS

Today's colorists have at their disposal three basic types of lighteners: oil, cream, and powder. Each classification has unique abilities, chemical characteristics, and formulation procedures.

Oil Bleaches

Oil bleaches are the mildest of the three types of lighteners and have the least amount of lightening action. This product is appropriate when only one or two levels of color lift are desired. Oil bleaches are generally milder than some high-lifting oxidative dyes when mixed with higher volumes of hydrogen peroxide. Oil bleach can be used as a single-application color to achieve moderate color change of the entire head or in a weaving to achieve a very subtle color change. It is also a popular product for presoftening resistant unpigmented hair prior to a tinting service. Because oil bleach is so mild, it is used professionally to lighten excessively dark facial and body hair.

Cream Lighteners

Cream lighteners are the most popular type because they are easy to apply and do not run, drip, or dry out easily. The weak hydrogen peroxide and ammonia solution of cream bleaches is strong enough to do pastel blonding, but gentle enough to be used on the scalp.

The benefits of cream lighteners are:

1. Conditioning agents give some protection to the hair and scalp.
2. Bluing agents help to drab gold tones.
3. Thickeners give more control during application.
4. Cream does not run or drip, which helps prevent overlapping during retouch.

Many manufacturers add a drabber to reduce brassy tones. Green, blue, and violet are effective, because these tones on the color wheel are complementary to and may help neutralize some of the red, orange, gold, and yellow tones that naturally occur as the melanin goes through decolorization. Other manufacturers prefer to leave their lighteners a pure white in color so that the colorist can monitor the lightening process without wiping the product off.

Cream lighteners are generally mixed with *accelerators*, sometimes called boosters, protinators, or activators, in the form of dry crystals to increase the lifting power. The greater the number of protinators, the greater the strength of the formula:

- 0 activator—formula comparable to oil bleach in mildness
- 1 activator—will lighten light brown hair
- 2 activators—will lighten medium to dark brown hair
- 3 activators—will lighten resistant dark brown hair
- 4 activators—equivalent of powder bleach; not used on scalp

The manufacturer's recommended amount of booster has the effect of doubling the strength of the hydrogen peroxide solution. It is for this reason that no higher than 20 volume is recommended for on-the-scalp application; this also protects the integrity of the hair fiber.

Powder Bleaches

Powder bleaches, like cream bleaches, are strong enough to do pastel blonding. However, powder bleach cannot be applied to the scalp because it does not contain the oil and conditioners that make a cream lightener safe for on-the-scalp application. Application to the scalp would result in severe skin irritation and possible chemical burns. Powder bleach lighteners are used exclusively for off-the-scalp applications and special effects, such as foil-wrapped weaving, highlighting with plastic caps, and hair painting.

Like oil and cream lighteners, powder bleaches contain ammonia. In this instance, however, it is in a dry form. The ammonia begins the oxidation process when it mixes with liquid or cream hydrogen peroxide.

Powder lighteners, also called quick lighteners, contain oxygen-releasing boosters for quicker and stronger action. They may dry out more quickly, but they do not run or drip. Most powder lighteners expand and spread out as processing continues and should not be used for retouch services. Powder lighteners are recommended for off-the-scalp applications on resistant hair. ✔

Completed:
Learning Objective
#6
TYPES AND USES OF LIGHTENERS

ACTION OF A LIGHTENER

One of the most frequent questions a colorist asks when lightening hair is, "Where does the color go?" It cannot be seen washing down the drain when the bleach is removed, nor does it appear to be absorbed into the bleach. In the early 1960s many cosmetologists were told that the bleaching agent "ate" the natural pigment. This theory was demonstrated and "proved " by the addition of a bottle of tint to a bleach formula. The color tint would disappear before your very eyes!

We now know that the addition of hydrogen peroxide to a bleach formula (the process known as oxidation) occurs within the cortical layer of the hair shaft. The gases crash into the melanin or pigment with enough force to diffuse the molecules of color.

Oxidation Causes Heat

The oxidation process that is occurring within the bleach formula causes heat, and this chemical heat is enhanced by body heat. Therefore, the stronger the chemical formula and the closer it is placed to the scalp, the greater the diffusion of melanin (decolorizing) within the shaft.

As soon as hydrogen peroxide is mixed into the bleach formula, it begins to release oxygen and the volume decreases. This process continues until the product either dries out or releases all available oxygen molecules.

Manufacturers of lighteners produce bleach mixtures in different degrees or strengths in a variety of formulas; but all diffuse, rather than remove, color. The eye interprets this diffusion of color, whether within the hair shaft or in a bowl of bleach to which tint has been added, as a lighter shade.

Structural Changes Caused by Lighteners

Lighteners cause the shaft to swell and lift the cuticle layer to allow penetration to the cortex. When the lightener is removed and the pH of the shaft is restored to normal, the shaft shrinks back down toward its prior size, but never quite reaches it. Some of the cuticle layer remains raised and thus each strand of hair becomes "fatter" or coarser.

Another structural change occurs with the breaking and restructuring of cortical bonds within the shaft. The weakening of these bonds makes the hair more pliable and less resistant. This additional pliability is considered an asset especially in conjunction with competition hair styling, finger waving, sculpture curling, roller setting, and back-combing.

The elasticity of the hair is also altered by lightening, and especially by bleaching. It is the most crucial factor to monitor during the lightening process. Healthy hair will stretch approximately $\frac{1}{5}$ of its length and then bounce back to normal.

If the hair is overlightened, moist strands will stretch more than $\frac{1}{5}$ of their length and not bounce back. They can even be stretched to the point where the hair snaps and breaks. In its dry form, the natural elasticity of over-lightened hair will appear to be decreased. In fact, in this condition, the hair becomes dry, brittle, and can snap just from normal combing and brushing.

With each level of color lift, the hair will exhibit signs of increased dryness, porosity, and pliability. The dryness is easily treated with moisturizers, and the porosity is treated with protein treatments so that the hair retains the benefits of increased pliability without becoming excessively dry, elastic, or porous.

THE DECOLORIZING PROCESS

A lightening product is used to diffuse pigment. (Fig. 12.46) The hair pigment goes through different stages of color as it lightens. The amount of change depends on how much pigment the hair has and the length of time the lightening product is processed.

The Degrees (or Stages) of Decolorizing

During the degrees of ***decolorizing***, hair can go through as many as 10 stages. (Fig. 12.47)

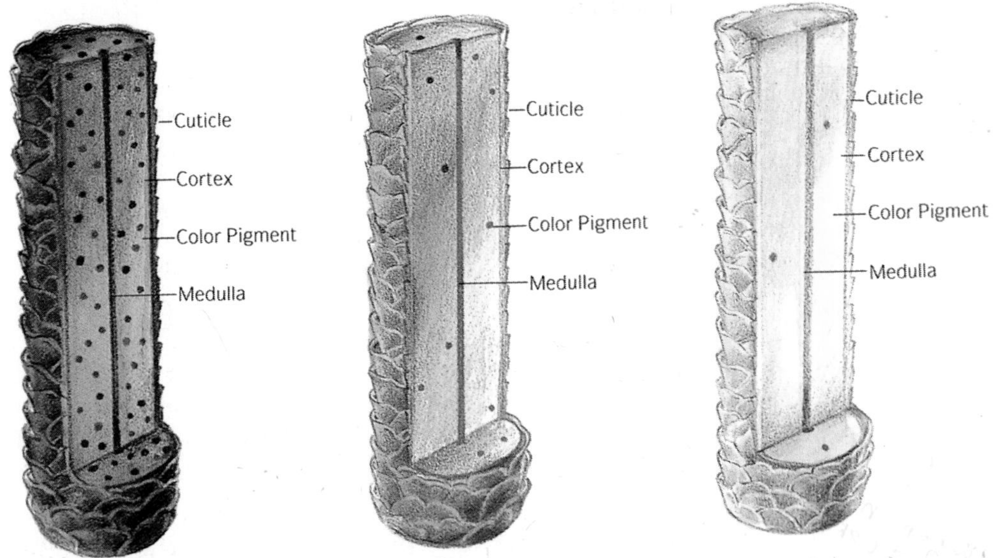

FIGURE 12.46 — Hair lighteners are used to diffuse pigment.

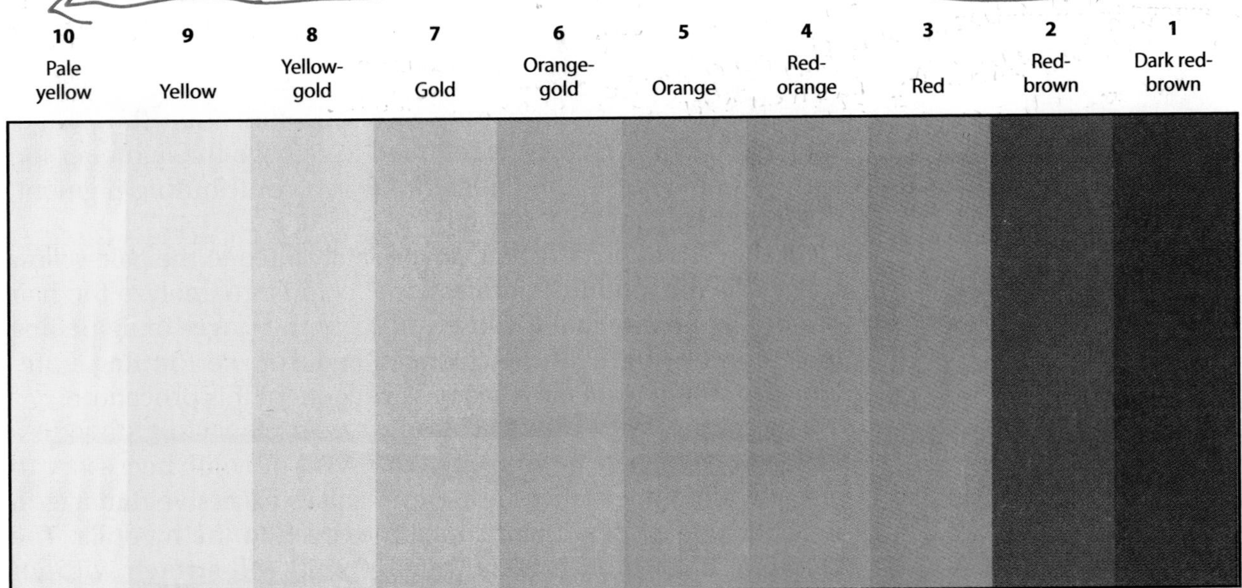

FIGURE 12.47 — Ten degrees of decolorization.

1. Dark Red-Brown
2. Red-Brown
3. Red
4. Red-Orange
5. Orange
6. Orange-Gold
7. Gold
8. Yellow-Gold
9. Yellow
10. Pale Yellow

Contribution of Underlying Pigment

Decolorizing the hair's natural melanin pigment allows the colorist to create the exact degree of contributing pigment needed for the final result. First, the hair is decolorized to the appropriate level. Then, the new color is applied to deposit the desired tonality and intensity. Lightening the hair to the correct degree is absolutely essential to a beautiful, controlled, final haircoloring result because the natural pigment that remains in the hair contributes to the artificial color that is added by the colorist, giving you the final result.

Generally, on-the-scalp lighteners are made to work for up to 2 hours. Since the strongest lightening action takes place within the first 60 minutes, it is sometimes helpful when decolorizing very resistant hair to remove the first lightening mixture after one hour and apply a fresh one.

It is extremely important to be patient. Red-orange (degree 4) and gold (degree 7) require the most decolorization time to get through. Often, a colorist is tempted to remove the lightener too early. When color is then added to warm contributing pigment, the results will not be as desired.

Most heads of healthy hair can be safely lifted to the pale yellow stage. It is the job of the professional colorist to analyze the hair prior to lightening and to closely observe the stages of lightening to determine how light the color can be taken. Performing a preliminary strand test takes the guesswork out of this procedure.

The hair is never safely lifted past the pale yellow stage to a white with bleach. The extreme diffusion of color necessary to give a white appearance to the eye causes excessive damage to the cuticle and cortex, and sometimes even to the medulla. The result is that wet hair feels "mushy" and will stretch without returning to its original length. When dry, the hair will be harsh and brittle. Such hair often suffers breakage and will not accept a toner properly. However, this does not mean that only those born with blonde hair can be a white blonde. The baby-blonde look can be achieved by lightening to pale yellow and neutralizing the unwanted undertone with a toner.

Not all hair will go through all 10 degrees of decolorization. Each natural hair color starts the decolorization process at a different stage. Only black hair will pass through all 10 degrees of lightening to reach pale yellow. Remember, the goal is to create the correct degree of contributing pigment as the foundation for the final haircolor result. (Fig. 12.48)

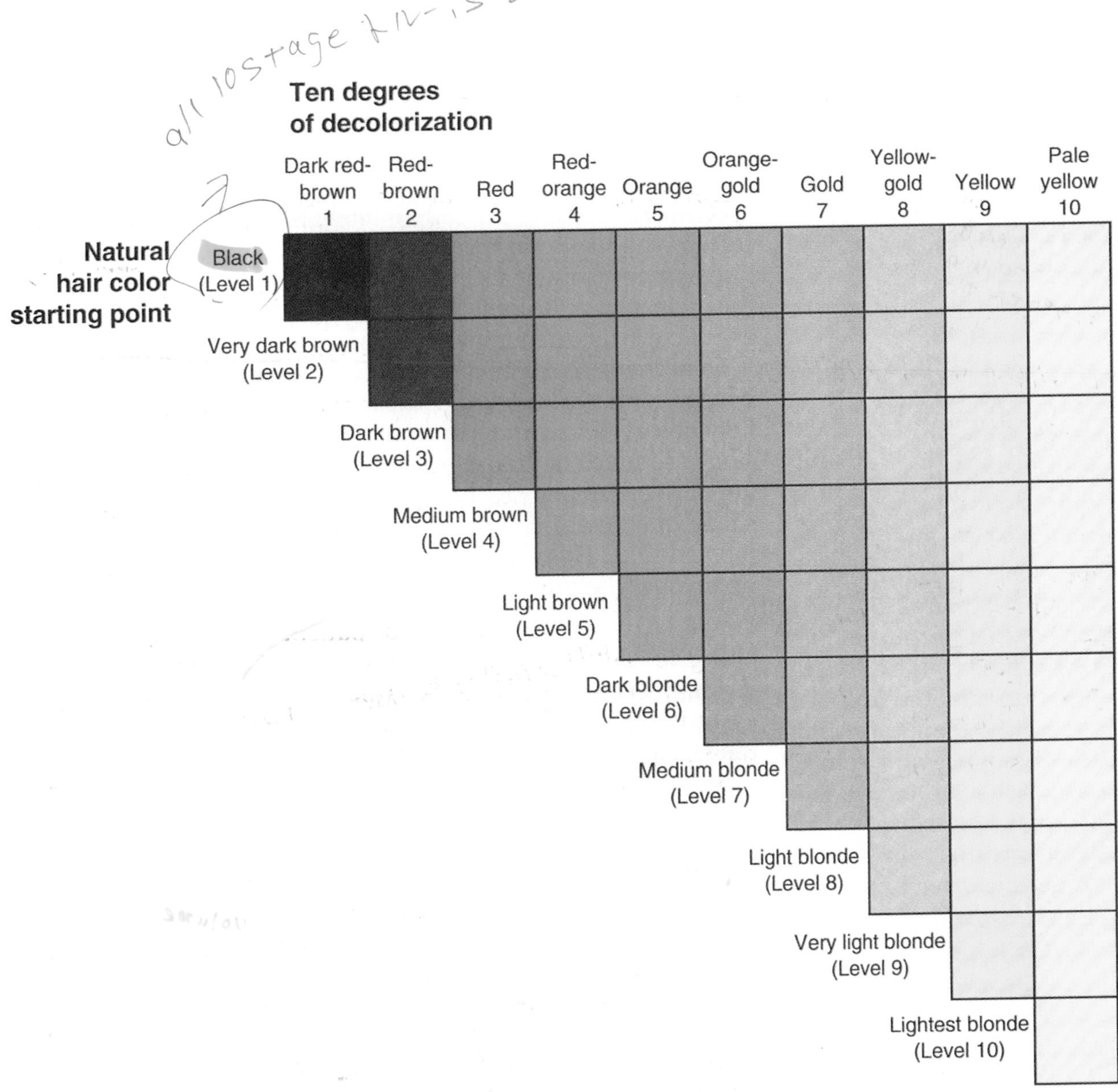

FIGURE 12.48 — Contribution of underlying pigment.

TIME FACTORS

The darker the natural hair color, the more melanin it has. The more melanin it has, the longer it takes to diffuse the color to give a lighter appearance to the hair. The amount of time needed to lighten the natural color is also influenced by the porosity. Porous hair of the same color level will lighten faster than hair that is nonporous because the bleaching agent can enter the cortex more rapidly.

Tone also influences the length of time necessary to lighten the natural hair color. The greater the percentage of red reflected in the natural color, the more difficult it is to achieve the pale, delicate shades of blonde. The ash blondes are especially difficult to achieve because the melanin must be diffused sufficiently to alter both the level and tone of the hair.

The strength of the product also affects the speed and amount of lightening. The stronger bleaches achieve the pale shades in the least amount of time.

Because heat, used in conjunction with lightening chemicals, softens the hair, creating a fragile state, caution must be exercised when using heat. Excessive heat can cause the motion of the molecules to become so great that extreme damage can occur as cuticle layers are removed and cortical bonds are destroyed.

Heat leads to quicker lightening, thus shortening the time needed for decolorization. The stages of lightening must be carefully observed to avoid excessive lift that could lead to the diffusion of so much natural pigment that the desired toner shade may not develop properly in the hair shaft. When this occurs, the toner shade may "grab" the base color, giving the hair an ashy, unpigmented tone. However, beautiful blondes can safely be achieved by anyone with proper analysis, products, and techniques.

LIGHTENING VIRGIN HAIR

A preliminary strand test is necessary before lightening in order to determine the processing time, the condition of the hair after lightening, and the end results. Carefully record all data on the client's record card.

Preliminary Test Results

1. If test shows the hair is not light enough:
   a) Increase strength of mixture, and/or
   b) Increase processing time.
2. If hair strand is too light:
   a) Decrease strength of mixture, and/or
   b) Decrease processing time.

3. Watch strand carefully for reaction to lightening mixture and for discoloration or breakage. Reconditioning may be required prior to toning.
4. If color and condition are good, proceed with lightening.

Note: A patch test must be taken 48 hours prior to the application of a toner containing aniline derivatives. To save the client's time, the strand test for lightening should be made the same day as the patch test.

Implements and Materials

Towels	Comb	Protective gloves
Plastic clips	Tint cape	Plastic or glass bowl
Shampoo	Peroxide	Acid or finishing rinse
Cotton	Record card	Applicator bottle or brush
Lightener	Timer	Protective cream

Procedure

The following general instructions may be changed by your instructor for particular lightening effects or products.

1. Prepare client. Protect client's clothing with towel and tint cape.
2. Analyze scalp and hair, and record on client's card. Do not perform the service if the client has abrasions or inflammation of the scalp.
3. Do not brush hair.
4. Check patch test area if toner is to be used. Proceed only if test results are negative.
5. Section hair into four quarters.
6. Apply protective cream around hairline and over ears.
7. Put on gloves to protect your hands.
8. Prepare lightening formula. Use immediately to prevent deterioration.
9. Apply lightener. Begin application where hair seems resistant or especially dark, usually the back of the head. Use ⅛" (.3125 cm) partings to apply lightener. Start ½" (1.25 cm) from the scalp and extend lightener up to, **but not through,** the porous ends. Apply lightener to top and underside of subsection in quick, rhythmic movements. (Fig. 12.49)

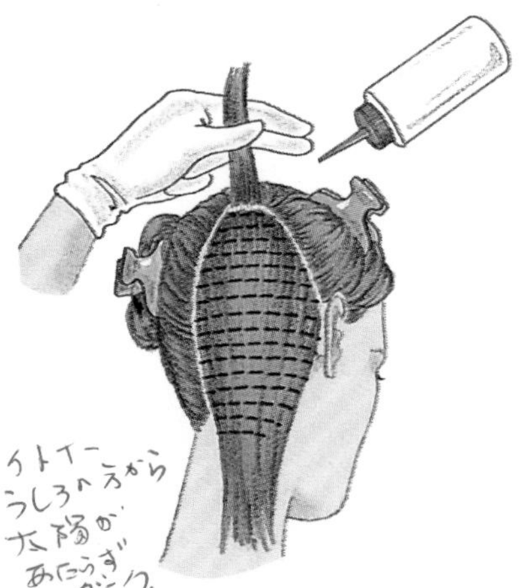

FIGURE 12.49 — Apply lightener to underside of strand.

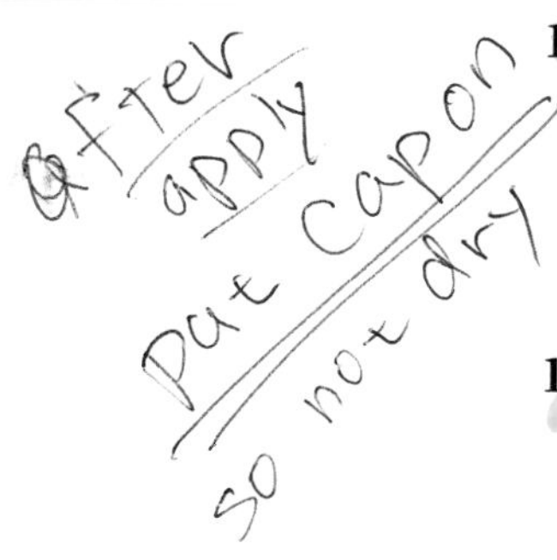

10. Continue to apply lightener. Double check application, adding more lightener if necessary. Do not comb lightener through hair. Keep lightener moist during development by misting the hair lightly with a spray bottle or reapplying lightener as the mixture dries.

11. Test for lightening action. Make first check about 15 minutes before time indicated by preliminary strand test. Remove mixture from strand with damp towel. Towel-dry and examine. If strand is not light enough, reapply mixture and continue testing frequently until desired level is reached.

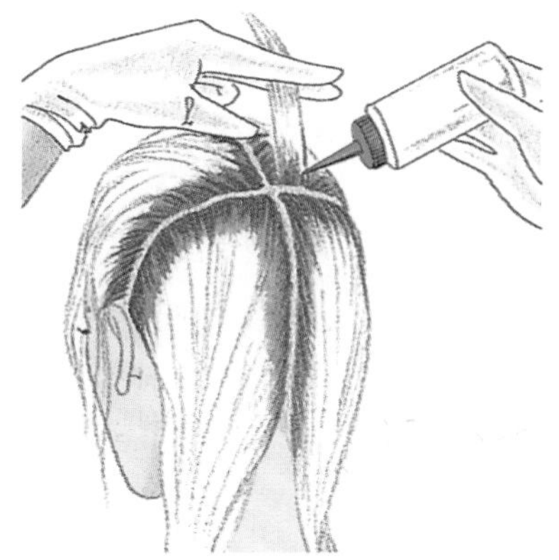

FIGURE 12.50 — Apply lightener at scalp.

12. Apply lightener to hair near scalp with ⅛" (.3125 cm) parting. (Fig. 12.50) If necessary, prepare fresh lightener. Process and strand test until entire shaft has reached desired stage.

13. Remove lightener. Rinse thoroughly with cool water. Shampoo gently with acid-balanced shampoo, with hands under hair to avoid tangling.

14. Neutralize the alkalinity of the hair with an acid or a normalizing rinse. Recondition if necessary.

15. Towel-dry hair, or dry completely under cool dryer if manufacturer requires it.

16. Examine scalp for abrasions. Analyze condition of hair.

17. Proceed with toner application.

18. Complete record card and file.

19. Clean up in usual manner.

LIGHTENER RETOUCH

As the hair grows, dark regrowth will be very obvious. A lightener retouch corrects this problem and matches the regrowth to the rest of the lightened hair. During retouch, the lightener is applied to the new growth only, with the following exceptions:

1. If another color is desired.
2. If a lighter shade is desired.
3. If color has become dull from repeated applications.

In each case, lighten the regrowth first. Then bring remaining lightener mixture gently through the hair shaft. Process for 1 to 5 minutes until problem is corrected.

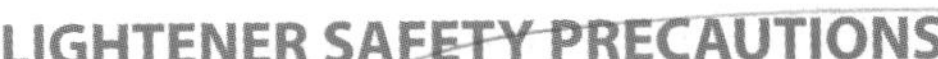

LIGHTENER SAFETY PRECAUTIONS

Always consult the client's record card to tell you about lightener formula, timing, and other pertinent information. The procedure for a lightener retouch is the same as that for lightening a virgin head of hair, except that the mixture is applied only to the new growth of hair. (Figs. 12.51–12.53)

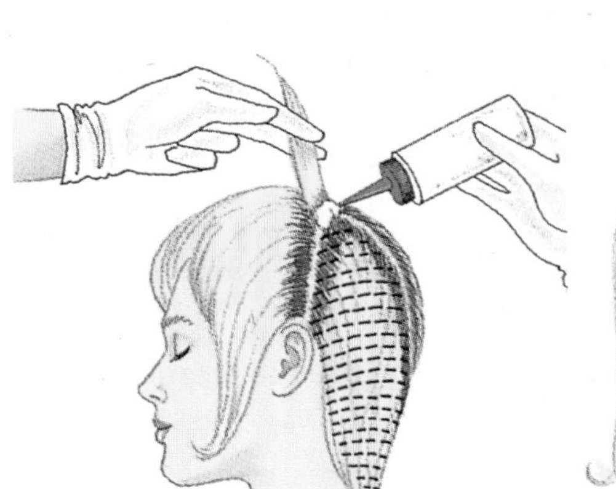

FIGURE 12.51 — Apply lightener to new growth.

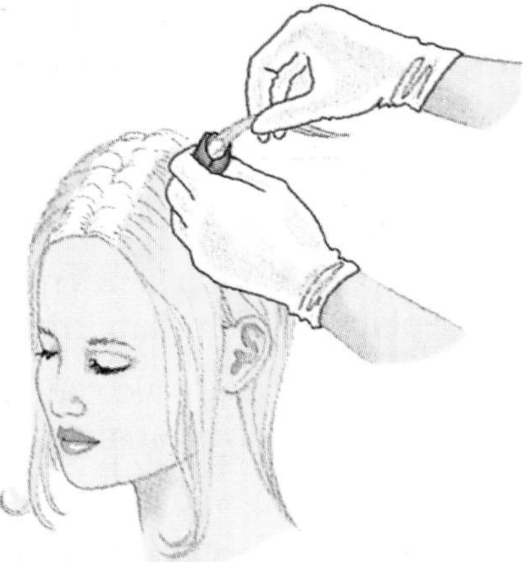

FIGURE 12.52 — Strand testing.

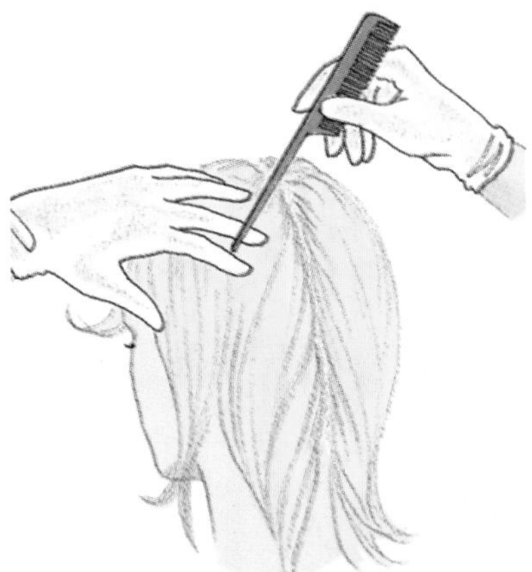

FIGURE 12.53 — Check for complete coverage.

A cream lightener is generally used for a lightener retouch because its consistency helps prevent overlapping of previously lightened hair, and it is gentler on the scalp. Overlapping can cause severe breakage and lines of demarcation.

Procedure

1. Give a patch test 48 hours before toner application.
2. Read manufacturer's directions before preparing lightener.
3. Always wash your hands before and after servicing a client.
4. Drape client properly to protect clothing.
5. Examine scalp carefully. Do not apply lightener if irritation or abrasions are present.
6. Do not brush hair. If shampoo is required, avoid irritating the scalp.
7. Analyze condition of hair and give any necessary reconditioning treatments.
8. Wear protective gloves.
9. Use only sanitized applicators and towels.
10. Conduct strand test prior to lightener retouch.
11. Cream lightener should be the thickness of whipped cream to avoid dripping, running, or overlapping.

12. Always use lightener immediately after mixing. Discard leftover lightener.
13. Apply lightener to resistant areas first. Use ⅛" (.3 cm) partings to ensure accurate coverage.
14. Apply rapidly and neatly for even lightening.
15. Give frequent strand tests until desired stage is reached.
16. Check skin and scalp after application and gently remove any lightener with cool, damp towel.
17. Lightener can be safely left on the scalp area for a maximum of 1 hour.
18. If towel around client's neck becomes saturated, remove and replace to avoid skin irritation.
19. Cool water and mild shampoo should be used to remove lightener. Avoid tangling fragile hair.
20. Cap all bottles to avoid contamination. Store carefully.
21. Complete record card and file.

SPOT LIGHTENING

Uneven lightening, streaking, or dark spots are usually due to careless lightener application. It is necessary to correct these areas to ensure even color. To correct streaked hair:

1. Prepare lightening formula.
2. Apply mixture only to darker areas.
3. Allow mixture to remain on hair until all streaks are removed.
4. Shampoo lightener from hair.

TONERS

Toners are aniline derivative tints and require a 48-hour patch test. They consist of pale and delicate colors, and are applied to the lightest degrees of contributing pigment from the decolorizing process.

Toners require a double-process application. The first process is the lightener; the second process is the toner.

Pre-Lightening to Create a Foundation for Toners

After the hair goes through decolorizing, the color left in the hair is known as its ***foundation***. Achieving the correct foundation is necessary to create the degree of porosity required for proper toner development.

Manufacturers of toners provide literature that recommends the proper foundation to achieve your desired color. As a general rule, the paler the desired color, the lighter the foundation must be. It is important to follow the guide closely because:

1. Overlightened hair will "grab" the base color of the toner.
2. Underlightened hair will appear to have more red, yellow, or orange than the intended color.

It is not advisable to prelighten past the pale yellow stage. This will create overporous hair with inadequate amounts of natural pigment left in the cortex for your toner to bond to. Refer to the Laws of Color to select a toner that will neutralize or tone the prelightened hair to the desired shade.

In addition to achieving the correct foundation stage for toning, you must also achieve a sufficient porosity for toner development. Occasionally, virgin blonde, unpigmented, or white hair reaches the correct color foundation without achieving sufficient porosity. You must then make adjustments in your color mixture to achieve the desired color.

Preliminary Toner Application

1. Give 48-hour patch test prior to toner application.
2. Strand test may be given on same day as patch test to save time.
3. Proceed with application only if test results are negative and hair is in good condition.

Implements and Materials

Towels
Protective gloves
Tint cape
Shampoo
Acid or finishing rinse
Protective cream
Toner
Timer
Comb
Plastic clips
Plastic or glass bowl
Peroxide
Cotton
Record card
Applicator bottle or brush

Preparation

1. Arrange all supplies.
2. Prepare client.
3. Wear protective gloves.

4. Prelighten hair to desired stage of decolorization.
5. Shampoo hair lightly, rinse, and towel dry.
6. Acidify and recondition as necessary.
7. Select desired toner shade (indicated by the degree of prelightening previously required to achieve desired tonal result).
8. Apply protective cream around hairline and over ears.
9. Strand test and record results on client's record card.
10. If using an oxidative toner, mix toner and developer in a nonmetallic bowl or bottle according to manufacturer's directions.

Procedure

Wear gloves for protection throughout the application. Speed and accuracy of application are crucial for good color results. Application of low or nonperoxide toners may vary. Your instructor will direct you.

1. Divide hair into four equal sections. Use the end of tail comb or tint brush. Avoid scratching the scalp.
2. At crown of a back quarter, part off ¼" (.6 cm) partings and apply toner from scalp up to, but not including, the porous ends.
3. When the strand test confirms proper color development, gently work toner through ends using brush or fingers.

Note: *Do not bring toner mixture through porous ends until the last, and then only if changing tonal value or significant fading has occurred. To do so will only make the hair even more porous and more susceptible to continued fading. If ends tend to absorb too much color, dilute remaining mixture with mild shampoo, conditioner, or distilled water before applying to ends.*

4. Apply additional mixture to hair, if needed, and blend. Leave hair loose to permit air circulation or cover hair with cap if required.
5. Time according to strand test results. Test frequently until desired shade is reached evenly throughout shaft and ends.
6. Remove toner by wetting hair and massaging toner to lather.

7. Rinse, shampoo gently, and rinse well again.
8. Apply finishing rinse to close cuticle, lower the pH, and help prevent fading.
9. Remove any toner stains from the skin, hairline, and neck.
10. Style as desired. Use caution to avoid stretching the hair.
11. Complete record card and file.
12. Clean up in usual manner.

Toner Retouch

A toner retouch requires careful analysis of the hair. The new growth must be prelightened to the same stage as the hair was for the first toner application. Based on your analysis and strand test, you will either apply the toner to the entire shaft, as in the original application, or you will apply toner only to the new growth. When that area is nearly processed, you can work diluted toner mixture through the remaining hair if necessary.

SPECIAL EFFECTS HIGHLIGHTING

Special effects ***highlighting*** involves any technique of partial lightening or coloring. Lightening for special effects is a fashion technique. As styles change, you only need to adapt placement of lightened strands and colors for the trend.

You may create special effects by strategically placing the light and dark colors in the hair. Some colors appear to advance; others appear to recede. Light colors will cause the area to advance toward the eye, appear larger, and make detail more visible. The contrasting dark areas will cause the area to recede, appear smaller, and make detail less visible.

Many do their own haircolor at home with a fair degree of success, but home haircoloring is limited. Special effects and advanced techniques cannot be achieved by an untrained person. It is for that reason that at-home haircolor will never replace professional haircoloring.

As you begin to expand your knowledge and expertise in haircoloring and lightening, you will find greater degrees of creativity in application techniques. Tone on tone, reverse highlighting, dimensional coloring, and scrunching are but a few ways to create special effects. Your instructor will assist you in mastering the basic techniques, and the rest is up to you. The possibilities are limited only by your imagination.

METHODS FOR HIGHLIGHTING

There are several methods for achieving highlights. The most frequently used are:

1. Cap technique
2. Foil technique
3. Freehand technique

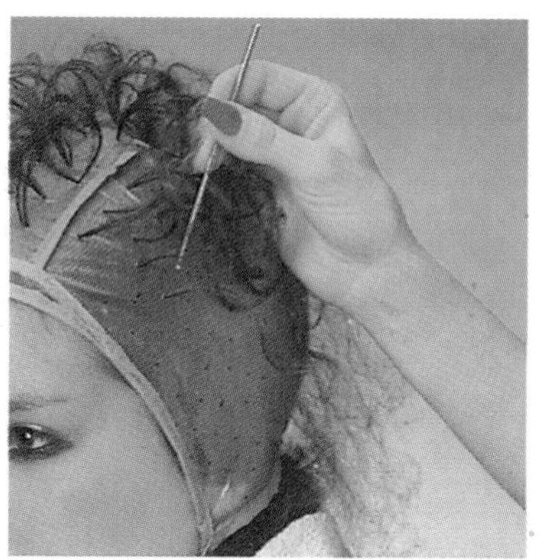

FIGURE 12.54 — Draw strands through holes in cap with hook.

The ***cap technique*** involves pulling clean strands of hair through a perforated cap with a hook. (Fig. 12.54) The amount of strands pulled through depends upon the amount of lightness desired. Pull small strands and leave holes empty for a subtle look. The lightening will be greater if all holes are used, and more dramatic if larger strands are pulled through the holes.

The hair is then lightened, usually with a powder or "quick" lightener, or with a tint that can lift a great deal. (Fig. 12.55) The lightener is removed by first rinsing with lukewarm water, then gently cleansing with an acid-balanced shampoo. After towel-blotting and conditioning, if necessary, the lightened hair is toned, if desired. (Figs. 12.56, 12.57)

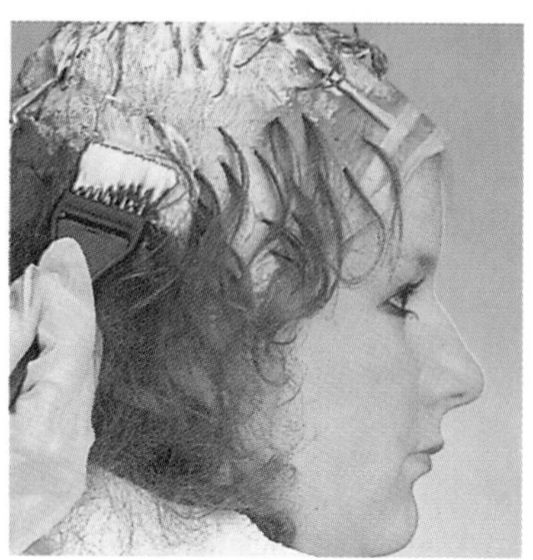

FIGURE 12.55 — Apply lightener to selected strands.

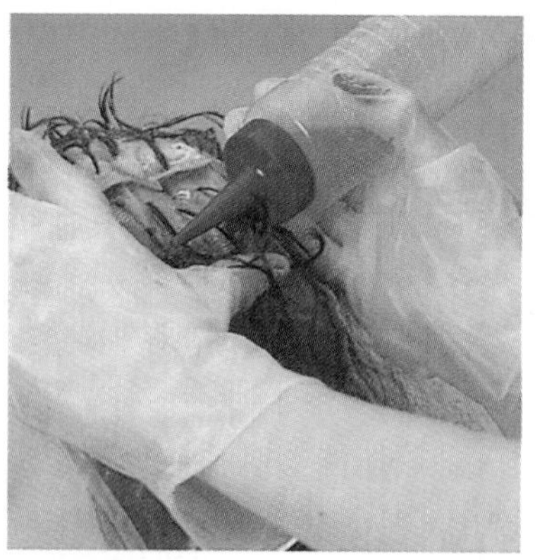

FIGURE 12.56 — Apply toner to prelightened strands.

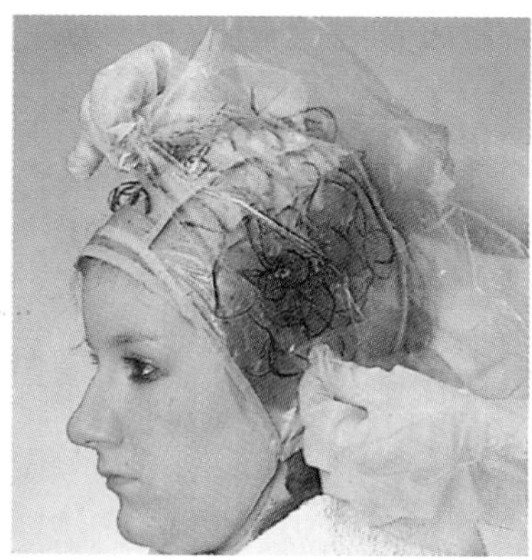

FIGURE 12.57 — Cover loosely with a plastic cap.

The ***foil technique*** involves weaving out (selecting) alternating strands from a subsection. (Fig. 12.58) The selected strands are then placed over foil or plastic wrap, and the appropriate lightener or high-lift tint is applied. The foil is folded to prevent lifting any unwoven hair. (Figs. 12.59a, b) With this technique, the colorist can strategically place highlights.

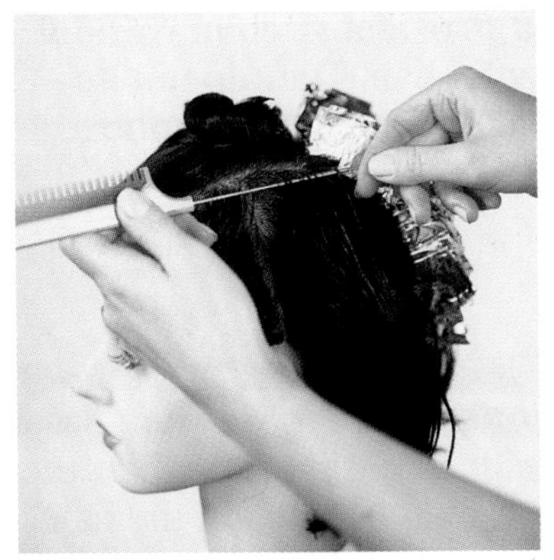

FIGURE 12.58 — Weave subsection with a tail comb.

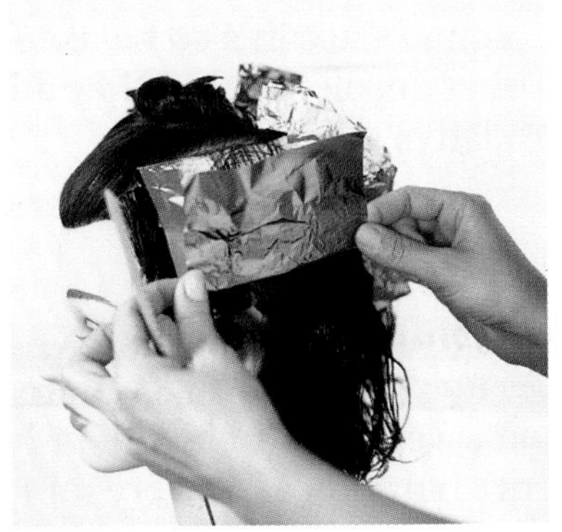

FIGURE 12.59a — Place hair in foil packet as shown.

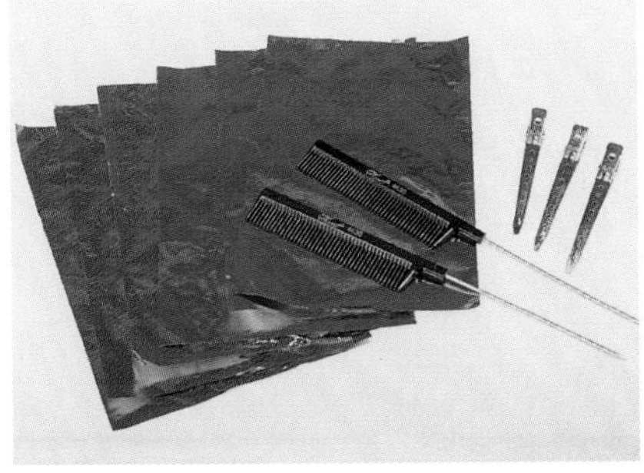

FIGURE 12.59b — Foils and combs.

Freehand techniques involve the placement of a lightening compound directly onto clean, styled hair. The lightener can be applied with a tint brush, an applicator bottle, or even with gloved fingers. Effects are extremely subtle and can be used effectively to draw attention to a waveline or an upsweep movement.

TONING OVERHIGHLIGHTED AND DIMENSIONALLY COLORED HAIR

When the hair is decolorized to the desired level and tonality during a highlighting service, the use of a toner is often eliminated. However, if a cool tonality is desired, then the use of a toner will cancel out the unwanted yellow contributing pigment.

When using a toner on highlighted hair, it is important to consider not only the varying degrees of porosity in the hair, but also the difference in pigmentation from strand to strand created by the lightening process. An oxidative toner would impart color into the highlighted strands, but it may also affect the natural, or pigmented, hair causing a slight amount of lift. The result may be an uneven tonality, with the underlying warmth brought out by the oxidative color. Strand test to ensure best results.

To avoid affecting the untreated hair, several choices are available:

1. A nonoxidative toner contains no ammonia, requires no developer (which produces no lift of the natural hair color), and is gentle on the scalp and hair. This is particularly useful for sensitive clients.
2. A semi-permanent color may be used to deposit tonality without lift. Not all colors will be delicate enough to avoid overpowering the prelightened hair. Always check the manufacturer's color chart for the base color of your chosen toner to make sure that when it combines with the contributing pigment in the hair you will have the exact tonality you wanted.

3. A deposit-only haircolor, which is an oxidative color without ammonia, can also be used to recolor hair. They do not further decolorize, but they are more permanent than nonoxidative toners.

HIGHLIGHTING SHAMPOOS

Highlighting shampoo tints are prepared by combining aniline derivative tints, hydrogen peroxide, and shampoo. They are used when a very slight change in hair shade is desired, or when the client's hair processes very rapidly. These tints highlight the hair's natural color in a single application. A patch test is required.

Highlighting shampoos are a mixture of shampoo and hydrogen peroxide. The natural color is slightly lightened. No patch test is required.

Procedure

Perform consultation and analysis as for a regular color procedure. If highlighting shampoo tint is to be used, a patch test must have been performed 48 hours before.

1. Drape client and take to shampoo bowl.
2. Distribute the color over clean, damp hair. Gently lather and process for 8 to 15 minutes.
3. Complete as for a regular tint procedure.

SPECIAL PROBLEMS IN HAIRCOLOR/CORRECTIVE COLORING

Each haircoloring service is unique. The colorist must carefully analyze the hair and consult with the client. Strand tests must be taken to ensure good results. But even the most skilled colorist will occasionally have a haircoloring problem. This may be due to the particular structure or condition of the client's hair or to the effects of prior treatments to the hair. Most haircoloring problems can be resolved or corrected if the colorist maintains calm.

UNPIGMENTED HAIR: CHALLENGES AND SOLUTIONS

Unpigmented, white, and salt-and-pepper hair have characteristics that create unique coloring problems. A major portion of salon coloring services are performed to either cover or enhance unpigmented hair.

Yellowed Unpigmented Hair

A yellow cast can occur from a variety of causes. Smoking, medication, exposure to the sun, and, to a lesser degree, hair sprays and styling aids can all cause the hair to turn yellow. Bleach and dye removers will remove yellow discoloration occurring from internal causes or the oxidation of melanin.

Undesired yellow can be overpowered by the artificial pigments deposited by tints of an equal or darker level than the yellow. Another option is to neutralize the yellow tones with a comparable level of violet.

Formulating for Unpigmented Hair

Level selection for white hair is relatively simple because it basically accepts the level applied. However, colors that are a level 9 or lighter may not give complete coverage because of the small percentage of artificial pigment for depositing in these shades. Generally, formulations from the levels 6, 7, or 8 will give better coverage and can be used to create pastel and blonde tones if desired.

For those clients who are 80% to 100% unpigmented, a haircolor within the blonde range is generally more flattering than a darker shade. This lighter level of artificial color may be selected to give a warm or cool finished product, depending upon the client's skin tone, eye color, and personal preference.

Another factor to consider when coloring the unpigmented in salt-and-pepper hair to a darker level is that color on color makes a darker color. The addition of dark artificial pigment to the natural pigment (peppered hair) results in a color that the eye perceives as darker. For this reason, when attempting to cover unpigmented hair in a salt-and-pepper head, a shade lighter than the naturally dark hair is generally selected.

A manufacturer's product color chart can be used in conjunction with the following formulation charts to select a color tonality within the proper level with which to perform a strand test.

SEMI-PERMANENT COLOR FORMULATION CHART FOR UNPIGMENTED HAIR

Percentage of Unpigmented Hair	Formulation
100%-90%	Desired level
90%-70%	Equal parts desired and 1 level lighter
70%-50%	1 level lighter than desired level
50%-30%	Equal parts 1 level lighter and 2 levels lighter
30%-10%	2 levels lighter than desired level

PERMANENT TINT FORMULATION CHART FOR UNPIGMENTED HAIR

Percentage of Unpigmented Hair	Formulation
100%-90%	Desired level
90%-70%	2 parts desired level and 1 part lighter level
70%-50%	Equal parts desired and lighter level
50%-30%	2 parts lighter level and 1 part desired level
30%-10%	1 level lighter

The unpigmented hair formulation chart will give you some basic general guidelines for formulating for unpigmented hair. Of course there are other considerations, such as the client's personality and his/her own personal preferences, as well as the amount of unpigmented hair and the location. You will note that in the chart there are no tones given in the formulations, only levels of haircoloring and various techniques.

Also note that in the chart there are no accommodations made for the location of the unpigmented hair. The chart is designed so the section that indicates 30% unpigmented presumes that the unpigmented hair is equally distributed throughout the entire head. If, for instance, the majority of the 30% unpigmented hair is located in the front section of the head, that section would be considered 80% unpigmented with the back portion containing just a sprinkling of unpigmented hair. In that instance you would have to determine what formulation would best suit the client—formulating for the 80% unpigmented or the sprinkling of unpigmented. If the unpigmented hair around the face is what the client sees, then you would be well advised to formulate for the 80% unpigmented hair. The section of hair that surrounds the face is what influences the client's self-perception.

Your client is accustomed to seeing a certain percentage of unpigmented hair. This unpigmented hair gives the client the perception of having lighter hair. This method of formulating is a method of determining how much lighter you should make the client's hair to give the illusion of the lightness he or she is accustomed to seeing.

The client would have to have at least 10% unpigmented hair before it is necessary to lighten the natural level. Once again it is the level of color, determined by the amount of unpigmented hair, that the client is accustomed to seeing.

This is where the creativity of color mixing comes in; first using a darker haircolor that will not bring out the undesirable undertones, then achieving the level of lightness by adding some highlights.

There are any number of techniques to aid in solving your haircolor challenges. The more techniques that you have at your disposal, the greater latitude you will have. Remember your knowledge and your techniques are your tools for successful haircoloring. Learning haircolor is not a destination; it is a journey that never ends.

Presoftening

Occasionally unpigmented hair is so resistant that even when formulation, application, and timing are correct, coverage is not satisfactory and presoftening becomes necessary. ***Presoftening*** is a two-step, or double-application, haircoloring in which two distinct and separate applications of product are necessary to achieve the desired shade. The presoftener is applied, processed, and removed. The second step is the application of the tint to complete the two-step process.

The purpose of presoftening is twofold: to soften and open the cuticle for improved penetration of color and to create missing yellow or gold tones in the hair so that the tint with a balance of color will adhere to the hair and process on-tone.

If the client's hair is unpigmented and resistant, the hair should be presoftened with gold-based tints or oil or cream bleaches. All will work to soften and open the cuticle. However, a gold-based tint will deposit missing yellow or gold into the hair, while a bleach will only diffuse and oxidize the remaining natural pigment within the shaft.

Follow the manufacturer's recommended directions to mix either an oil bleach or a lifting tint. The ammonia in these products is required to create the desired degree of porosity for color acceptance. However, if using a cream bleach, use no protinator, activator, or catalyst. White or unpigmented hair does not require high lift, and to do so will only cause unnecessary damage.

A gold-based tint one to two levels lighter than the desired level can be applied directly to the hair to be presoftened without mixing with developer, using only the ammonia content and staining ability in the product. Allow the tint to remain on the hair 5 to 10 minutes, then wipe gently with a cloth or paper towel to remove. Shampooing is not necessary as a little of the presoftening tint may remain on the hair, with the regular (desired) color formula applied directly over it.

Presoftening is also effective on pigmented resistant hair, but care must be given to leave the presoftening mixture on the hair only long enough to open the cuticle, rendering the hair porous enough to accept the tint. Otherwise, you may create more underlying warmth than you desired and will have to compensate for this added warmth in your color selection and formulation for deposit.

Presoftening Application Procedure

1. Mix product according to manufacturer's directions.
2. Apply with brush or bottle in most resistant areas first.
3. Process at room temperature for 5 to 20 minutes.
4. Rinse thoroughly and shampoo.
5. Apply tint in usual manner.

RULES FOR EFFECTIVE COLOR CORRECTION

1. Do not panic.
2. Establish the true problem.
3. Establish what caused the problem.
4. Establish the most suitable remedy.
5. Always take one step at a time.
6. Never guarantee an exact result.
7. Always strand test for accuracy.

HENNA REMOVAL

Henna has a coating that, if overused, can build up on the hair and prevent penetration of other chemicals. Henna also penetrates the cortex and attaches to the salt bonds. Both of these actions may leave the hair unfit for other professional treatments. Always perform a strand test prior to application.

It is sometimes possible to remove henna when it becomes excessively built up on the shaft or when it is incompatible with a future chemical service. Follow these steps for the removal of henna buildup.

Procedure

1. Apply 70% alcohol to the hair shaft, avoiding direct contact with the scalp. Allow to set 5 to 7 minutes.
2. Apply mineral oil directly over the alcohol, completely saturating each strand from the scalp to the ends.
3. Preheat hood dryer.

4. Tightly cover the head with a plastic bag.
5. Place under the dryer for 30 minutes.
6. Without rinsing, apply concentrated shampoo for oily hair and work into the oil.
7. Allow to set in for 3 minutes.
8. Massage the hair again.
9. Add comfortably hot water and rinse thoroughly.
10. Shampoo again. (Three shampoos may be necessary.)

Technically the alcohol should loosen the henna coating the hair shaft. However, more than one treatment may be necessary to loosen it enough to slide off. Always perform a strand test to determine if removal was successful before applying the next chemical treatment.

COMPOUND DYE TEST

Many clients use haircoloring products at home. Therefore, you must be able to recognize and understand their effects. Such coloring agents must be removed and the hair reconditioned prior to any other chemical service.

Hair treated with a metallic dye, or any other coating dye, looks dry and dull. It is generally harsh and brittle to the touch. These colorings usually fade to unnatural tones. Silver dyes have a greenish cast, lead dyes leave a purple color, and those containing copper turn red.

Test for Metallic Salts:

1. In a glass container, mix 1 ounce (30 ml) of 20 volume (6%) peroxide and 20 drops of 28% ammonia water.
2. Cut a strand of the client's hair, bind it with tape, and immerse in the solution for 30 minutes.
3. Remove, towel dry, and observe the strand.

Hair dyed with *lead* will lighten immediately. Hair treated with *silver* will show no reaction at all. This indicates that other chemicals will not be successful because they will not be able to penetrate the coating.

Hair treated with *copper* will start to boil and will pull apart easily. This hair would be severely damaged or destroyed if other chemicals, such as those found in permanent colors or perm solutions, were applied to it.

Hair treated with a *coating dye* either will not change color or will lighten in spots. This hair will not receive chemical services easily, and the length of time necessary for penetration may very well damage the hair.

Preparations designed to remove metallics and nonperoxide dye solvents may assist in the removal of metallic and coating dyes from the hair. Performing a strand test will indicate whether the metallic deposits have been removed. The most effective guarantee of future successful chemical services is to cut the tinted hair off.

Procedure for Removing Metallic and Coating Dyes

1. Apply 70% alcohol to hair and allow to stand for 5 minutes.
2. Without rinsing the alcohol, apply a heavy oil (mineral, castor, vegetable, or commercially prepared color removing oil) thoroughly to the hair.
3. Cover hair with a plastic bag and place under hot dryer for 30 minutes.
4. Remove mixture from hair using a concentrated shampoo for oily hair.
5. Work shampoo into oil for 3 minutes, then rinse with warm water.
6. Repeat shampoo steps until oil is completely removed.

DAMAGED HAIR

Blow-drying, wind, harsh shampoos, and chemical services all take their toll on the condition of the hair. Coating compounds such as hair sprays, styling agents, and some conditioners can prevent color penetration.

Hair is considered damaged when the hair has one or more of the following conditions:

- Rough texture
- Overporous
- Brittle and dry
- Breakage
- No elasticity
- Spongy, matted when wet
- Color fades or absorbs too rapidly

Any of these hair conditions will create problems during a tinting, lightening, permanent waving, or hair relaxing treatment. Therefore, damaged hair should receive reconditioning treatments prior to and after the application of these chemical processes.

Preventative and corrective steps that you should take include the following:

1. Incorporate reconditioning into any chemical service that you give.
2. Ensure that the client uses high-quality products at home. (Sell the best.)
3. Precondition hair if your analysis tells you it is damaged. Use a penetrating conditioner that can deposit protein, oils, and moisture regulators.
4. Complete each chemical service by normalizing the pH with a finishing rinse. This will restore the cuticle's protective capacity.
5. If hair is still unresponsive after a conditioning treatment, postpone any further chemical service until the hair is reconditioned.
6. Schedule the client for between-service conditioning.

Reconditioning Procedure

1. Always thoroughly analyze the hair to determine the problem. Consult with the client until you can discover the source of the damage. You can then correct the problem and avoid its recurrence.
2. Shampoo the hair with a mild shampoo. Use care to keep your hands underneath the hair, and only use gentle massage techniques to avoid tangling the fragile hair.
3. Rinse very well and towel blot gently.
4. Apply the conditioner as the manufacturer directs. If it is a liquid, use a spray bottle; if it is a cream, apply with a sanitized spatula or tint brush.
5. Blend the conditioner through the hair with a wide-toothed comb.
6. Cover the hair with a plastic cap, if required, and follow the manufacturer's directions for heat application and timing.
7. Rinse well. Re-examine the hair and proceed with the coloring service only if the hair's condition indicates that the treatment will be successful.

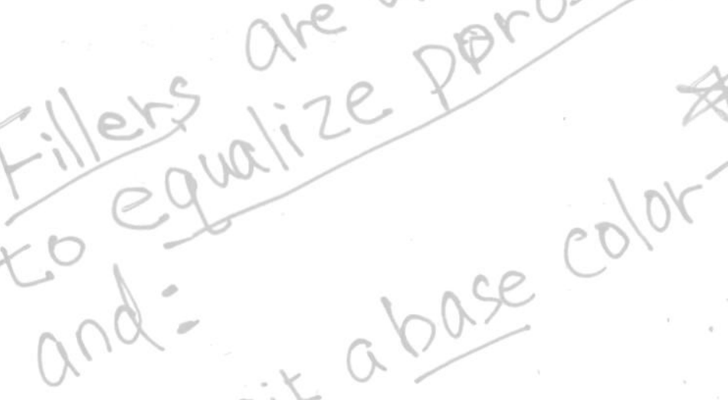

FILLERS

Fillers are specialized preparations that are designed to help equalize porosity and deposit a base color in one application. They can be a manufacturer's preparation or a mixture of tint and conditioner that your instructor will assist you in preparing.

Fillers are absorbed by the hair shaft on the basis of porosity. The greater the porosity, the greater the absorption of the filler. Inside the cortex, the filler molecules fill in the spaces left in the shaft from prior diffusion of melanin. This creates a base to which tint molecules can now attach, as well as a smooth and even surface on the shaft, which the eye perceives as warmth and sheen. Through this process, fillers help prevent the flat, dull color that can result when tinting damaged hair.

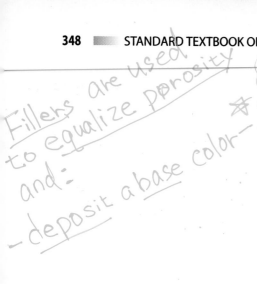

Conditioner fillers are used to recondition damaged hair before salon service. Conditioner fillers can be applied in a separate procedure or immediately prior to color application. The conditioner and the tint are then working at the same time.

Color fillers are recommended if the hair is in a damaged condition, and there is doubt that the color result will be an even shade.

Advantages of Using a Color Filler

1. Deposits color to faded ends.
2. Helps hair to hold color.
3. Helps color to develop uniformly from scalp to ends.
4. Prevents streaking.
5. Prevents off-color results.
6. Prevents dullness.
7. Produces more uniform, natural-looking color in a tint.

Selecting the Correct Color Filler

To obtain satisfactory results, select the color filler that will replace the missing primary color in your formulation. Always remember that all three primaries—red, blue, and yellow—must be present for natural-looking hair color. If you have blonde (yellow) hair, for example, that is being tinted back to an ash (yellow and blue) brown, you will need to use an orange-red filler so that the end result will be correct.

How to Use Color Fillers

Color fillers may be applied directly from their containers to damaged hair prior to tinting. Color fillers may also be added to the tint and applied to damaged ends. They may be used full strength or diluted with distilled water.

REDS FADING

Fading is a common problem of tinted red hair. The combination of ammonia and peroxide in the tinting formula diffuses the natural pigment, resulting in smaller molecules within the hair shaft. Artificial pigments then attach to the diffused melanin to create a new color. However, with every shampooing, blow-drying, permanent waving, and sun, chlorine, or salt water exposure, the artificial pigment is removed through porosity of the cuticle. This leaves behind the smaller, diffused melanin molecules and the warmth created by the oxidation process.

The first step to devising a solution to this situation is to determine the cause of the fading. A scarf, hat, or conditioner with UV absorbers all protect hair from the sun. Rinsing, preferably shampooing and conditioning, salt and chlorinated water from the hair immediately after swimming will lessen their damaging effects. Applying less heat to the hair will also help to prevent damage to the cuticle and diffusion of artificial and natural color. Also, a milder permanent waving solution should be advised for those clients who combine color and perming.

Use of a lower volume of hydrogen peroxide can also prevent excessive fading and brassiness. If the desired depth of red is of the same or deeper level than the natural color, the hue can be achieved through deposition without excessive lift. This technique can be particularly useful in achieving and retaining the violet-based reds.

For warmer or brighter (red-orange or gold) reds on darker natural levels, prelightening before application of your tint can have its advantages. The lightening process naturally brings out the warm contributing pigment, which serves as the ideal foundation for a vibrant red color. However, care must be taken to avoid over-lightening the hair, which will create the opposite reaction than you desire—dull, flat, lifeless color tonality.

Often, when using a single-process tint to achieve the desired red color tonality, a colorist may misjudge the natural hair color level and use a tint with too much lift and not enough depositing pigment to support the desired final result. This leads to the same diffusion of melanin and fading of tone.

When performing a retouch application with a red-based tint, the formula used to create the correct amount of lift at the new growth (utilizing the hair's natural contributing pigment) may produce too much lift if it is pulled through the ends to refresh the color. Better-lasting reds are created by using a separate formula with a deposit-only haircolor product for the hair ends. Your selection should correspond in tone and level to the formula used on the new growth. Strand testing will help indicate the correctness of your color choice.

CORRECTING BRASSINESS AND OTHER UNWANTED TONES IN THE HAIR

As the artificial pigment fades and brassiness becomes apparent, the natural tendency of the client is to request more frequent retouches. Scheduling retouches at closer and closer intervals causes greater porosity and diffusion of the natural pigment, leaving the hair brassier than before as the tint once again fades. A never-ending cycle begins.

The first step to camouflage excessive brassiness in either natural or tinted hair is to analyze it. Is it red, yellow, or orange? Locate the particular shade on the color wheel and use the complementary color to neutralize it. A number of options exist for solving the problem. Temporary rinses, a soap cap during retouches, fillers, and semi-permanent colors of a neutralizing shade all can be effective in correcting brassiness, depending on the situation. Your instructor will guide you in recommending the appropriate treatment for your situation.

TINT REMOVAL

Sometimes it is necessary to remove all or part of the tint from the hair in order to achieve the correct color. The client may want to change to a lighter shade (tint will not lift tint), or the present haircolor may have been a mistake. Occasionally color builds up or processes too dark due to an overporous condition of the hair shaft.

Commercial products are used to remove penetrating tints and are known as *tint, dye,* or *color removers.* Dye removers are not generally sold for use by nonprofessionals because the process is too complex for the untrained. Therefore, color removing is a professional service that can bring new clients into the salon and convert them to loyal customers.

Color removers may contain ingredients designed to diffuse pigment, both natural and artificial, and are sometimes mixed with hydrogen peroxide. Others have the option of being mixed with distilled water to create a milder color remover. Check the individual manufacturer's directions.

Color removers can, in certain situations, correct problems with brassiness. For instance, while bleach lightening mixtures are the most efficient products in lightening virgin hair, they are not the best product to use on hair that has been darkened or tinted red with an aniline derivative tint. Bleach locks in golds, oranges, and reds that occur as artificial haircolor decolorizes. Because bleach locks in and cannot remove brassiness in tinted hair, it often becomes impossible to lighten the hair to the desired shade without total destruction of the hair shaft. A dye solvent is chemically formulated to diffuse and dissolve these artificial color molecules without locking in brassiness. However, as the color remover lightens the artificial color molecules, it also lifts color from the natural pigment or melanin.

The removal of tint is always an advanced technique that requires careful analysis of the hair's condition and color. Reconditioning is often necessary after tint removal and before corrective coloring.

Procedure for Tint Removal

1. Prepare client.
2. Shampoo if required by manufacturer. Avoid manipulating the scalp.
3. Section hair into four quarters.
4. Wear gloves to protect your hands.
5. Mix preparation in glass or plastic bowl according to manufacturer's directions.
6. Immediately begin application where hair is darkest.
7. Apply mixture with tint brush. Saturate hair completely. (Fig. 12.60)
8. Work mixture through hair ends.
9. Pile hair loosely on top of head. (Fig. 12.61) Cover with plastic cap if required. (Fig. 12.62)
10. Strand test frequently. Lightening may happen quite rapidly.
11. When color is diffused, rinse thoroughly.
12. Shampoo gently but thoroughly to ensure that all of the chemical is removed from the hair. Any tint remover that remains in the hair will continue to process. (Fig. 12.63)

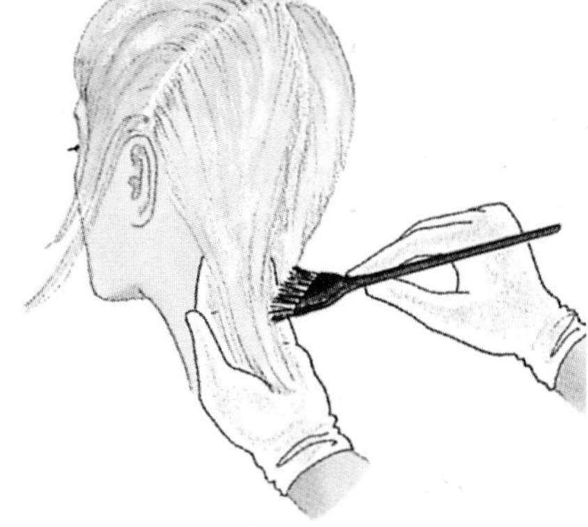

FIGURE 12.60 — Apply mixture.

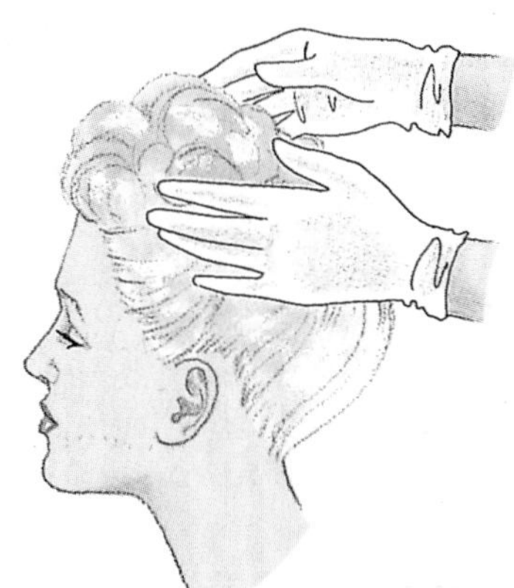

FIGURE 12.61 — Pile hair loosely on top of head.

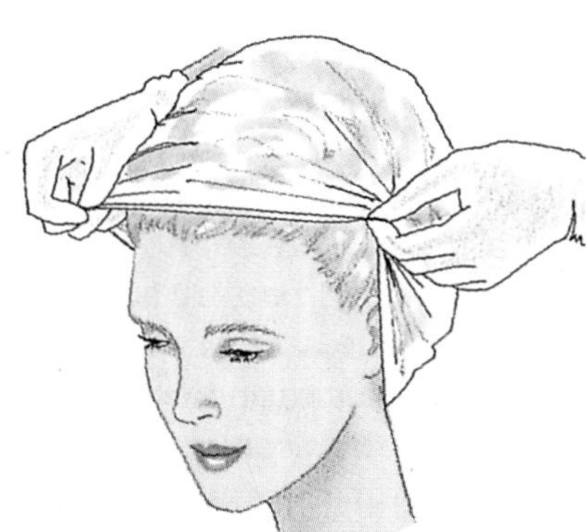

FIGURE 12.62 — Cover head with plastic cap if required.

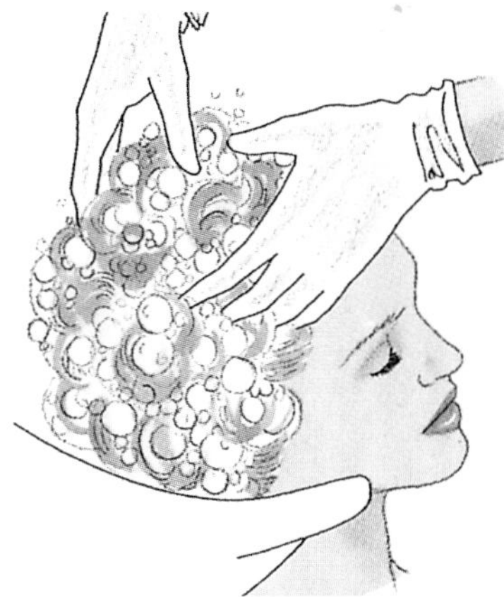

FIGURE 12.63 — Shampoo with tepid water.

13. Towel-dry hair.
14. Analyze hair strength. Condition as required.
15. Perform a strand test.
16. Proceed with the application of desired tint.

Alternate Procedure

1. Prepare client.
2. Analyze color to determine areas needing lightening.
3. Wear gloves to protect your hands.
4. Apply tint remover to hair keeping it away from the scalp by using foil.
5. Strand test frequently.
6. When desired lightness is achieved, remove foils and shampoo client.
7. Towel-dry hair.
8. Analyze hair strength. Condition as required.
9. Analyze the condition of the scalp.
10. Perform a strand test.
11. Proceed with the application of desired tint.

If color cannot be applied, style hair in the usual manner. Schedule reconditioning treatments until the hair can withstand tinting.

Tinting After Dye Removal

The use of a color remover does not, as a general rule, create a finished result. Double-application haircoloring is almost always necessary, because the color resulting from the dye solvent is rarely even and is usually red, orange, or gold. However, before continuing, analyze the hair and scalp to determine any sensitivity to further chemical services.

If the scalp appears reddened or irritated in any way, delay the second application of color until the scalp returns to normal. You may choose to use a temporary rinse at this point to achieve a toned-down appearance.

When you are ready to proceed with the next color service, remember, the hair has already been treated at least twice with chemicals. Application of a tint and a dye solvent cause the hair to become more porous. In this case, both chemicals have been applied to the hair.

A tint applied to porous hair will create a darker hue than on nonporous hair, so select a color at least one level lighter than desired. It's always easier to add more depth than to remove it.

Color will process cooler than it would on undamaged hair. The Law of Color must be used to add the missing foundation warmth when formulating the tint to be used after a color remover. A filler and/or a low volume developer used in tinting the hair is often desirable. Regardless of the chosen method, a strand test is a *must* before beginning this service.

Sometimes, the hair is so overporous that there are insufficient protein bonds and natural melanin left within the cortex for the artificial pigment to attach to. The hair may look "gun-metal gray," and this lighter-than-expected result is a real danger sign. Hair that is this porous is very fragile and may be close to the breaking point.

TINT BACK TO NATURAL COLOR

Clients who have been either tinting or bleaching will often want to return to their natural shade. Sun, chlorinated pool water, or prior chemical services can alter the hair color.

Each tint back to natural color must be handled as an individual problem. This type of hair is porous and may absorb color quickly and process darker and cooler than expected. It may also fade faster than normal. The natural pigment may be so diffused that it will not accept color at all. Carefully record all observations and treatments on the client's record card.

Check the hair for its natural color next to the scalp. After seeing their hair lighter than their natural color for any length of time, many clients may not realize how drastic a change they may be making. Discuss with your client options such as reverse highlighting (weaving strands of darker haircolor into the existing base color), or selection of a color 1 or 2 levels lighter than their natural color. Either of these options will enable you and your client to gradually add more depth if desired, as your client adapts to the new image. A strand test will be essential to ensure desired results.

The solution to a successful tint back to natural can lie in the use of a filler to even out the porosity and achieve color correction. Formulate to create the warmth necessary to prevent a drab, unnatural-looking color in the finished product. Milder color solutions that do no lifting as they deposit are less damaging. The symptoms and solutions are similar to tinting after color removal (discussed previously in this chapter). Refer to this service and the use of fillers for more information.

A ***soap cap*** is used in conjunction with a tint back to natural if the tint does not exactly match the natural color. A quick soap cap, using the addition of shampoo to the tint solution to create a milder formula, will break the line of demarcation.

Procedure

1. Assemble materials.
2. Prepare client in usual manner.
3. Check results of patch test. Proceed only if results are negative.
4. Shampoo hair as directed. Give conditioning treatments according to your analysis.
5. Perform a strand test. More than one test may be necessary to determine the correct formulation and timing for desired results.
6. Section hair into four quarters.
7. Apply filler as directed by your instructor. Remember to replace the missing primary.
8. Process filler according to manufacturer's directions. Proceed directly to tint application.
9. Resection the hair into four quarters.
10. Apply color formula to ¼" (.6 cm) subsections. Apply the tint as rapidly as possible to both sides of the subsection from the line of demarcation to the porous ends. Process according to your test strand results.
11. When correct color development has been confirmed by strand testing, apply tint to the porous ends. Continue processing.
12. (optional) A soap cap may be used after processing time is complete to blend color. For a soap cap add equal amounts of shampoo to the leftover tint and mix it thoroughly. The mixture is applied quickly and worked gently through the ends of the hair.
13. Remove tint from hair with a mild shampoo.
14. Use an acid rinse to close cuticle and help prevent fading.
15. Replace moisture with a finishing rinse.
16. Style as desired, using caution to avoid excessive heat or stretching.

17. Offer the client the opportunity to purchase high-quality salon products to prevent color stripping at home, and schedule the client for conditioning treatments.
18. Complete record card and file.
19. Clean work area in the usual manner.

Completed:
Learning Objective
#7
AVOIDING AND SOLVING HAIRCOLORING PROBLEMS

HAIRCOLORING SAFETY PRECAUTIONS

1. Give a patch test 48 hours prior to any application of aniline derivative.
2. Apply tint only if patch test is negative.
3. Do not apply tint if abrasions are present.
4. Do not apply tint if metallic or compound dye is present.
5. Do not brush hair prior to applying color.
6. Always read and follow manufacturer's directions.
7. Use sanitized applicator bottles, brushes, combs, and towels.
8. Protect client's clothing by proper draping.
9. Perform a strand test for color, breakage, and/or discoloration.
10. Use an applicator bottle or bowl (glass or plastic) for mixing the tint.
11. Do not mix tint before you are ready to use it; discard left-over tint.
12. Wear gloves to protect your hands.
13. Do not permit the color to come in contact with the client's eyes.
14. Do not overlap during a tint retouch.
15. Do not use water that is too hot; use lukewarm water for removing color.
16. Use a mild shampoo. If an alkaline or harsh shampoo is used, it will strip the color.
17. Always wash hands before and after serving a client.

Completed:
Learning Objective
#8
SAFETY PRECAUTIONS

HAIRCOLORING GLOSSARY

accelerator: (see *activator*)

accent color: (see *color additive*)

acid: An aqueous (water-based) solution having a pH less than 7.0 on the pH scale. The opposite of alkaline.

activator: An additive used to quicken the action or progress of a chemical. Another word for booster, accelerator, protenator, or catalyst.

alkaline: An aqueous (water-based) solution having a pH greater than 7.0 on the pH scale. The opposite of acid.

allergy: A reaction due to extreme sensitivity to certain foods or chemicals.

allergy test: A test to determine the possibility or degree of sensitivity. Also known as a patch test, predisposition test, or skin test.

amino acids: The group of molecules the body uses to synthesize protein. There are some 22 different amino acids found in living protein that serve as units of structure in protein.

ammonia: A colorless pungent gas composed of hydrogen and nitrogen; in water solution it is called ammonia water. Used in haircolor to swell the cuticle. When mixed with hydrogen peroxide, activates the oxidation process on melanin and allows the melanin to decolorize.

analysis (hair): An examination of the hair to determine its condition and natural color. (see *condition*; *consultation*)

ash: A tone or shade dominated by greens, blues, violets, or unpigmenteds. May be used to counteract unwanted warm tones.

base color: The predominant tonality of an existing color, i.e., gold-based brown or blonde with a neutral base.

bleeding: Seepage of tint/lightener from foil or cap due to improper application.

blending: A merging of one tint or tone with another.

blonding: A term applied to lightening the hair.

booster: (see *activator*)

brassy tone: Red, orange, or gold tones in the hair.

buildup: Repeated coatings on the hair shaft.

catalyst: A substance used to alter the speed of a chemical reaction.

certified color: A color that meets certain standards for purity and is certified by the FDA.

chemical change: Alteration in the chemical composition of a substance.

coating: Residue left on the outside of the hair shaft.

color: Visual sensation caused by light.

color additive: A concentrated color product that can be added to haircolor to intensify or tone down the color. Another term for concentrate.

color base: The combination of dyes that make up the tonal foundation of a specific haircolor.
color lift: The amount of change natural or artificial pigment undergoes when lightened by a substance.
color mixing: Combining two or more shades together for a custom color.
color priming: The process of adding pigments to prepare the hair for the application of a final color formula.
color refresher: 1. Color applied to midshaft and ends to give a more uniform color appearance to the hair. 2. Color applied by a shampoo-in method to enhance the natural color. Also called color wash, color enhancer.
color remover: A product designed to remove artificial pigment from the hair.
color test: The process of removing product from a hair strand to monitor the progress of color development during tinting or lightening.
color wheel: The arrangement of primary, secondary, and tertiary colors in the order of their relationships to each other. A tool for formulating.
complementary colors: A primary and secondary color positioned opposite each other on the color wheel. When these two colors are combined, they create a neutral color. Combinations are as follows: blue/orange, red/green, yellow/violet.
concentrate: (see *color additive*)
condition: The existing state of the hair; elasticity, strength, texture, porosity, and evidence of previous treatments.
consultation: Verbal communication with a client to determine desired result. (see *analysis* [*hair*])
contributing pigment: The current level and tone of the hair. Refers to both natural contributing pigment and decolorized (or lightened) contributing pigment. (see *undertone*)
cool tones: (see *ash*)
corrective coloring: The process of correcting an undesirable color.
cortex: The second layer of hair. A fibrous protein core of the hair fiber containing melanin pigment.
coverage: Reference to the ability of a color product to color unpigmented, white, or other colors of hair.
cuticle: The translucent protein outer layer of the hair fiber.
cysteine: The naturally occurring amino acid responsible for the development of pheomelanin.
D & C colors: Colors selected from a certified list approved by the FDA for use in drug and cosmetic products.
decolorize: A chemical process involving the lightening of the natural pigment or artificial color from the hair.
degree: Term used to describe various units of measurement. (see *stage*)

dense: Thick, compact, or crowded.
deposit: Describes the color product in terms of its ability to add color pigment to the hair. Color added equals deposit.
deposit-only color: A category of color products between permanent and semi-permanent colors. Formulated to only deposit color, not lift. Contains oxidation dyes and utilizes low-volume developer.
depth: The lightness or darkness of a specific hair color. (see *level*)
developer: An oxidizing agent, usually hydrogen peroxide, that reacts chemically with coloring material to develop color molecules and create a change in natural hair color.
development time (oxidation period): The time required for a permanent color or lightener to completely develop.
diffused: Broken down, scattered; not limited to one spot.
direct dye: A pre-formed color that dyes the fiber directly without the need for oxidation.
discoloration: The development of undesired shades through chemical reaction.
double process: A technique requiring two separate procedures in which the hair is decolorized or prelightened with a lightener before the depositing color is applied.
drab: Term used to describe hair color shades containing no red or gold. (see *ash; dull*)
drabber: Concentrated color, used to reduce red or gold highlights.
dull: A word used to describe hair or hair color without sheen.
dye: Artificial pigment.
dye intermediate: A material that develops into color only after reaction with developer (hydrogen peroxide). Also known as oxidation dyes.
dye solvents or dye remover: (see *color remover*)
elasticity: The ability of the hair to stretch and return to normal.
enzyme: A protein molecule found in living cells that initiates a chemical process.
fade: To lose color through exposure to the elements or other factors.
fillers: 1. Color product used as a color refresher or to fill damaged hair in preparation for haircoloring. 2. Any liquid-like substance to help fill a void. (see *color refresher*)
formulas: Mixtures of two or more ingredients.
formulate: The art of mixing to create a blend or balance of two or more ingredients.
granule: A minute particle in the hair containing melanin.
hair: A slender thread-like outgrowth of the skin of the head and body.
haircolor: (one word) An industry-coined term referring to artificial haircolor products.
hair color: (two words) The color of hair created by nature.
hair root: That part of the hair contained within the follicle, below the surface of the scalp.

hair shaft: Visible part of each strand of hair. It is made up of an outer layer called the cuticle, an innermost layer called the medulla, and an in-between layer called the cortex. The cortex layer is where color changes are made.

hard water: Water that contains minerals and metallic salts as impurities.

henna: A plant-extracted coloring that produces bright shades of red. The active ingredient is lawsone. Henna permanently colors the hair by coating and penetrating the hair shaft. (see *progressive dye*)

high-lift tinting: A single-process color with a higher degree of lightening action and a minimal amount of color deposit.

highlighting: The introduction of a lighter color in small selected sections to increase lightness of hair. Generally not strongly contrasting from the natural color.

hydrogen peroxide: An oxidizing chemical made up of 2 parts hydrogen and 2 parts oxygen (H_2O_2), used to aid the processing of permanent haircolor and lighteners. Also referred to as developer. Available in liquid or cream.

intensity: Used in haircoloring to describe the "strength" of the color's tonality. A tonality can be mild, medium, or strong in intensity.

keratin: The insoluble protein material that is the substance of hair.

level: A unit of measurement used to evaluate the lightness or darkness of a color, excluding tone.

Level System: A system colorists use to analyze the lightness or darkness of a hair color.

lift: The lightening action of a haircolor or lightening product on the hair's natural pigment.

lightener: The chemical compound that lightens the hair by dispersing, dissolving, and decolorizing the natural hair pigment. (see *prelighten*)

lightening: (see *decolorize*)

line of demarcation: An obvious difference between two colors on the hair shaft.

medulla: The center structure of the hair shaft that may not be present in every hair fiber. Very little is known about its actual function.

melanin: The tiny grains of pigment in the hair cortex that create natural hair color.

melanocytes: Cells in the hair bulb that manufacture melanin.

melanoprotein: The protein coating of a melanosome.

melanosome: Protein-coated granule containing melanin.

metallic dyes: Soluble metal salts such as lead, silver, and bismuth that produce colors on the hair fiber by progressive build-up and exposure to air.

molecule: Two or more atoms chemically joined together; the smallest part of a compound.

neutral: 1. A color balanced between warm and cool, which does not reflect a highlight of any primary or secondary color. 2. Also refers to a pH of 7.

neutralization: The process that counterbalances or cancels the action of an agent or color.

neutralize: Render neutral; counterbalance of action or influence. (see *neutral*)

new growth: The part of the hair shaft that is between previously chemically treated hair and the scalp.

nonalkaline: (see *acid*)

off-the-scalp lightener: Generally a stronger lightener usually in powder form, not to be used directly on the scalp.

on-the-scalp lightener: A liquid, cream, or gel form of lightener that can be used directly on the scalp.

opaque: Allowing no light to shine through.

outgrowth: (see *new growth*)

overlap: Occurs when the application of color or lightener goes beyond the line of demarcation.

overporosity: The condition where hair reaches an undesirable stage of porosity and requires correction.

oxidation: 1. The reaction of dye intermediates with hydrogen peroxide found in haircoloring developers. 2. The interaction of hydrogen peroxide on the natural pigment.

oxidative haircolor: A product containing oxidation dyes that require hydrogen peroxide to develop the permanent color.

para tint: A tint made from oxidation dyes.

para-phenylenediamine: An oxidation dye used in most permanent haircolors, often abbreviated as P.P.D.

patch test: A test required by the Food and Drug Act, made by applying a small amount of the haircoloring preparation to the skin of the arm or behind the ear to determine possible allergies (hypersensitivity). Also called predisposition or skin test.

penetrating haircolor: Color that enters or penetrates the cortex or second layer of the hair shaft.

permanent haircolor: A category of haircolor products mixed with developer that create a lasting color change.

peroxide: (see *hydrogen peroxide*)

peroxide residue: Traces of peroxide left in the hair after treatment with lightener or tint.

persulfate: In haircoloring, a chemical ingredient commonly used in activators. It increases the speed of the decolorization process. (see *activator*)

pH: The degree of acidity or alkalinity of any water solution. The pH scale is a numerical scale from 0 (very acidic) to 14 (very alkaline). A pH of 7 is neutral.

pheomelanin: Naturally occurring red/yellow pigment.

pigment: Any substance or matter used as coloring; natural or artificial hair color.

porosity: Ability of the hair to absorb water or other liquids.
powder lightener: (see *off-the-scalp lightener*)
prebleach: (see *prelighten*)
predisposition test: (see *patch test*)
prelighten: Generally the first step of double-process haircoloring, used to lift or lighten the natural pigment. (see *decolorize*)
presoften: The process of treating unpigmented or very resistant hair to allow for better penetration of color.
primary color: Pigment or color that is fundamental and cannot be made by mixing colors together. Red, yellow, and blue are the primary colors.
prism: A transparent glass or crystal solid that breaks up white light into its component colors, the spectrum.
processing time: The time required for the chemical treatment to react on the hair.
progressive dye or **progressive dye system**: 1. A coloring system that produces increased absorption with each application. 2. Color products that deepen or increase absorption over a period of time during processing.
regrowth: (see *new growth*)
resistant hair: Hair that is difficult to penetrate with moisture or chemical solutions.
retouch: Application of color or lightening mixture to new growth of hair.
salt-and-pepper: The descriptive term for a mixture of pigmented and unpigmented, or white, hair.
secondary color: Color made by combining two primary colors in equal proportion. Green, orange, and violet are secondary colors.
semi-permanent haircolor: Haircolor that lasts through several shampoos. It penetrates the hair shaft and stains the cuticle layer, slowly fading with each shampoo.
sensitivity: A skin highly reactive to the presence of a specific chemical. Skin reddens or becomes irritated shortly after application of the chemical. On removal of the chemical, the reaction subsides.
shade: 1. A term used to describe a specific color. 2. The visible difference between two colors.
sheen: The ability of the hair to shine, gleam, or reflect light.
single-process haircolor: Refers to an oxidative tint solution that lifts or lightens while also depositing color in one application. (see *oxidative haircolor*)
softening agent: A mild alkaline product applied prior to the color treatment to increase porosity, swell the cuticle layer of the hair, and increase color absorption. Tint that has not been mixed with developer is frequently used. (see *presoften*)
solution: A blended mixture of solid, liquid, or gaseous substances in a liquid medium.
solvent: Carrier liquid in which other components may be dissolved.

specialist: One who concentrates on only one part or branch of a subject or profession.
spectrum: The series of colored bands diffracted and arranged in the order of their wavelengths by the passage of white light through a prism. Shading continuously from red (produced by the longest wave visible) to violet (produced by the shortest): red, orange, yellow, green, blue, indigo, and violet.
spot lightening: Color correcting using a lightening mixture to lighten up darker areas.
stabilizer: General name for ingredient that prolongs lifetime, appearance, and performance of a product.
stage: A term used to describe a visible color change that natural hair color goes through while being lightened. (see *degree*)
stain remover: Chemical used to remove tint stains from skin.
strand test: Test given before treatment to determine development time, color result, and the ability of the hair to withstand the effects of chemicals.
stripping: (See *color remover*)
tablespoon: ½ ounce, 3 teaspoons, 15 milliliters.
teaspoon: ⅙ ounce, ⅓ tablespoon, 5 milliliters.
temporary haircolor or temporary rinses: Color made from preformed dyes that are applied to the hair, but are readily removed with shampoo.
terminology: The special words or terms used in science, art, or business.
tertiary color: The mixture of a primary and an adjacent secondary color on the color wheel. Red-orange, yellow-orange, yellow-green, blue-green, blue-violet, red-violet. Also referred to as intermediary colors.
texture, hair: The diameter of an individual hair strand. Termed: coarse, medium, or fine.
tint: Permanent oxidizing haircolor product having the ability to lift and deposit color in the same process.
tint back: To return hair back to its original or natural color.
tone or **tonality**: A term used to describe the warmth or coolness in color.
toner: A pastel color to be used after prelightening.
toning: Adding color to modify the end result.
touch-up: (see *retouch*)
translucent: The property of letting diffused light pass through.
tyrosinase: The enzyme (tyrosinase) that reacts together with the amino acid (tyrosine) to form the hair's natural melanin pigment.
tyrosine: The amino acid (tyrosine) that reacts together with the enzyme (tyrosinase) to form the hair's natural melanin pigment.
undertone: The underlying color that emerges during the lifting process of melanin, which contributes to the end result. When lightening hair, a residual warmth in tone always occurs. Also referred to as contributing pigment.

unpigmented hair: Hair with decreasing amounts of natural pigment. Hair with no natural pigment is actually white. White hairs look unpigmented when mingled with the still-pigmented hair.
urea peroxide: A peroxide compound occasionally used in haircolor. When added to an alkaline color mixture, it releases oxygen.
value: (see *depth*; *level*)
vegetable color: A color derived from plant resources.
virgin hair: Natural hair that has not undergone any chemical or physical treatment.
viscosity: A term referring to the thickness of the solution.
volume: The concentration of hydrogen peroxide in water solution. Expressed as volumes of oxygen liberated per volume of solution; 20 volume peroxide would thus liberate 20 pints (9.4 liters) of oxygen gas for each pint (liter) of solution.
warm: Containing red, orange, yellow, or gold tones.

REVIEW QUESTIONS

HAIRCOLORING

1. List the elements of an effective haircolor consultation.
2. What is the difference between primary, secondary, and tertiary colors?
3. What are the classifications of haircolor? How do they act on the hair?
4. What are some advantages of semi-permanent haircoloring?
5. What is the correct procedure for giving a strand test?
6. How is temporary haircolor applied?
7. What is the procedure for a single-process tint?
8. How does the procedure vary for a tint retouch?
9. What is the activity of hydrogen peroxide during haircoloring?
10. For what two purposes are hair lighteners used?
11. Name the types of lighteners and the uses of each.
12. What methods are available to achieve special effects highlighting?
13. What preventative and corrective steps avoid or solve haircoloring problems?
14. What are the safety precautions to follow during the haircoloring process?

CHAPTER

Chemical Hair Relaxing and Soft Curl Permanent

LEARNING OBJECTIVES

After completing this chapter, you should be able to:

1. Define the purpose of chemical hair relaxing.
2. List the different products used in chemical hair relaxing.
3. Explain the difference between sodium hydroxide relaxers and thio relaxers.
4. Describe the three basic steps of chemical hair relaxing.
5. Explain client analyzation for a chemical hair relaxing treatment.
6. Demonstrate the procedures used for a sodium hydroxide hair relaxing process.
7. Demonstrate the procedures used for an ammonium thioglycolate hair relaxing process.
8. Demonstrate the procedures used for a chemical blow-out.
9. Demonstrate the procedures used for a soft curl permanent.

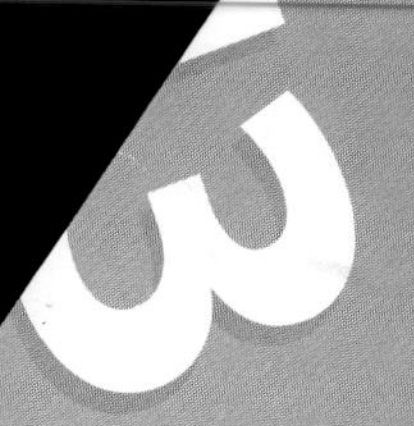

L STANDARDS

with the necessary information
dustry Skill Standards for Entry-Level Cosmetologists:

determine their needs and preferences

air relaxation and wave formation techniques in accordance with manufacturer's ections

- Providing styling and finishing techniques to complete a hairstyle to the satisfaction of the client
- Conducting services in a safe environment, taking measures to prevent the spread of infectious and contagious diseases

INTRODUCTION

Completed:
Learning Objective
#1
DEFINE PURPOSE OF CHEMICAL HAIR RELAXING

Chemical hair relaxing is the process of permanently rearranging the basic structure of overly curly hair into a straight form. When done professionally, it leaves the hair straight and in a satisfactory condition, to be set into almost any style.

CHEMICAL HAIR RELAXING PRODUCTS

Completed:
Learning Objective
#2
LIST CHEMICAL HAIR RELAXING PRODUCTS

The basic products that are used in chemical hair relaxing are a chemical hair relaxer, a neutralizer, a protein-rich moisturizer to stabilize the hair, and a petroleum cream, which is used as a protective base to protect the client's scalp during the sodium hydroxide chemical straightening process.

CHEMICAL HAIR RELAXERS

The two general types of hair relaxers are ***sodium hydroxide,*** which does not require pre-shampooing, and ***ammonium thioglycolate,*** which may require pre-shampooing.

Sodium hydroxide (caustic type hair relaxer) both softens and swells hair fibers. As the solution penetrates into the cortical layer, the cross-bonds (sulfur and hydrogen) are broken. The action of the comb, the brush, or the hands in smoothing the hair and distributing the chemical straightens the softened hair.

Manufacturers vary the sodium hydroxide content of the solution from 1½% to 3%, and the pH factor between 12 and 14. In general, the more sodium hydroxide used and the higher the pH, the quicker the chemical reaction will take place on the hair, and the greater the danger will be of hair damage.

> **CAUTION**
>
> *Because of the high alkaline content of sodium hydroxide, great care must be taken in its use.*

Although ammonium thioglycolate (thio type relaxer often called a softener, rearranger, or breakdown cream) is less drastic in its action than sodium hydroxide, it softens and relaxes overly curly hair in somewhat the same manner. You may recall that this is the same solution used in permanent waving.

Completed: Learning Objective #3

SODIUM HYDROXIDE VS. THIO RELAXERS

NEUTRALIZER

The ***neutralizer*** stops the action of any chemical relaxer that may remain in the hair after rinsing. The neutralizer for a thio type relaxer re-forms the cysteine (sulfur) cross-bonds in their new position and rehardens the hair.

BASE AND "NO BASE" FORMULAS

When using sodium hydroxide, there are two types of formulas, base and no base. The base formula is a petroleum cream that is designed to protect the client's skin and scalp during the sodium hydroxide chemical straightening process. This protective base also is important during a chemical straightening retouch. It is applied to protect hair that has been straightened previously, and to prevent over-processing and hair breakage.

Petroleum cream has a lighter consistency than petroleum jelly, and is formulated to melt at body temperature. The melting process ensures complete protective coverage of the scalp and other areas with a thin, oily coating. This helps to prevent burning and/or irritation of the scalp and skin. Previously treated hair should be protected with cream conditioner during the straightening process.

In recent years "no base" relaxers have become more commonly used. These relaxers have the same chemical reaction on the hair, although usually the reaction is milder. The procedure for the application of a "no base" relaxer is the same as for a regular relaxer except that the base cream is not applied. It is advisable to use a protective cream around the hairline and over the ears.

STEPS IN CHEMICAL HAIR RELAXING

All chemical hair relaxing involves three basic steps: ***processing, neutralizing,*** and ***conditioning.***

PROCESSING

As soon as the chemical relaxer is applied, the hair begins to soften so that the chemical can penetrate to loosen and relax the natural curl.

NEUTRALIZING

As soon as the hair has been sufficiently processed, the chemical relaxer is thoroughly rinsed out with warm water, followed by either a built-in shampoo neutralizer or a prescribed shampoo and neutralizer.

Completed: Learning Objective #4

THREE BASIC STEPS IN CHEMICAL HAIR RELAXING

CONDITIONING

Depending on the client's needs, the conditioner may be part of a series of hair treatments, or it may be applied to the hair after the relaxing treatment.

CAUTION

Overly curly hair that has been damaged from heat appliances or other chemicals must be reconditioned before a relaxer service is performed.

Hair treated with lighteners or metallic dyes must not be given a chemical hair relaxer, because it might cause excessive damage or breakage.

RECOMMENDED STRENGTH OF RELAXER

The strength of relaxer used is determined by the strand test. The following guidelines can help in determining which strength relaxer to use for the test.

1. Fine or tinted hair—Use mild relaxer.
2. Normal, medium-textured virgin hair—Use regular relaxer.
3. Coarse virgin hair—Use strong or super relaxer (but if the client has a sensitive scalp, use a regular or mild relaxer).

ANALYSIS OF CLIENT'S HAIR

It is essential that the cosmetologist have a working knowledge of human hair, particularly when giving a relaxing treatment. You will learn to recognize the qualities of hair by visible inspection, feel, and special tests. Before attempting to give a relaxing treatment to overly curly hair, the cosmetologist must judge its texture, porosity, elasticity, and the extent, if any, of damage to the hair. (For more complete information on hair analysis, refer to the chapter on permanent waving.)

CLIENT'S HAIR HISTORY

To help ensure consistent, satisfactory results, records should be kept of each chemical hair relaxing treatment. These records should include the client's hair history, products and conditioners used (see sample form below), and the client's release statement. The release statement is used to protect the cosmetologist, to some extent, from the responsibility for accidents or damages. You should be sure to find out if the client has ever had a hair relaxing. If so, was there any reaction? You must not chemically relax hair that has been treated with a metallic dye. To do so damages or destroys the hair. In addition, it is not advisable to use chemical relaxers on hair that has been bleached lighter.

Before starting to process the hair, you must know how the client will react to the relaxer. Therefore, the client must receive: (1) a thorough scalp and hair examination and (2) a hair strand test.

RELAXER RECORD

Name .... Tel ....

Address .... City .... State .... Zip ....

DESCRIPTION OF HAIR

Form	**Length**	**Texture**		**Porosity**	
□ wavy	□ short	□ coarse	□ soft	□ very porous	□ less porous
□ curly	□ medium	□ medium	□ silky	□ moderately porous	□ least porous
□ extra-curly	□ long	□ fine	□ wiry	□ normal	□ resistant

Condition

□ virgin □ retouched □ dry □ oily □ lightened

Tinted with ....

Previously relaxed with (name of relaxer) ....

□ Original sample of hair enclosed □ not enclosed

TYPE OF RELAXER OR STRAIGHTENER

□ whole head □ retouch

□ relaxer .... strength □ straightener .... strength

Results

□ good □ poor □ sample of relaxed hair enclosed □ not enclosed

Date	Operator	Date	Operator
....	....	....	....
....	....	....	....
....	....	....	....

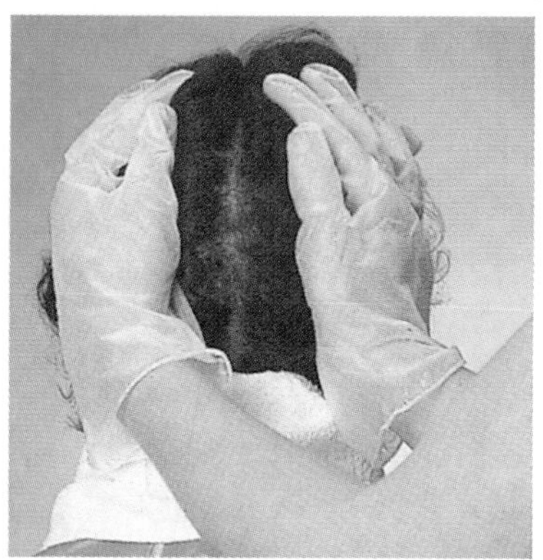

FIGURE 13.1 — Examining the scalp.

SCALP EXAMINATION

Inspect the scalp carefully for eruptions, scratches, or abrasions. To obtain a clearer view of the scalp, part the hair into ½" (1.25cm) sections. Hair parting may be done with the index and middle fingers or with the handle of a rat-tail comb. In either case, you must exercise great care not to scratch the scalp. Such scratches may become seriously infected when aggravated by the chemicals in the relaxer. (Fig. 13.1)

If the client has scalp eruptions or abrasions, or facial blemishes that extend into the scalp, do not apply the chemical hair relaxer until the scalp is healthy. If the hair is not in a healthy condition, prescribe a series of conditioning treatments to return it to a more normal condition. Then you may give a strand test.

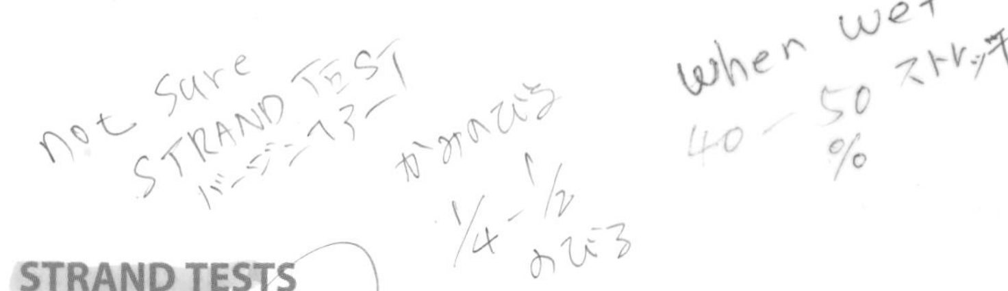

STRAND TESTS

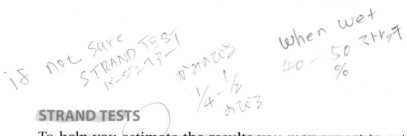

To help you estimate the results you may expect to get from a chemical relaxing, it is advisable to test the hair for porosity and elasticity. This can be done using one of the following strand tests:

Finger test. This test determines the degree of porosity in the hair. Grasp a strand of hair and run it between the thumb and index finger of the right hand, from the end toward the scalp. If it ruffles or feels bumpy, the hair is porous and can absorb moisture.

Pull test. This test determines the degree of elasticity in the hair. Normally, dry, curly hair will stretch about one-fifth its normal length without breaking. Grasp half a dozen strands from the crown area and pull them gently. If the hair appears to stretch, it has elasticity and can withstand the relaxer. If not, conditioning treatments are recommended prior to a chemical relaxing treatment.

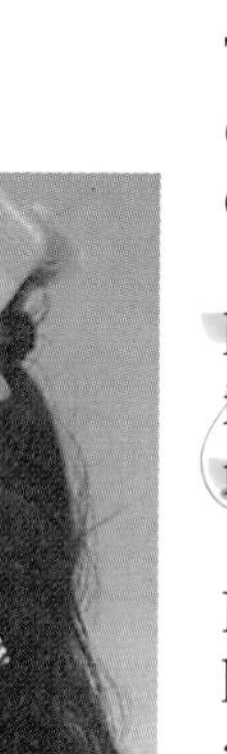

FIGURE 13.2 — Relaxer strand test.

Relaxer test. Application of the relaxer to a hair strand will indicate the reaction of the relaxer on the hair. Take a small section of hair from the crown or another area where the hair is wiry and resistant. Pull it through a slit in a piece of aluminum foil placed as close to the scalp as possible. Apply relaxer to the strand in the same manner as you would apply it to the entire head. Process the strand until it is sufficiently relaxed, checking the strand every 3 to 5 minutes. Make careful note of the timing, the smoothing required, and the hair strength. Shampoo the relaxer from the strand only, towel dry, and cover with protective cream to avoid damage during the relaxing service. If breakage has occurred, you should do another strand test using a milder solution. (Fig. 13.2)

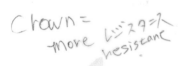

Completed:
Learning Objective
#5
CLIENT ANALYZATION FOR CHEMICAL HAIR RELAXING

CHEMICAL HAIR RELAXING PROCESS (WITH SODIUM HYDROXIDE)

The procedure outlined below is based primarily on products containing sodium hydroxide. For this, or any other kind of product, follow the manufacturer's directions and be guided by your instructor.

EQUIPMENT, IMPLEMENTS, AND MATERIALS

Chemical relaxer
Neutralizer or neutralizing shampoo
Shampoo and cream rinse
Shampoo cape
Protective base
Conditioner-filler
Protective gloves
Towels
Rollers
Comb and brush
Spatula
Timer
Conditioner
Absorbent cotton
Neck strip
Clips and picks
End papers
Setting lotion
Record card

PREPARATION

1. Select and arrange the required equipment, implements, and materials.
2. Wash and sanitize your hands.
3. Seat client comfortably. Remove earrings and neck jewelry; adjust towel and shampoo cape.
4. Examine and evaluate the scalp and hair.
5. Give a strand test and check results.
6. Do ***not*** shampoo hair. The relaxer will burn and irritate the scalp if the hair is shampooed prior to the procedure. (Hair ends may be trimmed after the application of the chemical relaxer.)
7. Have client sign release card.

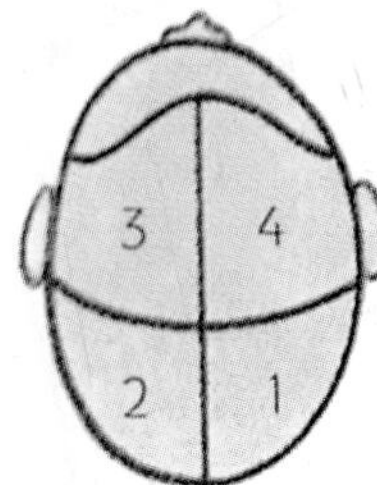

FIGURE 13.3 — Part hair into four sections.

PROCEDURE

1. Part hair into four or five sections, as recommended by your instructor. (Figs. 13.3, 13.4)
2. Dry hair. If moisture or perspiration is present on the scalp because of excessive heat or humidity, place the client under a cool dryer for several minutes.
3. If you're using a "no base" relaxer, it is recommended that a protective cream be applied on the hairline and around the ears.

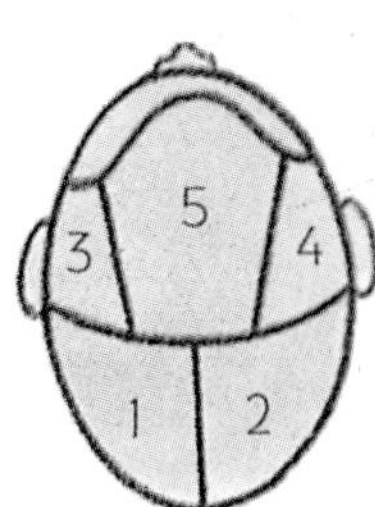

FIGURE 13.4 — Part hair into five sections; three sections in front area, two sections in back area.

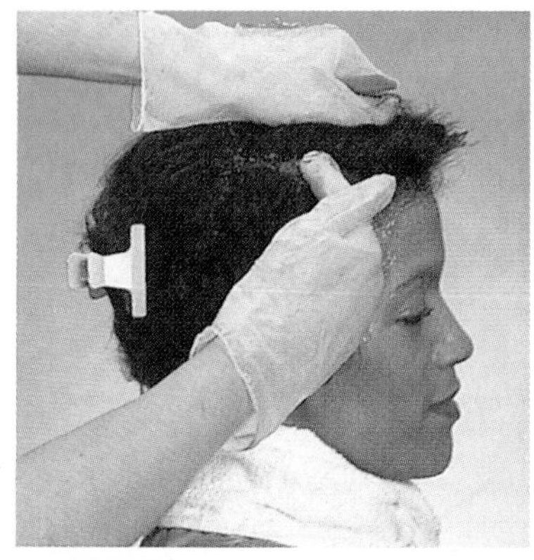

FIGURE 13.5 — Applying protective base.

If you're using a base formula, apply protective base to protect the scalp from the strong chemicals in the relaxer. To apply it properly, subdivide each of the four or five major sections into ½" to 1" (1.25 to 2.5 cm) partings, to permit thorough scalp coverage. (Fig. 13.5) Apply the base freely to the entire scalp with the fingers. The hairline around the forehead, nape of the neck, and area over and around the ears must be completely covered. Complete coverage is important to protect the scalp and hairline from irritation.

APPLYING THE CONDITIONER-FILLER

In many cases a conditioner-filler is required before the chemical relaxer can be used. The conditioner-filler, usually a protein product, is applied to the entire head of hair when dry. It protects over-porous or slightly damaged hair from being over-processed on any part of the hair shaft. It evens out porosity of the hair shaft, and permits uniform distribution and action of the chemical relaxer.

To give complete benefits from the conditioner-filler, rub it gently onto the hair from the scalp to the hair ends, using either the hands or a comb. Then towel dry the hair or use a cool dryer to completely dry the hair.

CAUTION

Avoid the use of heat, which will open the pores of the scalp and cause irritation or injury to the client's scalp.

Protective gloves must be worn by the cosmetologist to prevent damage to hands.

APPLYING THE RELAXER

Divide the head into four or five sections, in the same manner as for the application of the protective base.

The processing cream is applied last to the scalp area and hair ends. The body heat will speed up the processing action at the scalp. The hair is more porous at the ends and may be damaged. In both these areas, less processing time is required, and, therefore, the relaxer is applied last.

There are three methods in general use for the application of the chemical hair relaxer: the comb method, the brush method, and the finger method.

COMB METHOD

Remove a quantity of relaxing cream from the jar. Beginning in the back right section of the head, carefully part off ¼" to ½" (.66

to 1.25 cm) of hair, depending on its thickness and curliness. Apply the relaxer with the back of the comb, starting ½" to 1" (1.25 to 2.5 cm) from the scalp, and spread to within ½" (1.25 cm) of the hair ends. First apply the relaxer to the top side of the strand. (Fig. 13.6) Then, raise the subsection and apply the relaxer underneath. (Fig. 13.7) Gently lay the completed strand up, out of the way.

Complete the right back area and, moving in a clockwise direction, cover each section of the head in the same manner. Then, go back over the head in the same order, applying additional relaxing cream, if necessary, and spreading the relaxer close to the scalp and up to the hair ends. Avoid excessive pressure or stretching of the hair.

Smoothing the cream through the hair not only spreads the cream, but also gently stretches the hair into a straight position.

An alternate technique is to begin application at the nape, approximately 1" (2.5 cm) from the hairline, and continue toward the crown. The last place to apply relaxer is at the hairline. Be guided by your instructor's and the manufacturer's instructions.

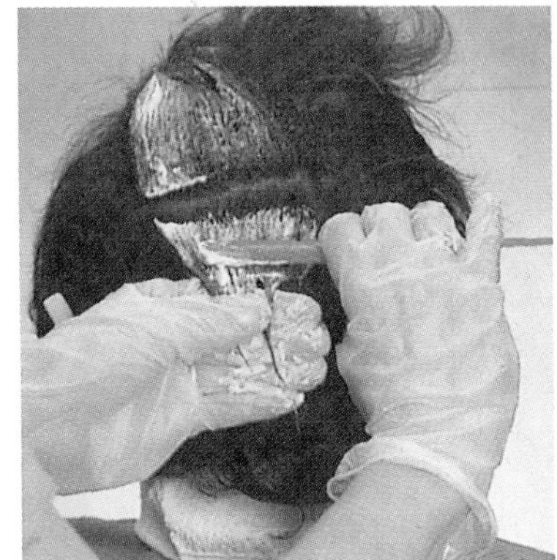

FIGURE 13.6 — Applying relaxer on top of strand.

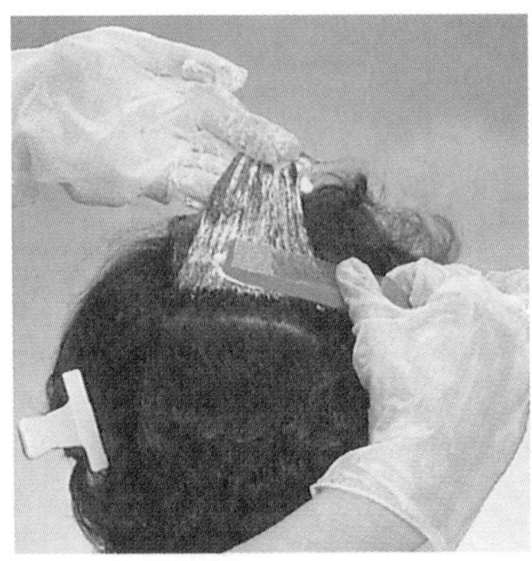

FIGURE 13.7 — Applying relaxer underneath strand.

BRUSH OR FINGER METHOD

The brush or finger method of applying the relaxer to the hair is the same as the comb method, except that a color applicator brush or the fingers and palms are used instead of the back of the comb. ***Wear protective gloves.***

PERIODIC STRAND TESTING

While spreading the relaxer, inspect its action by stretching the strands to see how fast the natural curls are being removed. Another method of testing is to press the strand to the scalp using the back of the comb or your finger. Examine the strand after your finger is removed. If it lies smoothly, the strand is sufficiently relaxed; if the strand reverts or "beads" back away from the scalp, continue processing.

RINSING OUT THE RELAXER

When the hair has been sufficiently straightened, rinse the relaxer out rapidly and thoroughly. (Fig. 13.8) The water should be warm, not hot. If the water is too hot, it may burn the client and cause discomfort because of the very sensitive condition of the scalp. The direct force of the rinse water should be used to remove the relaxer and avoid tangling the hair. Part hair with fingers to make sure no traces of the relaxer remain. Unless the relaxer is completely removed, its chemical action continues on the hair. The stream of water should be directed from the scalp to the hair ends.

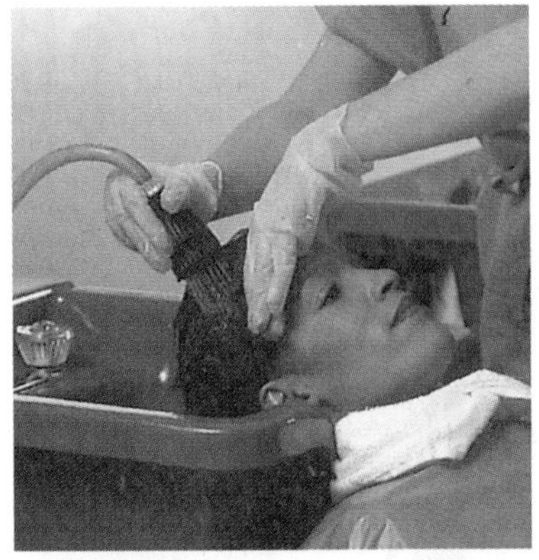

FIGURE 13.8 — Rinsing out relaxer.

CAUTION

Do not get relaxer or rinse water into the eyes or on unprotected skin. If the relaxer or rinse water gets into the client's eyes, wash it out immediately, and refer the client to a doctor without delay.

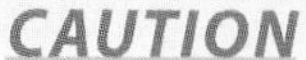

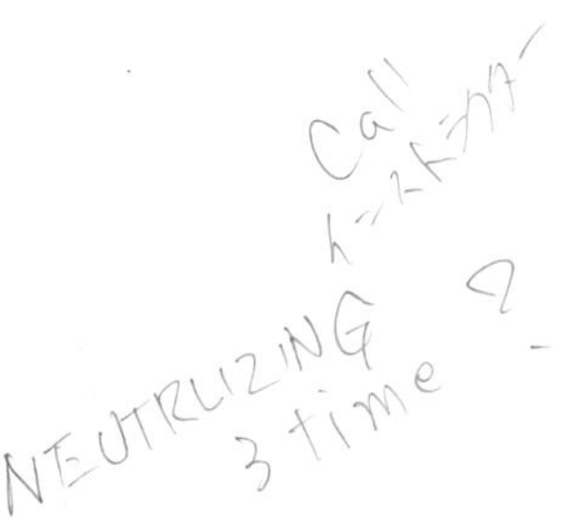

SHAMPOOING/NEUTRALIZING

When the hair is thoroughly rinsed, neutralize the hair as directed by your instructor. Most manufacturers provide a neutralizing shampoo that is applied to the hair after rinsing.

Completely saturate the hair with the neutralizing shampoo. Beginning at the nape, carefully comb with a wide-tooth comb, working upward, toward the forehead. Use the comb to:

1. Keep the hair straight.
2. Ensure complete saturation with the neutralizing shampoo.
3. Remove any tangles without pulling.

Time the neutralizer as directed and rinse thoroughly. Shampoo again to bring pH down to a safe level. Towel blot gently. Condition hair and proceed with styling. Discard used supplies. Cleanse and sanitize equipment. Wash and sanitize hands. Complete record of all timings and treatments during the service, and file the record card.

Note: *Different products used for relaxing require different methods. Always follow the manufacturer's directions.*

APPLYING THE CONDITIONER

Many manufacturers recommend that you apply a conditioner before setting the hair, to offset the harshness of the sodium hydroxide in the relaxer and to help restore some of the natural oils to the scalp and hair.

Two types of conditioners available are:

1. ***Cream-type conditioners*** are applied to the scalp and hair, then carefully rinsed out. The hair is then towel dried. Apply setting lotion; set the hair on rollers; dry and style the hair in the usual manner.
2. ***Protein-type (liquid) conditioners*** are applied to the scalp and hair prior to hairsetting and allowed to remain in the hair to serve as a setting lotion. Set the hair on rollers, dry, and style in the usual manner.

Note: *Because of the fragile condition of the hair, it is advisable to wind the hair on the roller without extreme tension.*

HOT THERMAL IRONS

Relaxed hair is in a weakened condition. To avoid hair breakage, excessive heat and excessive stretching should be avoided. Thermal curling with warm heat can be used to curl chemically relaxed hair. Conditioning treatments should be recommended and the hair dried completely before thermal curling. (See chapter on thermal hairstyling for a discussion of thermal irons.)

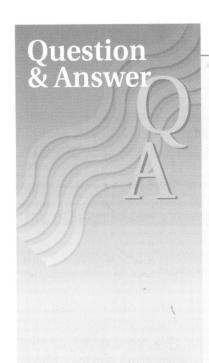

RELAXING TWO DEGREES OF CURL

Is it advisable to relax only half the head if excessive curl is in the front only?

It is not unusual for a person to have mixed hair textures. If you closely examine most Caucasian heads you'll find areas that are fine and straight while others are wavy to curly. It is no different with the hair of African-American clients. The reason for this is not thoroughly understood except to say each hair follicle controls the size, shape, and growth pattern of the hair growing from that particular root. Just as hair on different parts of the body differs in strength and structure, so can the hair on various portions of one's head.

It is not advisable to chemically re-structure only a portion of the hair on one head. Hair that has been chemically treated does not react the same as virgin hair and will make styling noticeably difficult.

Use a relaxer formulated with an ammonium thioglycolate base—widely called a curl re-arranger. The thio-based relaxer has a lower pH factor than sodium hydroxide relaxers; therefore they are not formulated to be used on kinky or wool-like hair. They are great for use on virgin hair with moderate curls or hair that must be relaxed for style control.

Inasmuch as the relaxer is thio-based, it is compatible with liquid thio-perm solution. The best solution for chemically treating hair that is only partially curly is to first apply a thio relaxer to the curly portion, then process and rinse. Then perm the entire head using large perm rods to relax and widen the original wave pattern for easier styling. All the hair, having been chemically treated, will react the same when dry.

—*From* Milady's Salon Solutions *by Louise Cotter*

Completed:
Learning Objective
#6
PROCEDURE FOR SODIUM HYDROXIDE HAIR RELAXING PROCESS

SODIUM HYDROXIDE RETOUCH

Hair grows about ¼" to ½" (.66 to 1.25 cm) per month. A retouch should probably be done every 6 weeks to 2 months, depending on how quickly the client's hair grows.

Follow all the steps for a regular chemical hair relaxing treatment, with one exception: ***apply the relaxer only to the new growth.*** In order to avoid breakage of previously treated hair, apply a cream conditioner over the hair that received the earlier treatment, thus avoiding overlapping and damage.

CHEMICAL HAIR RELAXING PROCESS (WITH AMMONIUM THIOGLYCOLATE)

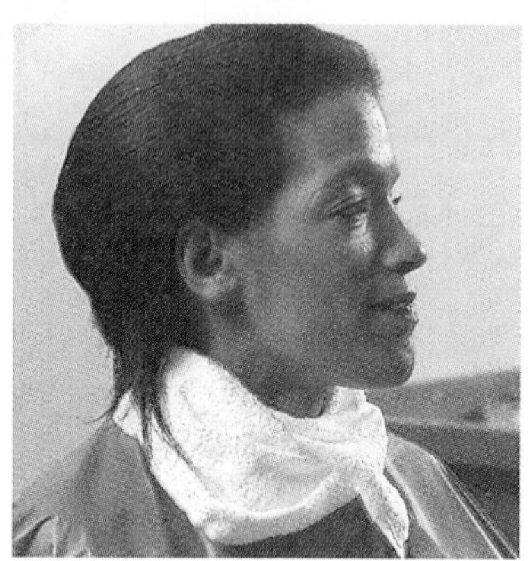

FIGURE 13.9 — Relaxed hair.

Ammonium thioglycolate (also called thio relaxer) is the same type of product used in cold waving, with a heavy cream or gel added to the formula in order to keep the hair in a straightened position. (Fig. 13.9)

As in cold waving, the relaxer breaks the sulfur and hydrogen bonds, softening and swelling the hair. The mechanical action of the hands, brush, or fingers smooths the hair and holds it in a straightened position.

Once the hair is straightened, the neutralizer is applied (serving the same purpose as the neutralizer in cold waving). It reforms the sulfur and hydrogen bonds and rehardens the hair in its newly straightened position.

Manufacturers vary their products according to the texture and condition of the hair. Tinted and lightened hair require a weaker formula than virgin hair.

Thio relaxers have a milder relaxing action on curly hair. You may choose to use them on fine-textured hair, or when it is desirable to remove less curl from the hair. Thio relaxers can also be used to reduce excessive curl formed in a permanent wave. Consult your instructor for directions and precautions for this specialized service.

Techniques for thio relaxers vary. The general procedure involves preparing the hair (gently shampooing if required), applying a base if necessary, applying the relaxer in the manner outlined under "Chemical Hair Relaxing Process (with Sodium Hydroxide)," and periodic strand testing. Directions at this point may vary greatly, so follow the manufacturer's directions *carefully.* Remove the relaxer from the hair and neutralize as directed, condition, and proceed with styling of the hair. As with any chemical service, exercise caution so that the hair is not excessively heated or stretched during styling as this may cause damage to both the hair and the desired curl formation.

THIO RETOUCH

As noted earlier, hair grows at the rate of ¼" to ½" (.66 to 1.25 cm) per month. A thio retouch should be given when there is a noticeable regrowth. Follow all steps for a regular thio hair relaxing treatment, with the exception of the relaxer, which is applied only to the new growth. A conditioner should be applied to the previously relaxed hair to protect it from damage.

Completed: Learning Objective #7

PROCEDURE FOR AMMONIUM THIOGLYCOLATE HAIR RELAXING PROCESS

OTHER RELAXERS

Researchers have also developed acid-based relaxers for the treatment of overly curly hair. Like acid permanent waves, the relaxer works with bisulfites rather than with thioglycolate acid. This type of relaxer is designed as a milder-acting one, much like the thio. Some can also be used as a pre-wrap preparation for performing a permanent wave on excessively curly hair.

CHEMICAL BLOW-OUT

To meet the needs of salon clients, great versatility in hairstyling may be achieved with the chemical blow-out. This technique removes only a small amount of the curl, leaving the hair in a more manageable condition. A chemical blow-out is a combination of chemical hair straightening and hairstyling, which creates a well-groomed style in the African-American tradition.

The chemical blow-out may be done with either the thio hair relaxer or the sodium hydroxide relaxer. The important consideration with either method is not to over-relax the hair to the point where the blow-out process becomes impossible to perform. Usually, when the thio relaxer is used, the hair is shampooed first. When the sodium hydroxide relaxer is used, the hair is shampooed after the hair is relaxed. (Follow the manufacturer's or your instructor's directions.)

EQUIPMENT, IMPLEMENTS, AND MATERIALS

Use the same equipment, implements, and materials as for a regular chemical relaxing, plus a wide-tooth comb (hair lifter or pick), scissors, clippers, and hand blower.

PROCEDURE

1. Prepare and drape client as for a regular hair relaxing treatment.
2. Apply scalp conditioner and/or base to the scalp.
3. Wear protective gloves; apply relaxer in the usual manner.

4. Stop the relaxing procedure by rinsing the relaxer from the hair with warm water before it is straightened and while it still shows a wave or curl formation.
5. Apply neutralizer or neutralizing shampoo.
6. Rinse out neutralizer and towel blot the hair.
7. Apply a conditioner to scalp and hair to help restore the natural oils removed by the relaxer.

Completed: Learning Objective #8 CHEMICAL BLOW-OUT PROCEDURE

If the blow-out style is desired, dry the hair with a hand dryer while lifting the hair with a hair lifter or pick. Dry from the scalp out to the ends. Distribute the dry hair evenly around the head and shape with clippers or shears. Continue to lift the hair out from the head to check progress of cut.

The hair can also be shaped while wet, then combed into place to let it dry naturally. For a softer look, the hair can be picked or combed when dry.

REVIEW OF SAFETY PRECAUTIONS

When giving a chemical relaxing treatment, you can never be too cautious. Here is a review of the safety measures that will ensure a comfortable and safe treatment for your client.

1. Examine the scalp for abrasions; if any are present, do not give a hair relaxing treatment.
2. Analyze the hair; give a strand test.
3. Do not relax damaged hair. Suggest a series of conditioning treatments. In extreme cases it may be advisable to cut off the damaged hair.
4. Do not shampoo the hair prior to the application of a sodium hydroxide product.
5. Do not apply a sodium hydroxide relaxer over a thio relaxer.
6. Do not apply a thio relaxer over a sodium hydroxide relaxer.
7. Never use a strong relaxer on fine hair, as it may cause breakage.
8. Cool or warm irons may be used on chemically relaxed hair. Do not use excessive heat, as it may cause damage to relaxed hair.
9. Apply a protective base, to avoid burning or irritating the scalp with the sodium hydroxide relaxer.
10. Wear protective gloves.
11. Protect client's eyes.

12. Use extreme care when applying the relaxer to avoid accidentally spreading it on the ears, scalp, or skin.
13. Strand test the action of the relaxer frequently to determine how fast the natural curl is being removed.
14. Be sure to thoroughly rinse the relaxer from the hair. Failure to do so permits the relaxer to continue to process, resulting in hair damage. Direct stream of warm water from scalp to hair ends.
15. Wear protective gloves until all the relaxer has been removed. When rinsing the shampoo from the hair, always work from the scalp to the ends, to prevent tangling the hair.
16. Use a wide-tooth comb and avoid pulling when combing the hair after the relaxation process is complete. Avoid scratching the scalp with comb or fingernails.
17. Apply a conditioner to the scalp and hair before setting the hair.
18. When retouching the new growth, do not allow the relaxer to overlap onto the hair already straightened.
19. Do not give a hair relaxing treatment to hair treated with a metallic dye.
20. At the completion of each treatment, fill out a complete record card.
21. Have the client sign a release statement to protect the salon and the cosmetologist.
22. It is not advisable to use chemical relaxers on lightened hair, which is already in a weakened condition.
23. Hair should not be relaxed or straightened more than 80%. To go beyond that point may severely damage the hair.

SOFT CURL PERMANENT

Soft curl permanent waving is a method of permanently waving overly curly hair. It is known by various names given by the manufacturers of the products.

> **CAUTION**
>
> *The product used contains ammonium thioglycolate (thio).*
>
> 1. *Do not use on hair that has been treated with sodium hydroxide products.*
> 2. *Do not use on hair that has been treated with metallic dye or compound henna.*

IMPLEMENTS AND MATERIALS

- Shampoo cape
- Neck strips and towels
- Mild shampoo
- Combs
- Gloves
- Protective cream
- Thio gel, cream, or lotion
- Applicators
- Curling rods
- Porous end papers
- Pre-wrap solution
- Waving lotion
- Cotton or neutralizing bands
- Plastic cap
- Neutralizer
- Styling lotion (curl activator)
- Finishing rinse
- Hair clips
- Scissors or razor
- Record cards

PROCEDURE

This procedure can be used for both men and women.

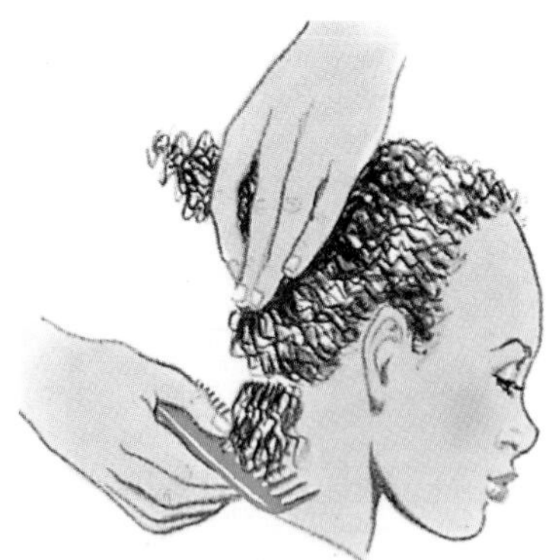

FIGURE 13.10 — Remove tangles from hair.

1. Examine the client's scalp. Do not use permanent waving gel or cream if the scalp shows signs of abrasions or lesions, or if the client has experienced an allergic reaction to a previous perm.
2. Shampoo and rinse hair thoroughly. Towel dry, leaving hair damp.
3. Remove tangles with a large-tooth comb. (Fig. 13.10)
4. Part hair into four to five sections, as recommended by your instructor. *(If the manufacturer requires it, put a protective cream on the entire scalp, including around the hairline.)*
5. Wear protective gloves.
6. Apply thio gel or cream to one section at a time, using the back of a comb, a haircoloring brush, or fingers. Use a tail comb to part hair and begin the application of thio gel or cream to the hair nearest the scalp, preferably starting at the nape area. Work the thio gel or cream to the ends of the hair. (Fig. 13.11)

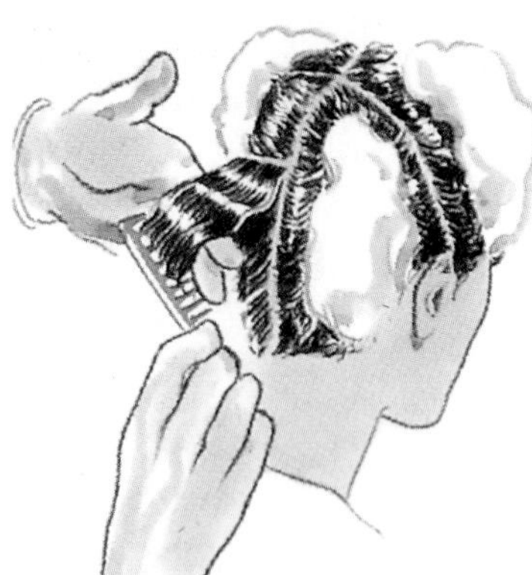

FIGURE 13.11 — Part hair into sections and coat with thio gel.

7. Comb the thio gel or cream through the entire head, first with a wide-tooth comb, then with a smaller-tooth comb. (Fig. 13.12)
8. When the hair becomes supple and flexible, rinse with tepid water and towel dry. Do not tangle the hair.

Note: *Always follow the manufacturer's instructions on the recommended procedure for rinsing off the chemical.*

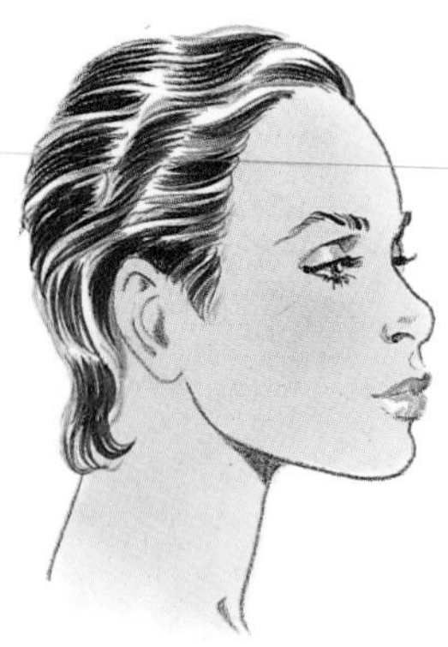

FIGURE 13.12 — Comb thio gel through hair.

9. Divide the hair into eight sections. (Fig. 13.13) Subsection as you wrap the hair. (Fig. 13.14)

10. Wrap hair as desired on curling rods. In order to rearrange the curl pattern of the hair, the rod selected must be at least two times larger than the natural curl. In order to achieve a good curl formation, the hair should encircle the rod at least 2½ times.
11. After the wrap has been completed, protect the client's skin by placing cotton around the hairline and neck. (Fig. 13.15)

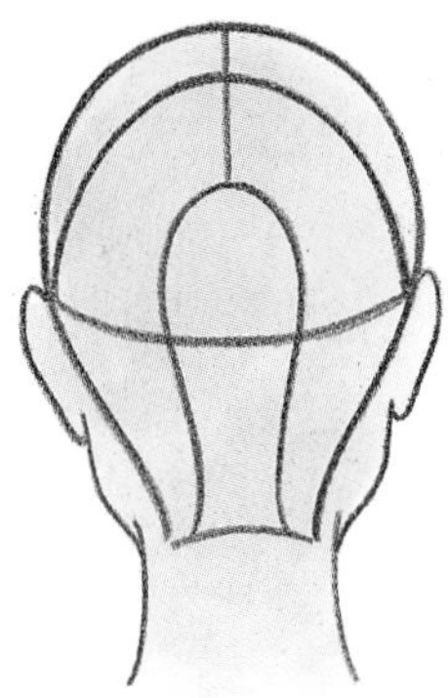

FIGURE 13.13 — Divide the hair into eight sections.

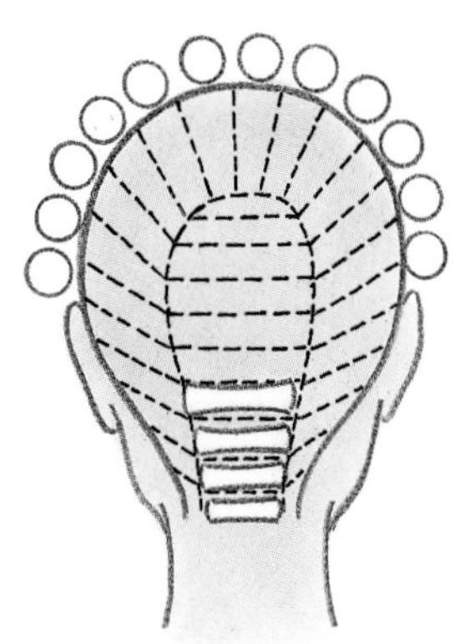

FIGURE 13.14 — Subsection as you wrap.

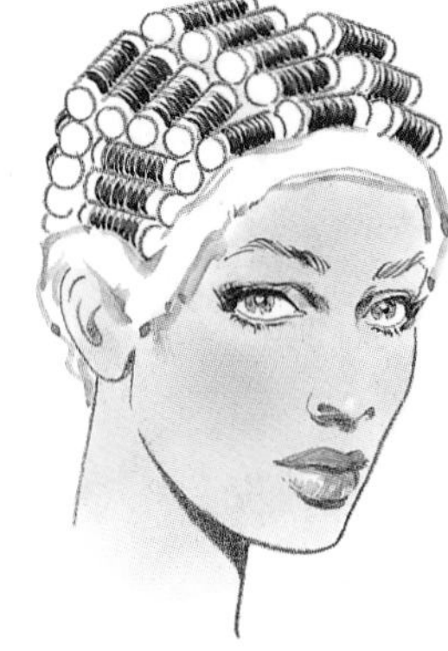

FIGURE 13.15 — Protect client's skin with cotton around hairline.

12. Apply thio gel, cream, or lotion to all the curls until they are thoroughly saturated. (Fig. 13.16) Replace saturated cotton.
13. Cover the client's head with a plastic cap.
14. Have the client sit under a pre-heated dryer for 15 to 25 minutes, or as recommended by the manufacturer. Wrapping the head with hot towels is another option. (Fig. 13.17)

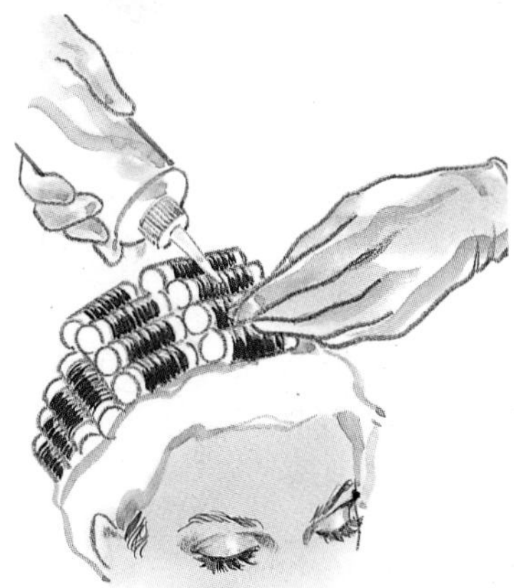

FIGURE 13.16 — Apply thio gel to curls.

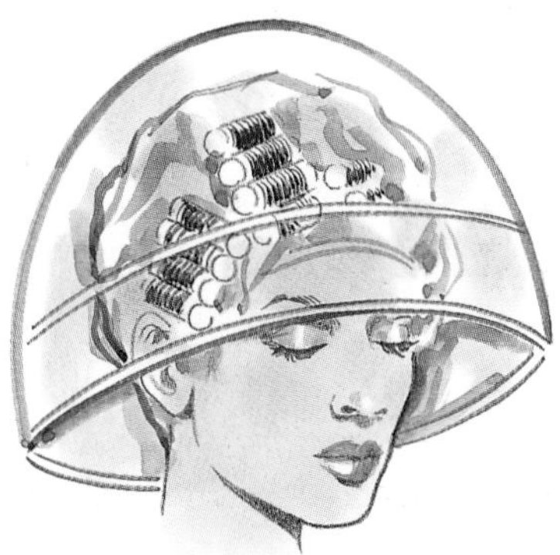

FIGURE 13.17 — Process under pre-heated dryer.

15. Take a test curl (Fig. 13.18), and if the desired curl pattern has not developed, have the client sit under the dryer for another 10 minutes or until a curl pattern develops.

16. When the desired curl pattern has been reached, rinse the hair thoroughly with warm (not hot) water. (Fig. 13.19) Blot each curl with a towel.

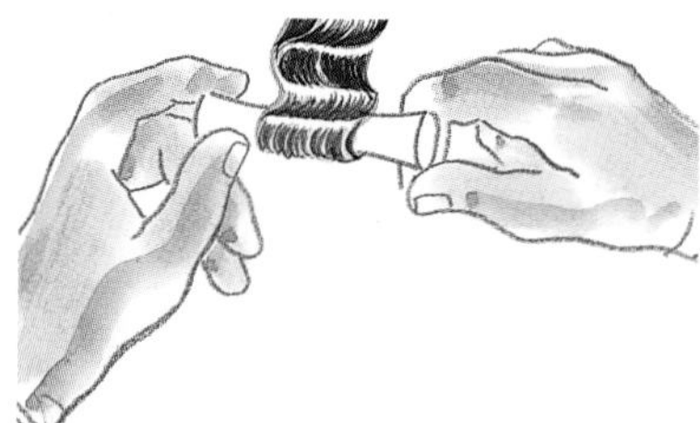

FIGURE 13.18 — Test a curl.

17. Use a prepared neutralizer, or mix neutralizer as directed by the manufacturer, and saturate each curl twice. (Fig. 13.20) Allow neutralizer to remain on the curls for 5 to 10 minutes, or as directed by the manufacturer.

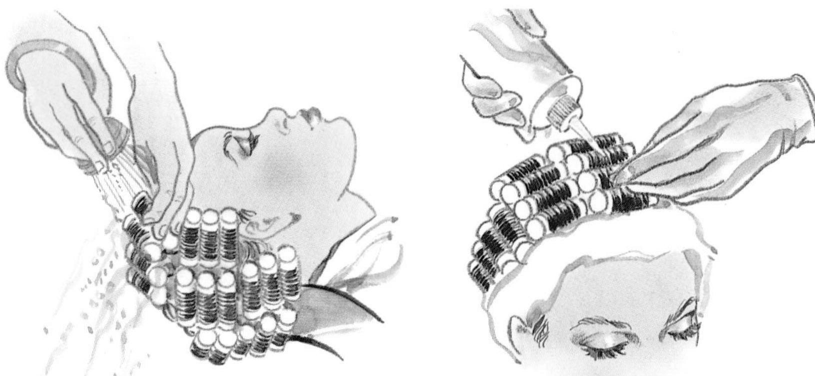

FIGURE 13.19 — Rinse the hair.

FIGURE 13.20 — Apply neutralizer.

18. Carefully remove rods and apply balance of neutralizer to the hair. Work neutralizer through with fingers for thorough distribution (Fig. 13.21), and allow it to remain on the hair for another 5 minutes.

19. Rinse hair thoroughly with warm water, then cool water, and towel blot.

20. Trim uneven hair ends. (Fig. 13.22)

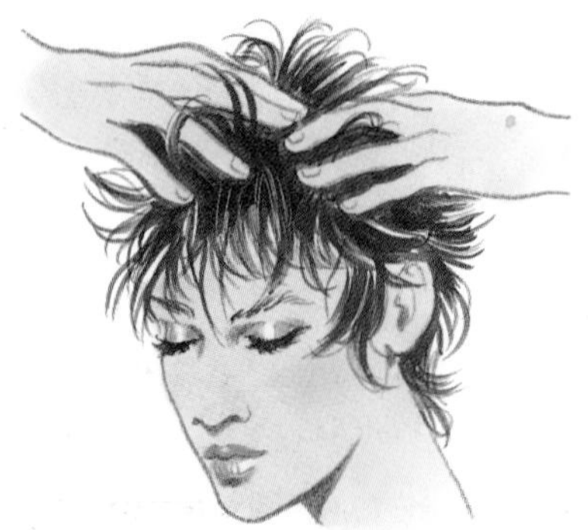

FIGURE 13.21 — Work neutralizer through hair.

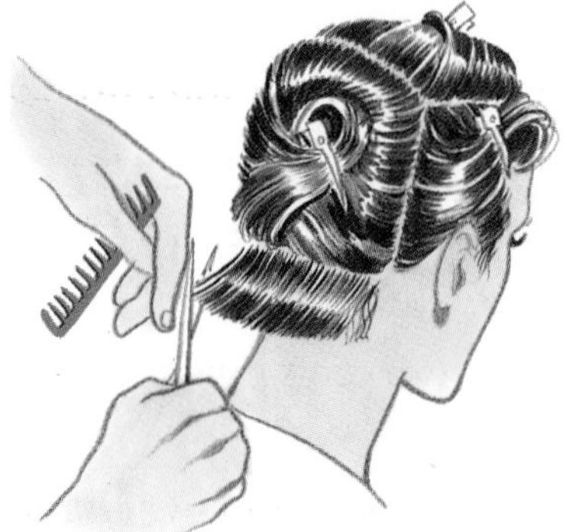

FIGURE 13.22 — Trim hair ends.

21. Apply conditioner as directed by the manufacturer.

22. Air dry hair or style as directed. (Fig. 13.23)

Completed: Learning Objective #9

SOFT CURL PERMANENT PROCEDURE

Figure 13.24 illustrates hairstyle *after* a soft curl permanent was given.

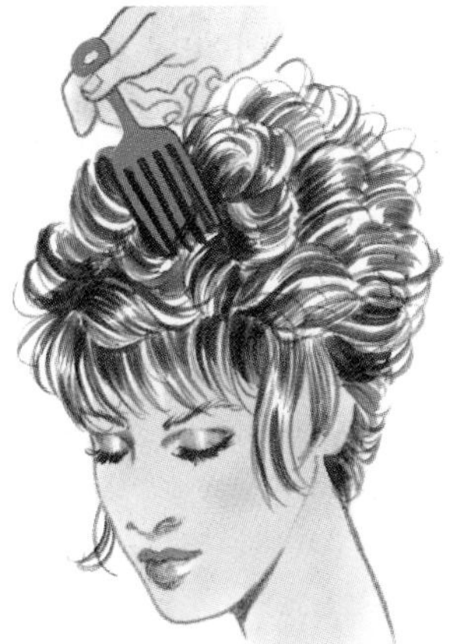

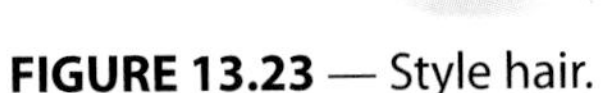

FIGURE 13.23 — Style hair.

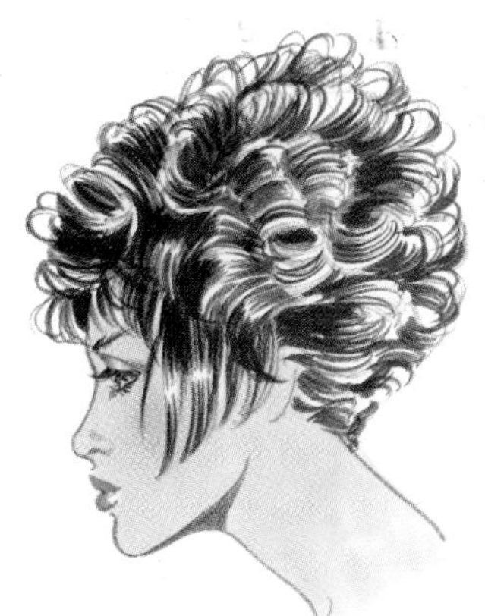

FIGURE 13.24 — Finished hairstyle.

AFTERCARE

1. Do not comb or brush the curls when wet; use a lifting pick instead.
2. Do not shampoo for at least five days. As with any chemical procedure, the hair takes time to return to a lower pH, and a shampoo with a higher pH may weaken the curl. Thereafter shampoo with a mild (acid-balanced) shampoo.
3. Conditioner or curl activator should be used daily to maintain flexibility, sheen, and proper moisture balance of the hair.

REVIEW OF SAFETY PRECAUTIONS

1. Do not give a soft curl permanent to hair treated with sodium hydroxide.
2. Do not give a soft curl permanent to hair that has been colored with a metallic dye or compound henna.
3. Thoroughly analyze the hair and scalp and record the information prior to giving a soft curl permanent.
4. Bleached, tinted, or damaged hair must be reconditioned until the hair is of sufficient strength to ensure that the soft curl service will not cause further damage.

5. If permanent waving lotion or neutralizer accidentally gets into the client's eye, flush the eye immediately with water and refer the client to a doctor.
6. Test curl frequently—but not the same curl—to ensure proper curl formation without damage.
7. Use protective cream around client's hairline and neck.
8. Complete client's record card carefully and accurately.

REVIEW QUESTIONS

CHEMICAL HAIR RELAXING AND SOFT CURL PERMANENT

1. What are the basic products used for chemical hair relaxing?
2. What are the two types of chemical hair relaxers?
3. What are the three steps of chemical hair relaxing?
4. What is the most important point to remember when performing a chemical service?
5. What type of hair relaxing technique achieves the greatest versatility in hairstyling?
6. List the three most important safety precautions for chemical hair relaxing.
7. What is the method of permanently waving overly curly hair?
8. If hair were treated with sodium hydroxide, what service could not be done?
9. If hair is damaged by an appliance or a chemical, what must you do before applying a chemical hair relaxer?

CHAPTER 14

Thermal Hair Straightening (Hair Pressing)

LEARNING OBJECTIVES

After completing this chapter, you should be able to:

1. Discuss the purpose served by hair pressing.
2. Explain how to analyze the client's hair and scalp condition prior to a hair pressing.
3. List the products required for a successful hair pressing.
4. Demonstrate the procedures involved in both soft pressing and hard pressing.
5. List the safety precautions that must be observed in hair pressing.

NATIONAL SKILL STANDARDS

This chapter provides you with the necessary information to master these National Industry Skill Standards for Entry-Level Cosmetologists:

- Consulting with clients to determine their needs and preferences
- Providing styling and finishing techniques to complete a hairstyle to the satisfaction of the client
- Conducting services in a safe environment, taking measures to prevent the spread of infectious and contagious diseases

INTRODUCTION

Completed: Learning Objective #1

PURPOSE OF HAIR PRESSING

Hair straightening, or ***pressing,*** is a profitable service that is popular in the beauty salon. When properly done, hair pressing temporarily straightens overly curly or unruly hair. A pressing generally lasts until the hair is next shampooed. (Permanent hair straightening is covered in the chapter on chemical hair relaxing.)

Hair pressing prepares the hair for additional services, such as thermal roller curling and croquignole thermal curling (the two-loop or "Figure 8" technique). A good hair pressing leaves the hair in a natural and lustrous condition and is not harmful to the hair.

There are three types of hair pressing:

1. *Soft press,* which removes about 50% to 60% of the curl and is accomplished by applying the thermal pressing comb once on each side of the hair.
2. *Medium press,* which removes about 60% to 75% of the curl and is accomplished by applying the thermal pressing comb once on each side of the hair using slightly more pressure.
3. *Hard press,* which removes 100% of the curl and is accomplished by applying the thermal pressing comb twice on each side of the hair. A hard press can also be done by passing a hot curling iron through the hair first. This is called a *double press.*

ANALYSIS OF HAIR AND SCALP

Before the cosmetologist undertakes to press the client's hair, there should be an analysis of the condition of the hair and scalp in order to evaluate the client's needs.

> **CAUTION**
>
> *Under no circumstances should hair pressing be given to a client who has a scalp abrasion, contagious scalp condition, scalp injury, or chemically treated hair.*

If the client's hair and scalp are not normal, the cosmetologist should give appropriate advice concerning preliminary corrective treatments. Relaxed hair should not be pressed. If the hair shows signs of neglect or abuse caused by faulty pressing, lightening, or tinting, the cosmetologist should recommend a series of conditioning treatments. Failure to correct dry and brittle hair can result in hair breakage during hair pressing. ***Burnt hair strands cannot be conditioned.***

You should also remember to check the elasticity and porosity of your client's hair. Under normal conditions, if a client's hair has good elasticity, it can be safely stretched about one-fifth of its length. If the ability of the hair to absorb water (porosity) is normal, then the hair returns to its normal curly appearance when it is wet or moistened.

A careful analysis of the client's hair and scalp should cover the following points:

1. Form of hair (curly or overly curly)
2. Length of hair (long, medium, or short)
3. Texture of hair (coarse, medium, fine, or very fine)
4. Feel of hair (wiry, soft, or silky)
5. Elasticity of hair (normal or poor)
6. Shade of hair (natural, faded, streaked, or gray)
7. Condition of hair (normal, brittle, dry, oily, damaged, or chemically treated)
8. Condition of scalp (normal, flexible, or tight)

It is important that the cosmetologist be able to recognize individual differences in hair texture, hair porosity, hair elasticity, and scalp flexibility. Guided by this knowledge, the cosmetologist can determine how much pressure the hair and scalp can tolerate without breakage, hair loss, or burning from a pressing comb that is not adjusted to the right temperature.

HAIR TEXTURE

Variations in hair texture can be traced to the following factors:

1. Diameter of the hair (coarse, medium, or fine). Coarse hair has the greatest diameter. Fine hair has the smallest diameter.
2. Feel of the hair (wiry, soft, or silky).

The client's hair texture also depends on how dry, oily, unpigmented, tinted, lightened, or curly it is. Touching the client's hair and asking specifically about hair characteristics will help you know how to treat the client's hair.

Coarse Hair

Coarse, overly curly hair has qualities that make it difficult to press. Coarse hair has the greatest diameter, and during the pressing process it requires more heat and pressure than medium or fine hair.

Medium Hair

Medium curly hair is the normal type of hair cosmetologists deal with in the beauty salon. No special problem is presented by this type of hair, and it is the least resistant to hair pressing.

Fine Hair

Fine hair requires special care. To avoid hair breakage, less heat and pressure should be applied than for other hair textures. Whereas coarse and medium hair have three layers (cuticle, cortex, and medulla), fine hair has only two layers (cortex and cuticle).

Wiry, Curly Hair

Wiry, curly hair may be coarse, medium, or fine. It feels stiff, hard, and glassy. Because of the compact construction of the cuticle cells, it is very resistant to hair pressing and it requires more heat and pressure than other types of hair.

SCALP CONDITION

The condition of the client's scalp can be classified as normal, tight, or flexible. If the scalp is normal, proceed with an analysis of the texture and elasticity of the hair. If the scalp is tight and the hair coarse, press the hair in the direction in which it grows to avoid injury to the scalp.

The main difficulty with a flexible scalp is that the cosmetologist might not apply enough pressure to press the hair satisfactorily.

Completed:
Learning Objective
#2
ANALYZING HAIR AND SCALP CONDITION

RECORD CARD

You should be sure to keep a record of all pressing treatments performed on a client. It also is advisable to question the client about any lightener, tint, color restorer (metallic), or other chemical treatment that was used on his or her hair.

CONDITIONING TREATMENTS

Effective conditioning treatments require special cosmetic preparations for the hair and scalp, thorough brushing, and scalp massage. These treatments usually help get better results from hair pressing. The use of an infrared lamp is optional, depending on the type of treatment being given.

A tight scalp can be rendered more flexible by the systematic use of scalp massage, hair brushing, and direct high-frequency current. The client benefits because there is better circulation of blood to the scalp.

PRESSING COMBS

There are two types of pressing combs: regular and electric. They are both constructed of either good quality stainless steel or brass. The handle is usually made of wood since wood does not readily absorb heat. The space between the teeth of the comb varies with the size and style of the comb. A comb with more space between the teeth produces a coarse-looking press. A comb with less space produces a smoother press. Pressing combs vary in size; some are short, to be used with short hair, while long combs are used with long hair. (Fig. 14.1)

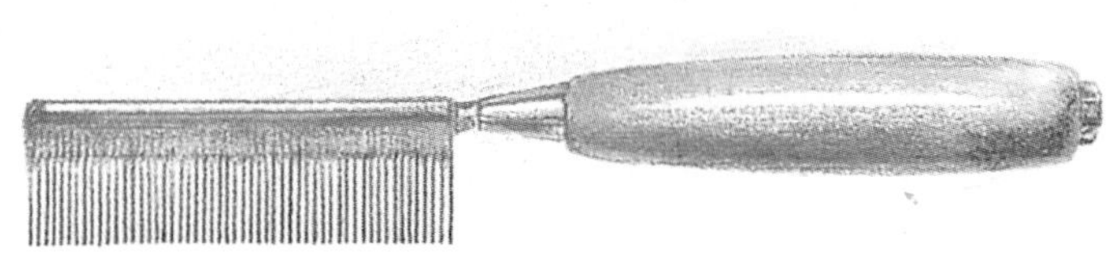

FIGURE 14.1 — Regular pressing comb.

It may be a good idea to *temper* a new pressing comb if it is made of brass. Tempering allows the brass to hold heat evenly along the length of the comb, with better results on your clients' hair. Another good reason to temper is to burn off any polish the manufacturer may have used to coat the comb. If the polish is not burned off, the comb may stick to the hair, causing scorching and breakage.

To temper, place the comb in the heating appliance until it is extremely hot. Remove the comb and submerge or coat it in petroleum or pressing oil. Let it cool down naturally, then rinse under hot running water to remove the oil.

Heating the Comb

Depending on their composition, combs vary in their ability to accept and retain heat. Regular pressing combs may be heated on gas stoves or electric heaters. (Fig. 14.2) While the comb is being heated, its teeth should face upward and the handle should be kept away from the fire. After heating the comb to the proper temperature, test it on a piece of light paper. If the paper becomes scorched, allow the comb to cool slightly before applying it to the hair.

Electric pressing combs are available in two forms: one comes with an "on" and "off" switch; the other is equipped with a thermostat, which has a control switch that indicates high or low degrees of heat.

There is also a straightening comb attachment that fits the nozzle of a standard hand-held dryer and is less damaging than an electric comb or an oven-heated comb.

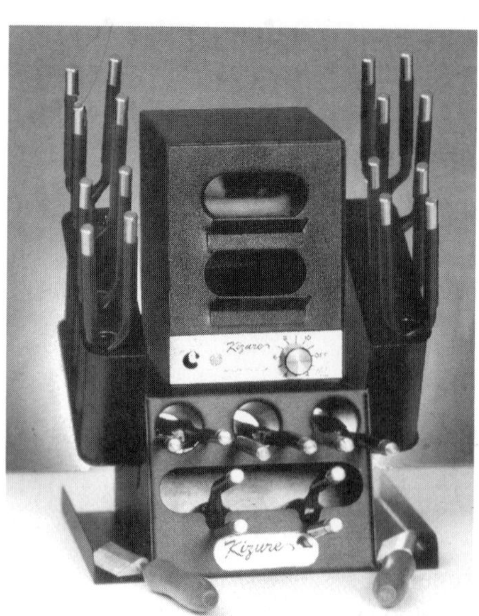

FIGURE 14.2 — Electric heater. *(Courtesy of Kizure Products)*

Cleaning the Comb

The pressing comb will perform more efficiently if it is kept clean and free of carbon. Wipe the comb clean of loose hair, grease, and dust before and after each use. The intense heat keeps the comb sterile when all loose hair or clinging dirt is removed.

Remove the carbon from the comb by rubbing its outside surface and between its teeth with one of the following: emery board, fine steel wool pad, or fine sandpaper. After using any of these cleaning methods, immerse the metal portion of the comb in a hot baking soda solution for about 1 hour; then rinse and dry. The metal will acquire a smooth and shiny appearance.

PRESSING OIL OR CREAM

Applying pressing oil or cream prior to a hair pressing treatment helps prepare the hair for pressing. Both of these products have the following beneficial effects:

1. Make hair softer
2. Prepare and condition hair for pressing
3. Help prevent hair from burning or scorching
4. Help prevent hair breakage
5. Help condition the hair after pressing
6. Add sheen to pressed hair
7. Help hair stay pressed longer.

Completed:
Learning Objective
#3
PRODUCTS REQUIRED FOR SUCCESSFUL HAIR PRESSING

PRESSING THE HAIR

HAIR SECTIONING

Divide the head into four main sections. Then subdivide these sections into 1" to 1½" (2.5 to 3.75 cm) partings. The size of the subsections depends on the texture and density of the hair.

1. For medium textured hair of average density, use subsections of average size.
2. For coarse hair with greater density, use smaller sections to ensure complete heat penetration and effectiveness.
3. For thin or fine hair with sparse density, use larger sections.

SOFT PRESSING PROCEDURE FOR NORMAL CURLY HAIR

The following procedure is one of several ways to give a hair pressing treatment and can be changed to meet your instructor's method.

Equipment, Implements, and Materials

Pressing comb
Heating appliance (gas or electric heater or attachment)
Pressing oil
Hairbrush and comb
Grease or pomade
Shampoo
Towels and cape
Spatula
Neck strips
Thermal irons

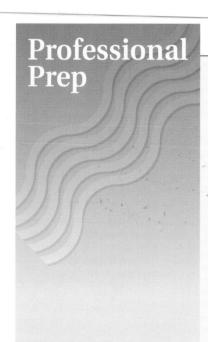

THE JOB INTERVIEW

Salon owners are looking for employees with good people skills, and you can demonstrate your attributes in this area during the job interview. Here are some tips for making the best impression:

- Call to confirm your interview. This establishes you as a professional who cares about keeping appointments.
- Pay particular attention to your appearance. After all, this is the beauty industry. Don't neglect one single aspect of your grooming or dress.
- Arrive 15 minutes early. This allows plenty of time for mishaps and eliminates rushing in at the last minute or, even worse, being late.
- Remain upbeat and positive. To most salon owners and managers, a positive attitude and pleasing personality are more important than technical skills.
- Answer the interviewer's questions honestly. If you are asked to name one of your weaknesses, admit what it is, but put yourself in a positive light by explaining how you are overcoming it.
- Ask questions of the interviewer. Take a list of questions and jot down the answers; this makes you appear organized and professional. Ask questions that display interest in the prospective employer, in the salon, and in your role, should you be hired.
- At the end of the interview, ask the interviewer for his or her business card, smile, shake hands, thank him or her, and leave promptly.

—*From* Communication Skills for Cosmetologists
by Kathleen Ann Bergant

Preparation

1. Select and arrange required materials.
2. Wash and sanitize hands.
3. Drape client.
4. Shampoo, rinse, and towel dry client's hair.
5. Apply pressing oil or cream. (Note: Some cosmetologists prefer to apply pressing oil or cream to the hair after it has been completely dried.)
6. Dry hair thoroughly. (Blow-drying will leave the hair more manageable than hood drying.)

7. Comb and divide hair into four main sections. Pin up four sections.
8. Place pressing comb in heater.

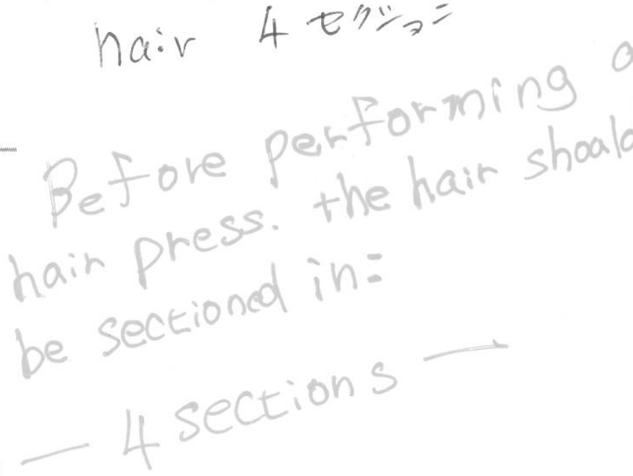

Procedure

1. Unpin one section of hair at a time and subdivide into small hair sections. Beginning at the right side of the head, work from front to back. (Some cosmetologists prefer to start at the back of the head and work forward.)
2. If necessary, apply pressing oil evenly and sparingly over the small hair sections.
3. Test the temperature of the heated pressing comb on a white cloth or white paper to determine heat intensity before you place it on the hair.
4. Lift the end of a small hair section with the index finger and thumb of the left hand and hold it upward away from the scalp.
5. Holding the pressing comb in the right hand, insert the teeth of the comb into the top side of the hair section. (Fig. 14.3)
6. Draw out the pressing comb slightly; make a quick turn so that the hair strand wraps itself partly around the comb. The back rod of the comb actually does the pressing.
7. Press the comb slowly through the hair strand until the ends of the hair pass through the teeth of the comb.
8. Bring each completed hair section over to the opposite side of the head.
9. Continue steps 4 to 8 on both sections on the right side of the head; then do the same on both sections on the left side.

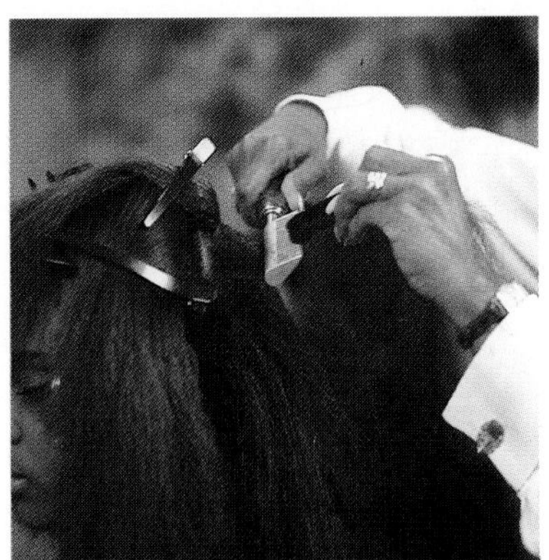

FIGURE 14.3 — Proper handling of pressing comb.

Completion

1. Apply a little pomade to the hair near the scalp and brush it through the hair.
2. If desired, thermal roller or croquignole curling can be given at this time. (The procedures and techniques are found in the chapter on thermal hairstyling.)
3. Style and comb the hair according to the client's wishes.
4. Place supplies in their proper places.
5. Sanitize implements and clean equipment.

HARD PRESS

A hard press is recommended when the results of a soft press are not satisfactory. The entire comb press procedure is repeated. Pressing oil may be added to hair strands only if necessary. A hard press is also known as a *double comb press.*

Completed:
Learning Objective
#4
SOFT PRESSING AND HARD PRESSING PROCEDURES

TOUCH-UPS

Touch-ups are sometimes necessary when the hair becomes curly again due to perspiration, dampness, or other conditions. The process is the same as for the original pressing treatment, with the shampoo omitted.

SAFETY PRECAUTIONS

The injuries that can occur in hair pressing are of two types:

1. Injuries that are the immediate results of hair pressing and cause physical damage, such as:
   a) Burnt hair that breaks off
   b) Burnt scalp that causes either temporary or permanent loss of hair
   c) Burns on ears and neck that form scars
2. Injuries that are not immediately evident but can subsequently cause physical damage, such as:
   a) Skin rash if the client is allergic to pressing oil
   b) Progressive breaking and shortening of the hair because of too frequent hair pressings

CAUTION

In case of a scalp burn, immediately apply 1% gentian violet jelly.

Good judgment should be used to avoid damage, with consideration always given to the texture of the hair and condition of the scalp. The client's safety is assured only when the cosmetologist observes every precaution and is especially careful during the actual hair pressing. The cosmetologist should avoid using the following:

1. Excessive heat or pressure on the hair and scalp
2. Too much pressing oil on the hair (it attracts dirt and makes the hair look greasy and artificial)

3. Perfumed pressing oil near the scalp if the client is allergic
4. Too frequent hair pressing, which weakens the hair

RELEASE STATEMENT

A release statement should be used for hair pressing, permanent waving, hair tinting, or any other service that might require the cosmetologist's release from responsibility for accidents or damages.

REMINDERS AND HINTS ON SOFT PRESSING

1. Keep the comb clean and free from carbon at all times.
2. Avoid overheating the pressing comb.
3. Test the temperature of the heated comb on a white cloth or white paper before applying it to the hair.
4. Adjust the temperature of the pressing comb to the texture and condition of the client's hair.
5. Use the heated comb carefully to avoid burning the skin, scalp, or hair.
6. Prevent the smoking or burning of hair during the pressing treatment by:
   a) Drying the hair completely after it is shampooed.
   b) Avoiding excessive application of pressing oil over the hair.
7. Use a moderately warm comb to press short hair on the temples and back of the neck. You may also use a temple comb, which is about half the size of a regular pressing comb.

Completed:
Learning Objective
#5
SAFETY PRECAUTIONS FOR HAIR PRESSING

SPECIAL PROBLEMS

PRESSING FINE HAIR

When pressing fine hair, follow the same procedure as for normal hair, being careful not to use a hot pressing comb or too much pressure. To avoid hair breakage, apply less pressure to the hair near the ends. After completely pressing the hair, style it.

PRESSING SHORT, FINE HAIR

When pressing short, fine hair, extra care must be taken at the hairline. When the hair is extra short, the pressing comb should not be too hot because the hair is fine and will burn easily; a hot comb can also cause accidental burns, which are very painful and can cause scars. In the event of an accidental burn, immediately apply 1% gentian violet jelly to the burn.

PRESSING COARSE HAIR

When pressing coarse hair, apply enough pressure so that the hair remains straightened.

PRESSING TINTED, LIGHTENED, OR UNPIGMENTED HAIR

Tinted, lightened, or unpigmented (gray) hair requires special care in hair pressing. Lightened or tinted hair might require conditioning treatments, depending on the extent to which it has been damaged. Unpigmented hair may be particularly resistant. To obtain good results, use a moderately heated pressing comb applied with light pressure.

Note: *Avoid excessive heat on tinted, lightened, or unpigmented hair as discoloration or breakage can occur.*

REVIEW QUESTIONS

THERMAL HAIR STRAIGHTENING (HAIR PRESSING)

1. What is another name for hair pressing?
2. What is the purpose of hair pressing?
3. Name the types of hair presses.
4. Under what circumstances should hair not be pressed?
5. How is an accidental scalp burn treated?
6. How do you test implements for your pressing service?
7. What types of hair require moderate heat?

CHAPTER 15

The Artistry of Artificial Hair

LEARNING OBJECTIVES

After completing this chapter, you should be able to:

1. List the reasons people wear wigs.
2. Identify the different types of wigs, extensions, and hairpieces.
3. Demonstrate the procedure for taking wig measurements.
4. Describe the method used when ordering wigs.
5. Demonstrate the procedures for blocking a wig and fitting a wig.
6. Demonstrate the procedure for cleaning a wig.
7. Demonstrate the procedure for shaping, setting, and styling a wig.
8. Demonstrate the procedure for coloring a wig.
9. Describe the various types of hairpieces and their uses.
10. List the safety precautions to be followed in handling wigs.

NATIONAL SKILL STANDARDS

This chapter provides you with the necessary information to master these National Industry Skill Standards for Entry-Level Cosmetologists:

- Consulting with clients to determine their needs and preferences
- Providing nonsurgical hair additions
- Effectively marketing professional salon products

INTRODUCTION

Throughout history, people have used wigs to beautify their appearance. The ancient Egyptians first wore wigs in 4000 B.C. for a very practical reason: to protect their hair from the sun. The wearing of wigs spread from Asia and Europe to America, where their use has become increasingly popular.

The use of wigs and hairpieces in hairstyling worldwide is a significant and exciting part of the beauty industry. The sale, styling, and servicing of artificial hair can be a source of increased salon income.

To offer the best possible service, the stylist must learn the following:

1. How wigs and hairpieces can improve the client's appearance.
2. How wigs and hairpieces are made and fitted.
3. How to select and style wigs and hairpieces to best benefit the client.
4. How to clean and service wigs and hairpieces.

WHY PEOPLE WEAR WIGS

People wear wigs for several reasons:

1. Personal choice—to cover up baldness due to heredity, and sparse or damaged hair.
2. Medical—to cover hair loss due to a health problem. Wigs have become popular hair replacements for use by people who have had hair loss due to illness, injury, or shock to the nervous system. Both men and women use wigs in these instances to replace lost hair and maintain their usual hairstyle.

3. Fashion—for changes in everyday hairstyles, to increase length and volume, and for decorative purposes and special occasions.
4. Practicality—for flexibility and ease of style change. For example, black clients might want to wear a straight style without chemically relaxing their hair, and a wig provides the flexibility to do so.

Completed: Learning Objective #1

THE REASONS PEOPLE WEAR WIGS

TYPES OF WIGS

Wigs can be made from human hair, synthetic hair (***modacrylic*** is the general term used to describe synthetic wig fibers), animal hair, or a blend of two or three types.

You can use a simple test to tell the difference between human hair and synthetic hair. Cut a small piece of hair from the back of the wig. With a lighted match, burn this hair and observe the following:

1. Human hair burns slowly and gives off a strong odor.
2. Synthetic hair burns quickly and gives off little or no odor. You can feel small, hard beads in the burnt ash of synthetic hair.

HUMAN HAIR WIGS

The quality of a wig depends largely on whether it is constructed by hand or by machine. Expensive, custom-made wigs are hand knotted into a fine mesh foundation. (Figs. 15.1, 15.2) In cheaper wigs, hair is sewn by machine into a net cap in circular rows. (Figs. 15.3–15.5)

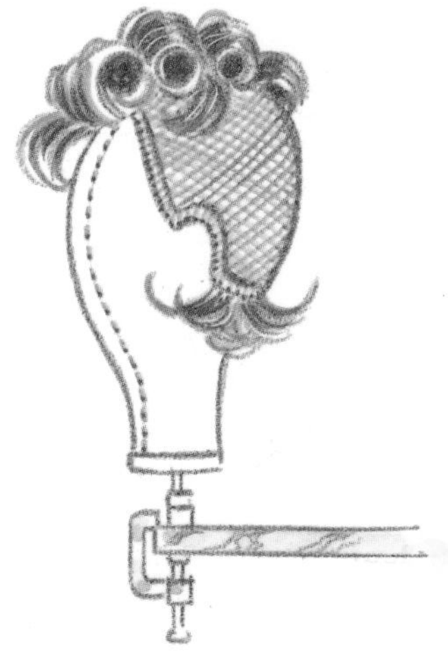

FIGURE 15.1 — Hand-knotted wig.

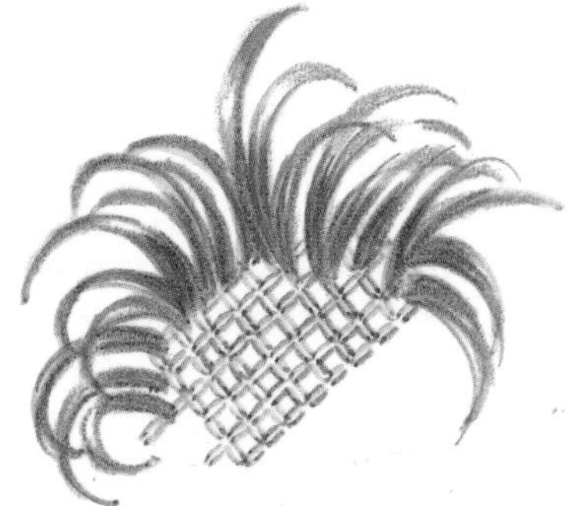

FIGURE 15.2 — Hair crocheted and hand knotted into mesh foundation.

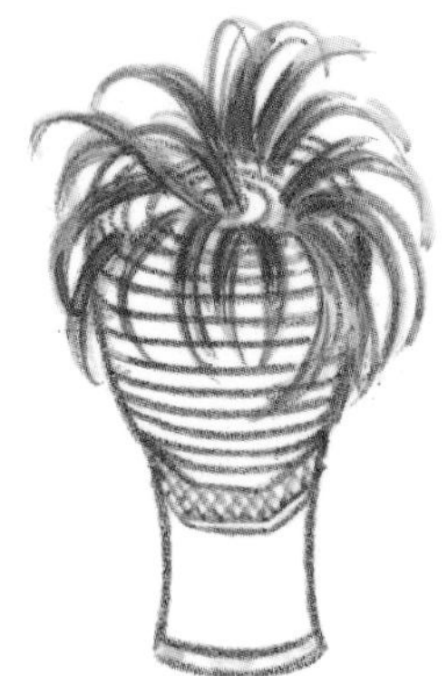

FIGURE 15.3 — Weft wig (top view).

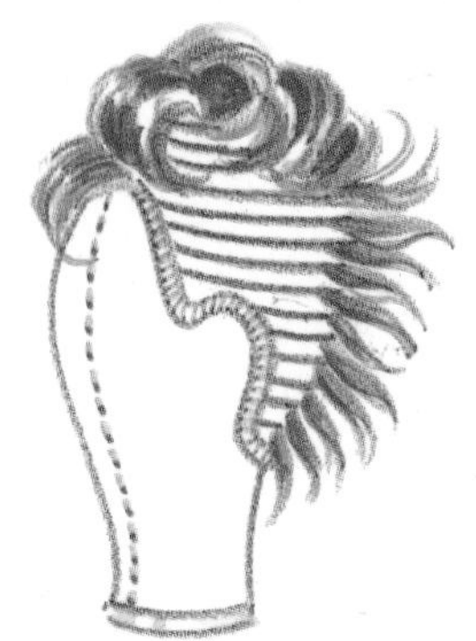

FIGURE 15.4 — Weft wig (side view).

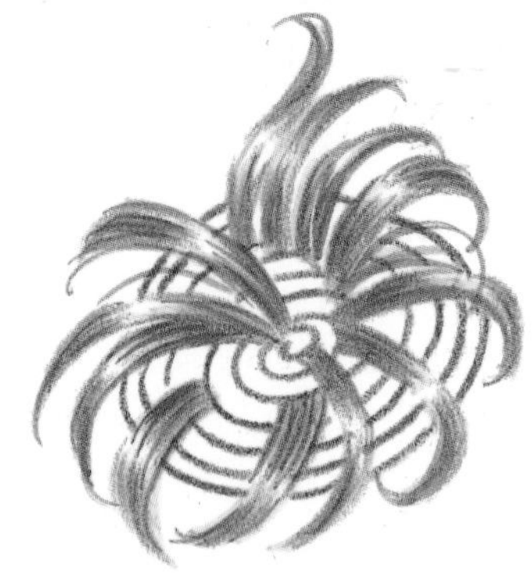

FIGURE 15.5 — Hair sewn by machine into net cap or weft in circular rows.

The quality of a wig also depends on the kind of hair it contains (human or synthetic), and how it is fitted to the client's measurements.

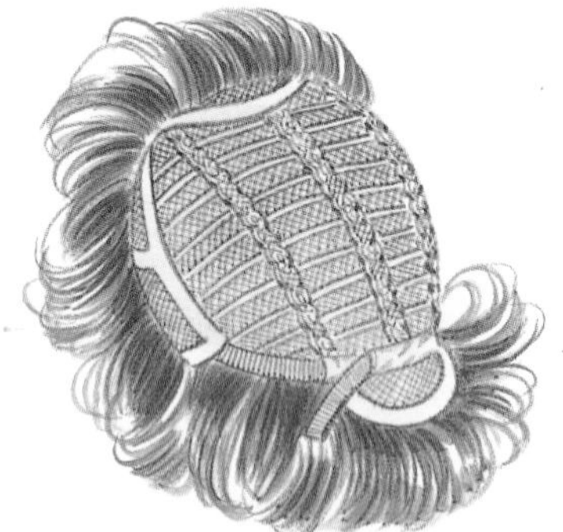

FIGURE 15.6 — Synthetic, handmade stretch wig.

SYNTHETIC WIGS AND HAIRPIECES

The manufacture of synthetic fibers has greatly improved. Modacrylic fibers, such as dynel, kanekalon, venicelon, and others, have eliminated most of the disadvantages of synthetic hair. Synthetic hair now closely resembles human hair in texture, resiliency, porosity, pliability, durability, sheen, and feel. These fibers can retain curl well, are nonflammable, and do not oxidize and change color in sunlight. In fact, some synthetic fibers appear so much like human hair that it is difficult to distinguish between them.

The many advantages of synthetic hair have led manufacturers to accept its use in wigs and hairpieces. Synthetically produced hair costs less than human hair and its supply is unlimited. It is also easier for the cosmetologist to use since synthetic hair is rolled on spools. Manufacturers weave synthetic wigs and hairpieces from long threads drawn from these spools.

You can find handmade synthetic stretch wigs, machine-made synthetic stretch wigs, and handmade synthetic fitted wigs. (Fig. 15.6) You must carefully select any type of wig for quality, proper fit, and good workmanship in order to satisfy your clients in terms of wear, comfort, and style.

Also available is the ***no-cap wig,*** composed of rows of wefting sewn to elastic bands. No-cap wigs are lighter and cooler to wear than other types of wigs. (Fig. 15.7)

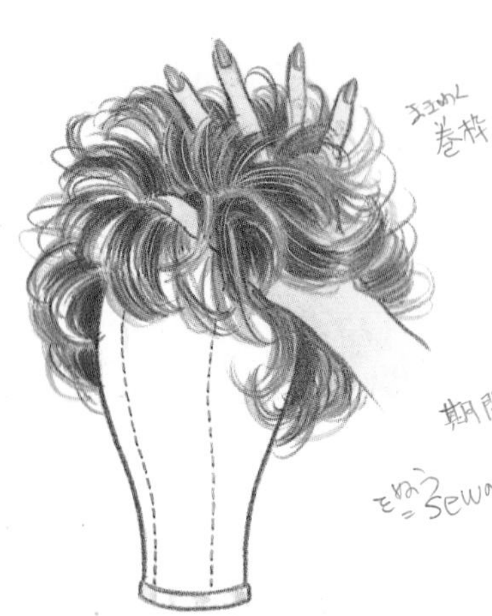

FIGURE 15.7 — No-cap wig.

Wig caps and hairpieces can be made of cotton, synthetic and cotton, all synthetic, or reinforced elastic. Hairpieces are generally made with a synthetic base that does not shrink when shampooed. Synthetic hairpieces come in wiglets, demi-wigs, braids, chignons, cascades, and falls.

HAIR EXTENSIONS

Hair extensions are permanent additions of hair that can make hair look longer, add thickness and volume, or vary an existing hairstyle. Extensions can be made from either human or synthetic hair, and can be affixed by gluing, fusing, or braiding the additional hair.

MEN'S WIGS

Many men now use wigs or toupees to compensate for hair loss. A toupee has adhesive applied to the base of the hairpiece so that the hairpiece sticks to the scalp.

To make men's hair appear fuller, many clients are using hair extensions. These extensions are interwoven or braided onto the existing hair, giving sparse areas the appearance of added thickness.

Once added, the extensions are styled to complement the client's hair type and facial features.

Completed:
Learning Objective
#2
TYPES OF WIGS

TAKING WIG MEASUREMENTS

To ensure a comfortable and secure fit, you must accurately measure the client's head. First, brush the hair down smoothly and pin it as flatly and tightly to the scalp as possible. Then, keeping close to the head without pressure, measure the head with a tape measure.

Procedure

1. Measure the circumference of the head. Place the tape completely around the head, starting at the hairline at the middle of the forehead; place the tape above the ears, around the back of the head, and return to the starting point. (Fig. 15.8)

2. Measure from the hairline at the middle of the forehead, over the top, to the nape of the neck. Bend the head back and measure to the point where the wig will ride on the base of the skull at the nape. (Fig. 15.9)

3. Measure from ear to ear, across the forehead. (Fig. 15.10)

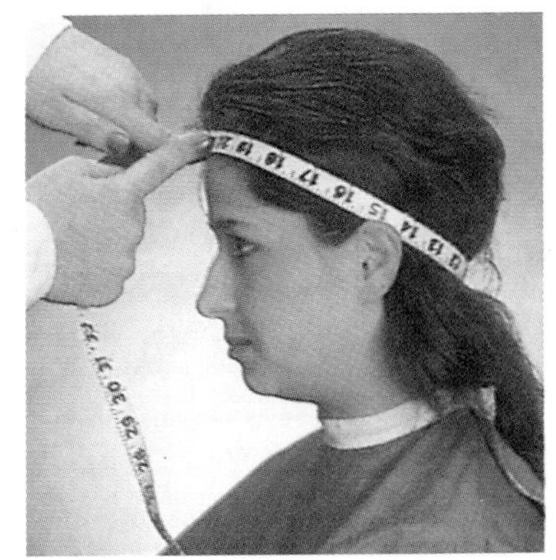

FIGURE 15.8 — Measure circumference of head.

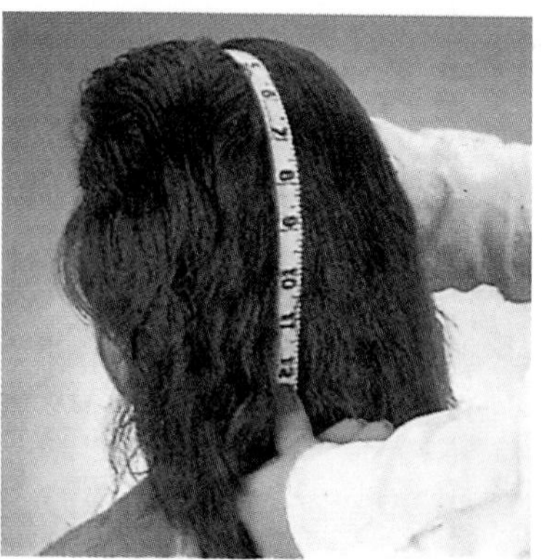

FIGURE 15.9 — Measure from hairline at middle of forehead to nape.

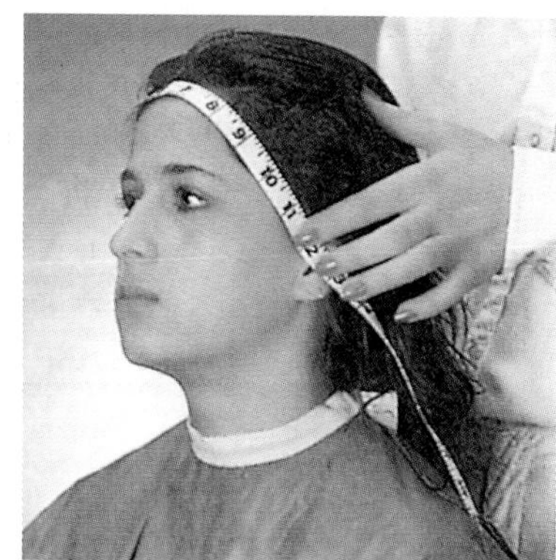

FIGURE 15.10 — Measure across forehead.

4. Measure from ear to ear, over the top of the head. (Fig. 15.11)
5. Place the tape across the crown and measure from temple to temple. (Fig. 15.12)
6. Measure the width of the napeline, across the nape of the neck. (Fig. 15.13)

Completed: Learning Objective #3

TAKING WIG MEASUREMENTS

Note: *Always check to make certain your measurements are accurate.*

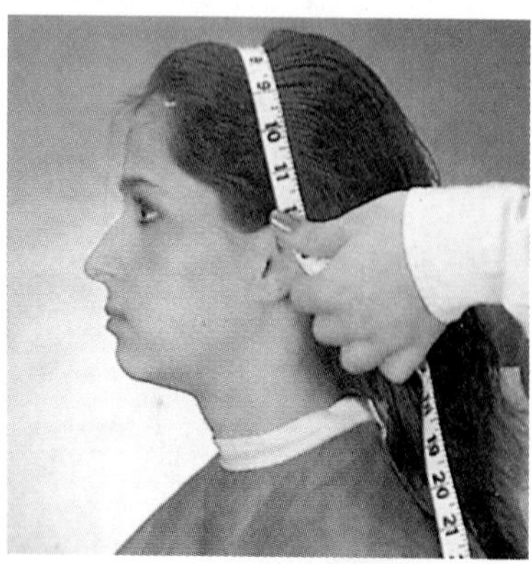

FIGURE 15.11 — Measure top of head.

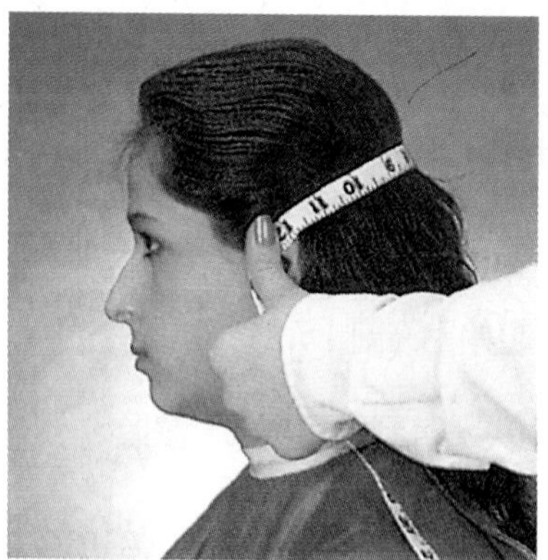

FIGURE 15.12 — Measure from temple to temple.

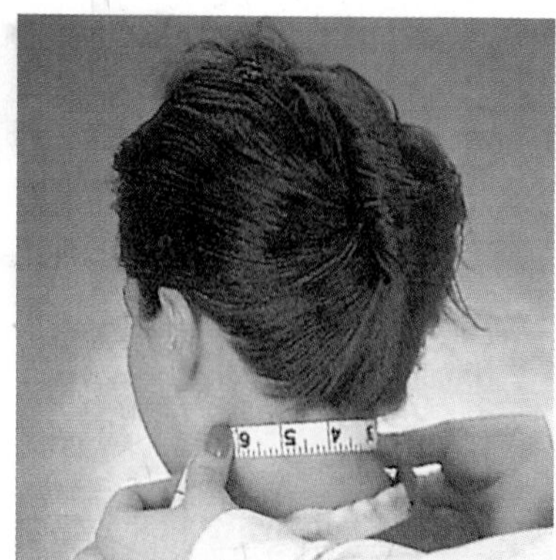

FIGURE 15.13 — Measure width of napeline.

ORDERING THE WIG

When ordering the wig, keep a written record of the client's head measurements and forward a copy to the wig dealer or manufacturer. Also specify what you desire as to:

1. Hair shade. If necessary, submit samples of the client's hair to the manufacturer. When you submit hair samples, you should use hair that has been freshly shampooed, tinted, or rinsed.
2. Quality of hair.
3. Length of hair.
4. Type of hair part and pattern.

Completed: Learning Objective #4
ORDERING WIGS

BLOCKING THE WIG

A block is a head-shaped form usually made of canvas-covered cork or styrofoam, to which a wig is secured for fitting, cleaning, and styling. Use properly protected canvas blocks for all professional wig services, because they stand up under continuous pinning and rough handling. T-pins ("T" shaped pins) are used to attach a hairpiece to a block. There are six sizes of canvas blocks available: 20", 20½", 21", 21½", 22", and 22½" (50, 51.25, 52.5, 53.75, 55, and 56.25 cm). A swivel clamp is used for better block control.

Good blocking gives you professional results when shaping, setting, and combing out a wig. It also reduces the possibility of disturbing the comb-out when you remove the T-pins.

Fit the wig comfortably on the right size block. Do not stretch a wig onto a block that is too big or let it hang too loosely on a block that is too small. If you stretch and pin a wig, it can expand if you wet the cap; when you hang a wig too loosely, it can shrink if you wet the cap (if made of cotton).

Mount the wig on the correct head size block and pin as follows:

1. At the center of the forehead.
2. At each side of the temple. (Fig. 15.14)
3. At the center of the nape.
4. At each corner of the nape. (Fig. 15.15)

(These illustrations show the proper placement of T-pins.)

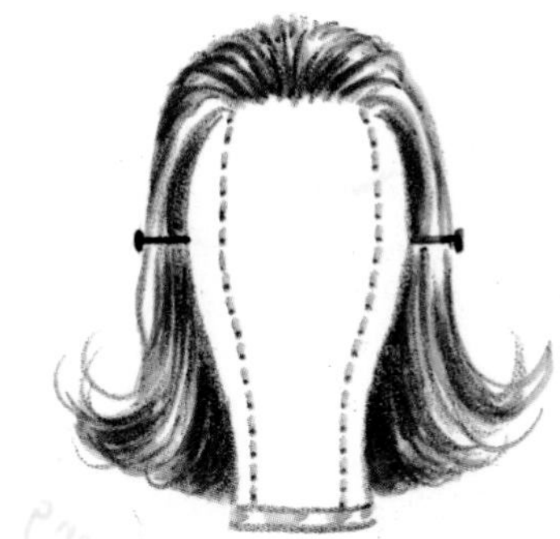

FIGURE 15.14 — Place one T-pin at center of forehead and one at each side.

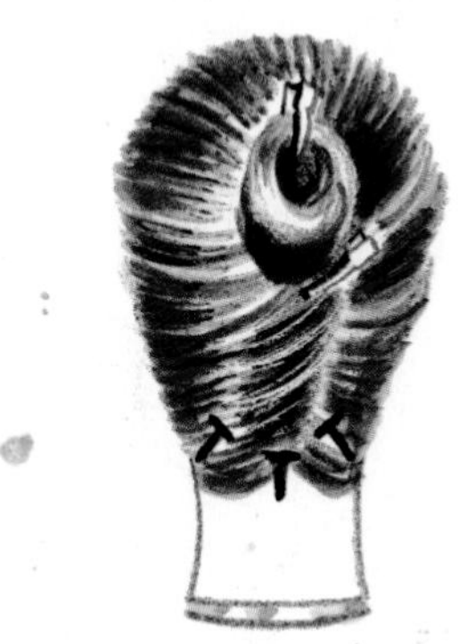

FIGURE 15.15 — Place one T-pin at center of nape and one at each corner.

Styrofoam blocks are used for storing or displaying the wig.

FITTING THE WIG

After the wig has been made according to specific measurements, you might have to adjust it to fit your client's head comfortably.

ADJUSTING THE WIG TO A LARGER SIZE

If the wig is too tight, you might have to stretch it. Turn the wig inside out and wet its foundation with hot water. Stretch the wig carefully (without ripping) onto a larger size block and pin it securely. Then allow the wig to dry naturally. (This process may have to be repeated more than once if the wig has to be enlarged more than one size.)

ADJUSTING THE WIG TO A SMALLER SIZE

If the wig is too loose, you must adjust it to fit properly.

Tucking

You can sew tucks to improve the fit of a wig that is too big.

1. ***Horizontal tucks*** shorten the wig from front to nape. They are made across the back of the wig to remove excess bulk, and shorten the length of the crown area of the wig. (Fig. 15.16)
2. ***Vertical tucks*** remove width at the back of the wig from ear to ear. (Fig. 15.17)

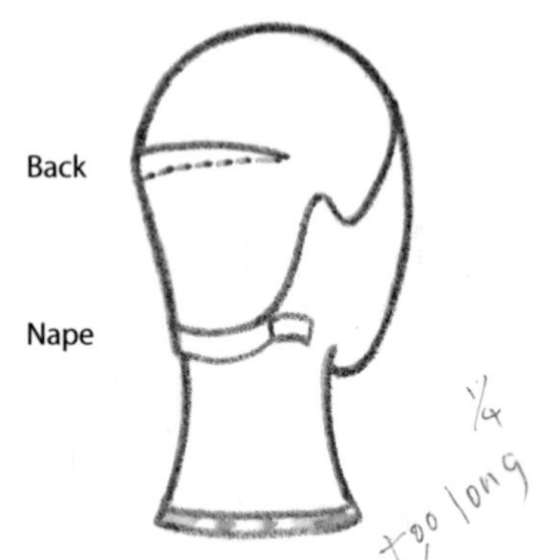

FIGURE 15.16 — Horizontal tuck.

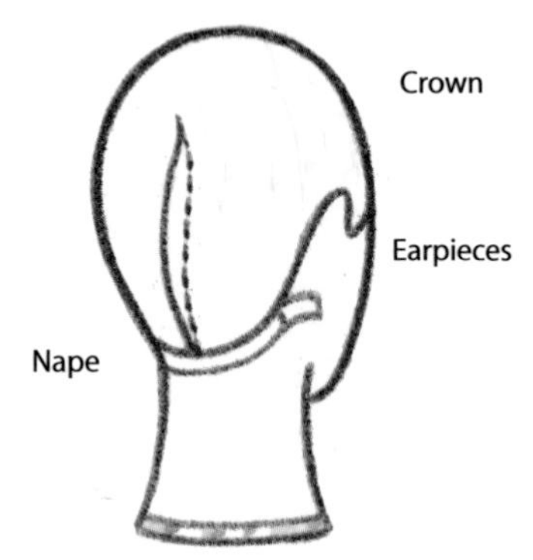

FIGURE 15.17 — Vertical tuck.

Check the cap fit after each tuck. Too much tucking can cause the wig to ride up and create new fitting problems.

Check both earpieces to be certain they are directly across from each other and do not touch the ears. If the wig touches the ear, make a small horizontal tuck over the ear to raise the wig. If the wig rubs or touches the side of the ear, make a small vertical tuck behind the ear to pull the wig back and eliminate the problem.

If a wig is too long from forehead to nape, make a tuck approximately ¼" (.625 cm) deep on the weft. Always sew a tuck toward the crown, never away from it, or hair will stand away from the wig when you comb it out. When tacking a tuck, be certain that you take out as much hair as possible before you complete the stitching process. The same applies if a wig is too large from the crown to the ear and it leans on the client's ears. You can correct this by stitching horizontally along the wefting.

Note: *When you adjust a ventilated or hand-tied wig, you should sew the tucks on the inside of the foundation. However, when you adjust a machine-made or wefted wig, you can sew horizontal tucks either inside or outside the wig.*

THE ELASTIC BAND

In the final step of the wig adjustment process, you must adjust the elastic band at the back of the wig. Pull the elastic band at the back of the wig to make the wig fit evenly and snugly at the back of the head and then fasten it. Some stylists favor pinning the ends of the elastic band with a small safety pin to allow for more convenience when making later adjustments or replacements. The elastic band does require periodic adjustment or replacement, because these bands stretch or deteriorate when exposed to body heat and cleaning fluids over a period of time. Other stylists believe that the band should be stitched securely and the stitches broken when adjustment or replacement is needed. (Fig. 15.18)

Completed:
Learning Objective
#5
BLOCKING AND FITTING WIGS

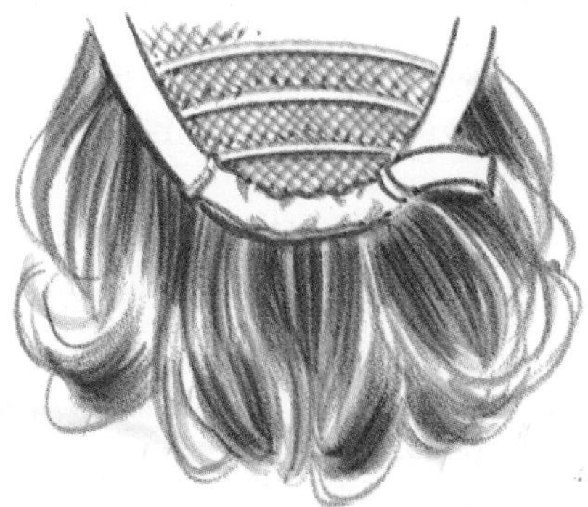

FIGURE 15.18 — Elastic band.

CLEANING WIGS

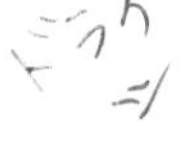

HUMAN HAIR WIGS

You should clean a human hair wig every 2 to 4 weeks, depending on how often it is worn or when you are ready to restyle it, using a nonflammable liquid cleanser. (Never wash in hot water.) Refer to the manufacturer's suggestions and cleaning instructions.

Procedure

1. Cover the block with a plastic cover to protect the canvas. (Fig. 15.19)
2. Block the wig. Remove back-combing, if necessary. Direct the hair off the hairline. Brush the hair to loosen dirt and hair spray.
3. Before you take the wig off the block to clean it, mark the size of the wig on the block so you can keep the wig the same size after you have finished cleaning it. You do this by placing a T-pin into the block on an angle next to the edge of the cap and directly in front of the six T-pins securing the wig. (Figs. 15.20, 15.21) Remove the wig and proceed with the cleaning.

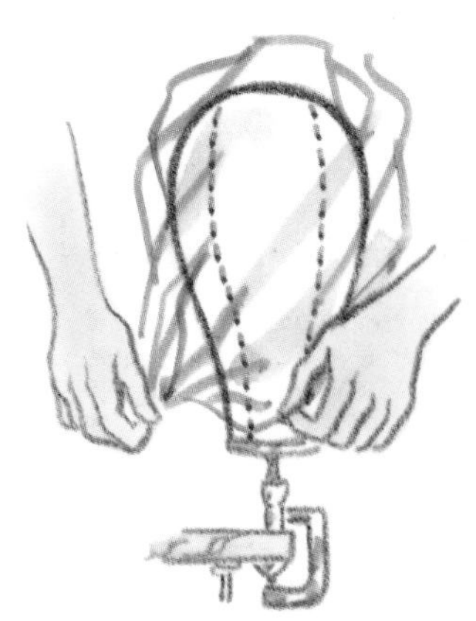

FIGURE 15.19 — Covering block.

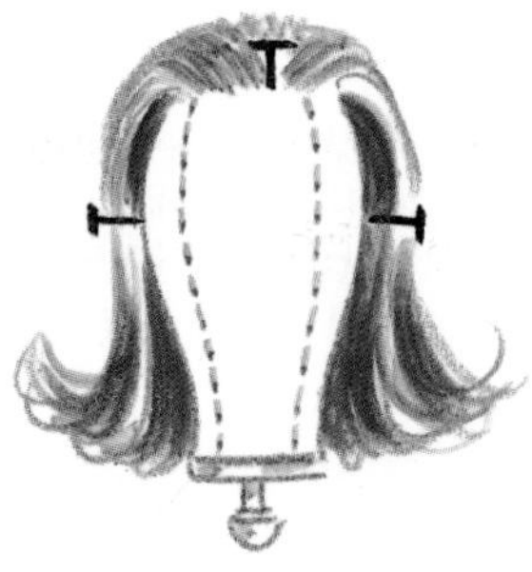

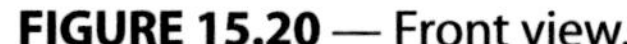

FIGURE 15.20 — Front view.

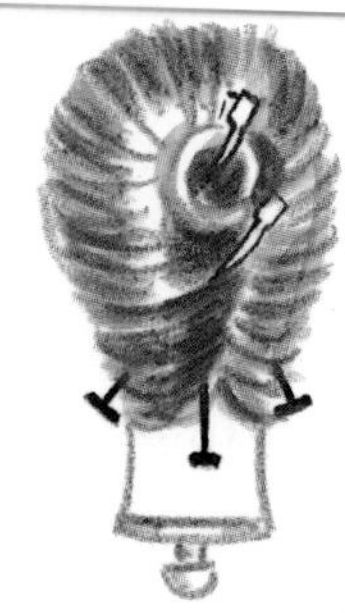

FIGURE 15.21 — Back view.

4. Wear rubber gloves to protect your hands. Saturate the wig in 3 ounces (90 ml) of nonflammable liquid cleanser in a large glass or porcelain bowl. With the hair side down, dip the wig up and down until it is clean. (Fig. 15.22)

   Alternate method: *Swirl the wig around in the liquid cleanser. If necessary, clean the edges and inside foundation with a cotton ball or toothbrush.*

5. Gently shake the wig to remove excess fluid. Place the wet wig immediately on the canvas block. Stretch the wig lightly and pin it securely to the block. (Fig. 15.23)
6. When the wig is dry, set and style it.

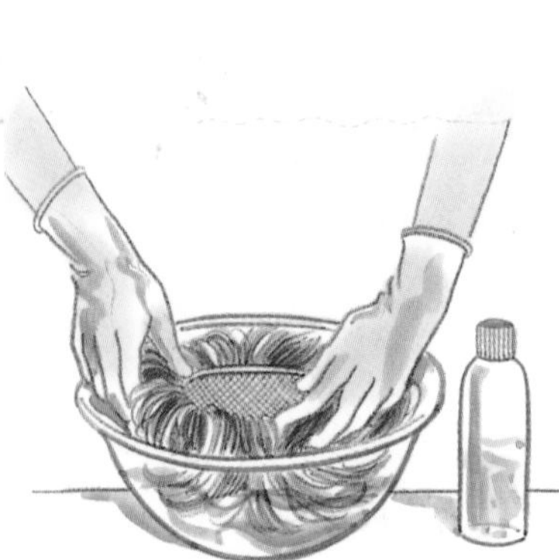

FIGURE 15.22 — Wash wig with nonflammable liquid cleanser.

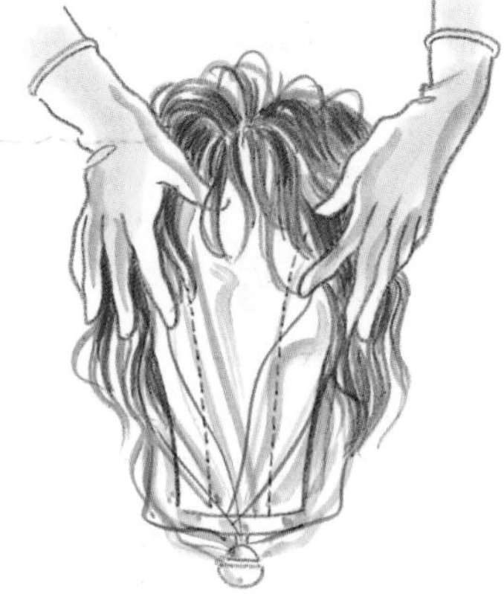

FIGURE 15.23 — Placing wig on block.

HAND-TIED WIGS

Since hand-tied wigs have a more delicate structure than machinemade wigs and cost much more, you should clean them on a block.

Procedure

1. Cover the canvas block with plastic to protect the canvas.
2. Clean the edges and inside foundation with a cotton ball or toothbrush.
3. Block the wig.
4. Saturate the wig in a large glass or plastic bowl containing liquid cleaner. (Fig. 15.24)
5. Soak the wig for 3 to 4 minutes.
6. Comb the cleaning solution through the length of hair with a wide-tooth comb.
7. Work the solution into the entire wig.
8. Carefully towel blot. (Fig. 15.25)
9. Allow to dry naturally on the block for about ½ hour.
10. Give a conditioning treatment, if necessary.
11. Set and style the wig.

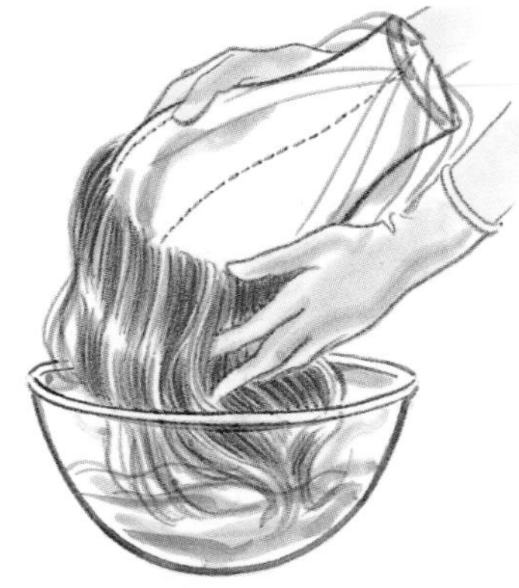

FIGURE 15.24 — Saturate wig and work solution through hair.

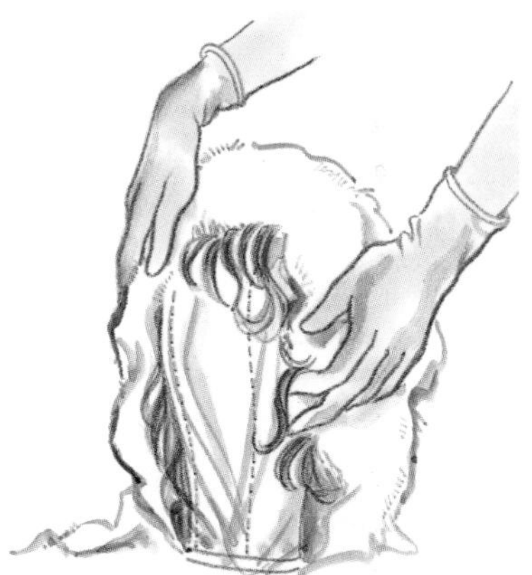

FIGURE 15.25 — Towel dry hair.

SYNTHETIC WIGS

Synthetic wigs and hairpieces need not be cleaned as often as human hair wigs. Synthetic fibers are nonabsorbent (lack porosity) and do not attract dust and dirt.

Clean and style synthetic wigs and hairpieces about every 3 months, depending on the amount of wear and styling. Use tepid or cool water to clean the wig; hot water takes the curl out of synthetic wigs. Do not comb or brush while wet.

Procedure

1. Cover the block with plastic to protect the canvas.
2. Mount the wig on the block and outline the size (as described earlier).
3. Brush the wig free of tangles and spray before cleaning.
4. Fill a container with mild shampoo or a specially formulated cleaner, according to the manufacturer's directions. Use tepid or cool water.
5. Remove the wig from the block. Swish the wig through cleaning solution for a few minutes. Rinse thoroughly in cool water.
6. Use a small brush or cotton to clean the mesh foundation.

7. Squeeze out excess water and towel blot. (Do not wring or twist wig.)
8. T-pin the wig on the proper size block and let dry naturally.
9. Do not brush a synthetic wig when it is wet; this can take out the curl.
10. Do not expose a synthetic wig to the excess heat of a hairdryer. This concentrated heat can cause the synthetic hair strands to stick together and lose their curl.
11. When the wig dries completely, brush out the hair and spray with conditioner to add luster.

Note: If you must reduce drying time, place the wig in a cool dryer using only the fan. Since most synthetic wigs are pre-styled, they require no further styling.

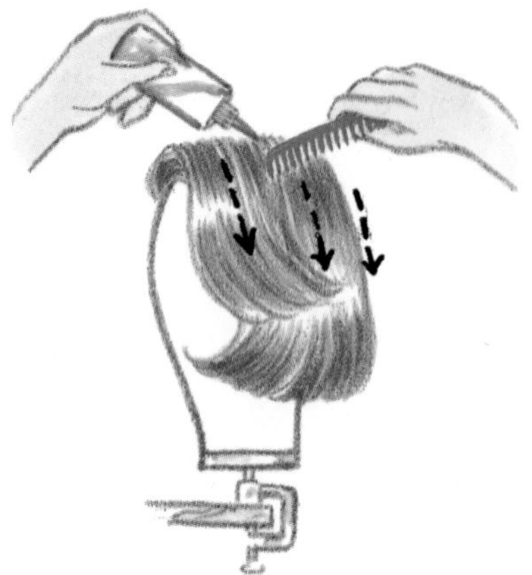

FIGURE 15.26 — Condition wig after cleaning.

CONDITIONING THE WIG

A wig differs from natural human hair in that it does not have its own supply of natural oils for self-lubrication. Since wig cleaners usually dry the hair excessively, use a conditioning treatment after each cleaning to keep the wig hair from drying and looking dull. This also keeps the wig in good condition. (Fig. 15.26)

Procedure

1. Cover the block with plastic and block the wig properly.
2. Apply conditioner. Distribute the conditioner evenly on clean, damp hair using a wide-tooth comb. Rinse conditioner out of hair according to product's instructions.
3. Set and style the wig. ✔

Completed:
Learning Objective
#6
CLEANING WIGS

SHAPING WIGS

HUMAN HAIR WIGS

You can shape (cut) a wig in the same way you cut natural hair on the head. However, you must consider the fact that a wig holds about twice as much hair as a human head. Thus, if you do not thin and taper the wig properly, it will look bulky and artificial. You can thin the wig with either a razor or thinning shears. Concentrate on removing bulk from the top hairline, in back of the ears, and around the face. You do not usually have to thin these areas on natural hair.

Cut as close to the wig foundation as possible, without damaging the cap itself. Thin hair close to the cap to remove additional bulk and to make sure you have not left hair spurs that will stick out when you style the wig later. Special care must be taken so that knots on the hand-knotted wig remain tight. Take equal care to not cut any of the wefts or sewing threads on the wefted wig. When you cut a wig, keep in mind that the hair will not grow back to cover an error in judgment. Proceed cautiously. Although it is more convenient to shape the wig on a canvas block, it is a good idea to cut the wig while it is on the client's head in order to suit the client's natural hair and facial features. Thus, you might find that the best technique is to cut a guideline on the client's head and then transfer the wig to the block. This ensures that the wig is being cut to the proper length. Then, you can move the wig to the block, secure it firmly, and avoid slippage during the rest of the shaping process. When you place the wig on the canvas block to cut it, set it carefully at the correct hairline distance and continue cutting the remaining hair evenly. Continue the shaping process, section by section, until the entire wig has been shaped. (Figs. 15.27–15.33)

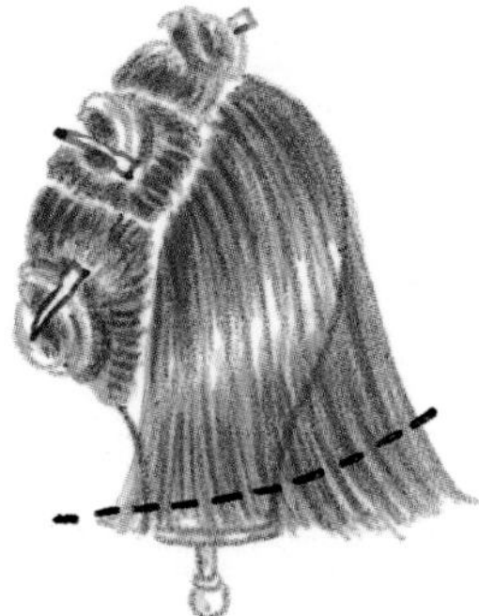

FIGURE 15.27 — Part off a 2″ (5 cm) guideline and cut to desired length.

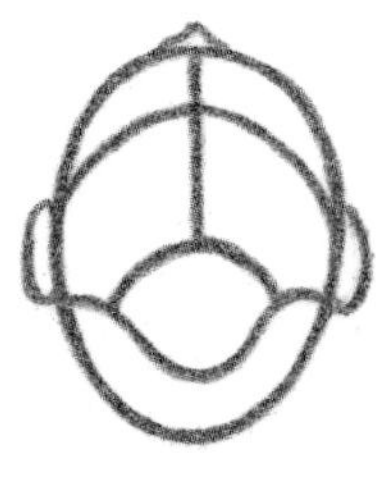

FIGURE 15.28 — Top front.

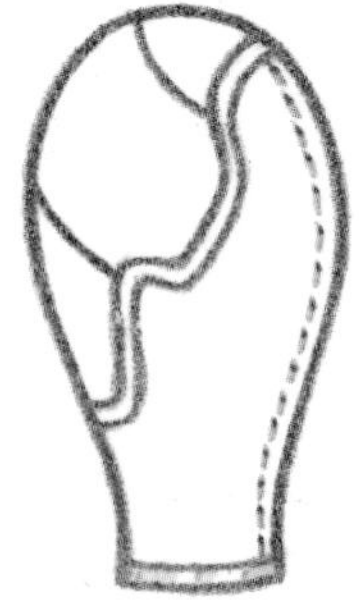

FIGURE 15.29 — Right side.

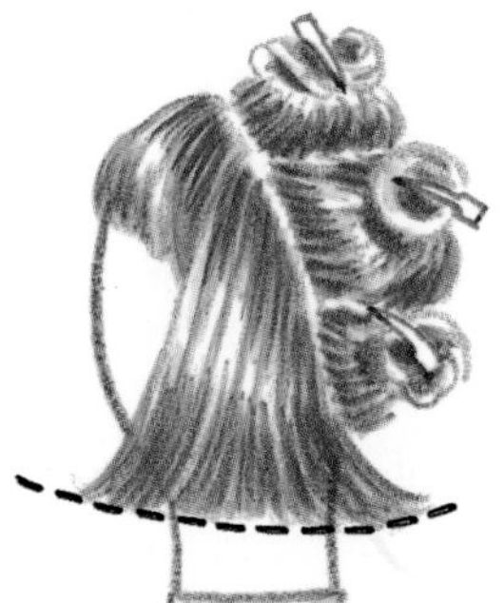

FIGURE 15.30 — Left side of head. This illustrates a completely cut guideline.

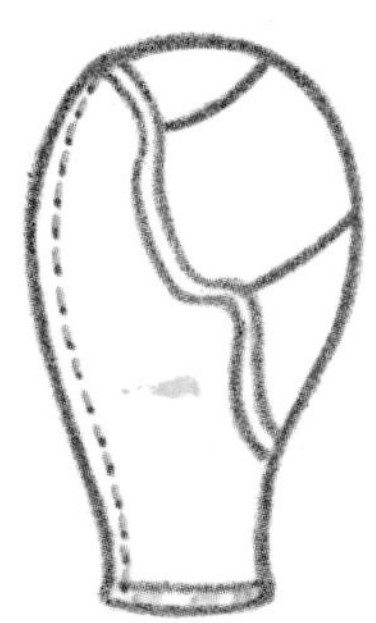

FIGURE 15.31 — Left side.

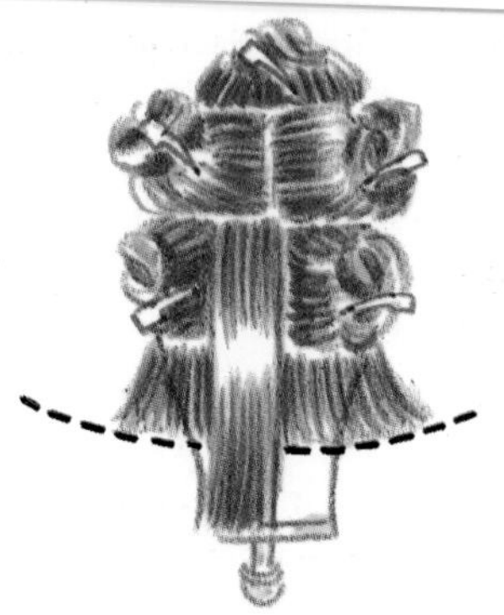

FIGURE 15.32 — Back of head. Let down center back hair. Cut to the same length as guideline.

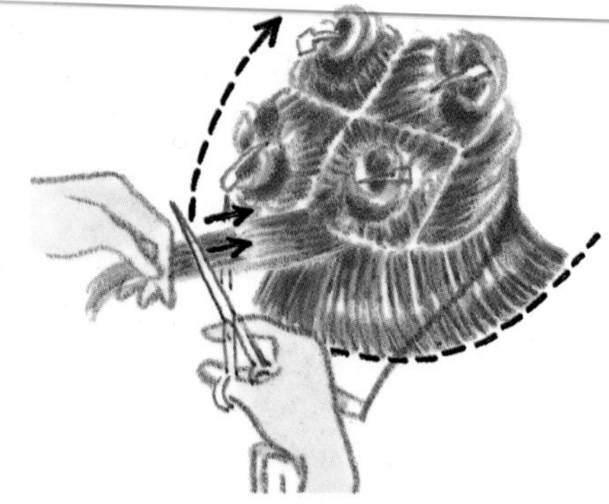

FIGURE 15.33 — Back of head. Pick up a strand of the guideline. With hands arched at a 45° (.785 rad.) angle, cut into longer hair. Proceed with a sweeping upward motion.

SYNTHETIC HAIR WIGS

Always cut synthetic wigs when dry, because the fibers can stretch out of shape if pulled when wet. Use only scissors and thinning shears on synthetic fiber or on a mixture of synthetic and human hair. Because synthetic fibers do not have the resiliency or flexibility of human hair, they can dull a razor badly. As a result, a razor can cause permanent damage to the wig.

SETTING AND STYLING WIGS

Setting wig hair resembles setting hair on the human head, except for hairline coverage and the need for a tight curl at the nape area. You must also consider the added fullness of the client's hair, plus the hair and foundation of the wig when setting and styling the wig. Wigs are always set and styled on the blocking. (Figs. 15.34, 15.35)

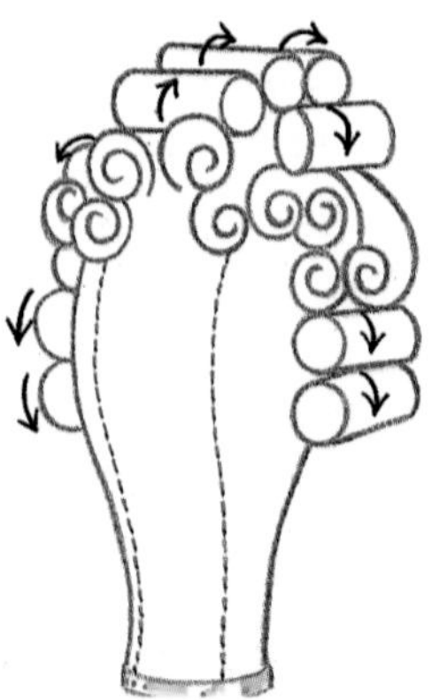

FIGURE 15.34 — Setting on block.

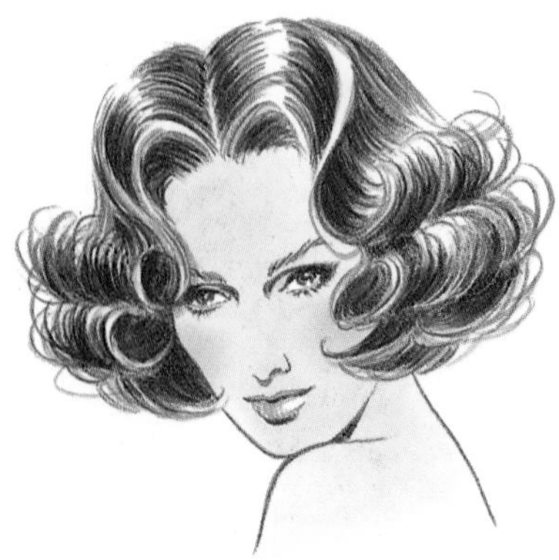

FIGURE 15.35 — Finished style.

Pin curls replace rollers in the front hairline, temple, and nape to keep the style close to the head. (Fig. 15.36) Use T-pins instead of clippies or bobby pins to hold both rollers and curls more securely. Set, dry, and style hair in the usual manner. (Fig. 15.37)

Cutting and styling synthetic wigs differs from cutting and styling human hair wigs in the following ways:

You may only tease or back comb wigs at the base of their fibers. Otherwise, you will damage the fibers that should be kept perfectly smooth at the wig surface. Damage to the hair shaft (by thinning) leaves you with a frizzy, fuzzy-looking wig.

Synthetic wigs are pre-cut into definite styles by their manufacturers. If the client desires a change, a good quality synthetic wig can be combed into different styles by a skilled stylist. These comb-out styles are all based on the basic pre-cut factory-created style. However, a stylist must be guided by the client's wishes.

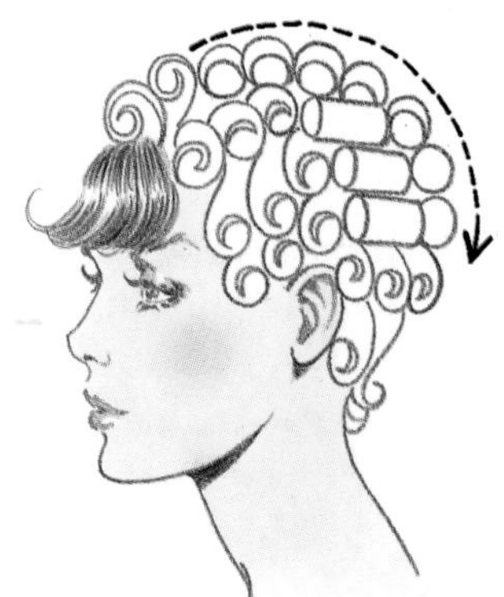

FIGURE 15.36 — How the setting would look on the head.

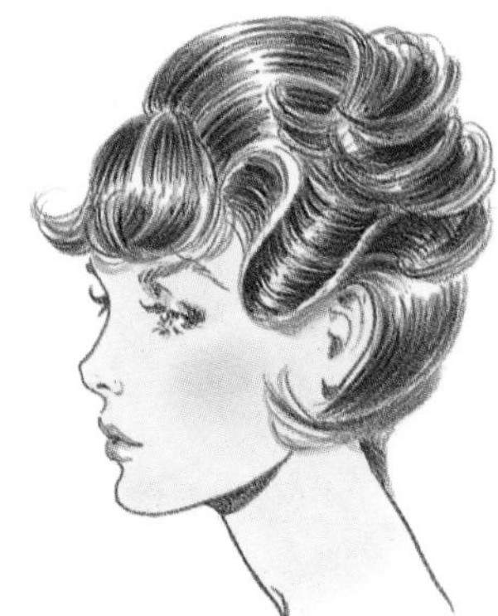

FIGURE 15.37 — Finished style.

PUTTING ON AND TAKING OFF A WIG

A simple but very important procedure is the way you remove a wig from a block and place it on the client's head. (Fig. 15.38) (It is a good idea to show the client the proper way to put on and take off the wig.)

COMBING CLIENT'S HAIR INTO A WIG

Depending on the style, set the client's hair that is to be blended with the wig in pin curls. When the wig is ready to be combined with the client's own hair, secure the wig starting either at the top or bottom depending on where you set the pin curls. When the wig is comfortably adjusted, comb and blend the client's hair into the style of the wig. (Fig. 15.39)

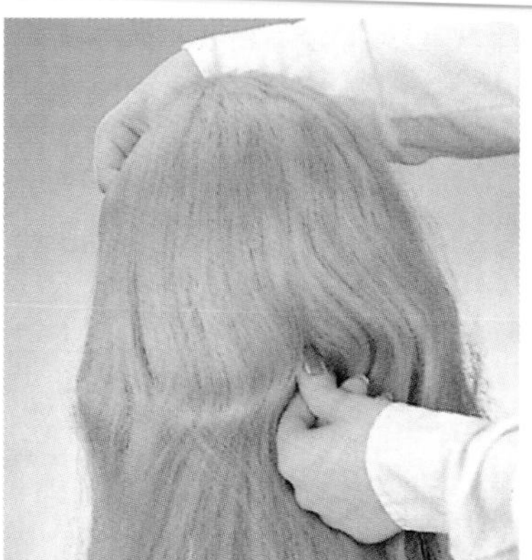

FIGURE 15.38 — Place wig on front of client's head. While holding wig securely on top, glide it back to nape. Pull securely over sides, front, and back.

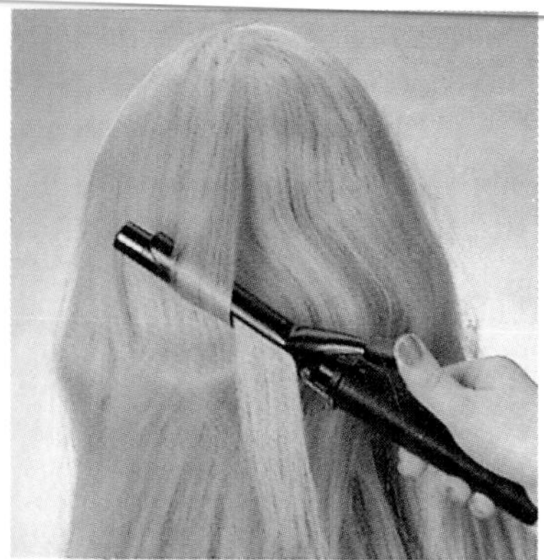

FIGURE 15.39 — Recomb, adjust, and style to suit client.

Completed:
Learning Objective
#7
SHAPING, SETTING, AND STYLING WIGS

REMOVING A WIG

To remove a wig, place only your thumb under the cap at the nape. ***Do not put your fingers into the hair.*** Have the client bend down his or her head. Then, slide the wig off.

WIG COLORING

COLOR RINSES

Color rinses temporarily color human hair wigs and must be reapplied whenever you clean the hair. Color rinses can only darken the hair; if the client desires a lighter color, a different wig must be worn.

Here is one way to apply a color rinse. (Your instructor's method may be equally correct.)

Procedure

1. Pin the wig securely on a plastic-covered block.
2. Dampen the clean hair, using a spray applicator bottle.
3. If you are unsure about which color to use, strand test the color rinse on the back of the wig.
4. Spray hair with the color rinse. Distribute it evenly with a downward motion, using a small brush and wide-tooth comb. (Fig. 15.40)
5. Apply setting lotion in the usual manner. (Fig. 15.41)

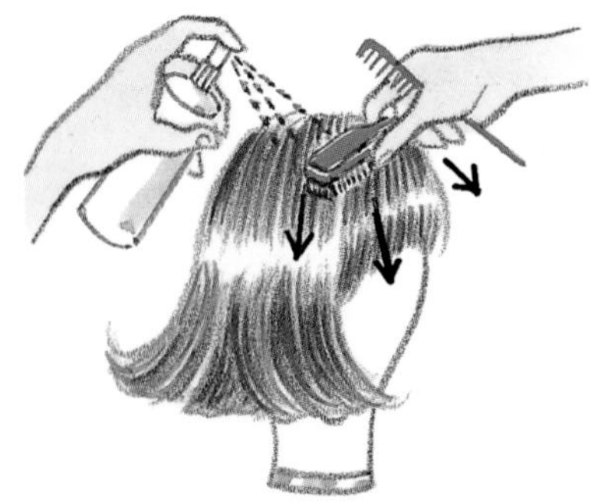

FIGURE 15.40 — Spray hair with color rinse.

6. Set, dry, (Fig. 15.42) and comb out the hair to the desired style.

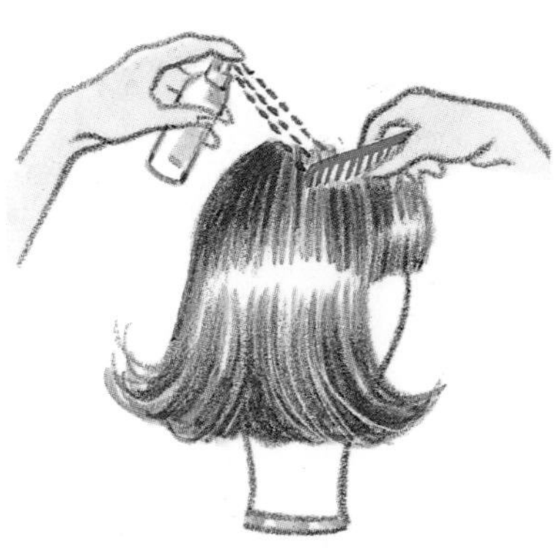

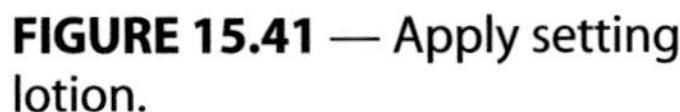

FIGURE 15.41 — Apply setting lotion.

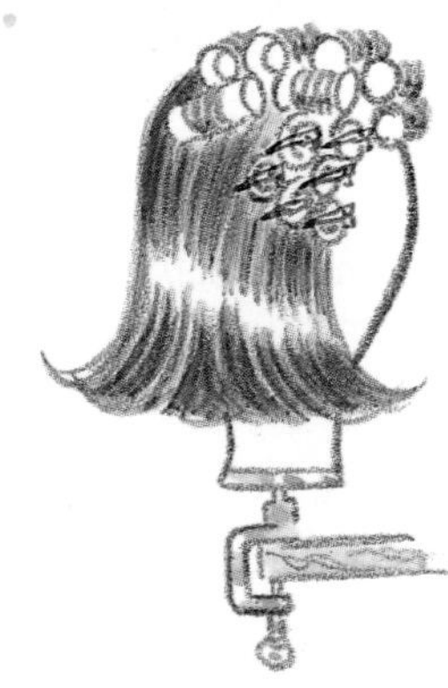

FIGURE 15.42 — Set, dry, and comb out.

Note: In addition to color rinses, you can color human hair wigs with a semi-permanent tint. However, you should never attempt to lighten (bleach) any wig or hairpiece.

SEMI-PERMANENT TINTS

Semi-permanent tints are referred to as 6-week tints. They are self-penetrating and require no peroxide. They do not change the basic structure of the hair.

Here is one way to apply semi-permanent tints to machine-made wigs:

Procedure

1. Mount the wig on the appropriate plastic-covered block and outline the size with T-pins.
2. Remove all teasing, tangles, and snarls.
3. Clean the wig and comb the hair smooth.
4. Remove the wig from the block.
5. Immerse the wig in a glass bowl of hot water and semi-permanent tint solution.
6. Leave it completely immersed for 10 minutes.
7. Remove it and rinse with cold water.
8. Apply conditioner.
9. Block, set, dry, and comb out in the usual manner.

Completed: Learning Objective #8 COLORING WIGS

PERMANENT TINTS

Since 100% human hair wigs and hairpieces have been subjected to extensive processing, applying a permanent tint to this kind of hair can be very risky and will result in uneven coloring.

CAUTION

When tinting wigs, be sure to follow the manufacturer's directions.

HAIRPIECES

You can create a variety of hairstyles with hairpieces, fashioning them for either daytime or evening wear. Hairpieces come in various forms, such as:

1. ***Switches.*** These are long wefts of hair mounted with a loop at the end. They are constructed with one to two stems of hair. Better switches are constructed with three stems to provide greater flexibility in styling and braiding. They can be worked into the hair or braided to create special styling effects. (Fig. 15.43)
2. ***Wiglets.*** These are hairpieces with a flat base that are used in special areas of the head. They are used primarily to blend with the client's own hair in order to extend the range of hair in a particular section of the head. Wiglets can be worked into the top of the hair in curls or under the hair to give height and body. They can also be used to create special effects. (Fig. 15.44)

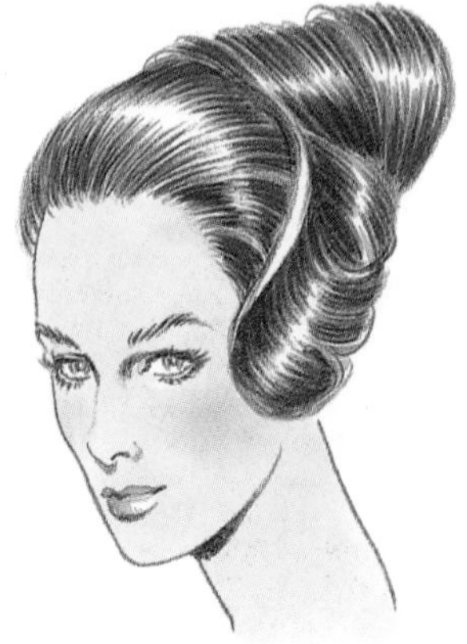

FIGURE 15.43 — Switch.

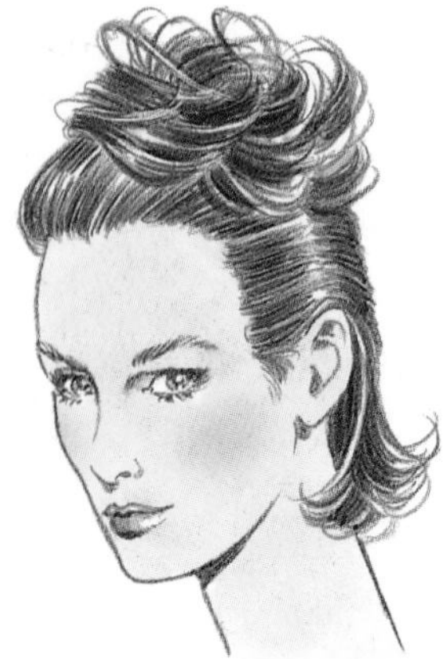

FIGURE 15.44 — Wiglet.

3. ***Bandeau.*** This is a hairpiece that is sewn to a headband. The headband, which is replaceable and comes in different colors, serves as an excellent disguise for the hairline. The bandeau hairpiece is usually worn over the hair and dressed casually. (Fig. 15.45)
4. ***Fall.*** This is a section of hair, machine wefted on a round base, running across the back of the head and available in various lengths. Falls have a thick, plushy look. *Short falls* range from 12" to 14" (30 to 35 cm) in length (Fig. 15.46); *demi-falls* from 15" to 20" (37.5 to 50 cm); and *long falls* from 18" to 24" (45 to 60 cm).
5. ***Demi-fall*** or ***demi-wig.*** This is a large-base hairpiece designed to fit the shape of the head. The demi-fall or demi-wig generally ranges in length from 15" to 20" (37.5 to 50 cm).
6. ***Cascade.*** This is a hairpiece on an oblong base that offers an endless variety of styling possibilities. Cascades can be styled in curls, braids, a pageboy, or used as a filler with the client's own hair. (Fig. 15.47)

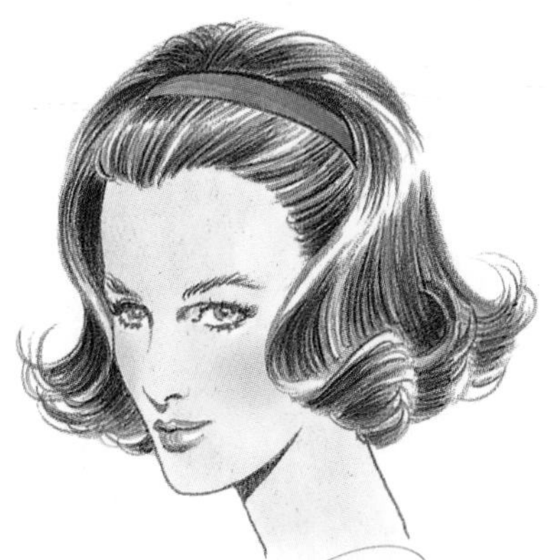

FIGURE 15.45 — Bandeau.

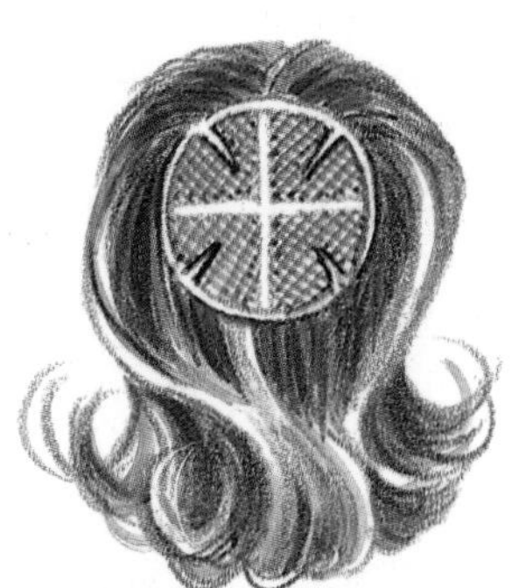

FIGURE 15.46 — Short fall.

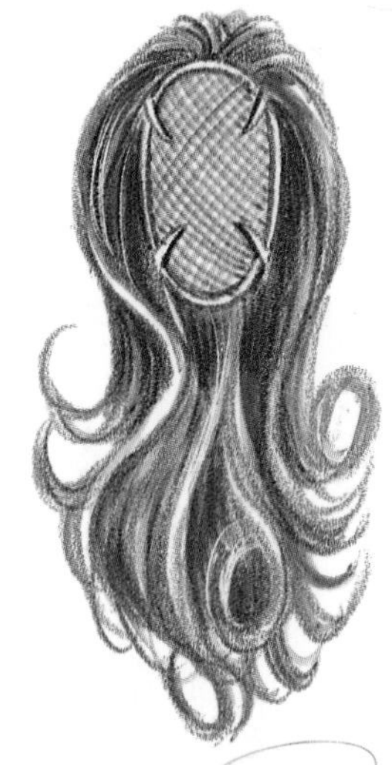

FIGURE 15.47 — Cascade.

7. ***Braid.*** This is a switch whose strands are woven, interlaced, or entwined. Some are prepared with a thin wire inside so that they can be formed into various shapes. Wireless braids hang loose on the head.
8. ***Chignon.*** This is a knot or coil of hair, created from synthetic hair, that is worn at the nape or crown of the head. A chignon works best when worn in combination with another hairpiece.
9. ***Crown curls.*** These are a group of light curls worn on top of the head.
10. ***Frosting curls.*** These are segments of frosted or blended hair pinned into natural hair to simulate frosted or streaked hair.

Completed:
Learning Objective
#9
TYPES OF HAIRPIECES

SAFETY PRECAUTIONS

1. Take great care when combing or brushing wigs to avoid matting.
2. When cleaning a wig or hairpiece, never rub or wring out the fluid.
3. When you shape (cut) a wig or hairpiece, use great care; once the hair has been cut, it cannot grow back.
4. When you comb a freshly set wig, use a wide-tooth comb to help you gain greater control and to avoid damaging the wig's foundation.
5. When you clean or work with a wet wig, always mount it on a block of the same head size as the wig to avoid stretching.
6. Take accurate measurements of the client's head to ensure a comfortable and secure fit.
7. Recondition wigs as often as necessary to prevent dry or brittle hair.
8. If needed, clean wigs before setting and styling.
9. Brush and comb wigs and hairpieces with a downward movement.
10. Never lighten (bleach) a wig or hairpiece.
11. Never give a permanent to a wig or hairpiece. ✔

Completed:
Learning Objective
#10
SAFETY PRECAUTIONS

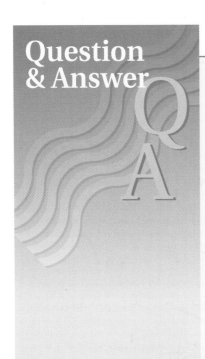

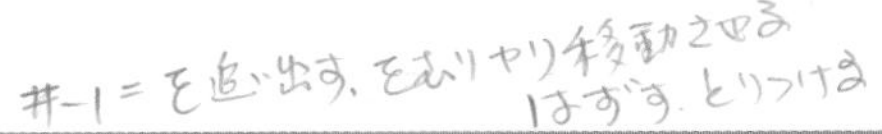

HAIR EXTENSIONS FOR FINE HAIR

I have a young client whose hair is very fine all over and quite thin in the crown and down the back. Which extension technique is best for this type of hair?

Your client is a good candidate for the "bonding" technique of attaching hair extensions. You must first determine whether or not the person is allergic to any type of adhesive. You must also determine the length of hair needed (or desired) by the client. It is not advisable to bond weft lengths longer than 15 inches. Another point to consider is whether or not your client has an excessively oily scalp, or if she requires hair-conditioning treatments that contain oil, since oil can dislodge bonding adhesive.

Cut the weft pieces into strips approximately two inches wide and attach them randomly throughout the hair. Even if you place them side-by-side, it takes the weight off any one spot. You may also consider combining both methods of attaching bonds if the situation calls for it. For instance, if a client wears a definite side part, a bonded strip just below the part will not be as obvious as a sewn weft. It serves as well to cover the wefts sewn beneath it.

Latex-based adhesive bond is easily removed from the natural hair and the weft extension. It comes out completely, allowing the extension to be readjusted as necessary.

—*From* Milady's Salon Solutions *by Louise Cotter*

REVIEW QUESTIONS

THE ARTISTRY OF ARTIFICIAL HAIR

1. List some of the reasons people wear wigs.
2. Name the different types of wigs, extensions, and hairpieces.
3. What is the purpose of a hair extension?
4. What is the purpose of blocking a wig?
5. How often should a human hair wig be cleaned?
6. Where should a wig be set and styled?
7. What effect does a color rinse have on a human hair wig?

CHAPTER

Manicuring and Pedicuring

LEARNING OBJECTIVES

After completing this chapter, you should be able to:

1. List the abilities of a good manicurist.
2. Identify the four natural nail shapes.
3. Demonstrate the proper use of implements, cosmetics, and materials used in manicuring.
4. Demonstrate the proper procedure and sanitary and safety precautions for a manicure.
5. Demonstrate massage techniques used when giving a manicure.
6. Define and demonstrate the different types of manicures.
7. Explain and demonstrate advanced nail techniques.
8. Demonstrate the procedure for a pedicure.

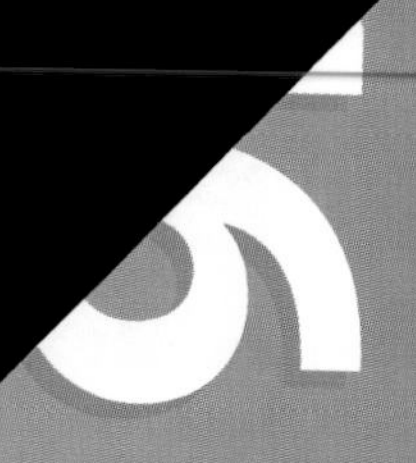

ILL STANDARDS

s you with the necessary information
nal Industry Skill Standards for Entry-Level Cosmetologists:

- s in a safe environment, taking measures to prevent the spread of infectious sease
- Providing basic manicure and pedicure

INTRODUCTION

The ancients regarded long, polished, and colored fingernails as a mark of distinction between aristocrats and common laborers. Manicuring, once considered a luxury for the few, is now a service used by many. In fact, many well-groomed women and men regularly use the services of a professional manicurist or nail technician. The services provided by a nail technician include the application of artificial nails, as well as pedicures.

The word ***manicure*** (**MAN**-i-kyoor) is derived from the Latin *manus* (hand) and *cura* (care), which means the care of the hands and nails. The purpose of a manicure is to improve the appearance of the hands and nails.

A client pleased with a professional manicure or other more advanced nail technique is more likely to become a regular client for these services, as well as for other beauty services.

A manicurist should have:

1. Knowledge of the structure of hands, arms, and nails.
2. Knowledge of the composition of the cosmetics used in manicuring.
3. The ability to give a good manicure efficiently.
4. The ability to care for the client's manicuring problems.
5. The ability to distinguish between disorders that may be treated in the salon and diseases that must be treated by a physician.
6. Knowledge of the structure of the foot and the ability to give a good pedicure.

Completed:
Learning Objective
#1
ABILITIES OF A GOOD MANICURIST

A nail technician should possess the above qualifications *and* be able to execute advanced nail techniques safely and professionally.

SHAPE OF NAILS

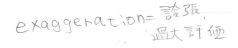

Nails naturally vary greatly in shape, but are usually classified into four general shapes: square, round, oval, and pointed. (Fig. 16.1)

Before you begin to work on a client's nails, both you and the client should agree on the best nail shape. The shape of the nail should conform to that of the fingertips for a more natural effect. In general the oval-shaped nail, nicely rounded at the base, and slightly pointed at the tips, fits most hands. Only an attractive hand can afford to direct attention to itself by exaggeration of shape and color. People who perform work with their hands usually require shorter, more round-shaped nails in order to avoid nail breakage and injury.

Completed:
Learning Objective
#2
SHAPES OF NAILS

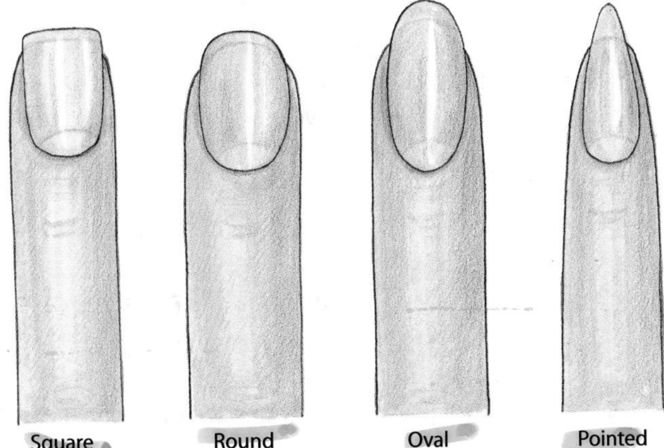

FIGURE 16.1 — Shapes of nails.

EQUIPMENT, IMPLEMENTS, COSMETICS, AND MATERIALS

The articles used in manicuring that are durable are referred to as equipment and implements. (Fig. 16.2) Cosmetics and materials refer to the supplies that are consumed and must be replaced.

EQUIPMENT

Manicuring table and *adjustable lamp*.

Client's chair and *manicurist's chair* or *stool*.

Cushion (8" x 12" [20 x 30 cm]), covered with a washable slipcover or sanitized towel, on which the client rests his or her arm. A towel, folded and covered by a small sanitized towel, may be used instead of the cushion.

Supply tray for holding cosmetics.

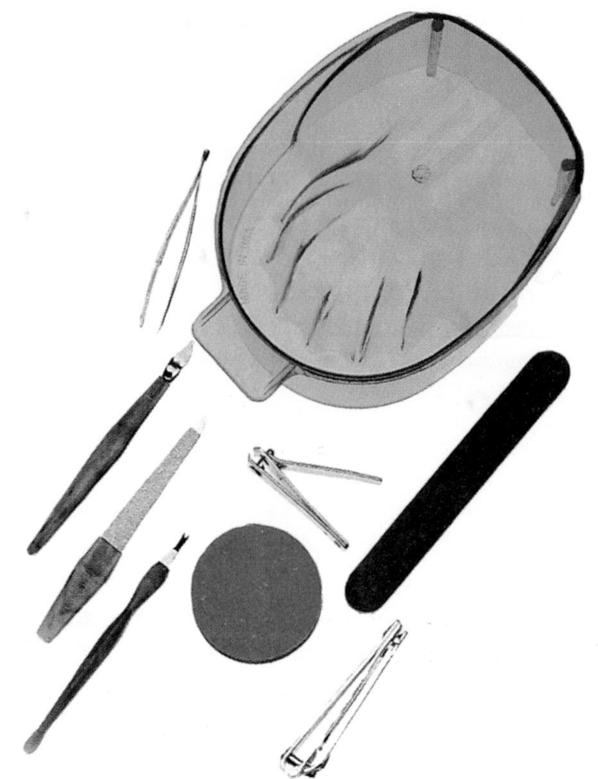

FIGURE 16.2 — Manicuring implements—clockwise, from top left: tweezers; finger bowl; fingernail clippers; emery board; toenail clippers; filing disk; cuticle pusher; large nail file; steel pusher. An antibacterial soap is recommended for the finger bath to eliminate germs and reduce the risk of infection.

Finger bowl (plastic, china, or glass) with removable paper cup for holding warm, soapy water.

Container for clean absorbent cotton.

Electric heater for heating oil when giving a hot oil manicure.

Wet disinfecting system for implements (jar or tray with disinfecting solution).

Glass containers for cosmetics and accessories.

IMPLEMENTS

Orangewood sticks (2) for loosening cuticle, for working around nail, and for applying oil, cream, bleach, or solvent to the nail and cuticle. (Fig. 16.3)

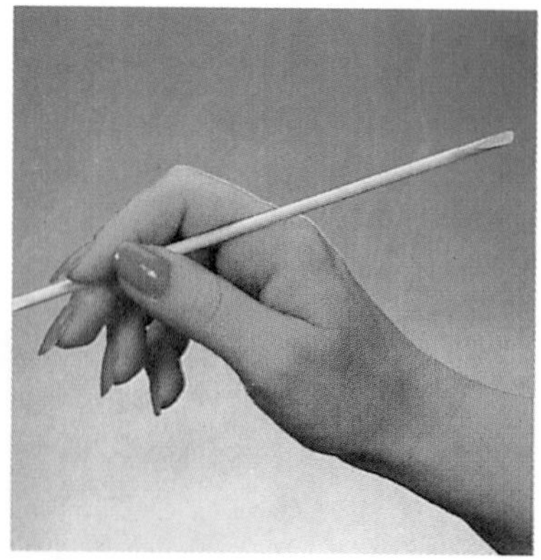

FIGURE 16.3 — The orangewood stick is held in the same manner as in writing with a pencil.

Nail file (7" or 8" [17.5 or 20 cm] long, thin and flexible) for shaping and smoothing the free edge of the nail. (Fig. 16.4)

Cuticle pusher for loosening and pushing back the cuticle. (Fig. 16.5)

Cuticle nippers or *cuticle scissors* for trimming the cuticle. (Fig. 16.6)

Nail brush for cleansing the nails and fingertips with the aid of warm, soapy water.

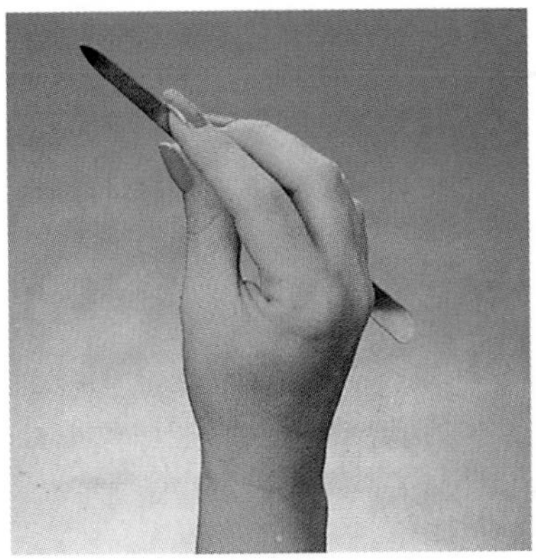

FIGURE 16.4 — Hold nail file in the right hand, with the thumb underneath it for support and the other four fingers on its upper surface.

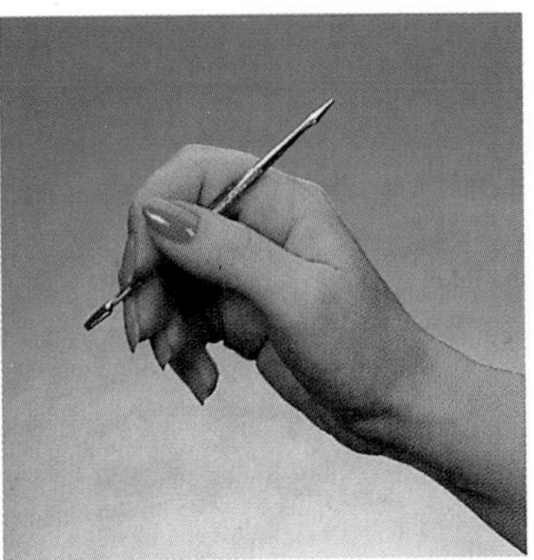

FIGURE 16.5 — The steel pusher is held in the same manner as in writing with a pencil. The dull side is used to push back and loosen the cuticle.

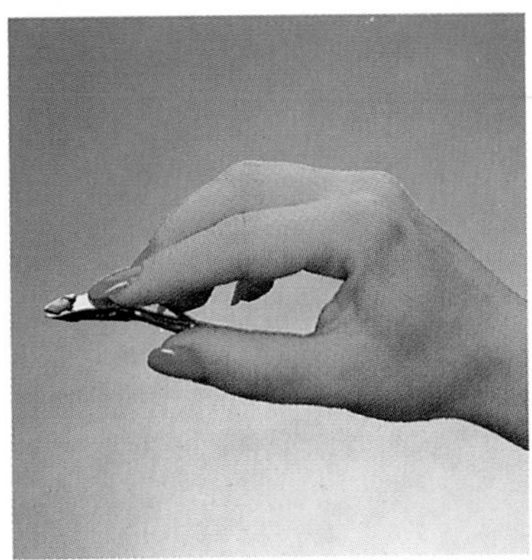

FIGURE 16.6 — Use cuticle nippers to trim cuticles.

Emery boards (2) for shaping the free edge of the nail with the coarse side, and for smoothing the nail with the finer side. (Fig. 16.7)

Nail buffer (designed with removable frame so the chamois cover can be changed for each client) for buffing and polishing the nails. (Figs. 16.8, 16.9) (Some states do not permit the use of a nail buffer. Some states recommend a disposable buffer that should be discarded after each use.)

Fine camel's hair brush for applying lacquer or liquid nail polish. (Camel's hair brush is usually attached to the top of the nail polish bottle.)

Tweezers for lifting small bits of cuticle.

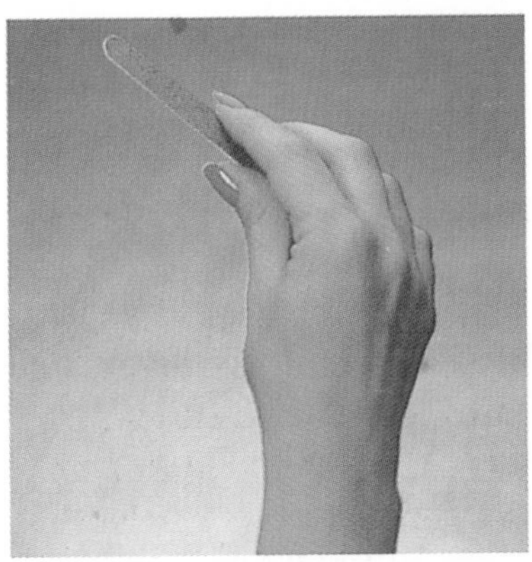

FIGURE 16.7 — The emery board is held in the same manner as the nail file.

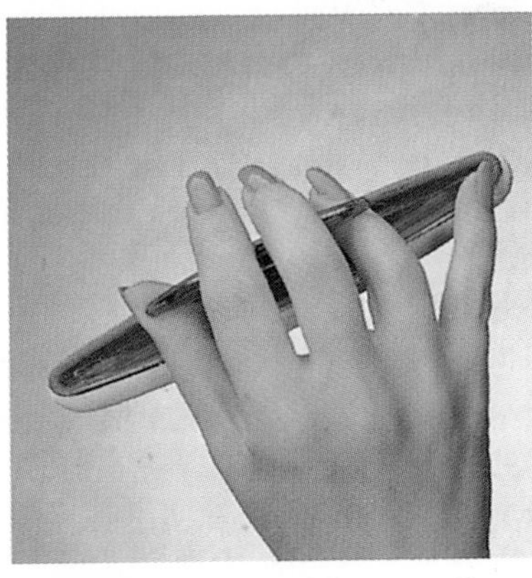

FIGURE 16.8 — Holding a nail buffer.

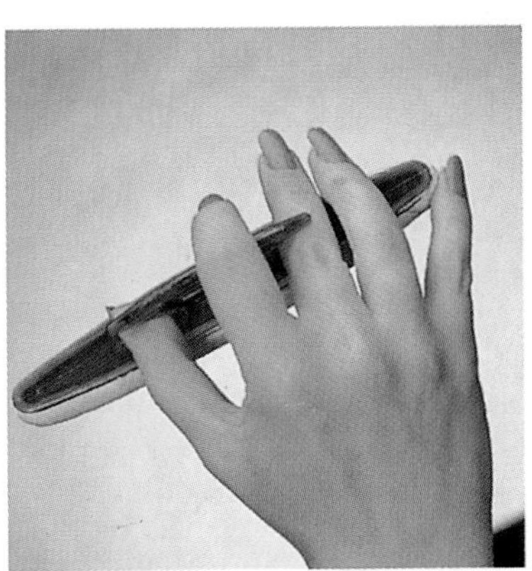

FIGURE 16.9 — Alternate way to hold a nail buffer.

COSMETICS

Nail and hand cosmetics vary in their composition and usage according to the purpose they serve.

Nail cleansers consist of detergent, usually cake, liquid, or flakes.

Nail polish removers contain organic solvents and are used to dissolve old polish on nails. To offset the drying action of the solvent, oil may be present in the nail polish remover.

Cuticle oil softens and lubricates the skin around the nails.

Cuticle creams are usually lanolin, petroleum, or beeswax based. They are used to prevent or correct brittle nails and dry cuticle.

Cuticle removers or *solvents* may contain 2% to 5% sodium or potassium hydroxide plus glycerine. Milder solutions may instead contain ***trisodium phosphate*** and ***triethanolamine*** or ***alkanolamines***. After the cuticle is softened with this liquid, it can be removed easily.

Nail bleaches contain hydrogen peroxide or diluted organic acids in a liquid form, or they can be mixed with other ingredients to form a white paste. When applied over nails, under the free edges, and on fingertips, they remove stains.

Nail whiteners are applied as a paste, cream, or coated string. They consist mainly of white pigments (zinc oxide or titanium dioxide). When applied under the free edges of the nails, they keep the tips looking white.

Dry nail polish usually is prepared in the form of powder or paste. The main ingredient is a mild abrasive, such as tin oxide, talc, silica, or kaolin. It smoothes the nail and gives it a gloss during buffing (where permitted).

An *abrasive* is available as a pumice powder and used with a buffer to smooth irregular nail ridges.

Liquid nail polish or *lacquer* is used to color or gloss the nail. It is a solution of nitro cellulose in ***volatile solvents,*** such as ***amyl acetate,*** together with a ***platiciser*** (castor oil), which prevents too rapid drying. Also present are resin and color.

Nail polish thinner, containing ***acetone*** or other solvent, is used to thin out nail polish when it has thickened.

A *base coat* is a liquid product applied before the liquid nail polish. It allows the nail polish to adhere readily to the nail surface. It also forms a hard gloss, which prevents the color in the nail polish from staining the nail tissue.

A *top coat,* or *sealer,* is a liquid applied over the nail polish. This product protects the polish and minimizes its chipping or cracking.

Nail hardeners or *strengtheners* are designed to prevent nails from splitting or peeling. Some are applied only to the tips of the nails, and others are applied over the entire nail. The nails must be thoroughly clean, free of oils or creams, and dry. Hardeners are applied before the base coat. There are four types of hardeners: protein hardeners, formaldehyde hardeners, nylon fiber hardeners, and nail conditioners. Protein hardeners are a combination of clear polish and a protein such as collagen. Formaldehyde hardeners utilize keratin fibers to strengthen and contain no more than 5% formaldehyde, because the ingredient can cause damage to the nail. Nylon fiber hardeners are a mixture of clear polish and nylon fibers applied first vertically, then horizontally over the entire nail. Nail conditioners are used independently of a manicure, usually overnight, on clean, dry nails. They contain moisturizing ingredients to combat dryness and brittleness.

A *nail dryer* is a solution that protects the nail polish against stickiness and dulling. It can be used either as a spray or brush-on, and it is applied over the top coat or directly on the nail polish.

Powdered alum or *alum solution* is used as a styptic to stop the bleeding of minor cuts.

Hand creams and *hand lotions* are recommended for dry, chapped, or irritated skin. Hand creams are made up of emollients, ***humectants*** (such as glycerine or propylene glycol), which promote the retention of water, emulsifiers, and preservatives. Hand lotions are similar in composition to hand creams, although they are a thinner consistency due to a higher oil content.

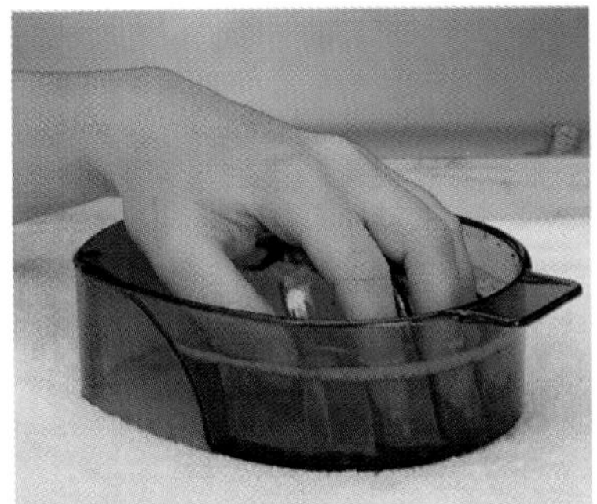

FIGURE 16.10 — An antibacterial soap is recommended for the finger bath to eliminate germs and reduce the risk of infection.

MATERIALS

Absorbent cotton for application of cosmetics to the nails.

Cleanser (liquid or other form) for finger bath. An antibacterial soap is recommended. (Fig. 16.10)

Warm water for finger bath.

Sanitized towel for each client.

Cleansing tissue for use whenever necessary.

Chamois for replacing soiled chamois on buffer.

Paper cups for replacing used paper cups in finger bowl.

Antiseptic to avoid infection when minor injuries to tissues surrounding the nails occur.

Disinfectant for sanitizing implements and for disinfecting the manicuring table.

Spatula for removing creams from jars.

Mending tissue, silk, linen, or *liquid nail wrap,* and *mending adhesive* for repairing or covering broken, split, torn, or weak nails.

Alcohol (70%) is used in a jar sanitizer where implements are kept during a manicure. It is also used to sanitize a client's fingers before a manicure. ✓

Completed: Learning Objective #3

THE USE OF IMPLEMENTS, COSMETICS, AND MATERIALS USED IN MANICURING

PREPARATION OF THE MANICURING TABLE

To give a professional manicure, all rules of sanitation must be followed. The table and the manicurist's hands must be perfectly clean. Everything, including containers, bowls, instruments, and materials, must be in perfect order. Disinfect manicuring implements after each use. Do not ask the client to sit at the table with the remains of the previous manicure in sight. Always clean the table immediately upon completion of a manicure so that it will be ready for the next client. This will make the manicure more pleasant for the client, and will put him or her in a more receptive mood for your advice and suggestions.

PROCEDURE

1. Spray the manicuring tabletop with a disinfectant and wipe with a damppaper towel.
2. Place a clean towel over the armrest or cushion.
3. Place a bowl of warm, soapy water to the left of the client.
4. Place the metal implements and orangewood sticks on a clean towel.
5. Arrange cream jars, lotion bottles, and nail polishes in the order to be used and place them to the left of the manicurist.
6. Place the nail file (which has been disinfected) and fresh emery boards to the right of the manicurist.
7. Attach a small plastic bag to the table with adhesive tape, on either the right or left side, for waste materials.
8. Prepare a fresh disinfectant solution for your implements daily.

The manicuring table drawer always should be clean and neat. Do not use it for waste materials; use the plastic bag. (Fig. 16.11)

PLAIN MANICURE

PREPARATION

The routine outlined in this text is one of several ways in which to give a manicure. Whatever routine your instructor outlines for you is equally correct.

1. Prepare manicuring table as previously outlined.
2. Seat client.
3. Wash your hands.
4. Examine client's hands.
5. Sanitize client's hands.

CAUTION

Be extremely careful to avoid cutting the client's skin. However, if this occurs, administer 3% hydrogen peroxide or powdered alum.

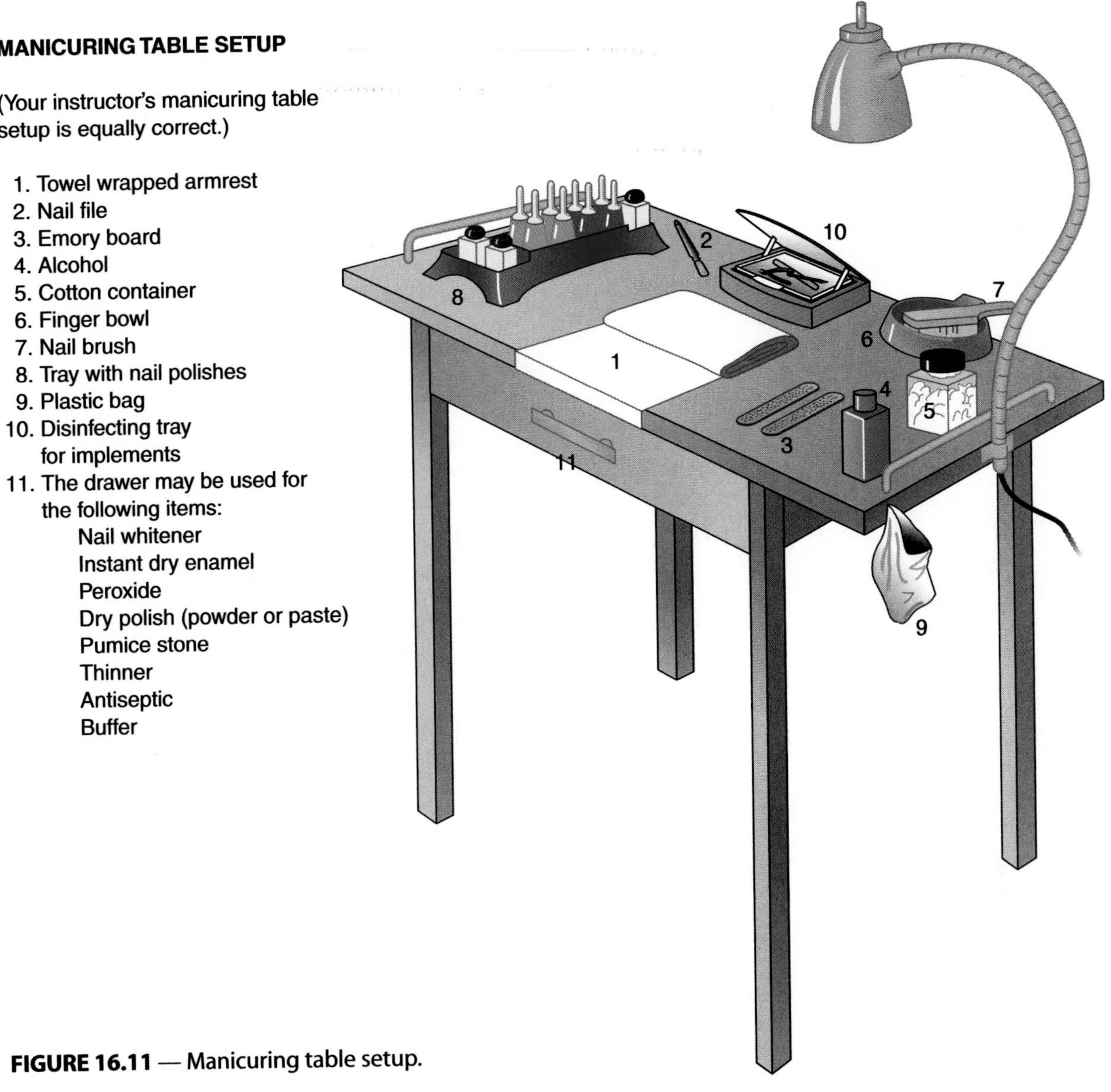

MANICURING TABLE SETUP
(Your instructor's manicuring table setup is equally correct.)
1. Towel wrapped armrest
2. Nail file
3. Emory board
4. Alcohol
5. Cotton container
6. Finger bowl
7. Nail brush
8. Tray with nail polishes
9. Plastic bag
10. Disinfecting tray for implements
11. The drawer may be used for the following items:
Nail whitener
Instant dry enamel
Peroxide
Dry polish (powder or paste)
Pumice stone
Thinner
Antiseptic
Buffer

FIGURE 16.11 — Manicuring table setup.

PROCEDURE

1. Remove old polish. (Start with the little finger of left hand.) Moisten cotton with nail polish remover and press over the nail for a few moments to soften the polish. With a firm movement, bring the cotton from the base of the nail to the tip. Do not smear the old polish into the cuticle or surrounding tissues. (An alternate method of removing nail polish is to moisten small pledgets of cotton with nail polish remover and press over old polish on each nail. Then moisten another pledget of cotton with nail polish remover and use it for removing the small pledgets on the nails. The pressed-on

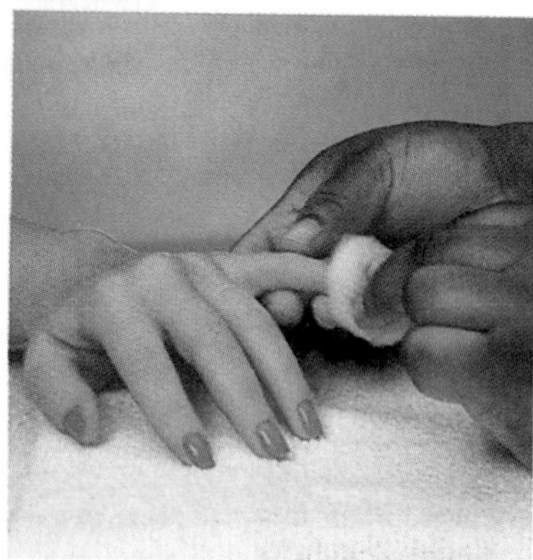

FIGURE 16.12 — Removing polish.

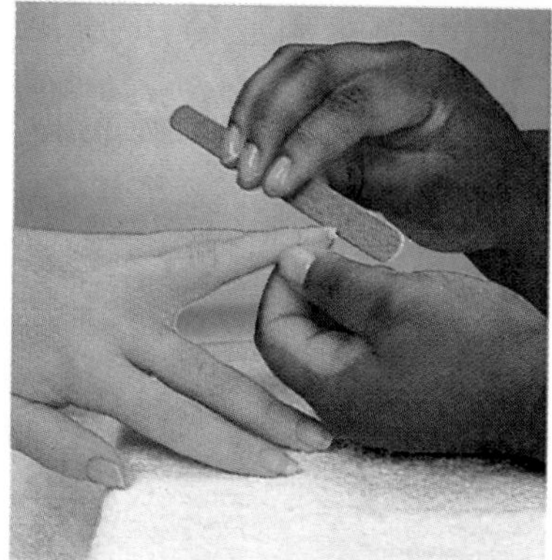

FIGURE 16.13 — Shaping nails.

pledget acts as a blotter and does not leave a polish smear on the cuticle.) (Fig. 16.12)

2. Shape nails. Discuss with the client the nail shape best suited for him or her. File the nails of the left hand, starting with the little finger and working toward the thumb, in the following manner:
   a) Hold the client's finger between the thumb and the first two fingers of the left hand.
   b) Hold the file or emery board in the right hand and tilt it slightly so that filing is confined mainly to the underside of the free edge.
   c) Shape nails as agreed with the client. Use the file or emery board to shape the nails. File each nail from corner to center, going from right to left and then from left to right. Filing nails according to the way the nail grows avoids splitting. Use two short, quick strokes and one long, sweeping stroke on each side of the nail. (Fig. 16.13)

Note: *Avoid filing deep into the corners of the nails. They will look longer and be stronger if permitted to grow out at the sides.*

3. Soften cuticle. After filing the nails of the left hand, file two nails of the right hand. Then, immerse the left hand into the finger bowl (soap bath) to permit softening of the cuticle. (*Note:* Use of an antibacterial soap in the finger bowl eliminates bacteria and allows you to work on a germ-free field.) Finish filing the nails of the right hand. Remove the left hand from the finger bowl. (Fig. 16.14)
4. Dry fingertips. Holding a towel with both hands, carefully dry the left hand, including the area between the fingers. With the towel, gently loosen and push back the cuticle and adhering skin on each nail. (Fig. 16.15)

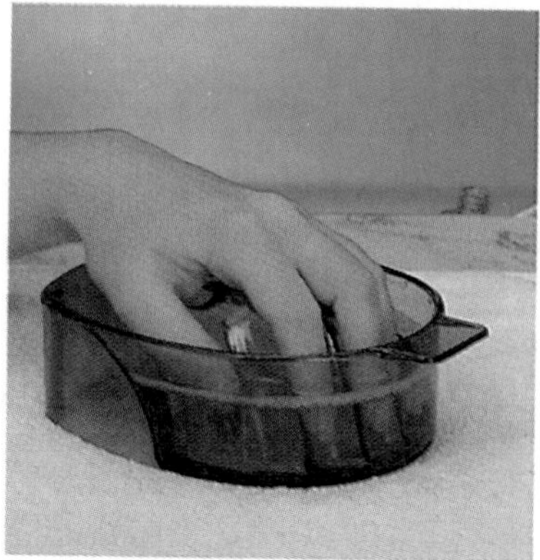

FIGURE 16.14 — Softening cuticle.

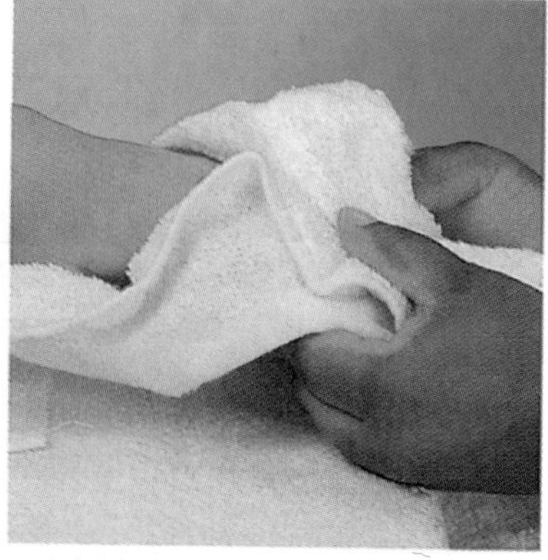

FIGURE 16.15 — Towel-drying fingertips.

5. Apply cuticle remover (solvent). Wind a thin layer of cotton around the blunt edge of an orangewood stick for use as an applicator. Apply cuticle solvent around the cuticle of the left hand.

6. Loosen cuticle. Use the spoon end of the cuticle pusher to gently loosen the cuticle. Keep the cuticle moist while working. Use the cuticle pusher, in a flat position, to remove dead cuticle adhering to the nail without scratching the nail plate. (Fig. 16.16) Push the cuticle back with a towel over the index finger.

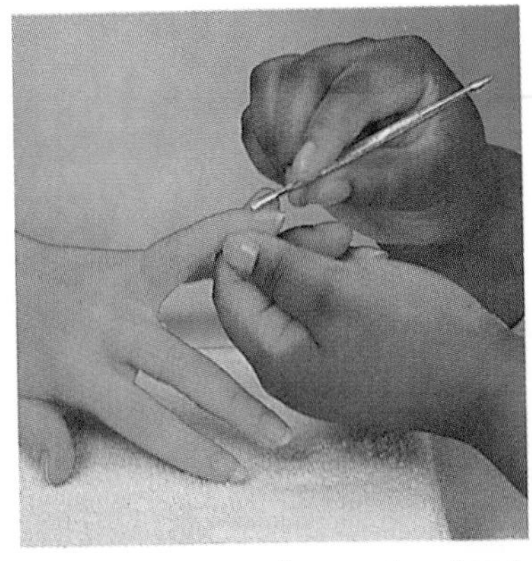

FIGURE 16.16 — Loosening dead cuticle with pusher.

Note: *Use light pressure when using a cuticle pusher or orangewood stick so the tissue at the root of the nail will not be injured.*

7. Clean under free edge. Use a cotton-tipped orangewood stick, dipped in soapy water, to clean under free edge, working from the center toward each side, employing gentle pressure. (Fig. 16.17)

8. Trim cuticle. If necessary, use cuticle nippers to remove dead cuticle, uneven cuticle, or hangnails. In cutting the cuticle, be careful to remove it as a single segment. (Fig. 16.18)

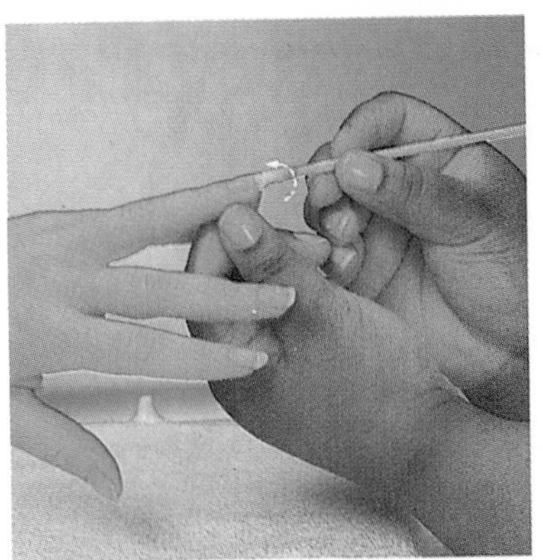

FIGURE 16.17 — Cleaning under free edge with cotton-tipped orangewood stick.

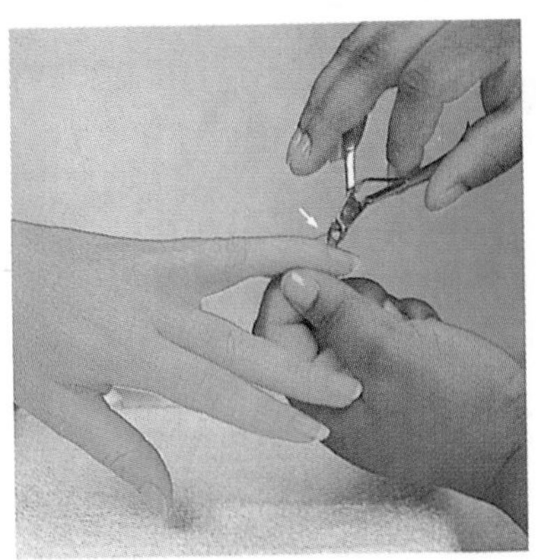

FIGURE 16.18 — Trimming cuticle with nippers.

9. When cutting the cuticle of the middle finger of the left hand, immerse fingers of the right hand into finger bowl, while continuing to manicure the left hand.

10. Bleach under free edge (optional). With a cotton-tipped orangewood stick, apply hydrogen peroxide or other bleaching preparation under the free edge of each nail.

11. Apply nail whitener under free edge of nails (optional). Use orangewood stick as applicator to apply chalk paste, or use a string treated with nail whitener.

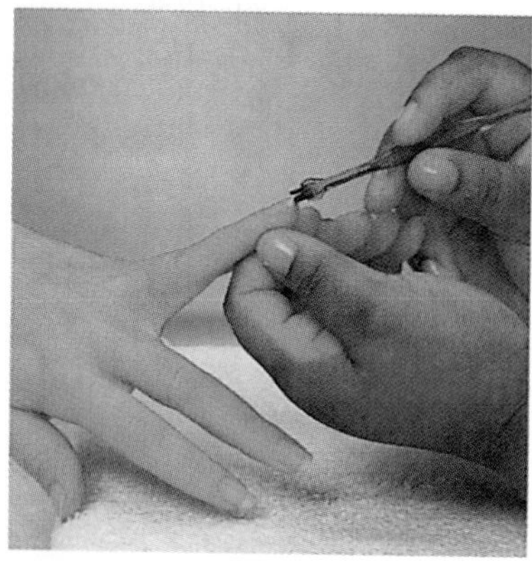

FIGURE 16.19 — Cleaning under nails with downward stroke.

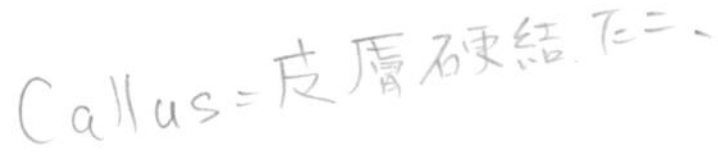

12. Apply cuticle oil or cream around the sides and base of the nail and massage with the thumb in a rotary movement.
13. Remove right hand from finger bowl. Manicure the nails and cuticles of right hand as described in steps 4 through 12.
14. Cleanse nails. Brush the nails over the finger bowl, using a downward movement, to clean the nails of both hands. (Fig. 16.19)
15. Dry hands and nails thoroughly.

NAIL PROBLEMS

A fringe of loose skin left around the nail after a manicure is caused by trimming the cuticle closer than necessary and then rolling back the epidermis. To prevent the occurrence of such loose skin, trim the cuticle only enough to allow a tiny margin of cuticle to remain.

Callus growth at the fingertips can be softened by the application of creams and lotions, and by removing the constant pressure that is causing it. Gentle rubbing with pumice powder also is helpful to start the removing process.

Stains on fingernails may be bleached with prepared nail bleach or peroxide. Slightly damp pumice powder also may be applied and the nails buffed to help remove stains.

COMPLETION

1. Re-examine nails and cuticles. Carefully re-examine the nails for defects. Use the fine side of an emery board to give the nails a smooth beveled edge. Remove remaining pieces of cuticle.
2. If required, repair split or broken nails.
3. As an added service, a hand massage or a hand and arm massage may be given at this time.
4. Apply base coat. Apply base coat to the left hand with long strokes, starting with the little finger and working toward the thumb. Allow it to dry until "slick to a light touch." (Fig. 16.20)
5. Apply liquid polish. Dip the camel's hair brush into the polish and wipe off excess by pressing it gently against the sides of the bottle.

   Apply the polish lightly and quickly, using sweeping strokes, from the base to the free edge of the nail, as shown in the illustrations. (Figs. 16.21–16.23) Always keep the polish thin enough to flow freely. If the polish is thick, add a little polish solvent and shake well.

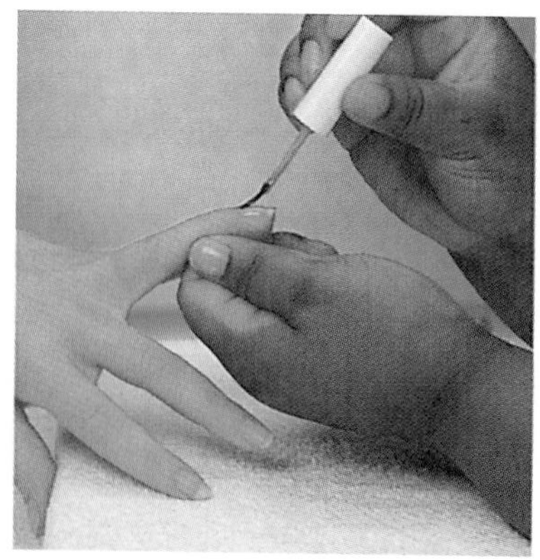

FIGURE 16.20 — Applying base coat.

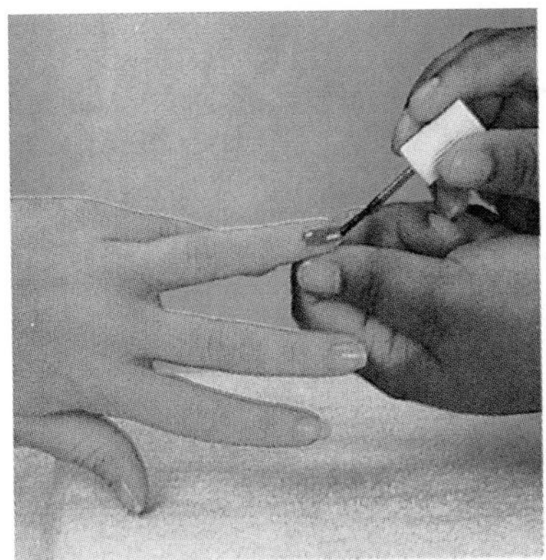

FIGURE 16.21 — Apply polish down center of nail.

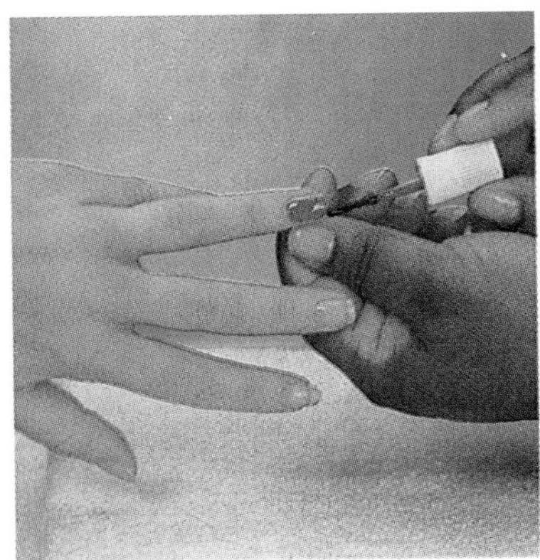

FIGURE 16.22 — Apply polish to right side of nail.

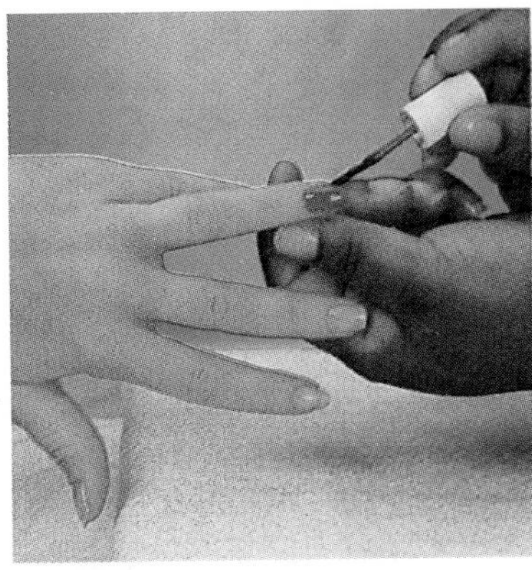

FIGURE 16.23 — Apply polish to left side of nail.

6. Remove excess polish. Dip a cotton-tipped orangewood stick into nail polish remover. Apply it carefully around the cuticles and nail edges to remove excess polish.
7. Apply top or seal coat. Apply top coat to the left hand with long strokes, and then apply it to the right hand in the same manner. Brush around and under tips of nails for added support and protection.
8. Apply hand lotion. As an additional service, after the top coat is completely dry, apply hand lotion with light manipulations over the hands, from wrists to fingertips.

FINAL CLEANUP

1. Disinfect used manicuring implements; place them in a clean, covered container.
2. Place used materials (tissues, cotton, emery board, etc.) into closed containers or plastic bag attached to manicuring table.
3. Spray manicuring table with disinfectant and wipe. Put everything in order.
4. Clean the tops of nail polish bottles with polish remover.
5. Inspect the manicuring table drawer for cleanliness and order.
6. Wash and dry your hands.

Career Path

NAIL TECHNICIAN

If you decide to become a nail technician, you will become part of a multi-billion-dollar industry. But if you want to do well in this business, you must be accomplished not only in giving manicures, pedicures, and artificial nail services, but in handling business matters.

Your first big decision will be whether to work in a full-service or nails-only salon. The full-service salon, unless it is very large, usually employs only one nail technician. In this situation, you will get all the salon's nail-care business, and most of your clients will be having their nails done in conjunction with other beauty services. The drawbacks are that you won't be able to share information with other nail technicians, and there will be no one to fill in for you when you are sick or on vacation. You may also be limited in the variety of artificial nail services you can provide.

In a nails-only salon, those disadvantages will not exist. Also, clients who patronize this type of salon are usually more serious about their nail care than the clients in a full-service salon. They may have special nail problems, or may want more creative artificial nail services. All of this gives you tremendous experience in your chosen field. Keep in mind, though, that there will be more competition for clients in the nails-only salon.

SAFETY RULES IN MANICURING

Observing safety rules in manicuring can be of great help in preventing accidents and injury to the client or nail technician. The following safety rules will guide the nail technician:

1. Keep all containers covered and labeled.
2. Hold or move containers with dry hands.
3. Handle sharp-pointed implements carefully and avoid dropping them.
4. Dull oversharpened cutting edges of sharp implements with an emery board.
5. Bevel a sharp nail edge with an emery board.
6. Do not file too deeply into nail corners.

7. Do not use a sharp, pointed implement to cleanse under the nail.
8. Avoid excessive friction in nail buffing (where permitted).
9. Apply an antiseptic immediately if the skin is accidentally cut.
10. Apply styptic powder or alum solution to stop the bleeding from a small cut. Never use a styptic pencil.
11. Avoid pushing the cuticle back too far.
12. Avoid too much pressure at the base of the nail.
13. Do not work on a nail when the surrounding skin is inflamed or is infected.
14. Any disposable sharp objects (files, etc.) or materials (such as cotton) that come in contact with blood or body fluids must be disposed of in a sealed plastic bag.
15. If blood is drawn during a procedure, stop the service until the implement is cleaned and disinfected, or use another implement. Do not risk cutting yourself with a sharp tool that has blood on it.

INDIVIDUAL NAIL STYLING

For a more natural effect, the shape of the nail should conform to that of the fingertip. A gracefully shaped nail adds beauty to the hands.

Nail shapes can be divided into four types:

1. Oval
2. Slender tapering (pointed)
3. Square or rectangular
4. Clubbed (round)

The oval nail is the ideal nail shape and can be styled by either covering the entire nail with polish, leaving the free edge white, or leaving the half moon at the base of the nail white. (Fig. 16.24)

The slender tapering nail is well suited for the thin, delicate hand. The nail should be tapered somewhat longer than usual to enhance the slender appearance of the hand. The nail can be completely polished, or a half moon can be left at the base. (Fig. 16.25)

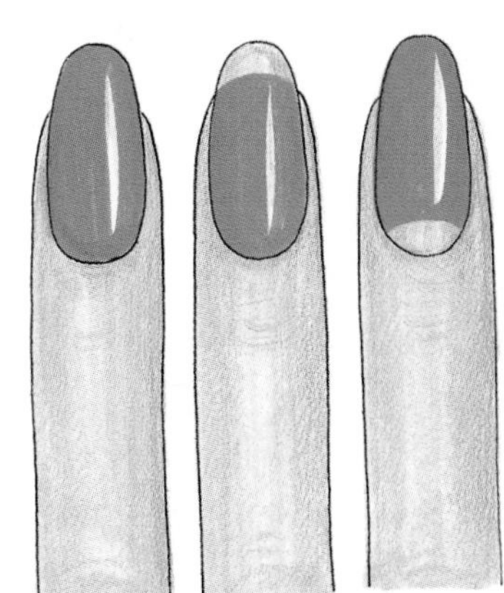

FIGURE 16.24 — Correct nail styling for oval nail.

Completed: Learning Objective #4

MANICURING PROCEDURES AND SANITARY AND SAFETY PRECAUTIONS

The square or rectangular nail should extend only slightly past the tip of the finger with the nail tip rounded off. The entire nail may be polished with a slight half moon left at the base and a white margin left at the sides of the nail. (Fig. 16.26)

The clubbed nail should be slightly tapered and extend just a bit past the tip of the finger. The entire nail should be polished with a thin white margin left at the sides. (Fig. 16.27)

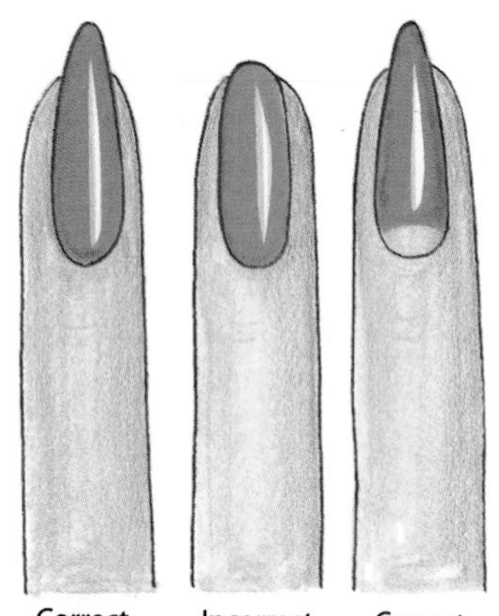

FIGURE 16.25 — Nail styling for slender nail.

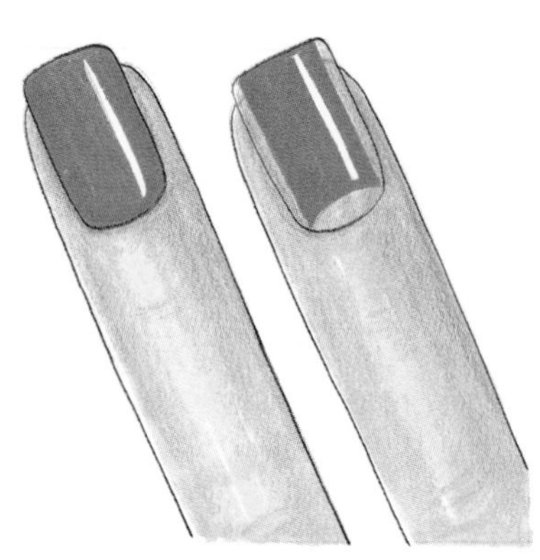

FIGURE 16.26 — Nail styling for square or rectangular nail.

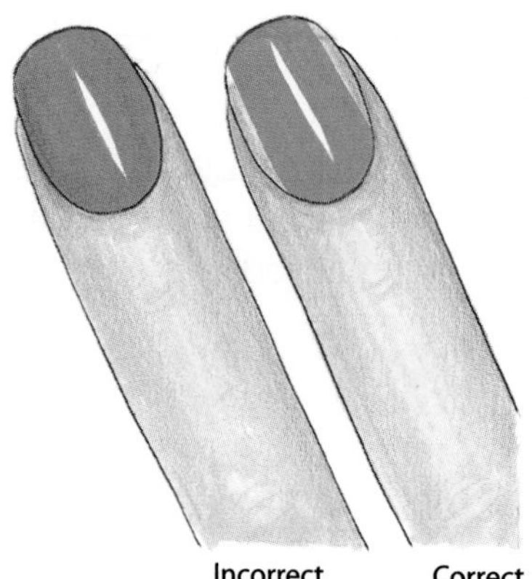

FIGURE 16.27 — Nail styling for clubbed nail.

HAND MASSAGE

Include a hand massage with each manicure. It keeps the hands flexible, well-groomed, and smooth.

PROCEDURE

1. Hold the client's hand in your hand. Place a dab of hand lotion on the back of the client's hand and spread it to the fingers and wrist.
2. Hold the client's hand firmly. Bend the hand slowly with a forward and backward movement to limber the wrist. Repeat three times. (Fig. 16.28)
3. Grasp each finger. Gently bend each finger, one at a time, to limber the top of the hand and finger joints. As the fingers and thumb are bent, slide your thumb down toward the fingertips. (Fig. 16.29)

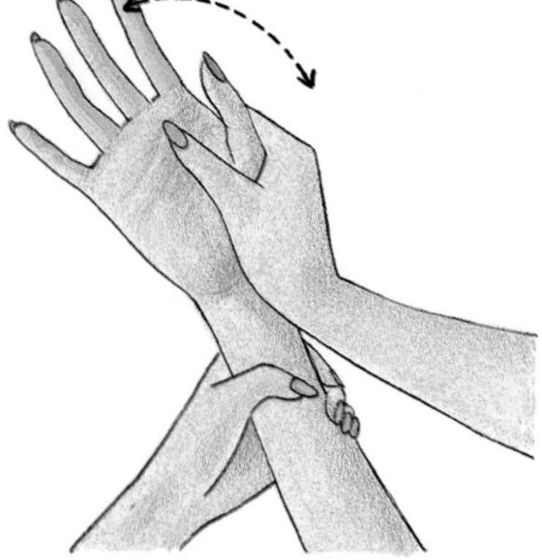

FIGURE 16.28 — Movement to limber the wrist.

4. With the client's elbow resting on the table, hold the hand upright. Massage the palm of the hand with the cushions of your thumbs, using a circular movement in alternate directions. This movement will completely relax the client's hand. (Fig. 16.30)
5. Rest client's arm on the table. Grasp each finger at the base, and rotate it gently in large circles, ending with a gentle squeeze of the fingertips. Repeat three times. (Fig. 16.31)
6. Hold the client's hand. Massage the wrist, then top of the hand with a circular movement. Slide back and with both hands wring wrist in opposite direction three times. Repeat movements three times. (Fig. 16.32)

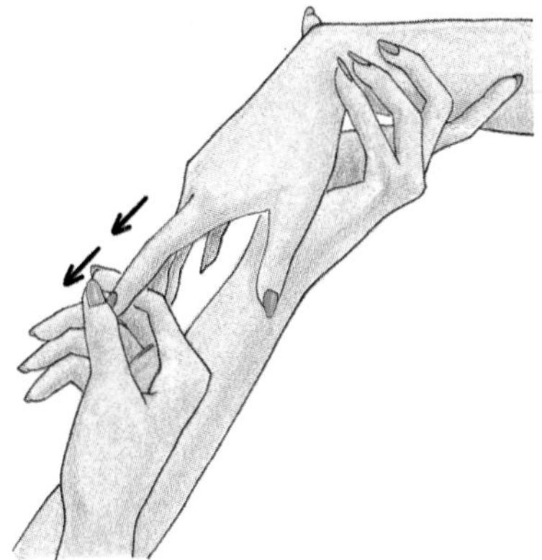

FIGURE 16.29 — Movement to limber the top of hand and finger joints.

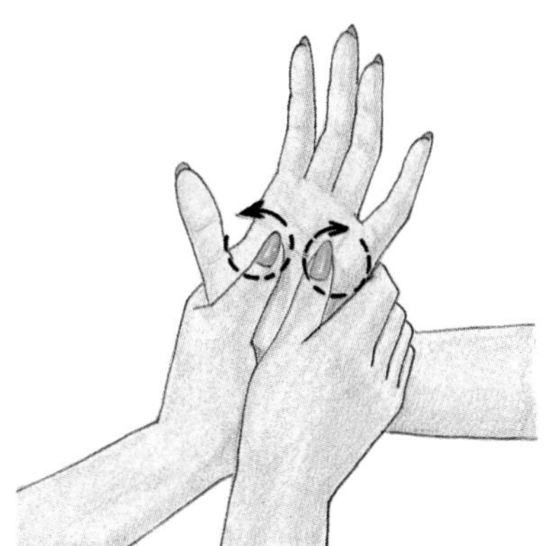

FIGURE 16.30 — Movement to relax the client's hand.

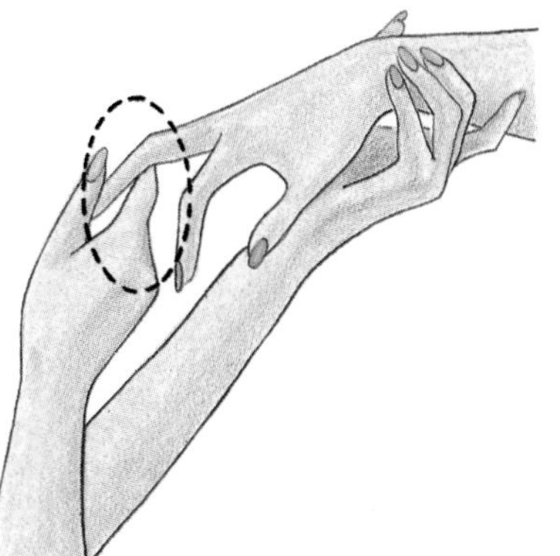

FIGURE 16.31 — Grasp each finger at base and rotate gently.

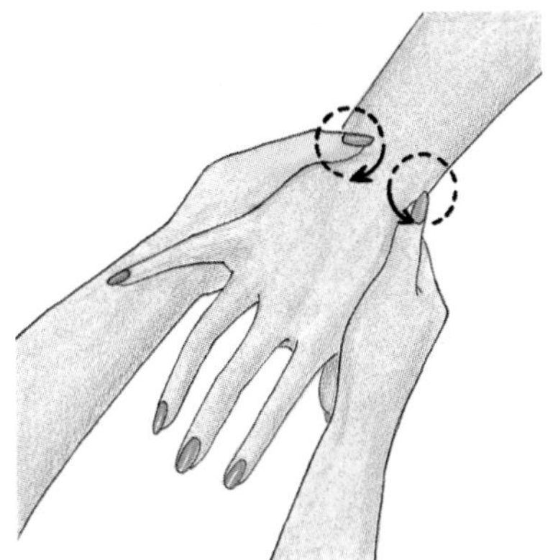

FIGURE 16.32 — Massage wrist and top of hand with a circular movement.

7. Finish massage by tapering each finger. Beginning at the base of each finger, rotate, pause, and squeeze with gentle pressure. Then, pull lightly with pressure until tip is reached. Repeat three times. (Fig. 16.33)
8. Repeat steps 1 to 7 on other hand.

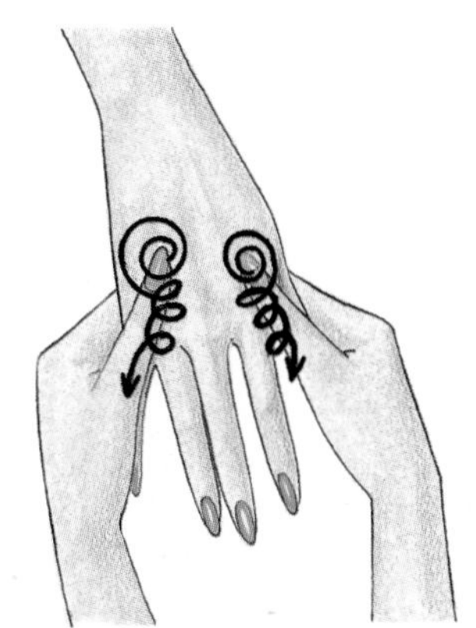

FIGURE 16.33 — Finish massage by tapering each finger.

HAND AND ARM MASSAGE

The hand and arm massage is a special service that may be added to the plain manicure. The procedure used is similar to the manicure with hand massage. However, all applications are extended to the forearm, including the elbow.

PROCEDURE

1. Complete hand massage as outlined.
2. Place client's arm on table, palm turned downward. Massage the arm from wrist to elbow, using a slow, circular motion in alternate directions. Repeat three times. Turn client's palm upward and repeat the same movements three times. (Fig. 16.34)
3. Firmly massage the underpart of the arm to the elbow, using fingers of each hand in alternate crosswise directions. Repeat three times. (Fig. 16.35)

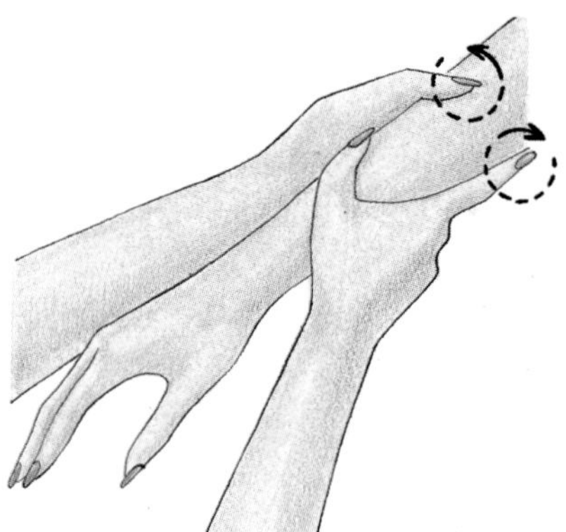

FIGURE 16.34 — Massage the arm from wrist to elbow.

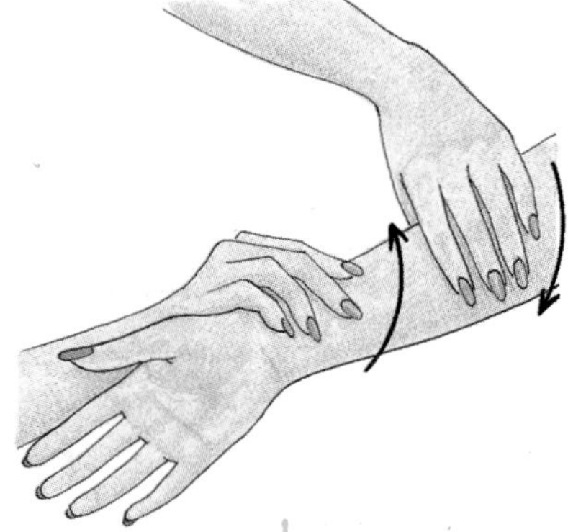

FIGURE 16.35 — Massage the underpart of the arm to the elbow.

4. Massage the top of the arm from the wrist to the elbow. Apply thumbs in opposite directions with a squeezing motion. Repeat three times. (Fig. 16.36)
5. Cup elbow joint in your hand. Massage the elbow with a circular motion. Repeat three times. (Fig. 16.37)
6. Stroke the arm firmly in opposite directions, from the elbow to wrist. (Fig. 16.38) Finally, stroke each finger, ending with a gentle squeeze of the fingertips.
7. Repeat steps 1 to 6 on the other arm. ✔

Completed:
Learning Objective
#5
MASSAGE TECHNIQUES

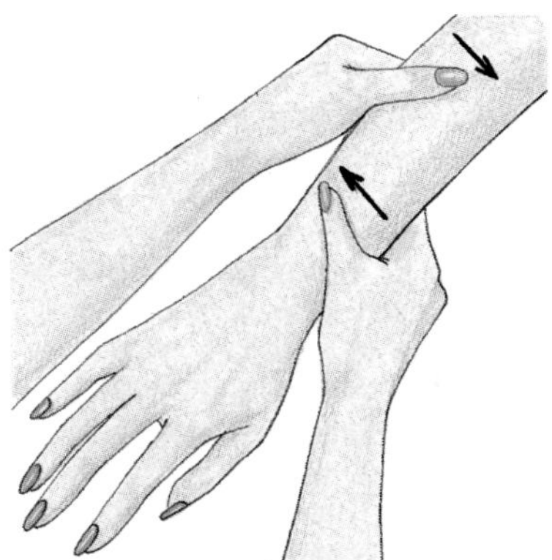

FIGURE 16.36 — Massage the top of the arm from wrist to elbow.

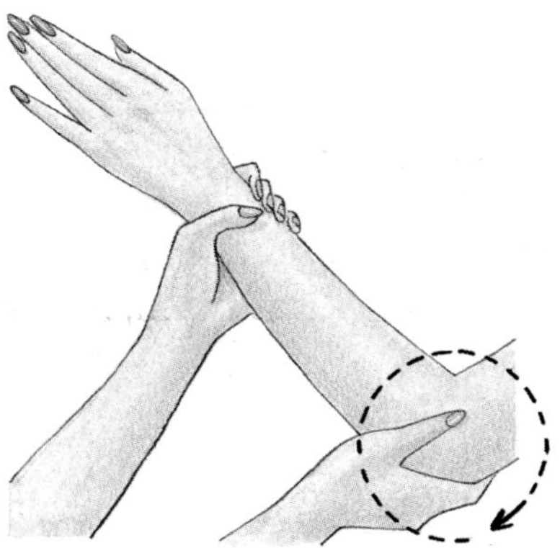

FIGURE 16.37 — Massage elbow with circular motion.

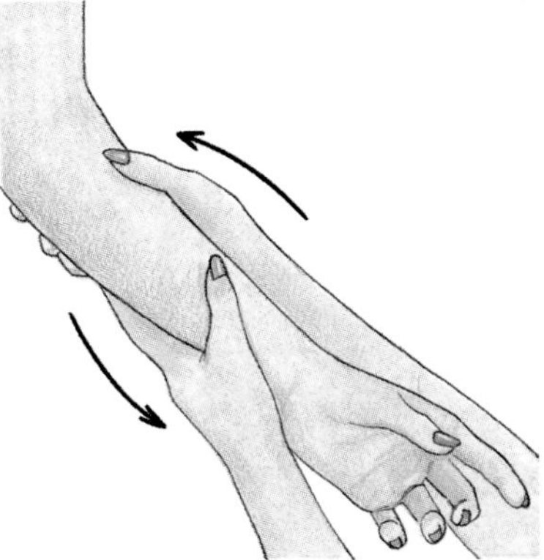

FIGURE 16.38 — Stroke arm firmly in opposite directions.

OTHER TYPES OF MANICURES

ELECTRIC MANICURE

The electric manicure is given with a portable device operated by a small motor. It uses a variety of attachments, including an emery wheel, cuticle pusher, cuticle brush, and buffer. Before using an electric manicure machine, read the manufacturer's instructions carefully. State regulations on this procedure may vary. Reminder: All drill bits must be properly disinfected after each client use.

OIL MANICURE

An oil manicure is beneficial for ridged and brittle nails and for dry cuticles. It also improves the hands by leaving the skin soft and pliable.

Procedure

1. Heat vegetable (olive) oil or commercial preparation to a comfortable temperature in an electric heater. (Fig. 16.39)
2. Perform a plain manicure to the point where you place the hand in the finger bowl; at that point, have client place his or her fingers in the heated oil.
3. Massage the hands and wrists with the oil; then treat the cuticles in the usual manner. Cuticle remover, cuticle oil, or cream is not needed.
4. Remove oil from the hands with a warm, damp towel.

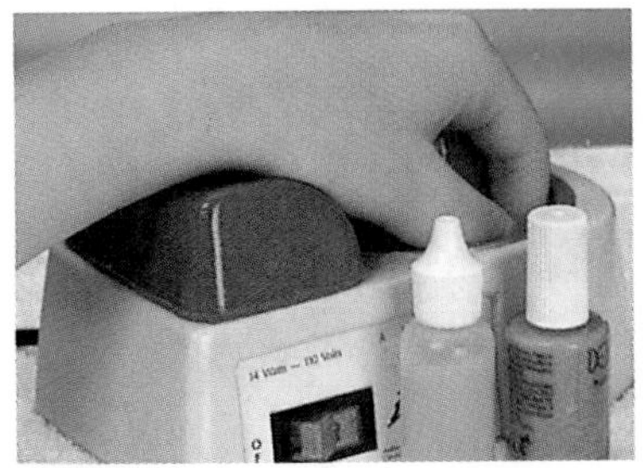

FIGURE 16.39 — Hot oil manicure heater.

5. Wipe each nail carefully with polish remover to remove all traces of the oil before applying the base coat.
6. Complete as you would a plain manicure.

MEN'S MANICURE

Men usually prefer a conservative manicure. File the nails either round or square. Apply a dry polish instead of a liquid polish.

Implements, materials, and supplies are the same as those used for a plain manicure. Follow the same procedure for a plain manicure up to the application of a base coat.

Buff nails (where permitted). Apply a small dab of paste polish over the buffer. Then buff the nails with downward strokes, from the base to the free edge of each nail, until a smooth, clear gloss has been obtained. To prevent a heating or burning sensation, lift the buffer from the nail after each stroke. Buffing the nails increases the circulation of the blood to the fingertips, smoothes the nails, and gives them a natural gloss or sheen.

Remove all residue from the nails by washing and drying the fingertips. If a clear liquid polish is used, buffing is not required. Apply polish in the same manner as for a plain manicure.

Completed:
Learning Objective
#6
DIFFERENT TYPES OF MANICURES

BOOTH MANICURE

A booth manicure is one that is given in the booth and not at the manicuring table. It is usually given while the client is receiving another service—for example, while a man is having his hair cut or styled.

ADVANCED NAIL TECHNIQUES

Clean, attractive hands and nails are an admirable part of anyone's top-to-toe grooming. When a person cannot grow natural nails of the desired length and strength, he or she could solve the problem with the help of advanced nail techniques, which include nail wrapping, sculptured nails, nail tipping, dipping, press-on nail caps, or acrylic overlays. When performed properly, these advanced nail techniques yield natural-looking artificial nails.

Artificial nails may be used for the following purposes:

1. To mend or conceal broken or damaged nails.
2. To improve the appearance of very short or badly shaped nails.
3. To help overcome the habit of nail biting.
4. To protect a nail or nails against splitting or breakage.

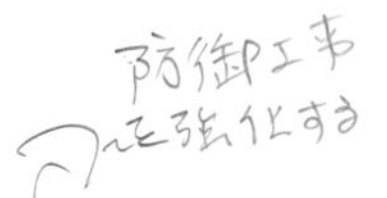

NAIL WRAPPING

Nail wrapping is done to mend torn, broken, or split nails, and to fortify weak or fragile nails. Mending tissue, silk, linen, or acrylic fiber are among the materials available for use in this procedure. Bolstering nails with silk will give a smooth, even appearance to the nail. Linen gives a more durable wrap; however, the coarseness of the material requires a colored polish to cover the completed nail.

The following two procedures are for use with materials that must be cut to fit the nail or nail fissure. Several manufacturers have recently made available pre-cut swatches of material that are adhesive backed and are attached only to the front of the nail.

Mending the Nail

1. Lightly file the split or chipped portion of the nail with the fine side of the emery board to help the mending material adhere to the nail.
2. Tear a small piece of mending material and saturate it with mending adhesive.
3. Place saturated mending material over the split or chipped area.
4. Tuck the material under the nail with an orangewood stick. The surface of the patch must be smoothed away from the nail edge with an orangewood stick dipped in polish remover.
5. If the split is deep, add a second patch for reinforcement.
6. Dry patch thoroughly before applying the base coat and polish.

Fortifying the Nail

1. Roughen the nail surface with the fine side of an emery board.
2. Tear or cut the wrapping material to fit the nail. If using mending tissue, tear into strips making sure edges of the tissue are feathered. (Fig. 16.40)
3. If using mending tissue, saturate each strip with mending adhesive. If using other material, place a line of mending adhesive down the center of the nail. (Fig. 16.41)
4. Using two fingers, place the wrapping material over the nail and hold until it adheres. Starting at the middle of the nail, use the orangewood stick to push the material in all directions, toward the edges and tip of the nail. Keep dipping the orangewood stick into the polish remover and patting the material until it is smooth. (Fig. 16.42)
5. Trim excess material extending past the free edge and sides of the nails. (Fig. 16.43)

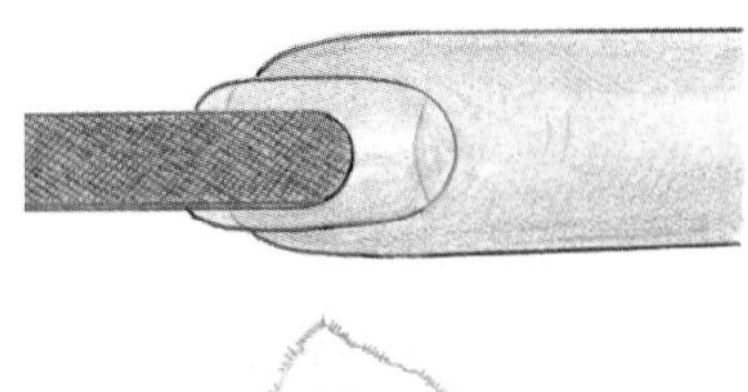

FIGURE 16.40 — Roughen nail surface and cut wrap to fit nail.

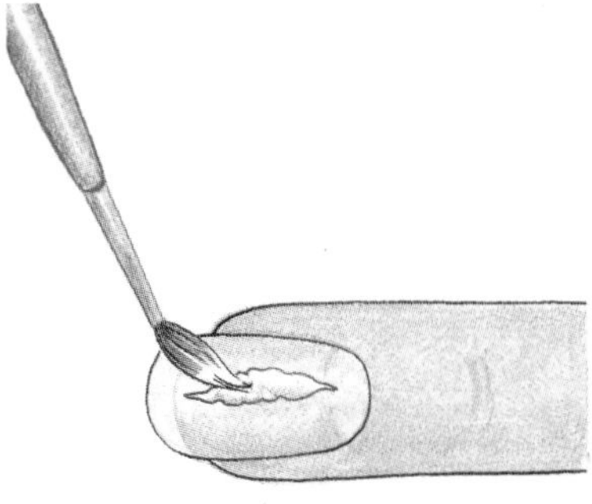

FIGURE 16.41 — Apply adhesive.

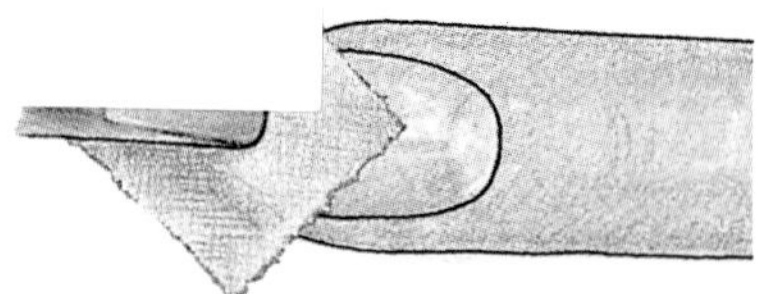

FIGURE 16.42 — Apply mending tissue.

6. If using mending tissue, turn the finger over and apply adhesive to the underside of the nail. Then, using the fingertips, fold the tissue over the nail edge and smooth out the tissue under the free edge with a pusher. If using other material, take the fine side of an emery board and lightly file the entire nail, top, sides, and free edge until smooth. (Fig. 16.44)
7. Apply one or two coats of adhesive on the top and underside of the free edge of the nail.
8. Apply a protective base coat to the top and underside of the free edge of the nail, and allow it to dry. Apply nail enamel and top coat or sealer, the same as for a plain manicure. (Fig. 16.45)

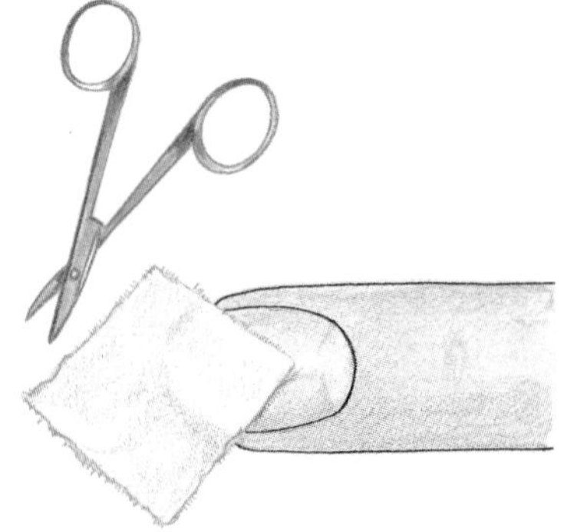

FIGURE 16.43 — Trim excess.

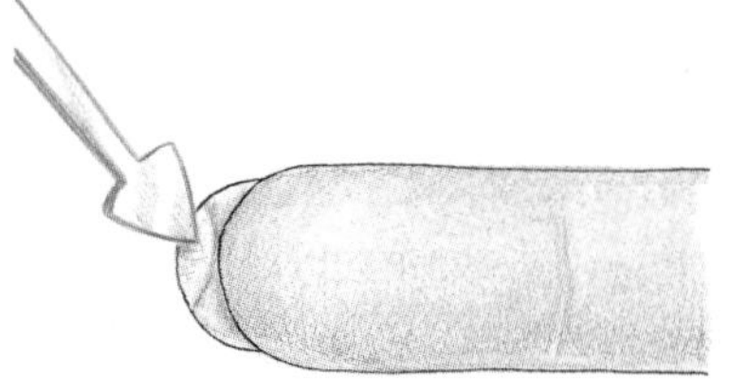

FIGURE 16.44 — Tuck tissue under free edge.

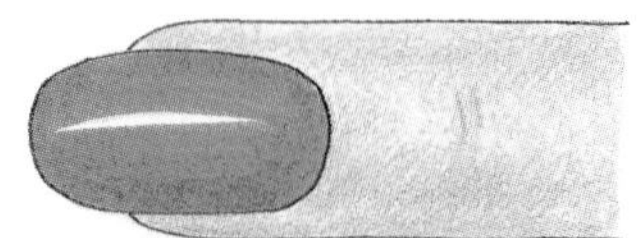

FIGURE 16.45 — Apply base and top coats.

Alternative Method

In step 3, when applying mending tissue, coat entire nail bed with adhesive and apply tissue.

Removing Nail Wraps

Remove polish from the client's right hand. To loosen the nail wrap, have the client place her fingertips in an approved type of solvent specified by the manufacturer's directions or recommended by your instructor.

After removing the polish from the left hand, have the client remove her right hand from the bowl, and ask her to place the fingertips of her left hand in the bowl of solvent. Gently remove the loosened wrap with an orangewood stick or metal pusher, and then place the fingertips in warm oil. Repeat the same procedure for the left hand.

Liquid Nail Wrap

Liquid nail wrap is a polish made of tiny fibers designed to strengthen and preserve the natural nail as it grows. It is brushed on to the nail in several directions to create a network that once hardened protects the nail. It is similar to nail hardener, though it is of a thicker consistency and contains more fiber.

SCULPTURED NAILS

Sculptured nails, also known as build-on nails, are used when one or more nails are to be lengthened. The manicurist should build the type of nail that best conforms to the shape of the client's fingers and hands.

Implements and Materials

Use all of the regular implements for manicuring plus the following:

Nail forms	Nail lengthener powder
Measuring spoon	Special liquid to dilute powder
Mixing cup	Brushes for application

Procedure

1. Give plain manicure up to but not including the application of polish. Scrub nails to remove oil from area.
2. Roughen nail slightly with emery board.
3. Dust the nail bed with a cosmetic brush or cotton swab.
4. Apply approved nail primer to the surface of the nail with a brush, according to the manufacturer's instructions.
5. Peel a nail form from its paper backing, and using the thumb and index finger of each hand, bend the tip to the desired nail shape. The adhesive tabs of the nail form grip the sides of the fingers when pressed with the thumb and index finger. Check to see that the form is snug under the free edge of the nail. (Fig. 16.46)
6. Dip the brush into the liquid mixture, wipe excess material on the side of the bowl and then immediately dip tip of brush into the powder, rotating it slightly as you draw it toward yourself to form a smooth ball of acrylic. (Fig. 16.47)
7. Place the ball of acrylic on the tip of the free edge of the nail. Form the new acrylic tip of the nail by dabbing and pressing material with the base of the brush. (Fig. 16.48)
8. Pick up additional acrylic material as in step 6 and place at the center of the nail and shape with the brush, making sure to avoid touching the cuticle. (Fig. 16.49)

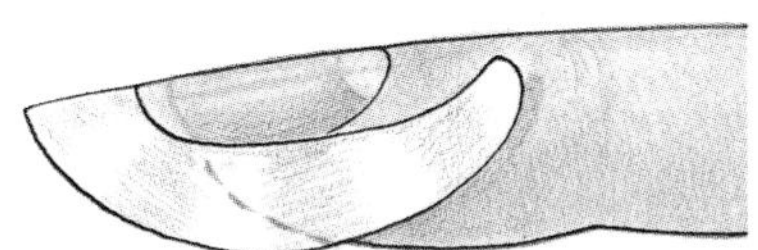

FIGURE 16.46 — Apply nail form.

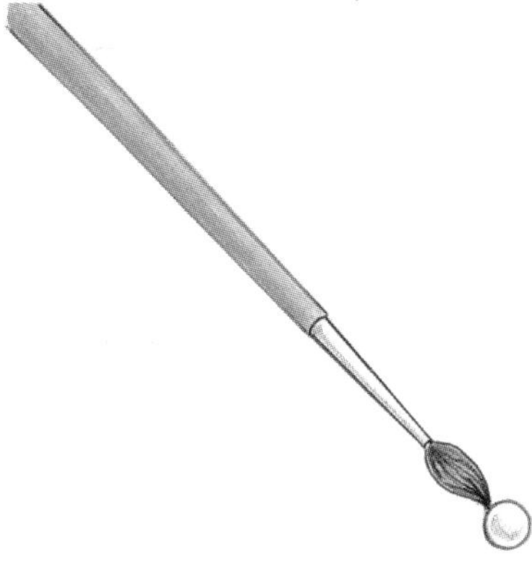

FIGURE 16.47 — Form a smooth ball of acrylic.

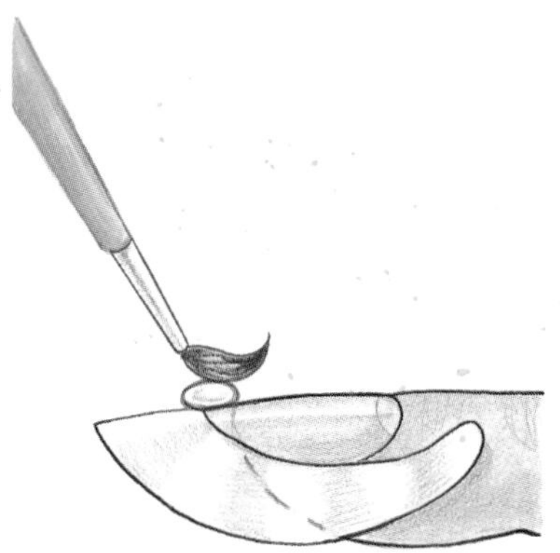

FIGURE 16.48 — Place ball of acrylic on tip of free edge.

9. Make an extremely wet acrylic mixture (very little powder) and place at the center of the lower half of the nail bed. Spread mixture to the sides of the nail bed, being careful not to touch the cuticle. (Fig. 16.50)

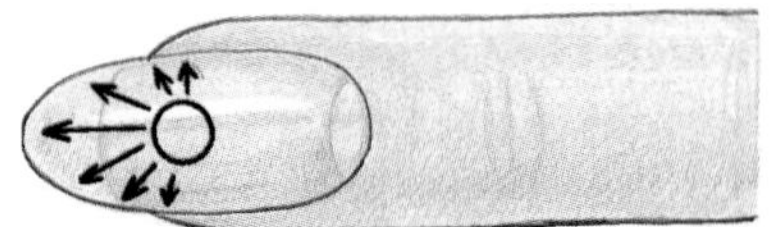

FIGURE 16.49 — Use additional acrylic material and shape with brush.

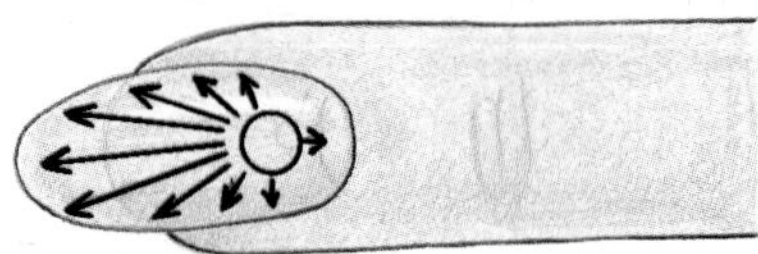

FIGURE 16.50 — Apply wet acrylic mixture.

10. Allow nails to dry and remove nail forms.
11. File new nail to desired shape and then buff nails until entire surface is smooth.
12. Wash the nail or nails thoroughly. Allow them to dry.
13. Apply a base coat, polish, and top coat sealer.

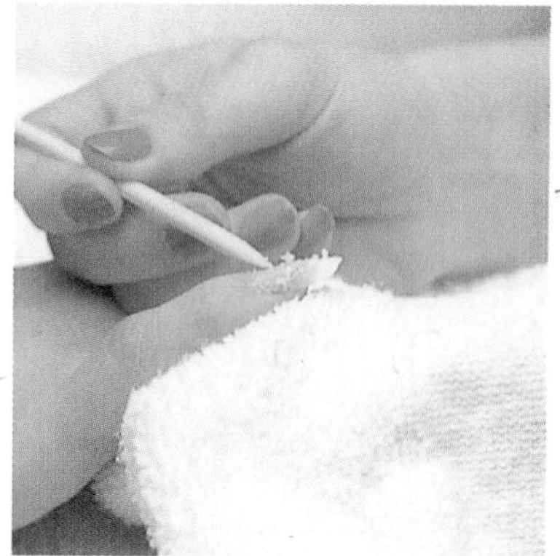

FIGURE 16.51 — Slide tip off with orangewood stick.

Removing Sculptured Nails

Soak nails in an approved solvent specified by the manufacturer or your instructor. Use orangewood stick and gently push off softened acrylic nail. Repeat until all acrylic has been removed. Do not pry off acrylic with nippers, as this will damage natural nail plate. (Fig. 16.51)

Repairs and Fill-ins for Sculptured Nails

1. Remove nail polish with non-acetone polish remover.
2. Use a medium/fine abrasive to smooth the ledge of acrylic in the new growth area so that it blends into nail bed.
3. Hold abrasive flat and glide it over entire nail to reshape and refine nail and thin out free edge.
4. Use buffer block to buff acrylic and blend it into new growth area.
5. Use a file to smooth out any acrylic that might have lifted.
6. Use fingerbowl filled with warm water and antibacterial soap and a nail brush to gently wash nails. Do not soak nails.
7. Use a cotton-tipped orangewood stick to gently push back cuticle.
8. Buff lightly over nail plate with medium/fine abrasive to remove the natural oil. Brush off filings.

9. Apply nail antiseptic to nails with cotton-tipped orangewood stick, cotton, or spray.
10. Brush exposed area with primer, following the manufacturer's instructions.
11. Dip tip of brush into liquid, then into powder to form a small acrylic ball.
12. Place acrylic material on exposed area, pressing and shaping it with the base of the brush until it blends into the existing sculptured nail. Let area dry. Reshape nail with emery board and buff for a smooth appearance.

If an acrylic nail is badly chipped or cracked, file a "V" shape into the crack or file flush to remove crack. A new nail form is then attached and acrylic material added to the free edge of the nail. A new tip is then formed and blended into the old material still adhering to the nail.

Acrylic Overlays

Acrylic overlays can strengthen weak nails or repair damaged ones. The acrylic material is used on sculptured nails, except that nails are reinforced on the top surface instead of extended.

Safety Precautions

1. Clean brush by dipping it into polish remover and wiping it clean.
2. Clean mixing dish by lifting hardened content out with pusher.
3. Make sure bottles are tightly capped when not in use.
4. Do not store product near heat, or use near open flame.
5. Do not apply to injured or inflamed skin.
6. Make sure work area is well ventilated.

When sculptured nails lift, crack, or grow out and are not attended to immediately, moisture and dirt become trapped under the nail, and fungus begins to grow. The spread of fungus can lead to nail injury or loss. Do not attempt to treat the condition yourself. It is very contagious and should be referred to a physician.

A change in the color of the natural nail after sculptured nails have been applied usually means that fungus has become trapped under the acrylic. Most primers have aseptic ingredients that disinfect the nail before acrylic is applied. To help ensure that contamination does not occur, *do not touch the nail after primer is applied.*

PRESS-ON ARTIFICIAL NAILS

Press-on nails are a convenient way to lengthen and beautify nails. They can be worn every day or on special occasions. Press-on nails are constructed of either plastic or nylon, and the manufacturer's instructions must be followed carefully.

Implements and Materials

Use all the regular implements and materials for manicuring, plus artificial press-on nails, nail adhesive, and adhesive remover.

Preparation

1. Remove polish from client's nails, and give a manicure up to, but not including, the application of polish.
2. Roughen the client's nails by going over them with an emery board.
3. Select the proper nail size for each finger. With sharp manicuring scissors, trim and then file the artificial nail at the cuticle end so that it fits to the shape of the natural nail. Artificial nails can be flattened by being firmly pressed down before application. They also can be reshaped by being held in warm water for a few seconds and molded to the desired shape.

Procedure

1. Apply a small amount of adhesive evenly on the edges of the client's nails. Do not apply adhesive on the center of the nails.
2. Apply adhesive on the inside of the artificial nail, excluding tip.
3. Allow the adhesive to dry thoroughly (about 2 minutes).
4. Press artificial nail gently onto the natural nail, with the base touching the cuticle or under it. As each nail is applied, hold it firmly in place for about a minute.
5. Carefully wipe away any excess adhesive from tips and around nails.
6. Allow the artificial nails to dry thoroughly. Advise the client to avoid disturbing the nails while they are drying.
7. Finish the manicure by applying base coat, polish, and top coat.

Removing Polish

To remove nail polish from nails constructed of plastic, use only nail polish remover that has an oily base and is non-acetone.

Reminder: Polish remover containing acetone will damage plastic artificial nails.

If nylon-constructed nails have been used, an acetone type of polish remover will not damage them.

Removing Press-on Artificial Nails

Apply a few drops of oily nail polish remover around the edge of the nail; then gently lift from the side with an orangewood stick. Do not attempt to pull or twist off the nail, as this could damage or injure the natural nail. Adhesive solvent can be used to remove press-on nails. It also can be used to remove any surplus adhesive from artificial nails and from natural nails. Press-on nails should be dried carefully and stored in a box. With proper care, they can be reused.

Reminders and Hints on Press-on Artificial Nails

1. Never apply artificial nails over sore or infected areas.
2. Most manufacturers suggest that artificial nails not be worn for more than 2 weeks at a time, in order to allow for natural growth of the nail.
3. Most artificial nail adhesives are flammable; be cautious with cigarettes, matches, and lighters.
4. When wearing artificial nails, do not subject them to a long period of immersion in water as they might tend to loosen.
5. Do not contaminate the adhesive with oil, cream, or powder.

OTHER ADVANCED TECHNIQUES

Following are several other advanced nail techniques you should be familiar with.

DIPPED NAILS

Dipped nails are artificial nail tips that are sprayed with an adhesive and then applied with glue to the ends of the natural nails. After filing and sanitizing, glue is applied down the center of the nail. The nail is then dipped for a short period of time into an acrylic mixture. When the acrylic dries, the nail is filed, buffed, and coated with adhesive. Dipped nails are removed with an adhesive solvent recommended by the manufacturer or your instructor.

NAIL TIPPING

Anyone can have long-looking nails by simply extending the natural nail artificially.

Procedure

1. Give manicure up to but not including polish.
2. Select proper sized tip to fit client's natural nail.
3. Slightly roughen the free edge of the nail.
4. File tip to fit the shape of the free edge of the nail only. (Fig. 16.52)
5. Hold nail tip with thumb and index finger and apply half a drop of glue to the free edge of the nail.
6. Press tip onto the free edge of the nail, and then hold until dry. (Fig. 16.53)

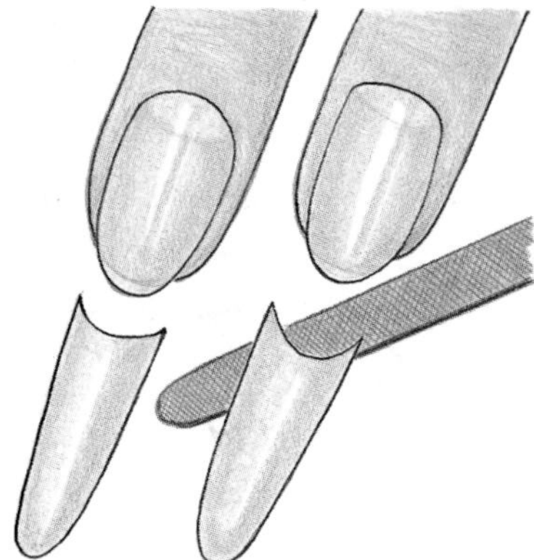

FIGURE 16.52 — Select size and shape nail.

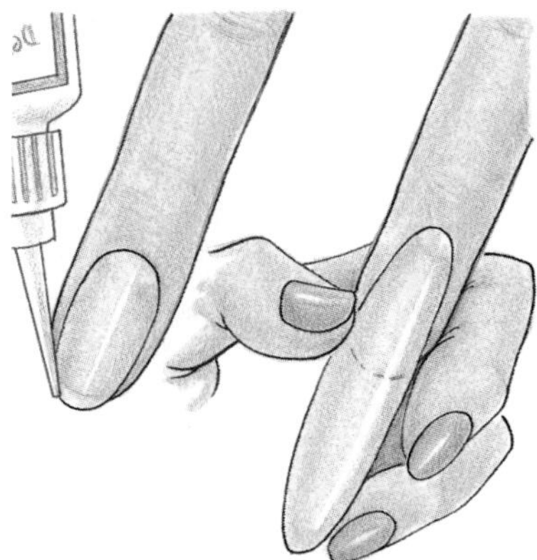

FIGURE 16.53 — Apply glue and affix nail.

7. Buff the nail where the free edge of the nail and the tip form a seam. Leave resulting dust on the nail. (Fig. 16.54)
8. Apply nail glue to seam where nail tip and free edge of nail meet. (Fig. 16.55) Glue placed over the nail dust will act as a bond and filler. Repeat glue application twice.
9. File sides of tip to blend with the natural nail. (Fig. 16.56) Cut nail to desired shape.

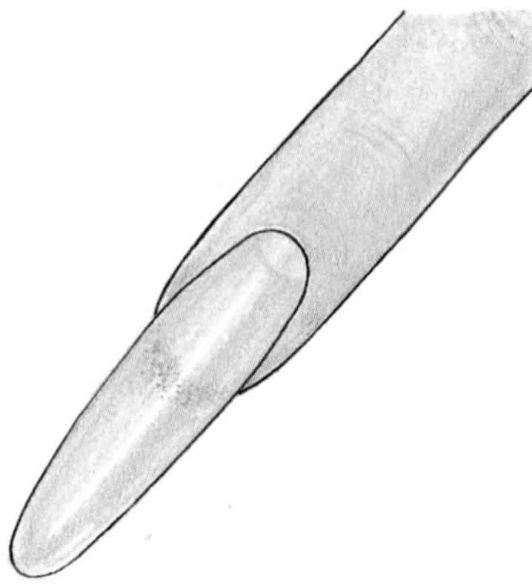

FIGURE 16.54 — Buff the nail.

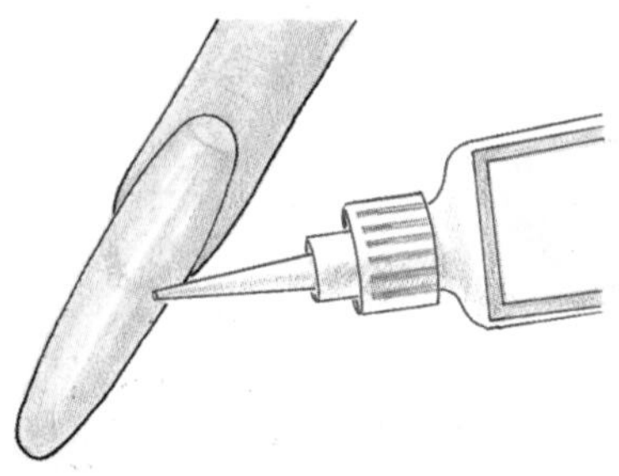

FIGURE 16.55 — Apply glue to seam.

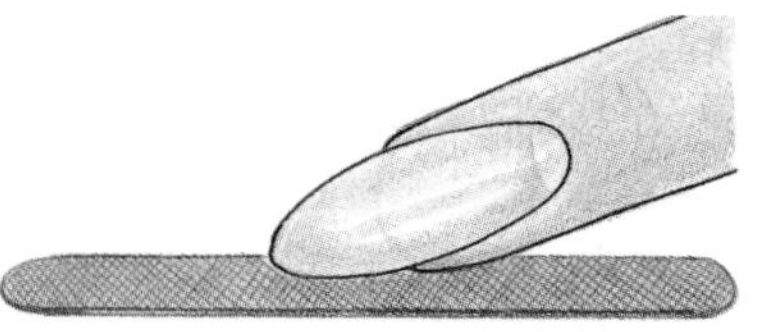

FIGURE 16.56 — File sides.

10. Apply glue from seam to the free edge of the nail tip. (Fig. 16.57) Buff seam and repeat procedure.

11. Apply nail polish as in a regular manicure. (Fig. 16.58)

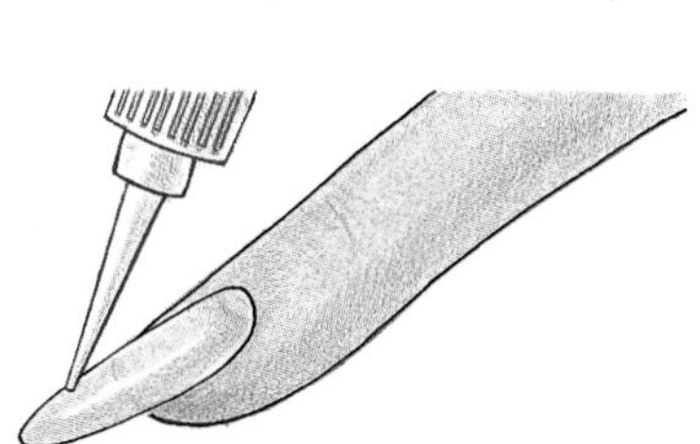

FIGURE 16.57 — Apply glue from seam to nail tip.

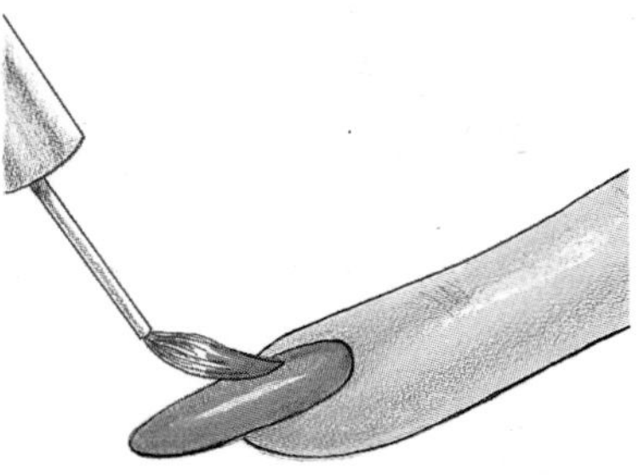

FIGURE 16.58 — Apply nail polish.

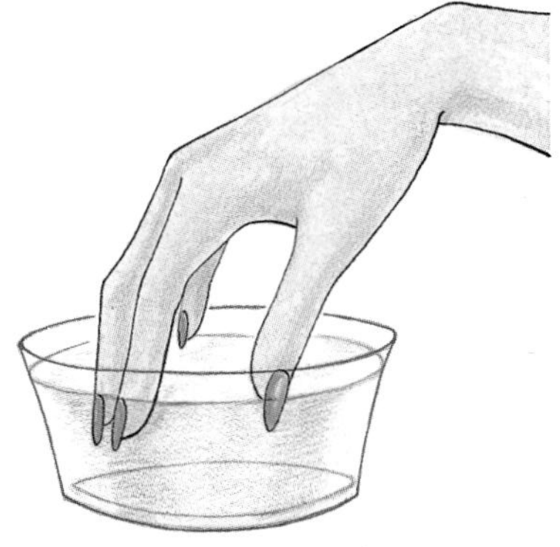

FIGURE 16.59 — Soak nail tips.

Removing Nail Tips

To remove nail tips, fill a small container with adhesive solvent recommended by the manufacturer or by your instructor. Soak nail tips until softened, and gently wipe fingers with a tissue. (Fig. 16.59)

Completed: Learning Objective #7

ADVANCED NAIL TECHNIQUES

PEDICURE

Pedicuring is the care of the feet, toes, and toenails. It has become an important salon service because of the shoe styles that expose various parts of the heel and toes. Neglected toenails and rough, harsh heels detract from the finest of footwear. Foot care not only improves personal appearance, it also adds to the comfort of the feet.

Abnormal foot conditions, such as corns, calluses, and ingrown nails, are best treated by a qualified podiatrist.

Ringworm of the foot (athlete's foot) is an infectious condition that can spread from one person to another. For an in-depth explanation of this disease, see the chapter on the nail and its disorders.

CAUTION

Do not administer a manicure or pedicure on hands or feet with a contagious disease or skin condition (for example, ringworm, or athlete's foot). Clients with such a condition should be referred to a physician.

EQUIPMENT, IMPLEMENTS, AND MATERIALS

The equipment, implements, and materials required for pedicuring are the same as those for manicuring, with the following additions:

Low stool for cosmetologist or pedicurist.

Ottoman on which to rest client's foot.

Two basins of warm water, each large enough for foot bath and rinse.

Waterproof apron, or an extra towel, to place over the lap to protect the uniform.

Two towels for drying client's feet.

Special toenail clippers.

Witch hazel or other *astringent.*

Paper towels.

Antibacterial soap or *antiseptic solution.*

Cotton pledgets and *foot powder.*

PREPARATION

1. Arrange required equipment, implements, and materials.
2. Seat client in chair; have client remove shoes and stockings.
3. Place client's feet on a clean paper towel on footrest.
4. Wash your hands.
5. Fill the two basins with enough warm water to cover the ankles.
6. Add antiseptic or antibacterial soap to one basin. Place both feet in bath for 3 to 5 minutes.
7. Remove feet from basin, rinse feet in second basin, and wipe dry.

PROCEDURE

1. Remove old polish from the nails of both feet. (Fig. 16.60)
2. File toenails of the left foot with an emery board. File the toenails straight across, rounding them slightly at the corners to conform to the shape of the toes. To avoid ingrown nails, do not file into the corners of the nails. Smooth rough edges with the fine side of an emery board. (Fig. 16.61)
3. Place the left foot in warm, soapy water. (Fig. 16.62)
4. Shape the nails of the right foot.
5. Remove the left foot from the basin and dry. (Fig. 16.63)
6. With a cotton-tipped orangewood stick, apply cuticle solvent to the cuticle and under the free edge of each toenail. (Fig. 16.64)

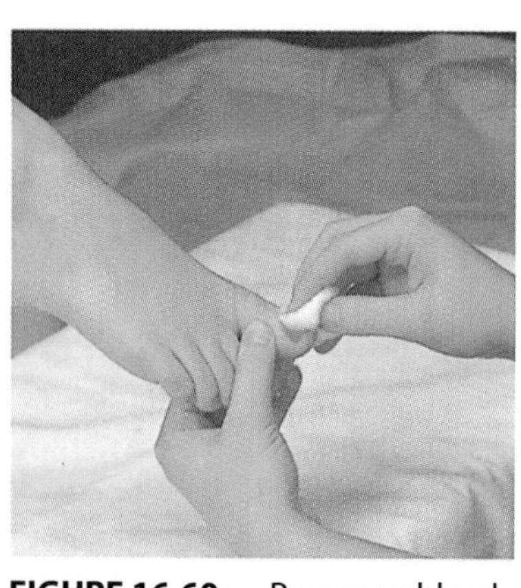

FIGURE 16.60 — Remove old polish.

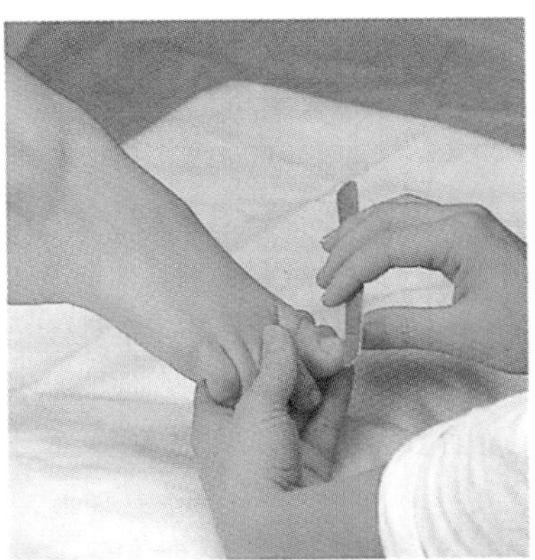

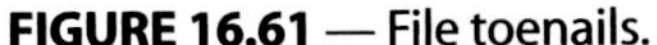

FIGURE 16.61 — File toenails.

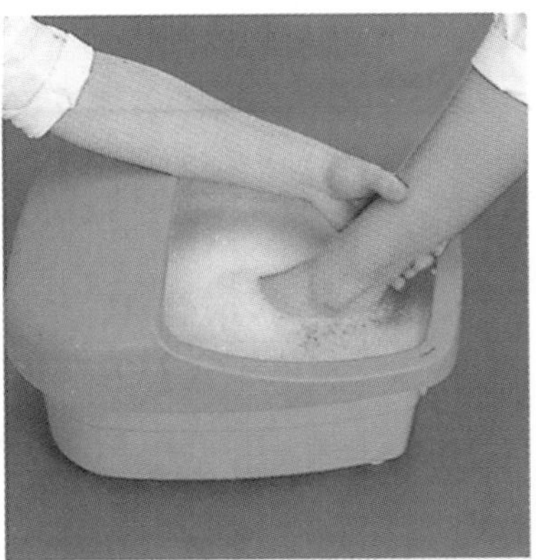

FIGURE 16.62 — Soak foot.

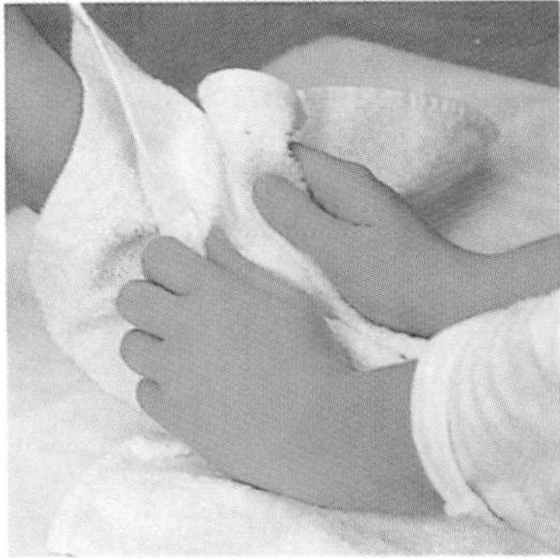

FIGURE 16.63 — Dry foot.

7. Place the right foot in the bath.
8. Loosen the cuticle gently on the left foot with a cotton-tipped orangewood stick. Keep the cuticle moist with additional lotion or water. Do not use excessive pressure. Avoid the use of the metal pusher.
9. Do not cut the cuticle. Only nip a large, ragged hangnail.
10. Rinse the left foot and dry. Massage each toe with cuticle cream or oil.
11. Repeat steps 5 to 10 on right foot.
12. Scrub both feet in warm, soapy water, rinse, and dry thoroughly.

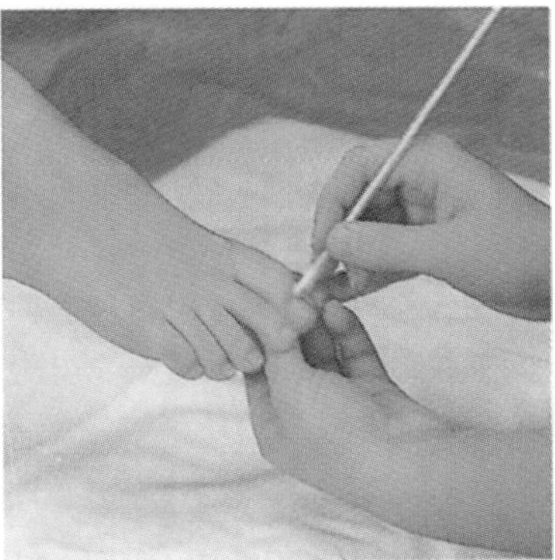

FIGURE 16.64 — Apply cuticle solvent.

FOOT MASSAGE

PROCEDURE

1. Apply lotion or cream over the foot to just above the ankle.
2. Start at the instep of the left foot and apply firm, rotary movements down to the center of the toes. (Fig. 16.65)
3. Slide the thumbs firmly back to the instep, and repeat same movement.
4. Slide the thumbs back to the hollow of the heel, and repeat same movement.
5. Slide the thumbs back to the base of the foot, and repeat same movement.

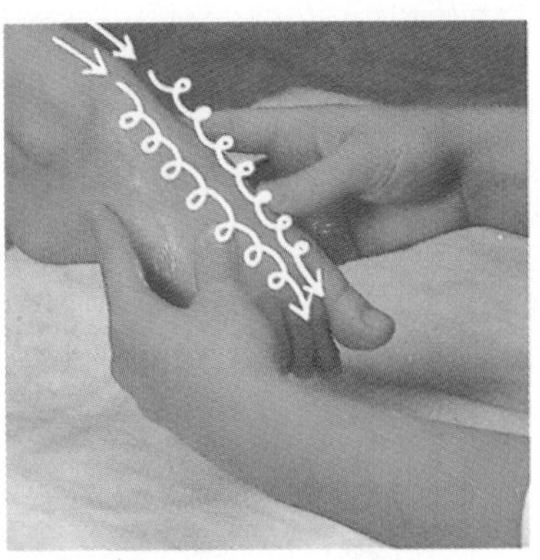

FIGURE 16.65 — Massage from instep to the center of the toes.

6. Start at the heel and work down to the center of the toes. (Fig. 16.66)
7. Slide firmly back to the heel, and repeat same movement up each side of the foot.
8. Hold one toe in one hand and the heel in the other hand, and apply three rotary movements; do the same with the other toes. (Fig. 16.67)
9. Slide the right hand to the ankle and the heel of your left hand to the ball of the foot, and apply six firm, rotary movements. (Fig. 16.68)
10. Repeat steps 2 to 9 with the right foot.

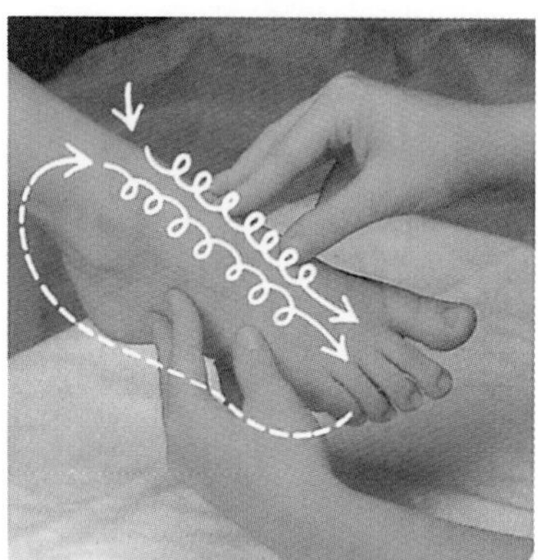

FIGURE 16.66 — Massage from heel down to the center of the toes.

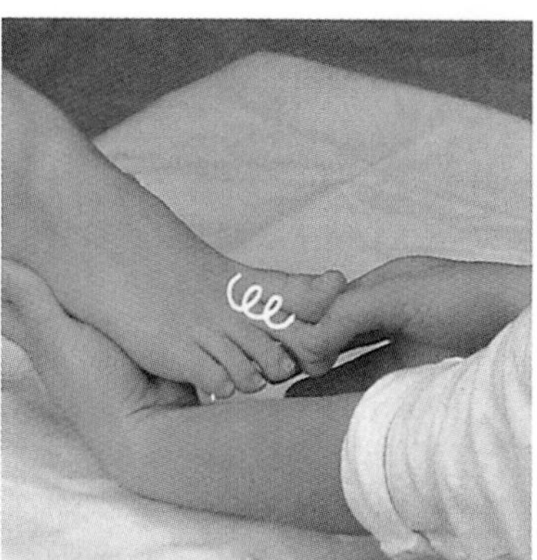

FIGURE 16.67 — Rotary movement of the toes.

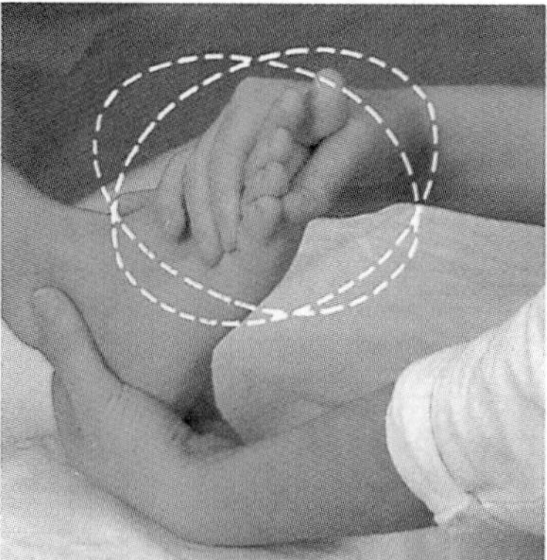

FIGURE 16.68 — Rotary movement of the foot.

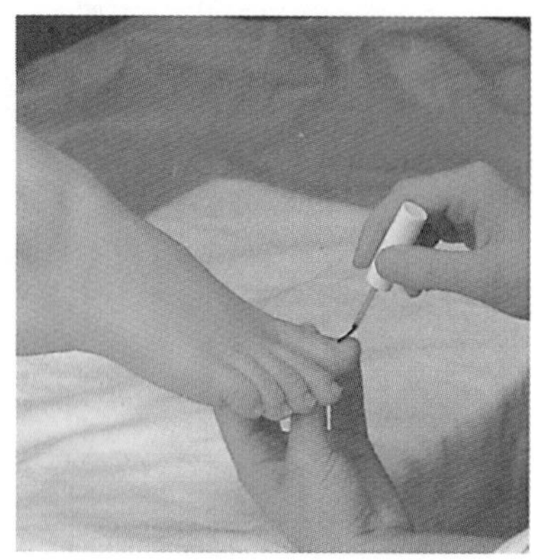

FIGURE 16.69 — Applying base coat.

COMPLETION

1. Remove lotion or cream from both feet with a warm towel.
2. Apply witch hazel or astringent to the feet with a large cotton pledget.
3. Dust lightly with talcum powder.
4. Wipe each toenail with polish remover to remove lotion or cream.
5. Apply a base coat, polish, and seal coat in the same manner as for a manicure. (Fig. 16.69)
6. Cleanup. Clean and sanitize implements, and place in dry sanitizer. Discard used materials. Wash your hands.

LEG MASSAGE

The foot massage may be extended up to and above the knee. When massaging from the ankle to the knee, do not massage over the shinbone and above the knee. It is advisable to keep the pressure to the muscular tissue on either side of the shinbone. On the calf area of the leg, you may use kneading upward movements up to the underpart of the knee.

Completed:
Learning Objective
#8
PEDICURING

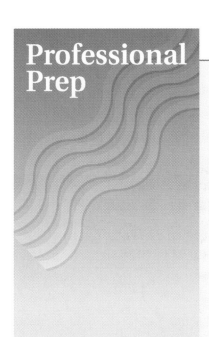

TELEPHONE TIPS

The way in which telephone calls are handled in a salon can affect the way your clients perceive you, especially if they are prospective clients. The telephone, when used properly, can be a powerful marketing tool, even in everyday transactions. Here are some hints on how to improve your telephone techniques:

- Keep your mouth empty; that means no candy, gum, food, or cigarettes.
- Smile or laugh just before answering the phone. When you are happy or smiling, your voice sounds more pleasant and energetic.
- Speak clearly and directly into the mouthpiece.
- Give your full attention to each caller; take notes to help you focus on what he or she is saying.
- Don't put callers on hold without asking first and waiting for an answer. Always give them a choice whether to hold or call back later. Never leave a caller on hold for more than two or three minutes.
- Avoid calling stylists to the phone when they are working on clients; instead take a message.
- Control your emotions. You must remain calm, even when a caller is upset or angry.
- Install an answering machine to take calls when the salon is closed.

—*From* Communication Skills for Cosmetologists
by Kathleen Ann Bergant

REVIEW QUESTIONS

MANICURING AND PEDICURING

1. What is the Latin word and definition for manicure?
2. What are the four general natural nail shapes?
3. What are some of the implements used in manicuring?
4. How do you file nails?
5. Why should a hand massage be included with a manicure?
6. List the different types of manicures.
7. List some of the advanced nail techniques available.
8. What is pedicuring and why is it an important client service?

CHAPTER 17

The Nail and Its Disorders

LEARNING OBJECTIVES

After completing this chapter, you should be able to:

1. Describe the structure and composition of nails.
2. Describe the structures adjoining and affecting nails.
3. Discuss how nails grow.
4. List the various disorders and irregularities of clients' nails.
5. Recognize diseases of the nails that should not be treated in the beauty salon.

NATIONAL SKILL STANDARDS

This chapter provides you with the necessary information to master this National Industry Skill Standard for Entry-Level Cosmetologists:

- Conducting services in a safe environment, taking measures to prevent the spread of infectious and contagious disease

INTRODUCTION

The *nail*, an appendage of the skin, is a horny, translucent plate that protects the tips of the fingers and toes. ***Onyx*** **(ON-iks)** is the technical term for the nail.

The condition of the nail, like that of the skin, reflects the general health of the body. The normal, healthy nail is firm and flexible and appears to be slightly pink in color. Its surface is smooth, curved, and unspotted, without any hollows or wavy ridges.

THE NAIL

The nail is composed mainly of ***keratin*** (**KER**-a-tin), a protein substance that forms the base of all horny tissue. The nail is whitish and translucent in appearance and allows the pinkish color of the nail bed to be seen. The horny nail plate contains no nerves or blood vessels.

NAIL STRUCTURE

The nails consist of three parts: nail body, nail root, and free edge. The ***nail body***, or ***plate***, is the visible portion of the nail that rests upon, and is attached to, the ***nail bed***. The nail body extends from the ***root*** to the ***free edge***.

Although the nail plate seems to be one piece, it is actually constructed in layers. This structure can be seen readily, in both length and thickness, when nails split.

The ***nail root*** is at the base of the nail and is embedded underneath the skin. It is attached to an actively growing tissue known as the ***matrix*** (**MAY**-triks).

The ***free edge*** is the end portion of the nail plate that reaches over the tip of finger or toe. (Figs. 17.1, 17.2)

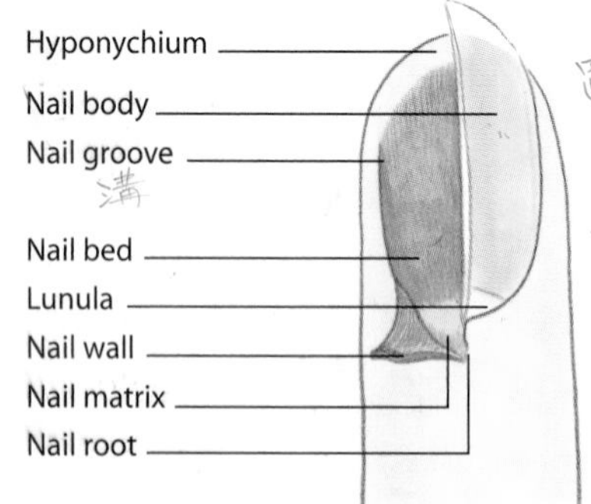

FIGURE 17.1 — Diagram of a nail.

Nail Bed

The ***nail bed*** is the portion of the skin upon which the nail body rests. It has many blood vessels that provide the nourishment necessary for the continued growth of the nail. The nail bed also is abundantly supplied with nerves. (Figs. 17.1, 17.2)

Matrix

The ***matrix*** is the part of the nail bed that extends beneath the nail root and contains nerves, lymph, and blood vessels to nourish the nail. The matrix produces cells that generate and harden the nail. The matrix will continue to grow as long as it receives nutrition and remains in a healthy condition.

Growth of the nails can be retarded if an individual is in poor health, if a nail disorder or disease is present, or if there is an injury to the nail matrix. (Figs. 17.1, 17.2)

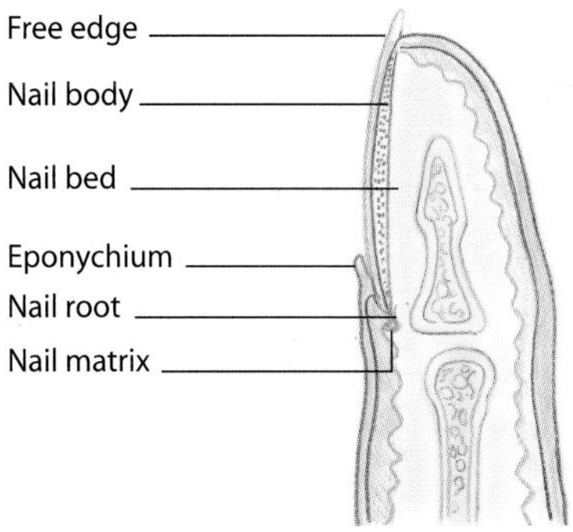

Free edge
Nail body
Nail bed
Eponychium
Nail root
Nail matrix

FIGURE 17.2 — Cross section of a nail.

LUNULA

The ***lunula*** (**LU**-noo-lah), or ***half-moon***, is located at the base of the nail. The light color of the lunula is caused by the reflection of light where the matrix and the connective tissue of the nail bed join. (Figs. 17.1, 17.2)

Completed: Learning Objective #1

NAIL STRUCTURE AND COMPOSITION

STRUCTURES SURROUNDING THE NAIL

The ***cuticle*** (**KYOO**-tih-kel) is the overlapping skin around the nail. A normal cuticle should be loose and pliable.

The ***eponychium*** (ep-oh-**NIK**-ee-um) is the extension of the cuticle at the base of the nail body that partly overlaps the lunula.

The ***hyponychium*** (heye-poh-**NIK**-ee-um) is that portion of the epidermis under the free edge of the nail.

The ***perionychium*** (**PER**-ee-oh-nik-ee-um) is that portion of the epidermis surrounding the entire nail border.

The ***nail walls*** are the folds of skin overlapping the sides of the nail.

The ***nail grooves*** are slits, or tracks, at either side of the nail upon which the nail moves as it grows.

The ***mantle*** (**MAN**-tel) is the deep fold of skin in which the nail root is embedded.

Completed: Learning Objective #2

STRUCTURES ADJOINING AND AFFECTING NAILS

NAIL GROWTH

The growth of the nail is influenced by nutrition, general health, and disease. A normal nail grows forward, starting at the matrix and extending over the tip of the finger. Normal, healthy nails can grow in a variety of shapes, according to the individual. (Fig. 17.3) The average rate of growth in the normal adult is about ⅛" (.3125 cm) per month. Nails grow faster in the summer than they do in the winter. Children's nails grow more rapidly, whereas those of

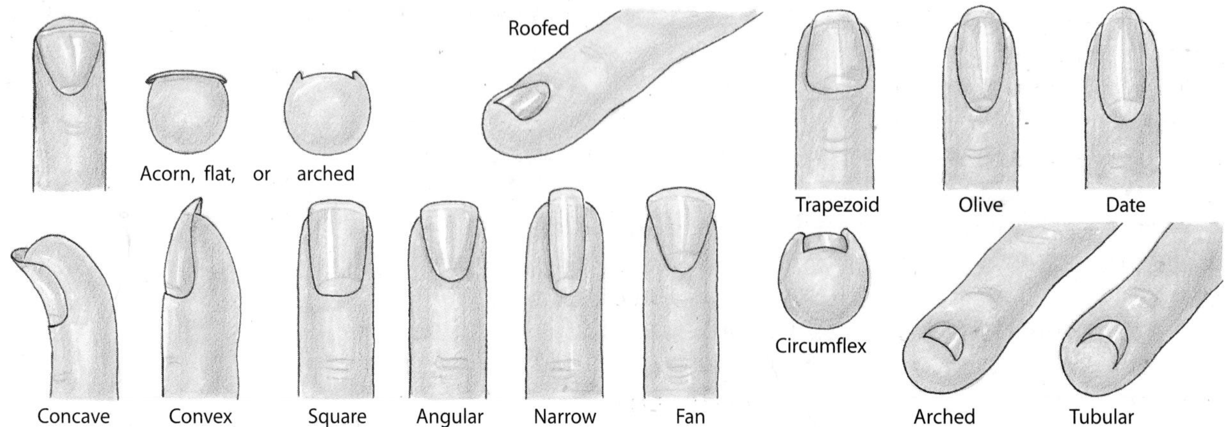

FIGURE 17.3 — Various shapes of nails.

Completed: Learning Objective #3
HOW NAILS GROW

elderly persons grow more slowly. The nail of the middle finger grows fastest and the thumbnail grows slowest. Although toenails grow more slowly than fingernails, they are thicker and harder.

NAIL MALFORMATION

If the nail is separated from the nail bed through injury, it becomes distorted or discolored. Should the nail bed be injured after the loss of a nail, the new nail will be badly formed.

Nails are shed neither automatically nor periodically, as is hair. They may be torn off accidentally or lost because of infection or disease. Nails lost under these conditions are frequently badly shaped when they grow back. This is due to interference at the base of the nail. A nail is replaced as long as the matrix remains in good condition. Ordinarily, replacement of the nail takes about four months.

NAIL DISORDERS

Diseases of the nail should never be treated by a nail technician. However, the technician should recognize normal and abnormal nail conditions, and understand the reasons for them. Simple nail irregularities and blemishes come within the province of cosmetology and can be treated by the technician. A client with an infection, soreness, or irritation should be referred to a physician.

NAIL IRREGULARITIES

Corrugations, or wavy ridges, are caused by uneven growth of the nails, usually the result of illness or injury. When manicuring a client with this condition, carefully buff the nails slightly with pumice powder. This helps to remove or minimize the ridges. Ridge filler used with colored polish can give a smooth look to the nail.

Furrows (depressions) in the nails can run either lengthwise or across the nail. (Fig. 17.4) These are usually the result of illness or an injury to the nail cells in or near the matrix. They can also be caused by pregnancy or stress. Since these nails are exceedingly fragile, great care must be exercised when giving a manicure. Avoid the use of the metal pusher; use a cotton-tipped orangewood stick around the cuticle.

Leuconychia (loo-koh-**NIK**-ee-ah), or white spots, appear frequently in the nails, but do not indicate disease. (Fig. 17.5) They can be caused by injury to the base of the nail. As the nail continues to grow, these white spots eventually disappear.

Onychauxis (on-ih-**KOK**-sis), or ***hypertrophy*** (heye-**PUR**-troh-fee), is an overgrowth of the nail, usually in thickness rather than length. (Fig. 17.6) It is usually caused by a local infection and can also be hereditary. If infection is present, the nail is not to be manicured. If infection is not present, the nail may be included in the manicure. File the nail smooth and buff with pumice powder.

Onychatrophia (on-ih-kah-**TROH**-fee-ah), atrophy, or wasting away, of the nail causes the nail to lose its luster, become smaller, and sometimes be shed entirely. (Fig. 17.7) Injury or disease might account for this nail irregularity. File the nail smooth with the fine side of the emery board. Advise the client to protect it from further injury or from exposure to strong soaps and washing powders.

Pterygium (te-**RIJ**-e-um) is a forward growth of the cuticle that adheres to the base of the nail. (Fig. 17.8) It can be caused by circulatory problems. Use the cuticle nippers carefully to remove the growth (if nipping is permitted by your state board). Suggest oil manicures.

Onychophagy (on-ih-**KOH**-fa-jee), or bitten nails, is a result of an acquired nervous habit that prompts the individual to chew the nail or the hardened cuticle. (Fig. 17.9) Advise the client that frequent manicures and care of the hardened cuticle often help to overcome this habit.

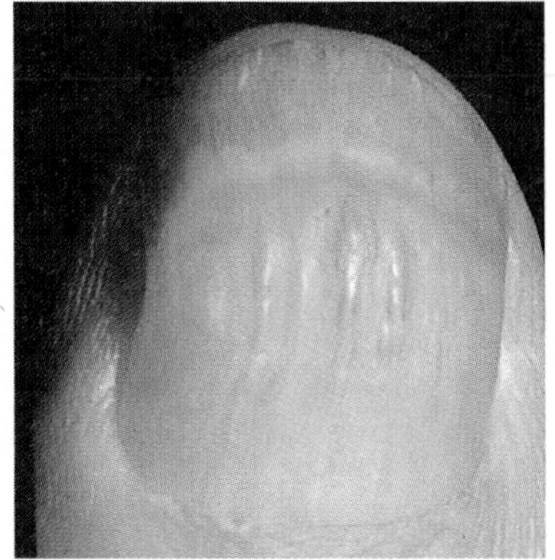

FIGURE 17.4 — Furrows.

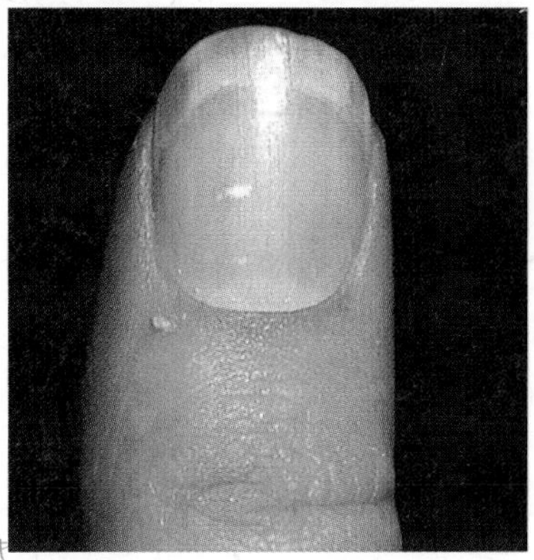

FIGURE 17.5 — Leuconychia.

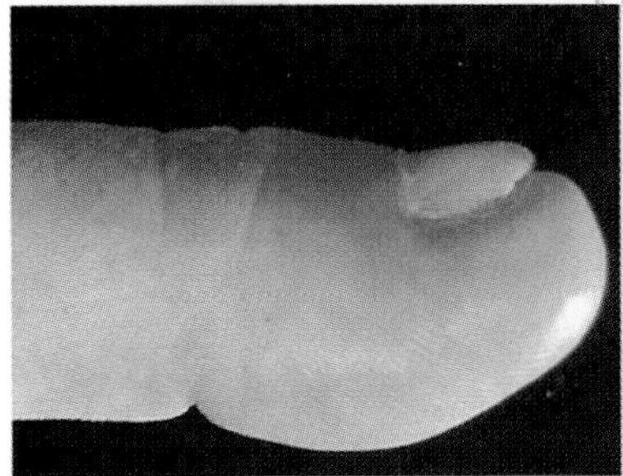

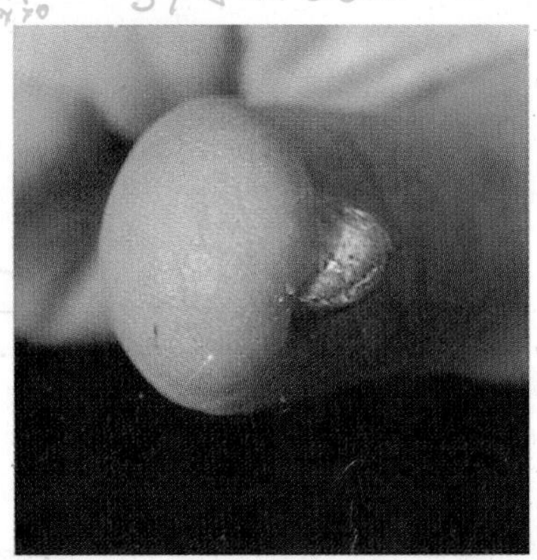

FIGURE 17.6 — Onychauxis or hypertrophy (above). Onychauxis end view (right).

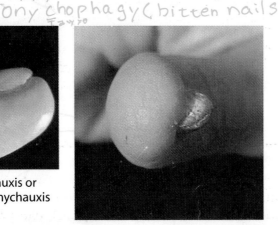

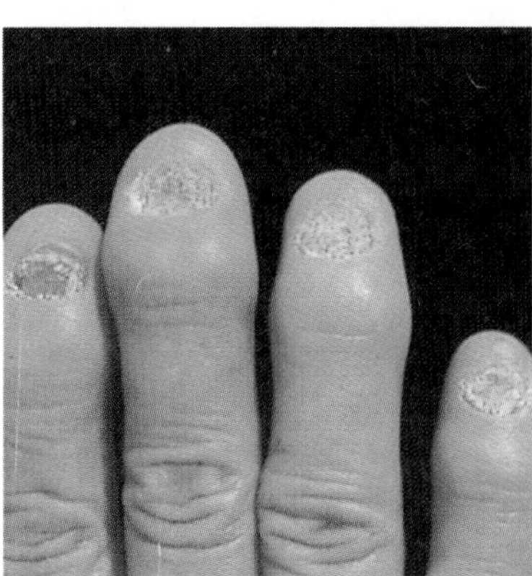

FIGURE 17.7 — Onychatrophia.

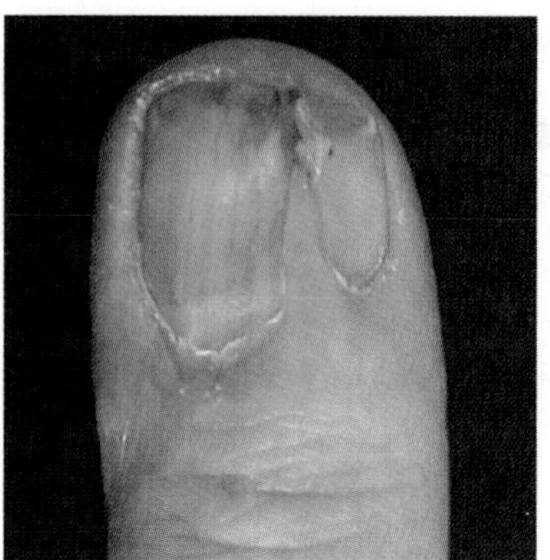
FIGURE 17.8 — Pterygium.

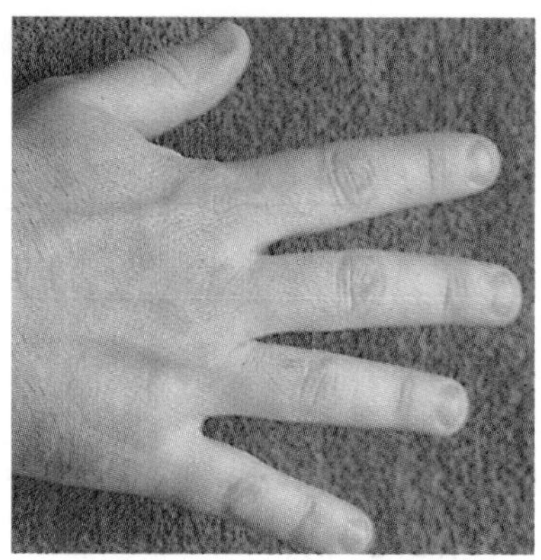
FIGURE 17.9 — Onychophagy.

Onychorrhexis (on-ih-koh-**REK**-sis) refers to split or brittle nails. (Fig. 17.10) Among the causes of split nails are injury to the finger, careless filing of the nails, vitamin deficiencies, illness, frequent exposure to strong soap and water, and excessive use of cuticle solvents and nail polish removers. Suggest oil manicures.

Hangnail (agnail) is a condition in which the cuticle splits around the nail. (Fig. 17.11) Dryness of the cuticle, cutting off too much cuticle, or carelessness in removing the cuticle can result in hangnails. Advise the client that proper nail care, such as hot oil manicures, will aid in correcting such a condition. If not properly cared for, a hangnail can become infected.

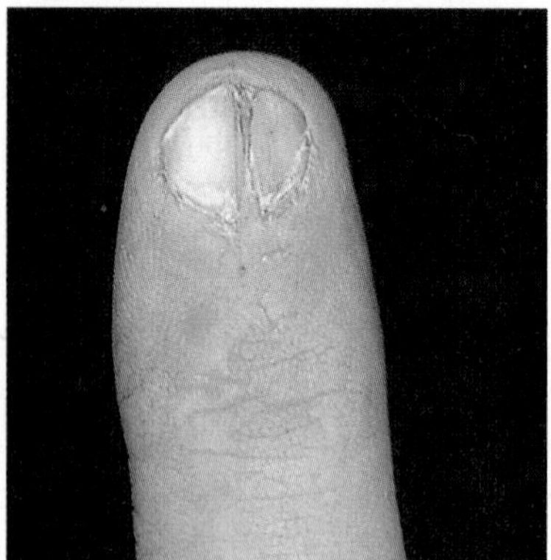
FIGURE 17.10 — Onychorrhexis.

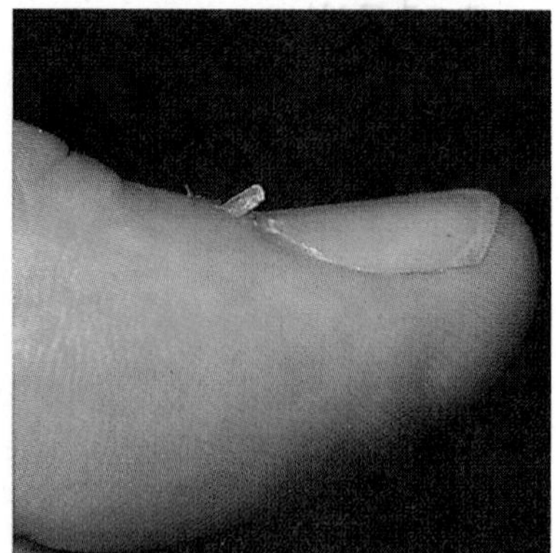
FIGURE 17.11 — Hangnail.

Eggshell nails are nails that have a noticeably thin, white nail plate and are more flexible than normal. (Fig. 17.12) The nail plate separates from the nail bed and curves at the free edge. This disorder can be caused by a chronic illness of systemic or nervous origin.

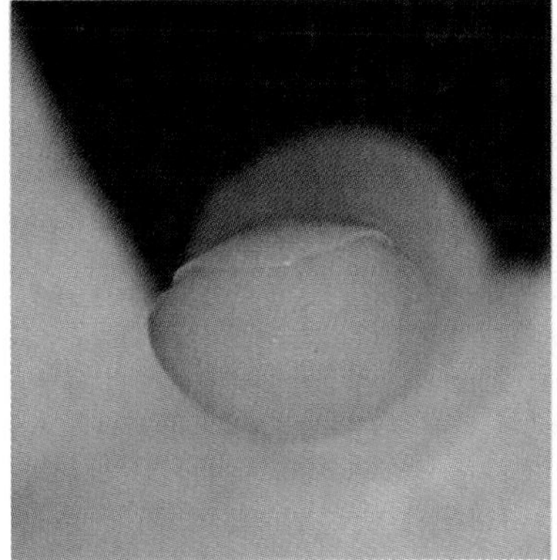
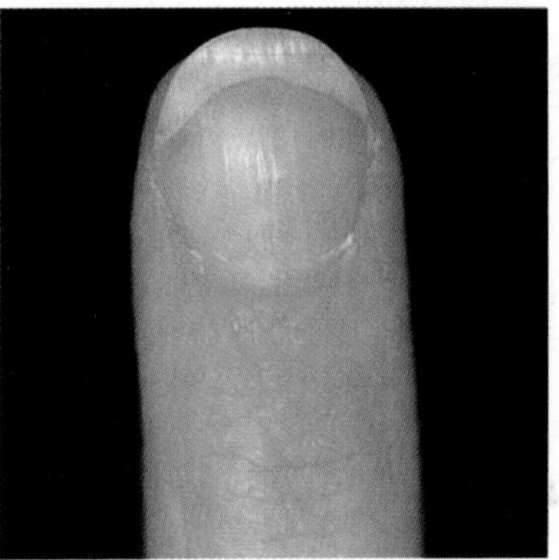

FIGURE 17.12 — Eggshell nail; end view (left), front view (right).

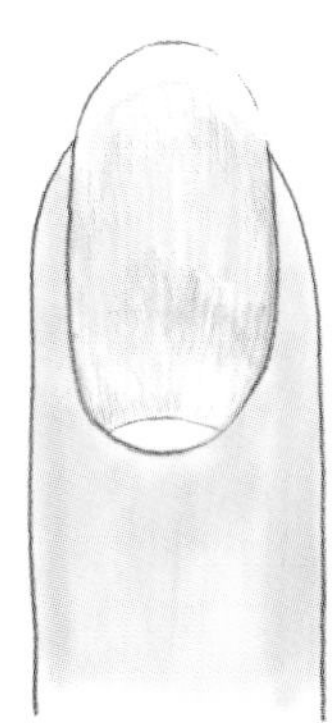

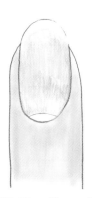

FIGURE 17.13 — Blue nail.

Blue nails can be caused by poor blood circulation or a heart disorder. (Fig. 17.13) However, a client with this condition may receive a regular manicure.

A ***bruised nail*** will have dark, purplish (almost black or brown) spots, usually due to injury and bleeding in the nail bed. The dried blood attaches itself to the nail and grows out with it. Treat this injured nail gently. Avoid pressure.

Treating cuts. If a client is accidentally cut during a manicure, apply an antiseptic immediately. Do not buff or apply nail polish to the injured finger. To protect against infection, apply a sterile bandage.

Infected finger. In the case of an infected finger, the client should be referred to a physician.

Completed:
Learning Objective
#4
NAIL DISORDERS AND IRREGULARITIES

FUNGUS AND MOLD

Fungi (FUN-geye) is the general term for vegetable ***parasites*** including all types of fungus and mold. The types of concern to the nail salon are nail fungus and nail mold. Both are contagious. They can spread from nail to nail on the client and from the client to the nail technician.

NAIL FUNGUS

Nail fungus usually appears as a discoloration in the nail that spreads toward the cuticle. (Fig. 17.14) As the condition matures, the discoloration becomes darker. Fungus may affect the hands, feet, and nails. Clients with nail fungus must be referred to a physician.

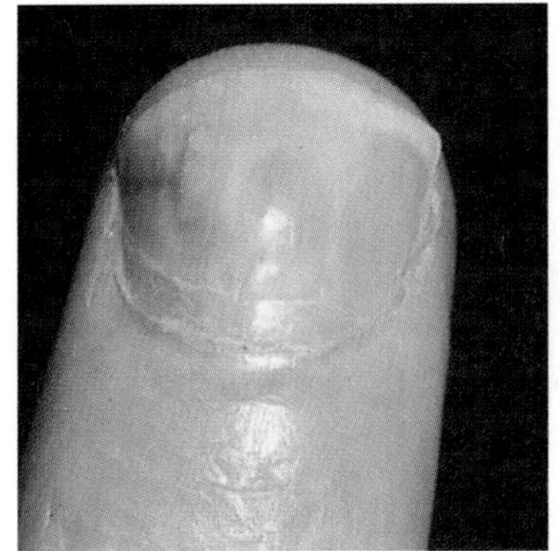

FIGURE 17.14 — Nail fungus (mold).

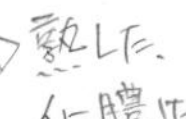

NAIL MOLD

Nail mold is a type of fungus infection caused when moisture is trapped between an unsanitized natural nail and products that are put over the natural nail, such as tips, wraps, gels, or acrylic nail products.

Nail mold can be identified in the early stages as a yellow-green spot that becomes darker in advanced stages. If the nail has been infected for a period of time, the discoloration becomes black and the nail softens and smells bad. If these conditions exist, the nail will probably fall off.

Exposing the Natural Nail

You should not provide nail services for a client who has nail fungus or nail mold, but the client may want you to remove any artificial nail covering to expose the natural nail. After the natural nail is exposed, the client should be referred to a physician.

You should wear gloves during removal of artificial nails and follow the manufacturer's directions for removal. When the artificial nail has been removed, discard orangewood sticks, abrasives, and any other porous product used. Completely sanitize all other implements, linen, and the table surface before and after the procedure.

Prevention

Nail mold and fungus may be avoided by following sanitary precautions. Do not perform nail services for a client who has discoloration on his or her nails. Do not take shortcuts or omit any of the sanitation steps when performing an artificial nail service.

NAIL DISEASES

There are several nail diseases that you may encounter. Any nail disease that shows signs of infection or inflammation (redness, pain, swelling, or pus) must not be treated in a beauty salon. Medical treatment is required for all nail diseases.

A person's occupation plays an important role in the cause of many nail infections. Infections develop more readily in people who regularly immerse their hands in alkaline solutions. Natural oils are removed from the skin by frequent exposure to soaps, solvents, and other substances. The cosmetologist's hands are exposed daily to chemical materials. Many of these are harmless, but some are potentially dangerous. A cosmetologist's hands and nails should be protected with gloves when working with chemicals.

Onychosis (on-ih-**KOH**-sis) is a technical term applied to nail disease.

Onychomycosis (on-ih-koh-meye-**KOH**-sis), ***tinea unguium*** (**TIN**-ee-ah **UN**-gwee-um), or ***ringworm*** of the nails is an infectious disease caused by a fungus (vegetable parasite). (Fig. 17.15) A common form is whitish patches that can be scraped off the surface. A second form is long, yellowish streaks within the nail substance. The disease invades the free edge and spreads toward the root. The infected portion is thick and discolored. In a third form, the deeper layers of the nail are invaded, causing the superficial layers to appear irregularly thin. These infected layers peel off and expose the diseased parts of the nail bed.

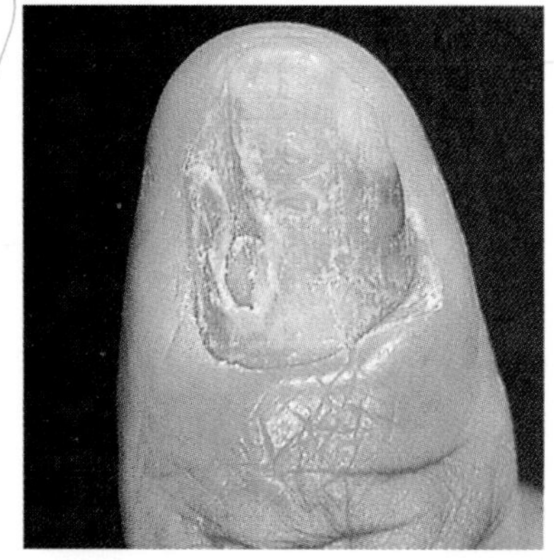

FIGURE 17.15 — Onychomycosis.

Ringworm (tinea) of the hands is a highly contagious disease caused by a fungus. (Fig. 17.16) The principal symptoms are red lesions occurring in patches or rings over the hands. Itching may be slight or severe.

Most cases of dermatitis of the hands resemble tinea but are actually a contact dermatitis, plus a staphylococcic infection. Only a physician can determine this condition.

Ringworm of the foot (athlete's foot) may also exits, and in acute conditions, deep, itchy, colorless ***vesicles*** (blisters) appear. (Fig. 17.17) These appear singly, in groups, and sometimes on only one foot. They spread over the sole and between the toes, perhaps involving the nail fold and infecting the nail. When the vesicles rupture, the skin becomes red and oozes. The lesions dry as they heal. Fungus infection of the feet is likely to become chronic.

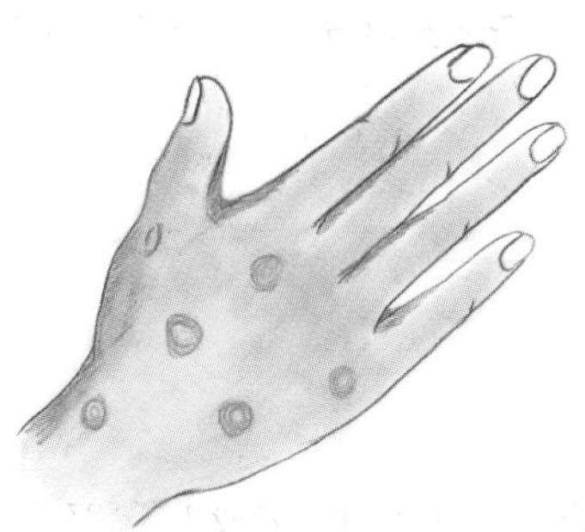

FIGURE 17.16 — Ringworm of the hand.

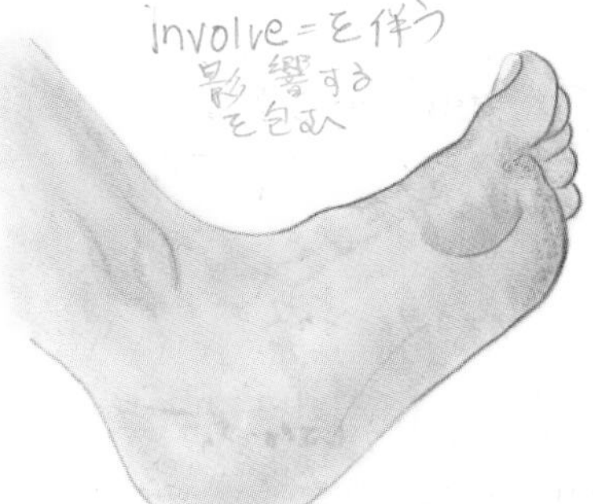

FIGURE 17.17 — Athlete's foot.

Prevention of infection and beneficial treatment are both accomplished by keeping the skin cool, dry, and clean.

Paronychia (par-oh-**NIK**-ee-ah), or ***felon*** (**FEL**-un), is an infectious and inflammatory condition of the tissues surrounding the nails. (Fig. 17.18) It is also characterized by gradual thickening and brownish discoloration of the nail plate. This condition can be traced to a bacterial infection.

Onychia (on-**NIK**-ee-ah) is an inflammation of the nail matrix, accompanied by pus formation. Improperly sanitized nail implements and bacterial infection can cause this disease.

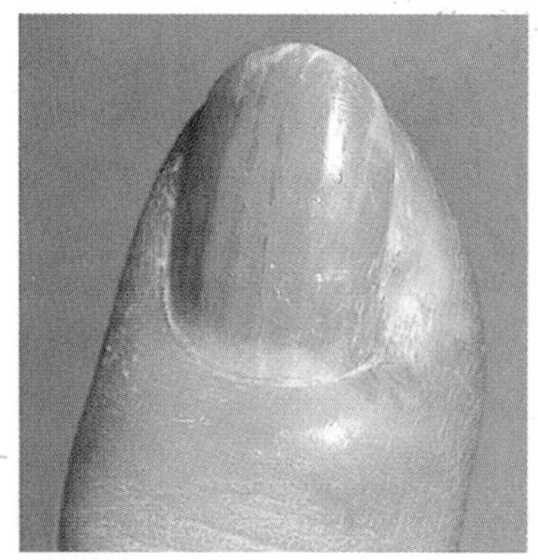

FIGURE 17.18 — Paronychia.

Onychocryptosis (on-ih-koh-krip-**TOH**-sis), or ***ingrown nails***, can affect either the finger or toe. (Fig. 17.19) In this condition, the nail grows into the sides of the flesh and can cause an infection. Filing the nails too much in the corners and failing to correct hangnails are often responsible for ingrown nails. Ill-fitting shoes can also cause ingrown nails.

Onychoptosis (on-ih-kop-**TOH**-sis) is the periodic shedding of one or more nails, either in whole or in part. (Fig. 17.20) This condition might follow certain diseases, such as syphilis.

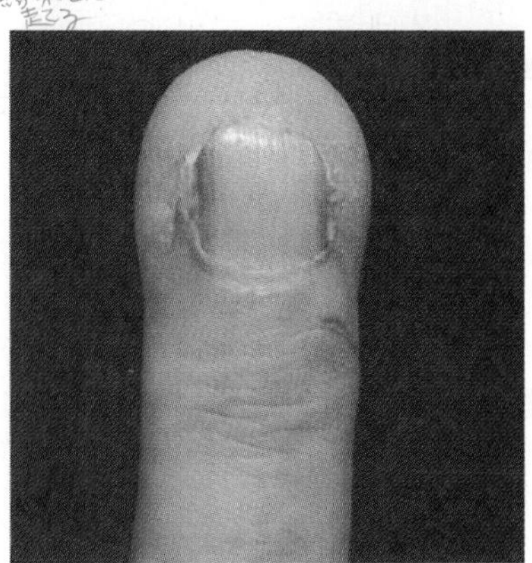

FIGURE 17.19 — Onychocryptosis.

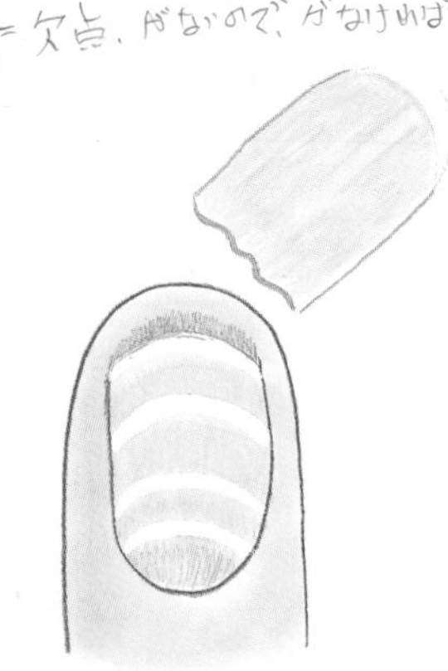

FIGURE 17.20 — Onychoptosis.

Onycholysis (on-ih-**KOL**-eye-sis) is a loosening of the nail, without shedding. (Fig. 17.21) It is frequently associated with an internal disorder.

Onychophyma (on-ih-koh-**FEE**-mah), more commonly referred to as onychauxis (see p. 457), denotes a swelling of the nail. (Fig. 17.22)

Onychophosis (on-ih-**KOH**-foh-sis) refers to a growth of horny epithelium in the nail bed. (Fig. 17.23)

Onychogryposis (on-ih-koh-greye-**POH**-sis), also known as ***onychogryphosis*** (on-ih-koh-greye-**FOH**-sis), pertains to enlarged and increased curvature of the nails. (Fig. 17.24)

Completed: Learning Objective #5

NAIL DISEASES NOT TO BE TREATED IN SALON

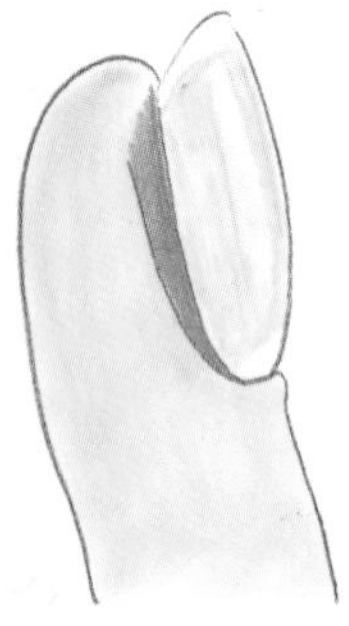

FIGURE 17.21 — Onycholysis.

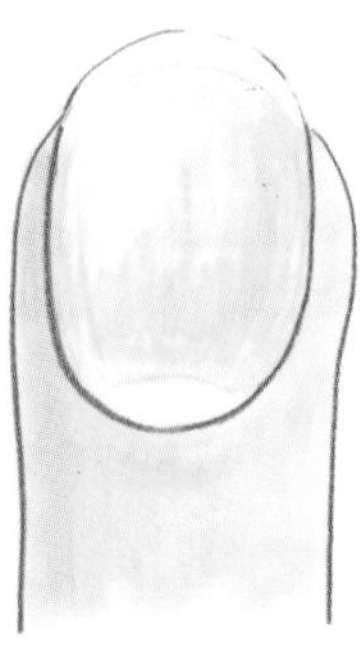

FIGURE 17.22 — Onychophyma.

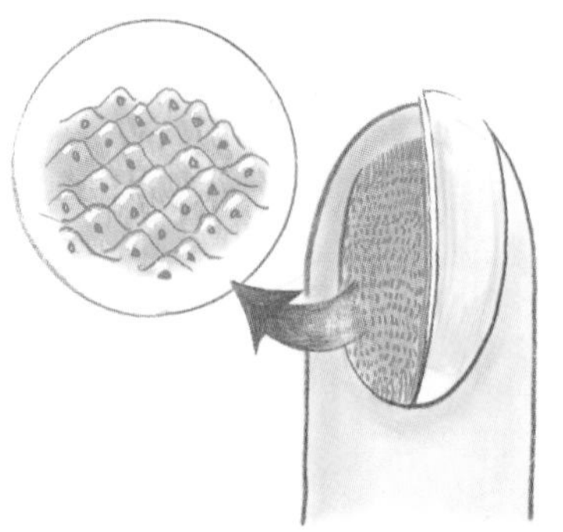

FIGURE 17.23 — Onychophosis.

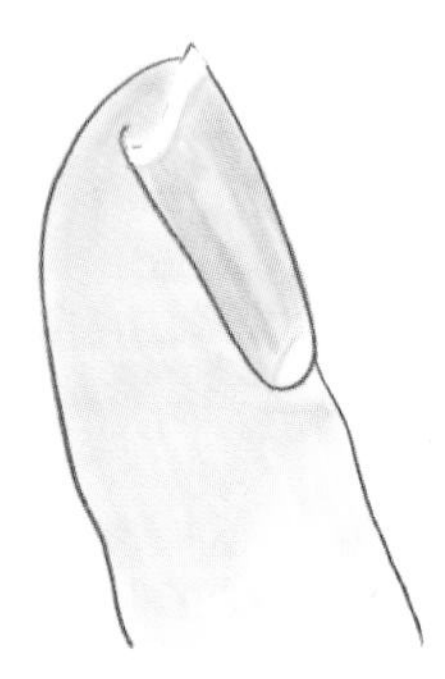

FIGURE 17.24 — Onychogryposis.

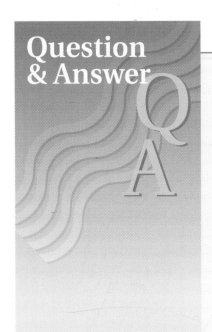

IS DISEASE A RISK IN NAIL SERVICES?

Since blood-transmitted diseases are such a concern for both clients and employees these days, why isn't it advisable for nail technicians to wear rubber gloves? If dentists' tools can contaminate, isn't there some danger in using metal tools in manicuring services?

There's no such thing as being too clean when it comes to the use of tools (instruments) used on more than one client. On the other hand, beyond using the prescribed methods for sanitation and sterilization, there is such a thing as having unwarranted fears and being overly cautious.

Many nail technicians have abandoned the use of sharp nippers to trim around the nail groove and cuticle. They have also replaced most metal cuticle pushers and other metal instruments with wood and plastic implements.

A good nail technician never draws blood by the careless use of instruments and abrasive buffers. The skin surrounding the nail plate is often thin and sensitive. It is far better to rely on softening creams and gels to remove dead skin than to use nippers of any kind.

The presence of rubber gloves, even the well-fitting surgical variety, would make the tedious task of nail care more difficult. The decision, of course, is yours. If it makes you and your clients feel better, why not do it? You'll be giving the message that you truly care about your clients' health.

One very high-profile nail technician suggests that you use a sterilizing system that is visible to your clients. Keep sterilizing solution on the manicuring table at all times. When your instruments are not in use, they should always be in that solution. The importance of cleanliness and safety precautions cannot be overestimated.

—*From* Milady's Salon Solutions *by Louise Cotter*

REVIEW QUESTIONS

THE NAIL AND ITS DISORDERS

1. Describe a normal healthy nail.
2. What is the technical term for nail?
3. What is the composition of a nail?
4. Describe the structure of the nail.
5. List the structures surrounding the nail.
6. What part of the nail contains the nerve and blood supply?
7. What are the diseases of the nails that should not be treated in the beauty salon?

CHAPTER 18

Theory of Massage

LEARNING OBJECTIVES

After completing this chapter, you should be able to:

1. Describe the purpose of massage.
2. Describe the manipulations used in massage and their benefits.
3. Identify the various types of massage movements and how they are applied.
4. Identify the motor nerve points of the face and neck.
5. List the physiological effects of massage.

NATIONAL SKILL STANDARDS

This chapter provides you with the necessary information to master this National Industry Skill Standard for Entry-Level Cosmetologists:

- Providing basic skin care services

INTRODUCTION

Completed: Learning Objective #1

THE PURPOSE OF MASSAGE

Massage is used to exercise facial muscles, maintain muscle tone, and stimulate circulation. Cosmetologists give massages to their clients to help them keep their skin healthy and muscles firm.

To master massage techniques, you must have a knowledge of anatomy and physiology, and considerable practice in performing the various movements.

Massage involves the application of external manipulations to the head and body. This is accomplished manually or with the use of electrical appliances, such as therapeutic lamps, high-frequency current, facial steamers, heating caps, scalp steamers, and vibrators.

Your services are limited to only certain areas of the body: scalp, face, neck, and shoulders; upper chest and back; hands and arms; and feet and lower legs.

To inspire confidence in a client it is important that you give a massage with a firm, sure touch. To do this, you must develop strong flexible hands, a quiet temperament, self-control, and the use of psychology.

Keep your hands soft by using creams, oils, and lotions. File and shape nails smooth so that you do not scratch the client's skin. Your wrists and fingers should be flexible, your palms firm, and warm.

Cream or oil should be applied to your hands to permit smoother and gentler hand movements and prevent drag or damage to the client's skin.

BASIC MANIPULATIONS USED IN MASSAGE

HOW MANIPULATIVE MOVEMENTS ARE ACCOMPLISHED

Every massage treatment combines one or more of the basic movements. Each manipulation is applied in a definite way for a particular purpose. It is used according to the client's condition and the desired results. The result of a massage treatment depends on the amount of pressure, the direction of movement, and the duration of each type of manipulation. Direction of movement is generally from the insertion of a muscle toward its origin. Massaging a muscle in the wrong direction (from its origin to its insertion) could result in loss of resiliency and the sagging of the skin and muscles.

The origin of a muscle is the fixed attachment of one end of that muscle to a bone or tissue.

The insertion is the attachment of the opposite end of the muscle to another muscle, or to a movable bone or joint.

Completed: Learning Objective

#2

THE ELEMENTS OF MASSAGE MANIPULATIONS

EFFLEURAGE

Effleurage (ef-**LOO**-rahzh) is a light, continuous stroking movement applied with the fingers (digital) and palms (palmar) in a slow and rhythmic manner. No pressure is used. The palms work over large surfaces, while the cushions of the fingertips work over small surfaces (around the eyes). Effleurage is frequently applied to the forehead, face, scalp, back, shoulders, neck, chest, arms, and hands for its soothing and relaxing effects.

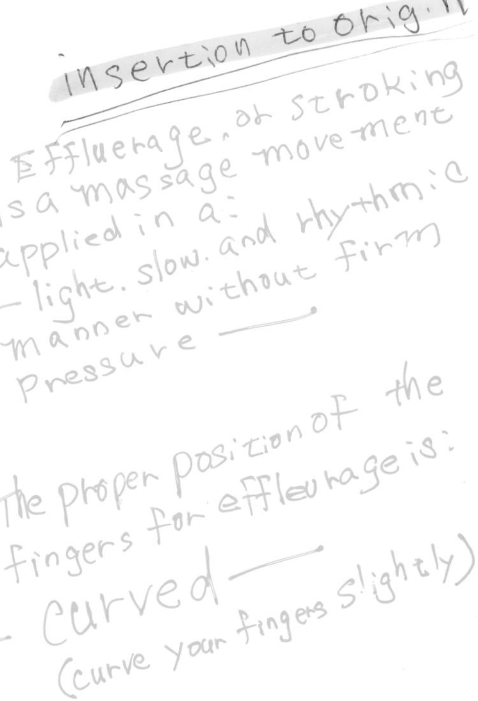

Position of Fingers for Stroking

Curve your fingers slightly, with just the cushions of the fingertips touching the skin. Do not use the ends of the fingertips for these massage movements. Since the tips of the fingers are pointier than the cushions, the effleurage will be less smooth, and the free edges of your fingernails are likely to scratch the client's skin. (Figs. 18.1 and 18.3)

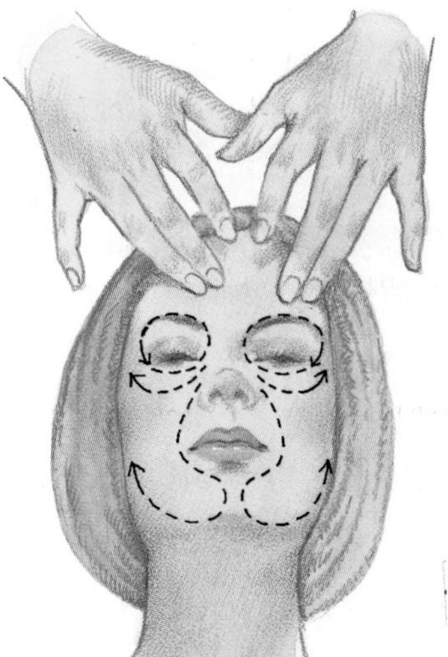

FIGURE 18.1 — Digital stroking of face.

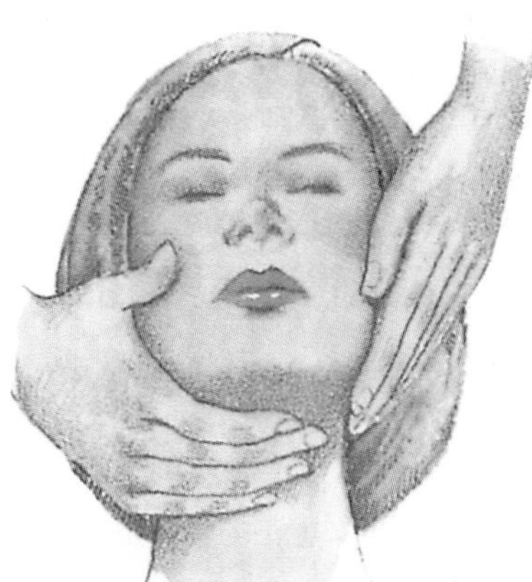

FIGURE 18.2 — Palmar stroking of face.

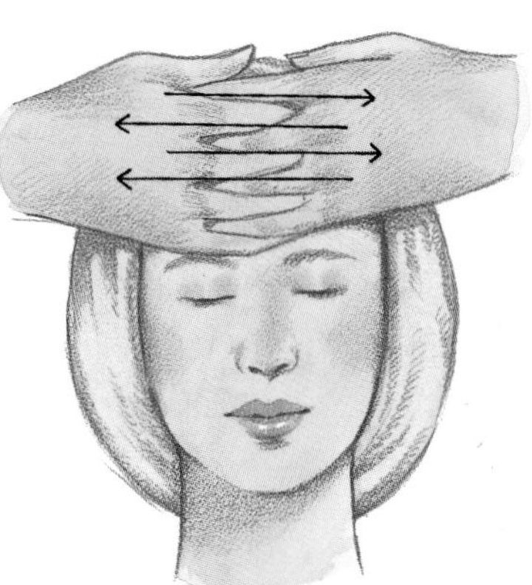

FIGURE 18.3 — Digital stroking of forehead.

Position of Palms for Stroking

Hold your whole hand loosely, keep your wrist and fingers flexible, and curve your fingers to conform to the shape of the area being massaged. (Fig. 18.2)

PETRISSAGE

Petrissage (**PAY**-tre-sahzh) is a kneading movement. Grasp the skin and underlying flesh between your fingers and palm of the hand. As you lift the tissues from their underlying structures, squeeze, roll, or pinch with a light, firm pressure. This movement invigorates the part being treated and is usually limited to back, shoulder, and arm massage.

Purpose of Kneading

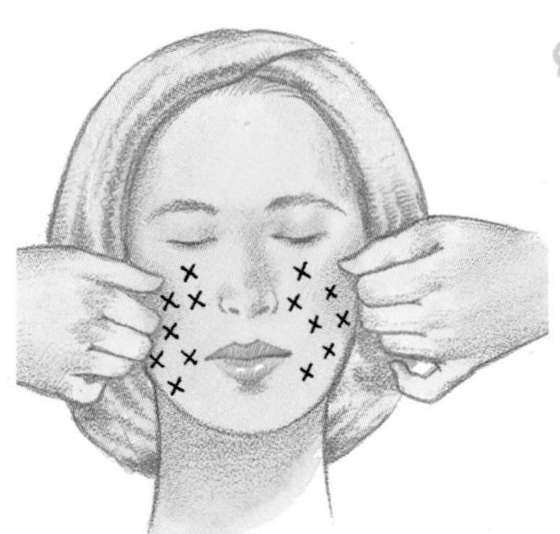

FIGURE 18.4 — Digital kneading of cheeks.

Kneading movements give deeper stimulation to the muscles, nerves, and skin glands, and improve the circulation. Digital kneading of the cheeks can be achieved by light pinching movements. (Fig. 18.4) The pressure should be light but firm. When grasping and releasing the fleshy parts, the movements must be rhythmic, never jerky.

Fulling

Fulling is a form of petrissage used mainly for massaging the arms. With the fingers of both hands grasping the arm, apply a kneading movement across the flesh. The kneading movement must be used with light pressure on the underside of the client's forearm, and between the shoulder and elbow.

FRICTION

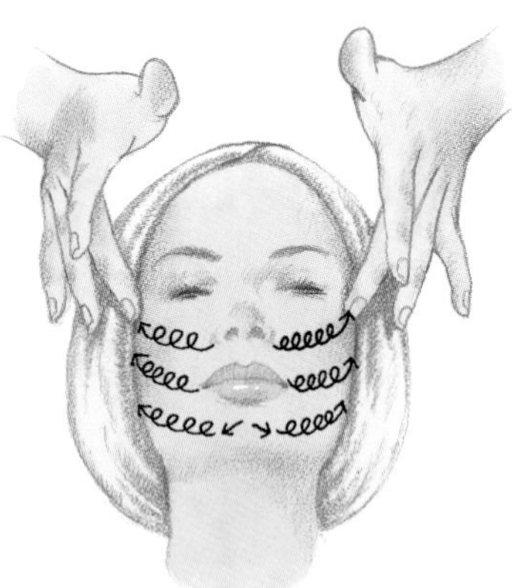

FIGURE 18.5 — Circular friction on face.

Friction (**FRIK**-shun) is a deep rubbing movement requiring pressure on the skin while moving it over the underlying structures. Use your fingers or palms. Friction has a marked influence on the circulation and glandular activity of the skin. Circular friction movements are usually used on the scalp, arms, and hands. Light circular friction movements are usually used on the face and neck. (Fig. 18.5) Chucking, rolling, and wringing are variations of friction and are used principally to massage the arms and legs.

The chucking movement is accomplished by grasping the flesh firmly in one hand and moving the hand up and down along the bone, while your other hand keeps the arm or leg in a steady position.

The rolling movement requires that the tissues be compressed firmly against the bone and twisted around the arm or leg. Both of your hands are active as you twist the flesh down the arm in the same direction.

Wringing is a vigorous movement in which your hands are placed a little distance apart on both sides of the client's arm or leg. While working your hands downward, apply a twisting motion against the bones in the opposite direction. (Fig. 18.6)

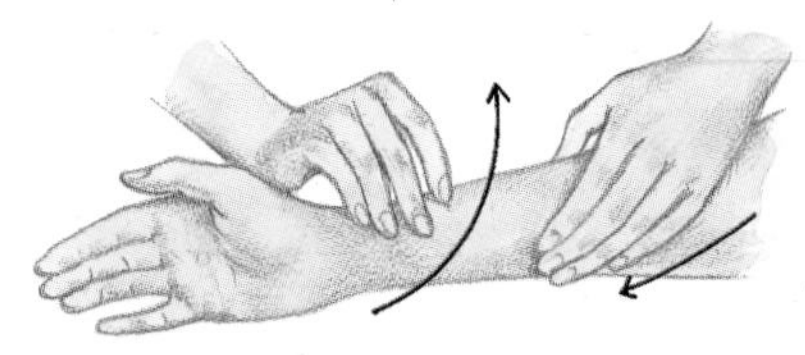

FIGURE 18.6 — Wringing movement of arm.

PERCUSSION OR TAPOTEMENT MOVEMENT

Percussion (per-**KUSH**-un), or ***tapotement*** (tah-**POHT**-mant), consists of tapping, slapping, and hacking movements. This form of massage is the most stimulating. It should be applied with care and discretion.

In facial massage, use only light digital tapping. In tapping, bring the fingertips down against the skin in rapid succession. Your fingers must be flexible, to create an even force over the area being massaged. (Fig. 18.7)

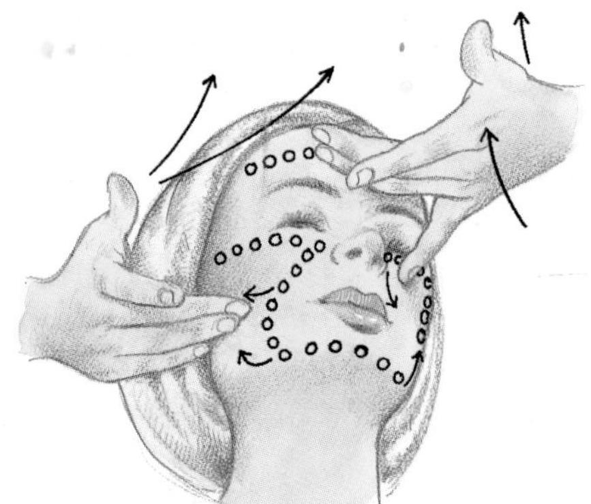

FIGURE 18.7 — Digital tapping on face.

In slapping movements, flexible wrists permit your palms to come in contact with the skin in light, firm, and rapid slapping movements. One hand follows the other. With each slapping stroke (which must be nothing more than a firm, light, and quick contact with the skin) lift the flesh slightly.

For hacking movements, use the wrists and outer edges of the hands. Both the wrists and fingers must move in fast, light, firm, flexible motions against the skin in alternate succession. Hacking and slapping movements are used mainly to massage the back, shoulders, and arms.

Percussion movements tone the muscles and impart a healthy glow to the part being massaged.

VIBRATION

Vibration (veye-**BRAY**-shun) is a shaking movement accomplished by rapid muscular contractions in your arms, while the balls of the fingertips are pressed firmly on the point of application. It is a highly stimulating movement, and should be limited to only a few seconds duration on any one spot. Muscular contractions also can be produced by the use of a mechanical vibrator. (Fig. 18.8)

Completed:
Learning Objective
#3
TYPES OF MASSAGE MOVEMENTS

JOINT MOVEMENTS

Joint movements are restricted to the massage of the arm, hand, and foot. These movements are applied either with or without resistance. (Fig. 18.9) (For information on joint movements, see the chapter on manicuring.)

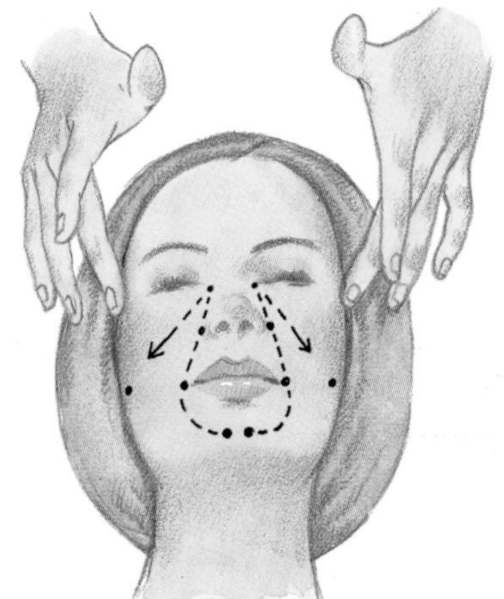

FIGURE 18.8 — Vibratory movement of face.

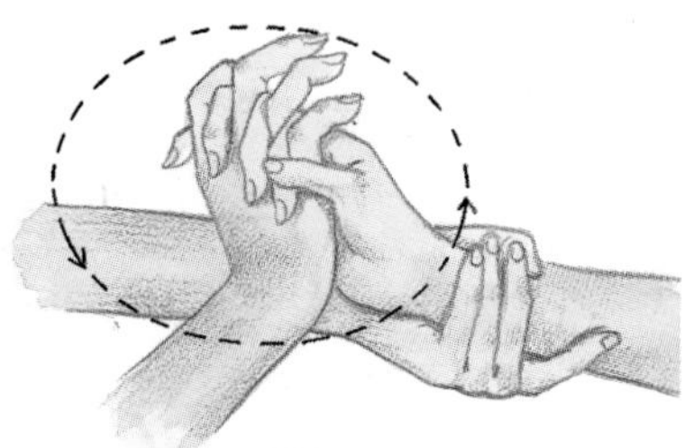

FIGURE 18.9 — Joint movement.

> **CAUTION**
>
> *Do not massage if client has high blood pressure, heart condition, or has had a stroke. Massage increases circulation and may be harmful to this client. Have client consult a physician first. Be very careful to avoid vigorous massage of joints if your client has arthritis. Talk with your client throughout the massage and adjust your touch to the client's needs.*

PHYSIOLOGICAL EFFECTS OF MASSAGE

To obtain proper results from a scalp or facial massage, you must have a thorough knowledge of all the structures involved: muscles, nerves, and blood vessels. Every muscle and nerve has a ***motor point***. Some examples are illustrated here. (Figs. 18.10, 18.11) In order to obtain the maximum benefits from a facial massage you must consider the motor nerve points that affect

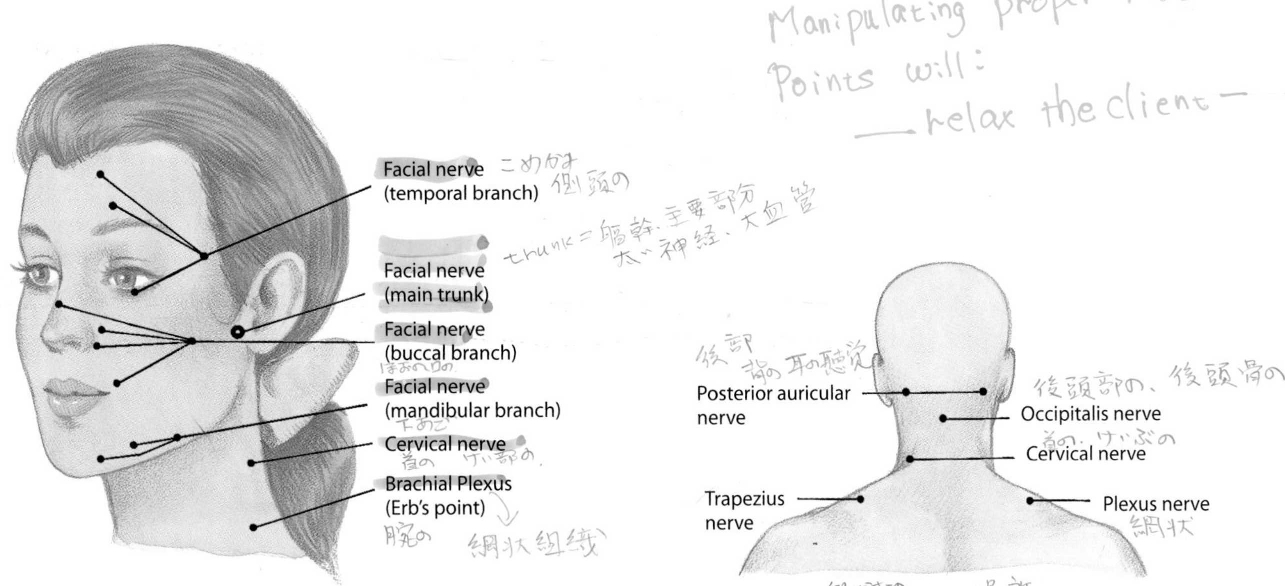

FIGURE 18.10 — Motor nerve points of the face.

FIGURE 18.11 — Motor nerve points of the neck.

the underlying muscles of the face and neck. The location of motor points varies among individuals due to differences in body structures. However, a few manipulations on the proper motor points will relax the client early in the massage treatment.

Completed:
Learning Objective
#4
MOTOR NERVE POINTS

Skillfully applied massage directly or indirectly influences the structures and functions of the body. The immediate effects of massage are first noticed on the skin. The part being massaged responds by increased circulation, secretion, nutrition, and excretion. The following beneficial results may be obtained by proper facial and scalp massage:

1. The skin and all its structures are nourished.
2. The skin is rendered soft and pliable.
3. The circulation of the blood is increased.
4. The activity of the skin glands is stimulated.
5. The muscle fiber is stimulated and strengthened.
6. The nerves are soothed and rested.
7. Pain is sometimes relieved.

Relaxation is achieved through light but firm, slow rhythmic movements, or very slow, light hand vibrations over the motor points for a short time. Another technique is to pause briefly over the motor points, using light pressure.

Body tissues are stimulated by movements of moderate pressure, speed, and time, or by light hand vibrations of moderate speed and time.

Body contours or fatty tissues are reduced by firm kneading, or by fast, firm, and light slapping movements over a fairly long period of time. Moderately fast hand vibrations with firm pressure also will accomplish this reduction.

Completed: Learning Objective #5 PHYSIOLOGICAL EFFECTS OF MASSAGE

The frequency of facial or scalp massage depends on the condition of the skin or scalp, the age of the client, and the condition to be treated. As a general rule, normal skin or scalp can be kept in excellent condition with the help of a weekly massage, accompanied by proper home care.

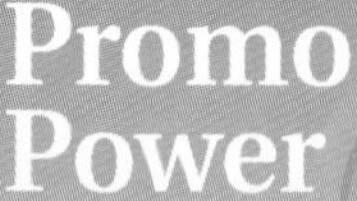

THE IN-SALON NEWSLETTER

You can keep your clients informed about and interested in your salon through regular newsletters. It's a great way to let them know important information as well as promote your stylists, your products, and your services. It can be as simple or elaborate as you want, but it should be attractive and interesting.

You don't want to get bogged down in too much publication, so it's good to release a newsletter twice a year or seasonally. One person should be placed in charge of collecting all the information you want to publish: special shows, charity events, awards, contests, promotions, etc. You may also want to include tips on the latest styles and fashions. You'll also need a staff member who can put the information in brief newsletter form. Decide on your format and logo, and get estimates on printing.

Here are some suggestions to get you started:

Topics, in addition to what's happening in your salon and news about current and upcoming specials and promotions, can include profiles or news on individual stylists, tips on hair care or makeup, healthful recipes, makeovers on some of your clients (including "before" and "after" photographs), or news about some of your regular clients.

Place coupons for products or services in the newsletter; this gives you feedback on who is reading it. Keep your articles short and to the point, and use photos and other art. Be sure to include the salon's name, address, and telephone number. If you plan to mail out the newsletter, leave one side blank for address labels.

Be sure to give yourself and your writer enough time. For example, a fall-winter release must be started in June or July to have time for collection of information, writing, layout, printing, and mailing.

—*From* The Salon Biz: Tips for Success *by Geri Mataya*

REVIEW QUESTIONS

THEORY OF MASSAGE

1. Describe the purpose of massage.
2. What is meant by massage?
3. Describe the origin of a muscle.
4. Describe the insertion of a muscle.
5. In which direction should a muscle be massaged?
6. What are some beneficial results of a proper facial and scalp massage?
7. Name the five types of massage manipulations.

21月

13、14、15、16、17、18

CHAPTER 19

Facials

LEARNING OBJECTIVES

After completing this chapter, you should be able to:

1. Describe the beneficial effects of a facial.
2. List the materials and equipment required for facial treatments.
3. Demonstrate basic procedure for a facial.
4. Demonstrate the required or optional manipulations for a facial.
5. Identify the various types of corrective facials given in the beauty salon.
6. Describe packs and masks and their possible ingredients.
7. Describe materials and procedures for various facial masks.
8. Identify reasons a client might find fault with a facial treatment.

NATIONAL SKILL STANDARDS

This chapter provides you with the necessary information to master these National Industry Skill Standards for Entry-Level Cosmetologists:

- Conducting services in a safe environment, taking measures to prevent the spread of infectious and contagious disease
- Providing basic skin care services

INTRODUCTION

A professional facial is one of the most enjoyable and relaxing services available to the salon client. Those individuals who have engaged in this very restful or stimulating experience do not hesitate to return for repeat facials. When taken regularly, facials result in very noticeable improvement in the client's skin tone, texture, and appearance.

FACIAL TREATMENTS

The cosmetologist does not treat skin diseases. However, you must be able to recognize the various skin ailments and you must also know when to advise the client to see a physician for treatment.

Facial treatments fall under two categories:

1. ***Preservative***—maintaining the health of the facial skin by using correct cleansing methods, increasing circulation, relaxing the nerves, and activating the skin glands and metabolism through massage.
2. ***Corrective***—correcting some facial skin conditions, such as dryness, oiliness, blackheads, aging lines, and minor conditions of acne.

Facial treatments are beneficial for:

1. Cleansing the skin.
2. Increasing circulation.
3. Activating glandular activity.
4. Relaxing the nerves.

5. Maintaining muscle tone.
6. Strengthening weak muscle tissue.
7. Correcting certain skin disorders.
8. Helping prevent the formation of wrinkles and aging lines.
9. Softening and improving skin texture and complexion.
10. Adding to the client's confidence.

Completed:
Learning Objective
#1
BENEFICIAL EFFECTS OF A FACIAL

FACIAL MASSAGE

PREPARATION FOR FACIAL MASSAGE

1. Help the client to relax by speaking in a quiet and professional manner. Explain the benefits of the products and service, and answer any questions the client may have.
2. Provide a quiet atmosphere; work quietly and efficiently.
3. Maintain neat, clean, sanitary conditions in the facial work area and an orderly arrangement of supplies.
4. For sanitary reasons you should never remove products from their containers with your fingers. Always use a ***spatula.*** Obtain and arrange in an orderly manner all the items you will be using for the facial *before* the client arrives.
5. Follow systematic procedures.
6. If your hands are cold, warm them before touching the client's face.
7. Keep your nails smooth so as not to scratch the client's skin.

EQUIPMENT, IMPLEMENTS, AND MATERIALS

The following is a basic list of items you will need to give a facial to a client. You can add other items that are beneficial to the client. (Also see chapter on electricity and light therapy for an explanation of light and electrical equipment used in facials.)

Cleansing cream/lotion
Moisturizer and protective lotion
Mask
Gauze (for mask)
Astringent
Freshening lotion (mild astringent)
Antiseptic lotion
Lubricating oil
Tissue strips
Headband or head covering
Towels
Clean sheet or other covering
Salon gown
Safety and bobby pins
Spatulas

Completed: Learning Objective #2

LIST OF FACIAL MATERIALS AND EQUIPMENT

Cleansing tissues
Absorbent cotton
Cotton swabs and pledgets
Cotton pads
Sponges
Facial steamer
Makeup tray
High-frequency machine
Infrared lamp
Magnifying lamp

PROCEDURE

The information given here may be changed to conform with your instructor's routine.

1. Prepare the client.
   a) Greet the client and say something complimentary. This puts the client at ease.
   b) Ask the client to remove any jewelry (such as necklace and earrings) and store it in a safe place. Clients might want to keep their handbags nearby during the facial.
   c) Show the client to the dressing room and offer assistance if needed.
   d) Place a clean towel across the back of the facial chair to prevent the client's bare shoulders from coming in contact with the chair.
   e) Seat the client in the facial chair (offer assistance, if needed). Then place a towel across the client's chest. Next, place the coverlet (or sheet) over the client's body and fold the top edge of the towel over the coverlet. Remove the client's shoes and tuck the coverlet around the feet. Some salons provide booties for the feet. These are worn to and from the dressing room.
   f) Fasten a headband lined with tissue, a towel, or other head covering around the client's head to protect the hair. There are several types of head coverings on the market. Some types are of a turban design; others are designed with elastic, similar to a shower cap. They are generally made of either cloth or paper towels. Draping the head with a towel is done in the following manner (for paper towel procedure, be guided by your instructor):
      1. Fold the towel lengthwise from one of the top corners to the opposite lower corner, and place it over the headrest with the fold facing down. Place the towel on the headrest before the client enters the facial area. When the client is in a reclined position, the back of the head should rest on the towel, so that one side of the towel can be brought up to the center of the forehead to cover the hairline. (Fig. 19.1)

2. With the other hand, bring the other side of the towel over the center and cross it over. (Fig. 19.2)

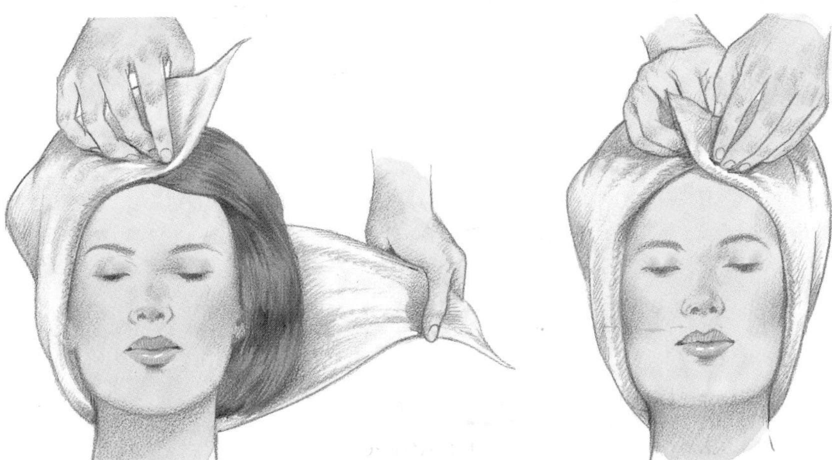

FIGURE 19.1 — Place towel around client's head.

FIGURE 19.2 — Join towel at center of client's head.

3. Use a regular bobby pin to hold the towel in place. Check to be sure that all strands of hair are tucked under the towel, earlobes are not bent, and the towel is not wrapped too tightly. (Fig. 19.3)

g) Remove lingerie straps from the client's shoulders. (*Alternate method:* If client is given a strapless gown to wear, tuck the shoulder lingerie straps into the top of the gown.)

h) Adjust the headrest, then lower the facial chair to a reclining position. (Fig. 19.4)

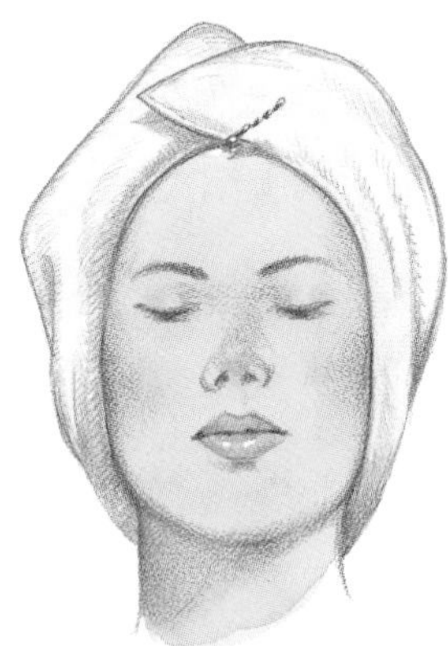

FIGURE 19.3 — Secure towel with a bobby pin.

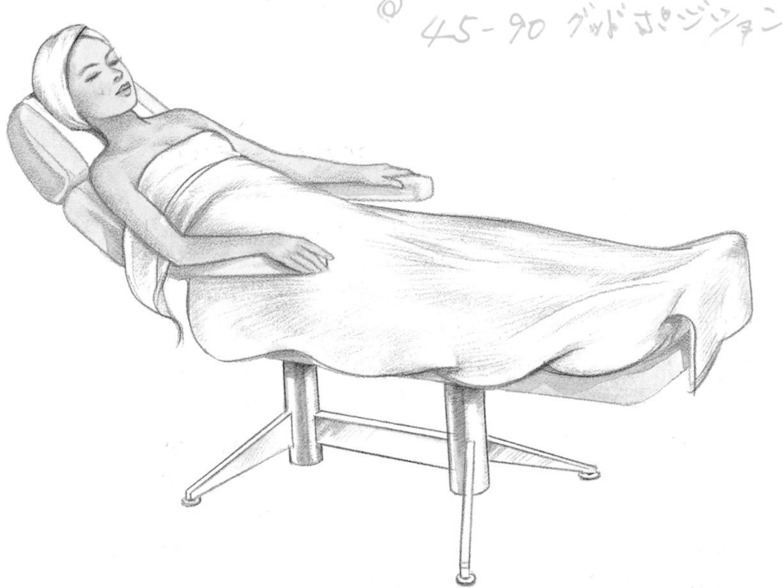

FIGURE 19.4 — Client is prepared for facial.

i) Wash your hands.

2. Analyze the client's skin.

a) Remove makeup to determine:

1. If the skin is dry, normal, or oily.
2. If fine lines or creases exist.
3. If blackheads (***comedones***) or acne are present.
4. If broken capillaries are visible.
5. If the skin texture is smooth or rough.
6. If the skin's color is even.

b) This analysis will determine:

1. The choice of products to use for the massage.
2. The areas of the face that need special attention.
3. The amount of pressure to use when giving the massage.
4. If lubricating oil or cream is needed around the eyes.
5. Equipment or apparatus to use.

3. Apply cleansing cream.

a) Remove about a teaspoon of cleansing cream or lotion from the container with a spatula. Blend the cream or lotion with your fingers to soften it. If the client is wearing heavy eye and lip makeup, use a small amount of cleanser and moist cotton pads or soft tissue to remove the excess makeup. Be very gentle when working around the eyes and on the mouth.

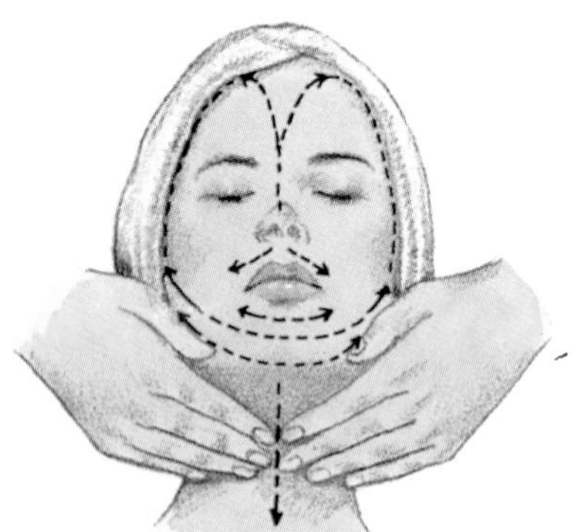

FIGURE 19.5 — Spreading cream over the face and neck.

b) Starting at the neck, use both hands in a sweeping movement to spread the cleansing product upward on the chin, jaws, cheeks, base of nose to temples, and along the sides and the bridge of the nose. (Fig. 19.5) Make small circular movements with your fingertips around the nostrils and sides of the nose. Continue the upward sweeping movements between the brows and across the forehead to the temples.

c) Take additional cleansing cream or lotion from the container with a spatula and blend. Smooth down the neck, chest, and back with long, even strokes.

d) Starting at the center of the forehead, move your fingertips in a circle lightly around the eyes to the temples and back to the center of the forehead.

e) Slide your fingers down the nose to the upper lip, to the temples and forehead, lightly down to the chin, then firmly up the jawline to the temples and forehead.

4. Remove the cleansing cream.

a) Remove the cleansing cream or lotion with tissues; warm, moist towels; moist cotton pads; or facial sponges. Start at the forehead and follow the contours of the face. Remove all the cream from one area of the face before proceeding to the next. Finish with the neck, chest, and back. (Fig. 19.6) (If eyebrows are to be arched, they should be done at this time.)

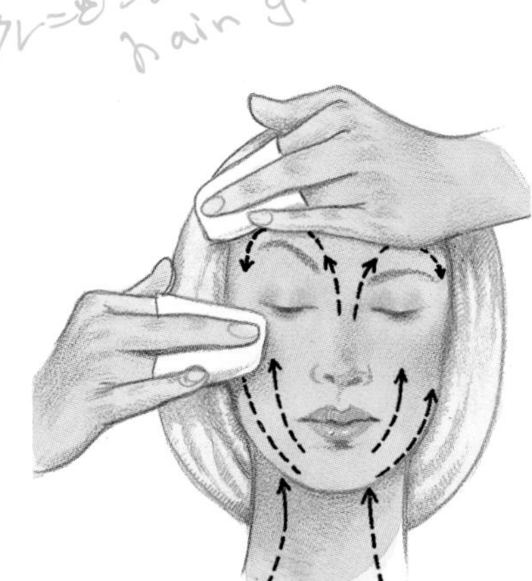

FIGURE 19.6 — Removing cleansing cream with tissues or with a warm, moist towel.

5. Steam the face (optional).

a) Steam the face mildly with warm, moist towels or with a facial steamer to open the pores so they can be cleansed of oil, blackheads, makeup, and other debris. Steam also helps to soften superficial lines and increases blood circulation to the surface of the skin.

6. Apply massage cream.

a) Select a massage cream for the client's skin type. Using the same procedure employed to apply cleansing cream, apply massage cream to face, neck, shoulders, chest, and back.

b) If needed, apply lubrication oil or cream around the eyes and on the neck.

7. Give facial manipulations.

a) Cover the client's eyes with cotton pads moistened with a mild astringent.

b) Massage the face using the facial manipulations described in this chapter.

8. Expose the face to infrared light. (Fig. 19.7) Infrared lamp may be given during or after facial manipulations.

a) Cover the client's eyes with cotton pads moistened with a mild astringent.

b) Place the lamp at a comfortable distance from the face.

c) Expose the face to infrared rays for 3 to 5 minutes.

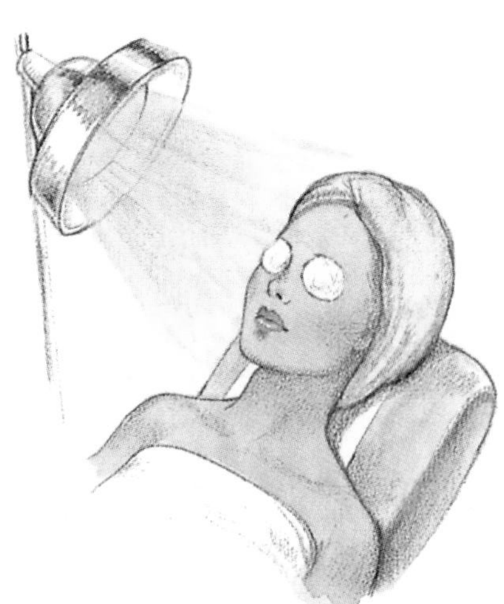

FIGURE 19.7 — Exposing the face to an infrared lamp.

9. Remove massage cream.

a) Remove cream with tissues; warm, moist towels; moist cleansing pads; or sponges. Follow the same procedure as for removing cleansing cream.

10. Apply astringent or mild skin freshening lotion.

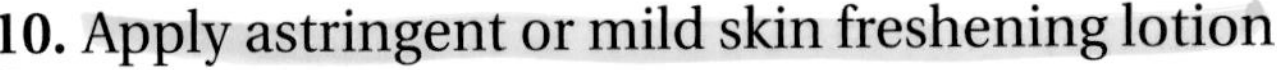

a) Sponge the face with cotton pledgets moistened with the lotion.

11. Apply a treatment mask formulated for the client's skin condition. Leave on the face for about 7 to 10 minutes.
12. Remove the mask with wet cotton pledgets or towels.
13. Wipe the face with pledgets saturated with a mild astringent.
14. Apply a moisturizer or protective lotion.
15. Completion.

a) Discard all disposable supplies and materials.

b) Close product containers tightly, clean them, and put them in their proper places. Return unused cosmetics and other items to the dispensary.

c) Place used towels, coverlets, head covers, and like items in appropriate containers

d) Tidy up the work area.

e) Wash and sanitize your hands.

Completed:
Learning Objective
#3
FACIAL PROCEDURE

FACIAL MANIPULATIONS

In giving facial manipulations, you must remember that an even tempo, or rhythm, induces relaxation. Do not remove your hands from the client's face once the manipulations have been started. Should it become necessary to remove your hands, feather them off, and then gently replace them with feather-like movements.

Note: *Each instructor may have developed his or her own routine in giving manipulations. The following illustrations merely show the different movements that may be used on the various parts of the face, chest, and back. Follow your instructor's routine.*

Massage movements are usually directed toward the origin of a muscle, in order to avoid damage to muscular tissues.

1. Chin movement. Lift the chin, using a slight pressure. (Fig. 19.8)
2. Lower cheeks. Using a circular movement, rotate from chin to ears. (Fig. 19.9)
3. Follow diagram for mouth, nose, and cheek movements. (Fig. 19.10)

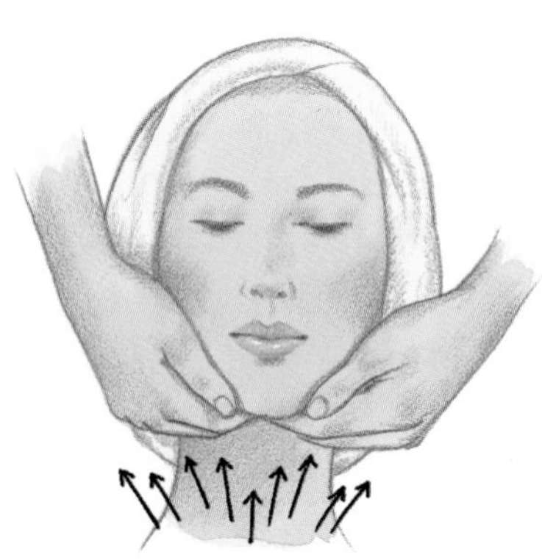

FIGURE 19.8 — Chin movement.

Note: *Many facial specialists prefer to start massage manipulations at the chin, while others prefer to start at the forehead. Both are correct. Be guided by your instructor.*

4. Linear movement over forehead. Slide fingers to temples; rotate with pressure on upward stroke; slide to left eyebrow; then stroke up to hairline gradually moving hands across forehead to right eyebrow. (Fig. 19.11)

5. Circular movement over forehead. Starting at eyebrow line, work across middle of forehead, and then toward the hairline. (Fig. 19.12)

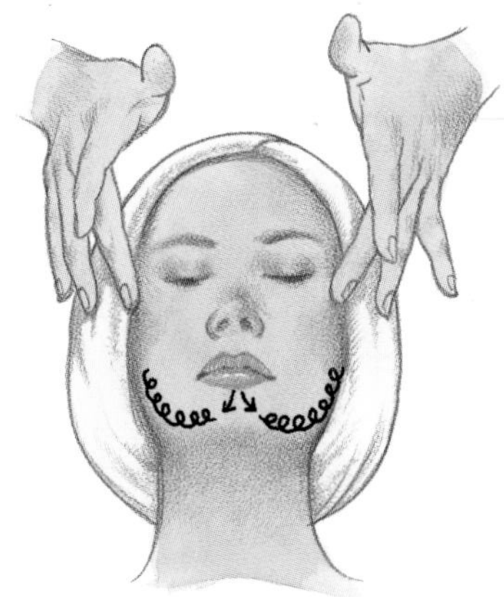

FIGURE 19.9 — Circular movement of lower cheeks.

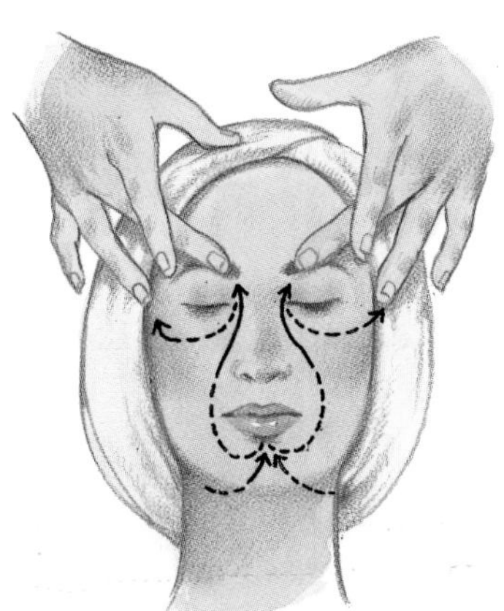

FIGURE 19.10 — Mouth, nose, and cheek movements.

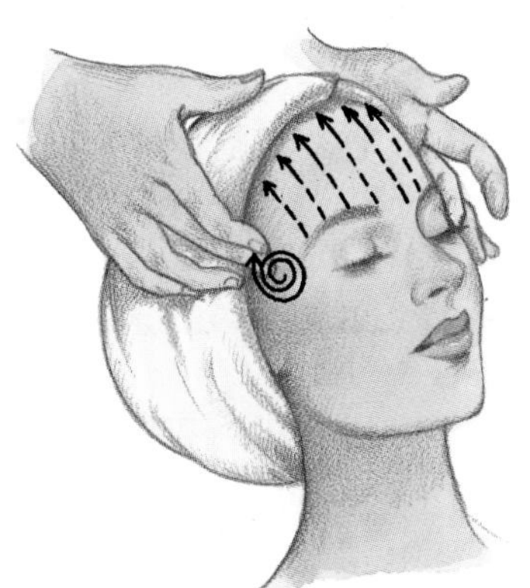

FIGURE 19.11 — Linear movement over forehead.

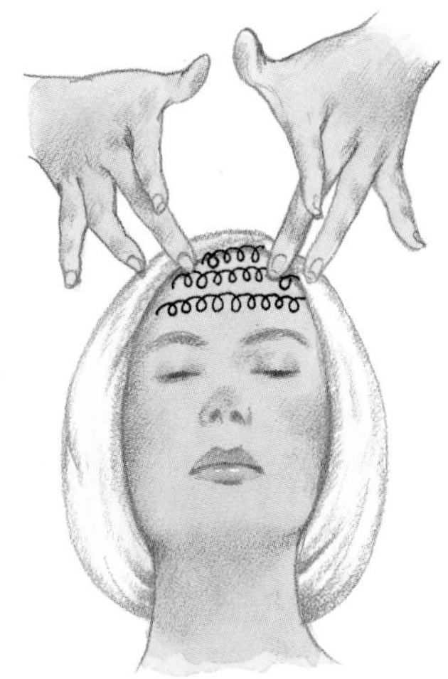

FIGURE 19.12 — Circular movement over forehead.

6. Crisscross movement. Start at one side of forehead and work back. (Fig. 19.13)

7. Stroking (headache) movement. Slide fingers to center of forehead; then draw fingers, with slight pressure, toward temples, and rotate. (Fig. 19.14)

8. Brow and eye movement. Place middle fingers at inner corners of eyes and index fingers over brows. Slide to outer corners of eyes, under eyes, and back to inner corners. (Fig. 19.15)

9. Nose and upper cheek movement. Slide fingers down nose. Apply rotary movement across cheeks to temples, and rotate gently. Slide fingers under eyes and back to bridge of nose. (Fig. 19.16)

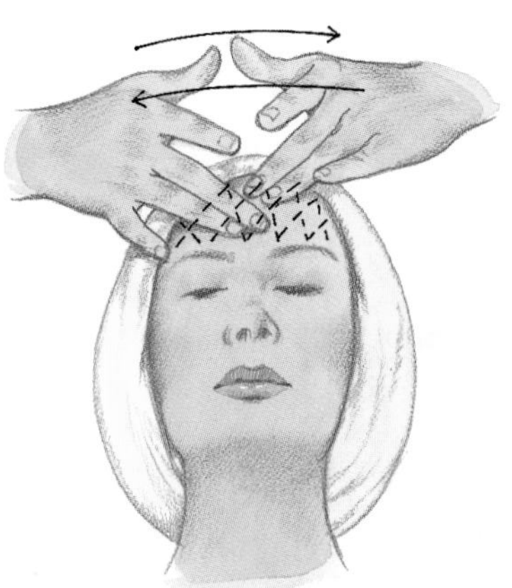

FIGURE 19.13 — Crisscross movement.

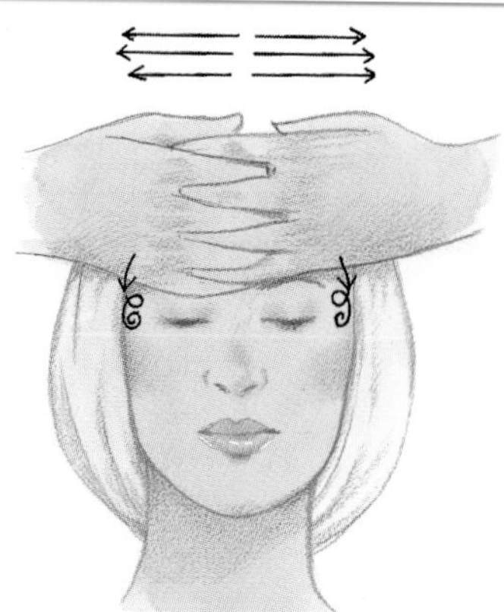

FIGURE 19.14 — Stroking (headache) movement.

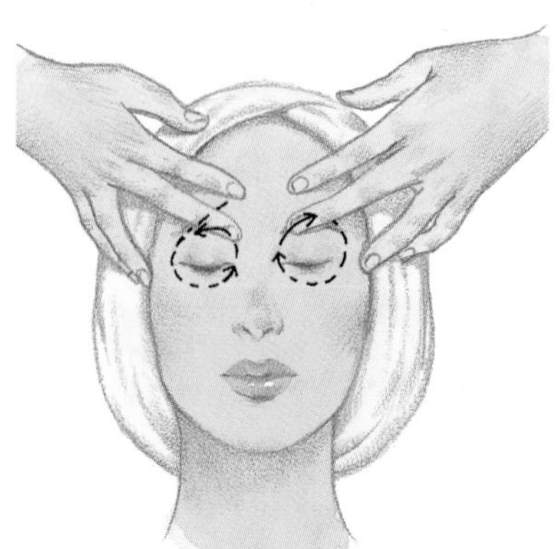

FIGURE 19.15 — Brow and eye movement.

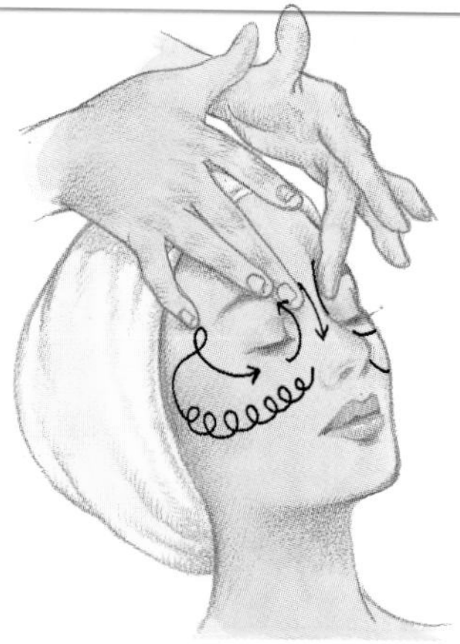

FIGURE 19.16 — Nose and upper cheek movement.

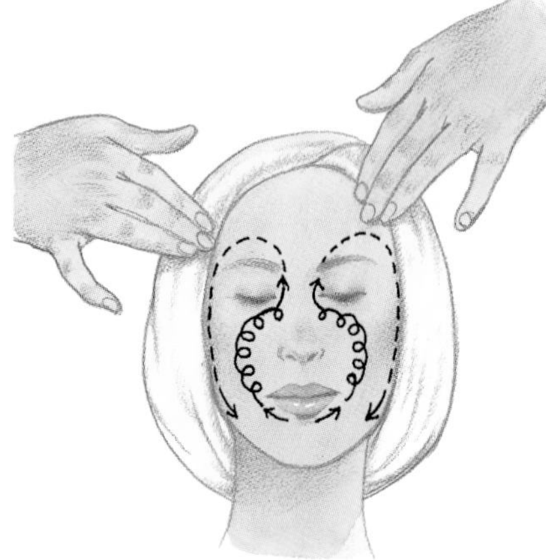

FIGURE 19.17 — Mouth and nose movement.

10. Mouth and nose movement. Apply circular movement from corners of mouth up sides of nose. Slide fingers over brows and down to corners of mouth. (Fig. 19.17)
11. Lip and chin movement. Draw fingers from center of upper lip, around mouth, going under lower lip and chin. (Fig. 19.18)
12. Optional movement. Hold head with left hand; draw fingers of right hand from under the lower lip, around mouth, to center of upper lip. (Fig. 19.19)
13. Lifting movement of cheeks. Proceed from the mouth to ears, and then from nose to top part of ears. (Fig. 19.20)

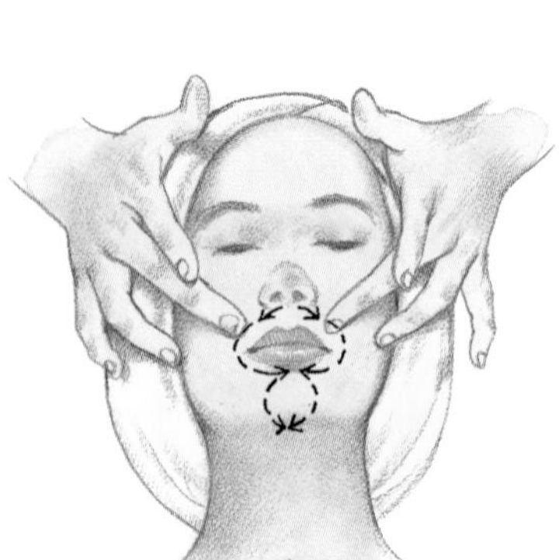

FIGURE 19.18 — Lip and chin movement.

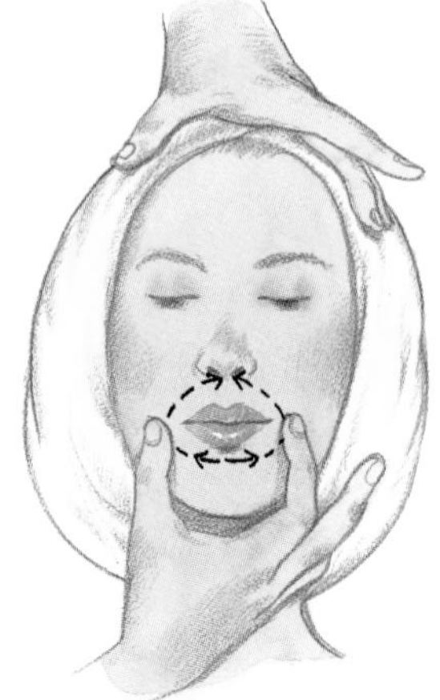

FIGURE 19.19 — Optional movement.

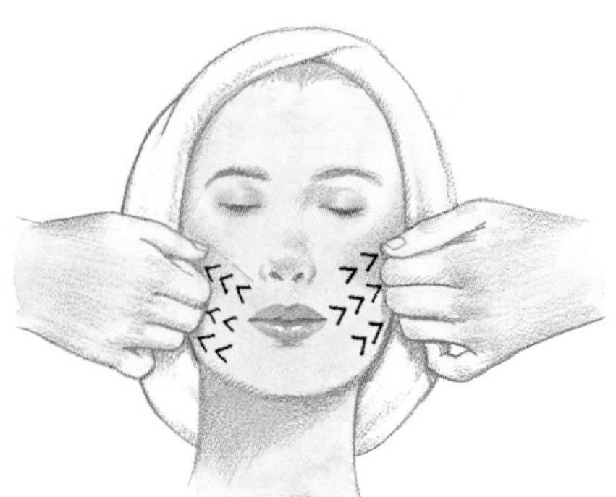

FIGURE 19.20 — Lifting movement of cheeks.

14. Rotary movement of cheeks. Massage from chin to ear lobes, from mouth to middle of ears, and from nose to top of ears. (Fig. 19.21)
15. Light tapping movement. Work from chin to earlobe, mouth to ear, nose to top of ear, and then across forehead. Repeat on other side. (Fig. 19.22)
16. Stroking movement of neck. Apply light upward strokes over front of neck. Use heavier pressure on sides of neck in downward strokes. (Fig. 19.23)

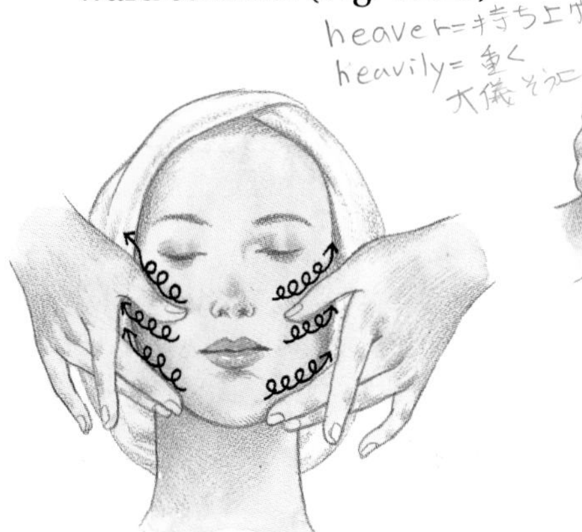

FIGURE 19.21 — Rotary movement of cheeks.

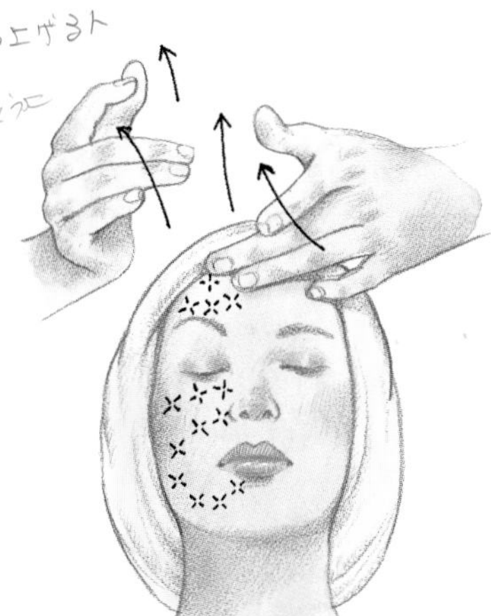

FIGURE 19.22 — Light tapping movement.

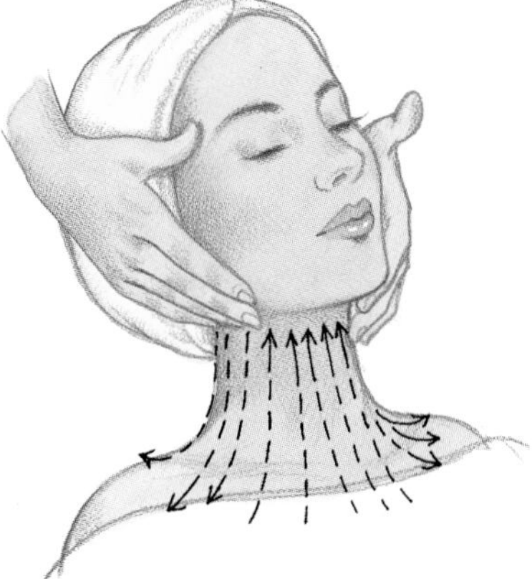

FIGURE 19.23 — Stroking movement of neck.

17. Circular movement over neck and chest. Starting at back of ears, apply circular movement down side of neck, over shoulders, and across chest. (Fig. 19.24).
18. Infrared lamp (optional). Protect eyes with eye pads; adjust lamp over client's face; leave on for about 5 minutes. (Fig. 19.25)

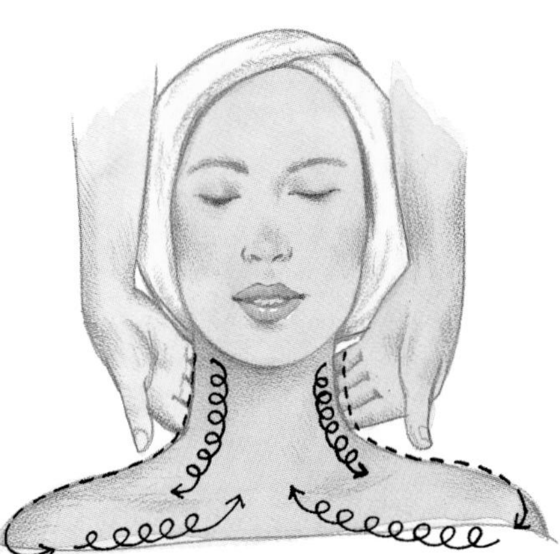

FIGURE 19.24 — Circular movement over neck and chest.

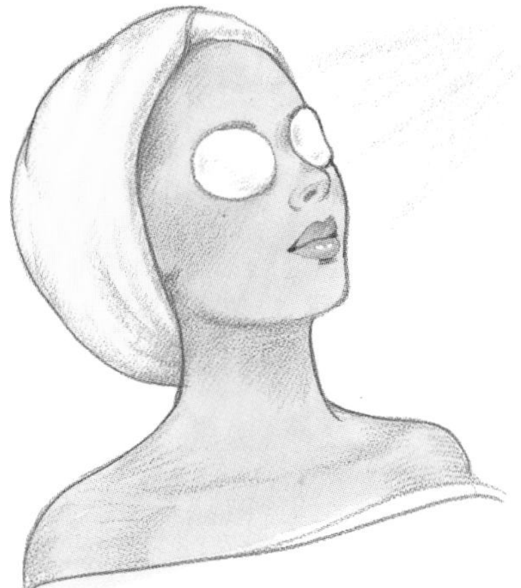

FIGURE 19.25 — Infrared lamp (optional).

CHEST, BACK, AND NECK MANIPULATIONS (OPTIONAL)

Some instructors prefer to treat these areas first before starting the regular facial. A suggested procedure is as follows:

1. Apply and remove cleansing cream.
2. Apply massage cream.
3. Give manipulations as outlined below.
4. Chest and back movement. Use rotary movement across chest and shoulders, then to spine. Slide fingers to base of neck. Rotate three times. (Fig. 19.26)
5. Shoulders and back movement. Rotate shoulders three times. Glide fingers to spine, then to base of neck. Apply circular movement up to back of ear, and then slide fingers to front of earlobe. Rotate three times. (Fig. 19.27)
6. Back massage (optional). To stimulate and relax client, use thumbs and bent index fingers to grasp the tissue at the back of the neck. Rotate six times. Repeat over shoulders and back to the spine. (Fig. 19.28)
7. Remove cream with tissues or warm, moist towel.
8. Dust the back lightly with talcum powder and smooth.

Completed: Learning Objective #4
POSSIBLE MANIPULATIONS DURING A FACIAL

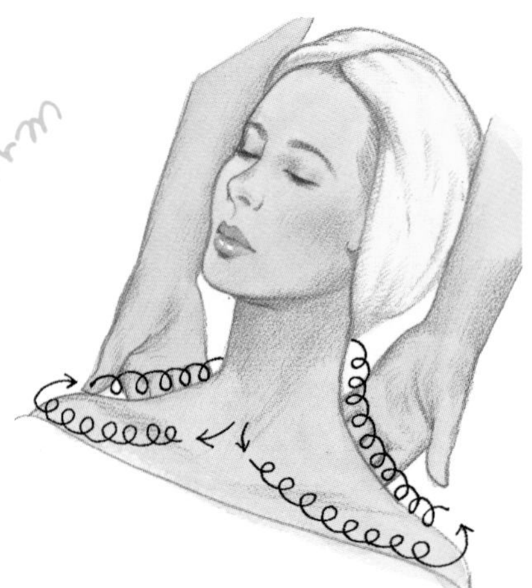

FIGURE 19.26 — Chest and back movement.

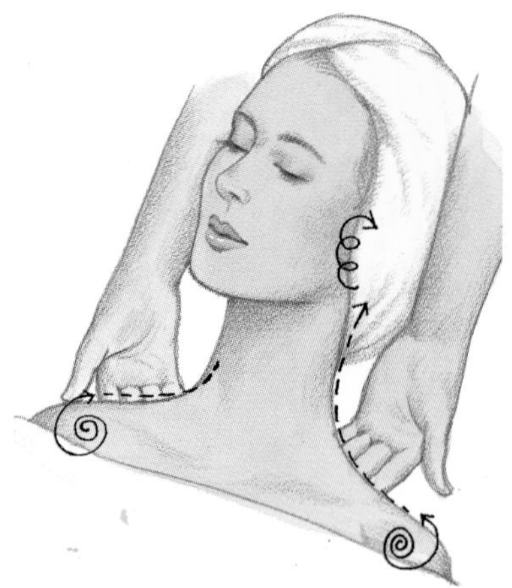

FIGURE 19.27 — Shoulders and back movement.

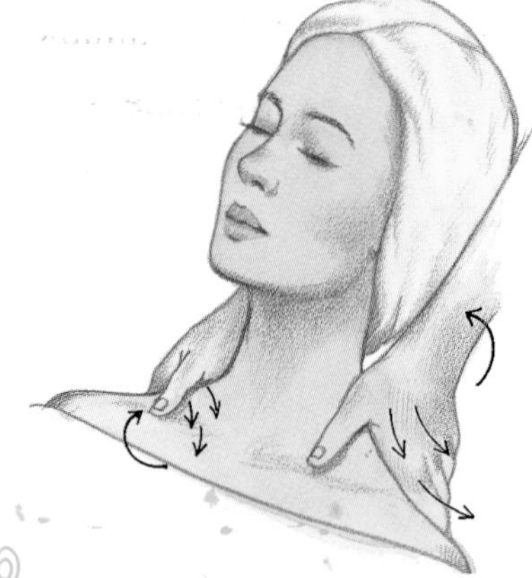

FIGURE 19.28 — Back massage (optional).

SPECIAL PROBLEMS

FACIAL FOR DRY SKIN

Dry skin is caused by an insufficient flow of sebum (oil) from the sebaceous glands. The facial for dry skin helps correct the dry condition of the skin. It may be given with or without an electrical current. For more effective results, the use of electrical current is recommended.

Procedure with Infrared Rays

1. Prepare the client as for a plain facial.
2. Apply cleansing cream; remove with tissues or with a warm, moist towel.
3. Sponge the face with cleansing lotion (for dry skin).
4. Apply massage cream.
5. Apply lubricating oil, or eye cream, over and under the eyes.
6. Apply lubricating oil over the neck.
7. Cover the client's eyes with cotton pads moistened with witch hazel and boric acid solution.
8. Expose the face and neck to infrared rays for not more than 5 minutes.
9. Give manipulation three to five times.
10. Remove massage cream and oil with tissues or with a warm, moist towel.
11. Apply skin lotion suitable for dry skin.
12. Blot face with tissues or towel.
13. Apply a base foundation suitable for the client's skin.
14. Complete and clean up as for a plain facial.

CAUTION

For dry skin, avoid using lotions that contain a large percentage of alcohol. Read the manufacturer's directions.

Procedure with Galvanic Current

The procedure for giving a dry skin facial with galvanic current is similar to the procedure for giving a dry skin facial with infrared rays, with a few changes:

1. Repeat steps 1 to 3 of the procedure with infrared rays.
2. Apply negative galvanic current for 3 to 5 minutes, to open the pores.

3. Repeat steps 4 to 11 of the procedure with infrared rays.
4. Apply positive galvanic current for 3 to 5 minutes, to close the pores.
5. Repeat steps 12 to 14 of the procedure with infrared rays.

Procedure with Indirect High-Frequency Current

1. Follow steps 1 through 8 of the procedure for a facial with infrared rays.
2. Give manipulations, using the indirect method of applying high-frequency current, for not more than 7 minutes. (Fig. 19.29)
3. Apply two to three cold towels to the face and neck.
4. Sponge the face and neck with skin freshener.
5. Apply a moisturizer of protective fluid.

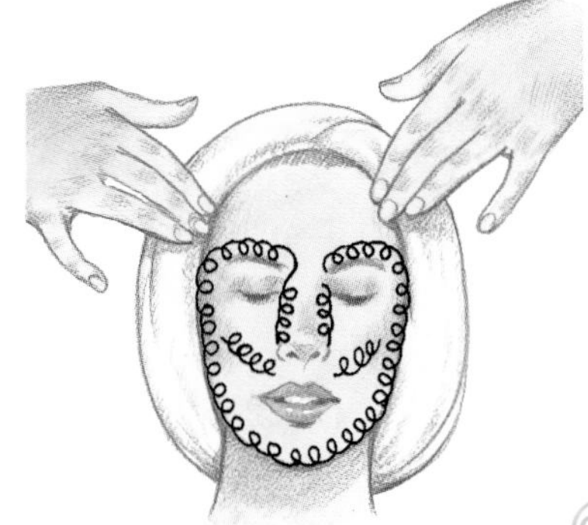

FIGURE 19.29 — High-frequency indirect method. (Client holds electrode.)

FACIAL FOR OILY SKIN AND BLACKHEADS (COMEDONES)

An oily skin and/or ***blackheads*** (***comedones***) are caused by a hardened mass of sebum formed in the ducts of the sebaceous glands. Sometimes the client's diet may be a factor in the condition. For an appropriate diet to help minimize oily skin and blackheads, the client should see a physician.

Procedure

1. Prepare the client as for a plain facial. Sanitize your hands.
2. Apply cleansing lotion and remove it with a warm, moist towel, moist cotton pads, or facial sponges.
3. Place the moistened eyepads on the client's eyes, then analyze the skin under a magnifying lamp.
4. Steam the face with three to four moist, warm towels, or with a facial steamer to open the pores.
5. Cover your fingertips with tissue and gently press out blackheads. Do not press so hard as to bruise the skin tissue.

CAUTION

If it is necessary to cleanse pimples that have come to a head and are open, use rubber or latex gloves. Do not attempt to deal with a skin problem that requires medical attention.

6. Sponge the face with astringent.
7. Cover the client's eyes with pads moistened with a mild astringent.
8. Apply blue light over the skin for not more than 3 to 5 minutes.
9. Apply massage cream suitable for the skin condition.
10. Give manipulations.
11. Remove cream with a warm, moist towel, cotton pads, or facial sponges.
12. Moisten a cotton pledget with an astringent lotion. Apply it to the face and neck with upward and outward movements to close the pores.
13. Blot the excess moisture with tissues.
14. Apply protective lotion if needed.
15. Complete and clean up, following proper sanitary procedures.

WHITEHEADS (MILIA)

Milia, or ***whiteheads***, is a common skin disorder, caused by the formation of sebaceous matter within or under the skin. It usually occurs in skin of fine texture. The surface openings of the skin may be so small that the sebum cannot pass out. As a result, it collects under the surface of the skin in small, round, hardened, pearl-like masses that resemble a small grain of sand. This condition may be treated under the supervision of a dermatologist.

FACIAL FOR ACNE

Acne is a disorder of the sebaceous glands; therefore it requires medical attention. If the client is under medical care, the role of the cosmetologist is to work closely with the client's physician to carry out instructions as to the kind and frequency of facial treatments.

Under medical direction, you must limit the cosmetic treatment of acne to the following measures:

1. Reducing the oiliness of the skin by local applications.
2. Removing blackheads, using proper procedures.
3. Cleansing the skin.
4. Using special medicated preparations.

Equipment, Implements, and Materials

Acne cream or lotion

Antiseptic lotion

Cleansing lotion

Astringent lotion for oily skin

Towels

Appropriate mask

High-frequency magnifying lamp

Procedure

Because acne skin contains infectious matter, it is advisable to use rubber or latex gloves and disposable materials such as cotton cleansing pads.

1. Prepare all materials to be used for the facial treatment.
2. Prepare the client.
3. Sanitize your hands.
4. Cleanse the client's face.
5. Place cotton eyepads over the client's eyes; then analyze the skin under the magnifying lamp.
6. Apply warm, wet towels to the face to open the pores for deep cleansing.
7. Extract blackheads and cleanse pimples.
8. Cleanse the face with a wet cotton pad that has been sprinkled with astringent.
9. Apply the acne treatment cream. Leave on the eyepads and turn on the infrared lamp for about 5 to 7 minutes to enable the treatment cream to penetrate the skin. Or, you can apply high-frequency current with direct application (facial electrode) over the affected area for not more than 5 minutes. (Fig. 19.30) Be guided by your instructor.

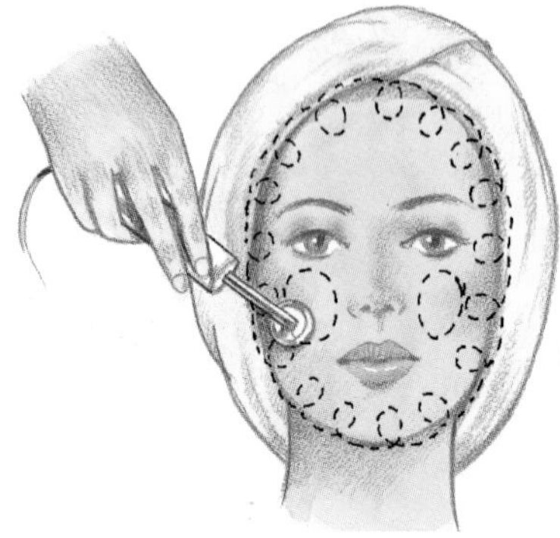

FIGURE 19.30 — Applying high-frequency current with facial electrode.

10. Leave the eyepads on and apply a treatment mask that is suitable for the skin condition. Leave it on the face for about 8 to 10 minutes.
11. Remove the mask with moist towels or cotton pads.
12. Apply astringent to the face with a wet cotton pad.
13. Apply protective fluid or special acne lotion.
14. Complete the cleanup procedures.

Completed:
Learning Objective
#5
CORRECTIVE FACIALS

DIET FOR ACNE

Modern studies show that acne might be due to hereditary and environmental factors. It can be aggravated by emotional stress and faulty diet. Acne is not believed to be caused by any particular food or drink, but foods high in fats, starches, and sugars tend to worsen the condition. The client should consult a physician for a prescribed diet. A well-balanced diet, drinking plenty of water, and following healthful personal hygiene habits are recommended.

PACKS AND MASKS

Masks and packs are somewhat the same, but generally the substances of a heavier consistency such as clay are referred to as packs. Pack facials are recommended for normal and oily skin and are usually applied directly to the skin. Mask facials are recommended for dry skin and are applied to the skin with the aid of gauze layers or masks. Masks are made of many ingredients and combinations such as vegetables, fruits, dairy products, herbs, and oils. Gauze is often used to aid in holding the mask preparation on the face.

CUSTOM-DESIGNED MASKS

You will usually use prepared masks, but there are times when a custom-designed mask prepared from fresh fruits, vegetables, milk, yogurt, or eggs might be preferred. These masks are generally beneficial unless the client is allergic to a particular substance. You should ask the client about allergies before applying a mask. Custom-designed masks are generally left on the face for 10 to 15 minutes during a one-hour treatment. The following is a list of ingredients used in custom-designed masks and their benefits to the skin:

1. *Fresh fruit mask.* Fresh strawberries can be crushed or sliced and applied to the face (usually over or between layers of gauze) for a mildly astringent and stimulating mask. Bananas can be sliced or crushed to make a mask for dry and sensitive skin, since they are rich in vitamins, potassium, calcium, and phosphorus and leave the skin soft and smooth.
2. *Fruits and vegetables that are mildly astringent* and have excellent soothing qualities are: tomatoes, apples, and cucumbers. These fruits or vegetables can be sliced very thin or crushed and applied to the face. Gauze helps to hold the mask in place.

Completed:
Learning Objective
#6
DESCRIBE PACKS AND MASKS

3. *The white of an egg* can be beaten until fluffy and applied to the face as a mask. Egg white has a tightening effect and clears impurities from the skin. It is beneficial to all skin types.
4. *Yogurt and buttermilk* are used for masks on all skin types. Their mildly astringent cleansing action leaves the skin feeling refreshed.
5. *Honey* is used for its toning, tightening, and ***hydrating*** effect.
6. Some ingredients such as honey and almond meal or oatmeal can be mixed into a paste with milk.

The Use of Gauze for Mask Application

Gauze is a thin, transparent fabric of loosely woven cotton, commonly called *cheesecloth*. Gauze is used to hold certain mask ingredients that do not cling or hold together on the face. Such is the case with sliced or crushed fruits or vegetables, which tend to run. These ingredients can be applied over a layer of gauze. The gauze holds the mask on the face but allows the ingredients to seep through to benefit the skin. In some cases, it is necessary to apply a second layer of gauze over the mask.

Procedure for Applying Gauze

1. Cut a piece of gauze large enough to cover the entire face and neck. (Fig. 19.31) Cut out spaces for the eyes, nose, and mouth. Although the client is able to breathe through the gauze, the cutout spaces will be more comfortable.
2. Apply the mask ingredients over the gauze. (Fig. 19.32) Start on the neck and apply upward on the face, ending on the forehead. Apply eyepads for the client's comfort.

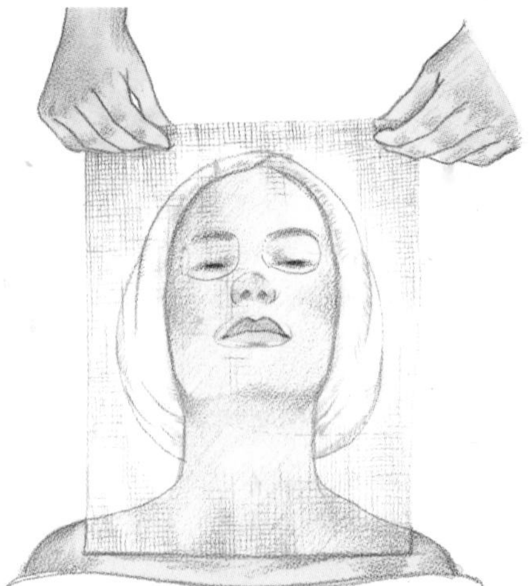

FIGURE 19.31 — Cover entire face and neck with gauze.

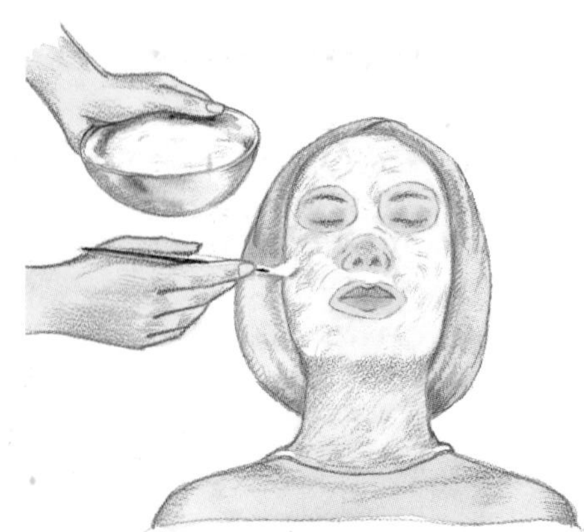

FIGURE 19.32 — Apply the mask ingredients over the gauze.

3. Allow the mask to remain on the face for the appropriate time; then lift and roll the gauze upward to remove most of the mask. (Fig. 19.33) Finish cleansing the face with moist cotton pads or facial sponges.

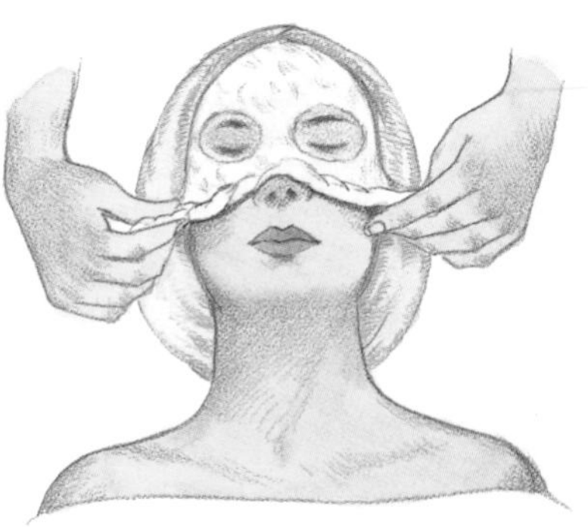

FIGURE 19.33 — Lift and roll the gauze upward to remove.

Equipment, Implements, and Materials for Custom-Designed Mask

Assemble all items needed for a plain facial and any special cosmetics or ingredients for the mask. Prepare the gauze.

Procedure for Custom-Designed Mask

1. Give a plain facial, including removal of massage cream after manipulations.
2. Place cotton pads moistened with mild astringent over the eyes.
3. Apply the gauze and the appropriate mask or mask ingredients for the skin condition. Keep the mask from getting into the client's eyes, nostrils, mouth, or on the hairline.
4. Allow the mask to remain on the skin 10 to 15 minutes or until it is dry. Follow the manufacturer's directions if using a prepared mask.
5. Remove the gauze mask carefully and finish cleansing the face with a warm, moist towel or cotton pads.
6. Apply a mild astringent or skin-freshening lotion.
7. Apply moisturizer or protective lotion.
8. Follow the usual completion and cleanup procedures.

HOT OIL MASK FACIAL

A hot oil mask facial is recommended for dry, scaly skin, or skin that is inclined to wrinkle. The mask is applied directly to the skin with the aid of gauze layers. Prepare the gauze in sections large enough to cover the face. Cut openings for the eyes, nose, and mouth.

Equipment, Implements, and Materials

Gather all items needed for a facial plus the following:

Prepared gauze facial mask

Hot oil preparation

Hot oil heater

Infrared lamp

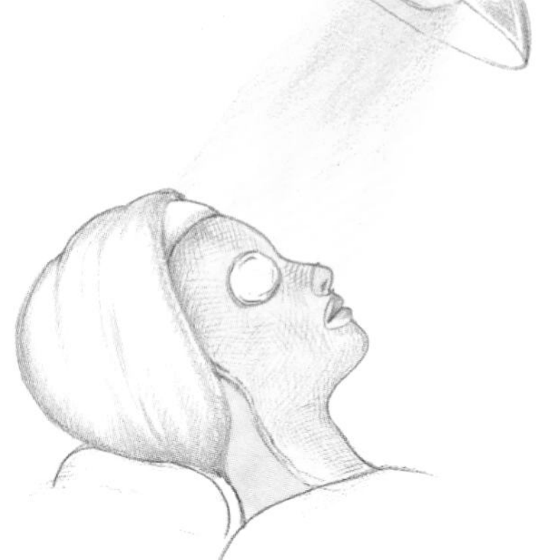

FIGURE 19.34 — Infrared lamp.

Completed: Learning Objective #7

MATERIALS AND PROCEDURES FOR FACIAL MASKS

Procedure

1. Give a plain facial, including the removal of massage cream.
2. Cover the eyes with eyepads moistened with mild astringent (skin-freshening lotion).
3. Moisten gauze facial mask with warm oil and place on the face, starting at the throat.
4. Place an infrared lamp about 24" (60 cm) from the client's face. (Fig. 19.34)
5. Allow the client to rest for 5 to 10 minutes under the lamp.
6. Remove the gauze facial mask.
7. Apply additional massage or moisturizing cream.
8. Give facial manipulations.
9. Remove cream with a warm, moist towel.
10. Apply an astringent lotion.
11. Apply moisturizer or protective lotion as needed.
12. Complete cleanup procedures.

REASONS A CLIENT MIGHT FIND FAULT WITH A FACIAL TREATMENT

A client might find fault with a facial treatment if you:

1. Fail to present yourself in a professional manner.
2. Have offensive breath or body odor.
3. Have rough nails that scratch the skin.
4. Have rough, cold hands.
5. Allow cream or other substances to get into the client's eyes, mouth, nostrils, or on the hairline.
6. Use towels that are too hot to be comfortable.
7. Apply substances or towels that are too cold.
8. Fail to follow sanitary procedures at all times.
9. Show no interest in the client's comfort and safety.
10. Fail to allow the client to relax by talking too much.

11. Give rough manipulations or massage muscles in the wrong direction.
12. Are disorganized and need to interrupt the facial to get supplies.
13. Fail to assist the client when necessary.
14. Fail to be courteous at all times.

Completed: Learning Objective #8

REASONS A CLIENT MIGHT FIND FAULT WITH A FACIAL TREATMENT

Career Path

ESTHETICIAN

An esthetician is a cosmetologist who specializes in skin care rather than in hairstyling. As highly trained specialists, they offer preventive care of the skin and give treatments to keep the skin healthy and attractive. They may also manufacture, sell, or apply cosmetics. Unless an esthetician is a licensed dermatologist, he or she cannot prescribe medication or give medical treatments. However, the esthetician is trained to detect skin problems and suggest that the client seek medical treatment from a physician. In some states, the esthetician must be a licensed cosmetologist with training in all areas of cosmetology; in others, one can attend a freestanding esthetics school and obtain a separate license.

There are many job opportunities for those who choose to specialize in esthetics. The possibilities for making a good living and for growth are greater than in any other field comparable in preparation time and expense.

In addition to becoming a skin care practitioner in a full-service salon, the licensed esthetician can become the owner of a skin care salon or day spa; the popularity of such establishments has soared in the past few years.

The merchandising field also has many possibilities for the esthetician: You can become a manager, salesperson or buyer in the cosmetics department of a large store. Another option is to become a manufacturer's representative, calling on salons or stores to explain or demonstrate the use of products. Estheticians can also sell directly to consumers as owners of their own line of cosmetics or skin care products.

The esthetician can also become a guest artist or demonstrator, traveling to conventions and other events to demonstrate products, techniques, and equipment to prospective buyers or to the general public.

—*From* Standard Textbook for Professional Estheticians *by Joel Gerson*

REVIEW QUESTIONS

FACIALS

1. What are the benefits of a facial?
2. Why should you analyze a client's skin before giving a facial?
3. Why is it important to use a spatula when removing a product from its container?
4. What causes dry skin?
5. What is another name for blackheads?
6. What causes oily skin or blackheads?
7. What is milia?
8. What is acne and how should it be treated?
9. For what type of skin are masks recommended?
10. For what type of skin are packs recommended?
11. For what type of skin is the hot oil mask recommended?

CHAPTER 20

Facial Makeup

LEARNING OBJECTIVES

After completing this chapter, you should be able to:

1. List the types of cosmetics used for facial makeup and their purposes.
2. Describe correct makeup application procedures.
3. Identify the different facial types.
4. Demonstrate the different procedures for basic corrective makeup.
5. Demonstrate the application and removal of artificial eyelashes.
6. List the safety precautions to be observed in the application of makeup.

NATIONAL SKILL STANDARDS

This chapter provides you with the necessary information to master these National Industry Skill Standards for Entry-Level Cosmetologists:

- Conducting services in a safe environment, taking measures to prevent the spread of infectious and contagious disease
- Applying appropriate cosmetics to enhance a client's appearance

INTRODUCTION

The main objective of a makeup application is to emphasize the client's most attractive facial features and to minimize less attractive features. There is no fixed pattern for applying facial makeup. It is important that you analyze each client's face carefully and consider individual needs.

When applying makeup, you must take into consideration the structure of the client's face; the color of the eyes, skin, and hair; how the client wants to look; and the results you can achieve.

Once you know the basic principles, you can use makeup to create optical illusions with shadowing, highlighting, and color. The client's natural beauty can be enhanced by the proper coordination of facial makeup, hairstyle, and clothing colors.

PREPARATION FOR MAKEUP APPLICATION

When the client is having hair care services and also wants makeup, the makeup should be applied just before the comb-out (after rollers and clips have been removed) or after the hair has been blown dry and/or curled. Fasten a protective strip of tissue, headband, or turban around the client's head to protect the hair.

The first step in a makeup procedure is to see that your work area is clean and neat and that all the items you use for applying and removing makeup are sanitized. Products must be removed from containers with a sanitized spatula or a clean applicator. Be sure to have disposable items and applicators available. Wash and sanitize your hands before touching the client's face.

EQUIPMENT, IMPLEMENTS, AND MATERIALS

Cleansing creams and lotions
Astringent and skin-freshening lotions
Moisturizer and protective lotion
Cream, liquid, or cake foundation in appropriate colors
Shading and highlighting cosmetics
Liquid, cream, and dry powder cheek colors
Face powder
Lip colors in a variety of colors
Assorted lip liners and brushes
A variety of eye colors (shadows)
Mascara and brushes
Eye makeup applicators (disposable)
Eyeliner pencils and brushes
Tissues
Disposable cotton-tipped applicators
Spatulas
Cotton pads and pledgets
Disposable towels
Draping sheets and towels
Makeup cape
Tissue neckbands
Headband or turban
Eyelash curler
Assorted brushes (eyebrow, powder, etc.)

When selecting and applying makeup, be sure to have a well-lighted makeup mirror and, when possible, check the makeup in natural light.

COSMETICS FOR FACIAL MAKEUP

FOUNDATION FOR MAKEUP

Probably no other item of makeup is as important as ***foundation***. Foundation, when properly applied, provides a base for color harmony, evens out the skin color, conceals minor imperfections, and protects the skin from soil, wind, and weather. Skin tones, or pigment, determine the selection of foundation color. Skin tones are generally classified with the following descriptions: very light or white, ivory, cream, pink, florid, sallow, olive, tan, brown, and ebony. Selecting the correct foundation color is of extreme importance to the success of the entire makeup application.

When choosing foundation color for light skin, a shade darker than the natural skin tone is usually best because it adds color. When choosing foundation for dark skin, foundation should be matched to the natural skin tone. For a sallow or pale skin tone, a rosy foundation will give a desirable glow to the skin. For a florid skin tone, a beige foundation will soften the reddish undertones.

For all other skin tones (fair, medium, or dark), select foundation and powder to blend with the lightness or darkness of the natural skin tone. If foundation is too light, it gives an artificial, pasty look to the skin.

When deciding on a foundation, place a small dot or two on the client's jawline and blend it upward on the jawline, then downward on the side of the neck. This will enable you to determine if the foundation color will blend well with the client's natural skin tone. Avoid creating a contrast between the color of the face and the color of the neck. When makeup is correctly matched in color and blended smoothly, no line of demarcation should be seen.

Selecting the Right Foundation

Liquid and cream foundations are the most widely used and give a slight sheen to the skin. Stick, water-base, or cake foundations give a matte (dull) finish.

1. Cream foundation gives the most natural look and is a long-lasting makeup. It is formulated for normal, dry, or oily skin types. Dot a small amount of foundation on the forehead, cheeks, and chin; then blend upward and outward for a smooth finish. A facial sponge can be used to finish the application and remove excess foundation.
2. Liquid (lotion) foundation is color suspended in a semi-liquid, delicate, light oil. For quick and effective blending, apply it on one area of the skin at a time, using long, smooth, upward strokes. A small facial sponge can be used to smooth the foundation and remove any excess.
3. Cake foundation adds color, gives a smooth velvety look, and helps conceal minor skin blemishes and discoloration. Cake foundation is effective for oily skin. If used on normal or dry skin, apply a moisturizer before applying cake makeup. To apply cake makeup, moisten a facial sponge and apply to one area of the face at a time, using upward strokes and smoothing carefully.
4. Stick foundation is particularly useful in concealing minor skin blemishes and discoloration. Because it is of thicker consistency, stick foundation can be patted over a blemish and then blended into the surrounding area for a more natural look. Use a facial sponge to smooth and finish the makeup.
5. Blemish-masking creams and sticks are available in a range of colors to coordinate with, or match, natural skin tones. Blemish-masking creams or sticks can be used to conceal blemishes and discolorations and may be applied before or after foundation. To apply, take a small amount of the product from the container with a spatula; then use your fingertips and a facial sponge to smooth and blend it over the desired area.

FACE POWDERS

Face powders improve the overall attractiveness of the skin by helping to conceal minor blemishes and discolorations and by toning down excessive color, gloss, or sheen. Face powder also enhances the skin's natural color and makes it soft and velvety to the touch.

Face powders come in cake or powder form, in a variety of tints and shades, and in different weights. Light and medium weights are generally best for dry and normal skin, and a heavier weight is effective on skin that tends to be oily. Face powder should coordinate with or match the natural skin tones and work well with the foundation. Powder may be slightly darker or lighter than the foundation if it achieves the desired effect, but it should never appear caked, spotted, or streaked on the face.

Note: *Translucent powder (colorless) blends with all foundations and will not turn to a color when applied.*

Apply face powder (after foundation) using a fresh cotton puff or pledget. Press the powder over the face in the desired areas; then use a powder brush or another puff or pledget to whisk off the excess. Face powder helps to set the makeup.

CHEEK AND LIP COLORS

The purpose of ***cheek color*** (also called rouge or blush) is to give a soft natural-looking glow of color to the face. It aids in creating more attractive facial contours.

Cheek color should coordinate with, or be the same color as, the lip color. However, when a deeper lip color is worn, generally, a lighter cheek color will appear more natural. Color on the cheeks should be less vivid in daylight than in artificial light. Bright colors call attention to that area of the face and the makeup looks artificial.

There are four types of cheek color: liquid, cream, dry, and brush-on.

1. Liquid cheek color blends well and is suitable for all skin types. Apply over the foundation before powdering the face.
2. Cream cheek color closely resembles pigmented foundation creams and cream makeup. It is generally preferred for dry and normal skin. Apply over the foundation before powdering the face.
3. Dry (compact) cheek color imparts a matte (dull) finish. Apply with a cotton puff or brush.

4. Brush-on powder (loose) cheek color comes in a variety of shades and tints, and is used to add color and to contour the cheeks. Apply over foundation and powder using a cotton puff or brush.

Lip color (also called lipstick or gloss) adds color to the lips and protects them from becoming dry and chapped. Lip color is also used to enhance or correct the shape of the lips.

Artistry and a keen sense of fashion are essential in selecting the appropriate lip color shade or tint. The prevailing fashion trend might call for a certain look, lighter or darker colors, or style of application. Consider the client's preferences before selecting and applying lip color.

Lip color must not be applied directly from the container unless it belongs to the client. Use a spatula to remove the lip color from the container; then take it from the spatula with a lip brush. Use the tip of the brush to line the lips, beginning at inner peak of the upper lip and working outward to the corner of the mouth. Do the other side, outline the lower lip, and then apply color on the lips staying within the outline. A lip lining pencil may be used when doing corrective makeup or when a more emphasized lip line is desired.

EYE MAKEUP

Eye makeup is available in a wide range of colors from pastels to deeper shades and tints of blue, gray, green, brown, beige, purple, and in colors with metallic silver and gold added.

When applied to the lids, ***eye color*** or ***shadow*** complements the eyes by making them appear brighter and more expressive. Eye colors can match the color of the eyes or be lighter or darker. Generally, a darker shade of eye color makes the natural color of the iris appear lighter, and a lighter shade makes the iris appear deeper. However, there are no set rules for selection of eye makeup colors except that they should enhance the client's eyes and be more subtle for daytime wear. Eye makeup colors may match or coordinate with the client's clothing color as desired.

Eye colors and shadows are available in stick, cream, cake, and dry powder form, and usually come with their own applicators. Remove the product from its container and use a fresh applicator. Unless you are doing corrective makeup, apply the eye color close to the lashes on the upper eyelid, sweeping the color slightly upward and outward. Blend to achieve the desired effect. More than one color may be used if a particular effect is desired.

Eyeliners are used to create a line on the eyelid close to the lashes to make the eyes appear larger and the lashes fuller. Eyeliners are manufactured in a variety of colors in pencil, liquid, or cake

Career Path

MAKEUP ARTIST

Some estheticians become professional makeup artists, either in full-service salons or in the fashion and entertainment industries. While few people attain fame and fortune as makeup artists, the successful salon artist is not expected to perform the miracles required for the stage, television, movies, or magazine covers. The salon artist's aim is to make any woman look her best for daytime or evening, and to recommend the right products for an individual's skin type and coloring. Occasionally clients will be men who need makeup for photographs or other occasions.

A salon or department store usually pays a makeup artist a salary with a commission on the products he or she sells. You can create outstanding makeups, but without the ability to sell products you won't be valuable to the salon. Often the makeup artist in a department store is called on to give free applications to customers to increase sales.

To be successful as a makeup artist, one should follow a few rules:

- Be honest and tactful when discussing skin care and makeup problems.
- Demonstrate what products can do without making exaggerated promises.
- Never pressure the client in any way.
- Suggest that the client return to the salon when she needs more cosmetics; if she likes the makeup, she will be a regular customer.
- Without giving false flattery, compliment the client on her good features and minimize her flaws.
- Never make derogatory remarks about your competitors or their products.
- Be sure that every service is given in the most sanitary and professional way.

—*From* Standard Textbook for Professional Estheticians
by Joel Gerson

form. Most clients prefer an eyeliner that is the same color as the lashes or mascara for a more natural look. More dramatic colors may be desired for evening wear. The same rules of sanitation apply to eyeliners as for other makeup application. No applicator may be used on more than one client unless it can be sanitized thoroughly before each use.

Using an eyelining pencil on the lower eyelids is a matter of choice. Some clients prefer lining both the upper and lower eyelids. Be extremely cautious when applying eyeliner. You must have a steady hand and should tell the client to remain still while the makeup is being applied.

Eyebrow pencils are used to modify the natural outline of the eyebrows, usually after tweezing. They can be used to darken the eyebrows, to fill in where the brow is too thin or devoid of hair, and to correct misshapen brows. Eyebrow pencils cannot be sanitized; therefore, a fresh pencil must be used for each client. Brush-on brow color comes in powdered form and is applied with a brush. Cream, liquid, and cake brow colors are also applied with a brush. Most brush applicators can be sanitized. Avoid harsh contrasts between hair and eyebrow color; for example, pale blonde or silver hair with black eyebrows.

Mascara is available in liquid, cake, and cream form. Mascara colors are available in a variety of shades and tints. The most popular colors are brown, black, and deep auburn, which enhance natural lashes and make them appear thicker and longer. Mascara is also used to darken eyebrows. Mascara and eyebrow pencils should be the same color or color coordinated so there is no harsh contrast. Usually the lashes should be darker than eyebrows.

Completed: Learning Objective #1
TYPES OF COSMETICS AND THEIR PURPOSES

PROCEDURE FOR APPLYING A PROFESSIONAL MAKEUP

1. Apply cleansing cream or lotion. Remove a small quantity of cleanser from the container with a spatula and place it in the palm of the left hand, or apply a dab of lotion to an applicator. With the fingertips of the right hand, place dabs of cleanser on the forehead, nose, cheeks, chin, and neck. Spread the cleanser over the face and neck with light upward and outward circular movements. (Fig. 20.1)

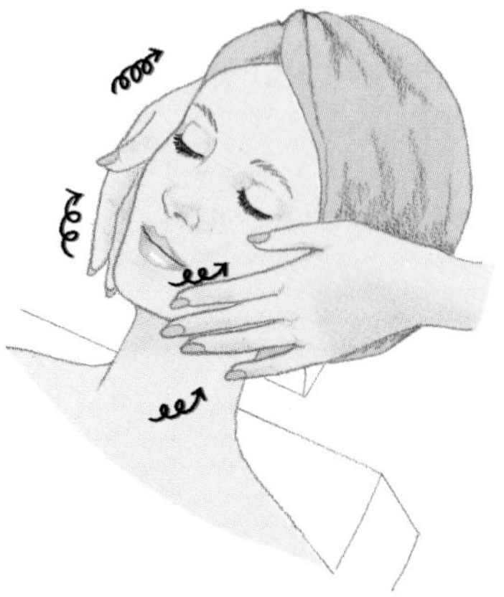

FIGURE 20.1 — Apply cleansing cream or lotion.

2. Remove the cleanser with tissue mitts or moistened cotton pads, using an upward and outward motion. Be especially gentle around the eyes. If necessary, apply cleanser a second time, to remove heavy makeup or color on the eyes and lips. (Fig. 20.2)

3. Apply astringent lotion or skin freshener (toner). For oily skin, apply astringent lotion; for dry skin, apply a skin freshener (mild astringent). Moisten a cotton pad with the lotion and pat it lightly over the entire face and under the chin and neck. Blot off excess moisture with tissues or a cotton pad. (Fig. 20.3)

4. Apply a moisturizing lotion when necessary, usually when the skin is dry and delicate. Dab a small amount of the moisturizer on the forehead, cheeks, and chin. Blend upward over the face. Remove excess with a tissue, cotton pad, or facial sponge.

5. Eyebrows. Eyebrow arching is a complete service in itself. The procedure for arching is given in another section of this chapter. However, you may remove a few straggly hairs before a facial makeup by tweezing the hair in the same direction in which it grows. (Fig. 20.4)

6. Apply foundation. Select the appropriate type and color of foundation. Test for color by blending the foundation on the client's jawline. Place a small amount of the foundation in the palm of your hand. With the tips of your fingers, apply sparingly and evenly over the entire face and around the neckline. Use gentle upward and outward motions. Blend near the hairline, and remove excess foundation with a cosmetic sponge or cotton pledget. When a moisturizer is needed, apply it in the same way, but before applying the foundation. (Fig. 20.5)

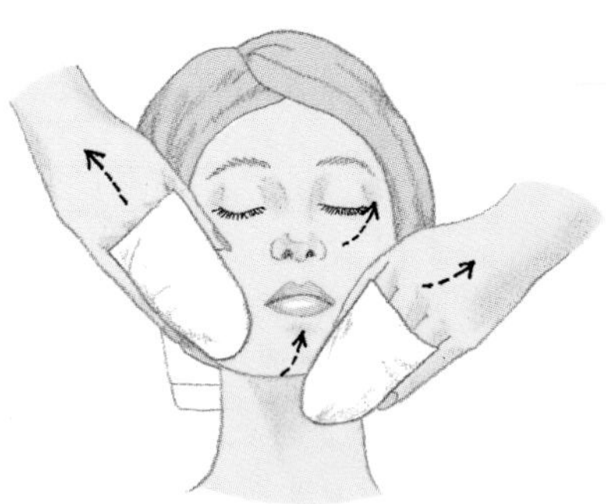

FIGURE 20.2 — Remove the cleanser.

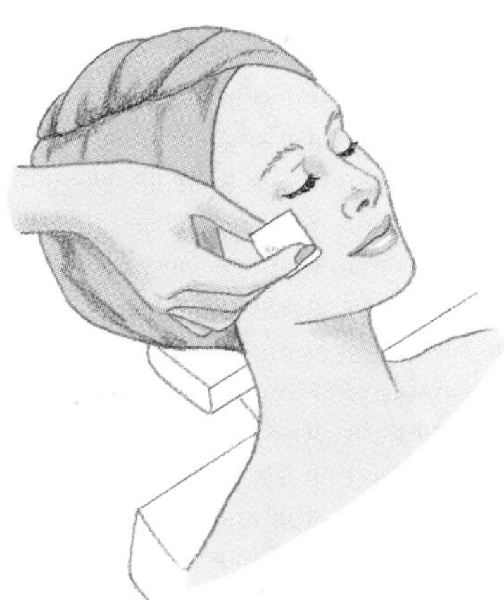

FIGURE 20.3 — Apply astringent lotion or skin freshener.

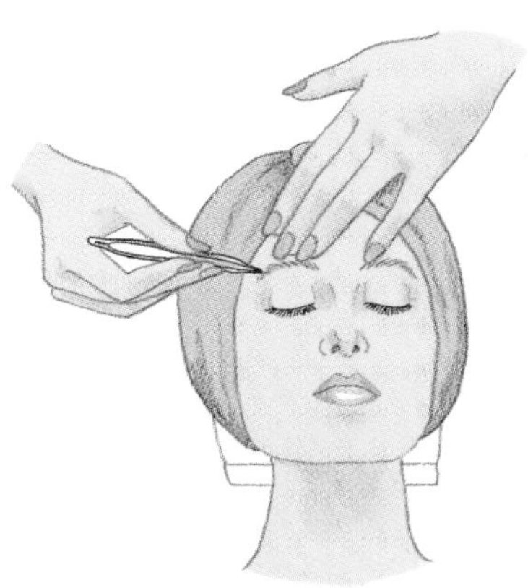

FIGURE 20.4 — Eyebrow arching.

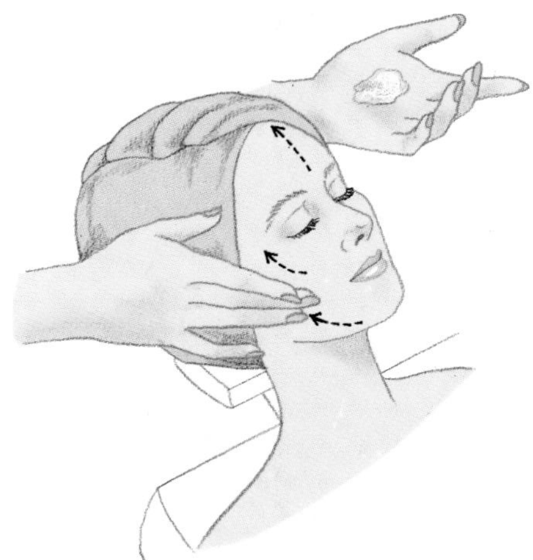

FIGURE 20.5 — Apply foundation.

7. Apply powder. Following the application of foundation, apply powder with a sanitary puff or cosmetic sponge. Press it over the face and whisk off the excess with a puff or powder brush. A moistened cosmetic sponge may be pressed over the finished makeup to give the face a matte look. (Fig. 20.6)

8. Apply cheek color. Cheek color is sometimes applied after the foundation and before powdering. Select the appropriate type and color. Have the client smile, to raise the cheeks. Apply liquid or cream cheek color with a sanitized applicator, and blend upward and outward toward the temples. Powder cheek color is brushed on following the application of powder. Use the same procedure as with a cream or liquid. (Fig. 20.7)

9. Apply corrective makeup, if desired. To minimize a feature, use a darker foundation or contouring makeup. To emphasize

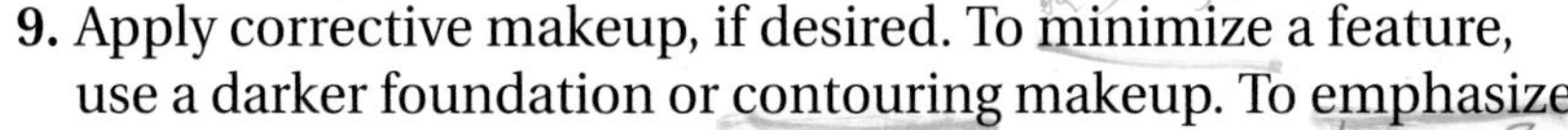

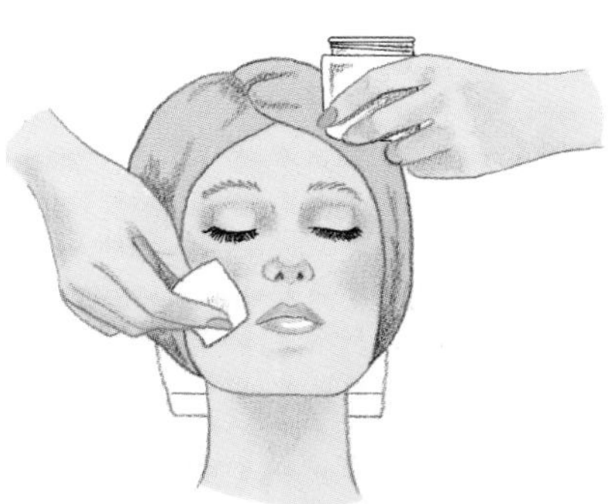

FIGURE 20.6 — Apply powder.

a feature, use a lighter foundation or a highlighting product. See corrective techniques in this chapter.

10. Apply eye color. Select the color to match or complement the eyes. Apply color lightly on the upper lid and softly blend outward with the color applicator or your fingertips. Shade a prominent puffy area beneath the brow, or highlight a small space between the eyelid and brow. (Fig. 20.8)
11. Apply eyeliner. Eyeliner is used to make the eyes look larger and lashes appear thicker. Select cake or liquid liner in a color to harmonize with the mascara you will apply. Pull eyelid taut, and gently draw a very fine line along the entire lid, as close to the lashes as possible. If eyeliner pencil is used, the point should be fine and care should be taken to avoid injury or discomfort to the client. (Fig. 20.9)

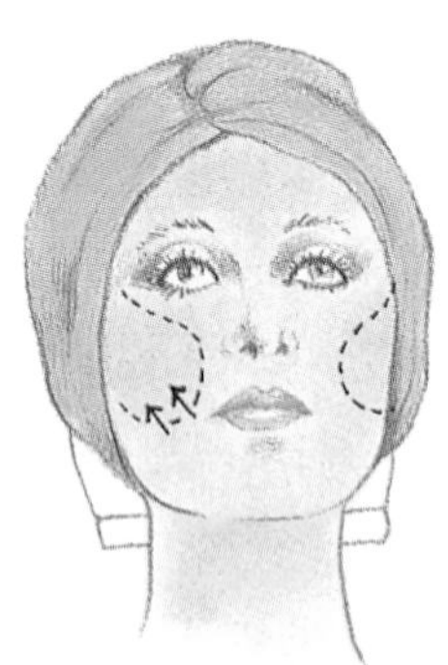

FIGURE 20.7 — Apply cheek color.

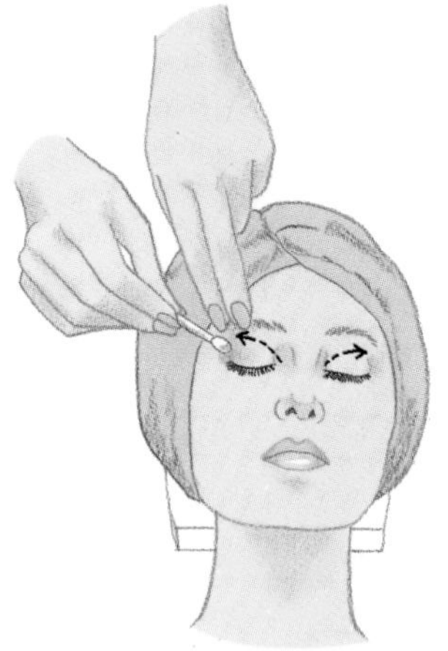

FIGURE 20.8 — Apply eye color.

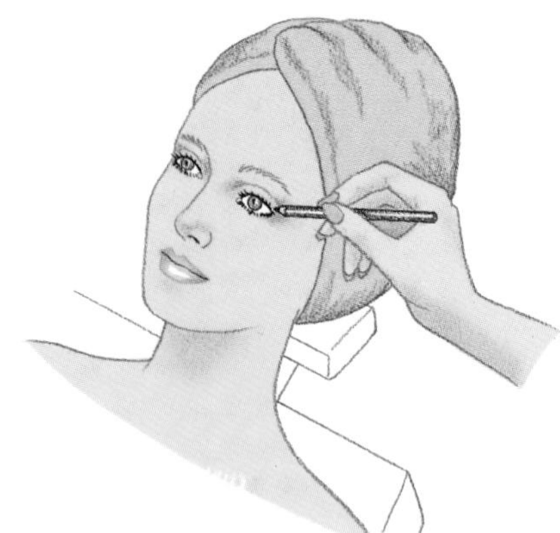

FIGURE 20.9 — Apply eyeliner.

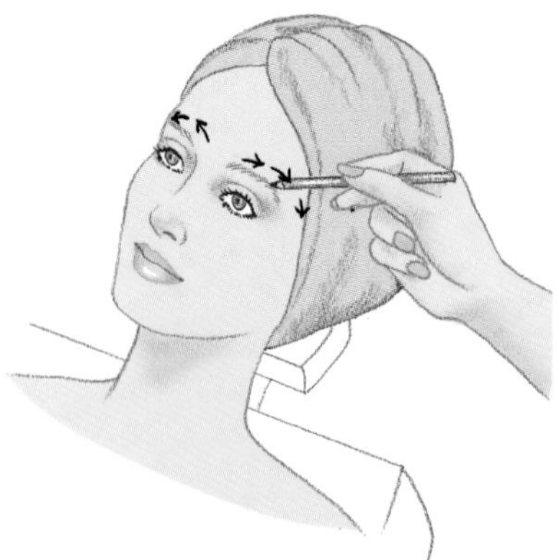

FIGURE 20.10 — Apply eyebrow makeup.

12. Apply eyebrow makeup. Brush the brows in place. With light feathery strokes, apply color with a fine pointed pencil. Brush the brows carefully. Excess color can be removed with a cotton-tipped swab. (Fig. 20.10)
13. Apply mascara to the top and underside of the upper lashes with careful, gentle strokes until the desired effect is achieved. Use a fresh brush or applicator to separate the lashes. Mascara may be applied to lower lashes if desired, but the effect should be subtle. (Fig. 20.11)
14. Apply lip color (lipstick). Lip color is removed from its container with a sanitized spatula. The lips are first outlined with a sanitized applicator such as a brush or pencil. Rest your

ring finger on the client's chin to steady your hand. Ask the client to relax her lips and part them slightly. Brush on the lip color. Ask the client to stretch her lips in a slight smile, to enable you to smooth the lip color in any small crevices. After the lip color application, blot the lips with tissue to remove excess. Blotting will also help to set the lip color. Powdering over the lips is not recommended, because the powder dries the lips and removes the attractive moist look. (Fig. 20.12)

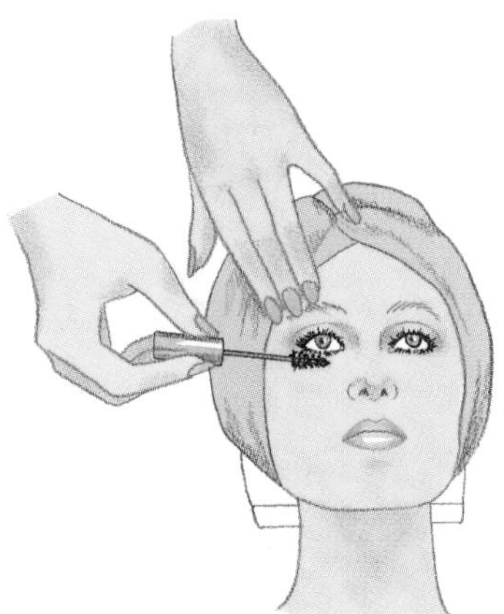

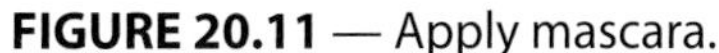

FIGURE 20.11 — Apply mascara.

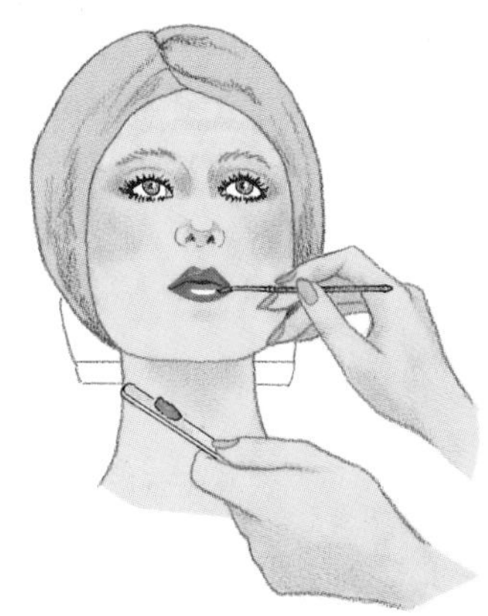

FIGURE 20.12 — Apply lip color.

MAKEUP TECHNIQUES FOR THE MULTICULTURAL CLIENT

When applying makeup to any face, many of the same techniques are used. The skin is analyzed and given a facial for its specific condition, and makeup is selected to enhance the client's skin, eyes, and hair color.

Before applying makeup, thoroughly cleanse the face, use an appropriate astringent, and apply a moisturizer, if needed.

PROCEDURE FOR MAKEUP APPLICATION

1. Choose an appropriate foundation shade and apply evenly. (Figs. 20.13, 20.14)
2. Apply translucent powder. (Fig. 20.15)

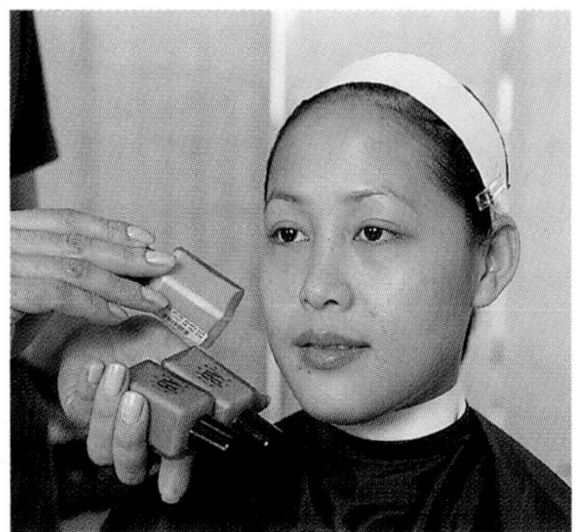

FIGURE 20.13 — Select foundation.

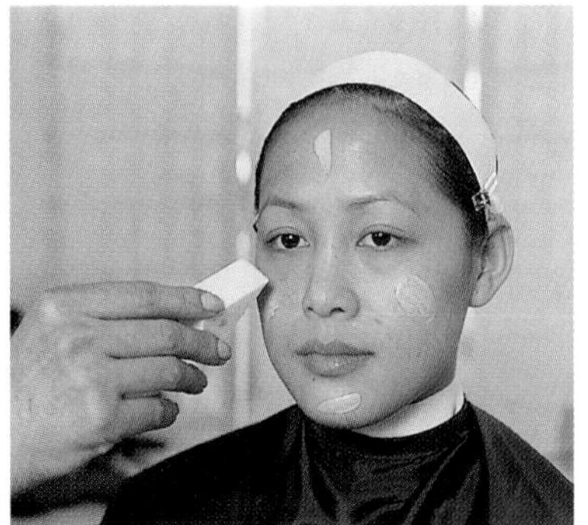

FIGURE 20.14 — Apply foundation.

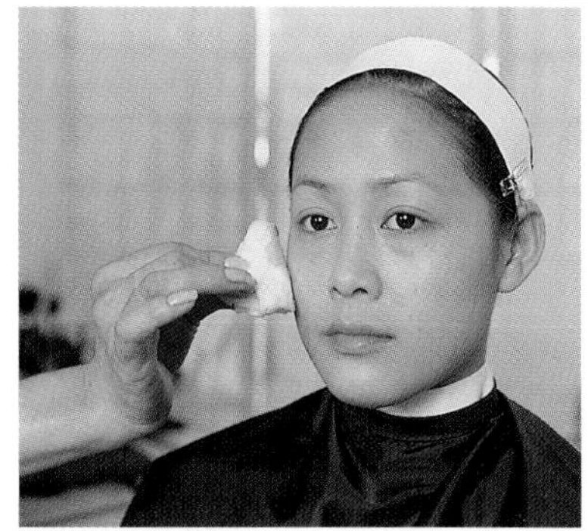

FIGURE 20.15 — Apply translucent powder using a disposable powder puff.

3. Apply a contouring (dark) blusher shade below the cheekbone. (Fig. 20.16) Now, using a lighter cheek color, apply blusher high on the cheekbone. (Fig. 20.17)
4. Apply eye shadow to eyelids and brow bone as desired. (Fig. 20.18)

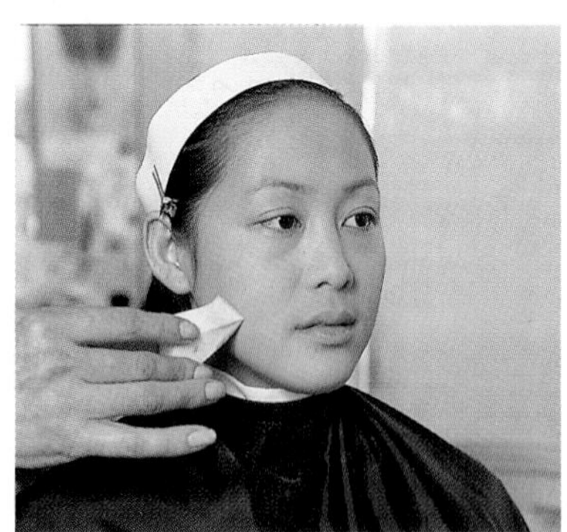

FIGURE 20.16 — Contour with blush.

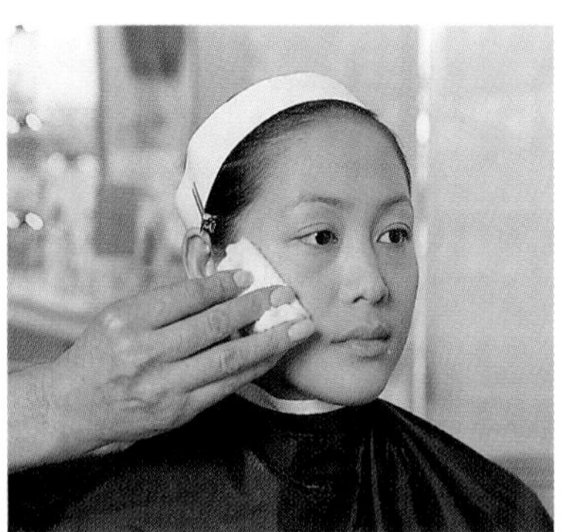

FIGURE 20.17 — Apply blusher.

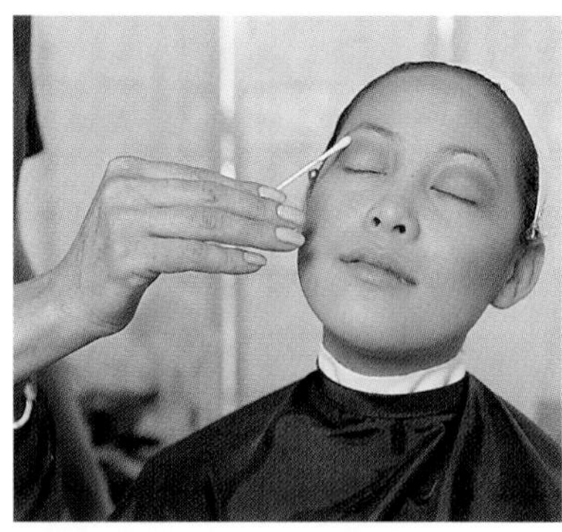

FIGURE 20.18 — Apply eye makeup.

5. Using an eyebrow brush, brush eyebrows and fill in sparse areas with an eyebrow pencil or brush. (Figs. 20.19, 20.20)
6. Line the eyes with an eyeliner pencil from the outer corner in toward the nose. (Fig. 20.21)
7. Apply mascara to top lashes, and then to bottom lashes. (Figs. 20.22, 20.23)
8. Line and fill lips with lip color. (Figs. 20.24, 20.25)
9. Complement a makeup application with hairstyle, clothing, and accessories. (Fig. 20.26)

Completed:
Learning Objective
#2
CORRECT MAKEUP APPLICATION PROCEDURES

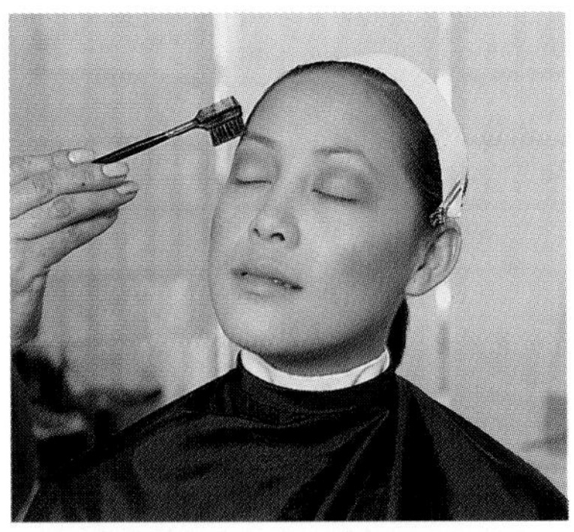
FIGURE 20.19 — Brush eyebrow.

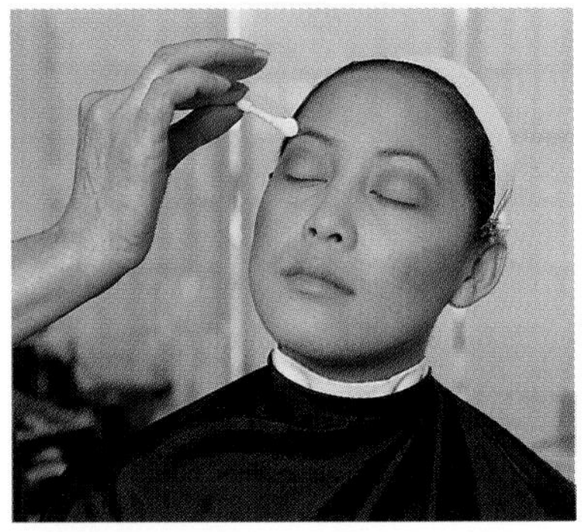
FIGURE 20.20 — Fill in eyebrows.

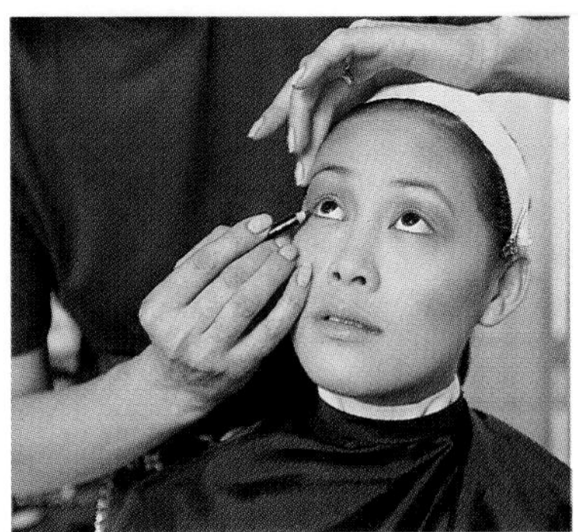
FIGURE 20.21 — Line eyes.

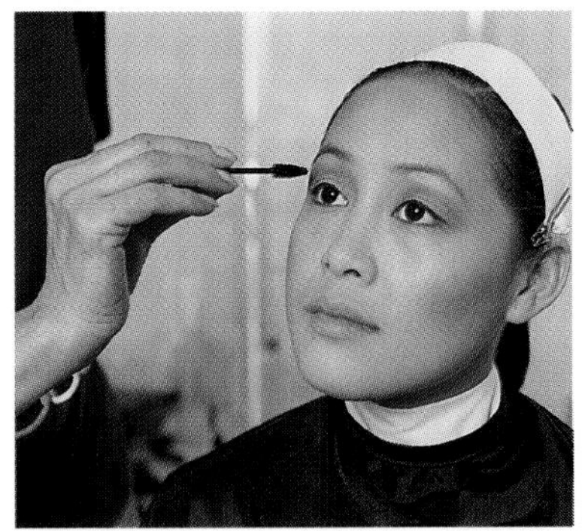
FIGURE 20.22 — Apply mascara to top lashes.

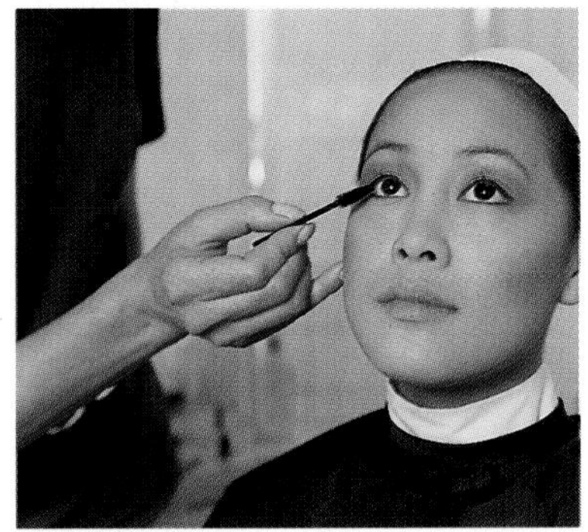
FIGURE 20.23 — Apply mascara to bottom lashes.

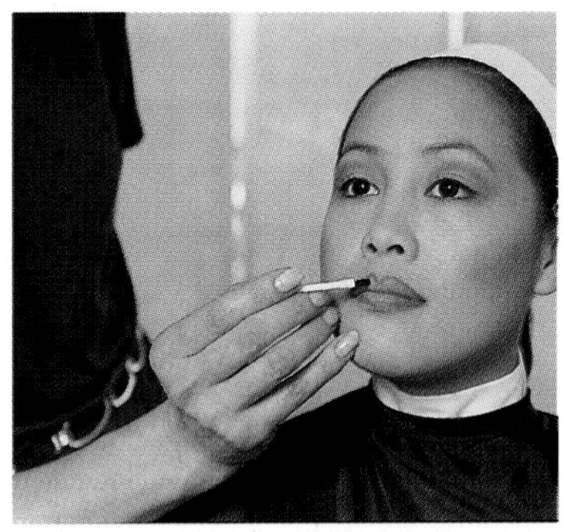
FIGURE 20.24 — Line lips.

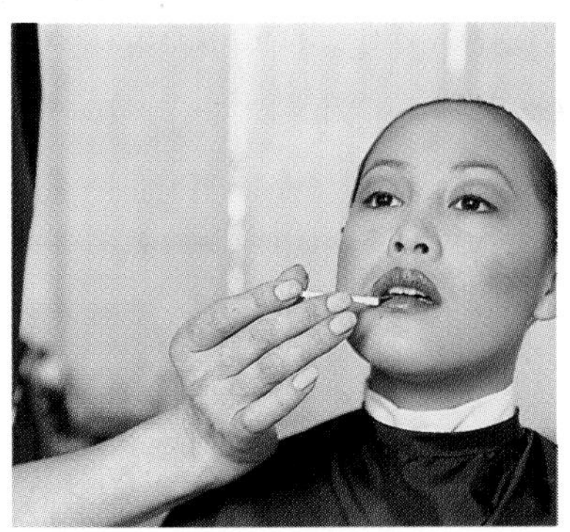
FIGURE 20.25 — Apply lip color.

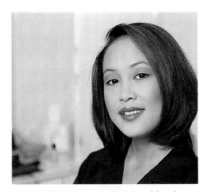

FIGURE 20.26 — Finished look.

FACIAL FEATURES

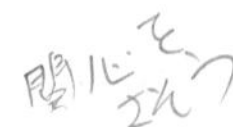

Faces are interesting, but few are perfect. When you analyze a client's face, you might see that the nose, cheeks, lips, or jawline are not the same on both sides, or that one eye might be larger than the other, and the eyebrows may not match. However, these subtle imperfections can make the face more interesting. Facial makeup can create the illusion of better balance and proportion when desired.

ANALYZING THE CLIENT'S FACIAL FEATURES AND FACE SHAPE

When applying makeup it is important to emphasize the client's attractive features while minimizing features that are out of proportion or unattractive in relation to the rest of the face. Learning to see the face and its features and to determine the best makeup for the individual takes practice. You might have an unsteady hand at first, especially when working with eye and lip colors. However, diligent practice and experience are the best ways to become proficient. The oval face with well-proportioned features has long been considered to be the ideal shape, but all face shapes are attractive when makeup is applied properly. What counts most is that the client's individuality is enhanced.

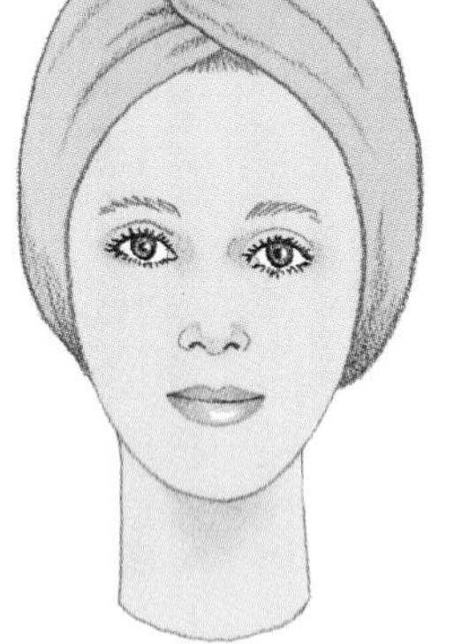

FIGURE 20.27 — The oval face.

CORRECTIVE MAKEUP TECHNIQUES

It is difficult to provide set rules for cheek color application because each person's facial structures are different. In addition, facial features as well as the shape of the face must be taken into consideration.

Oval-Shaped Face

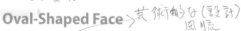

The artistically ideal proportions and features of the oval face are used to form the basis for corrective makeup application. The face is divided into three equal horizontal sections. The first third is measured from the hairline to the point between the eyebrows where they begin. The second third is measured from here to the end of the nose. The last third is measured from the end of the nose to the bottom of the chin.

The ideal oval face is approximately three-fourths as wide as it is long. The distance between the eyes is the width of one eye. (Figs. 20.27, 20.28)

The following suggestions can serve as a guide to face shapes and cheek color application.

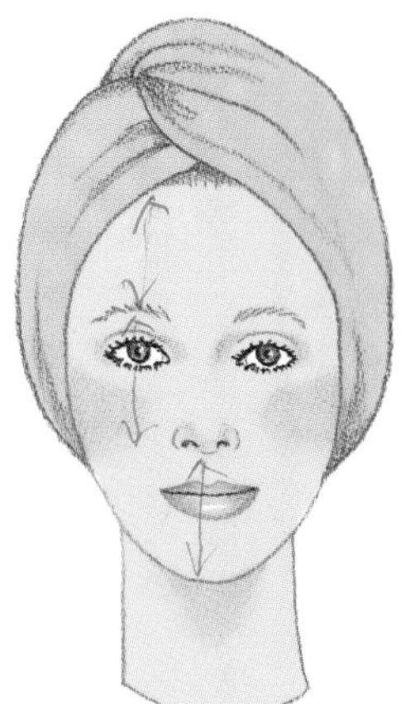

FIGURE 20.28 — Oval face with makeup applied.

Round-Shaped Face

The round face is usually broader in proportion to its length than the oval face. It has a rounding chin and hairline. Corrective makeup can be applied to slenderize and lengthen the face. (Figs. 20.29, 20.30)

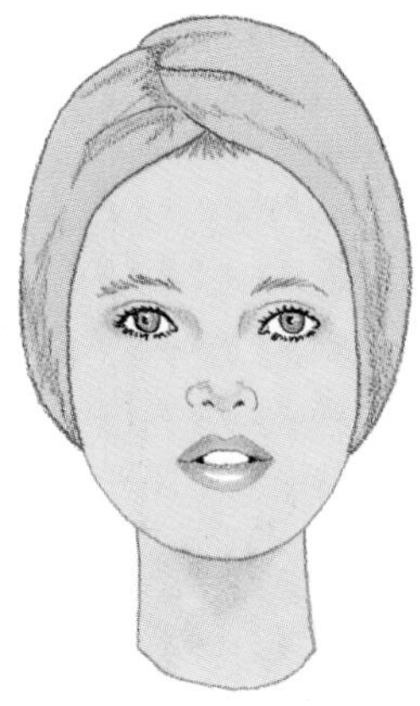

FIGURE 20.29 — The round face.

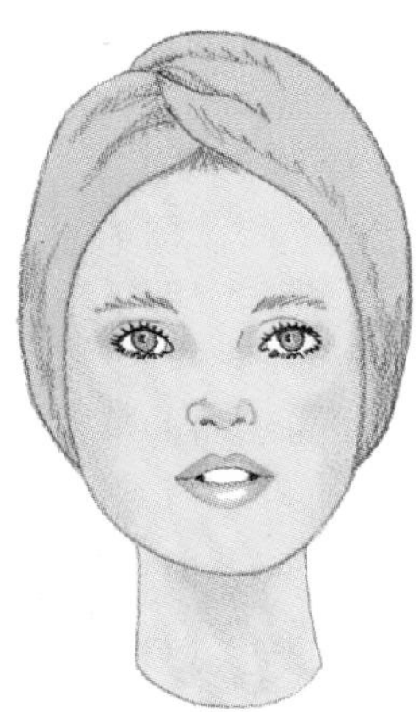

FIGURE 20.30 — Round face with corrective makeup.

Square-Shaped Face

The square face is composed of comparatively straight lines with a wide forehead and square jawline. Corrective makeup can be applied to offset the squareness and soften the hard lines around the face. (Figs. 20.31, 20.32)

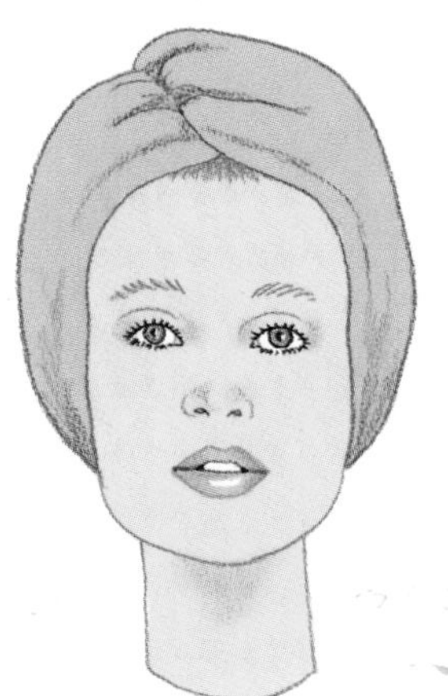

FIGURE 20.31 — The square face.

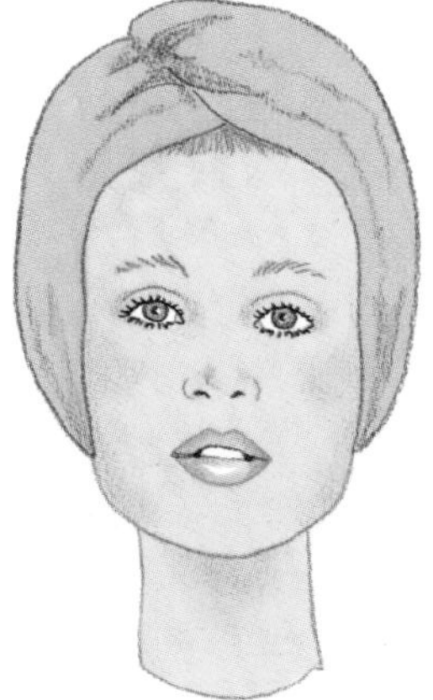

FIGURE 20.32 — Square face with corrective makeup.

Pear-Shaped Face

This face is characterized by a jaw that is wider than the forehead. Corrective makeup can be applied to create width at the forehead, to slenderize the jawline, and to add length to the face. (Figs. 20.33, 20.34)

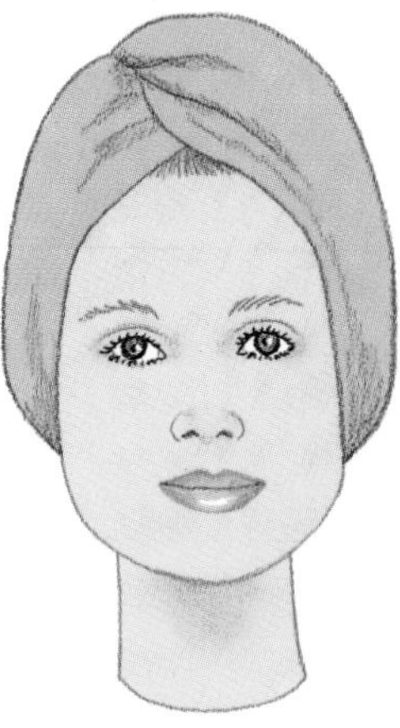

FIGURE 20.33 — The pear-shaped face.

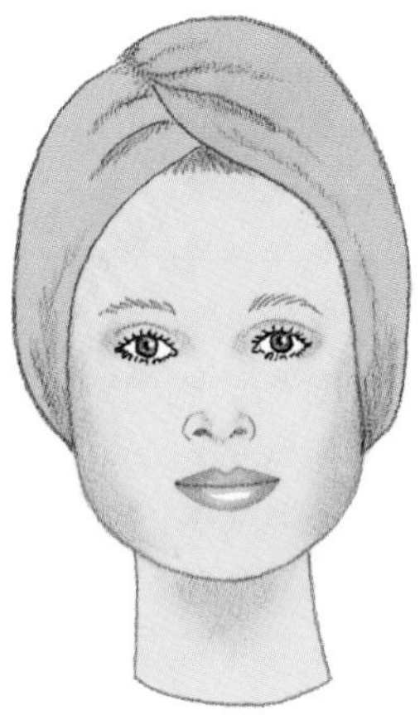

FIGURE 20.34 — Pear-shaped face with corrective makeup.

Heart-Shaped Face

The heart-shaped face has a wide forehead and narrow, pointed chin. Corrective makeup can be applied to minimize the width of the forehead and to increase the width of the jawline. (Figs. 20.35, 20.36)

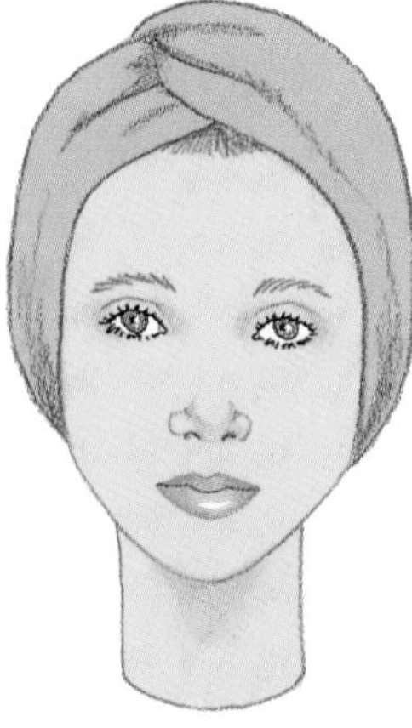

FIGURE 20.35 — The heart-shaped face.

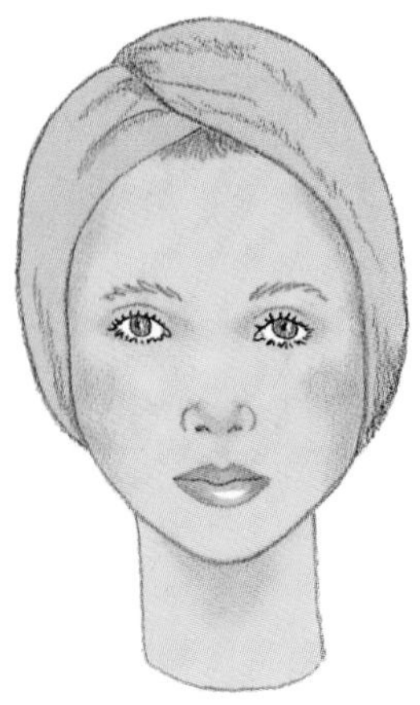

FIGURE 20.36 — Heart-shaped face with corrective makeup.

Diamond-Shaped Face

This face has a narrow forehead. The greatest width is across the cheekbones. Corrective makeup can be applied to reduce the width across the cheekbone line. (Figs. 20.37, 20.38)

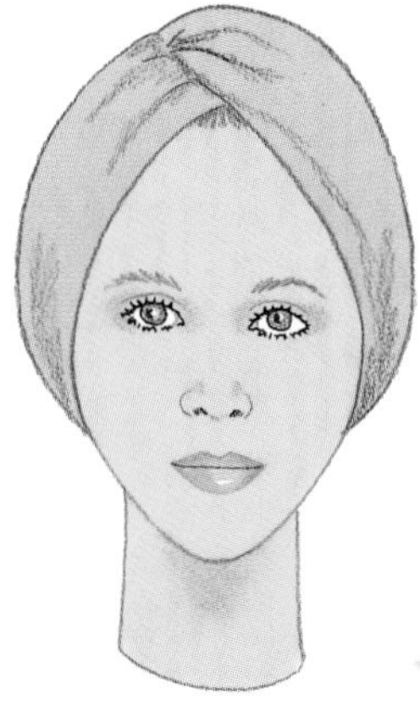

FIGURE 20.37 — The diamond-shaped face.

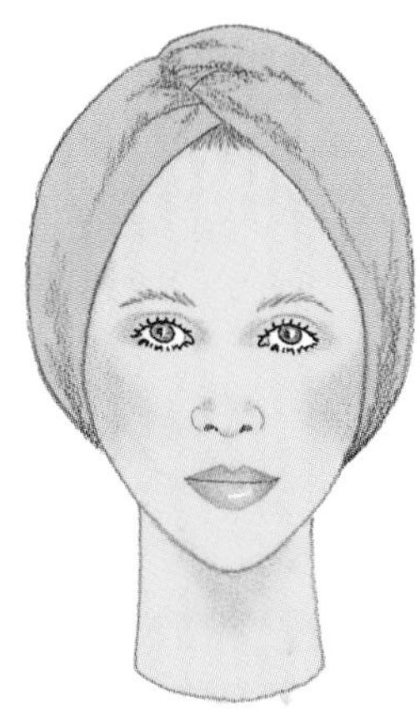

FIGURE 20.38 — Diamond-shaped face with corrective makeup.

Oblong-Shaped Face

This face has greater length in proportion to its width than the square or round face. It is long and narrow. Corrective makeup can be applied to create the illusion of width across the cheekbone line, making the face appear shorter. (Figs. 20.39, 20.40)

Completed:
Learning Objective
#3
IDENTIFYING DIFFERENT FACIAL TYPES

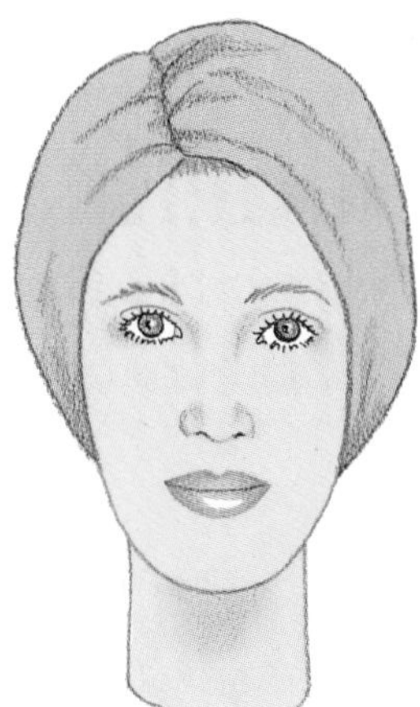

FIGURE 20.39 — The oblong-shaped face.

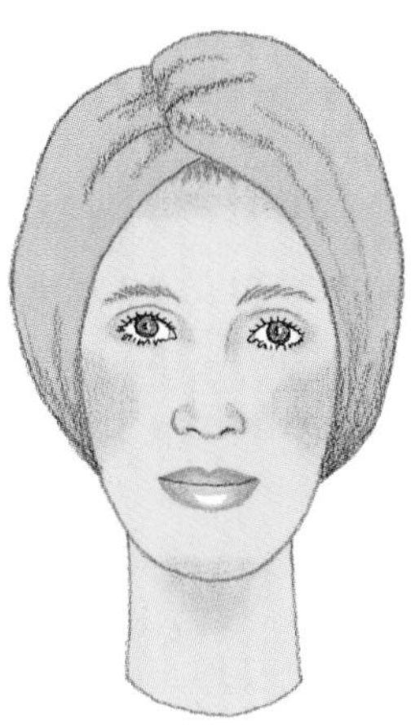

FIGURE 20.40 — Oblong-shaped face with corrective makeup.

TIPS FOR APPLYING CHEEK COLOR

Cheek color accents the part of the face where it is applied. The following are general rules for cheek color application:

1. Apply cheek color where natural color would normally appear in the cheeks. Do not apply the color in toward the nose beyond the center of the eye.
2. Keep color above the horizontal line at the tip of the nose.
3. Do not extend color above the outer corner of the eye.
4. Never apply color in a bright, round circle. Blend the color so that it fades softly into the foundation.

BASIC RULES FOR APPLYING CORRECTIVE BASE MAKEUP

The primary objective of corrective makeup is to minimize unattractive features and accent good features. Facial features can be accented with proper highlighting, subdued with correct shadowing or shading, and balanced with the proper hairstyle.

A basic rule for the application of makeup is that highlighting emphasizes a feature, while shadowing minimizes it. A highlight is produced when a shade lighter than the original foundation is used on a particular part of the face. A shadow is formed when the foundation used is darker than the original color. The use of shadows (dark colors and shades) minimizes or subdues prominent features so that they are less noticeable.

When two shades of foundations are used, care must be taken to blend them properly so that there will be no line of demarcation. Color harmony can be achieved when the makeup tones flatter the color of the client's eyes, hair, and skin. To determine what is best for each client, you must:

1. Analyze the color of the client's skin, hair, and eyes.
2. Examine the front and profile views of the facial features.
3. Select and apply those makeup highlights and/or shades that will produce the desired results.

Concealing Wrinkles with Foundation Cream

Age lines and wrinkles due to dry skin can be concealed with foundation cream. It should be used sparingly. Apply foundation cream evenly, in a light outward circular motion over the entire surface of the face. Care should be taken to remove any foundation cream that collects in lines and wrinkles of the face.

Corrective Makeup for Forehead

For a low forehead, applying a lighter foundation cream gives it a broader appearance between the brows and hairline. For a bulging forehead, applying a darker foundation over the prominent area gives an illusion of fullness to the rest of the face and minimizes the bulging forehead. With a suitable hairstyle, attention can be drawn away from the forehead. (Fig. 20.41)

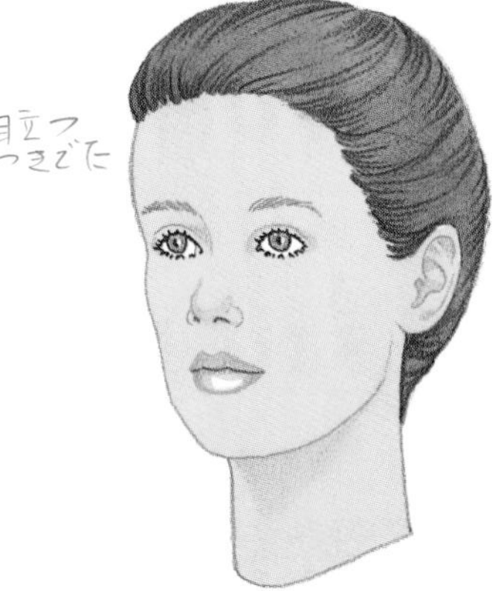

FIGURE 20.41 — Protruding forehead.

Corrective Makeup for Nose and Chin

For a *large or protruding nose*, apply a darker foundation on the nose and a lighter foundation on the cheeks at the sides of the nose. This will create fullness in the cheeks and make the nose appear smaller. Avoid placing the cheek color close to the nose.

For a *short and flat nose*, apply a lighter foundation down the center of the nose, stopping at the tip. This will make the nose appear longer and larger. If the nostrils are wide, apply a darker foundation to both sides of the nostrils. (Fig. 20.42)

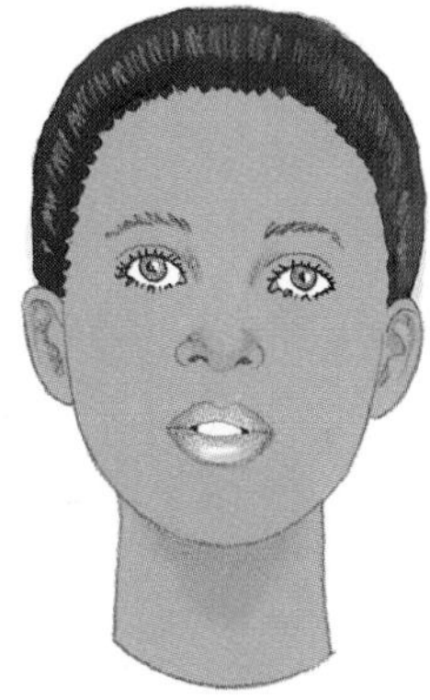

FIGURE 20.42 — Short flat nose.

For a *broad nose*, use a darker foundation on the sides of the nose and nostrils. Avoid carrying this dark tone into the laugh lines because it will accentuate them. The foundation must be carefully blended to avoid visible lines. (Fig. 20.43)

For a *protruding chin and receding nose*, shadow the chin with a darker foundation and highlight the nose with a lighter foundation.

For a *receding (small) chin*, highlight the chin by using a lighter foundation than the one used on the face. (Fig. 20.44)

For a *sagging double chin*, use a darker foundation on the sagging portion, and use a natural skin tone foundation on the face. (Fig. 20.45)

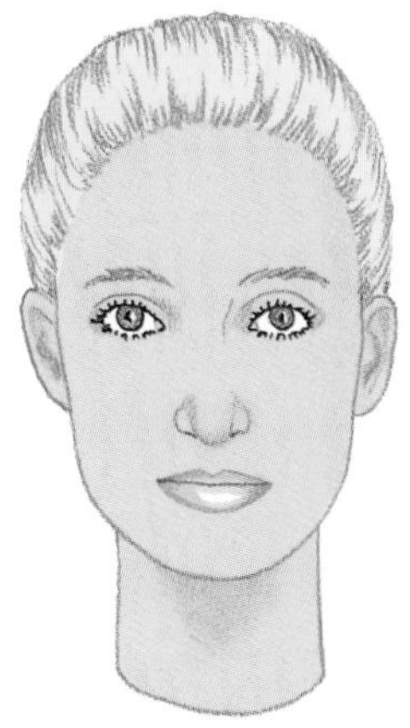

FIGURE 20.43 — Broad nose.

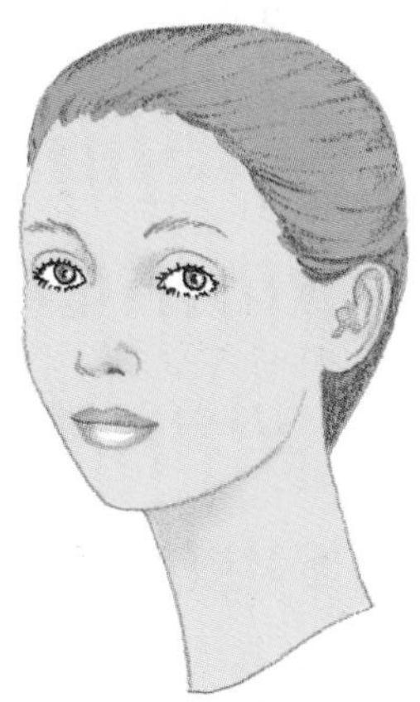

FIGURE 20.44 — Receding chin.

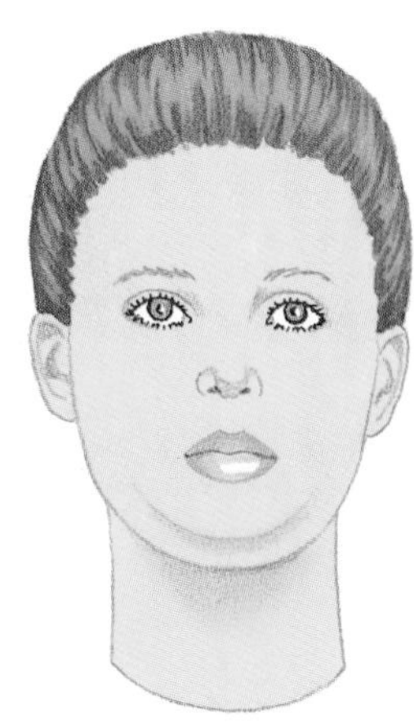

FIGURE 20.45 — Double chin.

Corrective Makeup for Jawline and Neck

The neck and jaw are just as important as the eyes, cheeks, and lips. When applying makeup, carry the foundation cream down below the neckline of the client's clothing to prevent the appearance of a line of demarcation.

To correct a *broad jawline*, apply a darker shade of foundation over the heavy area of the jaw, starting at the temples. This will minimize the lower part of the face and create an illusion of width in the upper part of the face. (Fig. 20.46)

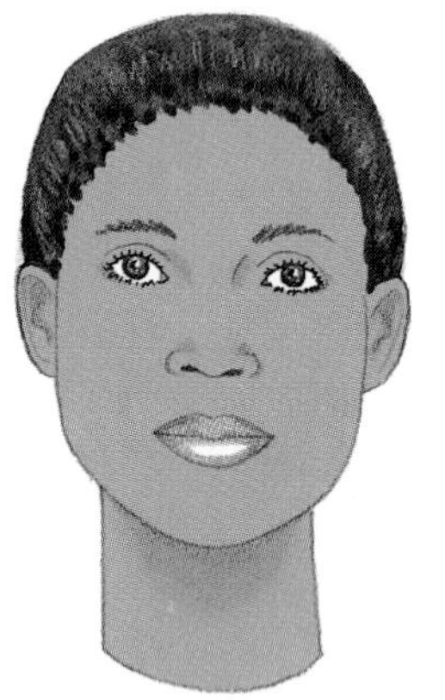

FIGURE 20.46 — Broad jawline.

A *narrow jawline* may be highlighted by using a lighter shade foundation than the one used on the rest of the face. (Fig. 20.47)

For a *round, square, or triangular face*, apply a darker shade of foundation over the prominent area of the jawline. By creating a shadow over this area, the prominent part of the jaw will appear softer and more oval.

For a *small face and a short and thick neck*, use a darker foundation on the neck than the one used on the face. This will make the neck appear thinner.

For a *long, thin neck*, apply a lighter shade foundation on the neck than the one used on the face. This will create fullness and counteract the long, thin appearance of the neck. (Fig. 20.48)

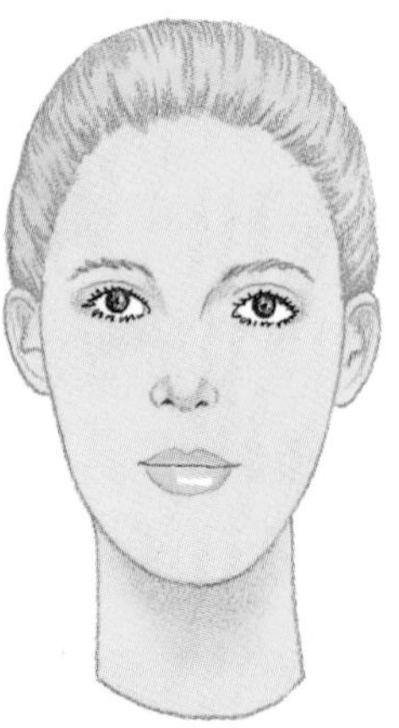

FIGURE 20.47 — Narrow jawline.

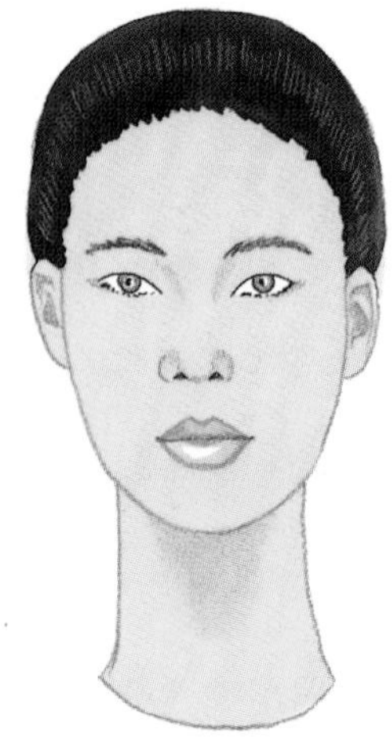

FIGURE 20.48 — Long, thin neck.

Corrective Makeup for Eyes

The eyes are very important features of correct facial balance. Applying eye colors and shadows properly can create the illusion of the eyes being larger or smaller, and enhance the overall attractiveness of the face.

Round eyes can be lengthened by extending the shadow beyond the outer corner of the eyes. (Figs. 20.49, 20.50)

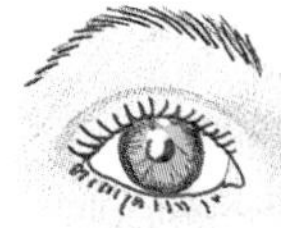
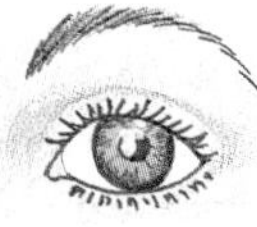

FIGURE 20.49 — Round eyes.

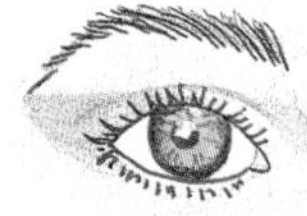
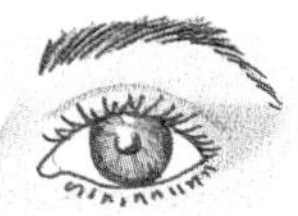

FIGURE 20.50 — Round eyes with corrective makeup.

Close-set eyes. For eyes that are set too close together, apply shadow lightly up from the outer edge of the eyes. (Figs. 20.51, 20.52)

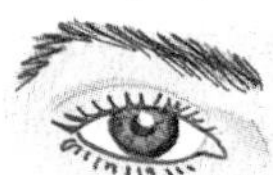
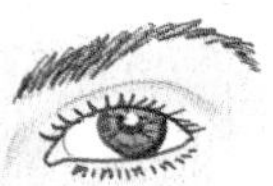

FIGURE 20.51 — Close-set eyes.

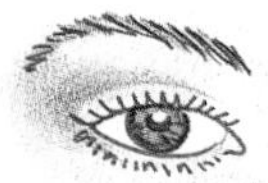
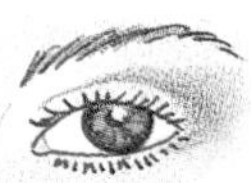

FIGURE 20.52 — Close-set eyes with corrective makeup.

Bulging eyes can be minimized by blending the shadow carefully over the prominent part of the upper lid, carrying it lightly to the line of the brow. Use dark shadow as in the illustration. (Figs. 20.53, 20.54)

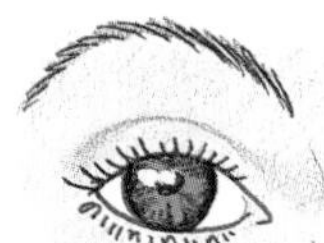
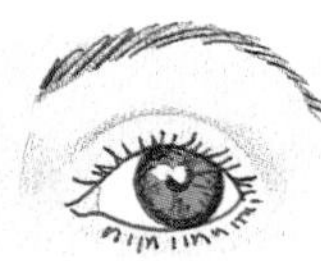

FIGURE 20.53 — Bulging eyes.

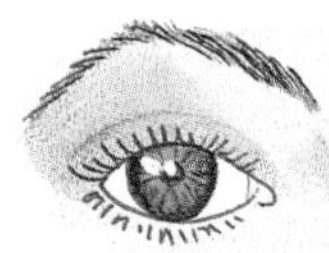
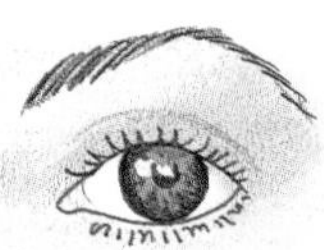

FIGURE 20.54 — Bulging eyes with corrective makeup.

Heavy-lidded eyes. Shadow evenly and lightly across the lid from the edge of the eyelash line to the small crease in the eye socket as in the illustration. (Figs. 20.55, 20.56)

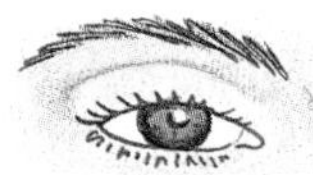
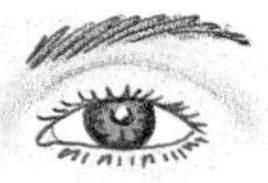

FIGURE 20.55 — Heavy-lidded eyes.

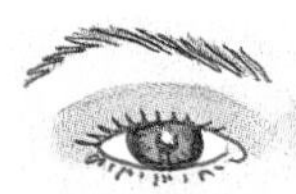
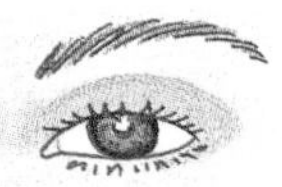

FIGURE 20.56 — Heavy-lidded eyes with corrective makeup.

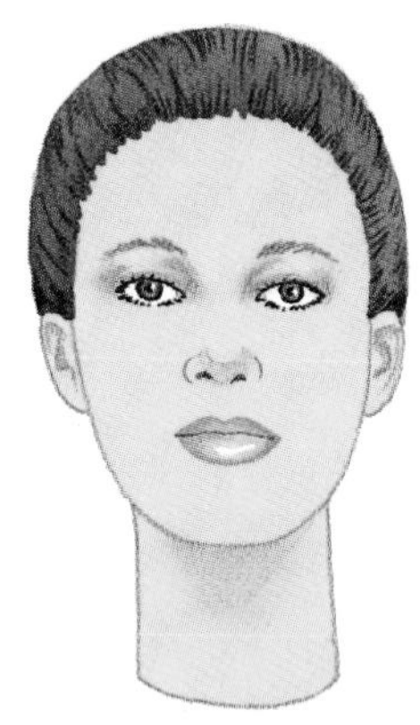

FIGURE 20.57 — Deep-sunken eyes.

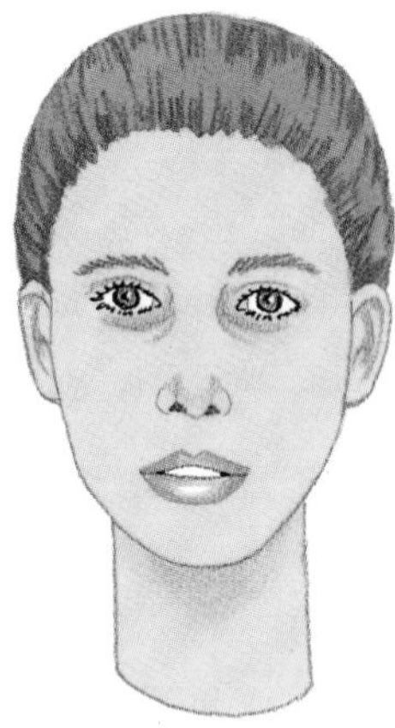

FIGURE 20.58 — Dark circles under eyes.

Small eyes. To make small eyes appear large, extend the shadow slightly above, beyond, and below the eyes.

Eyes set too far apart. When eyes are set too far apart, use the shadow on the upper inner side of the eyelid.

Deep-sunken eyes. Use very little shadow on the lids nearest the temples and leave untouched the part next to the nose and inner corner of the eyes. (Fig. 20.57)

Dark circles under eyes. Apply a lighter foundation cream over the dark area, blending and smoothing it into the surrounding area. (Fig. 20.58)

THE USE OF THE EYEBROW PENCIL

When a client wants to correct misshaped eyebrows, remove all unnecessary hairs and then demonstrate how to use the eyebrow pencil to draw short hair-like lines in the brows until the natural hairs have grown in again. When there are spaces in the brow devoid of hair, they can be filled in with hair-like strokes of an eyebrow pencil. Use an eyebrow brush to soften the pencil marks. (Figs. 20.59–20.62)

When the arch is too high, remove the superfluous hair from the top of the brow and fill in the lower part with eyebrow pencil. When the arch is too low, remove the superfluous hair from the lower part of the brow and build up the shape of the brow using the eyebrow pencil.

In the case of a high forehead, the eyebrow arch may be slightly elevated to detract from a high forehead. Avoid a too thin, too round line. This gives the client a "surprised" look.

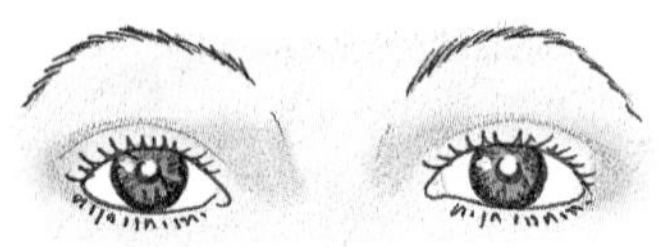

FIGURE 20.59 — Thin eyebrows.

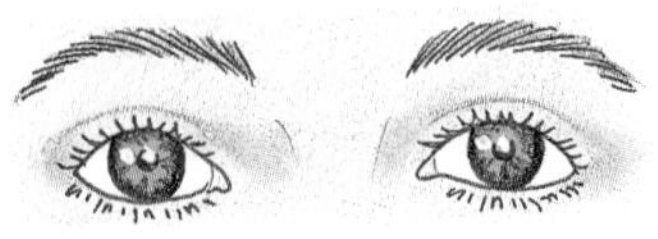

FIGURE 20.60 — Corrective technique for thin eyebrows.

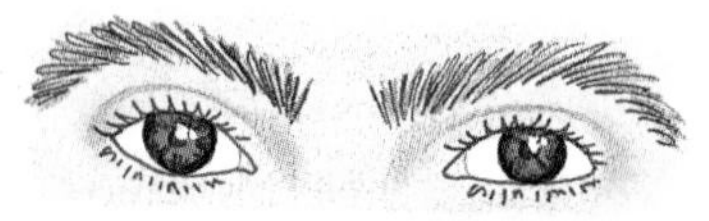

FIGURE 20.61 — Thick eyebrows.

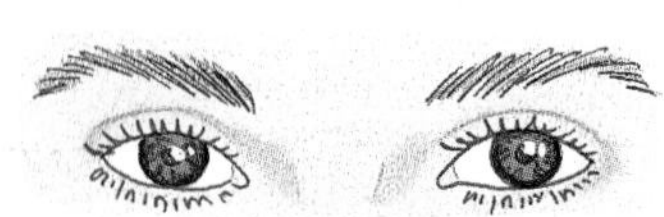

FIGURE 20.62 — Corrective technique for thick eyebrows.

Corrective Placing and Shaping of the Eyebrows

Low forehead. A low arch gives more height to a very low forehead.

Wide-set eyes. The eyes can be made to appear closer together by extending the eyebrow lines to the inside corners of the eyes. However, care must be taken to avoid giving the client a frowning look.

Close-set eyes. To make the eyes appear farther apart, widen the distance between the eyebrows; also slightly extend the brows outward.

Round face. Arch the brows high to make the face appear narrower. Start on a line directly above the inside corner of the eye and extend to the end of the cheekbone.

Long face. The illusion of a shorter face can be created by making the eyebrows almost straight. Do not extend the eyebrow lines farther than the outside corners of the eyes.

Triangular face. To offset a narrow forehead, arch the eyebrows slightly on the ends only. Start the lines directly above the inside corners of the eyes and continue to the ends of the cheekbones.

Square face. The face will appear more oval if there is a high arch on the ends of the eyebrows. Begin the lines directly above the corners of the eyes and extend them outward.

EYEBROW ARCHING

Correctly shaped eyebrows have a marked effect on the attractiveness of the face. The natural arch of the eyebrow follows the bony structure or the curved line of the ***orbit*** (eye socket). Most people have a disorderly growth of hairs both above and below the natural line. These hairs should be removed to give a clean and attractive appearance.

Because of the sensitivity of the skin around the eyes, some clients cannot tolerate tweezing. For them, shaving or a wax depilatory may be used. You will find a discussion of wax depilatory in the chapter on removing unwanted hair.

Implements, Supplies, and Materials

Emollient cream	Eyebrow brush	Astringent lotion
Cotton pledgets	Towels	Antiseptic lotion
Cleansing tissue	Tweezers	Eyebrow pencil

Procedure

1. Seat the client in a facial chair in a reclining position, as for a facial massage. Or, if you prefer, seat the client in a half-upright position and work from the side.
2. Discuss with the client the type of eyebrow arch suitable for that person's facial characteristics.

3. Cover the client's eyes with cotton pledgets moistened with witch hazel or a mild astringent.
4. Brush the eyebrows with a small brush to remove any powder or scaliness.
5. Soften brows. Saturate two pledgets of cotton or a towel with hot water and place over the brows. Allow them to remain on the brows long enough to soften and relax the eyebrow tissue. Brows and surrounding skin may be softened by rubbing emollient cream into them.
6. Remove the hairs between the brows. When tweezing, stretch the skin taut with the index finger and thumb (or index and middle finger) of the left hand. Grasp each hair individually with tweezers and pull with a quick motion in the direction in which the hair grows. (Fig. 20.63) Sponge the tweezed area frequently with cotton moistened with an antiseptic lotion to avoid infection. Hairs between the brows and above the brow line are tweezed first, because the area under the brow line is much more sensitive.
7. Remove hairs from above the eyebrow line. Brush the hair downward. Shape the upper section of one eyebrow; then shape the other. Frequently sponge the area with antiseptic. (Fig. 20.64)

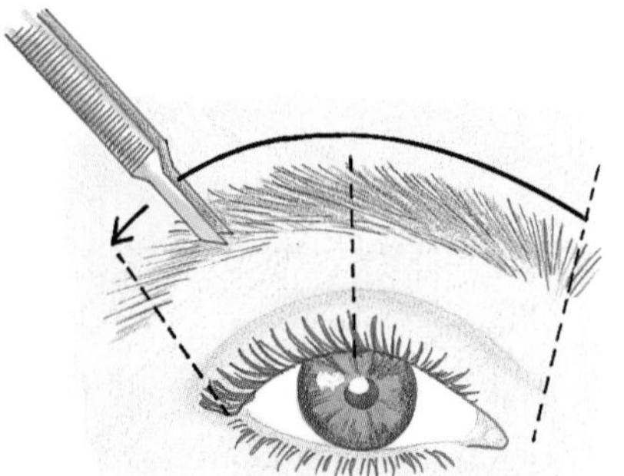

FIGURE 20.63 — Remove hair in this direction.

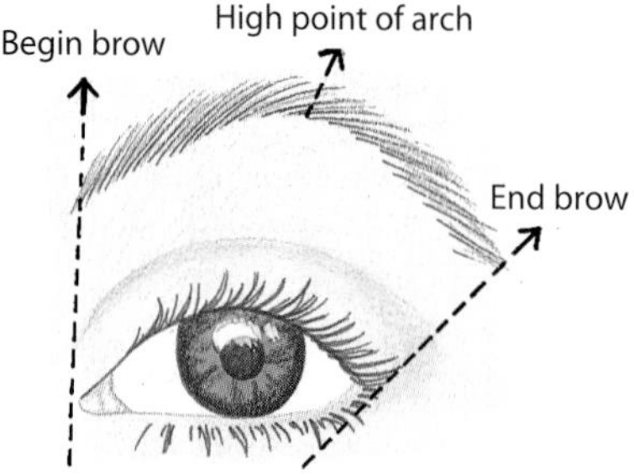

FIGURE 20.64 — Correct points for eyebrow arching.

8. Remove hairs from under the eyebrow line. Brush the hairs upward. Shape the lower section of one eyebrow; then shape the other. Sponge the area with antiseptic. (*Optional:* Apply emollient cream and massage brows. Remove cream with tissues.)
9. After the tweezing is completed, sponge the brows and surrounding skin with astringent to contract the skin.
10. Brush the brows, placing the hair in its normal position. Use an eyebrow pencil where necessary. The eyebrows should be treated about once a week.

CORRECTIVE MAKEUP FOR LIPS

Lips are usually proportioned so that the curves or peaks of the upper lip fall directly in line with the nostrils. (Fig. 20.65) In some cases, one side of the lips may differ from the other. Lips can be very full, very thin, or uneven. The following illustrations show various lip lines and how lip color can be used to create the illusion of better proportions. (Figs. 20.66–20.74)

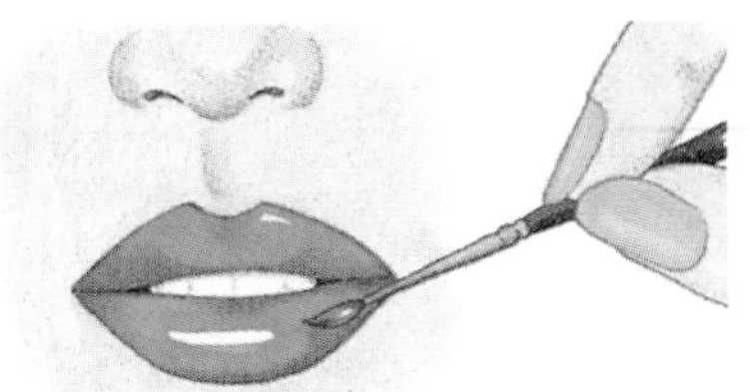

FIGURE 20.65 — Lip color application.

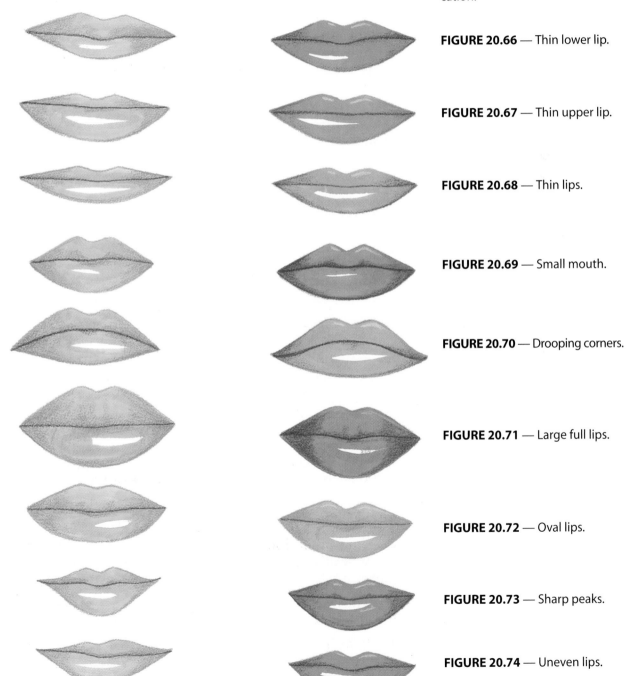

FIGURE 20.66 — Thin lower lip.

FIGURE 20.67 — Thin upper lip.

FIGURE 20.68 — Thin lips.

FIGURE 20.69 — Small mouth.

FIGURE 20.70 — Drooping corners.

FIGURE 20.71 — Large full lips.

FIGURE 20.72 — Oval lips.

FIGURE 20.73 — Sharp peaks.

FIGURE 20.74 — Uneven lips.

LASH AND BROW TINT

An aniline derivative tint should never be used for coloring eyebrows or eyelashes; to do so can cause blindness. Instead a harmless coloring agent can be used that usually consists of two solutions: one that allows the lashes to accept color and the other to deposit color. To temporarily color the lashes, mascara can be used.

The choice of color is limited to either brown or black. Although black is favored in most cases, brown is recommended for very light complexions with blonde hair. Follow the specific directions of the manufacturer when applying the coloring agent.

Materials and Implements

Petroleum jelly (Vaseline)
Lash and brow tinting solutions (solutions No. 1 and No. 2—Roux's Lash & Brow Tint Kit)
Stain remover
Dish of warm, soapy water
Dish of clear, cool water
Towels
Cotton
Paper eye shields
Applicator sticks and eye pads

Preparation

1. Follow sanitary measures.
2. Place the client in a partially reclining position in a facial or shampoo chair at approximately a 45° (.785 rad.) angle. Do not permit the client to lie in a straight position, because the tinting solution can enter the eyes more easily.

Procedure

1. Wash the lashes and brows with warm, soapy water, using a cotton pledget, and remove all traces of makeup.
2. Apply petroleum jelly below the lower lashes and place paper eye shields as close to the lower lashes as possible. These shields will protect the skin from stains.
3. Adjust the eye shields. Ask the client to look up, adjust the shield, and close the eye gently. Do the same with the other eye.
4. Apply the No. 1 solution to the lashes. Moisten a cotton-tipped applicator. Touch the tip to a towel to remove excess moisture. Apply over and under the lashes close to the skin. Moisten the lashes several times. Break the applicator stick and discard. Use a fresh applicator stick each time the solution is applied.

5. Apply the No. 1 solution to brows, following the natural brow line. Reapply against the natural growth, working the solution in thoroughly. Replace the cap on the No. 1 solution bottle. (If bottle caps are interchanged, oxidation starts and the liquids lose their value.) Moisten a fresh applicator with a stain remover and place it on the edge of the towel for future use. Replace the cap on the stain remover bottle.
6. Apply the No. 2 solution to lashes and brows in the same manner as the No. 1 solution. If stain gets on the skin, use stain remover immediately. Replace the cap on the No. 2 bottle.
7. Remove the eye shields and wash the lashes and brows with cool water, using cotton pledgets.
8. Place moist eye pads over the eyelids. Rewash the brows with soap and water, then remove eye pads. Place a small roll of cotton under the lashes and wash them from above with cool water.
9. Remove any stains with stain remover. Replace the bottle cap.
10. Soothe the skin with lotion or cream. Wash the eyes with a boric acid solution.
11. Clean up in the usual manner. ✓

Completed:
Learning Objective
#4
BASIC CORRECTIVE MAKEUP PROCEDURES

ARTIFICIAL EYELASHES

There are a number of reasons a client might want to wear artificial lashes. She might want to wear them for some special occasion because they enhance the eyes, making them appear larger and more expressive, or she might have extremely sparse eyelashes and want them to appear fuller and more natural. (Figs. 20.75, 20.76)

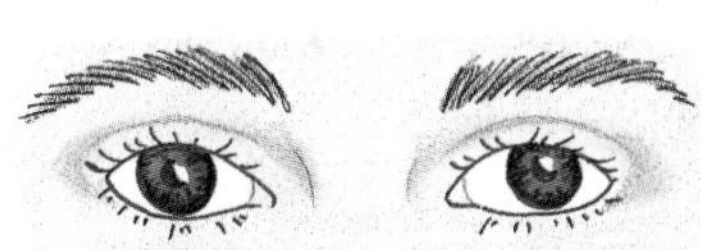

FIGURE 20.75 — Sparse eyelashes.

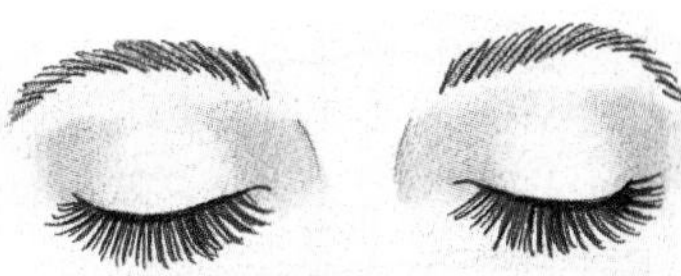

FIGURE 20.76 — False eyelashes attached.

Two basic types of artificial (false) eyelashes are in general use:

1. Strip eyelashes
2. Semi-permanent individual eyelashes (eye tabbing)

APPLYING STRIP EYELASHES

Strip eyelashes are available in a variety of types, sizes, and textures. They can be made from human hair or animal hair, such as mink, or synthetic fibers. Synthetic fiber eyelashes are made with a permanent curl and do not react to changes in weather conditions. Artificial eyelashes are available in colors ranging from light to dark brown and black or light to dark auburn to coordinate with the client's hair and brow color. Black and dark brown are the most popular choices.

Equipment, Implements, and Materials

Wet sanitizer for metal implements
Tweezers
Cotton swabs
Eyelash brushes
Eyelash curler
Hand mirror
Manicure scissors
Adjustable light (gooseneck lamp)
Lounge-style makeup chair
Lash adhesive
Adhesive tray
Eyelid and eyelash cleanser
Eyelash remover
Cotton pads
Eye makeup remover
Makeup cape

Procedure

1. Wash and sanitize your hands.
2. Check to see that all required supplies and sanitized implements are on hand.
3. Place the client in the makeup chair with her head at a comfortable working height.
4. The client's face should be well lighted, but avoid shining the light directly into her eyes.
5. If the client has not already done so, remove all eye makeup so that the lash adhesive will adhere properly. Work carefully and gently.
6. If the client wears contact lenses, they must be removed before starting the procedure.
7. Brush the client's eyelashes to make sure they are clean and free of foreign matter such as mascara particles. If the client's lashes are straight, they can be curled with an eyelash curler before you apply the artificial lashes.
8. Discuss with the client the desired length of lashes and the effect she hopes to achieve. Try to create an effect that makes the client's eyelashes fuller, longer, and more attractive without looking unnatural.

9. Work from behind or to the side of the client when applying artificial lashes. Avoid working directly in front of the client whenever possible.
10. Carefully remove the eyelash strip from the package.
11. Follow the manufacturer's directions carefully.
12. Start with the upper lash. If it is too long to fit the curve of the upper eyelid, trim the outside edge. Use your fingers to bend the lash into a horseshoe shape to make it more flexible so it fits the contour of the eyelid. (Fig. 20.77)
13. Feather the lash by nipping into it with the points of your scissors. This creates a more natural look.
14. Apply a thin strip of lash adhesive to the base of the lash and allow a few seconds for it to set. (Fig. 20.78)
15. Apply the lash. Start with the shorter part of the lash and place it on the inside of the eye. Position the rest of the artificial lash as close to the client's own lash as possible. Use the rounded end of a lash liner brush to press the lash on. (Fig. 20.79) Be very careful and gentle when applying the lashes. If eyeliner is to be used, the line is usually drawn on the eyelid before the lash is applied and retouched when the artificial lash is in place. (Fig. 20.80)

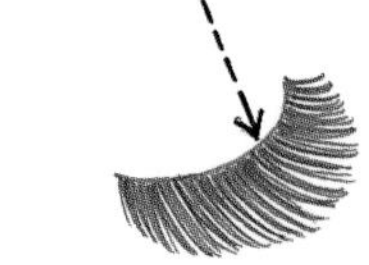

FIGURE 20.77 — Start with the upper lash.

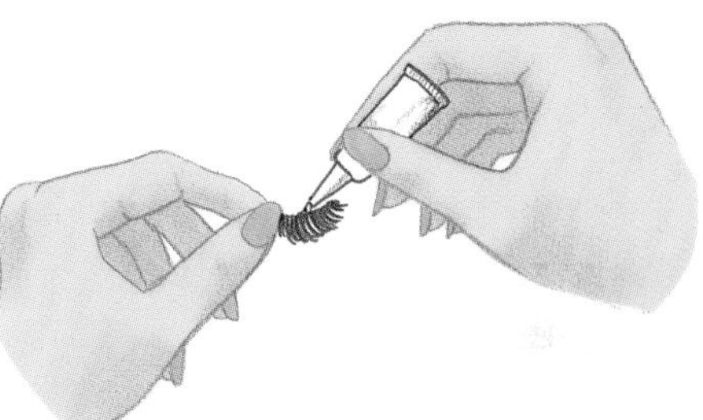

FIGURE 20.78 — Apply lash adhesive.

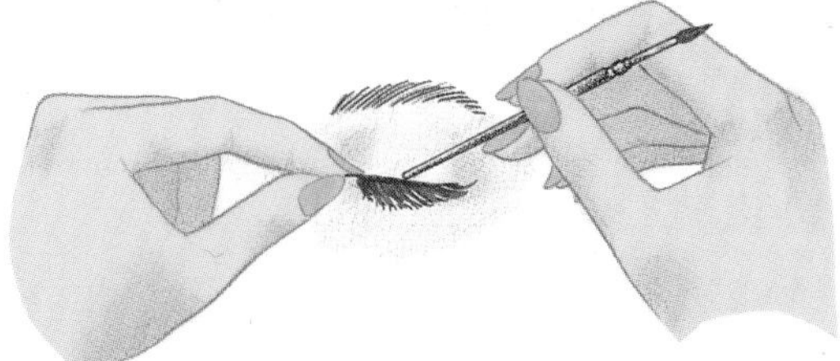

FIGURE 20.79 — Apply lash.

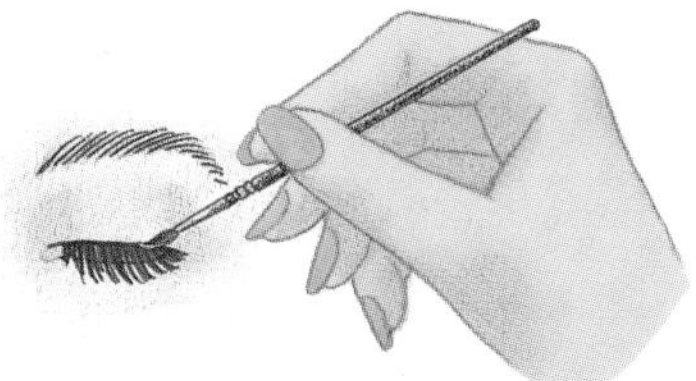

FIGURE 20.80 — Retouch the lash.

16. Apply the lower lash. Trim the lash as necessary and apply adhesive in the same way you did for the upper lash. Place the lash on top of the client's lower lash. Place the shorter lash toward the center of the eye and the longer lash toward the outer part of the lid.

Note: *Remind the client to be careful with lashes when swimming, bathing, or cleansing the face. Water or cleansing products will loosen the artificial lashes.*

REMOVING ARTIFICIAL STRIP EYELASHES

There are commercial preparations, such as pads saturated with specially prepared lotions, to facilitate the removal of false eyelashes. The lash base may also be softened by the application of a face cloth saturated with warm water and a gentle face soap or cleanser. Hold the pad or cloth over the eyes for a few seconds to soften the adhesive. Starting from the outer corner of the lashline, remove lashes carefully to avoid pulling out the client's natural lashes. Cotton tipped swabs may be used to remove makeup and adhesive remaining on the lid.

APPLYING SEMI-PERMANENT INDIVIDUAL EYELASHES (EYE TABBING)

Eye tabbing is the technique of attaching individual, synthetic eyelashes to a client's own eyelashes. Synthetic fibers are used in the manufacture of these false eyelashes because they can be easily curled.

Because synthetic lashes are attached to the client's own and become part of them, they last as long as the natural eyelashes, about 6 to 8 weeks. Hence, they are referred to as "semi-permanent eyelashes." However, due to the fact that natural eyelashes fall out regularly (a few each week), taking the attached false lashes with them, the false lashes should be filled in by periodic visits to the salon.

Equipment, Implements, and Materials

You will need the following for applying individual eyelashes. (Fig. 20.81)

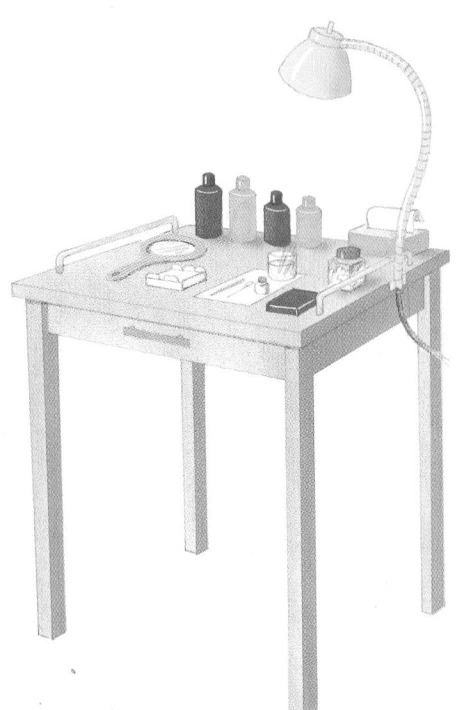

FIGURE 20.81 — False eyelash setup.

- Wet sanitizer to sanitize metal implements
- Tweezers
- Cotton swabs
- Eyelash brush
- Hand mirror
- Adhesive tray
- Eyelash remover
- Adhesive container
- Eye makeup remover (clear)
- Manicure table
- Adjustable light (gooseneck lamp)
- Makeup or facial chair
- Makeup cape
- Manicure scissors
- Tissues
- Trays of eyelashes
- Eyelash adhesive
- Eyelid and eyelash cleaner

Allergy Test

Some clients may be allergic to the adhesive. When in doubt it is advisable to give the client an allergy test before applying the lashes. This test may be accomplished by either one of the following methods:

1. Put a drop of the adhesive behind one ear; or
2. Attach a single eyelash to each eyelid.

In either case, if there is no reaction within 24 hours, it is probably safe to proceed with the application.

Lengths of False Lashes

False lashes usually come in three lengths: short, medium, and long. Some manufacturers have developed a fourth length, extra short. The different lengths are used separately or in combination, in order to achieve certain effects.

1. A natural effect is created by using short lashes intermingled with a few medium-size lashes.
2. A luxurious effect can be achieved by using a mixture of short and medium-length lashes with a few long ones added for glamour.
3. A very glamorous or high styling effect is achieved by using only long lashes.
4. The extra short lashes are used on lower lashes or in combination with others to achieve special effects.

Procedure for Upper Lashes

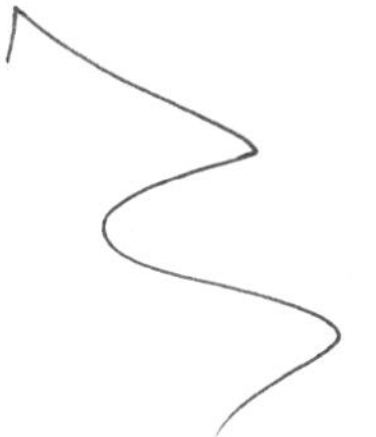

1. Wash and sanitize your hands.
2. Check and see that all required supplies and sanitized implements are on hand.
3. Place client in the makeup chair with her head at a comfortable working height.
4. Make sure that the client's face is well lighted, but avoid shining the light directly into the eyes.
5. If the client has not already done so, remove all eye makeup. If the eyelashes are not entirely clean, the adhesive will not adhere properly.
6. If the client wears contact lenses, they must be removed before you start the procedure.
7. Brush the client's lashes to make sure that they are clean and free from foreign matter. Brushing also separates lashes.
8. Discuss with the client the desired length of lashes and the effect she hopes to achieve. Try to create an effect that makes the eyelashes fuller, more attractive, without looking unnatural.

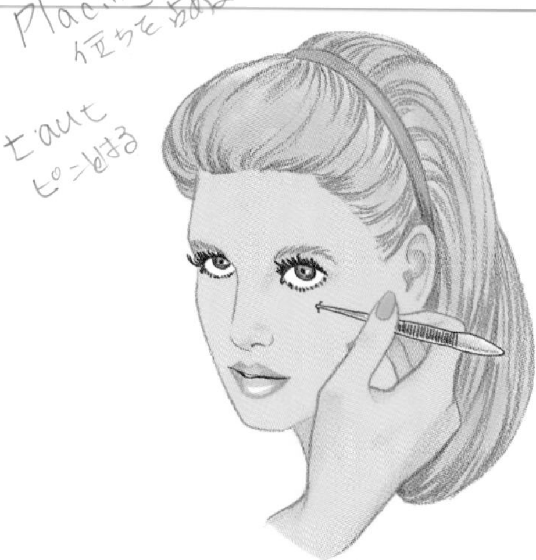

FIGURE 20.88 — Apply lower lashes.

Completed:
Learning Objective
#5
APPLICATION AND REMOVAL OF FALSE EYELASHES

Procedure for Lower Lashes

The application of the lower (bottom) lashes requires a different technique than when applying the upper lashes.

1. Have the client sit facing you. Work from the side rather than directly in front of the client whenever possible.
2. Ask the client to look upward with eyes wide open. (Fig. 20.88)
3. Use short lashes only.
4. Apply adhesive to the lash the same as for upper lashes. Remove excess adhesive.
5. Ask the client to keep her eyes open for a few extra seconds to permit the adhesive to dry.
6. You might have to use more adhesive when applying lower lashes in order to ensure a more lasting application.

Note: *Advise clients that natural oils from the eyelids tend to dissolve the adhesive. As a result, lower lashes will not stay on as long as upper lashes. Generally, lower lashes begin to fall off about one week after application.*

SAFETY PRECAUTIONS

1. Wash and sanitize your hands before and after every make-up application or after touching any object unrelated to the procedure.
2. Properly drape the client to protect her clothing and use hairline strip during the makeup procedure.
3. Protect the client's hair and skin from direct contact with the facial chair.
4. Keep your fingernails smooth to avoid scratching the client's skin.
5. Use only sanitized brushes and implements.
6. Use a shaker-type container for loose powder.
7. Pour all lotions from bottle containers.
8. Always use a clean spatula or cosmetic applicator to remove cosmetics from their containers.

9. Never apply lip color directly from the container to the client's lips. Use a spatula or special applicator to remove the product from the container; then use a brush to apply.
10. Use an antiseptic on tweezed areas of the eyebrow to avoid infection.
11. Place all used items that can be properly sanitized in a container until they can be sanitized.
12. Discard all disposable items, such as sponges, pads, spatulas, and applicators, after use.
13. Discard used pencils or applicators immediately following the makeup application so that they are not used on another client.
14. Place all towels, linens, makeup cape, or other washable items in the proper container until they can be washed and sanitized.
15. Keep your work area clean, neat, and well organized. ✓

Completed:
Learning Objective
#6
SAFETY PRECAUTIONS

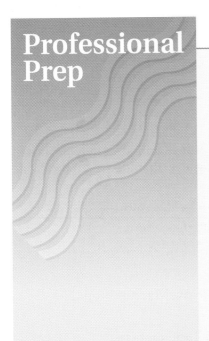

RETAILING

Selling products can be a major source of income for any salon, but too often retail items gather dust on the shelves. Yet selling takes very little extra effort. Here is an example of how selling can be done in the context of a full-service salon, with no pressure on the client:

When Ms. Jones comes in for her appointment, the stylist guides her to the shampoo area saying, "Ms. Jones, we have just gotten in some of the best shampoo I have ever used. It thoroughly cleans the scalp and hair and leaves the hair easy to manage. It's acid-balanced so it won't strip color or harm a permanent wave. It is also good for split ends. If you are looking for a shampoo for the whole family, I would certainly recommend it."

Later, when the stylist is working on Ms. Jones, she may say, "I have noticed that your hair spray seems to be building up on your hair shaft. This will eventually make your hair look dull. I'm going to use some water-soluble hair spray to finish styling your hair. It washes out completely when you shampoo your hair. Why don't you try a bottle and have some fun with it at home? I'll give you some pointers."

—*From* Salon Management for Cosmetology Students
by Edward Tezak

REVIEW QUESTIONS

FACIAL MAKEUP

1. What is the main objective of makeup application?
2. What factors must be taken into consideration when applying makeup?
3. Name the seven facial types.
4. Why is foundation (base) an important part of facial makeup?
5. How is a foundation color selected for a makeup application?
6. Name four types of cheek color.
7. When do you apply lipstick directly from the container?
8. Why do we use mascara?
9. What is the primary objective of applying corrective makeup?
10. Name two basic types of artificial eyelashes.

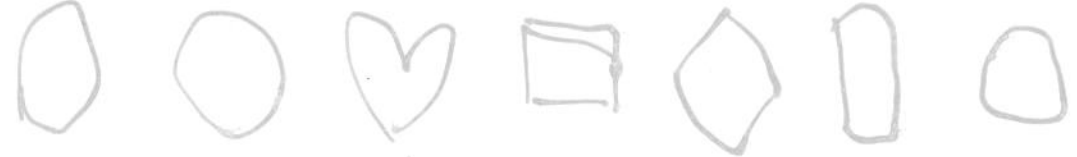

CHAPTER 21

The Skin and Its Disorders

LEARNING OBJECTIVES

After completing this chapter, you should be able to:

1. Describe the structure and composition of the skin (histology).
2. List the functions of the skin.
3. Define important terms relating to skin disorders.
4. Discuss which skin disorders may be handled in the beauty salon and which should be referred to a physician.

NATIONAL SKILL STANDARDS

This chapter provides you with the necessary information to master this National Industry Skill Standard for Entry-Level Cosmetologists:

- Conducting services in a safe environment, taking measures to prevent the spread of infectious and contagious disease

INTRODUCTION

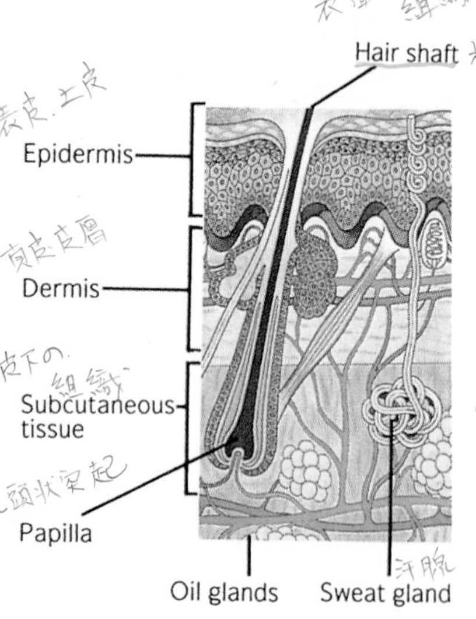

FIGURE 21.1 — Microscopic section of skin.

The skin is the largest and one of the most important organs of the body. The scientific study of the skin and scalp is important to the cosmetologist because it forms the basis for an effective program of skin care, beauty services, and scalp treatments. A cosmetologist who has a thorough understanding of skin, its structure, and functions is in a better position to give clients professional advice on scalp, facial, and hand care. (Fig. 21.1)

A healthy skin is slightly moist, soft, and flexible; possesses a slightly acid reaction; and is free from any disease or disorder. The skin also has immunity responses to organisms that touch or try to enter it. Its ***texture*** (feel and appearance) ideally is smooth and fine grained. A person with a good complexion has fine skin texture and healthy skin color. Appendages of the skin are hair, nails, and sweat and oil glands.

Skin varies in thickness. It is thinnest on the eyelids and thickest on the palms and soles. Continued pressure on any part of the skin can cause it to thicken and develop into a callus.

The skin of the scalp is constructed similarly to the skin elsewhere on the human body. However, the scalp has larger and deeper hair follicles to accommodate the longer hair of the head. (Fig. 21.2)

HISTOLOGY OF THE SKIN

The skin contains two main divisions: the epidermis and the dermis.

The ***epidermis*** (ep-ih-**DUR**-mis) is the outermost layer of the skin. This layer is commonly called the ***cuticle*** (**KYOO**-tih-kel), or ***scarf skin***. It is the thinnest layer of skin and forms a protective covering for the body. It contains no blood vessels, but it has many small nerve endings. The epidermis is made up of the following layers:

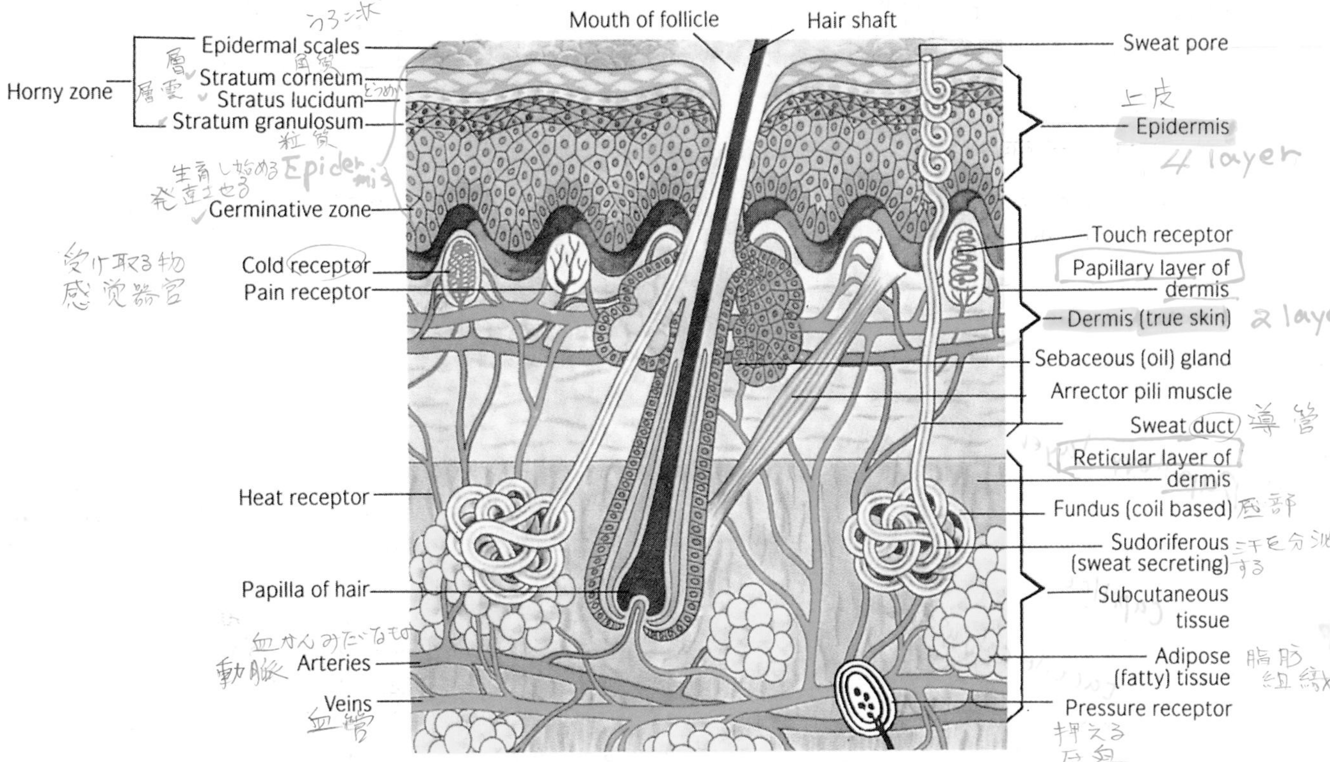

FIGURE 21.2 — Diagram of a section of the scalp.

1. The ***stratum corneum*** (**STRAT**-um **KOHR**-nee-um), or horny layer, is the outer layer of the skin. Its scalelike cells are continually being shed and replaced by underneath cells coming to the surface. These cells contain the protein keratin, and combined with a thin covering layer of oil help make the stratum corneum almost waterproof.
2. The ***stratum lucidum*** (**LOO**-sih-dum), or clear layer, consists of small, transparent cells through which light can pass.
3. The ***stratum granulosum*** (gran-yoo-**LOH**-sum), or granular layer, consists of cells that look like distinct granules. These cells are almost dead and are pushed to the surface to replace cells that are shed from the stratum corneum.
4. The ***stratum germinativum*** (jur-mih-nah-**TIV**-um), formerly known as the ***stratum mucosum*** (myoo-**KOH**-sum) and also referred to as the basal or Malpighian layer, is composed of several layers of different-shaped cells. The deepest layer is responsible for the growth of the epidermis. It also contains a dark skin pigment, called melanin, which protects the sensitive cells below from the destructive effects of excessive

ultraviolet rays of the sun or of an ultraviolet lamp. These special cells are called ***melanocytes*** (**MEL**-uh-noh-sights). They produce melanin, which determines skin color.

The ***dermis*** (**DUR**-mis) is the underlying, or inner, layer of the skin. It is also called the ***derma***, ***corium*** (**KOH**-ree-um), ***cutis*** (**KYOO**-tis), or ***true skin***. It is about 25 times thicker than the epidermis. It is a highly sensitive and vascular layer of connective tissue. Within its structure there are numerous blood vessels, lymph vessels, nerves, sweat glands, oil glands, hair follicles, arrector pili muscles, and papillae. The dermis is made up of two layers: the papillary, or superficial layer, and the reticular, or deeper layer.

1. The ***papillary layer*** (pah-**PIL**-ah-ry) lies directly beneath the epidermis. It contains small cone-shaped projections of elastic tissue that point upward into the epidermis. These projections are called ***papillae*** (pah-**PIL**-ee). Some of these papillae contain looped ***capillaries*** (**KAP**-ih-ler-ees); others contain nerve fiber endings, called ***tactile corpuscles*** (**TAK**-til **KOR**-pus-els), which are nerve endings for the sense of touch. This layer also contains some of the melanin skin pigment.
2. The ***reticular layer*** (reh-**TIK**-u-lar) contains the following structures within its network:

Fat cells	Sweat glands
Blood vessels	Hair follicles
Lymph vessels	Arrector pili muscles
Oil glands	

This layer also supplies the skin with oxygen and nutrients.

Subcutaneous tissue (sub-kyoo-**TAY**-nee-us) is a fatty layer found below the dermis. Some histologists consider this tissue as a continuation of the dermis. This tissue is also called ***adipose*** (**AD**-ih-pohs), or ***subcutis*** (sub-**KYOO**-tis) tissue and varies in thickness according to the age, sex, and general health of the individual. It gives smoothness and contour to the body, contains fats for use as energy, and also acts as a protective cushion for the outer skin. Circulation is maintained by a network of ***arteries*** and ***lymphatics***.

HOW THE SKIN IS NOURISHED

Blood and lymph supply nourishment to the skin. As they circulate through the skin, the blood and lymph contribute essential materials for growth, nourishment, and repair of the skin, hair, and nails. In the subcutaneous tissue are found networks of arteries and lymphatics that send their smaller branches to hair papillae, hair follicles, and skin glands.

NERVES OF THE SKIN

The skin contains the surface endings of many nerve fibers. They are:

1. *Motor nerve fibers,* which are distributed to the arrector pili muscles attached to the hair follicles. This muscle can cause gooseflesh when you are frightened or cold.
2. *Sensory nerve fibers,* which react to heat, cold, touch, pressure, and pain. These sensory receptors send messages to the brain. (Fig. 21.3)
3. *Secretory nerve fibers,* which are distributed to the sweat and oil glands of the skin. These nerves regulate the excretion of perspiration from the sweat glands and control the flow of sebum to the surface of the skin.

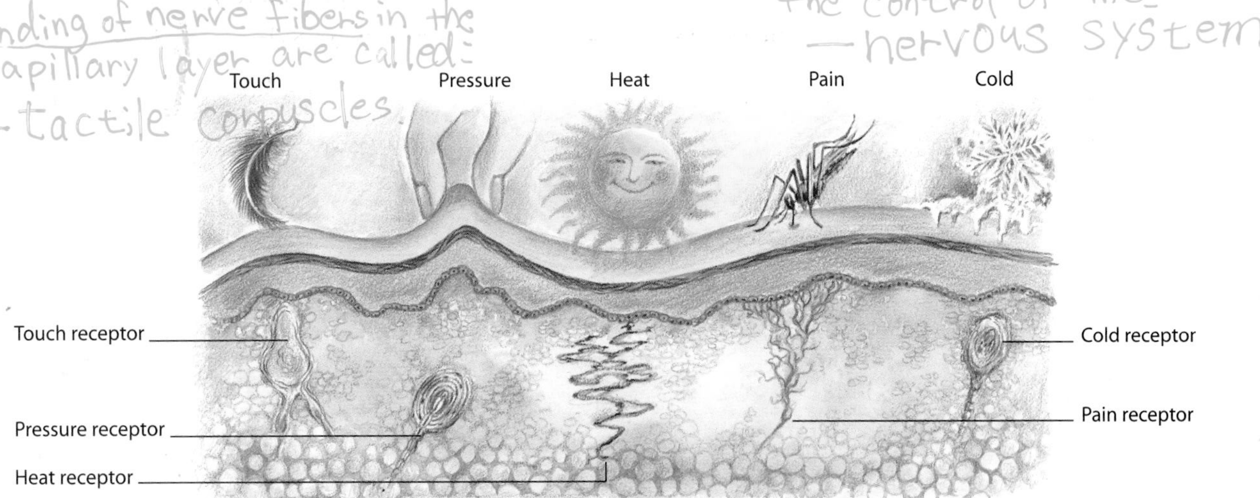

FIGURE 21.3 — Sensory nerves of the skin.

Sense of Touch

The papillary layer of the dermis houses the nerve endings that provide the body with the sense of touch. These nerve endings register basic sensations; touch, pain, heat, cold, pressure, or deep touch. Nerve endings are most abundant in the fingertips. Complex sensations, such as vibrations, seem to depend on the sensitivity of a combination of these nerve endings.

SKIN ELASTICITY

The pliability of the skin depends on the elasticity of the dermis. For example, healthy skin regains its former shape almost immediately after being expanded.

Aging Skin

The aging process of the skin is a subject of vital importance to everyone. Perhaps the most outstanding characteristic of the aged skin is its loss of elasticity. One factor that contributes to the loss of elasticity is that as we age subcutaneous tissue shrinks and is not as effective a support system in preventing the skin from wrinkling.

SKIN COLOR

The color of the skin, whether fair, medium, or dark, depends, in part, on the blood supply to the skin and primarily on melanin, the coloring matter that is deposited in the stratum germinativum and the papillary layers of the dermis. The color of pigment varies from person to person. The distinctive color of the skin is a hereditary trait and varies among races and nationalities. Melanin protects sensitive cells from sunburn and tanning beds with ultraviolet rays. A sun protection factor (SPF) should be used to help the melanin in the skin protect it from burning.

GLANDS OF THE SKIN

The skin contains two types of duct glands that extract materials from the blood to form new substances: the ***sudoriferous*** (soo-dohr-**IF**-er-us), or ***sweat glands***, and the ***sebaceous*** (sih-**BAY**-shus), or ***oil glands***. (Figs. 21.4–21.6)

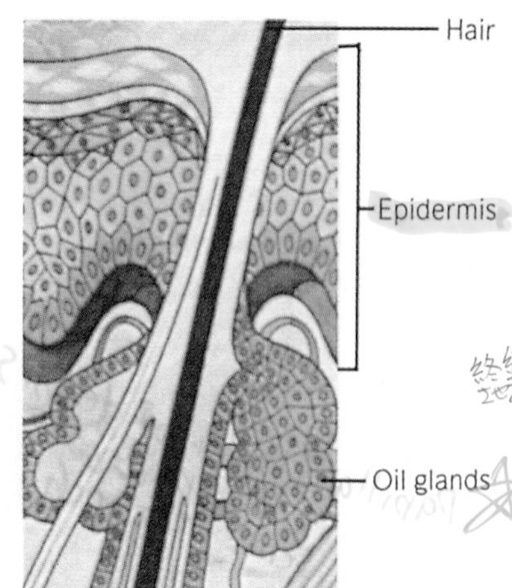

FIGURE 21.4 — Body hair and follicle.

Sweat Glands

The sweat glands (tubular type), which excrete sweat, consist of a coiled base, or ***fundus*** (**FUN**-dus), and a tubelike duct that terminates at the skin surface to form the sweat pore. Practically all parts of the body are supplied with sweat glands, which are more numerous on the palms, soles, forehead, and in the armpits.

The sweat glands regulate body temperature and help to eliminate waste products from the body. Their activity is greatly increased by heat, exercise, emotions, and certain drugs.

The excretion of sweat is controlled by the nervous system. Normally, 1 to 2 pints of liquids containing salts are eliminated daily through sweat pores in the skin.

Oil Glands

The oil glands (saccular type) consist of little sacs whose ducts open into the hair follicles. They secrete sebum, which lubricates the skin and preserves the softness of the hair. With the exception of the palms and soles, these glands are found in all parts of the body, particularly in the face and scalp where they are larger.

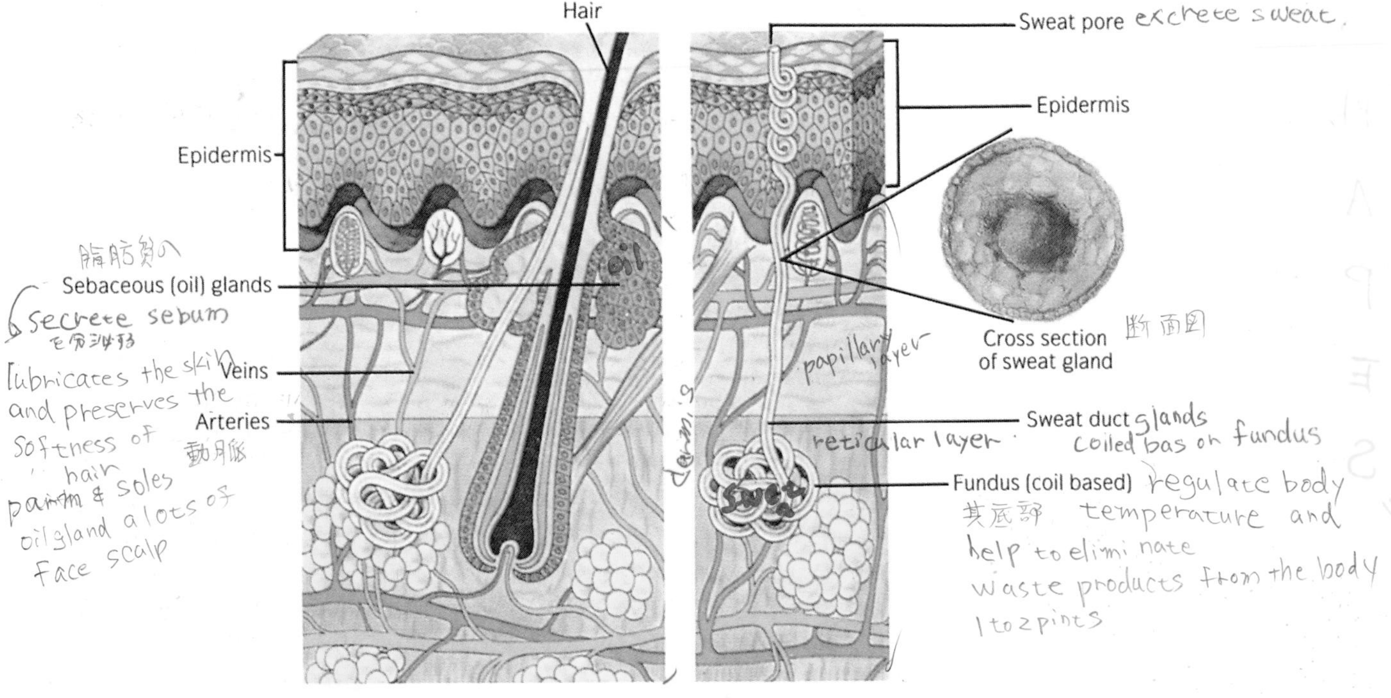

FIGURE 21.5 — Scalp hair, follicle, and oil glands.

FIGURE 21.6 — Sweat gland.

Sebum is an oily substance produced by the oil glands. Ordinarily, it flows through the oil ducts leading to the mouths of the hair follicles. However, when the sebum becomes hardened and the duct becomes clogged, a blackhead is formed.

Completed: Learning Objective #1

STRUCTURE AND COMPOSITION OF THE SKIN

FUNCTIONS OF THE SKIN

The principal functions of the skin are protection, sensation, heat regulation, excretion, secretion, and absorption.

1. *Protection*. The skin protects the body from injury and bacterial invasion. The outermost layer of the epidermis is covered with a thin layer of sebum, thus rendering it waterproof. It is resistant to wide variations in temperature, minor injuries, chemically active substances, and many forms of bacteria.
2. *Sensation*. By stimulating sensory nerve endings, the skin responds to heat, cold, touch, pressure, and pain. When the nerve endings are stimulated, a message is sent to the brain. You respond by saying "ouch" if you feel pain, by scratching an itch, or pulling away when you touch something hot.

Sensory nerve endings, responsive to touch and pressure, are located near hair follicles.

3. *Heat regulation* means that the skin protects the body from the environment. A healthy body maintains a constant internal temperature of about 98.6° Fahrenheit (37° Celsius). As changes occur in the outside temperature, the blood and sweat glands of the skin make necessary adjustments and the body is cooled by the evaporation of sweat.
4. *Excretion.* Perspiration from the sweat glands is excreted through the skin. Water lost through perspiration takes salt and other chemicals with it.
5. *Secretion.* Sebum, or oil, is secreted by the sebaceous glands. This oil lubricates the skin, keeping it soft and pliable. Oil also keeps hair soft. Emotional stress can increase the flow of sebum.
6. *Absorption* is limited, but it does occur. Female hormones, when an ingredient of a face cream, can enter the body through the skin and influence it to a minor degree. Fatty materials, such as lanolin creams, are absorbed largely through hair follicles and sebaceous gland openings. Research is being conducted with mink oil, turtle oil, and caviar as catalysts for absorption.

Completed:
Learning Objective
#2
FUNCTIONS OF THE SKIN

DISORDERS OF THE SKIN

In your work as a cosmetologist in a salon you will come in contact with skin and scalp disorders. You must be prepared to recognize certain common skin conditions and must know what you can and cannot do with them. Some skin and scalp disorders can be treated in cooperation with, and under the supervision of, a physician. Medicinal preparations, available only by prescription, must be applied in accordance with the physician's directions. If a client has a skin condition that the cosmetologist does not recognize as a simple disorder, the person should be referred to a physician.

Most important is that a client who has an inflamed skin disorder, infectious or not, should not be served in the beauty salon. The cosmetologist should be able to recognize these conditions and suggest that proper measures be taken to prevent more serious consequences. Thus, the health of the cosmetologist, as well as the health of the public, is safeguarded.

DEFINITIONS PERTAINING TO SKIN DISORDERS

Listed below are a number of important terms that should be familiar to the cosmetologist for an understanding of the subject of skin, scalp, and hair disorders.

Dermatology (dur-mah-**TOL**-oh-jee)—The study of the skin, its nature, structure, functions, diseases, and treatment.

Dermatologist (dur-mah-**TOL**-oh-jist)—A medical skin specialist.

Pathology (pa-**THOL**-oh-jee)—The study of disease.

Trichology (treye-**KOL**-oh-jee)—The study of the hair and its diseases.

Etiology (ee-ti-**OL**-oh-jee)—The study of the causes of disease.

Diagnosis (deye-ag-**NOH**-sis)—The recognition of a disease by its symptoms.

Prognosis (prog-**NOH**-sis)—The foretelling of the probable course of a disease.

LESIONS OF THE SKIN

A lesion is a structural change in the tissues caused by injury or disease. There are three types: primary, secondary, and tertiary. The cosmetologist is concerned with primary and secondary lesions only. If you are familiar with the principal skin lesions you will be able to distinguish between conditions that may or may not be treated in a beauty salon. (Fig. 21.7)

The symptoms or signs of diseases of the skin are divided into two groups:

1. *Subjective symptoms* are those that can be felt, such as itching, burning, or pain.
2. *Objective symptoms* are those that are visible, such as pimples, pustules, or inflammation.

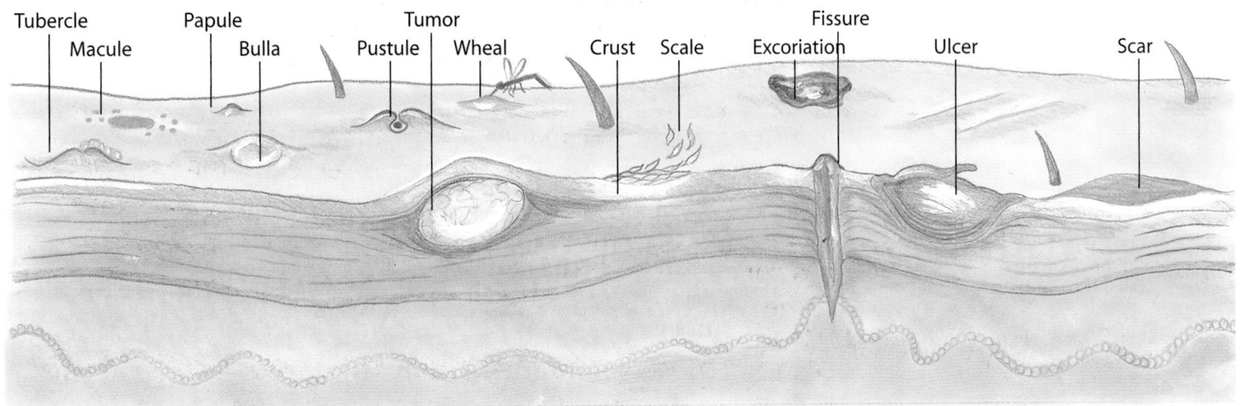

FIGURE 21.7 — Primary and secondary skin lesions.

DEFINITIONS PERTAINING TO PRIMARY LESIONS

The following is a list of important terms and definitions that should be familiar to the cosmetologist.

Macule (**MAK**-yool)—A small, discolored spot or patch on the surface of the skin, such as freckles. These are neither raised nor sunken.

Papule (**PAP**-yool)—A small, elevated pimple on the skin, containing no fluid, but which might develop pus.

Wheal (**HWEEL**)—An itchy, swollen lesion that lasts only a few hours. Examples include hives or the bite of an insect, such as a mosquito.

Tubercle (**TOO**-ber-kel)—A solid lump larger than a papule. It projects above the surface or lies within or under the skin. It varies in size from a pea to a hickory nut.

Tumor (**TOO**-mohr)—An abnormal cell mass, varying in size, shape, and color. ***Nodules*** are also referred to as tumors, but they are smaller.

Vesicle (**VES**-ih-kell)—A blister with clear fluid in it. Vesicles lie within or just beneath the epidermis; for example, poison ivy produces small vesicles.

Bulla (**BYOO**-lah)—A blister containing a watery fluid, similar to a vesicle, but larger.

Pustule (**PUS**-chool)—An elevation of the skin having an inflamed base, containing pus.

Cyst (**SIST**)—A semisolid or fluid lump above and below the skin.

DEFINITIONS PERTAINING TO SECONDARY LESIONS

Secondary skin lesions are those that develop in the later stages of disease. These are:

Scale—An accumulation of epidermal flakes, dry or greasy. (Example: abnormal or excessive dandruff)

Crust (scab)—An accumulation of sebum and pus, mixed perhaps with epidermal material. (Example: the scab on a sore)

Excoriation (ek-skohr-ee-**AY**-shun)—A skin sore or abrasion produced by scratching or scraping. (Example: a raw surface due to the loss of the superficial skin after an injury)

Fissure (**FISH**-ur)—A crack in the skin penetrating into the dermis, as in the case of chapped hands or lips.

Ulcer (**UL**-ser)—An open lesion on the skin or mucous membrane of the body, accompanied by pus and loss of skin depth.

Scar (cicatrix) (SIK-ay-triks)—Likely to form after the healing of an injury or skin condition that has penetrated the dermal layer.

Keloid (KEE-loyd)—A thick scar resulting from excessive growth of fibrous tissue.

Stain—An abnormal discoloration remaining after the disappearance of moles, freckles, or liver spots, sometimes apparent after certain diseases.

DEFINITIONS PERTAINING TO DISEASE

Before describing the diseases of the skin and scalp so that they will be recognizable to the cosmetologist, it is necessary to understand what is meant by disease.

Disease is any departure from a normal state of health.

Skin disease—Any infection of the skin characterized by an objective lesion (one that can be seen), which may consist of scales, pimples, or pustules.

Acute disease—One with symptoms of a more or less violent character, such as fever, and usually of short duration.

Chronic disease—One of long duration, usually mild but recurring.

Infectious (in-FEK-shus) ***disease***—One due to germs (bacterial or viral) taken into the body as a result of contact with a contaminated object or lesion.

Contagious disease—One that is communicable by contact.

Note: *The terms "infectious disease," "communicable disease," and "contagious disease" are often used interchangeably.*

Congenital disease—One that is present in the infant at birth.

Seasonal disease—One that is influenced by the weather, as prickly heat in the summer, and forms of eczema, which is more prevalent in cold weather.

Occupational disease (such as dermatitis)—One that is due to certain kinds of employment, such as coming in contact with cosmetics, chemicals, or tints.

Parasitic disease—One that is caused by vegetable or animal parasites, such as pediculosis and ringworm.

Pathogenic disease—One produced by disease-causing bacteria, such as staphylococcus and streptococcus (pus-forming bacteria), or viruses.

Systemic disease—Due to under- or over-functioning of the internal glands. It can be caused by faulty diet.

Venereal disease—A contagious disease commonly acquired by contact with an infected person during sexual intercourse.

Epidemic—The appearance of a disease that simultaneously attacks a large number of persons living in a particular locality. Infantile paralysis, influenza, or smallpox are examples of epidemic-causing diseases.

Allergy—A sensitivity that some people develop to normally harmless substances. Skin allergies are quite common. Contact with certain types of cosmetics, medicines, and tints or eating certain foods all can cause an itching eruption, accompanied by redness, swelling, blisters, oozing, and scaling.

Inflammation—A skin disorder characterized by redness, pain, swelling, and heat.

DISORDERS OF THE SEBACEOUS (OIL) GLANDS

There are several common disorders of the sebaceous (oil) glands that the cosmetologist should be able to identify and understand.

Comedones (KOM-e-donz), or blackheads, are wormlike masses of hardened sebum, appearing most frequently on the face, especially the forehead and nose.

Blackheads accompanied by pimples often occur in youths between the ages of 13 and 20. During this adolescent period, the activity of the sebaceous glands is stimulated, thereby contributing to the formation of blackheads and pimples. (Fig. 21.8)

When the hair follicle is filled with an excess of oil from the sebaceous gland, a blackhead forms and creates a blockage at the mouth of the follicle. Should this condition become severe, medical attention is necessary.

To treat blackheads, the skin's oiliness must be reduced by local applications of cleansers and the blackheads removed under sterile conditions. Thorough skin cleansing each night is a very important factor. Cleansing creams and lotions often achieve better results than common soap and water.

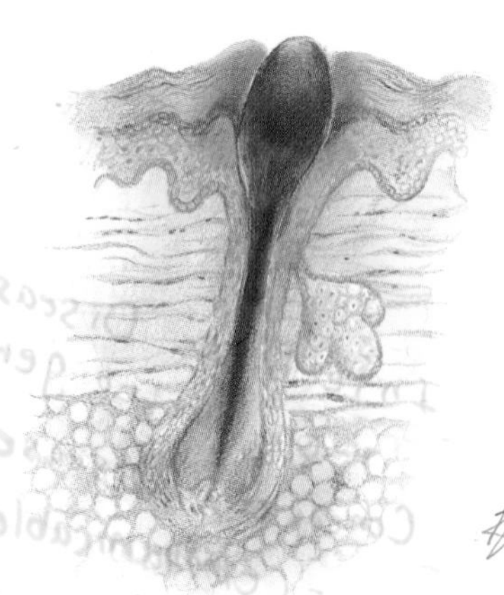

FIGURE 21.8 — Blackhead (plug of sebaceous matter and dirt) forming around mouth of hair follicle.

Milia (MIL-ee-uh), or whiteheads, is a disorder of the sebaceous (oil) glands caused by the accumulation of sebaceous matter beneath the skin. This can occur on any part of the face, neck, and, occasionally, on the chest and shoulders. Whiteheads are associated with fine-textured, dry types of skin.

Acne (AK-nee) is a chronic inflammatory disorder of the sebaceous glands, occurring most frequently on the face, back, and chest. The cause of acne is generally believed to be microbic, but predisposing factors are adolescence and perhaps certain foods in the diet. Acne, or common pimples, is also known as ***acne simplex*** or ***acne vulgaris.*** (Fig. 21.9)

Acne appears in a variety of different types, ranging from the simple (noncontiguous) pimple, to serious, deep-seated skin conditions. It is always advisable to have the condition examined and diagnosed by a physician before any service is given in a beauty salon.

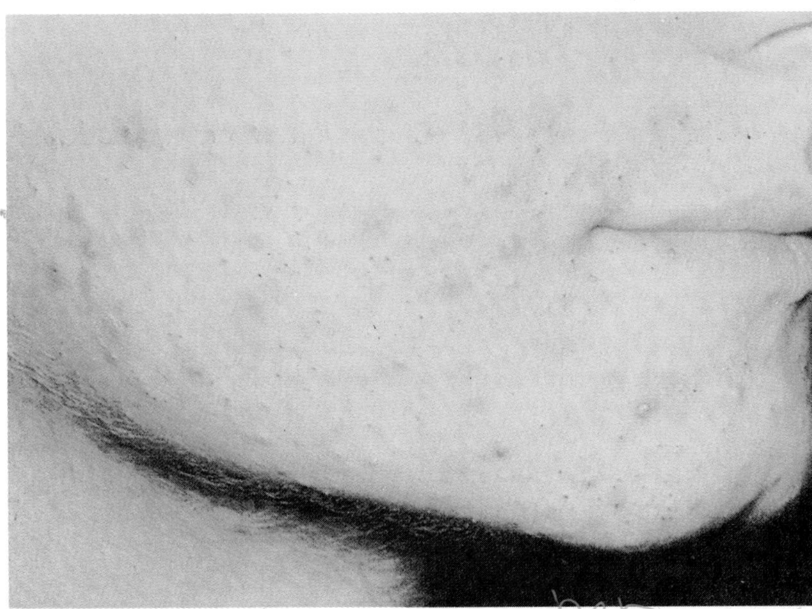

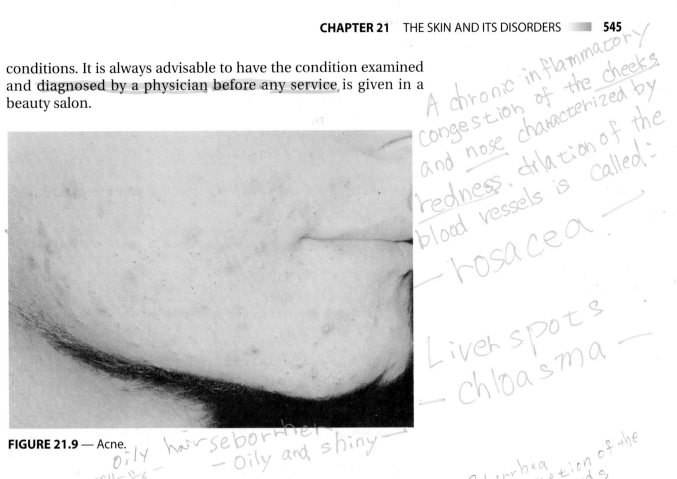

FIGURE 21.9 — Acne.

Seborrhea (seb-oh-**REE**-ah) is a skin condition caused by an excessive secretion of the sebaceous glands. An oily or shiny condition of the nose, forehead, or scalp indicates the presence of seborrhea. On the scalp, it is readily detected by an unusual amount of oil on the hair.

Asteatosis (as-tee-ah-**TOH**-sis) is a condition of dry, scaly skin, characterized by absolute or partial deficiency of sebum, due to senile changes (old age) or some bodily disorders. It can be caused by alkalis, such as those found in soaps and washing powders.

Rosacea (ro-**ZA**-see-ah), formerly called acne rosacea, is a chronic inflammatory congestion of the cheeks and nose. It is characterized by redness, dilation of the blood vessels, and the formation of papules and pustules. The cause of rosacea is unknown. Certain things are known to aggravate rosacea in some individuals. These include consumption of hot liquids, spicy foods or alcohol, being exposed to extremes of heat and cold, exposure to sunlight, and stress. (Fig. 21.10)

Steatoma (stee-ah-**TOH**-mah), or sebaceous cyst, is a subcutaneous tumor of the sebaceous gland. It is filled with sebum and ranges in size from a pea to an orange. It usually appears on the scalp, neck, and back. A steatoma is sometimes called a wen. (Fig. 21.11)

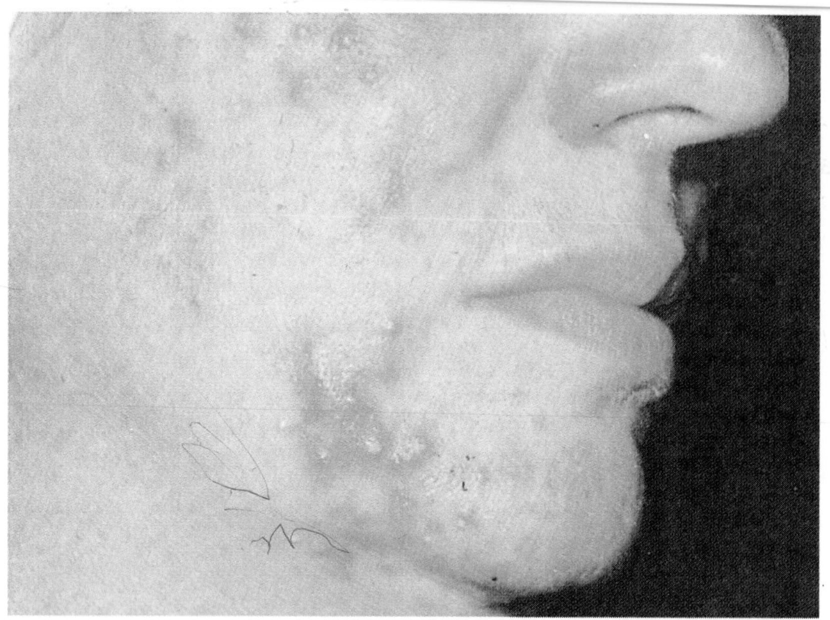

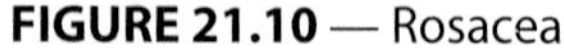

FIGURE 21.10 — Rosacea.

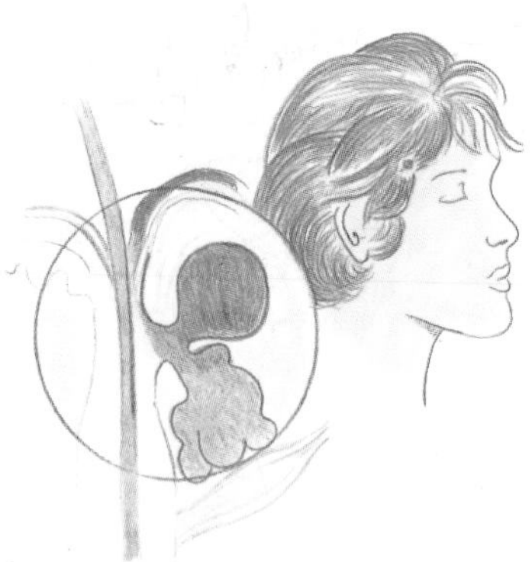

FIGURE 21.11 — Steatoma.

DEFINITIONS PERTAINING TO DISORDERS OF THE SUDORIFEROUS (SWEAT) GLANDS

Bromidrosis (broh-mih-**DROH**-sis), or ***osmidrosis*** (ah-smi-**DROH**-sis)—Foul-smelling perspiration, usually noticeable in the armpits or on the feet.

Anhidrosis (an-heye-**DROH**-sis), or lack of perspiration—Often a result of fever or certain skin diseases. It requires medical treatment.

Hyperhidrosis (heye-per-heye-**DROH**-sis), or excessive perspiration—Caused by excessive heat or general body weakness. The most commonly affected parts are the armpits, joints, and feet. Medical treatment is required.

Miliaria rubra (mil-ee-**AY**-ree-ah **ROOB**-rah), or ***prickly heat***—An acute inflammatory disorder of the sweat glands, characterized by an eruption of small red vesicles and accompanied by burning and itching of the skin. It is caused by exposure to excessive heat.

DEFINITIONS PERTAINING TO INFLAMMATIONS

Dermatitis (dur-mah-**TEYE**-tis)—A term used to indicate an inflammatory condition of the skin. The lesions come in various forms, such as vesicles or papules.

Eczema (**EK**-see-mah)—An inflammation of the skin, of acute or chronic nature, presenting many forms of dry or moist lesions. It is frequently accompanied by itching or a burning sensation.

All cases of eczema should be referred to a physician for treatment. Its cause is unknown.

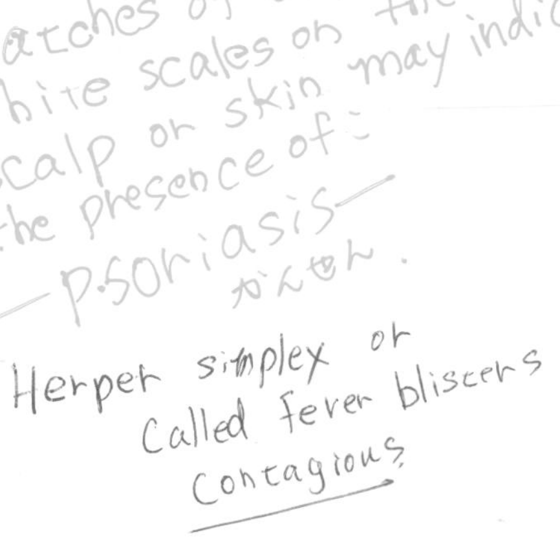

Psoriasis (soh-**REYE**-ah-sis)—A common, chronic, inflammatory skin disease whose cause is unknown. It is usually found on the scalp, elbows, knees, chest, and lower back, rarely on the face. The lesions are round, dry patches covered with coarse, silvery scales. If irritated, bleeding points occur. It is not contagious.

Herpes simplex (**HUR**-peez **SIM**-pleks)—A recurring virus infection, commonly called fever blisters. It is characterized by the eruption of a single vesicle or group of vesicles on a red swollen base. The blisters usually appear on the lips, nostrils, or other part of the face, and rarely last more than a week. It is contagious. (Fig. 21.12)

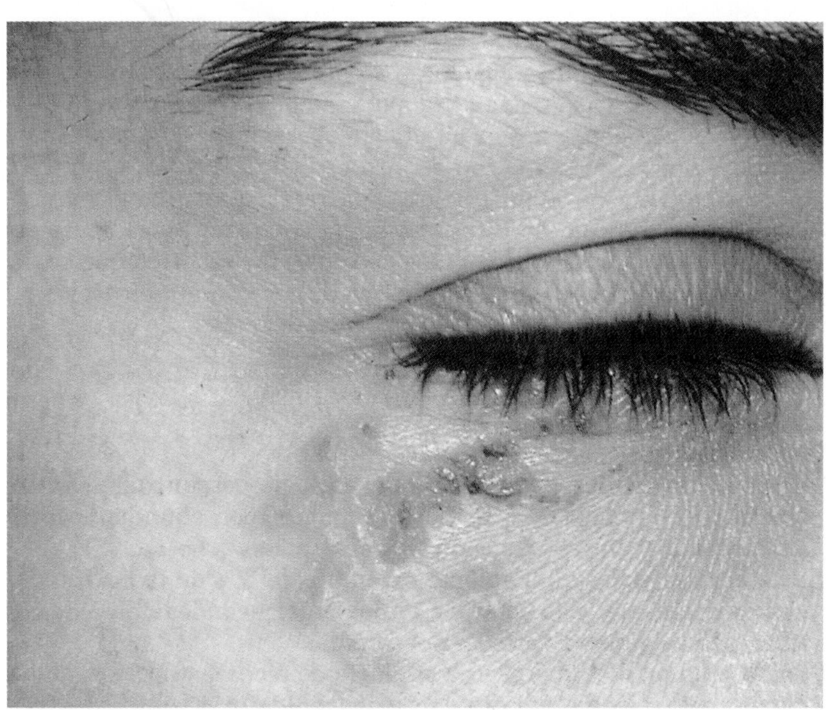

FIGURE 21.12 — Herpes simplex, or fever blisters.

Occupational Disorders in Cosmetology

Abnormal conditions resulting from contact with chemicals or tints can occur in the course of performing services in the beauty salon. Some individuals may develop allergies to ingredients in cosmetics, antiseptics, cold waving lotions, and aniline derivative tints. These can cause eruptive skin infections known as ***dermatitis venenata*** (**VEN**-eh-nay-tah). It is important that cosmetologists employ protective measures, such as the use of rubber gloves or protective creams whenever possible.

DEFINITIONS PERTAINING TO PIGMENTATIONS OF THE SKIN

In abnormal conditions, ***pigment*** can be affected from inside or outside the body. Abnormal colors accompany every skin disorder and many systemic disorders. A change in pigmentation is observed when certain drugs are being taken internally.

Tan—Caused by excessive exposure to the sun.

Lentigines (len-tih-**JEE**-neez) (singular, lentigo), or freckles—Small yellow-to-brown-colored spots on parts exposed to sunlight and air.

Stains—Abnormal brown skin patches, having a circular and irregular shape. Their permanent color is due to the presence of darker pigment. They occur during aging; after certain diseases; and after the disappearance of moles, freckles, and liver spots. The cause of these stains is unknown.

Chloasma (kloh-**AZ**-mah)—Characterized by increased deposits of pigment in the skin. It is found mainly on the forehead, nose, and cheeks. Chloasma is also called *moth patches* or *liver spots*.

Naevus (**NEE**-vus)—Commonly known as birthmark. It is a small or large malformation of the skin due to abnormal pigmentation or dilated capillaries.

Leucoderma (loo-koh-**DUR**-mah)—Abnormal white patches in the skin, due to congenital defective pigmentation. It is classified as:

Vitiligo (vit-ih-**LEYE**-goh)—An acquired condition of leucoderma, affecting the skin or the hair. The only treatment is a matching cosmetic color, making it less conspicuous. Must be protected from over-exposure to the sun.

Albinism (al-**BEYE**-niz-em)—Congenital absence of melanin pigment of the body, including the skin, hair, and eyes. The silky hair is white. The skin is pinkish white and will not tan. Eyes are pink. Skin ages early.

DEFINITIONS PERTAINING TO HYPERTROPHIES (NEW GROWTHS) OF THE SKIN

Keratoma (ker-ah-**TOH**-mah), or callus—An acquired, superficial, round, thickened patch of epidermis, due to pressure or friction on the hands and feet. If the thickening grows inward, it is called a corn.

Mole—A small, brownish spot, or blemish, on the skin. Moles are believed to be inherited. They range in color from pale tan to brown or bluish black. Some moles are small and flat, resembling freckles; others are more raised and darker in color. Large, dark hairs often occur in moles. Any change in a mole requires medical attention.

Melanotic sarcoma—Fatal skin cancer that starts with a mole.

> **CAUTION**
>
> *Do not treat or remove hair from moles.*

Verruca (veh-**ROO**-kah)—Technical term for ***wart***. It is caused by a virus and is infectious. It can spread from one location to another, particularly along a scratch in the skin.

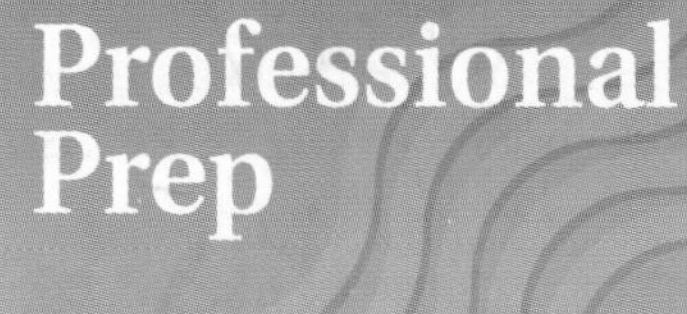

CHOOSING A SALON

Landing your first job in a salon is a two-way street. Many times we think of an employer choosing an employee, but in fact you must do the first choosing in deciding where you will apply for a job. A bit of research will help you target the salons where you would or would not like to work. Learning all about the salons where you apply will set you apart from the many applicants who don't bother to do this.

First of all, find out your prospective employer's name and how it is spelled and pronounced, and his or her position in the salon. Then find answers to the question, What are his or her needs and expectations?

Find out exactly what type of salon it is: its size and reputation, whether it is privately owned or part of a chain, and its atmosphere. Is it trendy and glitzy, or elegant and conservative? Is it relaxed or very high-pressure with a constant stream of clients?

Take a look at the clientele: Are they suburban housewives, professionals, lower-income people? What is the age range?

What services are offered in the salon, and what products are used?

Finally, is there a training program for new employees?

You can find the answers to these questions by talking to cosmetology instructors, salon employees, and clientele. You can call the salon and talk with the receptionist. If the salon is part of a chain or franchise, you can get information from trade journals, the library, the Chamber of Commerce, and the Better Business Bureau.

How do you start looking for a job? Remember that most job opportunities are not advertised in the classified sections of newspapers. Better ways of finding out who is hiring include word of mouth, membership in a professional organization, and unsolicited inquiry—in other words, send a resume and cover letter to a salon where you want to work.

—*From* Communication Skills for Cosmetologists
by Kathleen Ann Bergant

DEFINITIONS PERTAINING TO PLASTIC SURGERY

Estheticians are being added to the staff of many dermatologists and plastic surgeons. Estheticians are people who specialize in skin care. More specifically, they help clients preserve the youthful look of the face and neck. To be effective assisting in a medical office, you should be familiar with the following terms and procedures.

Rhytidectomy (rit-ih-**DECK**-tuh-mee)—A face-lift is an operation designed to diminish the changes of aging in the face and neck. It involves lifting and removing the excess skin of the face, neck, and temple.

Blepharoplasty (**BLEF**-uh-ro-plas-tee)—Eyelid surgery is the procedure often combined with a forehead or eyebrow lift to improve the overall appearance of the upper face. It involves incisions in the natural skin fold of the eyelids to remove skin and protruding fatty tissue.

Chemical peeling—A technique for improving the appearance when wrinkles of the skin are present. In this procedure, a specially formulated chemical solution is applied to the areas to be treated. The chemical causes a mild, controlled burn of the skin.

Rhinoplasty (**REYE**-no-plas-tee)—Plastic surgery of the nose. The procedure is sometimes performed in conjunction with a face-lift to adjust the aging nose's tendency to droop and lose definition. Incisions are hidden just inside the rim of the nostrils and sometimes across the skin between the nostrils. The cartilage and bone of the nose are then reshaped to give the nose a more pleasing appearance.

Mentoplasty (**MEN**-toh-plas-tee)—Chin surgery involves a small incision made either inside the mouth or just underneath and behind the most prominent part of the chin to change a person's profile by building up a small chin. It is often performed at the same time as plastic surgery of the nose.

Dermabrasion (dur-muh-**BRAY**-zhun)—A technique to smooth scarred skin by "sanding" irregularities so that scars blend better with the surrounding skin. This procedure is usually performed with a rotary abrasive instrument that actually thins the skin, making the sharp edges of facial scars less prominent.

Injectable fillers—When there are deep scars, severe acne scarring, or deep aging lines around the mouth or forehead, tiny injections of collagen may be used to raise depressions closer to the normal skin level. Collagen, a natural product derived from cowhide, blends well with skin tissue.

Retin-A™ (**RET**-in-ay)—***Retinoic*** (ret-ih-**NO**-ick) ***acid***, ***Tretinoin*** (treh-**TIN**-oh-in), ***Vitamin A acid*** are all names for *Retin-A*,™ which is a prescription cream used in the treatment of acne. Recently the general public has begun to use it as a sloughing off (shedding) agent to bring new cells to the epidermis more quickly. The purpose is to control and slow down the formation of wrinkles.

Completed:
Learning Objectives
#3 & #4
SKIN DISORDERS AND UNDERSTANDING MEDICAL VS. BEAUTY SALON TREATMENT

REVIEW QUESTIONS

THE SKIN AND ITS DISORDERS

1. What is skin?
2. Briefly describe healthy skin.
3. Name the two main divisions of the skin.
4. How is the skin nourished?
5. What determines the color of the skin?
6. What are the glands contained within the skin?
7. What are the six important functions of the skin?
8. Define dermatology.
9. What is a lesion of the skin?
10. Define acne.
11. Define herpes simplex. What is it commonly called?
12. Define albinism.
13. What is a mole?

CHAPTER 22

Removing Unwanted Hair

LEARNING OBJECTIVES

After completing this chapter, you should be able to:

1. List the two general classifications of unwanted hair removal.
2. Identify the three methods of permanent hair removal.
3. Demonstrate the techniques involved in the thermolysis method of permanent hair removal.
4. Demonstrate the methods of temporary hair removal.

NATIONAL SKILL STANDARDS

This chapter provides you with the necessary information to master these National Industry Skill Standards for Entry-Level Cosmetologists:

- Conducting services in a safe environment, taking measures to prevent the spread of infectious and contagious disease
- Performing hair removal services

INTRODUCTION

Hirsuties (hur-**SUE**-shee-eez) or ***hypertrichosis*** (heye-per-**TRIK**-oh-sis) means hairiness or superfluous hair. It is recognized by the growth of hair in unusual amounts or locations, as on the faces of women. Unwanted hair is not a new problem. It has plagued individuals throughout the ages. Unwanted hair is a problem that concerns many men as well as women.

One of the earliest methods of hair removal was the use of an abrasive, such as pumice stone to wear away the hair. Excavations of early Egyptian tombs revealed that abrasives were used for this purpose. Ancient Greek and Roman women were known to remove most of their body hair by abrasion. Native Americans used sharpened stones and seashells to rub off and pluck out hair.

History also records chemical means of removing excess hair. For example, the ancient Turks used *rusma*, a combination of yellow sulfide of arsenic, quicklime, and rose water, as a crude ***depilatory***. Most depilatories today also have an alkaline pH to assist in the decomposition of the hair.

Today, there are two types of hair removal: permanent and temporary. Several means of temporary hair removal are covered later in this chapter. This section covers the permanent hair removal method called ***electrolysis***.

Completed:
Learning Objective
#1
GENERAL CLASSIFICATIONS OF UNWANTED HAIR REMOVAL

PERMANENT METHODS OF HAIR REMOVAL

The first effective technique of permanent hair removal invented was electrolysis. This technique was devised by ophthalmologist Charles E. Michel of St. Louis, Missouri, in 1875 as he was trying to solve the problem of ingrown eyelashes. Michel attached a very fine conductor wire to a dry-cell battery. He then attached the wire to a surgical needle and inserted it into the follicle of the eyelash. In most cases, after the treatment, the hair did not grow back. History was made.

The electrolysis treatment devised by Michel used a ***galvanic*** or direct current of electricity. The galvanic current chemically decomposed the ***dermal papilla***, the lower hair root and source of nourishment of the hair follicle. The galvanic process was very time-consuming and tedious. In 1916 Professor Paul Kree developed a multiple galvanic machine or ***epilator***. This allowed the electrologist to insert up to ten needles in time sequence instead of spending several minutes on each hair.

In 1924, Dr. H. Brodier of Paris developed ***thermolysis*** (thur-**MOL**-e-sis), a method of hair removal using high-frequency or alternating current. This method created heat to destroy the papilla. It soon became popular because it was a much faster technique than the galvanic process.

In 1945, Henri St. Pierre and Arthur Hinkel successfully blended galvanic current with low-intensity high-frequency shortwave current running simultaneously through a single needle. Known as the blend method, the purpose was to destroy hair growth more quickly using galvanic current with the aid of the heat from high-frequency current.

Completed: Learning Objective #2

THE THREE PERMANENT HAIR REMOVAL METHODS

GENERAL INFORMATION

The importance of training. The electrologist is dealing with the skin, and an inefficient or unskilled operator could cause irreparable damage. Therefore, every electrologist must be thoroughly trained, both in the theory and in the practice of electrolysis. This means that she or he must use live models to practice on, under the direct supervision of an instructor, until proper skill, certificate (if required), and confidence are achieved.

Machines. Some shortwave machines have many safety factors. They are automatically timed and F.C.C. (Federal Communications Commission) approved. Pain is kept to a minimum by the rapid shut-off of current.

Areas that may be treated. Upper lips, chin, cheeks, arms, legs, eyebrows, hairline, and underarms may receive electrolysis treatments.

Areas that may not be treated. Do not treat the lower eyelids, inside the ears, or nostrils. Obtain permission from a physician before treating clients who have conditions such as diabetes or pregnancy, and those who have pacemakers or who are receiving hormone treatments.

Causes of unwanted hair. The growth of hair is due to hormonal imbalance in the body. No one knows the exact cause, although authorities agree that heredity often plays a large role in excessive hair growth. Certain drugs, pregnancy, and weight problems are also known to influence hair growth.

SHORTWAVE OR THERMOLYSIS METHOD

The shortwave method, also known as the thermolysis method, is the quickest of permanent hair removal methods and the one most generally used. (Fig. 22.1) In fact, because it is the overwhelming choice of electrologists today, we will describe it in detail. We will not discuss the other permanent removal methods.

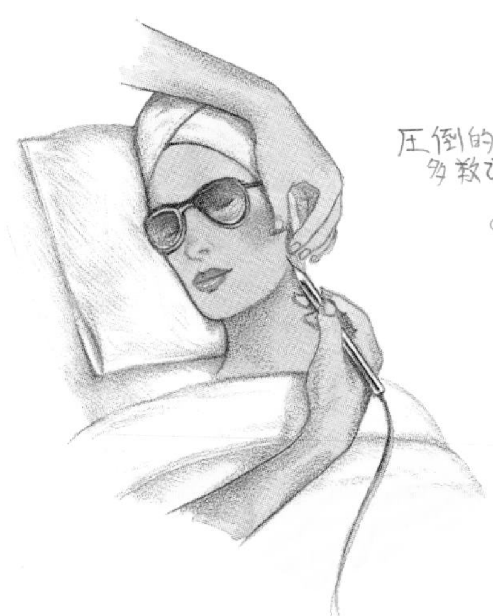

FIGURE 22.1 — Inserting needle in shortwave method.

Equipment, Implements, and Materials

You will need the following equipment and accessories to perform thermolysis treatment:

Shortwave epilator and stand (Fig. 22.2)
Needles
Patient chair or table
Electrologist's stool
Antiseptic solution
Sterilizer
Sterile cotton
Facial tissue
Protective eye shields
Magnification mirror and regular mirror
Magnification treatment lens lamp or glasses
Tweezers
Apron for client
After-treatment lotion
Small blunt-end scissors
Small treatment pillow
Covered waste container

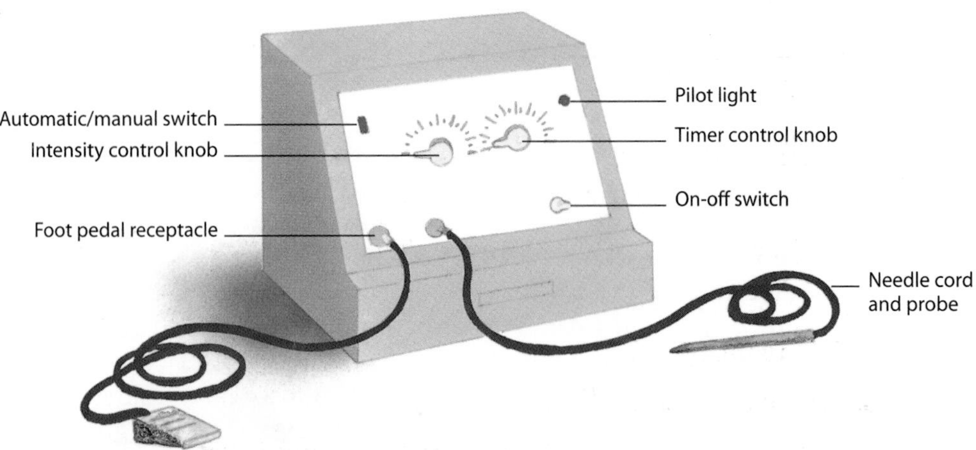

FIGURE 22.2 — Shortwave epilator.

Thermolysis Controls

Thermolysis epilators are also known as shortwave epilators. They use radio frequency and operate on alternating current (AC). All thermolysis epilators have the same control systems:

1. Plug to power source
2. On/off switch
3. Indicator light—indicates machine is on or off
4. Timer or manual switch
5. Intensity control—regulates current flow (rheostat)
6. Needle holder jack (negative electrode)
7. Foot pedal—on/off current flow
8. Intensity light—comes on when pedal is depressed
9. Timer light—stays on as long as pedal is depressed

Beyond the basic controls, manufacturers may add their own innovations. Some, for example, have incorporated two ***negative jacks*** to allow needle holders for different sized needles. Others may have radio frequency (RF) meters. Because machines may vary slightly, it is wise to follow the instruction manual provided by each manufacturer.

Client Comfort

The care and comfort of the client should always be of utmost importance to the electrologist. The comfort of the electrologist is also important. The treatment given will be of better quality if the electrologist is comfortable.

Procedure for Thermolysis

1. Position aproned client on chair.
2. Wash your hands.
3. Apply an astringent to the treatment area.
4. Sterilize tweezers.
5. Determine the size of needle required and sterilize it.
6. Turn on the epilator and wait 1 minute.
7. Set the timer on low.
8. Set the intensity on low.
9. Make the first insertion until slight resistance is felt.

10. Depress the foot switch.
11. Test the hair with tweezer for easy release.
12. Raise the intensity and timer controls accordingly, until hair is easily released.

Inserting the Needle into the Hair Follicle

Insertion is the most critical technique in electrolysis treatment. The size of the needle corresponds to the diameter of the hair being treated. Hold the needle holder as you would a pen or pencil, but not as firmly. The index finger and thumb must not touch. The needle holder may lean gently on the middle finger, which serves as a guide.

The angle at which the needle is inserted depends on the angle at which the hair is growing. For example, a hair that grows straight up requires that the needle be inserted straight down into the follicle. If a hair is growing at an angle, the needle should be inserted at an angle. (Figs. 22.3–22.6) When there is an excessive amount of hair and the hairs are long, it is difficult to see the hair follicle and the angle of growth. Simply cut the hair to a length where the follicle and angle of growth can be observed easily.

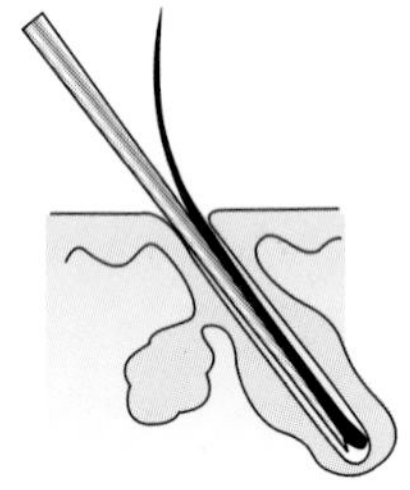

FIGURE 22.3 — Needle inserted correctly.

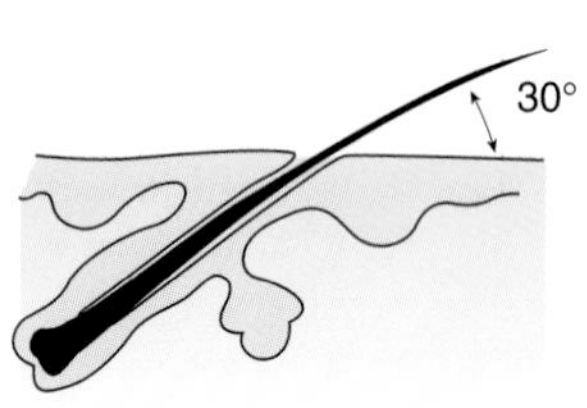

FIGURE 22.4 — Hair growing at a 30° (.523 rad.) angle on the neck.

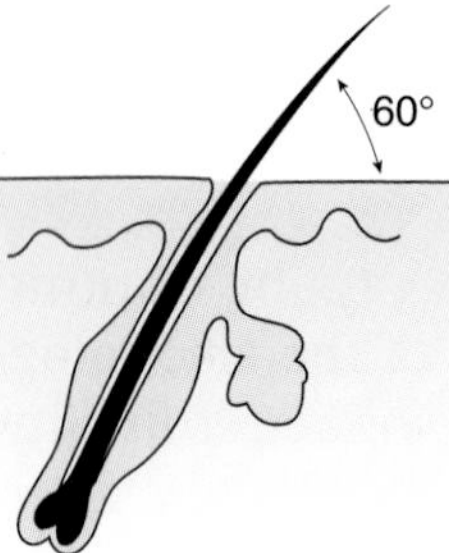

FIGURE 22.5 — Hair growing at a 60° (1.05 rad.) angle on the front of the chin.

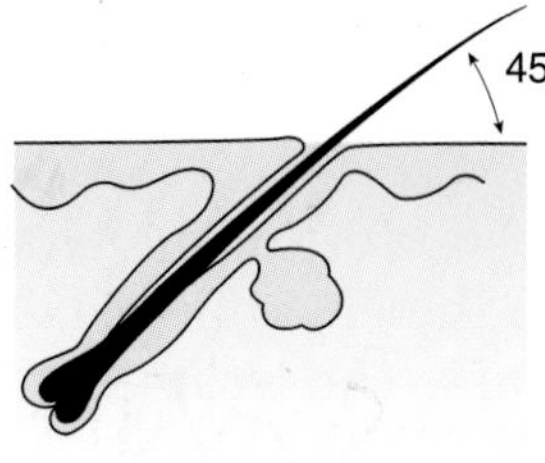

FIGURE 22.6 — Hair growing at a 45° (.785 rad.) angle on the face.

Tweezer Manipulation

It is necessary to use a tweezer to gently remove the hair. Once the current is turned off, remove the wire from the follicle and use your tweezer to remove the hair. You should not have to use any pressure. The needle holder and the tweezer should not be held tightly. You must practice a light touch and practice maneuvering the needle holder and tweezer in one hand while the fingers of the other hand hold the treatment area firmly but without causing discomfort to the client.

Developing an expert skill of insertion, tweezer manipulation, and correct intensity and timer judgments increase treatment efficiency.

After treatment is completed, turn the machine off. Saturate a pad of sterile cotton with a strong after-treatment lotion and press it gently on the area treated. This cools and soothes the skin and aids in the healing process.

Completed: Learning Objective #3

THERMOLYSIS METHOD OF PERMANENT HAIR REMOVAL

TEMPORARY METHODS OF HAIR REMOVAL

SHAVING

Shaving is usually recommended when the unwanted hairs cover a large area, such as under arms and on the legs. A shaving cream is applied before shaving.

An electric clipper may also be used. The application of a pre-shaving lotion helps to reduce any irritation. An electric clipper is most often used to remove unwanted hair at the nape.

Shaving does not cause the hair to grow thicker or stronger; it only seems that way because the razor blunts the hair ends and makes them feel stiff.

TWEEZING

Tweezing is commonly used for shaping the eyebrows. Tweezing can also be used for removing undesirable hairs from around the mouth and chin. (The procedure for tweezing the eyebrows will be found in the chapter on facial makeup.)

ELECTRONIC TWEEZER METHOD OF HAIR REMOVAL

Another method for the removal of superfluous hair that is used in salons is the electrically charged tweezer. This method transmits radio frequency energy down the hair shaft into the follicle area. It is claimed that the papilla is thus dehydrated and eventually destroyed.

The tweezer is used to grasp a single strand of hair. The energy is then applied, first at a low level to pre-warm and then at a higher level for up to 2 minutes to remove the hair. Most manufacturers suggest that the area be steamed first in order to increase efficiency.

The electronic tweezer is not a method of permanent hair removal. Further, the process of clearing any area of hair by this method is slow.

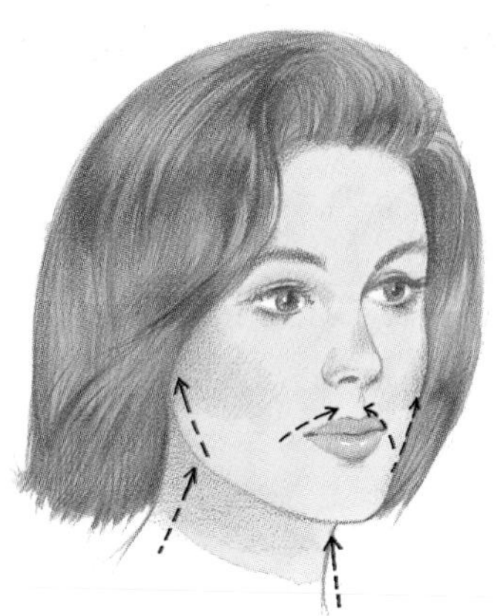

FIGURE 22.7 — Superfluous hair.

DEPILATORIES

Depilatories also belong to the group of temporary methods for the removal of superfluous hair. There are *physical* (wax) and *chemical* types of depilatories.

HOT WAX

The hot wax depilatory is applied either heated or cold as recommended by the manufacturer. It may be applied over such parts of the body as the cheeks, chin, upper lip, nape area, arms, and legs. Do not remove vellus (lanugo) hair; doing so may cause the skin to lose its softness. (Fig. 22.7)

Waxing and tweezing may cause the hair to grow stronger because it stimulates the circulation and increases the blood supply to the hair follicle.

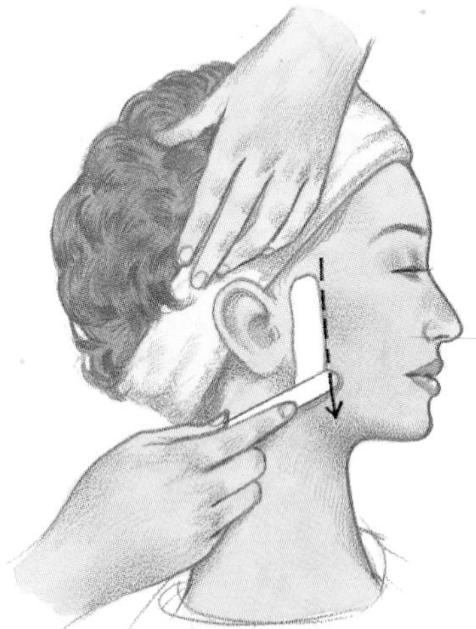

FIGURE 22.8 — Spread wax downward.

Procedure for Hot Waxing

1. Melt wax in a double boiler on a stove or in a heater.
2. Remove clothing from the area to be treated and seat the client comfortably.
3. Wash the skin area with a mild soap and water. Rinse thoroughly and dry.
4. Spread talcum powder over the skin surface.
5. Test temperature and consistency of heated wax by applying a little of it on your arm.
6. Using a spatula or brush, spread warm wax evenly over the skin surface in the same direction as the hair growth. Apply a sanitized cloth strip in the same direction as the hair growth. (Figs. 22.8, 22.10)
7. Allow the wax to cool and harden.

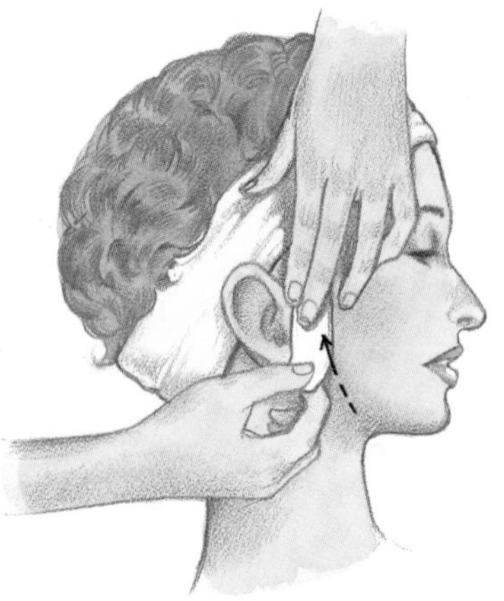

FIGURE 22.9 — Pull wax off upward.

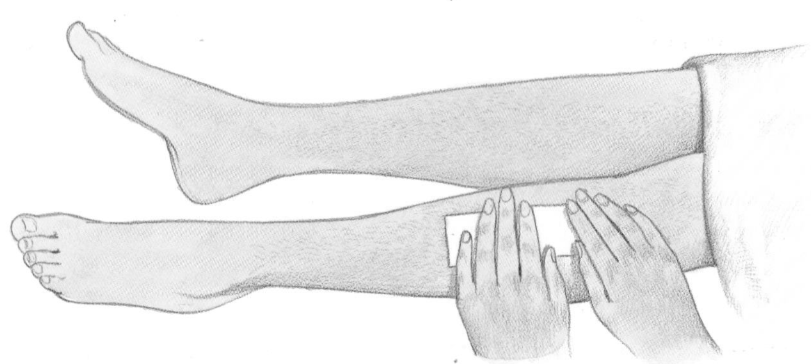

FIGURE 22.10 — Applying wax to skin.

8. Quickly pull off the adhering wax against the direction of hair growth. (Figs. 22.9, 22.11)
9. Gently massage treated area.
10. Dust off remaining powder from the skin.
11. Apply an emollient cream or antiseptic lotion to the treated area.

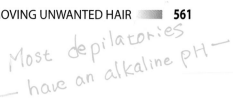

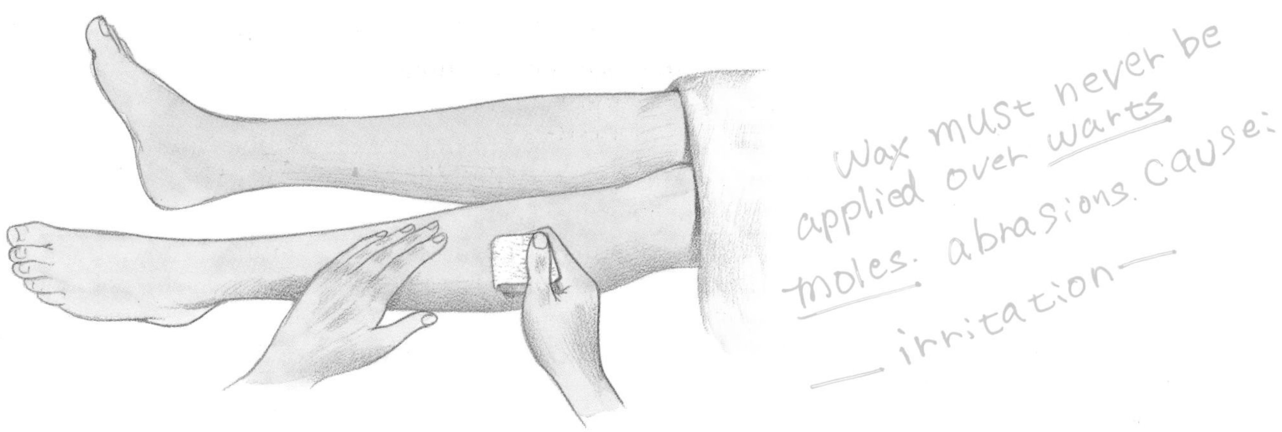

FIGURE 22.11 — Removing wax from skin.

Safety Precautions

1. To prevent burns, test the temperature of the heated wax before applying it to the client's skin.
2. Use caution so the wax does not contact the eyes.
3. Do not use a wax depilatory under the arms; if the client's skin is sensitive; over warts; on moles, abrasions, irritated or inflamed skin.

COLD WAX

For those clients who cannot tolerate heated wax, a cold wax method of hair removal also is available. This technique has all the advantages of hot wax in a ready-to-use form. It removes the hair in the same manner as warm wax, but needs no heating or special equipment.

Procedure for Cold Waxing

1. Apply wax at room temperature.
2. Using a spatula, spread a thin coat of wax in the direction of the hair growth.

3. Apply a strip of cellophane or cotton cloth and press down firmly so that the wax adheres correctly.
4. Holding the skin taut with one hand, use the other hand to grasp the wax strip, and with one fast movement, pull off the strip against the direction of the hair growth.

CHEMICAL DEPILATORIES

Chemical depilatories are available as a cream, paste, or powder mixed with water into a paste. These depilatories are generally used to remove hair from the legs.

A ***skin test*** is advisable to determine whether the individual is sensitive to the action of this type of depilatory.

To give such a test, select a hairless part of the arm, apply a portion of the depilatory according to the manufacturer's directions, and leave it on the skin from 7 to 10 minutes. If at the end of this time there are no signs of redness or swelling, the depilatory can probably be used with safety over a large area of the skin.

Procedure

1. The cream type is applied directly from the container, while the powder type is mixed to form a smooth paste according to the manufacturer's directions.
2. After the skin has been cleansed and dried, a thick layer of the depilatory is applied over the area where the hair is to be removed.
3. The surrounding skin is protected with petroleum jelly or cream.
4. The depilatory is kept on the hair for 5 to 10 minutes depending on the thickness of the hair. The thicker the hair, the longer the depilatory is kept on.
5. Wash off the depilatory and hair with warm water.
6. Pat the skin dry and apply cold cream.

Completed:
Learning Objective
#4
TEMPORARY METHODS OF HAIR REMOVAL

Career Path

ELECTROLOGIST

Electrology is a field which is often overlooked by students as a possible specialty. In this profession, you can help improve people's self-image by removing unwanted hair.

Starting your own practice as an electrologist involves careful planning, beginning with your location. Choose an office near other businesses or a shopping center, so people can make one stop to do several errands. An ideal location would be in a medical center near a mall. If you open a practice in your home, be sure the office has a separate entrance and is detached from your living quarters to ensure patient privacy. A full-service or skin care salon is not the best place to begin an electrology practice, because many patients feel uncomfortable walking past other customers to the electrologist's booth.

Once you begin, it is wise to allow yourself time for your practice to build. Patients who like your work will return and will recommend you to others. Much of your success will be determined not only by your mastery of the techniques of electrolysis, but even more by your ability to deal with people and to put them at ease.

The consultation, which occurs the moment a new patient walks in, is a crucial moment in your relationship. Be sure to create a positive, relaxed mood. Use brochures and pamphlets that answer the most commonly asked questions. Always explain that electrology takes time; with experience you will be able to give increasingly accurate estimates of the time and cost required to treat each individual case.

—*From* Modern Electrology: Excess Hair, Its Causes and Treatments *by Fino Gior*

REVIEW QUESTIONS

REMOVING UNWANTED HAIR

1. Define hirsuties.
2. What are two types of hair removal?
3. What was the first effective technique of permanent hair removal and who invented this method?
4. What is thermolysis?
5. What technique did Henri St. Pierre and Arthur Hinkel successfully develop in 1945?
6. Name three temporary methods of hair removal.
7. Name three areas that may not be treated by the electrologist.
8. What is the quickest method of permanent hair removal?
9. Name three safety precautions when waxing.

CHAPTER 23

Cells, Anatomy, and Physiology

LEARNING OBJECTIVES

After completing this chapter, you should be able to:

1. Define the functions of human cells.
2. Describe the various types of tissues.
3. Describe the structures and functions of the human body.
4. Demonstrate an understanding of the organs and systems of the human body and how they function.

KILL STANDARDS

vides you with the necessary information National Industry Skill Standard for Entry-Level Cosmetologists:

- basic skin care services

INTRODUCTION

In the first part of this chapter we discuss the cell, the basic structure from which all other body structures are made. In the second part of the chapter we discuss the body structures themselves, the anatomy and physiology of the human body, and its relationship to the cosmetology profession.

The human organism is made of a vast variety of parts that vary in complexity. These include organ systems, organs, tissues, cells. These cellular parts are composed of molecules, which are made of atoms or groups of atoms. And, as you will see in the chemistry chapter, atoms are made up of even smaller, submicroscopic particles called protons, neutrons, and electrons.

CELLS

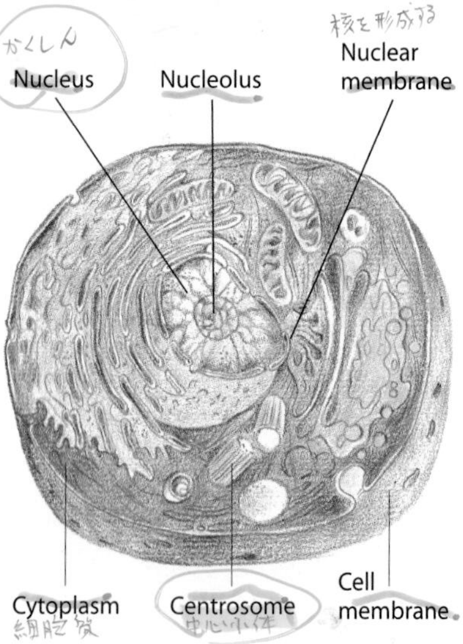

Nucleus
Nucleolus
Nuclear membrane
Cytoplasm
Centrosome
Cell membrane

FIGURE 23.1 — Cells consist of protoplasm and contain essential elements.

Cells are the basic units of all living things, including bacteria, plants, and animals. The human body is composed entirely of cells, fluids, and cellular products. As the basic functional units, the cells carry on all life processes. Cells also have the ability to reproduce, providing new ones for growth and replacement of worn and injured tissues. (Fig. 23.1)

Cells are made up of ***protoplasm*** (**PROH**-toh-plaz-em), a colorless, jellylike substance in which food elements such as protein, fats, carbohydrates, mineral salts, and water are present. The principal parts of a cell are the ***cytoplasm*** (**SEYE**-toh-plaz-em), ***centrosome*** (**SEN**-tro-sohm), ***nucleus*** (**NOO**-klee-us), ***nucleolus*** (new-**KLEE**-oh-lus), and ***cell membrane*** (**MEM**-brayn). The thin cell membrane or cell wall permits soluble (dissolvable) substances to enter and leave the protoplasm. The nucleus, near the center of the cell, is contained in a nuclear membrane. Outside of the nucleus are the cytoplasm and a centrosome. The nucleus and the cytoplasm are made of protoplasm. The centrosome and the nucleus control cell reproduction.

The protoplasm of the cells contains the following important structures:

Nucleus (dense protoplasm), found in the center, which plays an important part in the reproduction of the cell.

Nucleolus, a small spherical body, composed mostly of RNA (ribonucleic acid) and protein, within the cell nucleus.

Cytoplasm (less dense protoplasm), which is found outside of the nucleus and contains food materials necessary for the growth, reproduction, and self-repair of the cell.

Centrosome, a small, round body in the cytoplasm, which also affects the reproduction of the cell.

Cell membrane encloses the protoplasm. It permits soluble substances to enter and leave the cell.

CELL GROWTH

As long as the cell receives an adequate supply of food, oxygen, and water, eliminates waste products, and is favored with proper temperature, it will continue to grow and thrive. However, if these conditions do not exist and there is the presence of toxins (poisons) or pressure, then the growth and the health of the cells are impaired. Most body cells are capable of growth and self-repair during their life cycle. (Fig. 23.2)

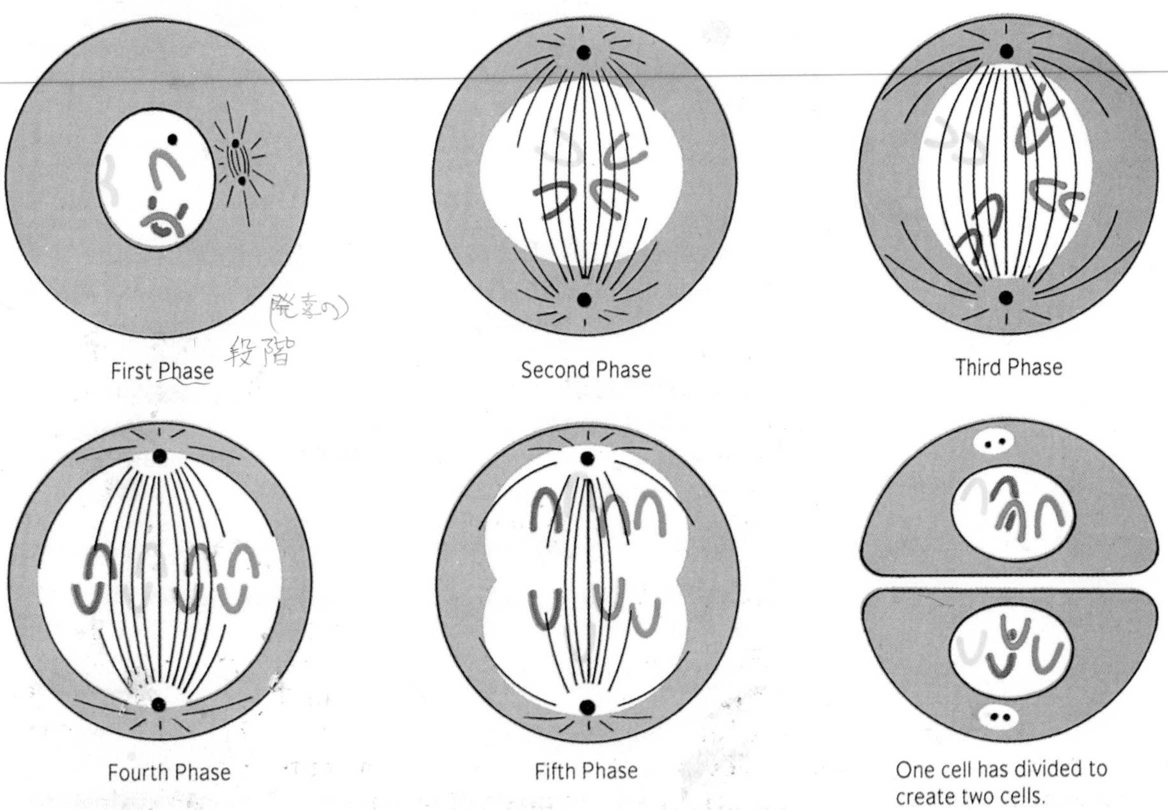

FIGURE 23.2 — Indirect division of the human cell.

CELL METABOLISM

Metabolism (meh-**TAB**-oh-liz-em) is a complex chemical process whereby the body cells are nourished and supplied with the energy needed to carry on their many activities.

There are two phases of metabolism:

1. ***Anabolism*** (ah-**NAB**-oh-liz-em) is the process of building up larger molecules from smaller ones. During this process the body stores water, food, and oxygen for the time when these substances are needed for cell growth and repair.
2. ***Catabolism*** (kah-**TAB**-oh-liz-em) is the breaking down of larger substances or molecules into smaller ones. This process releases energy that can be stored by special molecules to be used for muscle contraction, secretion, or heat production.

Anabolism and catabolism are carried out simultaneously and continuously in the cells. Their activities are closely regulated so that the breaking down, energy-releasing reactions are balanced with the building up, energy-consuming reactions. Therefore, ***homeostasis*** (**HOH**-mee-oh-**stay**-sis) (the maintenance of normal, internal stability in the organism) is maintained. However, if we use less energy than we manufacture, we may notice a weight gain. If molecules of energy are not used, they turn to fat. To get rid of the built-up fat, more energy must be used (exercise) or less energy (food) taken in.

Completed:
Learning Objective
#1
FUNCTIONS OF HUMAN CELLS

TISSUES

Tissues are composed of groups of cells of the same kind. Each tissue has a specific function and can be recognized by its characteristic appearance. Body tissues are classified as follows:

1. ***Connective tissue*** serves to support, protect, and bind together other tissues of the body. Bone, cartilage, ligament, tendon, fascia (separates muscles), and fat tissue are examples of connective tissue.
2. ***Muscular tissue*** contracts and moves various parts of the body.
3. ***Nerve tissue*** carries messages to and from the brain, and controls and coordinates all body functions.
4. ***Epithelial*** (ep-ih-**THEE**-le-al) ***tissue*** is a protective covering on body surfaces, such as the skin, mucous membranes, linings of the heart, digestive and respiratory organs, and glands.
5. ***Liquid tissue*** carries food, waste products, and hormones by means of the blood and lymph.

Completed:
Learning Objective
#2
TYPES OF TISSUES

ORGANS

Organs are structures designed to accomplish a specific function. The most important organs of the body are the brain, which controls the body; the heart, which circulates the blood; the lungs, which supply oxygen to the blood; the liver, which removes toxic products of digestion; the kidneys, which excrete water and other waste products; and the stomach and intestines, which digest food.

SYSTEMS

Systems are groups of organs that cooperate for a common purpose, namely the welfare of the entire body. The human body is composed of the following important systems. (These systems are discussed in detail later in the chapter.)

Integumentary (in-**TEG**-yoo-men-ta-ree) ***system***—skin

Skeletal (**SKEL**-eh-tahl) ***system***—bones

Muscular (**MUS**-kyoo-lahr) ***system***—muscles

Nervous (**NUR**-vus) ***system***—nerves

Circulatory (**SUR**-kyoo-lah-tohr-ee) ***system***—blood supply

Endocrine (**EN**-doh-krin) ***system***—ductless glands

Excretory (**EK**-skreh-tohr-ee) ***system***—organs of elimination

Respiratory (**RES**-pih-rah-tohr-ee) ***system***—lungs

Digestive (deye-**GES**-tiv) ***system***—stomach and intestines

Reproductive (ree-proh-**DUK**-tiv) ***system***—organs for reproducing

The ***integumentary system*** is made up of the skin and its various accessory organs, such as the oil and sweat glands, sensory receptors, hair, and nails, and is composed of two distinct layers, the dermis and epidermis. It functions as a protective covering, contains sensory receptors, and plays a major role in the body's heat regulation.

The ***skeletal system*** is the physical foundation or framework of the body. The function of the skeletal system is to serve as a means of protection, support, and locomotion (movement).

The ***muscular system*** covers, shapes, and supports the skeleton. Its function is to produce all the movements of the body.

Completed:
Learning Objective
#3
STRUCTURES AND FUNCTIONS OF THE HUMAN BODY

INTRODUCTION TO ANATOMY AND PHYSIOLOGY

Although you may have groaned when you saw a chapter on anatomy and physiology, these are important subjects in the practice of cosmetology. A basic understanding of the structure and functions of the human body forms the scientific basis for the proper application of cosmetic services. The cosmetologist should know which cosmetic service is best for a client's condition, and how to adjust and control the service for the best results.

Very generally, ***anatomy*** (ah-**NAHT**-oh-mee) is the study of the structure of the body and what it is made of, for example, bones, muscles, and skin. ***Physiology*** (fiz-i-**OL**-oh-jee) is the study of the functions or activities performed by those structures. The cosmetologist is concerned with ***histology*** (hi-**STOL**-oh-jee), the study of the minute structural parts of the body, such as tissues, hair, nails, sweat glands, and oil glands.

Although the names of bones, muscles, arteries, veins, and nerves are seldom used in the beauty salon, an understanding of body structures will help make you more proficient in performing many of the salon services such as facials and hand and arm massage.

THE SKELETAL SYSTEM

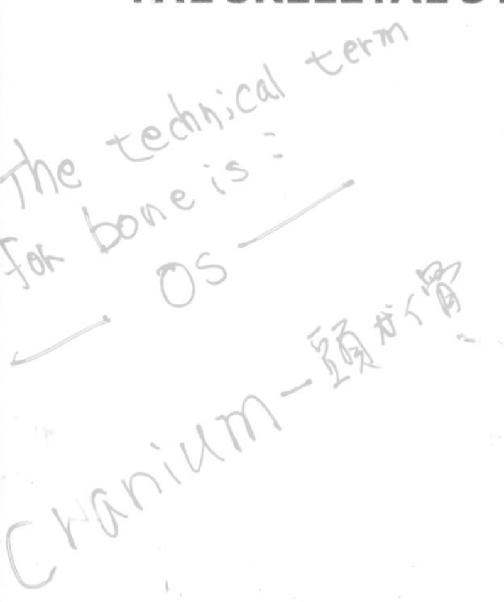

The ***skeletal system*** is the physical foundation of the body. It is composed of different shaped bones that are connected by movable and immovable joints.

Bone, except for the tissue that forms the major part of the tooth, is the hardest tissue of the body. It is composed of connective tissues consisting of about one-third animal matter, such as cells and blood, and two-thirds mineral matter, mainly calcium carbonate and calcium phosphate. The scientific study of bones, their structure, and functions is called ***osteology*** (os-tee-**OL**-oh-jee). ***Os*** is the technical term for bone.

The following are the primary functions of the bones:

1. Give shape and support to the body.
2. Protect various internal structures and organs.
3. Serve as attachments for muscles and act as levers to produce body movement.
4. Produce various blood cells in the red bone marrow.
5. Store various minerals such as calcium, phosphorus, magnesium, and sodium.

BONES OF THE SKULL

The ***skull*** is the skeleton of the head and is divided into two parts: the ***cranium***, an oval, bony case that shapes the top of the head and protects the brain, and the skeleton of the face, which is made up of fourteen facial bones. (Fig. 23.3)

Bones of the Cranium

Occipital (ok-**SIP**-i-tal) ***bone*** forms the lower back part of the cranium.

Two ***parietal*** (pah-**REYE**-eh-tal) ***bones*** form the sides and top (crown) of the cranium.

Frontal (**FRUNT**-al) ***bone*** forms the forehead.

Two ***temporal*** (**TEM**-poh-rahl) ***bones*** form the sides of the head in the ear region (below the parietal bones).

The ***ethmoid*** (**ETH**-moid) ***bone*** is a light spongy bone between the eye sockets and forms part of the nasal cavities.

Sphenoid (**SFEEN**-oid) ***bone*** joins together all the bones of the cranium. *(The ethmoid and sphenoid bones are not affected by massage.)*

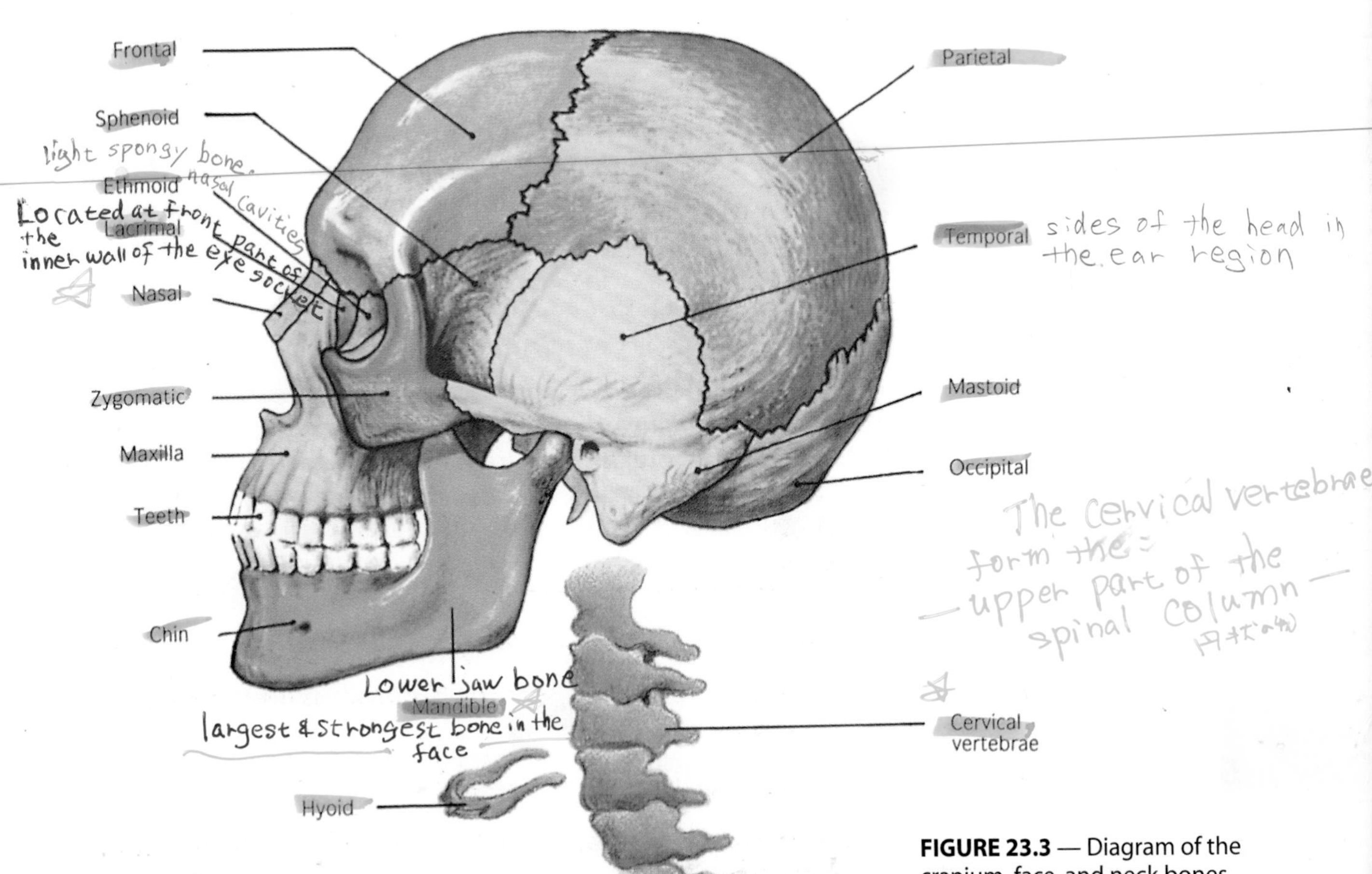

FIGURE 23.3 — Diagram of the cranium, face, and neck bones.

Bones of the Face

Two ***nasal*** (NAY-zal) ***bones*** form the bridge of the nose.

Two ***lacrimal*** (LAK-rih-mahl) ***bones*** are small fragile bones located at the front part of the inner wall of the eye sockets.

Two ***zygomatic*** (zeye-goh-MAT-ik), or ***malar bones***, form the prominence of the cheeks.

Two ***maxillae*** (mak-SIL-ee) are the upper jawbones that join to form the whole upper jaw.

Mandible (MAN-dih-bel) is the lower jawbone and is the largest and strongest bone of the face. It forms the lower jaw.

Facial bones that do not appear in Fig. 23.3 are two ***turbinal*** (TUR-bih-nahl) ***bones***, which are thin layers of spongy bone on either of the outer walls of the nasal depression; ***vomer*** (VOH-mer), which is a single bone that forms part of the dividing wall of the nose; two ***palatine*** (PAL-ah-teyen) ***bones***, which form the floor and outer wall of the nose, roof of the mouth, and floor of the orbits.

BONES OF THE NECK

(See Fig. 23.3)

Hyoid (HEYE-oid) ***bone***, a U-shaped bone, is located in the front part of the throat, and is referred to as the "Adam's apple."

Cervical vertebrae (SUR-vih-kal VER-te-bray) form the top part of the spinal column located in the neck region.

BONES OF THE CHEST (THORAX)

The ***thorax*** (THOH-racks), or chest, is an elastic bony cage that serves as a protective framework for the heart, lungs, and other delicate internal organs. This framework is constructed of twelve ***thoracic vertebrae***, twelve ribs on each side, the ***sternum*** (STUR-num) (breastbone), and the cartilage that connects the ribs to the sternum.

BONES OF THE SHOULDER, ARM, AND HAND

(See Figs. 23.4, 23.5)

The ***shoulder girdle***, each side of which is made up of one clavicle and one scapula.

Humerus (HYOO-mur-rus) is the uppermost and largest bone of the arm.

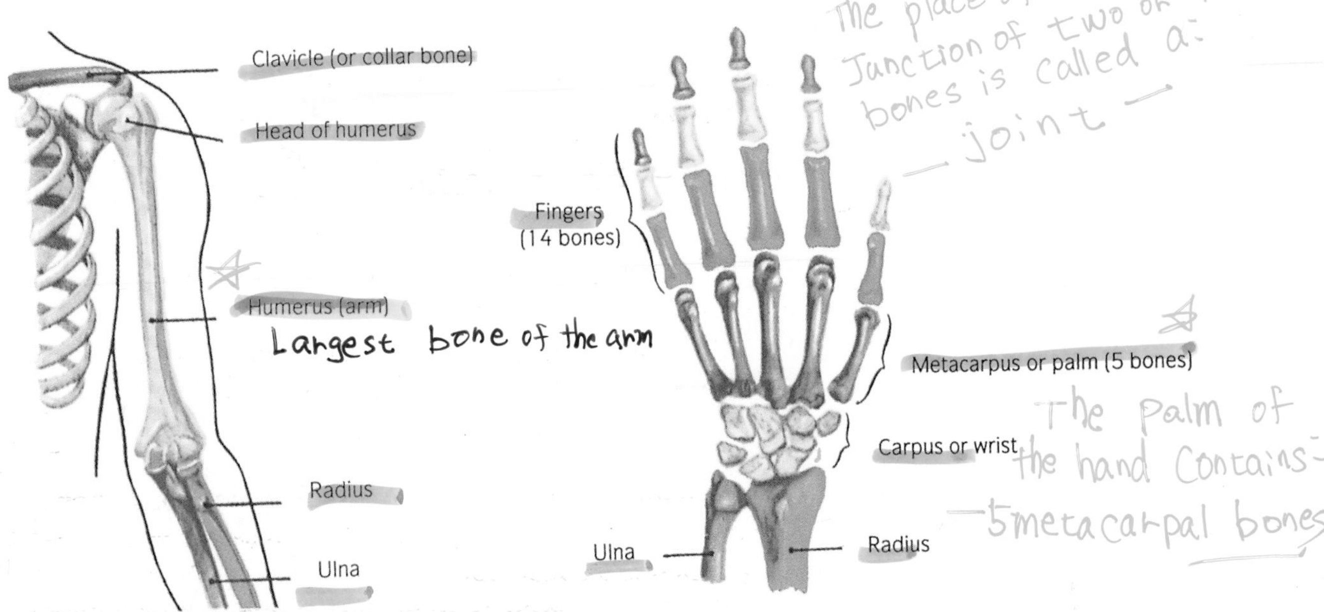

FIGURE 23.4 — Bones of the arm.

FIGURE 23.5 — Bones of the hand.

Ulna (**UL**-nah) is the large bone on the little finger side of the forearm.

Radius (**RAY**-dee-us) is the small bone on the thumb side of the forearm.

The ***wrist***, or ***carpus*** (**KAHR**-pus), is a flexible joint composed of eight small, irregular bones, held together by ligaments.

The ***palm***, or ***metacarpus*** (met-ah-**KAHR**-pus), consists of five long, slender bones, called metacarpal bones.

The ***fingers***, or ***digits*** (**DIJ**-its), consist of three ***phalanges*** (fah-**LAN**-jeez) in each finger, and two in the thumb, totaling fourteen bones.

THE MUSCULAR SYSTEM

The ***muscular*** (**MUS**-kyoo-lahr) ***system*** covers, shapes, and supports the skeleton. Its function is to produce all movements of the body. ***Myology*** (meye-**OL**-oh-jee) is the study of the structure, functions, and diseases of the muscles.

The muscular system consists of over 500 muscles, large and small, comprising 40% to 50% of the weight of the human body.

Muscles are fibrous tissues that have the ability to stretch and contract according to our movements. Different types of movements, for example, stretching and bending, depend on muscles to perform in specific ways.

There are three kinds of muscular tissue:

1. ***Striated*** (striped) or voluntary, which is controlled by will. Facial, arm, and leg muscles are voluntary muscles. (Fig. 23.6)
2. ***Non-striated*** (smooth) or involuntary muscles, such as those of the stomach and intestines. They function automatically. (Fig. 23.7)
3. ***Cardiac*** (heart muscle), which is the heart itself and is not found anywhere else in the body. (Fig. 23.8)

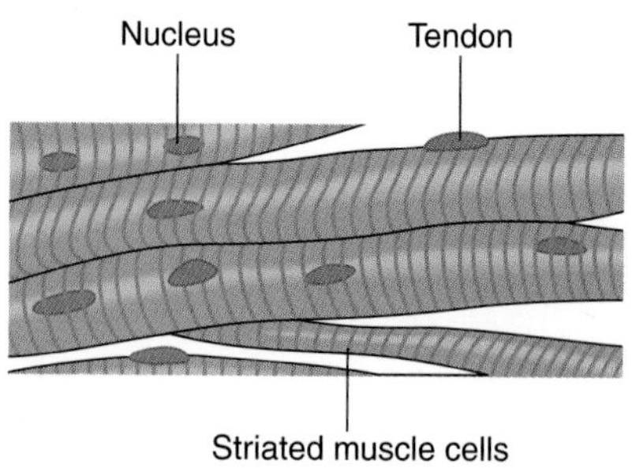

FIGURE 23.6 — Striated muscle cells.

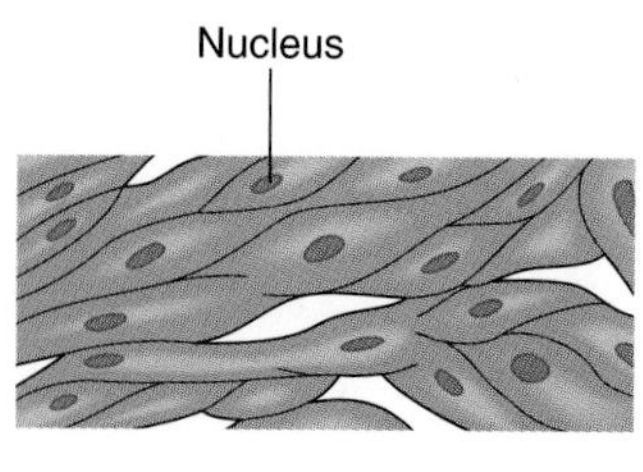

FIGURE 23.7 — Non-striated muscle cells.

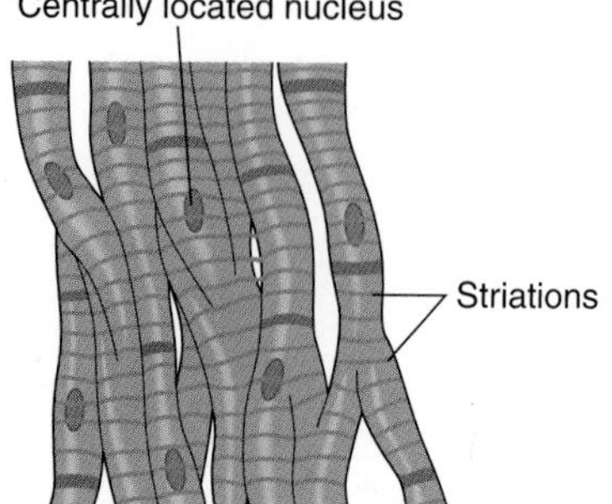

FIGURE 23.8 — Cardiac muscle cells.

MUSCLES

There are three parts to a muscle: the origin, the insertion, and the belly. The ***origin*** is the part that does not move. It is attached to the skeleton and is usually part of a skeletal muscle. The ***insertion*** is the part that moves, and the ***belly*** is the middle part.

Stimulation of Muscles

Muscular tissue can be stimulated by any of the following:

Massage (hand massage and electric vibrator)
Electric current (high-frequency and faradic current)
Light rays (infrared rays and ultraviolet rays)
Heat rays (heating lamps and heating caps)
Moist heat (steamers or moderately warm steam towels)
Nerve impulses (through the nervous system)
Chemicals (certain acids and salts)

Muscles Affected by Massage

The cosmetologist is concerned with the voluntary muscles of the head, face, neck, arms, and hands. It is essential to know where these muscles are located, and what they control. Pressure in massage is usually directed from the insertion to the origin. (Fig. 23.9)

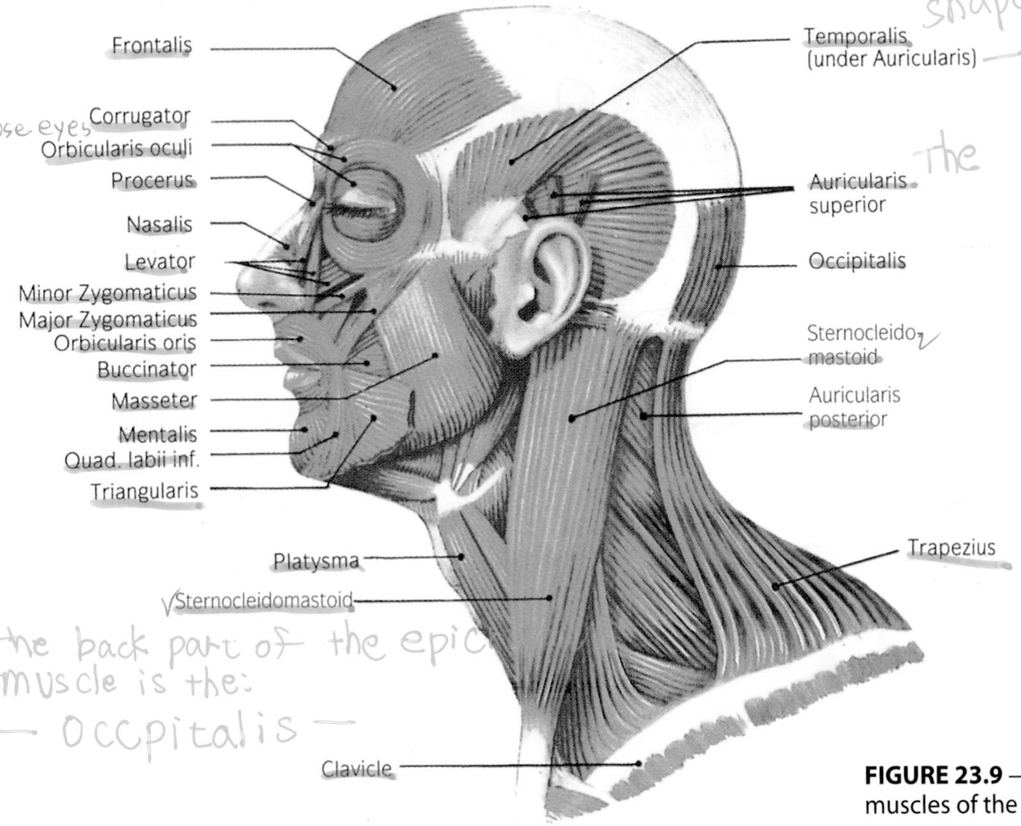

Frontalis
Corrugator
Orbicularis oculi
Procerus
Nasalis
Levator
Minor Zygomaticus
Major Zygomaticus
Orbicularis oris
Buccinator
Masseter
Mentalis
Quad. labii inf.
Triangularis
Platysma
Sternocleidomastoid
Clavicle
Temporalis (under Auricularis)
Auricularis superior
Occipitalis
Sternocleido-mastoid
Auricularis posterior
Trapezius

FIGURE 23.9 — Diagram of the muscles of the head, face, and neck.

Muscles of the Scalp

Epicranius (ep-i-**KRAY**-ne-us), or ***occipito-frontalis*** (ok-**SIP**-ih-toh-fron-**TAY**-lis), is a broad muscle that covers the top of the skull. It consists of two parts: the ***occipitalis*** (ok-**SIP**-i-ta-lis), or back part, and the ***frontalis*** (fron-**TAY**-lis), or front part. Both are connected by a tendon ***aponeurosis*** (ap-o-noo-**ROH**-sis). The frontalis raises the eyebrows, draws the scalp forward, and causes wrinkles across the forehead. (Fig. 23.10)

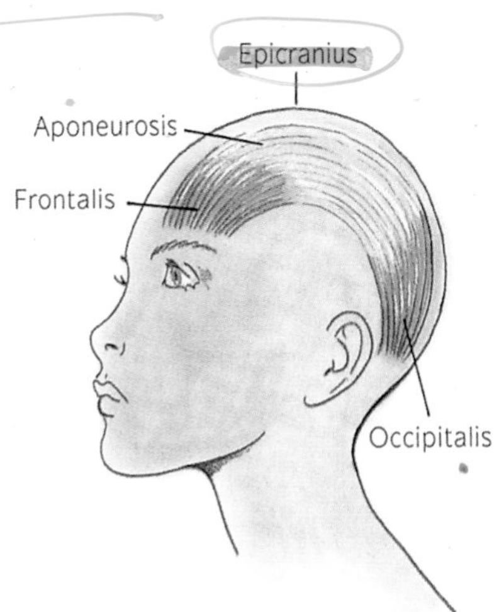

FIGURE 23.10 — Muscles of the scalp.

Muscles of the Eyebrow

Orbicularis oculi (or-bik-yoo-**LAY**-ris **OK**-yoo-leye) completely surrounds the margin of the eye socket and enables you to close your eyes.

Corrugator (**KOR**-oo-gay-tohr) muscle is beneath the frontalis and orbicularis oculi, and draws the eyebrow down and in. It produces vertical lines and is the muscle used for frowning. (Fig. 23.11)

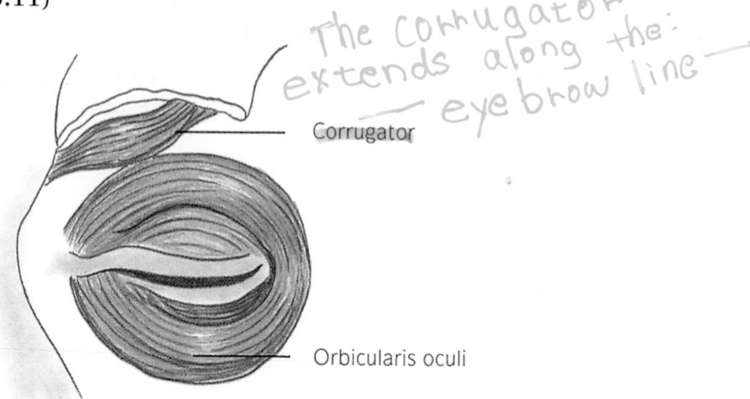

FIGURE 23.11 — Muscles of the eyebrow.

Muscles of the Nose

The ***procerus*** (proh-**SEE**-rus) covers the bridge of the nose, depresses the eyebrow, and causes wrinkles across the bridge of the nose. (Fig. 23.12)

(The other nasal muscles are small muscles around the nasal openings that contract and expand the openings of the nostrils.)

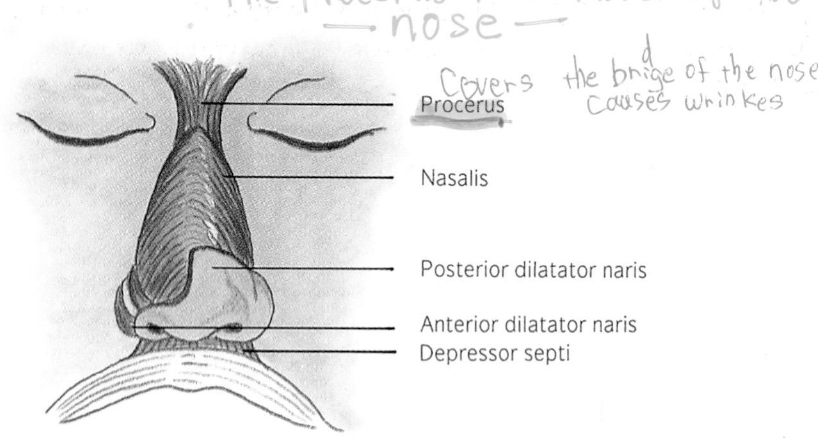

FIGURE 23.12 — Muscles of the nose.

Muscles of the Mouth

Quadratus labii superioris (kwah-**DRAY**-tus **LAY**-bee-eye soo-**PEER**-ee-or-is) consists of three parts. It surrounds the upper part of the lip, raises and draws back the upper lip, and elevates the nostrils, as in expressing distaste.

Quadratus labii inferioris (in-**FEER**-ee-or-is) surrounds the lower part of the lip. It depresses the lower lip and draws it a little to one side, as in the expression of sarcasm.

Buccinator (**BUK**-sih-nay-tor) is the muscle between the upper and lower jaws. It compresses the cheeks and expels air between the lips, as in blowing. (Fig. 23.13)

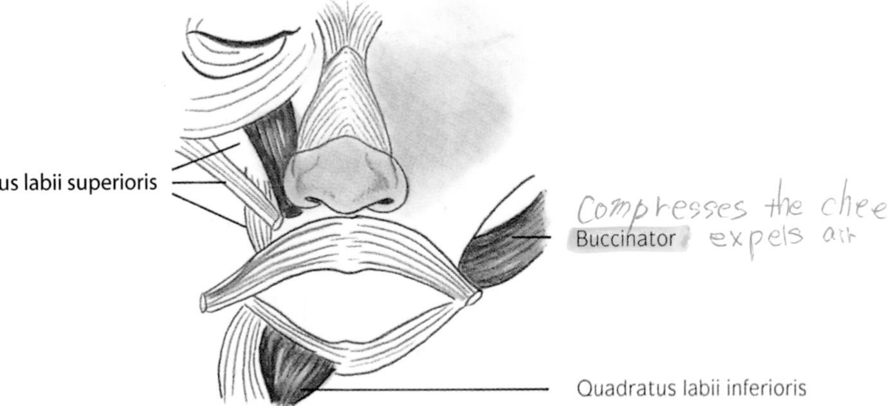

FIGURE 23.13 — Muscles of the upper and lower lips, and jaw.

Caninus (kay-**NEYE**-nus) lies under the quadratus labii superioris. It raises the angle of the mouth, as in snarling.

Mentalis (men-**TAL**-is) is situated at the tip of the chin. It raises the lower lip, causing wrinkling of the chin, as in doubt or displeasure. (Fig. 23.14)

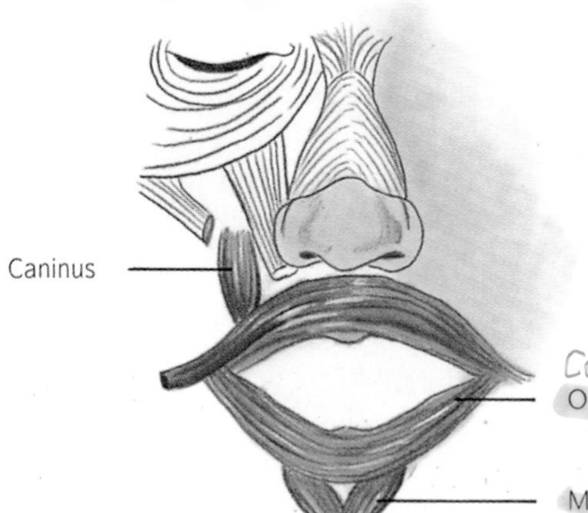

FIGURE 23.14 — Muscles of the mouth and chin.

Orbicularis oris (or-bik-yoo-**LAY**-ris **OH**-ris) forms a flat band around the upper and lower lips. It compresses, contracts, puckers, and wrinkles the lips, as in kissing or whistling.

Risorius (ri-**ZOHR**-ee-us) extends from the masseter muscle to the angle of the mouth. It draws the corner of the mouth out and back, as in grinning.

Zygomaticus (zeye-goh-**MAT**-ih-kus) extends from the zygomatic bone to the angle of the mouth. It elevates the lip, as in laughing.

Triangularis (treye-an-gyoo-**LAY**-ris) extends along the side of the chin. It draws down the corner of the mouth. (Fig. 23.15)

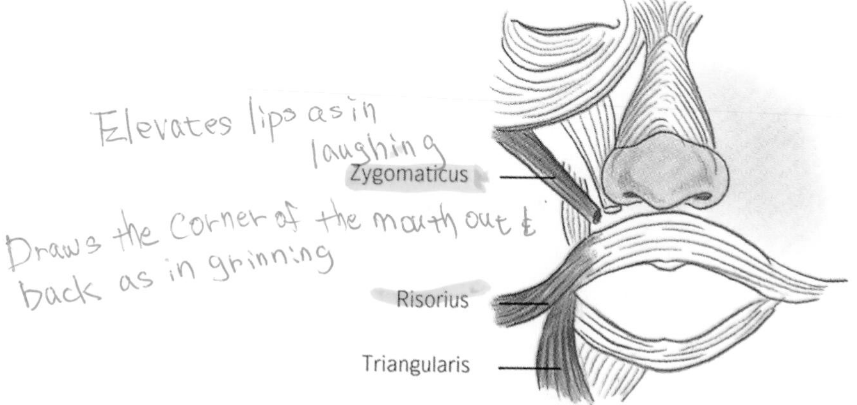

FIGURE 23.15 — Muscles of the jaw.

Muscles of the Ear

Three muscles of the ear are practically functionless:

Auricularis (aw-rik-yoo-**LAHR**-is) ***superior*** is above the ear.

Auricularis posterior is behind the ear.

Auricularis anterior is in front of the ear. (Fig. 23.16)

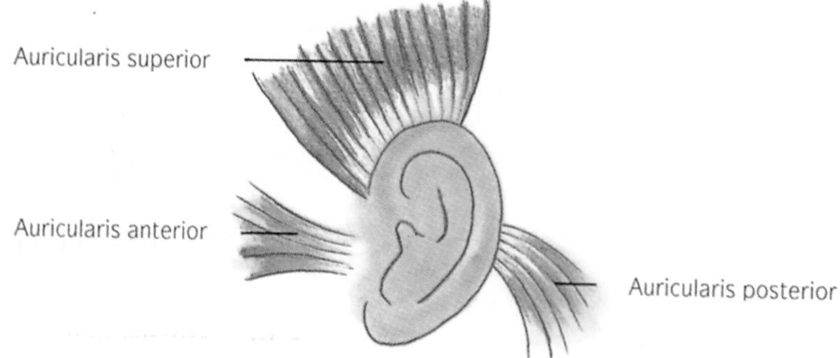

FIGURE 23.16 — Muscles of the ear.

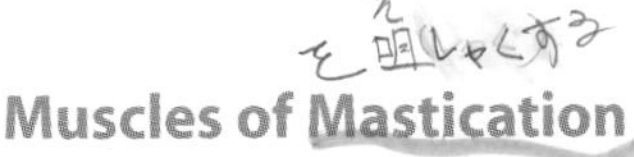

Muscles of Mastication

Masseter (ma-**SEE**-tur) and ***temporalis*** (tem-po-**RAY**-lis) are muscles that coordinate in opening and closing the mouth, and are referred to as chewing muscles. (Fig. 23.17)

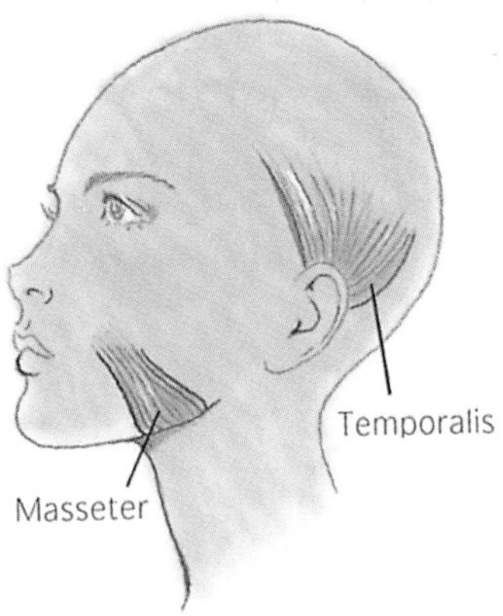

FIGURE 23.17 — Muscles of mastication.

Muscles of the Neck

Platysma (plah-**TIZ**-mah) is a broad muscle that extends from the chest and shoulder muscles to the side of the chin. It depresses the lower jaw and lip, as in the expression of sadness. (Fig. 23.18)

Sternocleidomastoid (**STUR**-noh-**KLEYE**-doh-**MAS**-toid) extends from the collar and chest bones to the temporal bone in back of the ear. It rotates and bends the head, as in nodding. (Fig. 23.19)

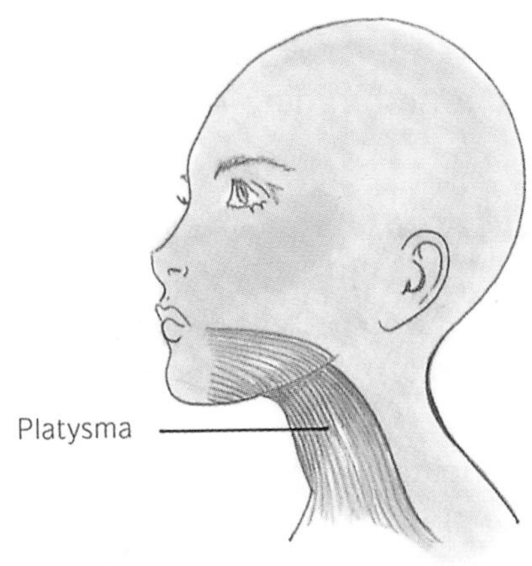

FIGURE 23.18 — Muscles of the jaw and neck.

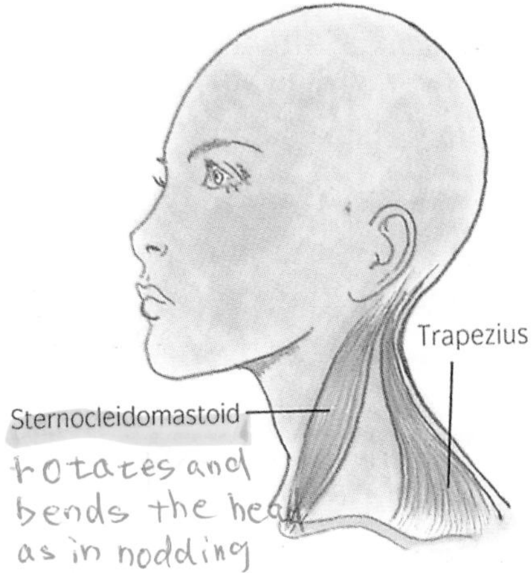

FIGURE 23.19 — Muscles of the neck.

Muscles that Attach the Arms to the Body

The principal muscles that attach the arms to the body and permit movements of the shoulders and arms are:

Trapezius (trah-**PEE**-zee-us) and ***latissimus dorsi*** (lah-**TIS**-ih-mus **DOR**-see) cover the back of the neck and upper and middle region of the back. They rotate the shoulder blade and control the swinging movements of the arm. (Fig. 23.20)

Pectoralis (pek-tor-**AL**-is) ***major*** and ***pectoralis minor*** cover the front of the chest. They also assist in swinging movements of the arm.

Serratus anterior (ser-**RAT**-us an-**TEER**-ee-or) assists in breathing and in raising the arm. (Fig. 23.21)

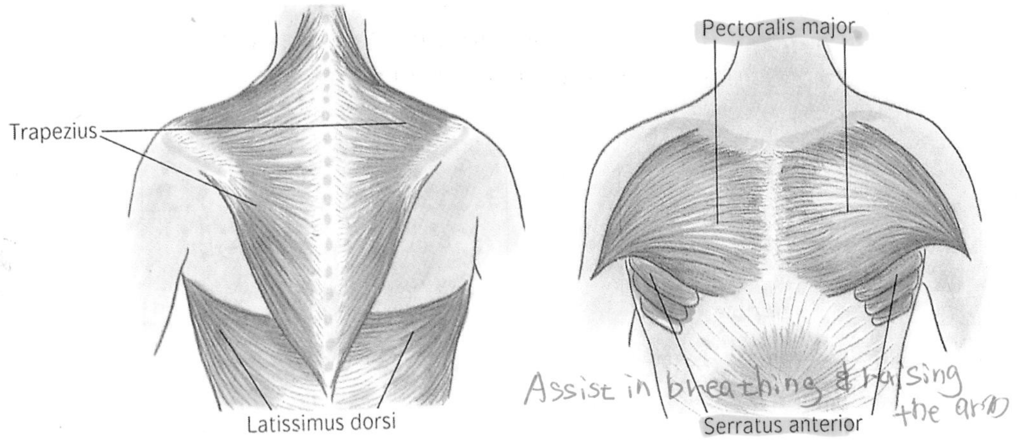

FIGURE 23.20 — Muscles of the back and neck.

FIGURE 23.21 — Muscles of the chest.

Muscles of the Shoulder, Arm, and Hand

The principal muscles of the shoulder and upper arm are given below. (Fig. 23.22)

Deltoid (**DEL**-toid) is the large, thick triangular-shaped muscle that covers the shoulder and lifts and turns the arm.

Biceps (**BEYE**-seps) is the two-headed and principal muscle in the front of the upper arm. It lifts the forearm, flexes the elbow, and turns the palm outward.

Triceps (**TREYE**-seps) is the three-headed muscle of the arm that covers the entire back of the upper arm and extends the forearm.

The forearm is made up of a series of muscles and strong tendons. The cosmetologist is concerned with the following:

Pronators (proh-**NAY**-tors) are found in the forearm and turn the hand inward, so that the palm faces downward.

Supinators (**SOO**-pi-nay-tors) turn the hand outward and the palm upward.

Flexors (**FLEKS**-ors) bend the wrist, draw the hand up, and close the fingers toward the forearm.

Extensors (ek-**STEN**-surs) straighten the wrist, hand, and fingers to form a straight line.

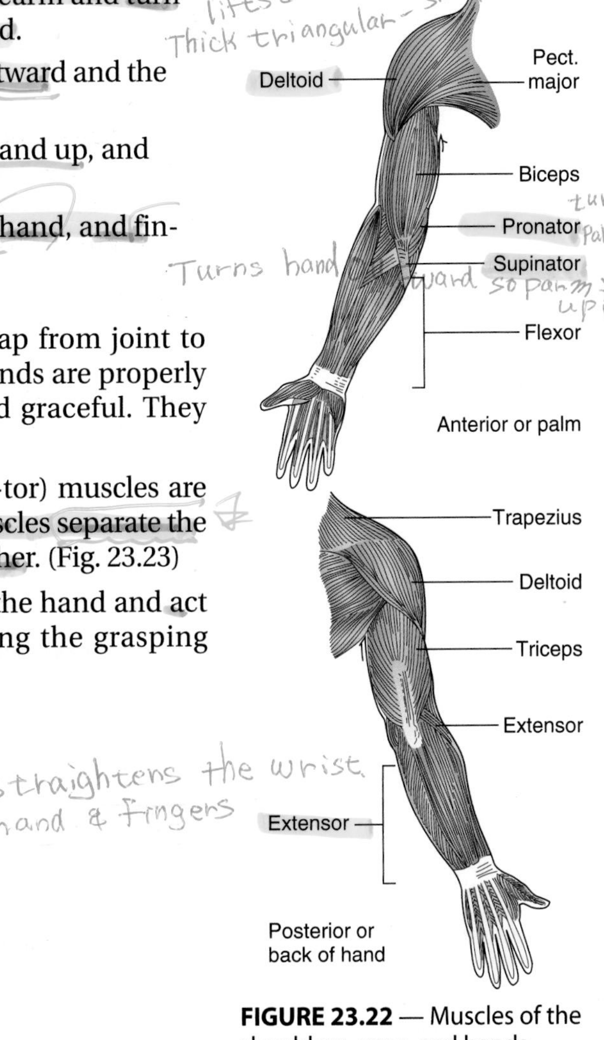

FIGURE 23.22 — Muscles of the shoulders, arms, and hands.

The hand has many small muscles that overlap from joint to joint, giving flexibility and strength. When the hands are properly cared for, these muscles will remain supple and graceful. They close and open the hands and fingers.

Abductor (ab-**DUK**-tor) and ***adductor*** (a-**DUK**-tor) muscles are located at the base of each digit. The abductor muscles separate the fingers and the adductor muscles draw them together. (Fig. 23.23)

Opponent muscles are located in the palm of the hand and act to bring the thumb toward the fingers, allowing the grasping action of the hands.

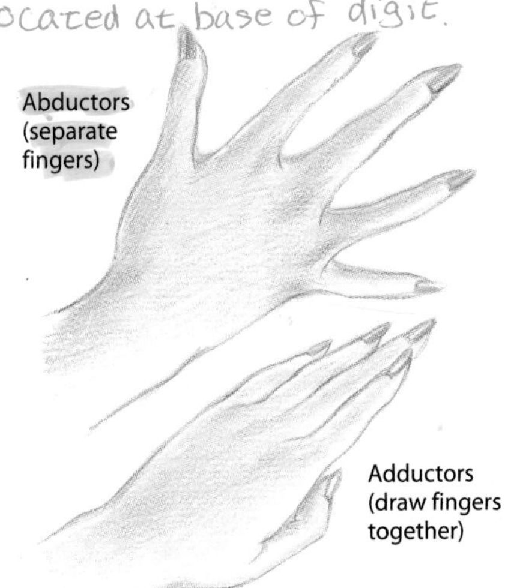

FIGURE 23.23 — Muscles of the hand.

THE NERVOUS SYSTEM

Neurology (noo-**ROL**-oh-jee) is the branch of anatomy that deals with the nervous system and its disorders.

The ***nervous*** (**NUR**-vus) ***system*** is one of the most important systems of the body. It controls and coordinates the functions of all the other systems and makes them work harmoniously and efficiently. Every square inch of the human body is supplied with fine fibers, which we know as ***nerves.***

The main purpose in studying the nervous system is to understand:

1. How the cosmetologist administers scalp and facial services for the client's benefit.
2. What effects these treatments have on the nerves in the skin and scalp, and on the body as a whole.

DIVISIONS OF THE NERVOUS SYSTEM

The principal parts that compose the nervous system are the brain and spinal cord and their nerves. Generally, the nervous system is composed of three main divisions:

1. The ***cerebro-spinal*** (ser-**EE**-broh **SPEYE**-nahl), or ***central,*** nervous system (CNS).
2. The ***peripheral*** (peh-**RIF**-er-al) nervous system.
3. The ***autonomic*** (aw-toh-**NAHM**-ik) nervous system (ANS), which includes the sympathetic (sim-pah-**THET**-ik) and parasympathetic (**PAH**-rah-sim-pah-**THET**-ik) systems.

The ***central nervous system*** consists of the brain and spinal cord. The following are its functions:

1. Controls consciousness and all mental activities.
2. Controls voluntary functions of the five senses: seeing, smelling, tasting, feeling, and hearing.
3. Controls voluntary muscle actions, such as all body movements and facial expressions.

The ***peripheral nervous system*** is made up of the sensory and motor nerve fibers that extend from the brain and spinal cord and are distributed to all parts of the body. Its function is to carry messages to and from the central nervous system.

The ***autonomic nervous system*** is the portion of the nervous system that functions without conscious effort and regulates the activities of the smooth muscles, glands, blood vessels, and heart. This system has two divisions: the ***sympathetic*** and ***parasympathetic systems,*** which act in direct opposition to each other to regulate such things as heart rate, blood pressure, breathing rate, and body temperature to aid the body in the maintenance of homeostasis (balance). The sympathetic division is primarily activated during stressful, energy-demanding, or emergency situations; the parasympathetic division is most active in ordinary restful situations.

THE BRAIN AND SPINAL CORD

The brain is the largest mass of nerve tissue in the body and is contained in the cranium. The weight of the average brain is 44 to 48 ounces (1232 to 1344 g). It is considered to be the central power station of the body, sending and receiving telegraphic messages. Twelve pairs of cranial nerves originate in the brain and reach various parts of the head, face, and neck.

The spinal cord is composed of masses of nerve cells, with fibers running upward and downward. It originates in the brain, extends the length of the trunk, and is enclosed and protected by the spinal column. Thirty-one pairs of spinal nerves, extending from the spinal cord, are distributed to the muscles and skin of the trunk and limbs. Some of the spinal nerves supply the internal organs controlled by the sympathetic nervous system. (Fig. 23.24)

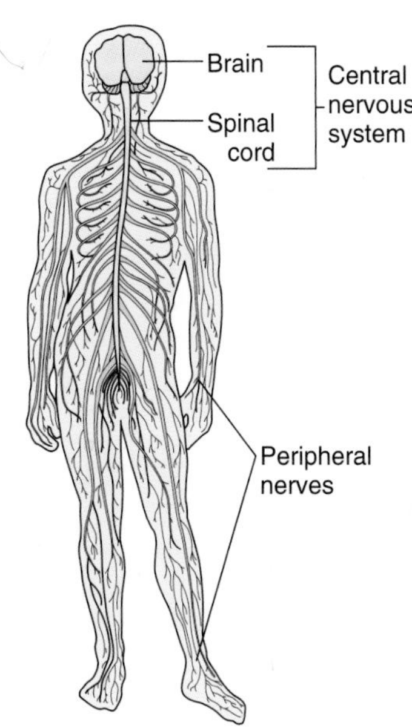

FIGURE 23.24 — Spinal cord.

NERVE CELLS AND NERVES

A ***neuron*** (NOOR-on), or ***nerve cell***, is the primary structural unit of the nervous system. (Fig. 23.25) It is composed of a cell body, ***dendrites*** (DEN-drights), which receive messages from other neurons, and an ***axon*** (AK-son) and ***axon terminal***, which send messages to other neurons, glands, or muscles.

Nerves are long, white cords made up of fibers that carry messages to and from various parts of the body. Nerves have their origin in the brain and spinal cord, and distribute branches to all parts of the body.

Types of Nerves

Sensory nerves, called ***afferent*** (AF-fer-ent) ***nerves***, carry impulses or messages from sense organs to the brain, where sensations of touch, cold, heat, sight, hearing, taste, smell, pain, and pressure are experienced.

Motor nerves, called ***efferent*** (EF-fer-ent) ***nerves***, carry impulses from the brain to the muscles. The transmitted impulses produce movement.

Mixed nerves contain both sensory and motor fibers and have the ability to both send and receive messages.

Sensory nerve endings called receptors are located near the surface of the skin. As impulses pass from the sensory nerves to the brain and back over the motor nerves to the muscles, a complete circuit is established and movement of the muscles results.

A ***reflex*** is an automatic response to a stimulus that involves the movement of an impulse from a sensory receptor along an

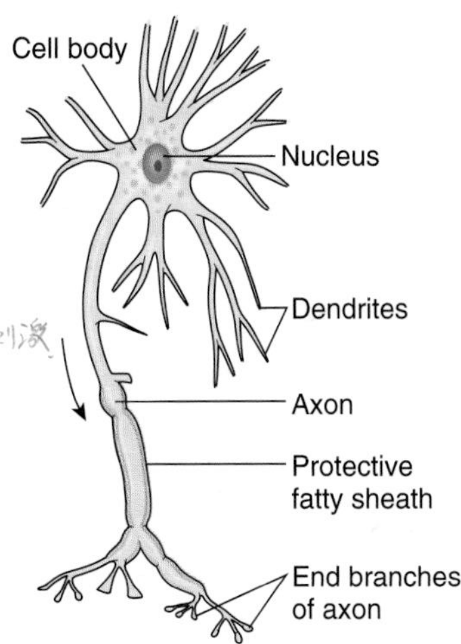

FIGURE 23.25 — A neuron or nerve cell.

afferent nerve to the spinal cord, and a responsive impulse along an *efferent* neuron to a muscle causing a reaction. (Example: the quick removal of the hand from a hot object.) A reflex act does not have to be learned.

Nerves of the Head, Face, and Neck

The ***fifth cranial, trifacial,*** or ***trigeminal nerve*** is the largest of the cranial nerves. It is the chief sensory nerve of the face, and the motor nerve of the muscles that control chewing. It consists of three branches: ***ophthalmic, mandibular,*** and ***maxillary.***

The following are the important branches of the fifth cranial nerve that are affected by massage. (Fig. 23.26)

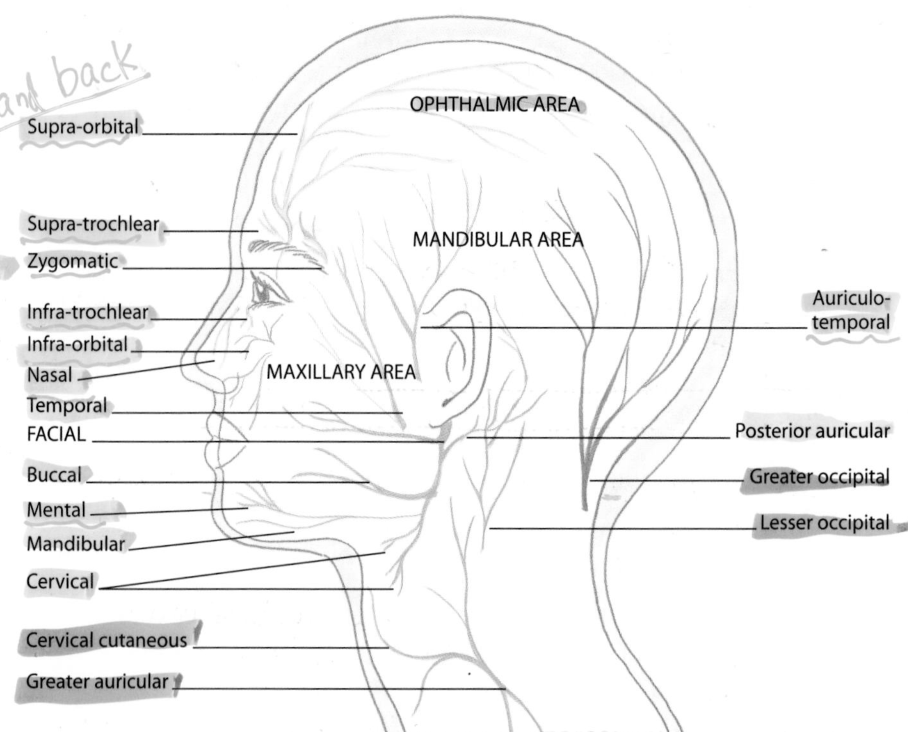

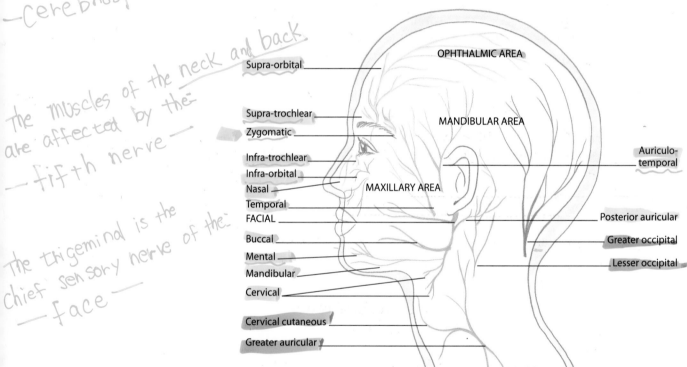

FIGURE 23.26 — Diagram of the nerves of the head, face, and neck.

1. ***Supra-orbital*** (soo-prah-**OHR**-bih-tahl) ***nerve*** affects the skin of the forehead, scalp, eyebrow, and upper eyelid.
2. ***Supra-trochlear*** (soo-prah-**TROK**-lee-ahr) ***nerve*** affects the skin between the eyes and upper side of the nose.
3. ***Infra-trochlear*** (in-frah-**TROK**-lee-ahr) ***nerve*** affects the membrane and skin of the nose.
4. ***Nasal*** (**NAY**-zal) ***nerve*** affects the point and lower side of the nose.

5. ***Zygomatic*** (zeye-goh-**MAT**-ik) ***nerve*** affects the skin of the temple, side of the forehead, and upper part of the cheek.
6. ***Infraorbital*** (in-frah-**OHR**-bih-tal) ***nerve*** affects the skin of the lower eyelid, side of the nose, upper lip, and mouth.
7. ***Auriculotemporal*** (aw-**RIK**-yoo-loh **TEM**-poh-ral) ***nerve*** affects the external ear and skin above the temple, up to the top of the skull.
8. ***Mental*** (**MEN**-tal) ***nerve*** affects the skin of the lower lip and chin.

The ***seventh (facial) cranial nerve*** is the chief motor nerve of the face. It emerges near the lower part of the ear; its divisions and their branches supply and control all the muscles of facial expression, and extend to the muscles of the neck.

The following are the most important branches of the facial nerve:

1. ***Posterior auricular*** (poh-**STEER**-ee-or o-**RIK**-yoo-lahr) ***nerve*** affects the muscles behind the ear at the base of the skull.
2. ***Temporal*** (**TEM**-poh-rahl) ***nerve*** affects the muscles of the temple, side of forehead, eyebrow, eyelid, and upper part of the cheek.
3. ***Zygomatic*** (zeye-goh-**MAT**-ik) ***nerve (upper and lower)*** affects the muscles of the upper part of the cheek.
4. ***Buccal*** (**BUK**-ahl) ***nerve*** affects the muscles of the mouth.
5. ***Mandibular*** (man-**DIB**-yoo-lahr) ***nerve*** affects the muscles of the chin and lower lip.
6. ***Cervical*** (**SUR**-vi-kal) ***nerve*** (branch of the facial nerve) affects the side of the neck and the platysma muscle.

The ***eleventh*** (accessory) ***cranial nerve*** (spinal branch) affects the muscles of the neck and back.

Cervical nerves originate at the spinal cord, and their branches supply the muscles and scalp at the back of the head and neck, as follows:

1. ***Greater occipital*** (ok-**SIP**-ih-tal) ***nerve***, located in the back of the head, affects the scalp as far up as the top of the head.
2. ***Smaller (lesser) occipital nerve***, located at the base of the skull, affects the scalp and muscles of this region.
3. ***Greater auricular*** (o-**RIK**-yoo-lahr) ***nerve***, located at the side of the neck, affects the external ear, and the area in front and back of the ear.

4. ***Cervical cutaneous*** (kyoo-TAY-nee-us), or ***cutaneous colli*** (CO-li) ***nerve***, located at the side of the neck, affects the front and side of the neck as far down as the breastbone.

Nerves of the Arm and Hand

The principal nerves supplying the superficial parts of the arm and hand are as follows. (Fig. 23.27)

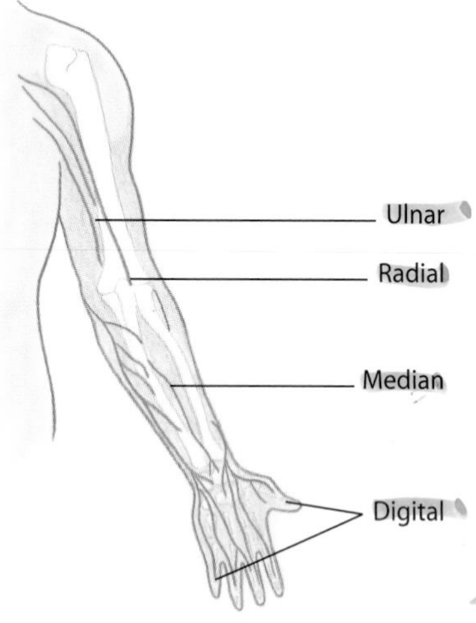

FIGURE 23.27 — Nerves of the arm and hand.

1. The ***ulnar*** (UL-nar) ***nerve*** (sensory-motor), with its branches, supplies the little finger side of the arm and the palm of the hand.
2. The ***radial*** (RAY-dee-al) ***nerve*** (sensory-motor), with its branches, supplies the thumb side of the arm and the back of the hand.
3. The ***median*** (MEE-dee-an) ***nerve*** (sensory-motor) is a smaller nerve than the ulnar and radial nerves. With its branches, it supplies the arm and hand.
4. The ***digital*** (DIJ-it-tal) ***nerve*** (sensory-motor), with its branches, supplies all fingers of the hand.

THE CIRCULATORY SYSTEM

The ***circulatory*** (SUR-kyoo-lah-tohr-ee), or ***vascular*** (VAS-kyoo-lahr), ***system*** is vitally related to the maintenance of good health. The vascular system controls the steady circulation of the blood through the body by means of the heart and the blood vessels (the ***arteries*** [AHR-te-rees], ***veins***, and ***capillaries*** [KAP-ih-lar-eez]).

The vascular system is made up of two divisions:

1. The ***blood-vascular*** (BLUHD VAS-kyoo-lahr) ***system*** consists of the heart and blood vessels (arteries, capillaries, and veins) for the circulation of the blood.
2. The ***lymph-vascular*** (LIMF VAS-kyoo-lahr), or ***lymphatic*** (lim-FAT-ik), ***system*** consists of lymph glands and vessels through which the lymph circulates.

These two systems are intimately linked with each other. Lymph is derived from the blood and is gradually shifted back into the bloodstream.

THE HEART

The heart is a muscular, conical-shaped organ, about the size of a closed fist. It is located in the chest cavity and is enclosed in a membrane, the ***pericardium*** (per-ee-**KAHR**-dee-um). It is an efficient pump that keeps the blood moving within the circulatory system. (Fig. 23.28) At the normal resting rate, the heart beats about 72 to 80 times a minute. The ***vagus*** (tenth cranial nerve) and nerves from the ***autonomic nervous system*** regulate the heartbeat.

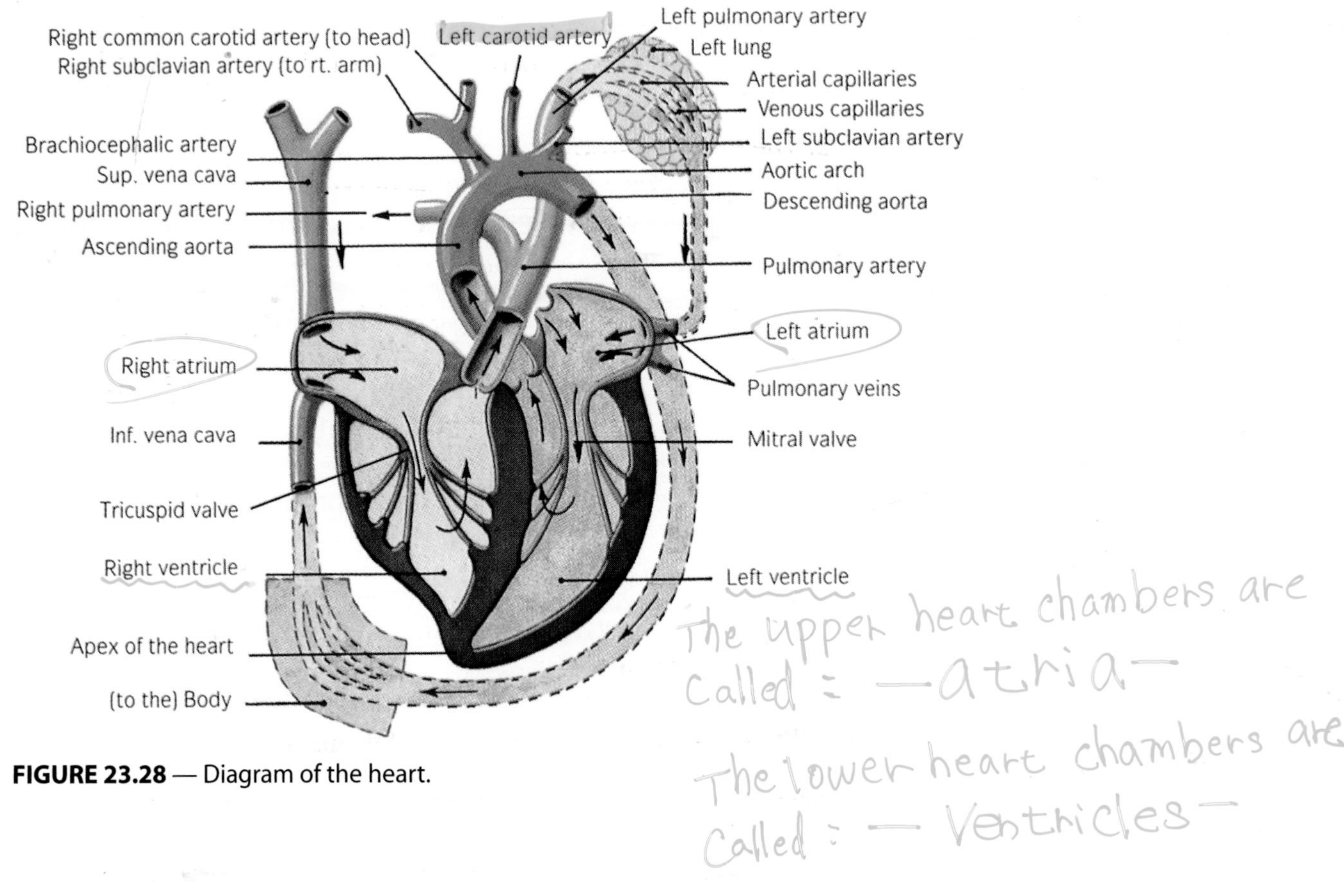

FIGURE 23.28 — Diagram of the heart.

The interior of the heart contains four chambers and four valves. The upper thin-walled chambers are the ***right atrium*** (**AY**-tree-um) and ***left atrium***. The lower thick-walled chambers are the ***right ventricle*** (**VEN**-trih-kel) and ***left ventricle***. ***Valves*** allow the blood to flow in only one direction. With each contraction and relaxation of the heart, the blood flows in, travels from the ***atria*** (**AY**-tree-ah) to the ventricles, and is then driven out, to be distributed all over the body. The atrium is also called the ***auricle*** (**OR**-ik-kel).

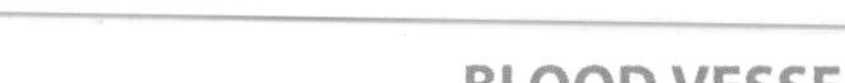

BLOOD VESSELS

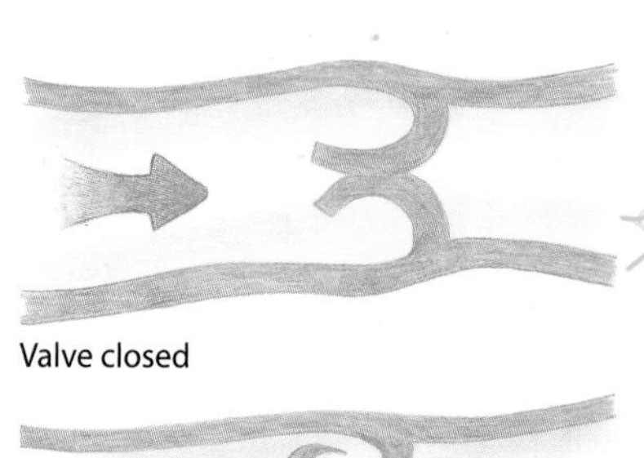

Valve closed

Valve open

FIGURE 23.29 — Cross sections of veins.

The arteries, capillaries, and veins are tube-like in construction. They transport blood to and from the heart and to various tissues of the body.

Arteries are thick-walled muscular and elastic tubes that carry pure blood from the heart to the capillaries.

Capillaries are minute, thin-walled blood vessels that connect the smaller arteries to the veins. Through their walls, the tissues receive nourishment and eliminate waste products.

Veins are thin-walled blood vessels that are less elastic than arteries. They contain cup-like valves to prevent back flow and carry impure blood from the various capillaries back to the heart. Veins are located closer to the outer surface of the body than arteries. (Fig. 23.29)

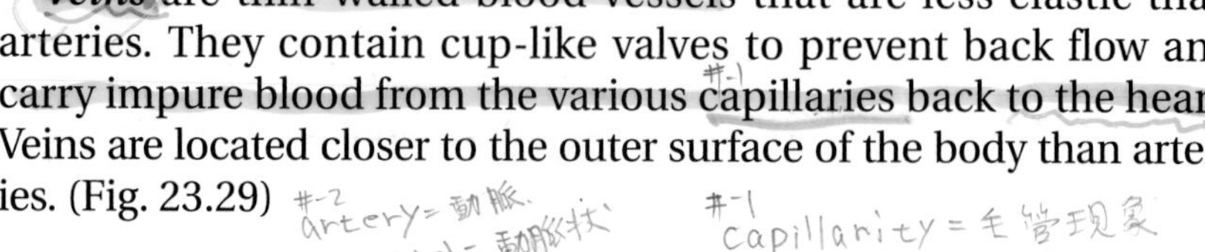

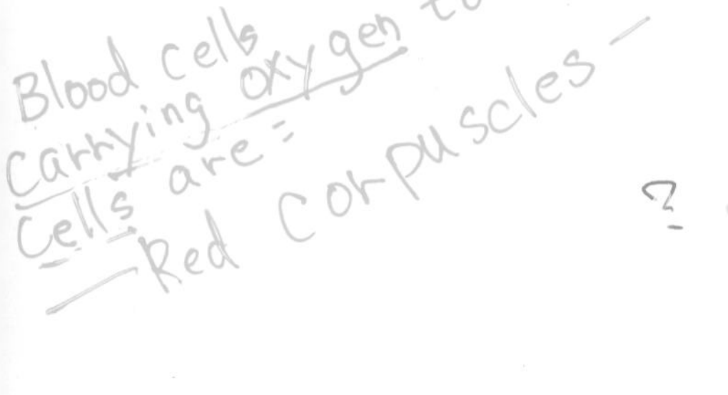

THE BLOOD

Blood is the nutritive fluid circulating through the circulatory system. It is a sticky, salty fluid with a normal temperature of 98.6° Fahrenheit (37° Celsius), and it makes up about one-twentieth of the weight of the body. Approximately 8 to 10 pints (3.76 to 4.7 l) of blood fill the blood vessels of an adult. Blood is bright red in color in the arteries (except in the pulmonary artery) and dark red in the veins (except in the pulmonary vein). This change in color is due to the exchange of carbon dioxide for oxygen as the blood passes through the lungs and the exchange of oxygen for carbon dioxide as the blood circulates throughout the body.

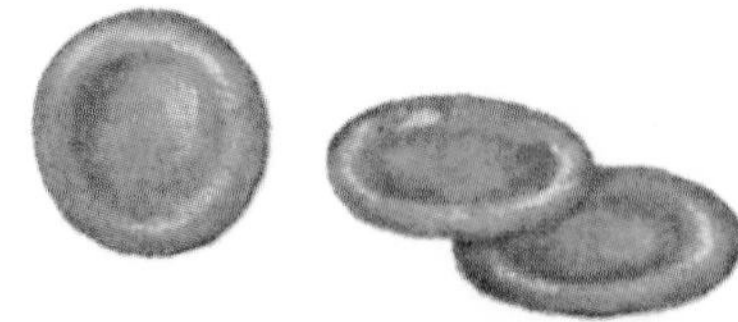

FIGURE 23.30 — Red corpuscles.

Circulation of the Blood

The blood is in constant circulation from the moment it leaves until it returns to the heart. There are two systems that take care of this circulation:

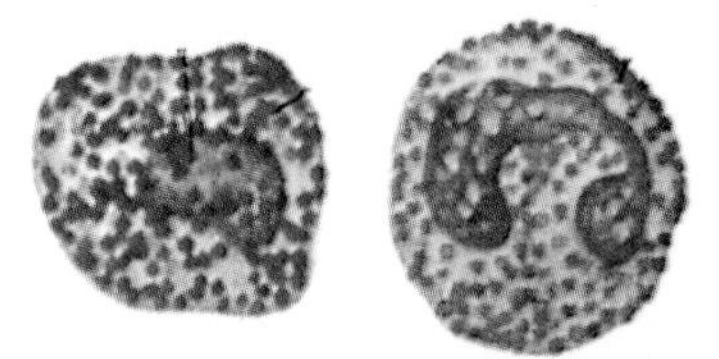

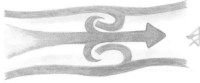

FIGURE 23.31 — White corpuscles.

1. ***Pulmonary*** **(PUL-moh-ner-ee)** ***circulation*** is the blood circulation that goes from the heart to the lungs to be purified.
2. ***Systemic*** or ***general circulation*** is the blood circulation from the heart throughout the body and back again to the heart.

Composition of the Blood

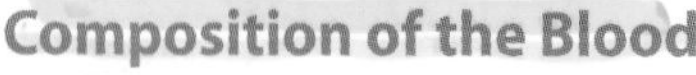

The blood is composed of red and white corpuscles, platelets, and plasma. (Figs. 23.30–23.32)

The function of ***red corpuscles*** (red blood cells) is to carry oxygen to the cells. ***White corpuscles*** (white blood cells), or ***leucocytes*** **(LOO-koh-sights)**, perform the function of destroying disease-causing germs.

Blood platelets are much smaller than the red blood cells. They play an important part in the clotting of the blood.

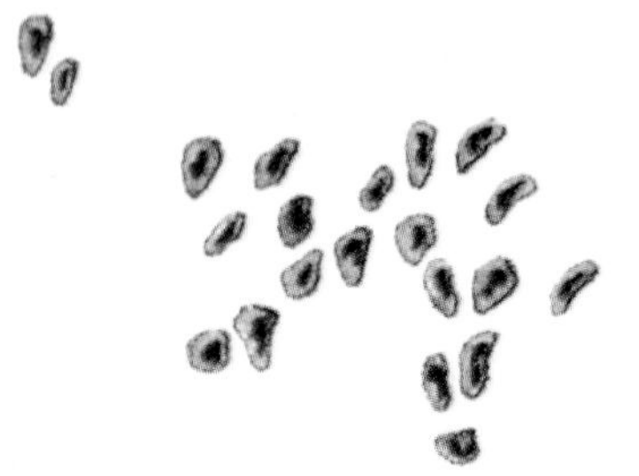

FIGURE 23.32 — Platelets.

Plasma is the fluid part of the blood in which the red and white blood cells and blood platelets flow. It is straw-like in color. About nine-tenths of plasma is water. It carries food and secretions to the cells and carbon dioxide from the cells.

Chief Functions of the Blood

The following are the primary functions of the blood:

1. Carries water, oxygen, food, and secretions to all cells of the body.
2. Carries away carbon dioxide and waste products to be eliminated through the lungs, skin, kidneys, and large intestine.
3. Helps to equalize the body temperature, thus protecting the body from extreme heat and cold.
4. Aids in protecting the body from harmful bacteria and infections, through the action of the white blood cells.
5. Clots the blood, thereby closing injured minute blood vessels and preventing the loss of blood.

THE LYMPH-VASCULAR SYSTEM

The ***lymph-vascular*** (**LIMF VAS**-kyoo-lahr) ***system***, also called ***lymphatic system***, acts as an aid to the blood system and consists of lymph spaces, lymph vessels, lymph glands, and ***lacteals*** (**LAK**-teels).

Lymph is a colorless, watery fluid that is derived from the plasma of the blood, mainly by filtration through the capillary walls into the tissue spaces. By bathing all cells, the tissue fluid acts as a medium of exchange, trading its nutritive materials to the cells in return for the waste products of metabolism. This fluid is absorbed into the lymphatics or lymph capillaries to become lymph and is then filtered and detoxified as it passes through the lymph nodes and is eventually reintroduced into the blood circulation.

The following are the primary functions of lymph:

1. Reaches the parts of the body not reached by blood and carries on an interchange with the blood.
2. Carries nourishment from the blood to the body cells.
3. Acts as a bodily defense against invading bacteria and toxins.
4. Removes waste material from the body cells to the blood.
5. Provides a suitable fluid environment for the cells.

ARTERIES OF THE HEAD, FACE, AND NECK

The ***common carotid*** (kah-**ROT**-id) ***arteries*** are the main sources of blood supply to the head, face, and neck. They are located on either side of the neck and divide into internal and external carotid arteries. The ***internal division*** of the common carotid artery supplies the brain, eye sockets, eyelids, and forehead, while the ***external division*** supplies the superficial parts of the head, face, and neck. (Fig. 23.33)

The external carotid artery subdivides into a number of branches, which supply blood to various regions of the head, face, and neck. Of particular interest to the cosmetologist are the following arteries:

Facial artery (external maxillary) (**MAK**-sih-ler-ee) supplies blood to the lower region of the face, mouth, and nose. Some of its branches are:

1. ***Submental*** (sub-**MEN**-tahl) ***artery*** supplies the chin and lower lip.
2. ***Inferior labial*** (**LAY**-bee-al) ***artery*** supplies the lower lip.
3. ***Angular*** (**ANG**-gyoo-lur) ***artery*** supplies the side of the nose.
4. ***Superior labial artery*** supplies the upper lip, septum, and wing of the nose.

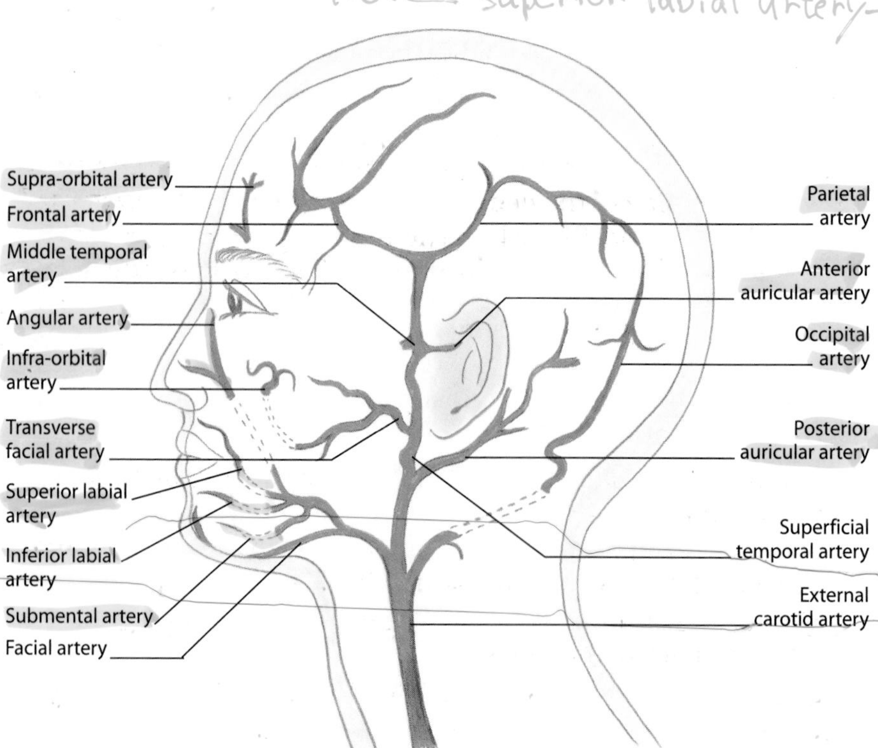

FIGURE 23.33 — Diagram of the arteries of the head, face, and neck.

Superficial temporal (**TEM**-poh-rahl) ***artery*** is a continuation of the external carotid artery, which supplies muscles, skin, and scalp to the front, side, and top of the head. Some of its important branches are:

1. ***Frontal*** (**FRUNT**-al) ***artery*** supplies the forehead.
2. ***Parietal*** (pah-**REYE**-eh-tal) ***artery*** supplies the crown and side of the head.
3. ***Transverse*** (trans-**VURS**) ***facial artery*** supplies the masseter.
4. ***Middle temporal*** (**TEM**-poh-ral) ***artery*** supplies the temples.
5. ***Anterior auricular*** (aw-**RIK**-yoo-lahr) ***artery*** supplies the anterior part of the ear.

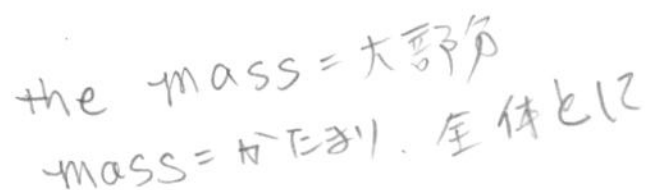

The ***supra-orbital*** (soo-prah-**OHR**-bih-tal) ***artery***, a branch of the internal carotid artery, supplies part of the forehead, the eye socket, eyelid, and upper muscles of the eye.

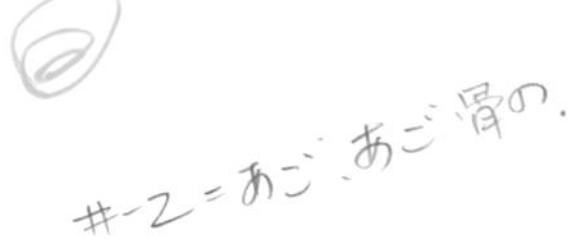

Infra-orbital (in-frah-**OR**-bi-tal) ***artery*** originates from the internal maxillary artery, and it supplies the muscles of the eye.

Occipital (ok-**SIP**-ih-tal) ***artery*** supplies the back of the head, up to the crown.

Posterior auricular (o-**RIK**-yoo-lahr) ***artery*** supplies the scalp, the area back and above the ear, and the skin behind the ear.

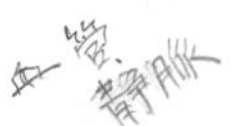

VEINS OF THE HEAD, FACE, AND NECK

The blood returning to the heart from the head, face, and neck flows on each side of the neck in two principal veins: the ***internal jugular*** and ***external jugular***. The most important veins of the face and neck are parallel to the arteries and take the same names as the arteries.

BLOOD SUPPLY FOR THE ARM AND HAND

The ***ulnar*** and ***radial*** arteries are the main blood supply for the arm and hand. (Fig. 23.34)

The ulnar artery and its numerous branches supply the little finger side of the arm and the palm of the hand.

The radial artery and its branches supply the thumb side of the arm and the back of the hand.

The important veins are located almost parallel with the arteries and take the same names as the arteries. While the arteries are found deep in the tissues, the veins lie nearer to the surface of the arms and hands.

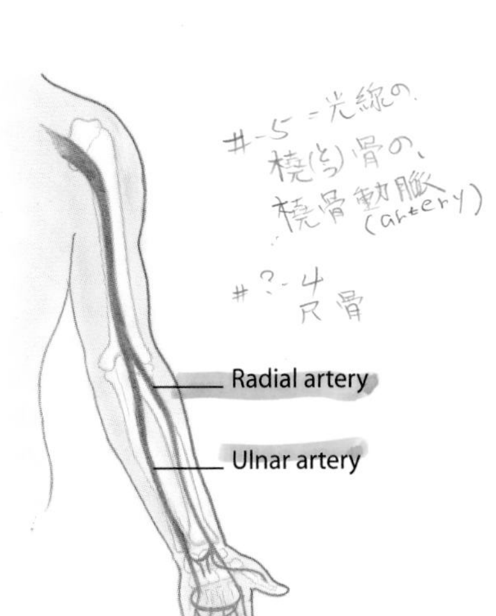

FIGURE 23.34 — Arteries of the hand and arm.

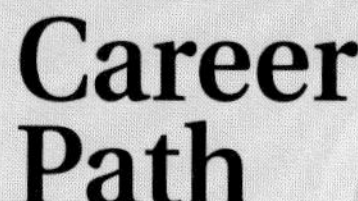

COSMETOLOGY TEACHER

If you have in-depth knowledge of the cosmetology field and a knack for getting information across to others, you may decide to become a cosmetology teacher, either in a private school or in a public vocational-technical institution.

A cosmetology teacher should have a high level of expertise in the practice of cosmetology. There is no way that a teacher can be effective without first mastering the techniques and knowledge required of a top-notch cosmetologist. The best way to achieve this is not only to complete your training, pass your boards, and take teacher training, but also to work in a salon for at least several years. The experience you gain in the practical aspects of surviving in the beauty industry—dealing with clients, competition, and selling products—will help you again and again in your teaching.

To be effective in the classroom, you must also have skill in the process of teaching: knowing how to give instruction to many different types of learners. These skills can be learned, thanks to educational research compiled in the past several decades. Educational training is a must.

A good teacher is also a well-rounded person who has interests outside of the classroom. A person who is well-read and knowledgeable in many areas (politics, the arts, social issues) will be an interesting teacher and a good role model.

In terms of attitude and personality, the successful teacher should have a calm, even temperament; a good sense of humor; an ability to adjust to changing conditions; a willingness to see different points of view; and, above all, patience.

Finally, if you are to remain at the top of your profession, you must constantly keep abreast of changes in the field of cosmetology in order to serve students entering this competitive industry. As a teacher, your own education never stops.

—*From* On Becoming a Cosmetology Teacher
by James K. Nighswander and A. Dan Whitley

THE ENDOCRINE SYSTEM

Glands are specialized organs that vary in size and function. The blood and nerves are intimately connected with the glands. The nervous system controls the functional activities of the glands. The glands have the ability to take certain elements from the blood and convert them into new compounds.

There are two main sets of glands:

1. One group is called the ***exocrine***, or ***duct glands***, with canals that lead from the gland to a particular part of the body. Sweat and oil glands of the skin and intestinal glands belong to this group.
2. The other group, known as ***endocrine***, or ***ductless glands***, have secretions called hormones delivered directly into the bloodstream, which in turn influences the welfare of the entire body.

THE EXCRETORY SYSTEM

The ***excretory*** (**EK**-skre-tohr-ee) ***system***, including the kidneys, liver, skin, intestines, and lungs, purifies the body by eliminating waste matter.

Each of the following plays a part in the excretory system:

1. The ***kidneys*** excrete urine.
2. The ***liver*** discharges bile.
3. The ***skin*** eliminates perspiration.
4. The ***large intestine*** evacuates decomposed and undigested food.
5. The ***lungs*** exhale carbon dioxide.

Metabolism of the cells of the body forms various toxic substances which, if retained, might poison the body.

THE RESPIRATORY SYSTEM

The ***respiratory*** (**RES**-pih-rah-tohr-ee) ***system*** is situated within the chest cavity, which is protected on both sides by the ribs. The ***diaphragm*** (**DEYE**-ah-fram), a muscular partition that controls breathing, separates the chest from the ***abdominal*** (ab-**DOM**-i-nal) region.

The ***lungs*** are spongy tissues composed of microscopic cells that take in air. These tiny air cells are enclosed in a skin-like tissue. Behind this, the fine capillaries of the vascular system are found.

With each respiratory, or breathing cycle, an exchange of gases takes place. During ***inhalation*** (in-hah-**LAY**-shun), oxygen is absorbed into the blood, while carbon dioxide is expelled during ***exhalation*** (eks-hah-**LAY**-shun). Oxygen is more essential than either food or water. Although a man or woman may live more than 60 days without food, and a few days without water, if they are deprived of oxygen, they will die in a few minutes.

Nose breathing is healthier than mouth breathing because the air is warmed by the surface capillaries, and the bacteria in the air are caught by the hairs that line the ***mucous*** (**MYOO**-kus) membranes of the nasal passages.

The rate of breathing depends on the activity of the individual. Muscular activities and energy expenditures increase the body's demands for oxygen. As a result, the rate of breathing is increased. A person requires about three times more oxygen when walking than when standing.

THE DIGESTIVE SYSTEM

Digestion (deye-**JES**-chun) is the process of converting food into a form that can be assimilated by the body. The ***digestive*** (deye-**JES**-tiv) ***system*** changes food into ***soluble*** (**SOL**-yu-bel) form, suitable for use by the cells of the body. Digestion begins in the mouth and is completed in the small intestine. From the mouth, the food passes down the ***pharynx*** (**FAR**-ingks) and the ***esophagus*** (i-**SOF**-a-gus), or food pipe, and into the stomach. The food is completely digested in the stomach and small intestine and is assimilated or absorbed into the bloodstream. The large intestine (colon) stores the refuse for elimination through the rectum. The complete digestive process of food takes about nine hours.

Responsible for the chemical changes in food are the ***enzymes*** (**EN**-zighms) present in the digestive secretions. ***Digestive enzymes*** are chemicals that change certain kinds of food into a form capable of being used by the body. Intense emotions, excitement, and fatigue seriously disturb digestion. On the other hand, happiness and relaxation promote good digestion.

Completed: Learning Objective #4

THE ORGANS AND SYSTEMS OF THE HUMAN BODY AND HOW THEY FUNCTION

REVIEW QUESTIONS

CELLS, ANATOMY, AND PHYSIOLOGY

1. What are the functions of human cells?
2. How do cells grow?
3. What is metabolism?
4. What are the functions of organs?
5. What are systems?
6. What is anatomy?
7. What is physiology?
8. What is histology?
9. What are the primary functions of the bones?
10. What is the structure of the muscular system and what is its function?
11. Give two reasons why the cosmetologist should study the nervous system.
12. What is the function of the heart?
13. What is the composition of blood?
14. What is lymph?
15. What are the two types of glands in the endocrine system?
16. Name the five important organs of the excretory system.
17. Describe a respiratory cycle.
18. What is the function of the digestive system?

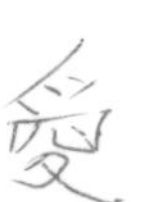

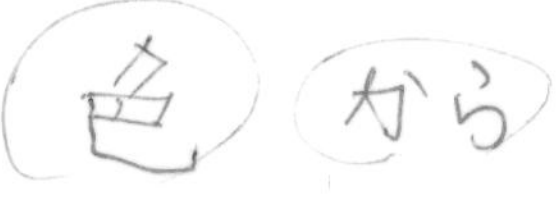

CHAPTER 24

Electricity and Light Therapy

LEARNING OBJECTIVES

After completing this chapter, you should be able to:

1. Define the nature of electricity and name two forms of electricity.
2. Explain the proper use of the different types of electricity and the safety precautions that must be followed when using electricity.
3. Define the four types of current and explain the benefits derived from the various currents.
4. List and describe electrical appliances available for use in the salon.
5. Explain light therapy.
6. Demonstrate the proper uses of light therapy.

NATIONAL SKILL S

This chapter provides you with the necessary information to master these National Industry Skill Standards for Entry-Level Cosmetologists:

- Using appropriate methods to insure personal health and well-being
- Providing basic skin care services

INTRODUCTION

The beneficial effects of electricity have long been recognized to be valuable to the cosmetology profession. When used intelligently and safely, electricity can be a valuable tool. It supplies light and heat, operates appliances, and is essential to the operation of a modern salon.

Electricity is a form of energy that produces *magnetic, chemical,* and *heat* effects. There are some basic terms that you should learn and some that you may already be familiar with. An ***electric current*** is the movement of electricity along a conductor.

A ***conductor*** is a substance that permits electric current to pass through it easily. Metals like copper, silver, and aluminum are good conductors of electricity, as are carbon, wet cotton, the human body, and water solutions of acids and salts. A ***nonconductor*** or ***insulator*** is a substance that resists the passage of an electric current, such as rubber, silk, dry wood, glass, cement, or asbestos. An ***electric wire*** is composed of twisted fine metal threads (conductor) covered with rubber or silk (insulator or nonconductor).

USING ELECTRICITY

There are two types of electricity:

1. ***Direct current*** (DC) is a constant, even-flowing current, traveling in one direction. This current produces a chemical reaction. A battery-operated instrument, such as a portable radio or a flashlight, uses direct current.
2. ***Alternating current*** (AC) is a rapid and interrupted current, flowing first in one direction and then in the opposite direction. This current produces a mechanical action. When you plug an appliance, such as a hair dryer, into a wall socket, you are using an alternating current.

If necessary, one type of current can be changed to the other type by means of a converter or rectifier. A ***converter*** is used to change direct current into alternating current. A ***rectifier*** is used to change alternating current to direct current.

A ***complete circuit of electricity*** is the path traveled by the current from its generating source through the conductors (wire, electrode, or body) and back to its original source. ✔

Completed:
Learning Objective
#1
THE NATURE AND FORMS OF ELECTRICITY

ELECTRICAL MEASUREMENTS

Electrical measurements are expressed in terms of the following units:

A ***volt*** (V) is a unit for measuring the pressure that forces the electric current forward. A higher voltage increases the strength of the current. If the voltage is lower, the current is weaker.

An ***amp*** (A), short for ***ampere*** (**AM**-peer), is the unit of measurement for the amount of current running through a wire. A cord must be heavy duty enough to handle the amps put out by the appliance. For example, an appliance that puts out 40 amps of current requires a cord that is thicker than the one for an appliance that puts out 20 amps of current. If the current—or number of amps—is too strong, your appliances can overheat or the wires can even burn out. If the current is not strong enough, your appliance will not operate at full strength or might not operate at all.

A ***milliampere*** (mil-i-**AM**-peer) is 1/1000th part of an ampere. The current for facial and scalp treatments is measured in milliamperes by a milliamperemeter (mil-i-**AM**-peer-**MEE**-ter); an ampere current would be much too strong.

An ***ohm*** (O) is a unit for measuring the resistance of an electric current. Unless the force (volts) is stronger than the resistance (ohms), current will not flow through the wire.

A ***watt*** (W) is a measurement of how much electric energy is being used in one second. A 40-watt bulb uses 40 watts of energy per second.

A ***kilowatt*** (K) equals 1000 watts. The electricity in your house is measured in kilowatt hours (kwh).

SAFETY DEVICES

A ***fuse*** is a safety device that prevents the overheating of electric wires. It blows out or melts when the wire becomes too hot from overloading the circuit with too much current from too many appliances or if faulty equipment is used. To reestablish the circuit, you must disconnect the appliance and insert a new fuse.

The ***circuit breaker*** has largely replaced the fuse in modern electric wiring. This device has all the safety features offered by the fuse and does not require replacement every time it shuts off. It is a switch device that automatically shuts down at the first indication of overheating or circuit trouble. When the problem is corrected, the switch is simply reset, and all the safety factors are restored.

CAUTION

If, after resetting the circuit breaker, it continues to shut down, call in a licensed electrician to check for further problems.

Safety of Electrical Equipment

The protection and safety of the client is the primary concern of the cosmetologist. All electrical equipment should be inspected regularly to determine whether or not it is in safe working condition. If you are careless when making electrical connections or if you do not check that you use the right amount of current, a shock or a burn can result. Observing safety precautions helps to eliminate accidents and ensure greater satisfaction to the client. (Figs. 24.1–24.4) Here is a list of useful hints about using electricity:

1. Study the instructions before using any electrical equipment.
2. Disconnect appliances when you have finished using them.
3. Keep all wires, plugs, and equipment in good repair.
4. Inspect all electrical equipment frequently.
5. Avoid wetting electrical cords.
6. When using electrical equipment, protect the client at all times.
7. Do not touch any metal while using an electrical appliance.
8. Do not handle electrical equipment with wet hands.
9. Do not allow the client to touch any metal surfaces while being treated with electrical equipment.
10. Do not leave the room when your client is connected to an electrical device.
11. Do not attempt to clean around an electric outlet while equipment is plugged in.
12. Do not touch two metallic objects at the same time if either is connected to an electric current.
13. Do not step on or set objects on electrical cords.

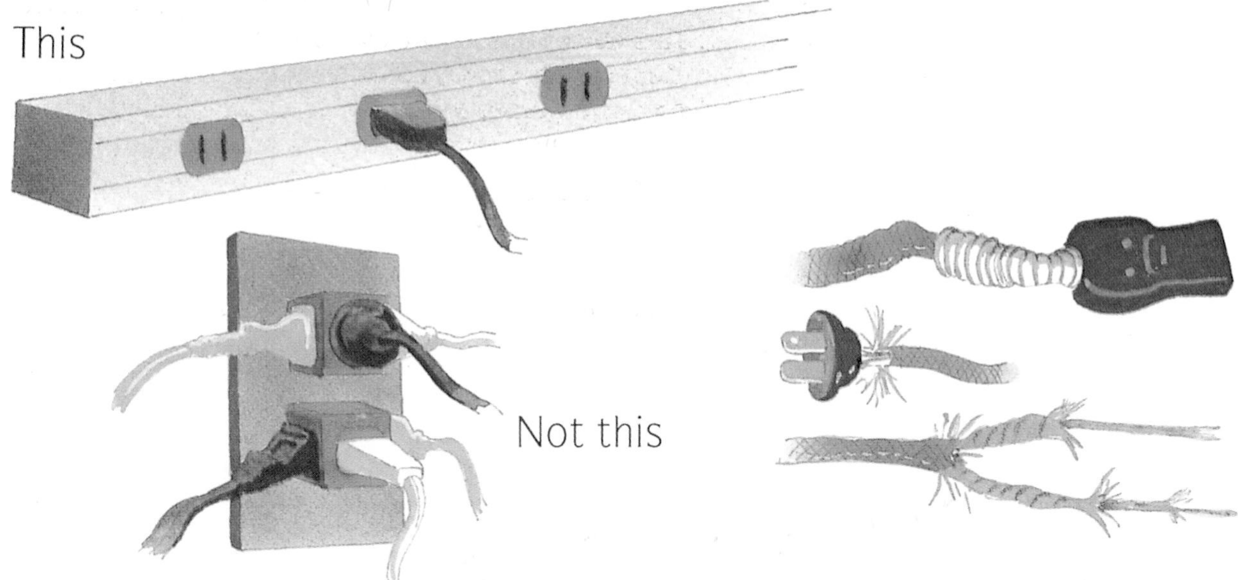

FIGURE 24.1 — Use only one plug to each outlet. Overloading, as in illustration on the bottom, may cause fuse to blow out.

FIGURE 24.2 — Examine cords regularly.

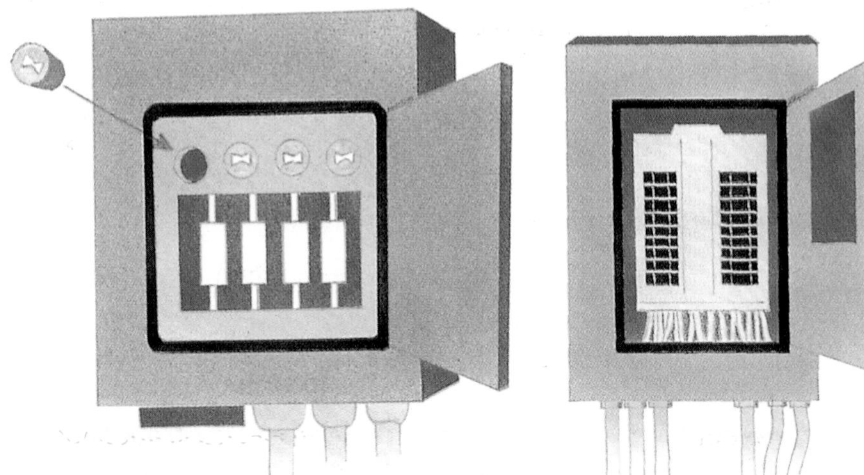

FIGURE 24.3 — Carefully replace blown-out fuses.

FIGURE 24.4 — Circuit breakers automatically disconnect any current of a defective appliance.

14. Do not allow electrical cords to become twisted or bent; the fine wires inside the cord will break and the insulation will wear away from the wires.
15. Disconnect the appliance by pulling on the plug, not the cord.
16. Do not repair electrical appliances unless you are qualified to do so.

Completed:
Learning Objective
#2
THE USE AND SAFETY PRECAUTIONS OF ELECTRICITY

ELECTROTHERAPY

A ***wall plate*** (facial stimulator) is an instrument that, when plugged into an ordinary socket, can produce particular currents used for electronic facial treatments. An electronic facial treatment is called ***electrotherapy***. These currents are referred to as ***modalities***. Each produces a different effect on the skin. There are many types of modalities, but cosmetologists are concerned with only the ***galvanic*** (gal-**VAN**-ik), ***sinusoidal*** (seye-nu-**SOID**-al), ***faradic*** (fah-**RAD**-ik), and the ***Tesla high-frequency*** (**TES**-lah heye-**FREE**-kwen-see). Some wall plates have all four currents and some have only the galvanic current.

An ***electrode*** is an apparatus that conducts the electric current from the machine to the client's skin. It is usually made of carbon, glass, or metal. Each of the modalities requires two electrodes (one negative and one positive) to conduct the flow of electricity through the body, except the Tesla high-frequency.

MODALITIES

Polarity

Before discussing the various modalities, it will be useful to discuss the test for polarity. ***Polarity*** is the negative or positive state of electric current. Electrotherapy equipment has a negatively charged pole and a positively charged pole. If the electrodes are not marked with negative or positive indicators, a simple test will tell you which is which.

1. Separate the tips of two conducting cords from each other and immerse them into a glass of saltwater. Turn the selector switch of the appliance to galvanic current, and then turn up the intensity. As the water is decomposed, more active bubbles will accumulate at the negative pole than at the positive pole.
2. Place the tips of two conducting cords on two separate pieces of blue moistened litmus paper. The paper under the positive pole will turn red, while the paper under the negative pole will stay blue. If you use red litmus instead of blue, the positive pole will keep the red litmus the same and the negative pole will turn the red litmus blue.

CAUTION

Do not let the tips of the cords touch or you will cause a short circuit.

Galvanic Current

The most commonly used modality is the ***galvanic* current**. It is a constant and direct current (DC), reduced to a safe, low-voltage level. Chemical changes are produced when this current is used. Galvanic current produces two different chemical reactions depending on the polarity (negative or positive) used on the area treated. A positive electrode is called an ***anode,*** is red, and is marked with a "P" or a plus (+) sign. A negative electrode is called a ***cathode,*** is black, and is marked with an "N" or a minus (–) sign.

The positive pole:

Produces acidic reactions

Closes the pores

Soothes nerves

Decreases blood supply

Contracts blood vessels

Hardens (firms) tissues

Forces alkaline solutions into the skin

The negative pole:

Produces alkaline reactions

Opens the pores

Stimulates (irritates) the nerves

Increases the blood supply to the skin

Expands the blood vessels

Softens tissues

Softens and liquifies grease deposits in the hair follicles and pores

Note that the effects to the body of the positive pole are just the opposite of those produced by the negative pole.

> **CAUTION**
>
> *Do not use the negative galvanic current on skin with broken capillaries, pustular acne conditions, or on a client with high blood pressure or metal implants.*

The effects of the galvanic current are experienced by your client as the current passes through the body from one electrode to the other and completes a circuit. Both the active and inactive (positive and negative) poles must be functioning to complete the circuit. Both the active and inactive carbon (ball and cylinder) electrodes must be lightly wrapped with a moistened cotton pledget.

The ***active electrode*** is the electrode used on the area to be treated. For instance, if negative reactions (e.g., opened pores, softened tissue) are desired on the face, the negative pole is the active electrode. Apply the carbon ball or carbon roller to the active electrode.

The ***inactive electrode*** is the opposite pole from the active electrode. Either your client can hold the carbon stick (inactive electrode) wrapped in a moistened cotton pledget or you can place the wet pad somewhere on the client's body.

Procedure to Close Pores

1. Wrap the carbon ball electrode (active) in cotton moisturized with astringent.
2. Wrap the cylinder electrode (inactive) in cotton moisturized with water.
3. Have the client hold the inactive electrode or place the wet pad on a comfortable spot on the client's body.
4. After a good contact is established with the two electrodes, slowly turn up the current to the desired strength.
5. When the treatment is completed, slowly turn down the current before breaking contact with the client.

Phoresis

The process by which chemical solutions are forced into the unbroken skin using a galvanic current is called ***phoresis*** (foh-**REE**-sis). ***Cataphoresis*** (**KAT**-ah-foh-ree-sis) is the use of the positive pole to pull a positively charged substance (an acid pH astringent solution) into the skin. ***Anaphoresis*** (**AN**-ah-foh-ree-sis) is the use of the negative pole to force, or push, a negatively charged substance (an alkaline pH solution) into the skin. ***Disincrustation*** is a process used to soften and liquefy grease deposits (oil) in the hair follicles and pores. This process is used frequently to treat acne, milia, and comedones.

Faradic Current

The ***faradic*** current is an alternating and interrupted current that produces a mechanical reaction without a chemical effect. The faradic current is used during scalp and facial manipulations to cause muscular contractions that tone the facial muscles. In some states it is illegal to cause visible muscle contractions with the faradic or sinusoidal currents.

Benefits derived from the use of the faradic current include:

1. Improves muscle tone.
2. Promotes removal of waste products.
3. Increases circulation of the blood.
4. Relieves congested blood.
5. Increases glandular activity.
6. Stimulates hair growth.
7. Increases metabolism.

Sinusoidal Current

The ***sinusoidal*** current is similar to the faradic current and is used also during scalp and facial manipulations. It is an alternating current that produces mechanical contractions that tone the muscles. The manner of application is the same as that for the faradic current.

The sinusoidal current has the following advantages:

1. It supplies greater stimulation, deeper penetration, and is less irritating than the faradic current.
2. It soothes the nerves and penetrates into the deeper muscle tissue.
3. It is best suited for the nervous client.

Caution When Using Faradic and Sinusoidal Currents

Do not use the faradic current if it causes pain or discomfort, if the face is very florid, or if your client has any of the following: many gold-filled teeth, high blood pressure, broken capillaries, or pustular conditions of the skin. The faradic and sinusoidal currents are never used longer than 15 to 20 minutes.

Application of Faradic and Sinusoidal Current

Two electrodes (one negative and one positive) are required to complete the faradic or sinusoidal circuit.

Indirect method. In the indirect method, you wear a wrist electrode covered with a moistened pad while your client holds the carbon stick electrode wrapped in damp absorbent cotton, or you can place the wet pad on the client's body. Before turning on the current, establish contact with the client's forehead. During treatment, use your fingertips to perform the massage movements. When you have completed the treatment, slowly turn down the current before breaking contact with your client.

Direct method. In the direct method of applying the faradic and sinusoidal currents, two felt-tipped electrodes are used. The cosmetologist should move the two electrodes around the face in circular movements without allowing them to touch. The circuit is completed between the two felt disks.

High-Frequency Current

The ***high-frequency (Tesla)*** current is characterized by a high rate of oscillation, or vibration. It is commonly called the ***violet ray*** and is used for both scalp and facial treatments. The Tesla current may be used to treat thinning hair, itchy scalp, and excessively oily or dry skin and scalp. The primary action of this current is thermal or heat producing. Because of its rapid vibration, there are no muscular contractions. The physiological effects are either stimulating or soothing, depending on the method of application.

The electrodes for high-frequency current are made of glass or metal, and you only need one electrode to perform a service. The facial electrode is flat, and the scalp electrode is rake shaped. As the current passes through the glass electrode, tiny violet sparks are emitted. Some units use a neon gas in the tube, which produces an orange glow. Both units produce the same effects. All treatments given with high-frequency current should start with a mild current and gradually increase to the required strength. The length of the treatment depends on the condition to be treated. Allow about 5 minutes for a general facial or scalp treatment. (Figs. 24.5–24.7)

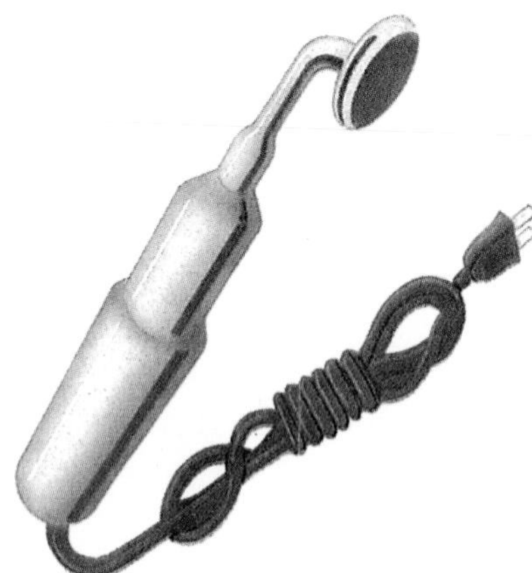

FIGURE 24.5 — Facial electrode using Tesla current.

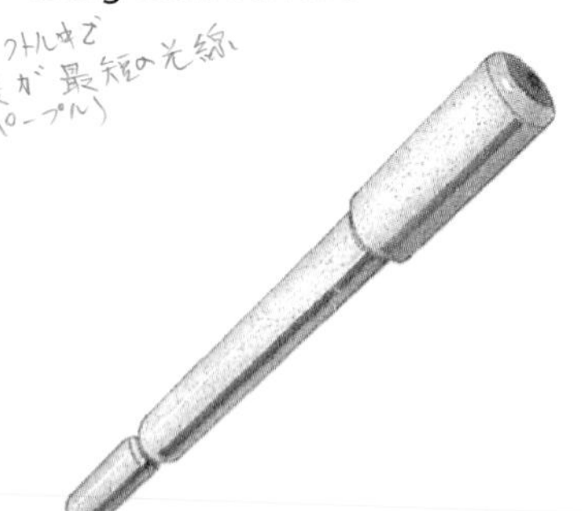

FIGURE 24.6 — Metal electrode attachment for Tesla current.

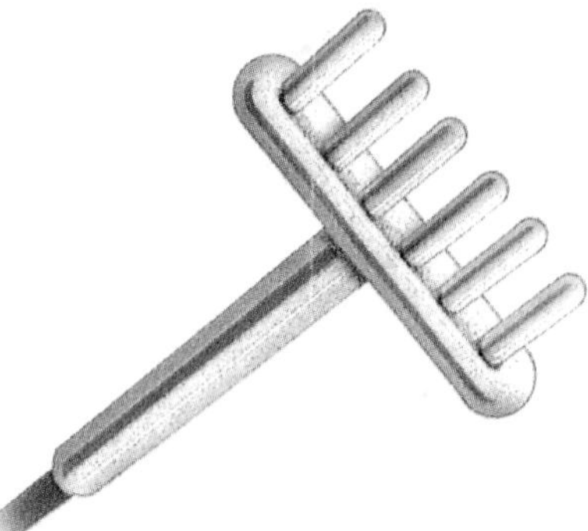

FIGURE 24.7 — Scalp electrode attachment for Tesla current.

Note: For proper use, follow the instructions provided by the manufacturer of Tesla equipment.

Application of High-Frequency Current

There are three methods for using the Tesla current:

1. ***Direct surface application.*** Apply a nonalcohol, noncombustible facial cream to the client's face. The cosmetologist holds the electrode and applies it directly to the client's skin. To obtain a stimulating effect, lift the electrode slightly from the area to be treated and apply the current through gauze or a towel. The direct method is more drying to the skin and is recommended for acne-prone and oily skin. When you apply and remove the electrode from the skin, you must hold your finger on the electrode to prevent shock. Remove your finger once the electrode has been placed on the skin. (Figs. 24.8, 24.9)

2. ***Indirect application.*** The client holds the electrode while you use your fingers to massage the surface being treated. At no time do you hold the electrode. To prevent shock, turn on the current after the client has firmly grasped the electrode.

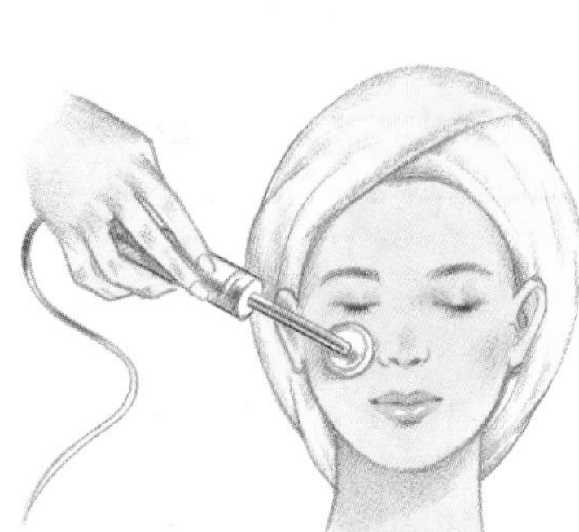

FIGURE 24.8 — Applying high-frequency current to face using facial electrode.

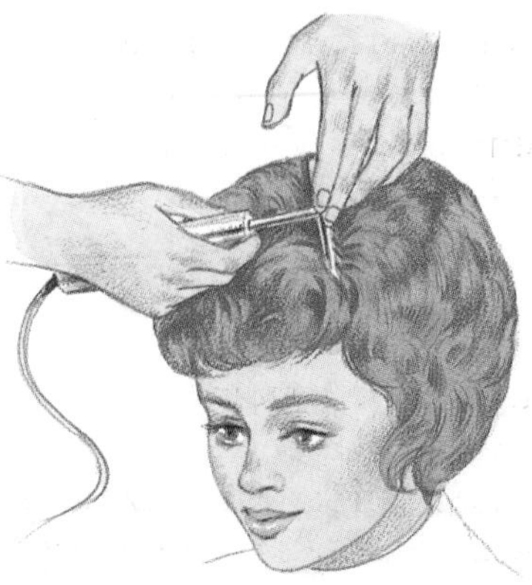

FIGURE 24.9 — Applying high-frequency current to scalp using rake electrode.

Turn the current off before you remove the electrode from the client's hand.

> **CAUTION**
>
> *The client should avoid any contact with metal, such as chair arms and stools. A burn may occur if such contact is made.*

3. ***General electrification.*** Place the electrode in the client's hand and turn on the unit. The client's body will be charged with a small amount of electricity.

Benefits derived from the use of Tesla high-frequency current are as follows:

1. Stimulates circulation of the blood.
2. Increases glandular activity.
3. Aids in elimination and absorption.
4. Increases metabolism.
5. Germicidal action occurs during use.
6. Relieves congestion.

Completed: Learning Objective #3

THE TYPES OF CURRENT AND THEIR USES

> **CAUTION**
>
> *High-frequency current should not be used with clients who are pregnant, epileptic, asthmatic, who have high blood pressure, excessive fillings in the teeth, sinus blockage, a pacemaker, or metal implants.*

OTHER ELECTRICAL EQUIPMENT

The ***vibrator*** is an electrical appliance used in massage to produce a mechanical succession of manipulations. It has a stimulating effect on the muscular tissues, increases the blood supply to the areas treated, is soothing to the nerves, and increases glandular activities.

By attaching the vibrator to the back of the hand the vibrations are transmitted through the hand or fingers to the areas being treated. The vibrator is used over heavy muscular tissue, such as the scalp, shoulders, and upper back. It is never used on a woman's face, but can be used on a man's face.

CAUTION

The vibrator should never be used when there is heart disease or when fever, abscesses, or inflammation are present.

The ***steamer***, or ***vaporizer***, is applied over the head or face to produce a moist, uniform heat. The steamer may be used instead of hot towels to cleanse and steam the face. The steam warms the skin, inducing the flow of both oil and sweat. It thus helps to cleanse the skin, clean out the pores, and soften any scaliness on the surface of the skin.

The steamer also may be used for scalp and hair conditioning treatments. When fitted over the scalp, it produces controlled moist heat. Its action is to soften the scalp, increase perspiration, and promote the effectiveness of applied scalp cosmetics. Another use for the steamer is to speed up the action of a lightener.

Electrically heated curling irons come in various types and sizes. They have built-in heating elements and operate from electric outlets. One type has perforations. Oil is injected into the barrel of the curling irons where it is vaporized. The vapor is released through small perforations in the irons and conditions the hair as it curls.

Heating caps are electrical devices, which, when placed on the head, provide a uniform source of heat. Their main use is as part of corrective treatments for the hair and scalp. They recondition dry, brittle, and damaged hair, and also serve to activate a sluggish scalp.

The ***processing machine***, or ***accelerating machine***, has been designed as an aid to the professional haircolorist. Its function is to reduce the processing time for lightening and tinting the hair. The machine accelerates the molecular movement of the chemicals in the color so that they work much faster.

Accelerating machines may be used efficiently and successfully for various haircoloring treatments, such as hair lightening, tinting, frosting, tipping, streaking, and stripping. Accelerating machines must not be used with powdered lighteners.

The ***electric chair hair dryer*** delivers hot, medium, or cold air for the proper drying of the hair. It consists of an adjustable hood, or helmet, with deflectors that distribute the air evenly, and is capable of drying heavy hair in a relatively short time. The ***hand dryer*** also delivers hot, medium, and cold air.

The ***small electric oil heater*** is used to heat oil and to keep the oil warm when giving an oil manicure.

Completed:
Learning Objective
#4
ELECTRICAL APPLIANCES IN THE SALON

LIGHT THERAPY

Light therapy refers to skin treatment using light rays. The sun is the basic source of light rays. In salon work we are concerned with the white rays of the visible spectrum, which make up 12% of natural sunlight, and the invisible infrared and ultraviolet rays, which respectively make up 80% and 8% of natural sunlight. The infrared rays produce heat, and the ultraviolet rays produce chemical and germicidal reactions. When the white light of the visible spectrum is passed through a prism, it produces the colors of the rainbow: red, orange, yellow, green, blue, indigo, and violet. These colors are referred to as the visible spectrum. (Fig. 24.10) We are concerned with the white, blue, and red lights. Each of these produces a different effect on the skin.

Completed:
Learning Objective
#5
LIGHT THERAPY

HOW LIGHT RAYS ARE REPRODUCED

Artificial light rays are produced by using an electrical apparatus called a ***therapeutic*** (ther-ah-**PYOO**-tik) ***lamp***. These lamps or bulbs are capable of producing the same rays that are originated by the sun. The lamp used to reproduce these light rays is usually a dome-shaped reflector mounted on a pedestal with a flexible neck. The dome usually has a highly polished metal lining capable of reflecting the rays from the different types of light.

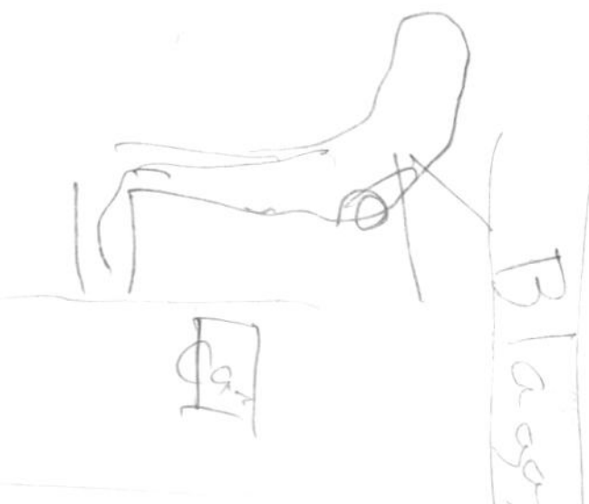

PROTECTING THE EYES

The client's eyes always should be protected during any light ray treatment. Use cotton pads saturated with boric acid solution, witch hazel, or distilled water. The eyepads protect the eyes from the glare of the reflecting rays.

CAUTION

The cosmetologist and the client always should wear safety goggles when using ultraviolet rays to avoid damage to the eyes.

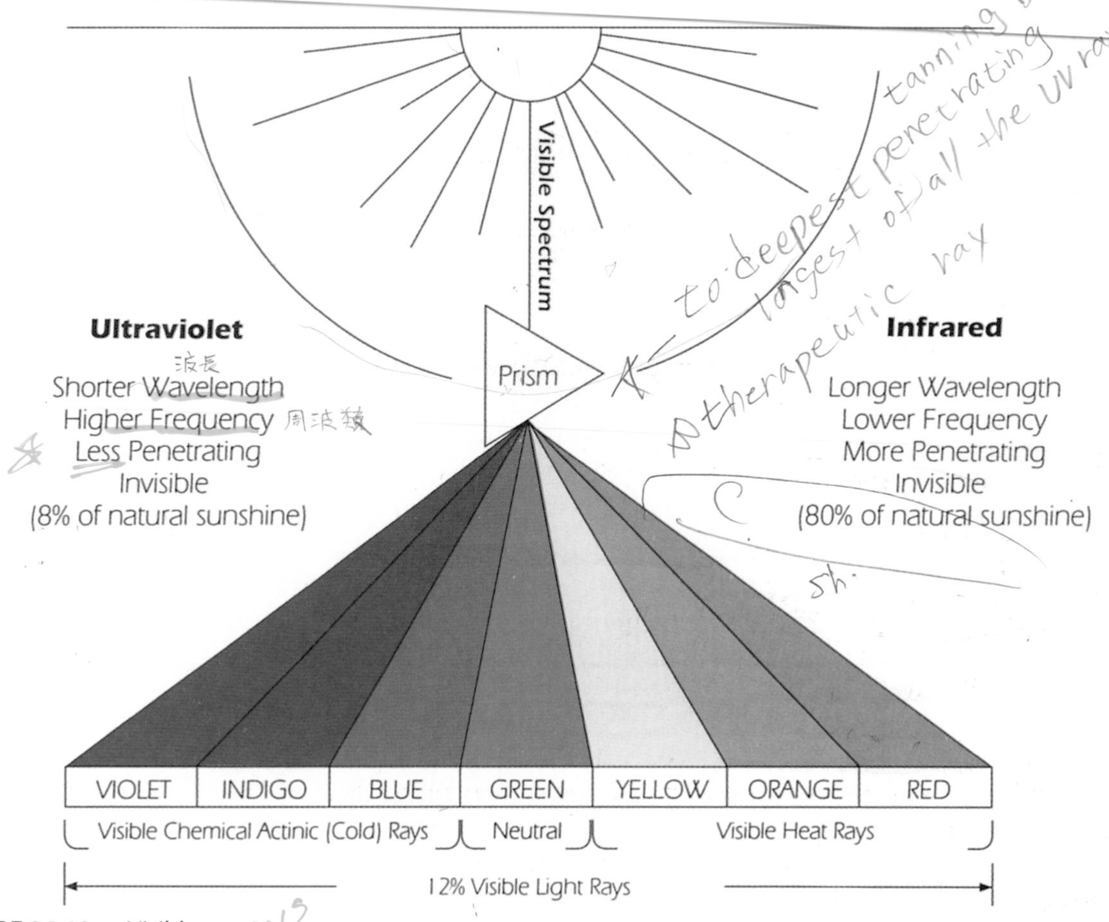

FIGURE 24.10 — Visible spectrum.

INFRARED RAYS

Infrared rays are located beyond the visible red rays of the spectrum. Infrared rays are long, have the greatest (deepest) penetration, and can produce the most heat. The infrared lamp is red and produces a reddish glow when turned on. Infrared lamps can also be white.

The lamp should be operated at an average distance of 30" (76.2 cm). Check the comfort of your client frequently.

CAUTION

NEVER leave your client unattended during the exposure time. The exposure time should be about 5 minutes.

Use and Effects of Infrared Ray Treatment

1. Heats and relaxes the skin without increasing the temperature of the body as a whole.
2. Dilates blood vessels in the skin, thereby increasing the blood circulation.
3. Increases metabolism and chemical changes within the skin tissues.
4. Increases the production of perspiration and oil on the skin.
5. Relieves pain in sore muscles because of the ray's deep penetration.
6. Is soothing to the nerves.

ULTRAVIOLET RAYS

Ultraviolet rays are located beyond the visible spectrum. They are the shortest and least penetrating of the light rays. The ultraviolet ray is also referred to as the ***cold ray*** or ***actinic ray.*** Ultraviolet (UV) rays are divided into three categories: UVA, UVB, and UVC. The farther away from the visible light spectrum, the shorter and less penetrating the ultraviolet rays. UVC rays are the most germicidal and chemical of the ultraviolet rays, as well as being the farthest away from the visible spectrum. These rays cause the most burning to the skin. UVC rays are destructive to bacteria as well as to skin tissue if the skin is exposed to them for too long a period of time.

The UVB rays are the therapeutic rays in the middle of the UV range, which produce some effects from both ends of the ultraviolet rays. This ray will also burn if the skin is left exposed too long. The UVA ray is the tonic UV ray. It is closest to the visible spectrum, is the deepest penetrating, and is the longest of all the UV rays. The UVA ray is used in tanning booths. This ray does not burn the skin but penetrates deeply into the skin tissue and can destroy the elasticity of the skin, causing premature aging and wrinkling.

It was once thought that the slightest obstruction would keep the ultraviolet rays from reaching the skin. Recent studies have proved that ultraviolet rays can penetrate up to 3 feet (91.4 cm) below the water and that approximately 50% of the ultraviolet rays can penetrate to the skin through a wet T-shirt. It you want to receive full benefit from ultraviolet rays, the area treated should be bare and no cream or lotion should be applied so that you can receive the full benefits of the rays.

Application of Ultraviolet Rays

Ultraviolet rays are applied with a lamp at a distance of 30" to 36" (76.2 to 91.4 cm) from the skin. If the shorter rays are needed, the lamp can be held as close as 12" (30.4 cm) from the skin. Extra precautions must be used when the lamp is held at such a close range to avoid damage to skin tissue.

Time Limit

The average exposure can produce redness of the skin and overdoses will cause blistering. It is well to start with a short exposure of 2 to 3 minutes and gradually increase the exposure over a period of days to 7 to 8 minutes.

Benefits of Ultraviolet Rays

Ultraviolet rays increase resistance to disease by increasing iron and vitamin D content and the number of red and white cells in the blood. They also increase elimination of waste products, restore nutrition where needed, and stimulate the circulation by improving the flow of blood and lymph. The rays also have a tendency to increase the fixation of calcium in the blood. Ultraviolet rays are used to treat acne, tinea, seborrhea, and to combat dandruff. They also promote healing and can stimulate the growth of hair, as well as produce a tan by increasing skin pigment if the skin is exposed in short doses over a long period of time.

Disadvantages of Ultraviolet Rays

Ultraviolet rays destroy hair pigment. Continued exposure to the sun's rays causes premature aging of the skin, painful sunburn, and a higher risk of skin cancer, especially for fair- or light-skinned individuals.

VISIBLE LIGHT RAYS OR VISIBLE SPECTRUM

The visible lights are the primary source of lights used for facial and scalp treatments. The bulbs used for the visible light therapy are available in white, red, or blue.

White Light

White light is referred to as a combination light because it is a combination of all the visible rays of the spectrum. White light also has the benefits of all the rays of the visible spectrum. Used for normal skin, the benefits of the white light include: it relieves pain, especially in congested areas, and more particularly, around the nerve centers, such as in the back of the neck and across the shoulders; has some chemical and germicidal actions; and is slightly relaxing to the muscles.

Blue Light

Blue light is used on oily skin that is bare. The blue light contains few heat rays, is soothing to the nerves, produces good skin tone, has some germicidal and chemical effects, and is used for mild cases of skin eruptions. Blue light does not penetrate.

Red Light

Red light is used on dry skin in combination with oils and creams. The red light is the deepest penetrating of the visible spectrum, is good for dry, scaly wrinkled skin, and relaxes tissues.

Completed: Learning Objective #6

THE PROPER USE OF LIGHT THERAPY

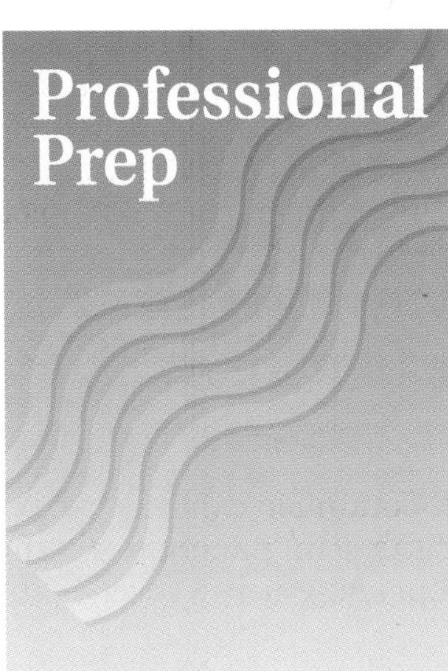

Professional Prep

CUSTOMER SERVICE

There simply is no more important issue pertaining to your success as a cosmetologist than customer service. How you treat people is far more important to most salon owners than how fast you wrap a perm or how perfect your haircuts are.

Here are some tips for improving your customer service:

- Focus on your clients. Clients buy services to satisfy their needs, not yours.
- Maintain a professional image. Taking care of your appearance and your work station conveys that you care about details and about others.
- Treat each client as a unique individual. Everyone wants to feel special.
- Listen to your clients. This cannot be stressed enough.
- Respond to your clients' needs. Be ready to help them with problems they have with their hair, skin, and nails.
- Give clients more than they expect. Example: an extra massage during the shampoo or manicure.
- Be honest and forthright, but tactful.
- Don't make any promises you can't keep, and always fulfill the ones you do make.
- Educate your clients. Teach them about products suitable for home use and show them how to maintain their new look.
- Treat all clients with respect and courtesy.
- Focus all of your attention on the client sitting in your chair. Refrain from talking with co-workers, their clients, or others in the salon.

If you follow these suggestions you'll find that clients will return to you, because not only are you improving their appearance, but you're also building a relationship with them.

—*From* Communication Skills for Cosmetologists *by Kathleen Ann Bergant*

REVIEW QUESTIONS

ELECTRICITY AND LIGHT THERAPY

1. What is electricity?
2. What is a conductor?
3. What is a nonconductor or insulator? Give six examples.
4. What is a direct current (DC)?
5. What is an alternating current (AC)?
6. Describe galvanic current.
7. Give the chemical action of the positive pole; the negative pole.
8. Name three effects of the positive pole on the body.
9. Name three effects of the negative pole on the body.
10. In what cases should faradic current never be used?

CHAPTER 25

Chemistry

LEARNING OBJECTIVES

After completing this chapter, you should be able to:

1. Define organic and inorganic chemistry and know the differences between them.
2. Discuss the types of matter.
3. Describe the composition of elements, compounds, and mixtures.
4. Describe the properties of matter, elements, compounds, and mixtures.
5. Define acids and alkalies and know the differences between them.
6. Describe the chemistry of water.
7. Describe the classification of shampoos and types of conditioners.
8. Describe the composition of hair before, during, and after permanent waving and chemical hair relaxing.
9. Describe the composition of hair before, during, and after haircoloring.
10. Describe the physical and chemical classifications of cosmetics.
11. Discuss the basic chemistry, types, and action of professional products.

NATIONAL SKILL STANDARDS

This chapter provides you with the necessary information to master these National Industry Skill Standards for Entry-Level Cosmetologists:

- Marketing professional salon products
- Using a variety of salon products while providing client services
- Applying appropriate cosmetics to enhance a client's appearance
- Providing styling and finishing techniques to complete a hairstyle to the satisfaction of the client
- Performing hair relaxation and wave formation techniques in accordance with manufacturer's directions

INTRODUCTION

Professional cosmetologists are more than just practicing technicians. You will be working with chemicals and performing services that change the hair both chemically and physically. For your client's protection as well as your own, you must understand the safety and health standards of the chemicals you will be working with.

A basic knowledge of modern chemistry is an essential requirement for an intelligent understanding of the multitude of products and cosmetics currently used in the salon. In addition, the science of chemistry brings us a constant flow of new and advanced products. It is important for you, as a professional, to understand these products and learn to use them in a way that is beneficial to your clients.

THE SCIENCE OF CHEMISTRY

Chemistry (KEM-ih-stree) is the science that deals with the composition, structure, and properties of matter and how matter changes under different chemical conditions. The broad subject of chemistry is divided into two areas: organic chemistry and inorganic chemistry.

Organic (or-GAN-ik) ***chemistry*** is the branch of chemistry that deals with all substances in which carbon is present. Carbon can be found in all plants, animals, petroleum, soft coal, natural gas, and in many artificially prepared substances.

Most organic substances will burn. They are not soluble (not able to be liquefied) in water, but they do dissolve in organic solvents, such as alcohol and benzene.

Examples of organic substances are grass, trees, gasoline, oil, soaps, detergents, plastics, and antibiotics.

Inorganic (in-or-GAN-ik) ***chemistry*** is the branch of chemistry that deals with all substances that do not contain carbon. Inorganic substances will not burn and are usually soluble in water. Examples of inorganic substances are water, air, iron, lead, minerals, and iodine.

Completed: Learning Objective

#1

DIFFERENCE BETWEEN ORGANIC AND INORGANIC CHEMISTRY

MATTER

Since chemistry is the science that deals with matter, it is essential that we develop an understanding of what matter really is. ***Matter*** is defined as anything that occupies space, has physical and chemical properties, and exists in one of the following three forms: solids, liquids, or gases.

Solids. Look around your classroom and note what you see: hair, students, teachers, desks, chairs, walls. These are all matter in a solid state.

Liquids. In the clinic area of your school you see water, shampoos, lotions, and hydrogen peroxide. These are matter in a liquid state.

Gases. Take a deep breath. The air you have just brought into your lungs also is matter. It is in a gaseous state.

It is not the purpose of this text to train you to be a scientist. But it will help you learn enough about matter so that you are comfortable talking about it in relation to your profession. Therefore, we will briefly examine the nature and structure of matter.

Completed: Learning Objective

#2

TYPES OF MATTER

FORMS OF MATTER

Matter exists in the form of elements, compounds, and mixtures.

Elements. An ***element*** is the basic unit of all matter. An element, being composed of a single part or unit, cannot be reduced to a more simple substance. There are more than 109 known elements.

Each element is identified by a letter symbol, which is generally made up of the principal letter or letters of either the English or Latin name of the element. For example, the letter symbol that identifies sulfur is S; oxygen, O; carbon, C; iron, Fe; lead, Pb; and silver, Ag. The symbols for each element can be obtained by referring to the Periodic Table of Elements found in almost any chemistry textbook.

Atoms

An ***atom*** (AT-om) is the smallest particle of an element that is capable of showing the properties of that element. If you took a piece of gold (an element) and divided it into smaller and smaller pieces, you would eventually come to a particle so small that it no longer showed the properties of the element.

Molecules

A ***molecule*** is two or more atoms that are joined together chemically.

When two of the *same* atoms are joined, the result is an element. When two *different* atoms are joined, the result is a compound.

Compounds. A ***compound*** is any substance made up of two or more different elements chemically joined together in definite proportions by weight. When joined, each element loses its characteristic properties and a new set of properties called a compound is created. For example, the combining of nitrogen (N) and hydrogen (H) at a ratio of 1 nitrogen molecule for every 3 hydrogen molecules (NH_3) creates ammonia. A compound can be altered only by chemical means, not by mechanical methods.

Compounds can be divided into four classes.

1. ***Oxides*** are compounds of any element combined with oxygen. For example, a combination of elements you will work with as a cosmetologist is 2 parts hydrogen and 2 parts oxygen, which create the compound known as hydrogen peroxide.

ELEMENTS AND COMPOUNDS

Matter	Types and Definition	Smallest Particle
Solids Gases Liquids	Elements: Simplest form of matter	Atom: (Cannot be broken down by simple chemical reactions.) About 100 different kinds.
	Compounds: Formed by combination of elements.	Molecule: (Consists of 2 or more atoms chemically combined.) Unlimited kinds possible.

Elements Found in Skin or Hair	Compounds Used on Skin or Hair
Carbon	Water
Nitrogen	Hydrogen peroxide
Oxygen	Ammonium thioglycolate
Sulfur	Alcohol
Hydrogen	Alkalies
Phosphorus	

2. ***Acids*** are compounds of hydrogen, a nonmetal, and sometimes oxygen that release hydrogen in a solution. For example, nitrogen + hydrogen + oxygen = nitric acid (NHO), which is used in making dyes. You can test for acidity with litmus paper. Acids turn blue litmus paper red. Acids also have a sour taste, for example, vinegar and lemons.
3. ***Alkalies***, also known as ***bases***, are compounds of hydrogen, a metal, and oxygen. For example, sodium + oxygen + hydrogen = sodium hydroxide (NaOH), which is used in making soap and hair relaxers. Alkalies neutralize acids and turn red litmus paper blue.
4. ***Salts*** are substances formed when the hydrogen part of an acid is replaced by a metal. For example, when copper replaces the hydrogen in sulfuric acid, the result is salt copper sulfate. The most common salt is sodium chloride (NaCl) or table salt.

Mixtures. A mixture is a substance made up of elements combined *physically* rather than chemically. The ingredients do not change their properties as in a compound, but retain their individual characteristics. For example, concrete is a mixture of sand, gravel, and cement. Upon examination, you will notice that although the grains of sand and gravel are held together by the cement, they retain their identity and can be picked apart. Although concrete is a mixture having its own functions, its ingredients never lose their characteristics.

Completed: Learning Objective #3

ELEMENTS, COMPOUNDS, AND MIXTURES

CHEMICAL AND PHYSICAL CHANGES IN MATTER

Matter can be changed in two ways, either through physical or chemical means.

A ***physical change*** refers to a change in the form (solid, liquid, gas) of a substance without the formation of any *new* substance. For example, ice, a solid substance, melts at a certain temperature and becomes a liquid (water), and water freezes at a certain temperature and becomes a solid (ice). There is no change in the inherent nature of the water; merely a change in its form. An example of a physical change in the cosmetology industry is the physical change in the outside of the hair shaft when a temporary color rinse is applied. The hair has a different appearance because color molecules have been physically added to the surface of the hair. However, there has been no inherent change in the nature of the hair shaft.

A ***chemical change*** is one in which a new substance or substances are formed, having properties different from the original substances. For example, when you mix hydrogen peroxide into a para dye, a chemical change occurs. The chemical reaction known as oxidation creates color within the cortex of the hair (within the bottle if you are too slow with your application). The chemical reaction between the two has created a new substance (in this case, a color) with its own characteristic properties.

PROPERTIES OF MATTER

Properties of matter refer to how we distinguish one form of matter from another. Substances have two kinds of properties: physical and chemical.

Physical properties refer to characteristics such as density, specific gravity, hardness, odor, and color.

1. ***Density*** of a substance refers to its weight divided by its volume. For example, the volume of 1 cubic foot (0.03 m^3) of water weighs 62.4 pounds (28.08 kg). Therefore, its density (weight) is 62.4 pounds (28.08 kg) divided by (volume) (0.03 m^3), or water has a density of 62.4 pounds (28.08 kg) per cubic foot (0.03 m^3).

2. ***Specific gravity*** of a substance is its "lightness" or "heaviness." Using water as the basis for comparison, substances are either more or less dense than water. If "zero" is assigned as the density of water, and if copper is 8.9 times as dense as water, the specific gravity (or relative density) of copper is 8.9.

3. ***Hardness*** refers to the ability of a substance to resist scratching. A substance will scratch any other substance that is softer. Scientists use the ***MOH Hardness Scale*** as a basis for comparing the hardness and softness of substances; low numbers indicate softness and high numbers indicate hardness. Some of these ratings might surprise you. For example, the diamond is rated a 10, the average knife blade is rated a 6.2, but asphalt is rated a 1.3.

4. ***Odor*** helps to identify many substances. For example, the characteristic odor of ammonium thioglycolate, known as the thio odor, helps you identify this product. **(Caution: Sniffing products can result in damage to mucous membranes.)**

5. ***Color*** also helps to identify many substances. For example, we easily recognize the colors of gold, silver, and copper. White substances are usually described as colorless.

Chemical properties allow a substance to change and form a new substance. The change is called a ***chemical change*** or ***chemical reaction***. Knowing the chemical properties of a substance allows you to know what happens when that substance is combined with another one. For example, combining 1 atom of carbon with 2 atoms of oxygen produces the gas exhaled by humans and animals known as carbon dioxide (CO_2).

PROPERTIES OF COMMON ELEMENTS, COMPOUNDS, AND MIXTURES

Knowledge about the properties of the most common elements, compounds, and mixtures can help you understand why certain chemical reactions take place.

Oxygen (O) (**OK**-sih-jen) is the most abundant element. It can be found either by itself or as one element of a compound. It makes up about 50% of the solid crust of the earth, 20% of the atmosphere, and 89% of water. Oxygen is a colorless, odorless, tasteless, gaseous substance that can be combined with most other elements to form an infinite variety of compounds called oxides.

When a substance is combined with oxygen, the substance is always oxidized. Combining a substance with oxygen creates heat energy. When the rate of reaction is slow and only heat energy is given off, the process is known as ***slow oxidation***. Oxidation tints and perm neutralizers are examples of slow oxidizers. When oxygen combines with other substances so rapidly that light energy as well as heat is created, the process is known as ***combustion***. Lighting a match or burning wood is an example of ***rapid oxidation*** or combustion.

Hydrogen (H) (**HEYE**-droh-jen) is a colorless, odorless, and tasteless gas. It makes up about 1% of the earth's crust. In total numbers of atoms, hydrogen is probably the second most abundant element on earth (oxygen is most abundant) and the most abundant element in the *universe*. In the laboratory, hydrogen is prepared by the action of active metals on water or an acid.

Pure hydrogen peroxide (H_2O_2) (peh-**ROK**-sighd) is an oily liquid compound of hydrogen and oxygen. Solutions of 30% are used to bleach fabric, hair, and feathers. Solutions of 12% cause the chemical reaction in oxidation tints, and a solution of 3% is used as an antiseptic.

Oxidizing (**OK**-sih-deye-zing) ***agents*** are substances that readily release oxygen. Hydrogen peroxide releases oxygen, which oxidizes both melanin and artificial pigments found in para dyes. The releasing of oxygen is known as ***reduction*** and the substance that attracts the oxygen is the ***reducing agent***. Thus melanin and artificial pigments are oxidized and the solution left on the outside of the hair shaft is reduced (now missing the extra oxygen element).

Nitrogen (N) (**NEYE**-troh-jen) is a colorless, gaseous element that makes up about 78% of the earth's atmosphere. It is found in nature chiefly in the form of ammonia and nitrates.

Completed: Learning Objective #4

PROPERTIES OF MATTER, ELEMENTS, COMPOUNDS, AND MIXTURES

Acidity and Alkalinity

You may recall from the chapter on permanent waving that the pH of a solution is a chemical measure of its acidity or alkalinity. The pH scale ranges from zero to 14. (Fig. 25.1) Pure water is considered neutral and represented by the number 7 in the middle of the scale. Recall that if a solution has a pH of less than 7, it has an acid pH. If a solution has a pH of more than 7, it has an alkaline pH. Also remember that an alkaline solution softens and swells hair; an acid solution contracts and hardens hair.

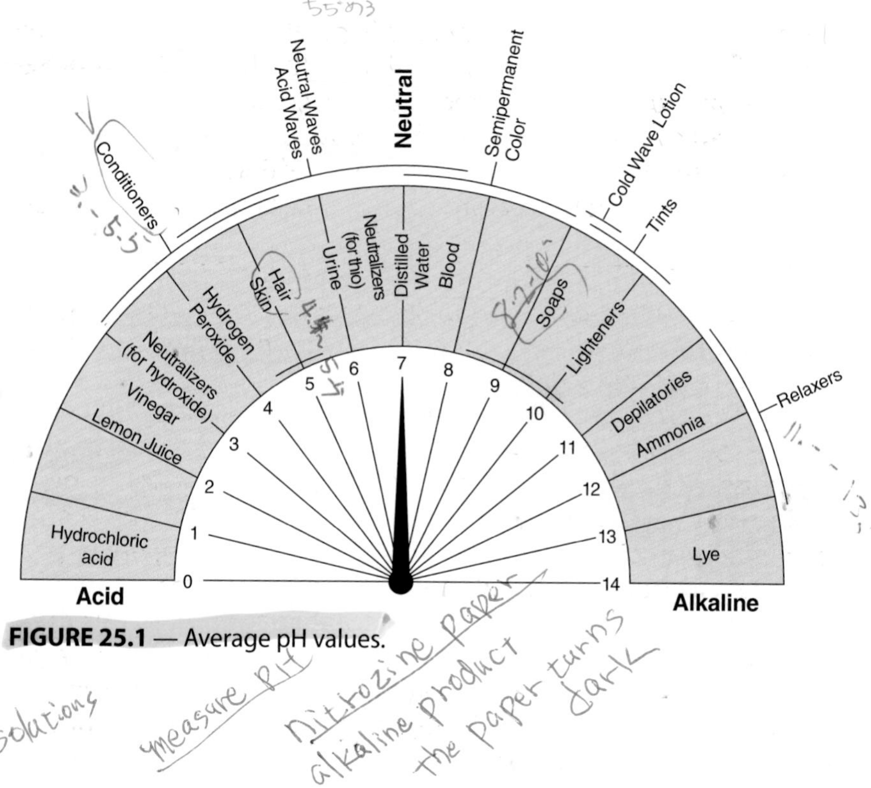

FIGURE 25.1 — Average pH values.

There are meters and other indicators such as ***nitrozine paper*** available so you can measure the pH of the products you use. If a product is more alkaline, the paper turns dark; if it is more acid, there is not much, if any, change in color.

If you wet hair with water and test the pH balance, it is normally between 4.4 to 5.5; it is slightly acid (remember that 7 is neutral). Shampoos normally have a pH of about 8 (more alkaline); chemical waving solutions have a pH of about 9 (also more alkaline). Color rinses have a pH of about 2; neutralizers about 3 (both are more acidic). Until you become familiar with a client's hair and history, and until you are sure of what you're doing, you should try to use solutions that are close to a pH balance of 7. Otherwise, you can unknowingly damage your client's hair.

Completed:
Learning Objective
#5
DIFFERENCE BETWEEN ACIDS AND ALKALIES

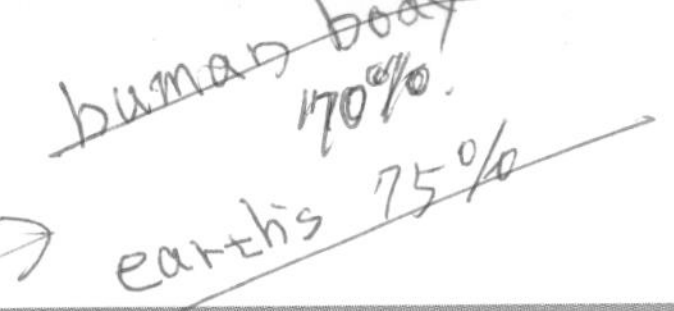

CHEMISTRY OF WATER

Water (H_2O) is the most abundant and important chemical on the earth. It is essential to the life process. The human body is made of approximately 70% water, and water covers almost 75% of the earth's surface. Water is a solvent, meaning that it has the ability to dissolve another substance.

WATER PURIFICATION

Fresh water from lakes and streams is purified by sedimentation (a treatment that causes mass to sink to the bottom) and filtration (passing through a porous substance, such as a filter paper or charcoal) to remove suspended clay, sand, and organic material. Small amounts of chlorine are then added to kill bacteria. Boiling water at a temperature of 212° Fahrenheit (100° Celsius) will also destroy most microbic life.

Water can be further treated by distillation, which is a process of heating water so that it becomes a vapor, then condensing the vapor so that it collects as a liquid. This process is often used in the manufacture of cosmetics.

Why is water so important in the cosmetology industry? Although the answer is obvious—water is used for shampooing, mixing solutions, and other functions—it is interesting to learn more about what water is made of. How does water help chemical or other solutions that are used in the salon? Water is made of protons and electrons (also neutrons, but here we are only concerned with protons and electrons), which contain power that gives them electrical charges. Protons are positive charges; electrons are negative charges. If you add a solid particle to water, for example, salt, the positive and negative charges work together to pull apart, or dissolve, the salt. The same process occurs when you combine other solids or liquids with water. Only oil and wax cannot be dissolved with water.

Completed: Learning Objective #6
CHEMISTRY OF WATER

CHEMISTRY OF SHAMPOOS

To determine which shampoo will leave your client's hair in the best condition for the intended service you must understand the chemical ingredients of shampoos. Most shampoos have many common ingredients. It is often the small differences in formulation that make one shampoo better for a particular hair texture or condition.

The ingredient that most shampoos have in common, and it usually is number one on the list to show that there is more of it than any other ingredient, is water. Generally, it is not just plain water, but purified or de-ionized water. From there, ingredients are listed in descending order according to the percentage of each ingredient in the shampoo.

CLASSIFICATIONS OF SHAMPOOS

The second ingredient that most shampoos have in common is the ***base surfactant*** (sur-**FAK**-tant) or ***base detergent***. These two terms, surfactant and detergent, mean the same thing, cleansing or "surface active agent." The term surfactant describes organic compounds brought together by chemical synthesis (combining chemical elements to form a whole) to create wetting, dispersing, emulsifying, solubilizing, foaming, or washing agents (detergents).

The base surfactant or combination of surfactants determines into which class a shampoo will fall. The base surfactants used in shampoos fall into four broad classifications: ***anionic*** (an-eye-**ON**-ik), ***cationic*** (**KAT**-i-on-ik), ***nonionic*** (non-eye-**ON**-ik), and ***ampholytic*** (**AM**-foh-lih-tik).

Most manufacturers use detergents from more than one classification. It is customary to use a secondary surfactant to complement or offset the negative qualities of the base surfactant. For example, an ***amphoteric*** (**AM**-foh-ter-ik) that is nonirritating to the eyes can be added to a harsh anionic to create a product that is more comfortable to use.

Anionics. Sodium lauryl sulfate and sodium laureth sulfate, which fall into the first classification known as *anionic surfactants*, are the most commonly used detergents. Sodium lauryl sulfate is a relatively harsh cleanser that produces a rich foam. It is suitable for use in hard or soft water because it rinses easily from the hair. Sodium laureth sulfate is also a strong, rich, foaming detergent. However, because it is less alkaline than the lauryl sulfates, it is often used in shampoos that are designed to be milder or less drying to the hair shaft. Other anionics commonly used in shampoos are:

- Disodium oleamide sulfosuccinate
- Coconut sulfated monoglycerides
- Sodium dioctyl sulfosuccinate
- Sodium lauryl isoethionate
- Triethanolamine (TEA) lauryl sulfate
- Alcohol sulfates
- Magnesium salt
- Potassium salt
- Sarcosine

Cationics. The second classification of detergents or surfactants, cationics, is made up almost entirely of quarternary ammonium compounds or ***quats.*** Practically all the quarternary compounds have some antibacterial action; therefore, they are sometimes included in the chemical composition of dandruff shampoos. Other cationics commonly used in shampoos are:

Benzalkonium chloride
N-2 ethylaminoformylmethylpyridinium

Nonionics. The third classification, nonionics, are valued as surfactants for their versatility, stability, and ability to resist shrinkage, particularly in cold temperatures. They have a mild cleansing action and low incidence of irritation to human tissues. Cocamide (DEA, MEA) is one of the most widely used nonionics in the industry, not only in shampoos but also in lipstick and permanent waving lotions. Other nonionics commonly used in shampoos are:

Diethanolamide	Monoethanolamide
Polysorbate 20 & 40	Sorbitan laurate
Palmitate	Stearate

Ampholytes. The fourth type of cleanser, the ampholyte, is important commercially because it can behave as an anionic or a cationic substance depending on the pH of the solution. The ampholytes have a slight tendency to cling to hair and skin and thus are conducive to hair manageability. They possess germicidal properties that vary between derivatives. Amphoteric surfactants are used in several baby shampoos because they do not sting the eyes. Many amphoterics are identified on the ingredient list by Amphoteric 1-20. Other ampholytes commonly used in shampoos are:

Cocamidopropyl betaine	Cocamide betaine
Sodium lauraminopropionate	
Triethanolamine (TEA) lauraminopropionate	

A familiarity with these four classifications of detergents or surfactants and their use in shampoo products will enable you to make a professional decision when selecting a product to use on a client.

Action of Surfactants in Shampoos

A surfactant molecule has two ends: ***hydrophilic*** (heye-droh-FIL-ik) (head) and ***lipophilic*** (lip-oh-FIL-ik) (tail). During the shampooing process, the hydrophilic, or water-loving, end attracts water and the lipophilic, or oil-loving end, attracts oil. This creates a push-pull process that causes the oils, dirt, and deposits to roll up into little balls that can be lifted off in the water and rinsed from the hair. (Figs. 25.2–25.5)

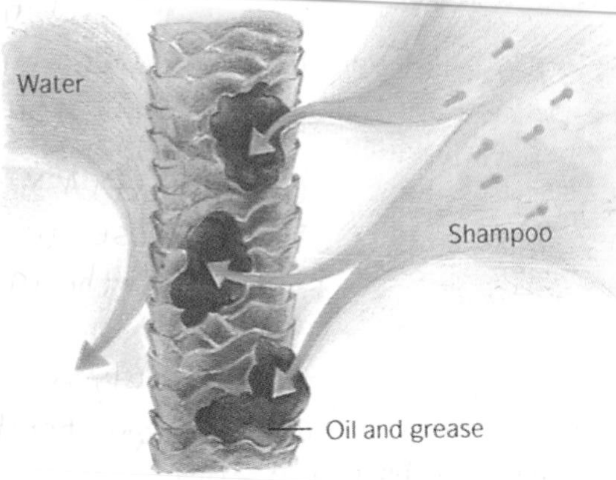

FIGURE 25.2 — Tail of shampoo molecules is attracted to hair, grease, and dirt.

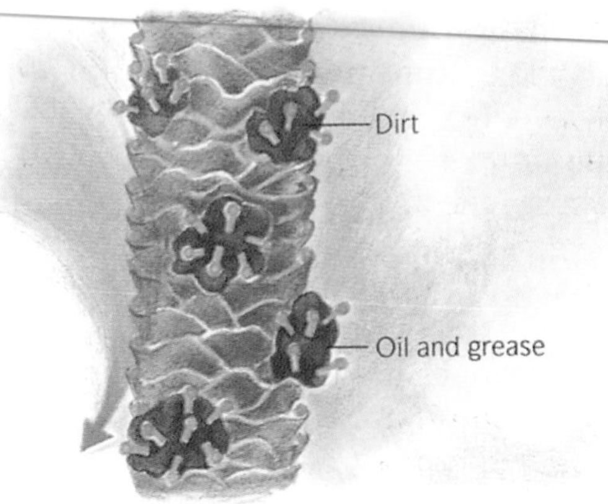

FIGURE 25.3 — Shampoo causes grease and oils to roll up into small globules.

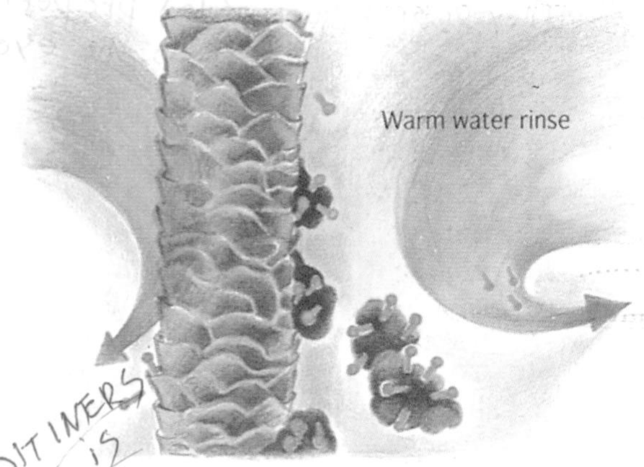

FIGURE 25.4 — While rinsing, shampoo heads attach to water molecules and cause debris to roll off.

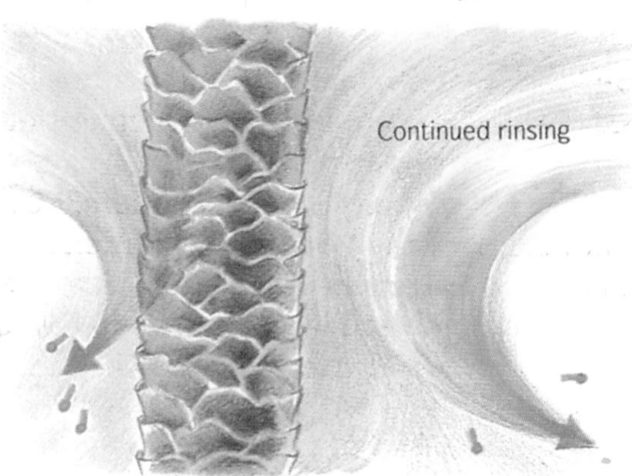

FIGURE 25.5 — Thorough rinsing ensures that debris and excess shampoo are washed away.

Other Shampoo Ingredients

Other ingredients are added to the base surfactants to create a multitude of chemical formulations. Moisturizers, oils, proteins, preservatives, foam enhancers, and perfumes are all standard components of shampoo.

CONDITIONERS

The best conditioner is only a temporary remedy for problem hair. It cannot "heal" damaged hair, nor can it improve the quality of the new hair growth. Heredity, health, and diet control the texture and structure of the hair. However, a conditioner is valuable because it can minimize the damage to hair during a cosmetology service, and it can restore luster, shine, manageability, and strength while the damaged hair grows long enough to be cut off and replaced by new hair.

Instant Conditioners

Within the classification of ***instant conditioners*** fall those products that either remain on the hair for a very short period (1 to 5 minutes) or are left in the hair during styling. Instant conditioners contain humectants to improve the appearance of dry, brittle hair. ***Humectants*** (hew-**MECK**-tants) are chemical compounds that absorb and hold moisture from the hair. Sorbitol, ethylene glycol, butylene glycol, and propylene glycol are humectants that work effectively on the hair to temporarily lock moisture into the hair.

Cetyl alcohol and stearyl alcohol, common ingredients in instant conditioners, work as pearlizing agents and lubricants to leave the hair with a glossy finish.

Chemical ingredients of lanolin derivatives, such as acetylated lanolin, lanolin acid, or lanolin oil, are often included in conditioning formulas for fine hair because of their light molecular weight.

Silicone oils, such as simethicone and dimethicone, are effective lubricants and emollients, but they have little staying power and are almost completely removed during the next shampooing.

Most conditioners fall in the pH range of 3.5 to 6.0. Therefore, they have the ability to restore the pH balance after an alkaline chemical treatment. Those conditioners designed primarily to balance pH are considered instant because of their short application time. They generally contain an acid that counteracts the alkalinity of a prior chemical service.

Moisturizers

Moisturizers are a heavier, creamier formulation than instant conditioners, and they also have a longer application time (10 to 20 minutes). They contain many of the same ingredients as instant conditioners but are formulated to be more penetrating and have longer staying power. Some moisturizers incorporate the application of heat, others do not. Stearatkonium chloride is a white paste used in moisturizers to counteract the drying effects of anionic detergents and chemical treatments.

The quarternary ammonium compounds (quats) are included in the chemical formulation of moisturizers for their ability to attach themselves steadfastly to hair fibers and provide longer lasting protection than the instant conditioners.

Protein Conditioners

Proteins are ***polymers*** (substances formed by combining many small molecules, usually in a long chain-like structure) composed of combinations of any of 23 different amino acids (used to recondition damaged hair), ranging in molecular weight. In the cosmetology industry, hydrolysis (chemical process of decomposition, involving splitting of a bond with the addition of the elements of water) and chemical modification are used to change natural protein into a usable substance. The size of the molecule, the distribution of molecular weights, how much salt the product contains, and how the protein is hydrolyzed all determine a product's effectiveness on the hair.

Setting lotions have protein-based conditioners that are part of the hair setting process. A little water, added during the hair setting procedure, facilitates setting by keeping the hair soft and manageable. This type of conditioner is designed to slightly increase hair diameter with its coating action and to give it body. It is available in several strengths to accommodate the texture, condition, and quality of hair.

Concentrated protein conditioners can be recognized by their brown liquid appearance. They are used to increase the tensile strength of the hair and to temporarily close split ends. These conditioners utilize hydrolized protein (very small fragments) and are designed to pass through the cuticle, penetrate into the cortex, and replace the keratin that has been lost from the hair. They improve texture, equalize porosity, and increase elasticity. The excess conditioner must be rinsed from the hair before setting. Concentrated protein treatments generally are not given immediately after a chemical treatment, because they can alter the freshly completed and desirable rearrangement of protein bonds after a permanent wave, relaxer, or haircoloring.

Packs

Conditioning packs are chemical mixtures of concentrated protein in the heavy cream base of a moisturizer. They penetrate several cuticle layers and are utilized when an equal degree of moisturizing and proteinizing is required.

Completed: Learning Objective #7 SHAMPOOS AND CONDITIONERS

Other Conditioning Agents

A large variety of conditioning agents in addition to the ones highlighted in this chapter are currently used in cosmetology products. Each one is designed to deal with one or more of the hair and scalp problems that will be encountered in the salon.

PERMANENT WAVING

Permanent waving makes physical and chemical changes in the structure of the hair shaft. Therefore, in order to understand the actions of permanent waving, we will review the composition of the hair and hair bonds.

COMPOSITION OF HAIR

Hair is made of a hard protein called *keratin*. The hair shaft has three layers: the *cuticle*, *cortex*, and *medulla*. Since permanent hair waving takes place in the cortical layer, you should understand the complex structure of the cortex.

The cortex is composed of numerous parallel fibers of hard keratin, referred to as ***polypeptide chains***. These parallel fibers are twisted around one another in a manner resembling the twisting of the fiber strands in a rope.

Peptide Bonds

Each amino acid is joined to another ***peptide bond*** (end bonds), forming a chain as long as the hair. They are the strongest bonds in the cortex and most of the strength of hair is due to their properties. Peptide bonds are chemical bonds, and if even a few are broken, the hair is weakened or damaged. If too many of these bonds are broken, the hair will break off.

Chemical Bonds

Three types of chemical bonds attract hair proteins to each other. The presence of these bonds or links gives hair the ability to be permanently waved. To become an expert, you should have a working knowledge of these three chemical bonds:

1. Sulfur bonds called S bonds
2. Hydrogen bonds called H bonds
3. Disulfide bonds called S-S bonds

Sulfur bonds are formed by the attraction of opposite electric charges. When two atoms of hydrogen are attracted to each other they form a ***hydrogen bond***. Both sulfur and hydrogen bonds help to hold the protein molecules of the hair together. They are relatively weak and can be broken by water. However, because there are thousands of them, they are the main bonds between protein chains and account for most of the hair's resistance to change. (Fig. 25.6)

The ***disulfide bond*** is formed by the joining of two sulfur atoms. It is the material that surrounds the spiral proteins in the cortex. The number of disulfide bonds is smaller than hydrogen and sulfur bonds, but they are much more stable.

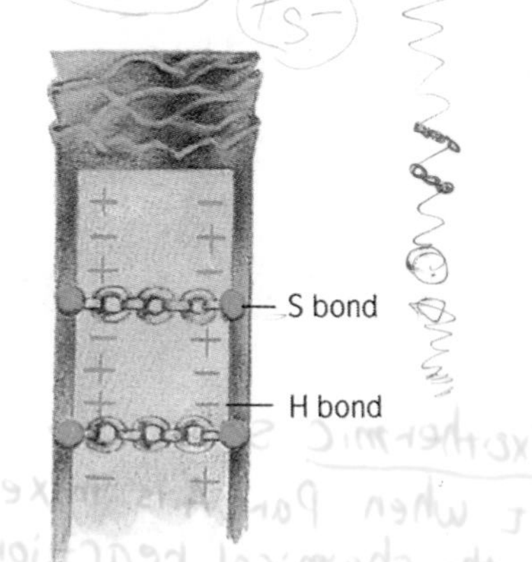

FIGURE 25.6 — Sulfur and hydrogen bonds.

Changes in Hair Bonds: Wet Waving and Curling

A temporary hair set is produced by physical changes that occur within the hair cortex. The physical changes are a result of using water, stretching techniques, and heat application and are the basis of finger waving, pin curling, roller curling, and blow-dry styling. Because of the nature of these physical changes, you can style hair as frequently as desired.

You can use water alone, because it has the ability to break down the hydrogen bonds in the cortex. The hydrogen bonds are held in place by the polypeptide chains, and you must cause these chains to slip before a strong wave can be formed.

Stretching or ribboning the hair strand causes a temporary rearrangement of the chains. Water lubricates the chains so that they can move relative to one another. However, even though the hydrogen bonds are broken, the total amount of movement is very small, because the strong disulfide bonds are completely unaffected by the water and continue to resist the slippage of the polypeptide chains.

THE PERMANENT WAVING PROCESS

To permanently wave the hair, the disulfide bonds within the cortex must be broken and rearranged. (Figs. 25.7a–e) Permanent waving lotion causes the cuticle of the hair to swell and the imbrications to open, allowing the solution to penetrate into the cortex. The solution breaks the disulfide bonds found within the cortex. Different perm solutions achieve that goal in different ways. In acid waves, also known as neutral waves, heat and tension are used along with the solution to break down the disulfide

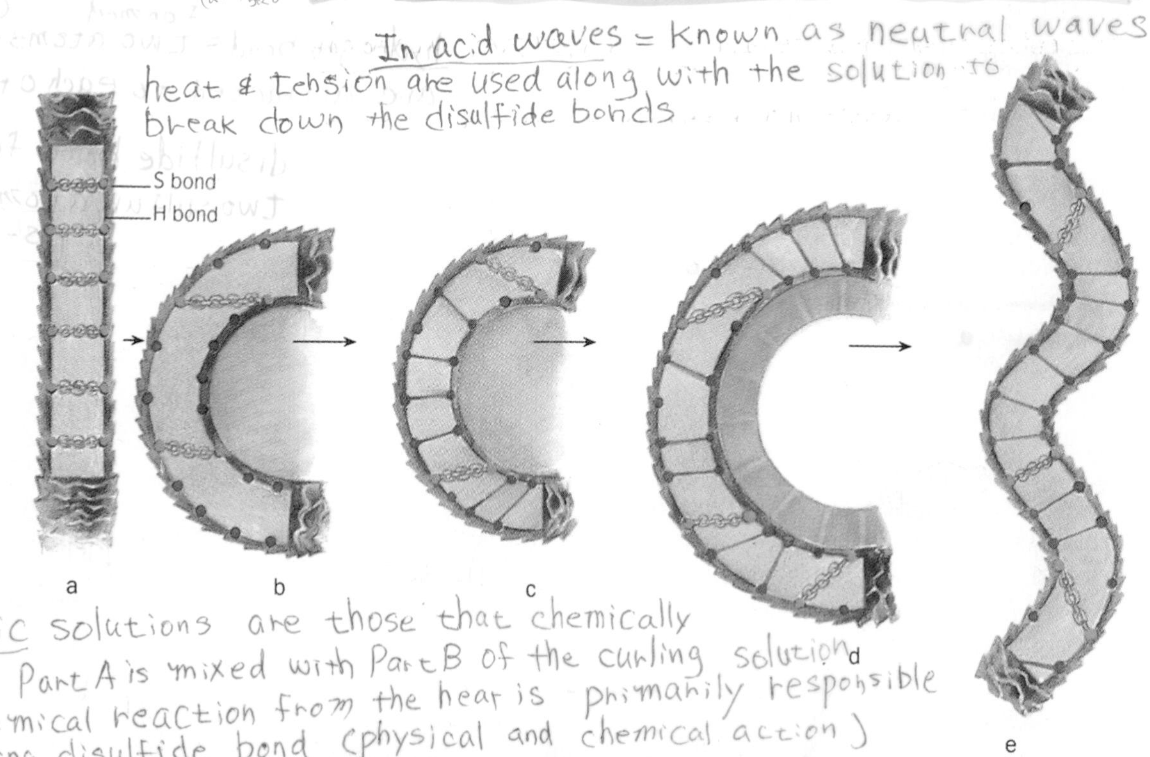

FIGURE 25.7a — H and S bonds in straight position.
FIGURE 25.7b — H bonds and nearly all S bonds broken.
FIGURE 25.7c — Some H bonds and many S bonds re-formed.
FIGURE 25.7d — Most H bonds and S bonds re-formed.
FIGURE 25.7e — Original S bonds stretched into waved positions.

bonds. In thio solutions (containing ammonium thioglycolate), the chemical is primarily responsible for breaking the bonds. Exothermic solutions are those that chemically create heat when Part A is mixed with Part B of the curling solution and the chemical reaction from the heat is primarily responsible for breaking disulfide bonds. However, with all three solutions, breaking the bonds is a physical and chemical action.

Neutralizer

When sufficient processing has taken place, the solution is rinsed from the hair and a neutralizer is applied. The neutralizer, also known as stabilizing lotion, is a neutral solution with a pH between 6.5 and 7.5. This solution is a chemical neutralizing and stabilizing agent that re-forms the disulfide bonds in their new shape and closes the cuticle of the hair shaft. The main active ingredient in neutralizers that works to re-form the disulfide bonds is generally either hydrogen peroxide, sodium bromide, or sodium bromate.

CHEMICAL HAIR RELAXING (STRAIGHTENING)

Chemical hair relaxing is the process of straightening excessively curly hair. In this process, the disulfide bonds are broken, which leaves the hair in a relaxed and straightened form. (Figs. 25.8a–d)

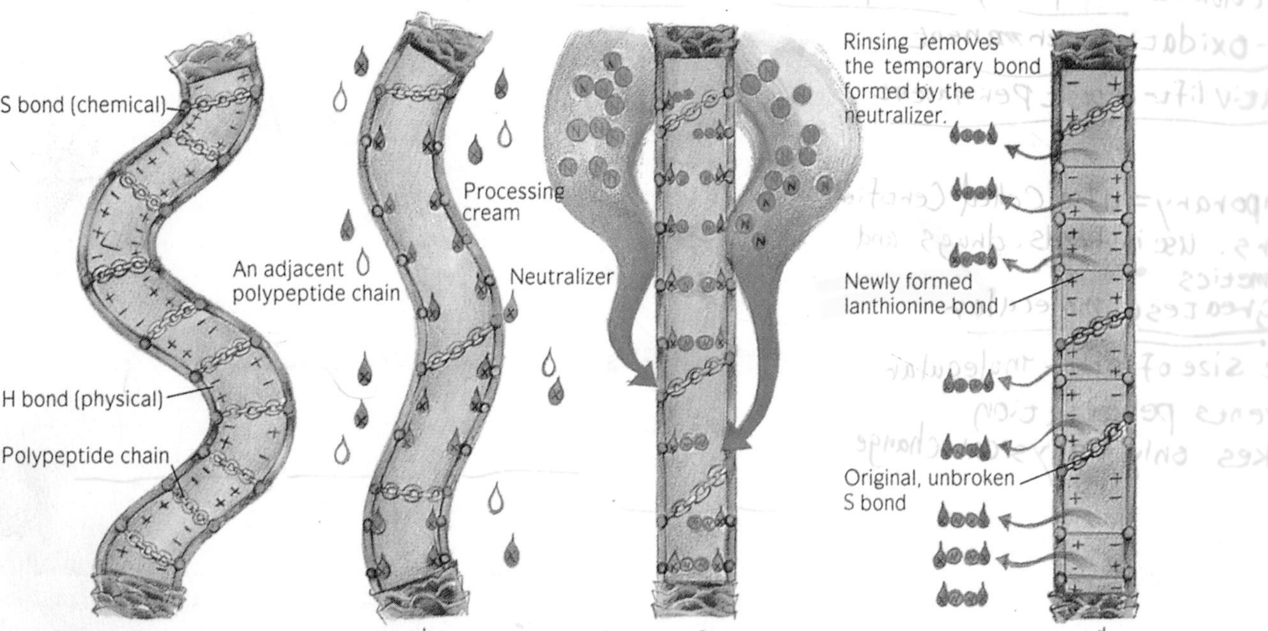

FIGURE 25.8a — Both H and S bonds holding polypeptide chains in position.
FIGURE 25.8b — All H bonds broken and most S bonds broken.
FIGURE 25.8c — Neutralizer returns hair to its normal pH.
FIGURE 25.8d — Straightened hair.

Professional cosmetologists have two types of chemical hair relaxers available for use in the salon: ***sodium hydroxide*** and ***thio***.

Sodium hydroxide works by chemically and permanently altering the disulfide bonds, leaving the hair softened in preparation for straightening. Because the bonds are permanently altered, the hair is unfit for other types of permanent waving services. In other words, you will not be able to put curl back in hair that is straightened with sodium hydroxide. The straightened hair must grow out.

Sodium hydroxide relaxers are alkaline in reaction with an approximate pH of 13. These relaxers should be handled with caution, because sodium hydroxide is considered a caustic chemical.

Completed:
Learning Objective
#8
HAIR COMPOSITION THROUGHOUT PERMANENT WAVING AND CHEMICAL HAIR RELAXING

SOFT PERMANENT WAVES

A thio cream or gel-based ammonium thioglycolic product is used to straighten the hair by breaking the disulfide bonds. This allows the hair to take on a relaxed and straightened form. After the hair is straightened with the thio relaxer, the hair can be permanently waved in the manner normally used in permanent waving the hair. It is neutralized in the same way as a normal cold wave perm.

THE CHEMISTRY OF HAIRCOLORING

Haircolor is divided into five classifications: *temporary*, *semi-permanent*, *oxidative deposit-only (demi)*, *non-oxidative permanent*, and *oxidative/lift-deposit (permanent)*. These classifications indicate color fastness or ability to remain on the hair. These characteristics are determined by chemical composition and molecular weight of the pigments and dyes within the products found in each classification.

TEMPORARY HAIRCOLORS

Temporary colors are also called certified colors because they contain colors accepted by the government for use in foods, drugs, and cosmetics. Temporary colors for the hair come in various forms, such as color rinses, color sprays, color mousses, and color shampoos. They are available in a wide range of colors and are easily applied.

Temporary colors utilize dye molecules of the greatest molecular weight. The large size of this color molecule prevents penetration of the cuticle layer of the hair shaft and allows only a coating action on the outside of the strand.

The chemical composition of a temporary color is acid in reaction and makes only a physical change rather than a chemical change in the shaft. This creates a color that is designed to be removed completely with the next shampooing.

SEMI-PERMANENT HAIRCOLOR

Two types of semi-permanent colors are available to the professional cosmetologist: *traditional* and *polymer*.

Traditional semi-permanent colors are designed to last 3 to 4 weeks. They utilize pigment and dye molecules that are of a lesser molecular weight than those of temporary colors. These smaller molecules have the physical capability to penetrate the hair shaft somewhat. The chemical composition of semi-permanent colors is mildly alkaline. This makes the hair shaft swell and the cuticle rise, allowing some penetration into the cortex. Traditional semi-permanent colors make a mild chemical change, as well as a physical change, in the hair shaft.

A polymer is a substance that has long-chain structural units created from the combining of many small molecules. These chains have tensile strength, elasticity, and hardness. Other examples of polymers are vinyl, plastic, and human tissue. Polymer semi-permanent colors are classified as semi-permanent colors because they require no oxidation process or the addition of an oxidizer for color development. However, the colorfastness of polymer colors differs from traditional semi-permanent colors. The long-chain structure of the polymer inhibits its penetration of the cuticle and ability to adhere to the keratin of the hair shaft. Therefore, heat is applied to deepen the color penetration and extend the colorfastness. (Fig. 25.9)

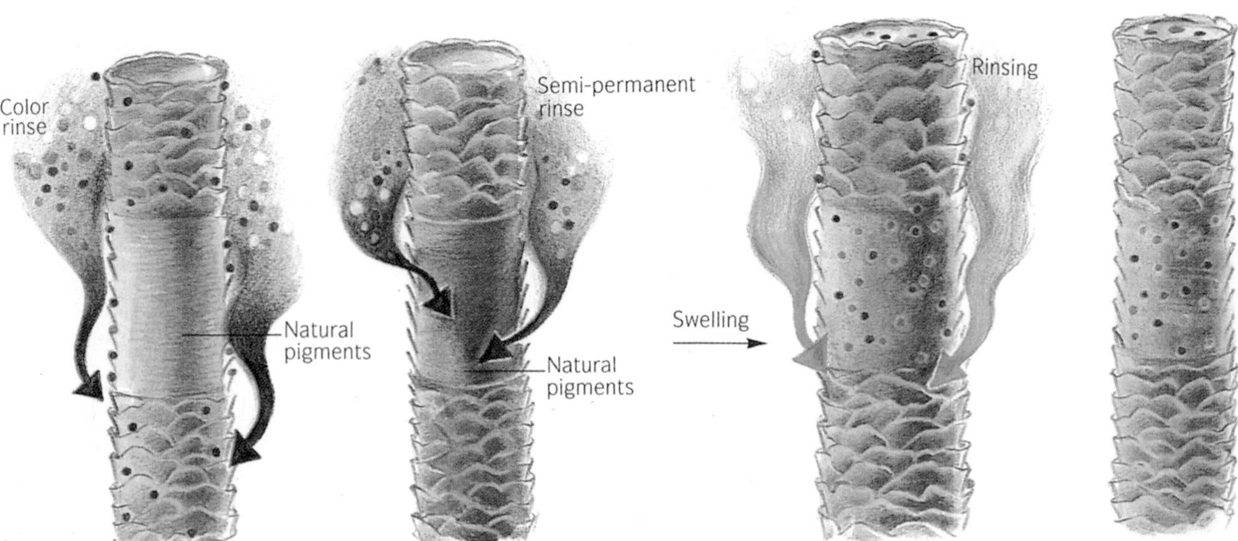

FIGURE 25.9 — Action of semi-permanent haircolors.

OXIDATIVE DEPOSIT-ONLY HAIRCOLOR

Oxidative deposit-only, or ***demi***, colors are the newest type of haircolor products on the market. This type of haircolor is formulated using mostly oxidation or aniline derivative dyes. The primary difference is that deposit-only colors utilize a different type of alkalizing agent that does not lift the natural melanin. These are either methylethylamine or AMP aminomethypropanol. These chemicals contribute the alkaline pH to the haircolor product without lift. The alkalinity is necessary to create an oxidation reaction with the developer, which allows the dyes to develop. The developer for deposit-only products is usually 10 volume peroxide.

These products penetrate the cuticle and deposit color in the cortex of the hair shaft. They are generally milder on the hair than permanent lift-deposit haircolor and longer wearing than semi-permanent colors.

NON-OXIDATIVE PERMANENT HAIRCOLOR

Three types of products fall within the classification of permanent hair tints: *vegetable tints*, *metallic tints*, and *compound dyes*. (Figs. 25.10a–d)

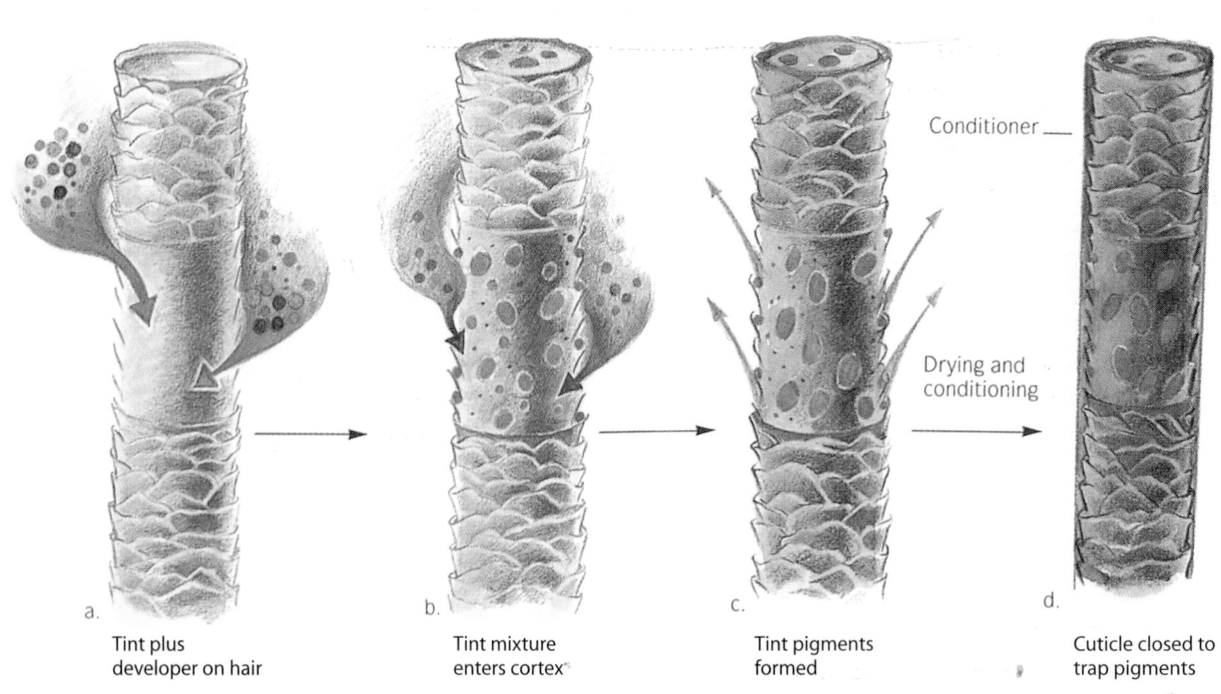

FIGURE 25.10a — Tint and peroxide on hair.
FIGURE 25.10b — Tint mixture enters into cortex.
FIGURE 25.10c — Tint pigments formed.
FIGURE 25.10d — Shrinking of cuticle scales to trap pigment.

Vegetable Tints

In the past, many vegetable materials such as logwood, indigo, chamomile, and henna were used as haircoloring ingredients. Both logwood and indigo are also used to color fabric. Apigenin is the pigment distilled from an herb known as chamomile. The chamomile flowers can be ground into a powder and used as a paste to give a lighter, brighter effect to the hair. Although vegetable henna has been used for haircoloring since the days of the early Egyptians, its use is very limited in the modern professional practice of haircolor.

Henna owes its hair dyeing abilities to the presence of a chemical known as *lawsone*. Lawsone is soluble in water and a substantial amount in an acid solution will adhere to the keratin of the hair shaft. Citric or other acids are added to create a pH of 5.5, which is optimum for henna after it is mixed and ready for application.

Henna penetrates into the cortical layer, as well as coating the cuticle of the shaft when the pigment molecule of the henna and the S-bonds are combined in the cortex. Henna has a coating action that can process unevenly on hair that has uneven porosity, and it can build up on hair to the point that solutions cannot penetrate properly. Although it is considered permanent, henna eventually fades with shampooing.

Metallic Dyes

Metallic hair dyes make up a small portion of the home haircoloring market and currently are not used professionally. However, it is important for you to be informed of the chemical composition and characteristics of metallic dyes, because metals react adversely with the oxidation solutions commonly used in the professional salon.

The colors produced by metallic salts are due to sulfides formed by the reaction between the sulfur in the keratin and the metallic salts, and to the metallic oxides formed by the keratin reducing the metal salts. The metallic salts react with the sulfur of the hair keratin and turn the protein brown.

Metallic salts (lead, silver, copper) have been known to cause headaches, scalp irritation, contact dermatitis, facial swelling, hair breakage and loss, lead poisoning, and can cause bottles of dye to explode. If you do use these dyes, it is important to wash your hands thoroughly because ingestion through oral contact or contamination of food can be fatal.

Compound Dyes

Compound dyes are a combination of vegetable and metallic dyes. Metallic salts are added to the vegetable dyes as a fixative, thus creating a formulation that lasts longer. The addition of metallic salts also creates colors that are new and different from those available with pure vegetable tints. The most common example of this is compound henna, which is the combination of pure vegetable henna and a metallic salt. Like metallic dyes, compound dyes are not used professionally.

OXIDATIVE/LIFT-DEPOSIT HAIRCOLOR

Oxidative permanent haircolor. As a professional cosmetologist, the permanent color you will use most often is known as ***oxidation,*** or ***aniline derivative,*** haircolor. The dye molecules of oxidation haircolors have the lowest molecular weight, the smallest used in the five classifications of haircolor.

Oxidative haircolors are composed of primary intermediates and couplers. The primary intermediates are composed of aromatic (fragrant) compounds obtained almost exclusively from coal. They are synthetic, organic ingredients that, when mixed with an oxidizer, work together to create artificial color. The couplers are ingredients added to obtain a variety of colors. For example, a brown primary intermediate can be varied by the addition of different couplers. The same primary will become greenish brown, yellow brown, or violet brown depending on the coupler used.

When you mix oxidation tints with the oxidizing agent (hydrogen peroxide), an oxidation-reduction reaction occurs at an alkaline pH. This causes the cuticle to swell, raising and separating the cuticle layers. The small dye precursors enter the cortex and couple and bond to the hair structure, creating the new color. At the same time, the oxidation-reduction reaction causes the natural melanin to break apart and diffuse, creating a lighter, warmer effect from the natural color.

The Professional Hair Care and Beauty Trades Division of the United Food and Commercial Workers International Union cites studies that indicate that some of the chemicals found in oxidation tints do penetrate the skin and can be harmful to health. They advise handling these products with care, which means that wearing gloves during the mixing, application, and removing of oxidation tints is recommended.

COLOR REMOVERS

Two basic types of products are available to remove artificial pigment from the hair: ***oil-based color removers*** and ***dye solvents.***

Oil-based color removers are products that gently remove color buildup or stain from the cuticle layer of the hair shaft. They make no structural or chemical change in the hair.

Dye solvents are designed to diffuse (break apart) artificial color molecules deposited by aniline derivative tints. However, as a dye solvent lightens the artificial color molecules, it also diffuses the melanin of the hair shaft.

HAIR LIGHTENING

Very simply, the oxidation of melanin in the hair is what causes hair color to lighten. How does this take place? When hydrogen peroxide is added to a bleach formula (the oxidation process), it releases molecules of gas. These molecules of gas are in constant motion. When the bleach formula is applied to the client's hair, the gases crash into the hair melanin with enough force to break apart, or diffuse, the melanin. This action oxidizes the melanin in the hair shaft, making it lighter.

In the salon, three basic classifications of bleach are used: ***oil, cream,*** and ***powder***. Each classification has unique uses, abilities, and chemical characteristics.

Oil bleaches are the mildest of the three types and have the least amount of lightening action. Oil bleach is a shampoo-based product containing sulfonated oils (oils treated with sulfuric acid or castor oil) to slow down the bleaching action. These bleaches contain a hydrogen peroxide and ammonia solution that creates an alkaline pH strong enough to soften and open the cuticle allowing the bleach to gently lighten the hair.

Career Path

COSMETIC CHEMIST

Cosmetic and product manufacturers are constantly developing new and better products. Since competition among these companies is keen, a good cosmetic chemist can usually find employment. This is a perfect field for an esthetician with additional background in science. More advanced education in chemistry and biology may be required for some jobs; occasionally a company will offer on-the-job training to an esthetician who wishes to enter this field.

A director of cosmetic research usually has a background in chemistry, physics, biology, and other sciences. The research director and his or her assistants are responsible for running tests in the laboratory to determine the safety of products before they are distributed. For many years, animals have been used to test products; since many people are opposed to such tests, more companies are beginning to use human volunteers and other methods of testing cosmetics for allergic reactions. Facial treatments, cosmetics, and most other products must be extensively tested before they are marketed. Products labeled "hypoallergenic" must be thoroughly tested, and the manufacturers are required by the FDA to document their claims.

A research director or assistant may also be involved in conducting consumer surveys and writing reports for scientific journals.

—*From* Standard Textbook for Professional Estheticians *by Joel Gerson*

Cream bleaches are similar to oil bleaches in that both have a shampoo base containing sulfonated oil. However, the cream bleach has other ingredients that make it strong enough to do pastel blonding, yet gentle enough to be used on the scalp. When a cream bleach is mixed for use, it is the addition of protinators or activators containing an alkali, such as sodium metasilicate, or oxidizers, such as urea peroxide, potassium persulfate, and ammonium persulfate, that give it the extra lightening power. Cream bleaches have an average pH of 10 and contain a solution of hydrogen peroxide that can be as great as 6%.

Powder bleaches, like cream bleaches, are strong enough to do pastel blonding. Powder bleach is similar to oil bleach in chemical composition, but powder bleach cannot be applied to the scalp, because it does not contain the oil and conditioners that make a cream bleach safe for on-the-scalp application. Like oil and cream bleaches, powder bleaches contain ammonia; however, in this instance it is in a dry form. The ammonia begins the oxidation process when it mixes with liquid or cream hydrogen peroxide.

TONERS

Toners are permanent aniline derivative colors designed for pre-lightened hair. The difference between a tint and a toner is that the dye load of a toner is less. This creates pale, delicate shades of color used to "tone" pre-lightened hair.

COLOR FILLERS

As a professional cosmetologist, you might use fillers to equalize the porosity of abused or damaged hair and to create a color base in the hair. Fillers are absorbed by the hair according to its porosity; the greater the porosity, the greater the absorption. Filler molecules fill in spaces left in the shaft from prior diffusion of melanin, creating a base to which tint molecules can attach.

Protein fillers are made from a variety of sources, both animal (tallow protein) and vegetable (soy protein). These proteins are hydrolyzed into small chains of polypeptides that form protein salt bonds, which will attach to the protein in the hair.

Nonprotein fillers are made of oil and water emulsions that are thickened with a mildly acid pH of approximately 3.5 to 4.0. These fillers use cationic compounds as the active ingredient, which cause the product to adhere to the shaft.

Completed:
Learning Objective
#9
COMPOSITION OF HAIR AND HAIRCOLORING

COSMETIC CHEMISTRY

Cosmetic chemistry is the scientific study of the cosmetics used in our industry. You will find yourself better equipped to incorporate the art and science of cosmetics into your professional services after you acquire an understanding of the chemical composition, preparation, and use of cosmetics. Cosmetics can be classified according to their physical and chemical nature and the characteristics by which we identify them.

PHYSICAL AND CHEMICAL CLASSIFICATIONS OF COSMETICS

1. Powders
2. Solutions
3. Suspensions
4. Emulsions
5. Ointments
6. Soaps

Powders

Powders are a uniform mixture of insoluble substances (inorganic, organic, and colloidal) that have been properly blended, perfumed, and/or tinted to produce a cosmetic that is free from coarse or gritty particles. Mixing and sifting are used in the process of making powders.

Solutions

A ***solution*** (soh-LOO-shun) is an evenly dispersed mixture of two or more kinds of molecules. For example, a solution is made by mixing a solute (for example, a sugar cube) into a solvent (for example, water). A ***solute*** (SOL-yoot) is any substance that dissolves into a liquid and forms a solution. A ***solvent*** (SOL-vent) is any substance that is able to dissolve another substance.

Solutions are clear mixtures of a solute and solvent that do not separate when left standing. Solutions are easily prepared by dissolving a powdered solute in a warm solvent and stirring at the same time. The solute can be separated from the solvent by applying heat and evaporating the solvent. A good solution should be clear and transparent; thus filtration is often necessary if the solution is cloudy.

Water is a universal solvent. It is capable of dissolving more substances than any other solvent. Oils, grain alcohol, and glycerine are frequently used as solvents. Solvents are classified as ***miscible*** (MIS-eh-bel) or ***immiscible***. Water, glycerine, and alcohol readily mix with each other; therefore, they are miscible (mixable). On the other hand, water and oil do not mix with each other; hence, they are immiscible (nonmixable).

The solute can be either a solid, liquid, or gas. For example, boric acid solution is a mixture of a solid in a liquid; glycerine and rose water is a mixture of two miscible liquids; ammonia water is a mixture of a gas in water.

Solutions containing ***volatile*** (VOL-ih-til) (easily evaporated) substances, such as ammonia and alcohol, should be stored with lids tightly secured in a cool place to discourage evaporation. If excessive evaporation takes place, the solution may become flammable.

There are three methods of expressing concentration of solutions:

A *dilute* (deye-**LOOT**) *solution* contains a small quantity of the solute in proportion to the quantity of the solvent.

A *concentrated solution* contains a large quantity of the solute in proportion to the quantity of solvent.

A *saturated* (**SACH**-oo-rayt-ed) *solution* will not dissolve or take more of the solute than it already holds at a given temperature.

Suspensions

Suspensions are mixtures of one type of matter in another type of matter. The particles might have a tendency to separate on standing, making it necessary to shake or stir the product before use. Some skin lotions, such as calamine lotion, are suspensions. Other examples are whipping cream, salad dressing, clouds, and smoke.

Emulsions

Emulsions (ee-**MUL**-shuns) are formed when two or more immiscible (nonmixable) substances, such as oil and water, are united with the aid of a binder (gum) or an emulsifier (soap). If a suitable emulsifier and the proper techniques are used, the resulting emulsion will be stable. A stable emulsion can hold as much as 90% water. Depending on the balance between the liquids and solids, the emulsion may be cream, liquid, or semi-solid in character.

Emulsions are prepared by hand or with the aid of a grinding and cutting machine called a ***colloidal mill***. In the process of preparing the emulsion, the emulsifier forms a protective film around the microscopic globules of either the oil or water. The smaller the globules, the thicker and more stable the resulting emulsion.

Emulsions basically fall into two different classes: *oil-in-water (O/W)* and *water-in-oil (W/O)*.

Oil-in-water (O/W) emulsions are made of oil droplets suspended in a water base. In addition to the emulsifier, which coats the oil droplets and holds them in suspension, there may be a number of additional ingredients present that are designed to cause certain reactions in the hair, for example, permanent wave solutions, lighteners (bleaches), neutralizers, and tints.

Water-in-oil (W/O) emulsions are formed with drops of water suspended in an oil base. These are usually much thicker and oilier than the O/W emulsions, for example, hair grooming creams, cleansing creams, and cold creams.

Ointments

Ointments (**OINT**-ments) are semi-solid mixtures of organic substances (lard, petrolatum [Vaseline], wax) and a medicinal agent. No water is used. For the ointment to soften upon application, its melting point should be lower than body temperature (98.6° Fahrenheit [37° Celsius]).

Sticks are similar to ointments in that they are a mixture of organic substances (oils, waxes, petrolatum) poured into a mold to solidify. Sticks are firmer and harder than ointments. No water is present. (Examples: lipstick, color crayons)

Pastes are soft, moist cosmetics that have a thick consistency. They are bound together with gum, starch, and sometimes water. If oils and fats are present, water is generally absent. The colloidal mill assists in the removal of grittiness from the paste. (Example: cream rouge)

Mucilages (***MYOO***-sih-lij-ez) are thick liquids containing either natural gums (tragacanth or karaya) or synthetic gums mixed with water. Since mucilages undergo decomposition, a preservative is required. (Example: hair setting lotions)

Soaps

Soaps are compounds formed when a mixture of fats and oils is fed into a tank of superheated water (which converts the mixture into fatty acids) and then purified by distillation. Potassium hydroxide is mixed with the fatty acids to make soft soap or with sodium hydroxide to make hard soap. During the process of making soap, glycerine is given off as a by-product. A high-quality soap is made from pure oils and fats and does not contain excessive alkalies.

Completed:
Learning Objective
#10
PHYSICAL AND CHEMICAL CLASSIFICATIONS OF COSMETICS

INFORMATIONAL REFERENCES

As a professional cosmetologist, you should become familiar with the United States Pharmacopeia (U.S.P.), a book that defines and standardizes drugs; the Federal Drug Administration (FDA), which also regulates cosmetics and colorings; the Professional Hair Care and Beauty Trades Division of the United Food and Commercial Workers International Union; the health and safety codes of your state; the Material Safety Data Sheets (MSDS) from each manufacturer; and commercially available cosmetic dictionaries. All provide information that is of great importance to you as a professional cosmetologist.

The following are examples of some of the terms used in the cosmetology industry:

Alcohol, also known as grain or ethyl alcohol, is a colorless liquid obtained by the fermentation of starch, sugar, and other carbohydrates. It is no longer used as a skin sanitizer because of current classification as a hazardous chemical and because it does not kill bacteria.

Alum is aluminum potassium or ammonium sulphate, supplied in the form of crystals or powder. It has a strong astringent action and is used in aftershave and astringent lotions, as well as in powder form as a styptic (to stop bleeding).

Ammonia water is ammonia gas dissolved in water. It is a colorless liquid with a pungent, penetrating odor that can be irritating to the eyes and mucous membranes. Ammonia water is used in cosmetology in hair straighteners, aniline and metallic hair dyes, and alone as a 28% ammonia water solution.

Boric acid is used for its bactericidal and fungicidal properties in baby powder, eye creams, mouthwashes, soaps, and skin fresheners. It is a mild healing and antiseptic agent although the American Medical Association warns of possible toxicity. Severe irritation and poisonings have occurred after application to *open* skin wounds.

Ethyl methacrylate is an ester (compound) of ethyl alcohol and methacrylic acid used in the chemical formulation of many sculptured nails. Daily inhalation of fumes is not recommended for health reasons.

Formaldehyde is a colorless gas manufactured by an oxidation process of methyl alcohol. It is used as a disinfectant, fungicide, germicide, and preservative, as well as an embalming solution. In the industry, formaldehyde is used in soap, cosmetics, nail hardeners, and polishes. It should be used with caution because National Cancer Institute studies indicate that it is toxic, can lead to DNA damage, and can react with other chemicals to become carcinogenic.

Glycerine is a sweet, colorless, odorless, syrupy liquid formed by the decomposition of oils, fats, or molasses. It is used as a skin softener in cuticle oil, facial creams, and a variety of lotions.

Petrolatum, commonly known as *Vaseline*, petroleum jelly, or paraffin jelly, is a yellowish to white semi-solid greasy mass that is almost insoluble in water. It is used in wax epilators, eyebrow pencils, lipsticks, protective creams, cold creams, and many other cosmetics for its ability to soften and smooth the skin.

Phenylenediamine, derived from coal tar, has a succession of derivatives known to penetrate the skin and believed to cause cancer.

Potassium hydroxide (caustic potash) is prepared by electrolysis of potassium chloride. It may be used for its emulsifying abilities in the formulas for hand lotions, liquid soaps, protective creams, and cuticle softeners.

Quaternary ammonium compounds (quats) are found in many antiseptics, surfactants, preservatives, sanitizers, and germicides. Quats are synthetic derivatives of ammonium chloride. Although quats can be toxic, they are considered safe in the proportions used in the industry.

Sodium bicarbonate (baking soda) is a precipitate made by passing carbon dioxide gas through a solution of sodium carbonate. The resulting white powder is used as a neutralizing agent and (when mixed in shampoo) to remove hair spray buildup.

Sodium carbonate (soda ash or washing soda) is found naturally in ores and lake brines or seawater. It is used in shampoos and permanent wave solutions. Sodium carbonate absorbs water from the air.

Witch hazel is a solution of alcohol, water, and powder ground from the leaves and twigs of the *Hamamelis virginiana.* It works as an astringent, local anesthetic, and skin freshener. Because of the alcohol content it should not be applied directly to an open wound or the delicate membranes of the eye. (See ***alcohol.***)

Zinc oxide is a heavy white powder that is insoluble in water. It is used cosmetically in face powder and foundation creams for its ability to impart opacity.

COSMETIC BODY CLEANSERS

Cosmetics that are designed to cleanse and beautify the skin, hair, and nails are important to the industry. To provide clients with professional services, you need an understanding of these products designed to remove dirt, hair, or foreign odors from the skin. The classifications of these products are soaps, depilatories, and epilators.

Kinds of Soaps

There are two methods of making soap: *traditional* and *synthetic.* ***Traditional soap*** is a mixture of various types of fatty acids and sodium salts manufactured through a process of adding alkalies to the fats with glycerol. The ***synthetic*** process is a chemical combination of oils and fatty acids.

The soaps currently used in the beauty industry fall into three classifications: deodorant, beauty, and medicated.

Deodorant soaps include a bactericide that remains on the body to kill the bacteria responsible for odors. The most common antiseptic and antibacterial agent is probably triclocarban. Triclocarban, often listed in the ingredients as TCC, is prepared from aniline. Aniline additives have been known to increase the skin's sensitivity to the sun, which can inflame some types of skin.

Beauty soaps are intended for the more delicate tissues of the face. They are more acid in pH, less drying to the skin, yet able to remove dirt and debris from the skin's surface. Many beauty soaps are transparent and contain large quantities of glycerine. Other beauty soaps contain larger amounts of oils that leave an emollient film on the skin.

Medicated soaps are designed to treat skin problems such as rashes, pimples, and acne. Many contain small percentages of cresol, phenol, or other antiseptics. Resorcinol is often used as a drying agent in medicated products designed to treat oily conditions. The strongest medicated soaps can only be obtained with a physician's prescription.

Depilatories

Depilatories are preparations used for the temporary removal of superfluous hair by dissolving it at the skin line. Depilatories contain detergents to strip the sebum from the hair and adhesives to hold the chemicals to the hair shaft for the 5 to 10 minutes necessary to remove the hair. During the application time, swelling accelerating agents, such as urea or melamine, expand the hair, helping to break hair bonds. Finally, chemicals, such as sodium hydroxide, potassium hydroxide, thioglycolic acid, or calcium thioglycolate, destroy the disulfide bonds. These chemicals turn the hair into a soft, jelly-like mass of hydrolyzed protein that can be scraped from the skin. Although depilatories are not commonly used in salons, you should be familiar with them in case your clients have used them.

Epilators

Epilators remove the hair by pulling it out of the follicle. Two types of wax are currently used for professional epilation: cold and hot. Both products are made primarily of resins and beeswax. Beeswax has a relatively high incidence of allergic reaction; therefore, it is advisable to give a small patch test of the product to be used. Recently, electrical apparatus made for the home market has become available.

COSMETICS FOR SKIN AND FACE

The cosmetic industry has made available a vast array of products designed to improve the condition and appearance of the skin.

Creams

The creams you will be using for professional skin treatments fall into four main categories: *cleansing*, *wrinkle treatments*, *moisturizers*, and *massage cream*.

The action of ***cleansing cream*** is, in part, caused by the oil content of the cream, which has the ability to dissolve other greasy substances. Older formulas, such as cold cream, contain relatively few ingredients: vegetable or mineral oil, beeswax, water, preservatives, and emulsifiers. The new cleansing formulations are much more complicated and may contain additional degreasers such as lemon juice, synthetic surfactants, emollients (oils), and humectants (water retainers).

Wrinkle treatments are designed to conceal lines on aging skin in two ways. One is with a crease-filling capacity and the other is through a plumping up of the tissues. Among the many possible ingredients in these treatments are hormones, hyaluronic acid, and collagen. Some are made of herbs and other natural ingredients; others are entirely synthetic.

Moisturizing creams are designed to treat dryness. They contain humectants, which create a barrier that allows the natural water and oil of the skin to accumulate in the tissues. This barrier also works to protect the skin from air pollution, dirt, and debris. Moisturizers contain a variety of emollients, ranging from simple ingredients, such as peanut, coconut, or a variety of other oils, to more complex chemical compounds, such as cetyl alcohol, cholesterol, dimethicone, or glycerine derivatives.

Massage creams are used to help the hands glide over the skin. They are formulations of cold cream, lanolin or its derivatives, and possibly casein (a protein found in cheese).

Lotions

Lotions are used professionally in a variety of hair and facial treatments. The lotions you will work with generally are available in clear or lightly tinted solutions.

Cleansing lotions serve the same purposes as cleansing creams but are of a lighter oil content. They come in formulations for dry, normal, and oily skin conditions. Some ingredients common to cleansing lotions are cetyl alcohol, cetyl palmitate, and sorbitol combined with perfumes and colorings to enhance their marketing value.

Astringent lotions are designed to remove oil accumulation on the skin. The alcohol content of the product also "irritates" the skin, causing it to swell slightly and appear to "close" the pores. Astringent lotions contain a large percentage of alcohol and small percentages of some or all of the following: alum, boric acid, sorbitol, water, camphor, and perfumes.

Freshener lotions are similar to astringent lotions; however, they are designed to be gentler for dry to normal skin types. The formulation of a freshener typically includes some or all of the following: witch hazel, alcohol and camphorated alcohol, citric acid, boric acid, lactic acid, phosphoric acid, aluminum salts, menthol, chamomile, and floral scents.

Eye lotions are generally formulas of boric acid, bicarbonate of soda, zinc sulfate, glycerine, and herbs. They are designed to soothe and brighten the eyes.

Medicated lotions are prescribed by a physician for skin problems, such as acne, rashes, or other eruptions.

Suntan lotions are designed to protect the skin from the harmful ultraviolet rays of the sun. They are rated with a sun protection factor (SPF) that enables sunbathers to calculate the time they can remain in the sun before the skin begins to burn. Suntan lotions are emulsions that might contain para-aminobenzoic acid (PABA), a variety of oils, petrolatum, sorbitan stearate, alcohol, ultraviolet inhibitors, acid derivatives, preservatives, and perfumes.

COSMETICS FOR MAKEUP

The wide range of cosmetics available today meets the needs of every skin type. Figure 25.11 shows some examples.

Face Powder

Two forms of face powder are widely used in the salon: ***loose*** and ***compact (cake)***. Both types have the same basic composition; compact powders are simply compressed and held together with binders so the cake will not crumble.

Face powder consists of a powder base, mixed with a coloring agent (pigment) and perfume. A good face powder for normal skin should possess the following qualities:

1. ***Slip***—gives a smooth feel to the skin. This quality is gained primarily (35% to 79%) by the talc content, but zinc stearate or magnesium stearate may be added for additional slip.
2. ***Covering power***—the balance between opacity (covering defects and skin shine) and transparency (allowing the natural appearance of the skin to show through). The two ingredients that provide the balance in most powders are zinc oxide and titanium dioxide.

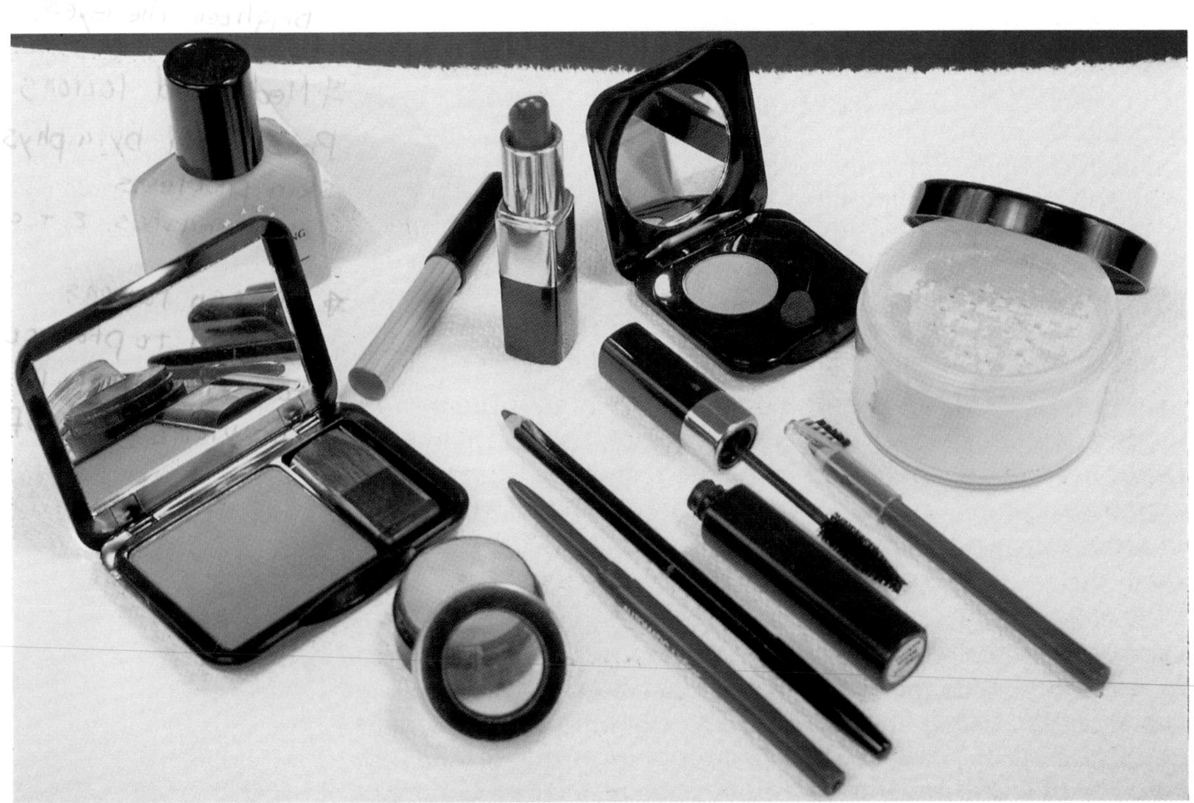

FIGURE 25.11 — A variety of cosmetics are available on the market.

3. ***Adherency***—determines how long the powder will remain on the face without needing to be touched up. Talc, zinc stearate, magnesium stearate, kaolin, and chalk have adhesive qualities.

4. ***Bloom***—ability to impart a velvet-like appearance to the skin. Starches and chalk are used to create bloom.

5. ***Other ingredients***—include bactericides, color, and perfume. Bactericides are added to inhibit growth of bacteria and preserve the product. The colors listed on the ingredient list should be FD&C (Food, Drug, and Cosmetic) or D&C (Drug and Cosmetic) approved, indicating that the colors have been certified by the Food and Drug Administration. Perfumes are added to increase the marketability of the product.

CAUTION

Although talc is generally considered safe for use in powders, the FDA has received reports of tissue swelling upon use. Talc has also been linked to coughing, vomiting, pneumonia, and even ovarian cancer when inhaled. Miners of talc frequently suffer from a lung disease called talcosis.

Foundation Makeup

The purpose of foundation makeup is to improve the appearance of the complexion by blending skin tones, covering blemishes, and creating a smooth, healthy glow. Many foundations contain barrier agents, such as UV inhibitors, cellulose derivatives, and silicone, to protect the complexion from light rays (artificial and natural), the wind and cold, and from dirt and debris.

Cream foundations are predominantly water, mineral oil, stearic acid, cetyl alcohol, propylene glycol, triethanolamine, lanolin derivatives, borax, and insoluble pigments. Foundations may also contain surfactants (detergents), emulsifiers, humectants, perfume, and preservatives, such as paraben. The formulation of this product is generally suited for dry to normal skin and gives good coverage.

Liquid foundations are suspensions of organic and inorganic pigments in an alcohol and water solution. Most liquid foundations must be shaken before use, but bentonite is added to help keep the product blended. The formulation of this product is generally suited for clients with oily to normal skin conditions desiring light to natural-looking coverage.

Cheek Color (Blush)

Cheek color is available in powder and cream form.

Powder cheek color is simply compact or cake powder with coloring added. The pigment ranges from 5% to 20% of the product.

Cream cheek colors fall into two categories: oil-based and emulsions. The oil-based formulations are combinations of pigments dispersed in an oil or fat base. Blends of waxes (carnauba wax and ozokerite) and oily liquids (isopropyl myristate and hexadecyl stearate) create a water-resistant product. In addition, cream cheek colors contain water, thickeners, and a variety of surfactants or detergents that enable particles to penetrate the hair follicles and cracks in the skin.

Lip Color

Lip color is available in a variety of forms: creams, glosses, pencils, gels, and sticks. All are formulas of oils, waxes, and dyes. Castor oil is the primary ingredient in lipsticks, accounting for approximately 65% of the product. Other oils used are olive, mineral, sesame, cocoa butter, petroleum, lecithin, and hydrogenated vegetable oils. Waxes commonly included in the ingredients are paraffin, beeswax, carnauba (also used in car waxes), and candelilla wax. Bromic acid, D&C Red No. 27, D&C Orange No. 17 Lake, and related dyes are examples of those often used as coloring agents.

Eye Makeup

Eye pencils consist of a wax (paraffin) or hardened oil base (petrolatum) with a variety of additives to create color. They are available in both soft and hard form for use on the eyebrow, as well as the upper and lower eyelid. According to the American Medical Association, eye pencils should not be used to color the inside border of the eyes, because this can lead to infection of the lacrimal duct, tearing, blurring of vision, and permanent pigmentation of the mucous membrane lining inside the eye.

Eye shadows are available in cream and powder form. The cream shadows are water-based with oil, petrolatum, thickener, wax, perfume, preservatives, and color added. Water-resistant shadows have a solvent base, such as mineral spirits. Powder shadows are composed much the same as pressed face powder and powdered cheek color.

Mascara is available in tube and wand applicators. Both are polymer products that include water, wax, thickeners, film-formers, and preservatives in their formulation. The pigments in mascara must be inert (unable to combine with other elements) and usually are carbon black, carmine, ultramarine, chromium oxide, and iron oxides. Coal tar dyes are not permitted. Some wand mascaras contain rayon or nylon fibers to lengthen and thicken the hair fibers.

> **CAUTION**
>
> *Apply mascara carefully. The most common injury with mascara is poking the eye with the applicator.*

Eyeliners are available in liquid and cake form, as well as the pencil form described earlier. In the ingredient list you will find alkanolamine (a fatty alcohol), cellulose, ether, polyvinylpyrrolidone, methylparaben, antioxidants, perfumes, and titanium dioxide.

Eye makeup removers fall into two categories: oil-based and non-oil-based. Oil-based removers are generally mineral oil with a small amount of fragrance added. Non-oil-based removers are a water solution to which acetone, boric acid, oils, lanolin or lanolin derivatives, and other solvents have been added. Because most eye makeup products are water-resistant, plain soap and water is less effective for removal.

Cosmetics for eye and face makeup comprise an important segment of the beauty industry. As a professional cosmetologist, you will be called upon to use, recommend, and sell these cosmetics.

Miscellaneous Cosmetics

Greasepaint is a mixture of fats, petrolatum, and a coloring agent and is used for theatrical purposes.

Cake or ***pancake makeup*** is generally composed of kaolin, zinc, talc, titanium oxide, mineral oil, fragrances, precipitated calcium carbonate, finely ground pigments, and inorganic pigments, such as iron oxides. Cake makeup is used to cover scars and pigmentation defects.

Masks and ***packs*** are available to serve many purposes and skin conditions—deep cleansing, pore reduction, tightening, firming, moisturizing, wrinkle reduction. Clay masks typically contain varying combinations of kaolin (china clay), bentonite, purified siliceous (fuller's) earth or colloidal clay, petrolatum, glycerine, proteins, SD alcohol, and water. The prime ingredients typically found in peel-off masks are SD alcohol 40, polysorbate-20, and polymers, such as polyvinyl alcohol or vinyl acetate.

Scalp Lotions and Ointments

Scalp lotions and ointments usually contain medicinal agents for the purpose of correcting a scalp condition, such as itching and flakiness. An astringent lotion may be applied to the scalp before shampooing to control oiliness, as well as the itching and flakiness of dry scalp conditions. Medicated lotions and ointments for severe scalp conditions must be prescribed by a physician.

Hair Dressings

Hair dressings give shine and manageability to dry or curly hair. They may be applied to either wet or dry hair. Such dressings typically consist of lanolin or its derivatives, petrolatum, oil emulsions, fatty acids, waxes, mild alkalies, and water.

Styling Aids

As a professional cosmetologist, you will utilize a variety of styling gels and mousses. Both of these products are typically polymer and resin formulations designed to give the hair body and texture. Many incorporate the same ingredients found in hair sprays but add moisturizers and humectants, such as cetyl alcohol, panthenol, hydrolyzed protein, quats, or a variety of oils to the ingredient list.

Hair Sprays

Hair spray is used to hold the finished style. Many new formulations for hair spray contain a variety of polymers, such as acrylic/acrylate copolymer, vinyl acetate, crotonic acid copolymer, PVM/MA copolymer, and polyvinylpyrrolidone (PVP); plasticizers, such as acetyl triethyl citrate, benzyl alcohol; and silicones as stiffening agents. Additional ingredients might include silicone, shellac, perfume, lanolin or its derivatives, vegetable gums, alcohol, sorbitol, and water.

Completed:
Learning Objective
#11
BASIC CHEMISTRY, TYPES AND ACTION OF PROFESSIONAL PRODUCTS

CAUTION

Careless use of hair spray can cause eye and lung damage and throat irritation.

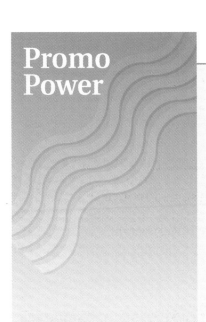

SILENT ADVERTISING

Some advertising for the salon can be done without saying a word; in fact, clients may not even be conscious that anything is happening. But these methods of selling your services are effective and easy to use:

- Operators' hairstyles: Your stylists' hair should be done once a week and be professionally combed when needed. Uncombed hair and boring styles send the wrong message about what kind of styling is done in your salon. If possible, have all your female stylists wear some type of haircolor, so they can give firsthand information on what haircolor can do.
- Pictures in the styling area: These should be in color, and should be changed at least once a month. Two or three large photos are better than many small ones.
- Magazine articles: An article from a magazine on display in the salon can help sell products. The article can be written by a beauty specialist, consultant, salon owner, or manager. The nice thing about this type of advertising is that the person is already sold before the sales attempt has begun.
- Styling aids and cosmetic items: Products used on a client's hair are easy to sell because the client has seen the stylist use the product. Everything the stylist uses should be retailed in the salon and prominently displayed.

—*From* Salon Management for Cosmetology Students
by Edward Tezak

REVIEW QUESTIONS

CHEMISTRY

1. Why is it important to understand basic chemistry to be successful as a cosmetologist?
2. What is the difference between organic and inorganic chemistry?
3. List the three forms of matter.
4. Define physical change and give one example.
5. Define chemical change and give one example.
6. What is pH?
7. List the four classifications of shampoo.
8. What are polypeptide chains?
9. List the three types of chemical bonds in the cortex.
10. What changes occur in the hair cortex during permanent waving?
11. Define the following terms as they relate to oxidation tints: primary intermediate, coupler, oxidizer.
12. List the six physical and chemical classifications of cosmetics.
13. Why must you be concerned with the application of concentrated alcohol on the skin?
14. What causes hair removal when using a depilatory?
15. List the four main types of creams you will be using as a professional cosmetologist.
16. What is the action of an astringent?
17. What are some of the common chemical ingredients in foundation makeup?

CHAPTER 26

The Salon Business

LEARNING OBJECTIVES

After completing this chapter, you should be able to:

1. List some facts you need before opening a beauty salon.
2. Discuss financial considerations involved in operating a beauty salon.
3. Explain the importance of maintaining accurate business records.
4. Explain the importance of good business operation and personnel management.
5. Discuss the principles and practices of good selling.
6. Explain the importance of advertising.

NATIONAL SKILL STANDARDS

This chapter provides you with the necessary information to master these National Industry Skill Standards for Entry-Level Cosmetologists:

- Consulting with clients to determine their needs and preferences
- Interacting with co-workers as part of a team
- Managing your time to provide efficient client service
- Taking necessary steps to develop and retain clients
- Marketing professional salon products
- Maintaining business records on client development, income, and expenses
- Managing product supply for salon use and retail sales
- Participating in lifelong learning to stay current with trends, technology, and techniques pertaining to cosmetology

INTRODUCTION

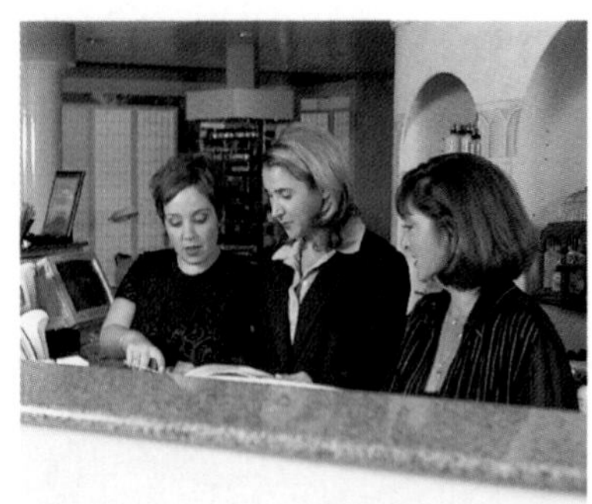

FIGURE 26.1 — Active salon managers.

Numerous management opportunities exist in the field of cosmetology. Many cosmetology school graduates want to advance themselves and become owners or managers of salons. However, only if you are adequately prepared to manage a business will you be able to realize your ambitions. (Fig. 26.1)

Starting your own business is a big responsibility and not a step to be taken without serious planning. A knowledge of business principles, bookkeeping, business laws, insurance, salesmanship, and psychology is crucial to the cosmetologist who aspires to be an owner and/or manager of a salon. This chapter covers some of the areas you must know about before becoming an owner/manager of a business.

WHAT YOU SHOULD KNOW ABOUT OPENING A SALON

When planning to open a salon, give careful consideration to every aspect of running a business, including location, written agreements, business regulations, laws, insurance, salon operation, record keeping, and salon policies.

LOCATION

A good location is one that has a population large enough to support the salon. When possible, the salon should be located near other active businesses, such as restaurants, department stores, or specialized clothing stores, shoe stores, and other fashion-related shops or supermarkets. People are drawn to shopping areas where they can make one stop serve several purposes, and unless you can afford to do a great deal of advertising, it is difficult to operate a successful salon in a low traffic area.

In general, the location you select should reflect your target market. If you are targeting a high-income client, your location should reflect that. If you plan to appeal to middle-income clients, you should consider a high-traffic area with access to public transportation.

Study the Area

Determine the area's demographics. Find out about the size, income, and buying habits of the population. Talk to other business owners to see how well they think a salon would do in the area.

Be Visible

The salon should be clearly visible and eye catching to attract the attention of people walking or driving by.

Parking Facilities

When selecting a site for a new business, or when planning to take over an established business, you must consider parking facilities. People hesitate to patronize a business that is inconvenient to reach during bad weather. Convenience of parking should be a major consideration. If your salon is open for evening service, the parking area should be well lighted. In larger cities, consider locating the salon near public transportation to attract clients who do not drive or for easy access when the weather is bad.

Competition

Avoid too much direct competition in the immediate area. It is better to locate in an area where yours is the only salon of its type. Salons can be located near each other, provided that each has a different clientele. For example, an up-scale salon can operate close to a budget salon and both may be successful because they attract different markets.

WRITTEN AGREEMENTS

Written agreements for building alterations and repairs will prevent disputes over who must pay for what.

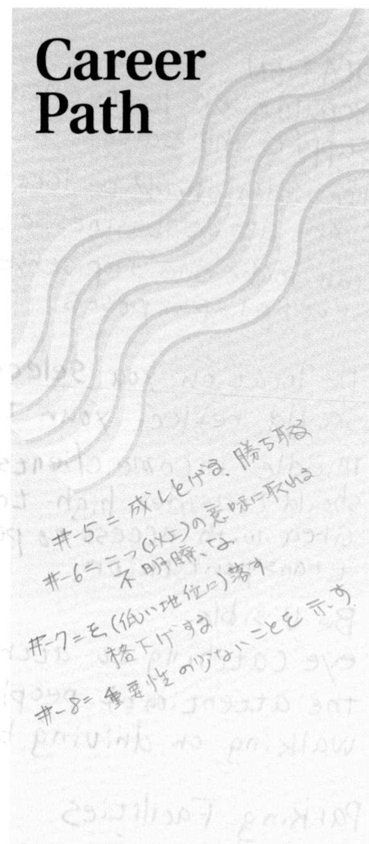

Career Path

SALON OWNER

The primary factor at the core of nearly every salon failure, and the chief reason stylists fail to build a solid, profitable following, is poor communication. We are either not taught good communication skills or have not learned their importance in achieving success in the beauty industry. We focus so much time, energy, and effort into developing technical skills and expertise that we relegate the art of effective communication to a lesser role. But to be a successful salon owner, you must be sure that communication is paramount for you and all of your employees.

We know that too large a percentage of people patronizing salons go away unhappy. This is not so much related to poor styling skills or dirty salons or rudeness, although these problems should be taken care of as well, but the chief reason for their unhappiness is that they didn't bridge the gap between the style they wanted and the style they got.

The reason that didn't happen, usually, was that we failed to communicate well. Our TV set was tuned to channel 5 while they were watching channel 21. We must recognize that our professional language is ambiguous, and we need to establish common definitions between ourselves and the person sitting in the chair.

—*From* You and Your Clients
by Leslie Edgerton

Completed: Learning Objective
#1
FACTS FOR OPENING A BEAUTY SALON

Study the Lease

Before signing a ***lease***, be certain you understand all provisions that pertain to the landlord and to the tenant. The lease should provide for alterations that must be made by the landlord. Most leases provided by the landlord are written in favor of the landlord. To protect your interests, hire a lawyer to help with your negotiations.

BUSINESS PLAN

It is very important that you develop a business plan before you open a salon. It is a necessary tool to obtain financing and to provide a blueprint for future growth. The plan should include a general description of the business and the services it will provide; a statement of the number of personnel to be hired; their salaries and other benefits; an operations plan that includes your price structure, expenses such as equipment, supplies, repairs, advertising, taxes, and insurance, and a financial plan that includes a profit and loss statement. If you are uncertain about developing a business plan, consult a professional.

In addition, it is important to have enough working capital when you open a salon. It often takes time to build a clientele, so you must have enough money available for your expenses.

REGULATIONS, BUSINESS LAWS, AND INSURANCE

When running a business you must comply with local, state, and federal regulations and laws.

Local regulations usually cover building renovations (local business codes).

Federal law covers Social Security, unemployment compensation or insurance, and cosmetics and luxury tax payments. OSHA requires that ingredients of cosmetic preparations (including permanent wave solutions and hair tints) be displayed prominently for clients. OSHA distributes MSDS sheets for this purpose.

State laws cover sales taxes, licenses, and employee compensation.

Income tax laws are covered by both the state and federal governments.

Insurance covers malpractice, premises liability, fire, burglary and theft, and business interruption. Also, check into Key Man Insurance (an insurance policy that safeguards against the loss of work of an important employee or yourself) and disability policies and make sure you are covered for everything your lease demands.

TYPES OF SALON OWNERSHIP

A salon can be owned and operated by an ***individual***, a ***partnership***, or a ***corporation***. Before deciding which type of ownership is most desirable, you should be acquainted with the relative merits and shortcomings of each.

Individual Ownership

1. The proprietor is owner and manager.
2. The proprietor determines policies and makes decisions.
3. The proprietor receives all profits and bears all losses.

Partnership

1. Ownership is shared (not necessarily equally) by two or more people. One purpose of this type of arrangement is to have more capital available for investment.

2. The abilities and experience of each partner make it easier to share work and responsibilities and to make decisions.
3. Each partner assumes each other's unlimited liability for debts.

Corporation

1. Ownership is shared by three or more people called ***stockholders***.
2. A ***charter*** is required by the state.
3. A corporation is subject to taxation and regulation by the state.
4. The management is in the hands of a board of directors who determine policies and make decisions in accordance with the corporation's charter.
5. The division of profits is proportionate to the number of shares owned by each stockholder.
6. The stockholders cannot lose more than their original investment in the corporation.

Purchasing an Established Salon

An agreement to buy an established salon should include the following:

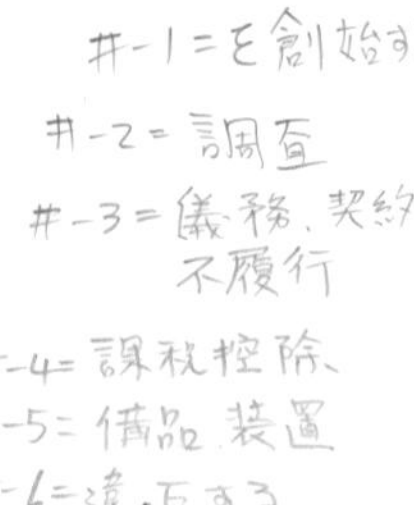

1. A written purchase and sale agreement to avoid any misunderstandings between the contracting parties.
2. A complete and signed statement of inventory (goods, fixtures, etc.) indicating the value of each article.
3. If there is a transfer of a note, chattel mortgage, lease, and bill of sale, the buyer should initiate an investigation to determine if there is any default in the payment of debts.
4. Identity of owner.
5. Use of salon's name and reputation for a definite period of time.
6. A statement that the seller will not compete with the new owner within a specified distance from the present location.
7. Additional guidance provided by your lawyer.

Drawing Up a Lease

1. Secure exemption of fixtures or appliances that might be attached to the salon so that they can be removed without violating the lease.
2. Secure an agreement about necessary renovations and repairs, such as painting, plumbing, fixtures, and electrical installation.

3. Secure an option from the landlord to assign the lease to another person. In this way, the obligations for the payment of rent are kept separate from the responsibilities of operating the business.

PROTECTION AGAINST FIRE, THEFT, AND LAWSUITS

1. Keep the premises securely locked.
2. Purchase liability, fire, malpractice, and burglary insurance.
3. Do not violate the medical practice law of your state by attempting to diagnose, treat, or cure a disease.
4. Become thoroughly familiar with all laws governing cosmetology and with the sanitary codes of your city and state.
5. Keep accurate records of the number of workers, the amount of salaries, lengths of employment, and Social Security numbers required by various state and federal laws that affect the social welfare of employees.

Note: *Ignorance of the law is no excuse for its violation.*

BUSINESS OPERATION

The owner or manager must have business sense, knowledge, ability, good judgment, and diplomacy. Smooth salon management depends on:

1. Sufficient investment capital.
2. Efficiency of management.
3. Good business procedures.
4. Cooperation between management and employees.
5. Trained and experienced salon personnel.

If there is failure in one or more of these categories, you probably will have difficulty staying in business.

Allocation of Money

As a good business operator you must always know where your money is being spent. A good accountant and accounting system are highly valuable.

The following figures may vary in different localities. In large towns and cities items such as rent might run higher, while in small towns rent might be lower and utilities and telephone higher. The figures are suggested merely as a general guide.

Average Expenses for Salons in the United States

(Based on total gross income)	Percent
Salaries and commissions (including payroll taxes)	53.5
Rent	13
Supplies	5
Advertising	3
Depreciation	3
Laundry	1
Cleaning	1
Light and power	1
Repairs	1.5
Insurance	.75
Telephone	.75
Miscellaneous	1.5
Total expenses	85
Net profit	15
	100%

Completed: Learning Objective #2

FINANCIAL CONSIDERATIONS FOR OPERATING A BEAUTY SALON

Clearly, the largest expense items are salaries, rent, supplies, and advertising. The first three merit your closest attention. Advertising can be adjusted at your discretion.

THE IMPORTANCE OF RECORD KEEPING

Good business operation requires that you have a simple and efficient record system. Proper business records are necessary to meet the requirements of local, state, and federal laws regarding taxes and employees. Records are of value only if they are correct, concise, and complete. Bookkeeping includes keeping an accurate record of all income and expenses. Income is usually classified as receipts from services and retail sales. Expenses include rent, utilities, insurance, salaries, advertising, equipment, and repairs. A professional accountant is recommended to help keep records accurate. Retain check stubs, canceled checks, receipts, and invoices.

All business transactions must be recorded for the following reasons:

1. To determine income, expenses, profit, or loss.
2. To assess the value of the salon for prospective buyers.
3. To arrange a bank loan or financing.
4. For reports on income tax, Social Security, unemployment and disability insurance, accidents, and for percentage payments of gross income required in some leases.

Weekly Records

A weekly or monthly summary helps to:

1. Make comparisons with other years.
2. Detect any changes in demands for services.
3. Check on the use of materials according to the type of service rendered.
4. Control expenses and waste.

Daily Records

Keeping daily records enables the owner or manager to know just how well the business is functioning. Each expense item affects the total gross income. Accurate records show the cost of operation in relation to income. Keep daily sales slips, appointment book, and a petty cash book for at least six months. Payroll book, canceled checks, and monthly and yearly records are usually held for at least seven years. Service and inventory records are also important to keep.

Purchase and Inventory Records

Purchase records help to maintain a perpetual inventory that can be used to:

1. Prevent overstock of needed supplies.
2. Prevent running short of needed supplies.
3. Help establish the net worth of the business at the end of the year.

Keep a running inventory of all supplies. Classify them according to their use and retail value. Those to be used in the daily business operation are ***consumption supplies***. Those to be sold to clients are ***retail supplies***.

Inventory records can tell you which merchandise is selling most quickly and which items do not sell well. You will then be able to judge how much of each product to order so that it can be used or sold within a reasonable period of time. It is better to have slightly more than enough supplies. Try to plan major purchases of supplies around times when dealers offer special prices.

Service Records

A service record should be kept of treatments given and merchandise sold to each client. A card file system or memorandum book kept in a central location should be used for these records.

All service records should include the name and address of the client, date of each purchase or service, amount charged, products used, and results obtained. Also, note the client's preferences and tastes.

Completed:
Learning Objective
#3
MAINTAINING BUSINESS RECORDS

PLANNING THE SALON'S LAYOUT

The layout of a salon should be well planned to achieve maximum efficiency. Most professional product suppliers will be happy to help you plan your layout, usually at a reasonable fee, or perhaps for no fee at all. (Fig. 26.2)

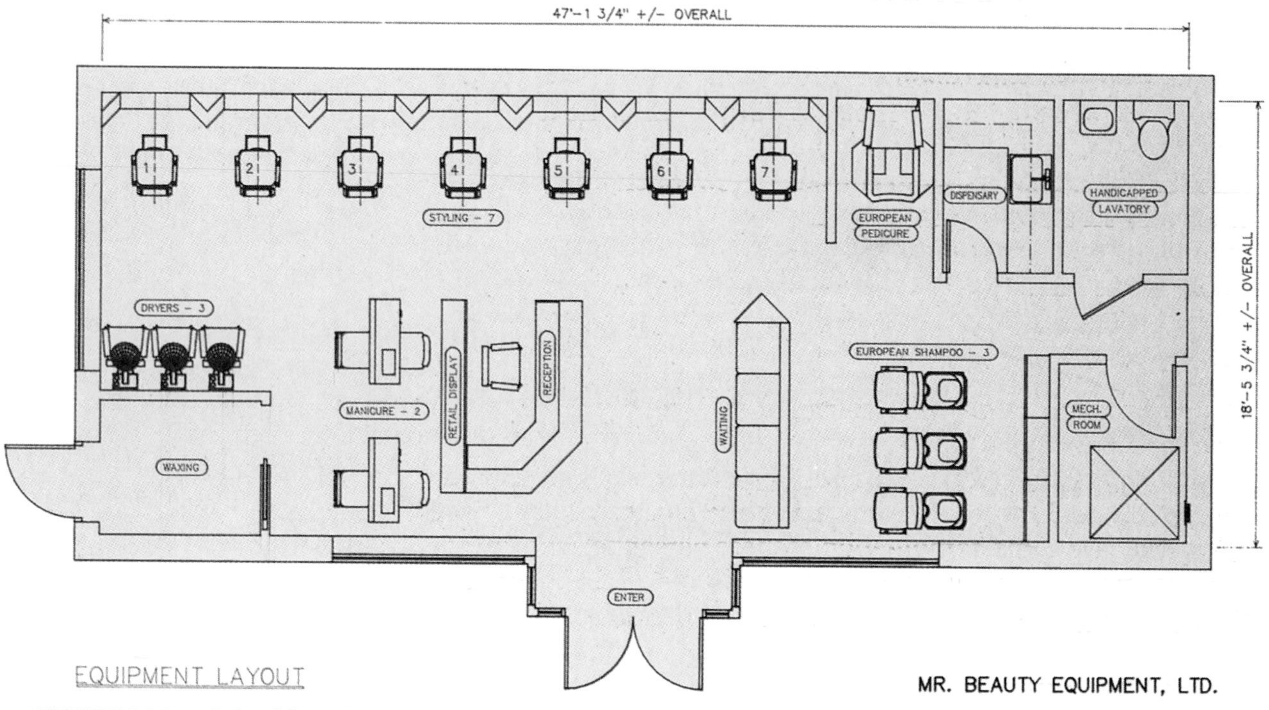

FIGURE 26.2 — Salon blueprint.

To obtain maximum efficiency when planning the physical layout of a salon, you should consider the following:

1. Flow of operational services to and from the reception area.
2. Adequate aisle space.
3. Space allotment for equipment.
4. Furniture, fixtures, and equipment chosen on the basis of cost, durability, utility, and appearance. The purchase of standard and guaranteed equipment is a worthwhile investment.
5. A color scheme that is restful and flattering.
6. A dispensary.
7. Adequate storage space.
8. A clean restroom with a toilet and basin.

9. Good plumbing and sufficient lighting for satisfactory services.
10. Good ventilation, air conditioning, and heating.
11. Adequate clothing closet and changing area for clients.

OPERATING A SALON

Clients who visit your salon should feel that they have been well taken care of and should look forward to their next visit. To accomplish this goal, your salon needs to be well organized and smoothly run. The factors to consider about operating your salon efficiently on a day-to-day basis are your personnel, policies and practices, price structure, advertising and promotion, and the "look" of the salon.

PERSONNEL

The size of your salon will determine the size of your staff. For example, large salons have receptionists, hair stylists, manicurists, shampoo persons, colorists, masseurs and masseuses, people who give facials, and those who do waxing and electrolysis. A smaller salon will have some combination of these personnel who are able to perform more than one service. For example, in a smaller salon, the stylist might also be the colorist and give permanents.

Hiring Your Staff

The success of a salon depends on the quality of the work done by the staff. A satisfied client returns for more services and recommends the salon to others. When interviewing potential employees, you should consider their personality, level of skill, personal grooming, and the clients they will bring with them.

SALON POLICIES AND PRACTICES

It is important that all salon personnel are aware of policies and practices in order to maintain a smooth day-to-day operation.

Pricing of Services

Cost of services is generally established according to the location of the salon and the type of clientele you expect to serve. A price list should be posted in a place where it can be seen by all clients—probably at the reception desk.

The Reception Area

First impressions count, and since the reception area is the first thing clients see, you should make your reception area attractive, appealing, and comfortable. Remember that your receptionist, phone system, dressing area, and retail merchandise may be located in this area. You should also have a supply of business cards with the address and phone number of the salon on the reception desk. Most important to you, this is also the place where the client's financial transactions are handled.

The Receptionist

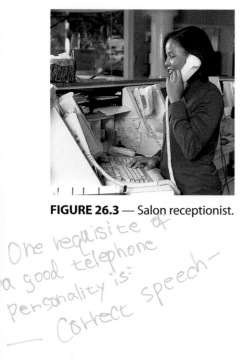

FIGURE 26.3 — Salon receptionist.

Second only in importance to your cosmetologists is your receptionist. A good receptionist is the "quarterback" of the salon. This is the first person seen by the arriving client. The receptionist should be pleasant, greet each client with a smile, and call him or her by name. Efficient service creates goodwill, confidence, and satisfaction. Favorable impressions begin with the courteous reception of the client. These impressions last as long as the client obtains the desired results from salon services. (Fig. 26.3)

The receptionist handles many important functions including answering the phone, booking appointments, informing the stylist that a client has arrived, preparing the daily appointment information for the cosmetologists, recommending other services, and reminding the client of retail products.

The receptionist should be especially attentive on the hour and then every 15 minutes after the hour because these are the times clients are scheduled to arrive. Incidental duties and activities, such as cleaning, maintaining inventory and daily reports, personal calls, or any other reason to be away from the desk, should be carried out during the slowest periods of the hour.

Booking Appointments

Booking appointments must be done with care, because services are sold in terms of time on the appointment page. Appointments must be scheduled so that there is the most efficient use of the time of all salon personnel. A client should not have to wait for a service, and a cosmetologist should not have to wait for the next client.

The size of the salon determines who books the appointments. This can be done by a full-time receptionist, the owner or manager, or any of the cosmetologists working in the salon.

A receptionist with a pleasing voice and personality is a valuable asset to the beauty salon. In addition, he or she must have:

1. An attractive appearance.
2. Knowledge of the various beauty services, their cost, and how much time they require.
3. Unlimited patience with both clients and salon personnel.

Appointment Book

The use of an appointment record helps the cosmetologist arrange working time to suit the client's needs. The salon appointment book accurately reflects what is taking place in the salon at a given time. The appointment schedule allows the cosmetologist to see how many clients will be coming in during the day and how much time is needed to deliver the appropriate services. In most salons, the receptionist prepares the appointment schedule for staff members; in smaller salons, however, each person may prepare his or her own schedule. (Fig. 26.4)

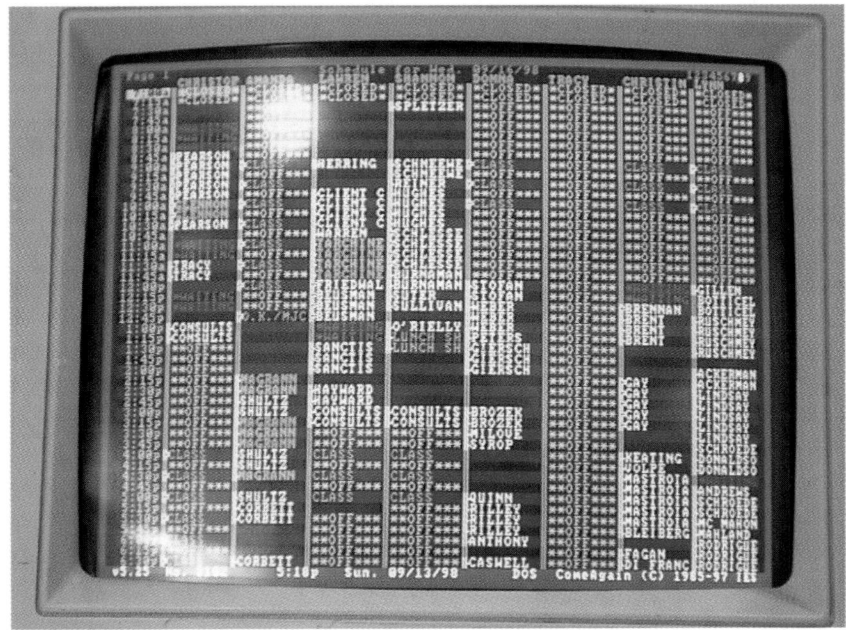

FIGURE 26.4 — Appointment book.

USE OF THE TELEPHONE IN THE SALON

An important part of the salon business is handled over the telephone. Good telephone habits and techniques make it possible for the salon owner and cosmetologist to increase business and improve relationships with clients and suppliers. With each call, you have a chance to build the salon's reputation by providing high-caliber service.

The telephone can be used to:

1. Make or change appointments.
2. Seek new business, or find out why you've lost a client.
3. Remind clients of needed services.

4. Answer questions and provide friendly service.
5. Handle complaints to the client's satisfaction.
6. Receive messages.
7. Order equipment and supplies.

Business in the salon can be promoted effectively over the phone, provided there is:

1. Good planning.
2. Good telephone usage.

Good Planning

Good planning consists of assigning the right person to a telephone task and providing the necessary information with which to perform the task. A reliable substitute should be trained to make outgoing and answer incoming calls when the regular person is not in.

The phone is usually located at the reception desk since this is where the salon appointment book is located. Because it can be noisy at the reception desk, outgoing business calls to clients and suppliers should be made at a quiet time of the day or from a telephone placed in a quieter area of the salon.

Provide a comfortable seat by the phone. There should also be an appointment book, client's record cards, pencil or ball-point pen, and paper pad readily accessible. An up-to-date list of frequently called telephone numbers and a recent telephone directory should also be available.

The person using the telephone should:

1. Have a pleasant telephone voice. Speak clearly, use correct grammar, and put a "smile" in his/her voice.
2. Show interest and concern when talking with a client or a supplier.
3. Be polite, respectful, and courteous to all, even though some people test the limits of your patience.
4. Be tactful. Do not say anything to irritate the person on the other end of the phone.
5. Plan what is to be said during the call. Make a list of the main points you want to discuss. Knowing what you want to say helps you to project an image of confidence and efficiency. It is also useful to jot down key points of the other person's responses or questions. That can help you address yourself to the speaker's concerns and interests.

Incoming Phone Calls

Incoming phone calls are the lifeline of a salon. Clients usually call ahead for appointments with a preferred cosmetologist, or they might call to cancel or reschedule an appointment. The person answering the phone, usually the receptionist, should develop telephone skills to handle the different types of incoming calls. As mentioned, always answer the phone with a smile in your voice, speak clearly, use correct grammar, concentrate on listening to the person you are speaking with, and be polite, respectful, and tactful. In addition, here are some guidelines to remember when answering the telephone:

1. When you answer the phone, say, "Good morning (afternoon or evening), Milady Salon. May I help you?" Some salons also require that you give your name to the caller. The first words you say tell the caller something about your personality. Let that person know that you're glad he or she called. (Fig. 26.5)
2. Answer the phone promptly. Nothing is more irritating than calling a place of business and having to wait four or five rings before somebody answers the phone. On a multi-line system, when a call comes in while you are talking on another line, ask to put the person on hold, answer the second call, and ask that person to hold while you complete the first call. Take callers in the order that they phone.
3. If you do not have the information requested by the caller, you can do one of two things: put the caller on hold and get the information or offer to call the person back with the information as soon as you have it.
4. Do not talk with someone standing nearby while you are speaking with someone on the phone. You are doing a disservice to both clients.

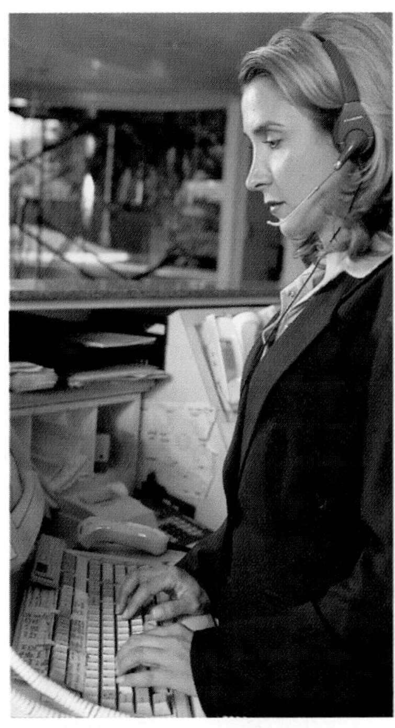

FIGURE 26.5 — The telephone is an important part of the salon business.

Booking Appointments by Phone

1. When booking appointments, you should be familiar with all services and products available in the salon and their costs.
2. Be fair when making assignments. Do not schedule six appointments for one cosmetologist and two for another, unless, of course, a client has requested a particular cosmetologist. Assign four clients to each cosmetologist.
3. If someone calls asking for an appointment with a particular cosmetologist at a particular day and time and that technician is not available then, there are several ways to handle the situation:

a) If the client regularly uses one cosmetologist, suggest other times the cosmetologist is available.

b) If the client cannot come in at any of those times, suggest another cosmetologist.

c) If the client is unwilling to try another cosmetologist, offer to call the client if there is a cancellation at the desired time.

Handling Complaints by Telephone

Handling complaints, particularly over the phone, is a difficult task. The caller is probably upset and short-tempered. Try to use self-control, tact, and courtesy, no matter how trying the circumstances may be. Only then will the caller be made to feel that he or she has been fairly treated.

Remember that the tone of your voice must be sympathetic and reassuring. Your manner of speaking should make the caller believe that you are really concerned about the complaint. Do not interrupt the caller. Listen to the entire problem. After hearing the complaint in full, you should try to resolve the situation quickly and effectively. The following are suggestions for dealing with some problems. If other problems arise, follow the policy of the salon or check with the owner/manager for advice.

1. Tell the unhappy client that you are sorry for what happened and explain the reason for the difficulty. Tell the client that the problem will not happen again.
2. Sympathize with the client by saying that you understand and that you regret the inconvenience suffered. Express thanks that the person called this matter to your attention.
3. Ask the client how the salon can remedy the situation. If the request is fair and reasonable, check with the owner/manager for approval.
4. If the client is dissatisfied with the results of a service, suggest a visit to the salon to see what can be done to remedy the problem.
5. If a client is dissatisfied with the behavior of a cosmetologist, call the owner/manager to the phone.

Completed: Learning Objective #4

GOOD BUSINESS OPERATION AND PERSONNEL MANAGEMENT

SELLING IN THE SALON

As more products are added to salon operations, selling is becoming an increasingly important responsibility of the cosmetologist. The cosmetologist who is equally proficient as hairstylist and salesperson is most likely to be the one to succeed in business. Advising clients about the proper products to use in their beauty regimen will not only add dollars to your income, but will better enable the clients to maintain the look you worked so hard to achieve.

No attempt is made here to cover all aspects of selling, but if you use this material as a basis upon which to build, effective selling techniques will become part of your repertoire of skills.

To be successful in sales you need ambition, determination, and a good personality. The first step in selling is to sell yourself. Clients must like and trust you before they will purchase beauty services, cosmetics, skin care items, shampoos and conditioners, or other merchandise.

Every client who enters the salon is a prospective purchaser of additional services or merchandise. The manner in which you treat that person lays the foundation for suggestive selling. Recognizing the needs and preferences of clients makes the intelligent use of suggestive selling possible. (Fig. 26.6)

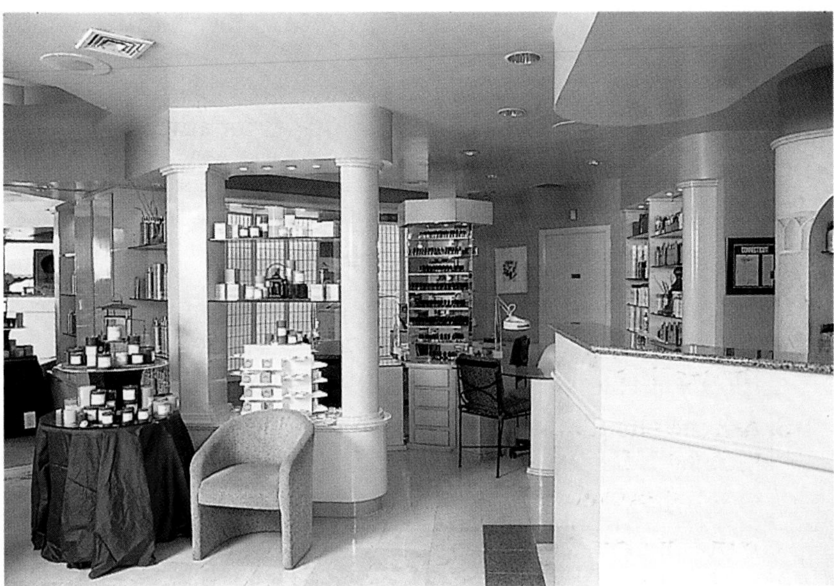

FIGURE 26.6 — Salon retail display.

SELLING PRINCIPLES

To become a proficient salesperson you must understand and be able to apply the following principles of selling:

1. Be familiar with the merits and benefits of each service and product.
2. Adapt your approach and technique to meet the needs of each client.

3. Be self-confident.
4. Generate interest and desire, which are the steps leading to a sale.
5. Never misrepresent your service or product.
6. Use tact when selling to a client.
7. Don't underestimate the client or the client's intelligence.
8. To sell a product or service, deliver a sales talk in a relaxed, friendly manner and, if possible, demonstrate its use.
9. Recognize the right psychological moment to close any sale. Once the client has offered to buy, quit selling—don't oversell, except to praise the client for the purchase and assure her that she will be happy with it.

TYPES OF CLIENTS

The cosmetologist who is most likely to be successful in selling additional services or merchandise to clients is one who can recognize the many different types of people and knows how to deal with each type.

The following material describes seven of the most common types you are likely to meet and suggests ways each type might be treated.

1. ***Shy, timid type.*** Make the client feel at ease. Lead the conversation. Don't force the conversation. Be cheerful.
2. ***Talkative type.*** Be a good, patient listener. Tactfully switch the conversation to beauty needs.
3. ***Nervous, irritable type.*** Does not want much conversation. Wants simple, practical hairdo and a fast worker. Get started and finished as quickly as possible.
4. ***Inquisitive, over-cautious type.*** Explain everything in detail. Show him or her facts—sealed bottles, brand names. Ask for the client's opinion.
5. ***"Know-it-all" type.*** Suggest things in question form. Don't argue with this person. Offer compliments.
6. ***Teenager.*** Usually interested in current fashions. Give special advice on hair care and other beauty needs.
7. ***Mature*** (60 and older). Be extra courteous. Suggest hairstyles that give this person a younger look without looking too young (and foolish).

THE PSYCHOLOGY OF SELLING

Each person who enters a salon is an individual with specific wants and needs. No matter how good a beauty service or product may be, you will find it difficult to make a sale if the client has no need for it. Thus, your first task is to determine whether the client has a need for or an interest in a service or product.

Motives for Buying

What are the motives that prompt clients to purchase services and products? Very often the motivations are vanity, personal satisfaction, and esthetic gratification. In our society people try to look youthful with a trim figure, fresh complexion, and a contemporary hairstyle.

Helping Your Client Decide

If a client is doubtful or undecided about a service or a product, help the decision along with honest and sincere advice. For example, if a client is thinking about coloring her hair and she already has had a permanent, you might advise her about the extra care that is needed with both treatments.

It is important that you tell the client about the beauty service and what it can mean in terms of results and benefits. Always keep in mind that the best interests of the client should be your first consideration. Careful consideration will acquaint you with the client's needs, and those needs can be fulfilled to the complete satisfaction of the client, as well as to your financial advantage.

SELLING PRODUCTS

Many salons offer a wide range of products from jewelry to cosmetics. In order to satisfy the varied needs and desires of clients, the salon should stock a wide range of inventory. The person in charge of these accessories must be familiar with all products and their comparative merits.

Completed: Learning Objective #5

PRINCIPLES AND PRACTICE OF GOOD SELLING

ADVERTISING

Advertising includes all activities that promote the salon favorably. Advertising must attract and hold the reader's, listener's, or viewer's attention and create a desire for the service or product.

A pleased client is the best form of advertising. Some salons hire an advertising firm rather than develop their own advertising, but this can be expensive.

An advertising budget should run about 3% of your gross income. Plan at least 6 months to a year ahead, and concentrate most of your advertising on traditionally slow periods. Also, plan for holidays and special yearly events. Here are some suggested ways to advertise:

1. Newspapers.
2. Direct mail for closer contact with the potential client.
3. Classified advertising in the yellow pages of your telephone book is relatively inexpensive. For a yellow pages display ad, consult with your suppliers as to the availability of ***co-op advertising*** with certain major product lines.
4. A window display attracts passersby.
5. Radio advertising is more expensive, but is very effective.
6. TV is a dramatic, but expensive, medium of advertising.
7. Personal public appearances are an excellent means of advertising, especially at women's and men's clubs, church functions, political gatherings, charitable affairs, and on TV and radio talk shows.
8. Contacting clients who have not been in the salon for a while and inviting them back can be very effective.
9. Telemarketing your products and services can also be very effective, and can be done by stylists with "down time."
10. Taped promotions shown on a VCR in the salon can also be developed.

Completed: Learning Objective #6
IMPORTANCE OF ADVERTISING

REVIEW QUESTIONS

THE SALON BUSINESS

1. What things should be considered when opening a beauty salon?
2. Under what three types of ownership may a beauty salon be operated?
3. What purpose do accurate records serve?
4. What two types of supplies make up a beauty salon's inventory?
5. Why is the reception area of a beauty salon important?
6. How will the use of good telephone techniques help a salon?
7. What are the main principles and practices of good selling?
8. Define advertising.
9. What is the best form of advertising?

Answers to Review Questions

Chapter 1
YOUR PROFESSIONAL IMAGE

(Answers to Questions on Page 22)

1. rest, exercise, relaxation, nutrition, personal hygiene, and personal grooming
2. posture, walk, and movements
3. Personality is the outward reflection of inner feelings, thoughts, attitudes, and values.
4. listening skills, voice, speech, manner of speaking, and conversational skills
5. the psychology of getting along well with others
6. A professional attitude is expressed by self-esteem, confidence in one's profession, and respect for others.
7. the study of standards of conduct and moral judgment

Chapter 2
BACTERIOLOGY

(Answers to Questions on Page 31)

1. Bacteriology is necessary to protect individual and public health.
2. Bacteriology is the science that deals with the study of microorganisms called bacteria.
3. Bacteria are minute, one-celled vegetable microorganisms found nearly everywhere.
4. Bacteria can exist almost anywhere, for example, on the skin, in water, air, decayed matter, secretions of body openings, on clothing, and beneath the nails.
5. a) nonpathogenic bacteria—helpful, harmless, perform useful functions such as decomposing refuse b) pathogenic bacteria—harmful, produce disease when they invade plant or animal tissue
6. Parasites are harmful pathogenic bacteria that require living matter for their growth. Saprophytes are helpful nonpathogenic bacteria that live on dead matter and do not produce disease.
7. a) Cocci are round-shaped organisms that appear singly. b) Bacilli are rod-shaped organisms. They are the most common bacteria and produce diseases. c) Spirilla are curved or corkscrew-shaped organisms.
8. a) Staphylococci are pus-forming organisms that grow in bunches or clusters. They cause abscesses, pustules, and boils. b) Streptococci are pus-forming organisms that grow in chains. They cause infections such as strep throat. c) Diplococci grow in pairs and cause pneumonia.
9. Bacteria grow and reproduce under favorable conditions with sufficient food. When they reach their largest size, they divide into two new cells by a process called mitosis.
10. During the active or vegetative stage, bacteria grow and reproduce. During the inactive, spore-forming stage, no growth or reproduction occurs.
11. by hairlike projections called flagella or cilia
12. a) A local infection is indicated by a boil or pimple that contains pus. b) A general infection results when the bloodstream carries the bacteria to all parts of the body, as in syphilis.
13. one that can be spread from one person to another by contact
14. Infections can be prevented and controlled through personal hygiene and public sanitation.
15. a) Plant parasites can produce contagious diseases, such as ringworm and favus (a skin disease of the scalp). b) Animal parasites can produce contagious diseases, such as scabies and pediculosis (infection of the scalp by lice).
16. Immunity is the ability of the body to destroy bacteria that have gained entrance and thus to resist infection. The two types are natural immunity and acquired immunity.
17. Bacteria can be destroyed by disinfectants and by intense heat.

Chapter 3
DECONTAMINATION AND INFECTION CONTROL

(Answers to Questions on Page 46)

1. removing pathogens and other substances from tools or surfaces
2. Sterilization completely destroys all living organisms on a surface, even bacterial spores, the most resistant form of life on Earth.
3. Sanitation means to significantly reduce the number of pathogens found on a surface. Salon tools and other surfaces are sanitized by cleaning with soaps or detergents.

4. Antiseptics can kill bacteria or slow their growth. Antiseptics are weaker than disinfectants and are safe for application to skin. Disinfectants kill microbes on contaminated tools and other non-porous surfaces. Disinfectants are not for use on human skin, hair, or nails.

5. All disinfectants must be approved by the EPA and each individual state. The disinfectant's label must also have an EPA registration number.

6. MSDSs (Material Safety Data Sheets) provide all pertinent information on products, ranging from content and associated hazards, to combustion levels and storage requirements. They are available from a product's distributor.

7. They must be bactericides to kill harmful bacteria and fungicides to destroy fungus.

8. a) quaternary ammonium compounds (quats) b) phenolic disinfectants (phenols) c) bleach (sodium hypochlorite)

9. Bar soap can actually grow bacteria. It is much more sanitary to provide pump-type liquid, antibacterial soaps.

10. Formaldehyde, the gas released from formalin tablets or liquids, is a suspected human cancer-causing agent. It is poisonous to inhale and is extremely irritating to the eyes, nose, throat, and lungs.

11. Universal precautions are the use of gloves and safety glasses, disinfectants and detergents in conjunction with personal hygiene and salon cleanliness.

Chapter 4
PROPERTIES OF THE SCALP AND HAIR

(Answers to Questions on Page 80)

1. The chief purposes of hair are adornment and protection of the head from heat, cold, and injury.

2. Hair is an appendage of the skin, a slender, threadlike outgrowth of the skin and scalp.

3. Hair is composed chiefly of the protein keratin, which is found in all horny growths, including the nails and skin.

4. the hair root and the hair shaft

5. The rate of growth of human hair differs on specific parts of the body, between sexes, among races, and with age. Hair growth is also influenced by seasons of the year, nutrition, health, and hormones.

6. anagen, or growing phase; catogen, or transitional phase; telogen, or resting phase

7. heredity, hormones, age, physical stress

8. cleanliness and stimulation

Chapter 5
DRAPING

(Answers to Questions on Page 84)

1. the comfort and protection of the client

2. Draping is the means of protecting clients' skin and clothing with the use of neck strips, towels, and capes.

3. to protect skin and clothing from water, chemicals, and bacteria

4. It is used for sanitary reasons to prevent the cape from coming into direct contact with the client's skin.

5. a) prepare materials b) sanitize hands c) ask the client to remove all neck and hair jewelry and remove objects from the client's hair d) turn collar to the inside

6. For wet services, use a towel over and under the cape. For dry services, use neck strip only. For chemical services, use a towel under and above the cape.

Chapter 6
SHAMPOOING, RINSING, AND CONDITIONING

(Answers to Questions on Page 97)

1. It lets your client know that you can perform all hair services with professional competency and concern.

2. to cleanse the hair and scalp and as a preliminary step for other hair services

3. Hair should be shampooed as often as necessary to remove the accumulation of oil and perspiration, which can offer a breeding place for disease-producing bacteria.

4. Select the shampoo according to the condition of the hair.

5. hard and soft

6. It stimulates blood circulation to the scalp; helps remove dust, dirt, and hair spray; and gives hair added sheen.

7. before giving a chemical service or if scalp is irritated

8. potential hydrogen

9. The amount of hydrogen in a solution is measured on a pH scale ranging from 0 to 14; the more hydrogen present, the more alkaline the shampoo (7 to 14); the less hydrogen, the lower the pH (0 to 6.9).

10. The lower pH or acid balance prevents excessive dryness and hair damage. The higher pH or alkaline balance can leave the hair dry and brittle.

11. It is a mixture of water with a mild acid, coloring agent, or ingredients designed to serve a particular purpose.

12. It removes soap scum from the hair and restores the hair's pH balance.
13. a cream rinse
14. an acid-balanced rinse
15. by closing the cuticle and trapping color molecules
16. It is formulated to control minor dandruff conditions.
17. to highlight or add temporary color to the hair

Chapter 7
HAIRCUTTING

(Answers to Questions on Page 126)

1. Haircutting serves as a foundation for attractive hairstyles and for other services.
2. head shape, facial contour, neckline, and hair texture
3. haircutting scissors, thinning shears, straight razors, clippers, edgers, combs, and clippies
4. sectioning the hair properly
5. Four sections are used for one-length and low-elevation haircuts, five sections for high-elevation haircuts.
6. The guide creates the line we see around the perimeter of a haircut.
7. head forward and down: hair is undercut; head upright: ends are graduated, slightly longer underneath; head pulled back: ends are graduated, longer underneath
8. low or zero-degree elevation, high or 90-degree elevation, reverse or 180-degree elevation, and blended elevation
9. Slide cutting is a method of cutting or thinning the hair with nonserrated, razor-sharp shears.
10. around the visible portions of the hairline and along the part
11. Clippers are used primarily for short haircuts.
12. to avoid pulling the hair and dulling the razor
13. It should be cut dry.

Chapter 8
ARTISTRY IN HAIRSTYLING

(Answers to Questions on Page 158)

1. The five elements of design are form, space, line, color, and texture.
2. The five art principles are proportion, balance, rhythm, emphasis, and harmony.
3. A body that is not in proportion is more obvious if the hair form is too large or too small.
4. Harmony is the most important art principle in hair design, because it holds all the elements of the design together.
5. The seven facial shapes are oval, round, square, oblong, pear-shaped, heart-shaped, and diamond-shaped.
6. true
7. forehead, eyes, nose, jaw, chin, neck
8. side part, center part, diagonal back part, and zigzag part

Chapter 9
WET HAIRSTYLING

(Answers to Questions on Page 196)

1. Hairstyling is the process of creating wearable art.
2. to learn the technique of moving and directing hair
3. Waving lotion makes the hair more pliable and keeps it in place during the procedure.
4. horizontal finger waving, vertical finger waving, and shadow waving
5. base, stem, and circle
6. A shaping is a section of hair that is molded into a design to serve as a base for a curl or wave pattern. It is classified as forward and reverse; diagonal, vertical, or horizontal; oblong or circular.
7. Stem direction determines which way the curls will be turned—toward the face, away from the face, upward, downward, or diagonally.
8. The most commonly shaped bases are rectangular, triangular, arc, and square.
9. on base, one-half base, and off base

Chapter 10
THERMAL HAIRSTYLING

(Answers to Questions on Page 221)

1. the art of waving and curling straight or pressed hair
2. a) conventional b) electric self-heated c) electric self-heated, vaporizing
3. Place a comb between iron and scalp.
4. drying and styling damp hair in one operation
5. dryer, brushes, and combs
6. styling lotion, hair conditioner, and hair spray

Chapter 11
PERMANENT WAVING

(Answers to Questions on Page 259)

1. It provides a long-lasting style; makes home styling easy; adds volume and fullness to fine hair; and gives greater control over coarse, wiry, and hard-to-manage hair.
2. wrapping hair from scalp to ends
3. wrapping hair from ends toward scalp
4. A cold wave is a perm that does not require heat.
5. a) A waving lotion softens or breaks the internal structure of the hair. b) A neutralizer rehardens or rebonds the internal structure of the hair.
6. a mild perm with pH levels ranging from 4.5 to 7.9, which penetrates the hair more slowly and uses heat to shorten the processing time
7. a process incorporated into many waving lotions to ensure optimum curl development within a fixed time, without risk of overprocessing or damaging the hair
8. a strong perm with pH levels ranging from 8.2 to 9.6, which processes at room temperature within 5 to 20 minutes, producing a strong curl
9. a) ammonium thioglycolate b) glyceryl monothioglycolate
10. exothermic
11. hydrogen peroxide, at an acidic pH
12. physical action and chemical action
13. a) cuticle—outer covering protecting the hair b) cortex—where physical and chemical action takes place; gives hair flexibility, elasticity, strength, resilience, and color c) medulla—innermost section, function unknown
14. keratin
15. disulfide bonds
16. Evaluate and analyze client's hair, and consult with client about expectations (tight or loose curl).
17. to determine if it is safe to perm and what products and technique to use
18. It is the hair's capacity to absorb liquids.
19. lotion specifically designed to even out the porosity so that even curl patterns result
20. Hair texture is the thickness or thinness (in diameter) of each individual strand.
21. a) texture b) porosity
22. It is the ability of hair to stretch and contract.
23. It refers to the number of hairs per square inch.
24. the size of the rod
25. a) concave b) straight
26. a) amount of curl desired b) physical characteristics of the hair
27. Sectioning and blocking makes work easier because it creates an overall pattern for rod placement.
28. a) The average parting should match the diameter of the rod. b) The length of blocking should be the same or a little shorter than the length of the rod.
29. It should be wrapped smoothly and neatly without stretching.
30. End wraps ensure smooth, even wrapping and minimize the danger of breakage.
31. a) double end paper wrap b) single end paper wrap c) book end wrap
32. It is a test to determine optimum curl development. Unwind the rod and check for the "S" pattern foundation.

Chapter 12
HAIRCOLORING

(Answers to Questions on Page 364)

1. Perform the consultation in a well-lighted room, preferably with natural lighting. Use haircolor swatches, magazines, or picture books to help you and your client agree on a color choice. Observe your client's hair and scalp, skin tone, and eye color, and practice reflective listening. Discuss your client's expectations, hair limitations, and lifestyle. Advise the client on the benefits of using good-quality shampoos and conditioners. Always record the consultation on a client record card.
2. Primary colors are basic or true colors that are not created by combining other colors. The three primary colors are yellow, red, and blue. Secondary colors are created by mixing equal amounts of two primary colors. Tertiary colors are created by mixing equal amounts of one primary color with one of its adjacent secondary colors.
3. The classifications of haircolor are: temporary, semi-permanent, oxidative deposit-only (demi), non-oxidative permanent, and oxidative permanent. Temporary color only deposits color; it does not lighten. Semi-permanent color has a mild penetrating action that results in a gentle addition of color in the cortex, as well as some coating on the cuticle. It does not lighten the natural color or change the structure of the hair. Oxidative deposit-only (demi) color swells the cuticle and penetrates into the cortex, depositing

artificial color inside the hair shaft. The structure of the hair is affected very little. Non-oxidative permanent colors are vegetable or metallic in composition. These products are not used professionally. They coat the hair and can prevent the penetration of conditioners. Oxidative permanent color swells the cuticle and penetrates into the cortex. It lightens the natural pigment and then deposits artificial color. The hair structure is changed and the cuticle remains slightly shifted after the haircolor service.

4. The color is self-penetrating. It is applied the same way each time. Retouching is not necessary. Color does not rub off on pillow or clothing. Hair returns to its natural color after 4 to 6 shampoos.
5. Mix ½ tsp. of color with hydrogen peroxide. Apply mixture to a ½" section. Process. Rinse strand, shampoo, towel-dry, and examine results. Adjust formula, timing, or preconditioning necessary and proceed with tinting on entire head. If results are unsatisfactory, adjust the formula and repeat process on a new test strand. Record results on client record card.
6. Apply with applicator bottle. Apply rinse through entire hair shaft and comb through. Blend the color with a comb, applying more color as necessary.
7. Section hair. Prepare tint. Begin where color change will be greatest. Part off ¼" subsection. Apply tint to hair ½" from scalp up through ends. Process according to strand test results. Check for color development by removing color from strand. Apply tint mixture to hair at scalp. Blend tint to hair ends. Massage color to lather and rinse thoroughly. Remove stains. Shampoo. Apply an acid or finishing rinse.
8. Client is consulted. Hair is analyzed and conditioned. Tint is applied to new growth only. Diluted color formula is applied to hair ends. Diluted tint mixture is applied to entire head if ends have faded.
9. Hydrogen peroxide serves as an oxidizing agent that causes oxygen to combine with another substance, such as melanin. As the oxygen and melanin combine, the peroxide solution diffuses and lightens the melanin within the hair shaft.
10. a) as a color treatment, to lighten the hair to the final shade desired b)as a preliminary treatment, to prepare the hair for the application of a toner or tint
11. Oil bleaches are used for lightening the entire head. Cream lighteners are popular for all types of lightening services. Powder lighteners are generally used for special effects lightening.
12. cap, foil, and freehand techniques
13. Incorporate reconditioning. Ensure that the client uses high-quality products at home. Precondition hair that is damaged. Use a penetrating conditioner. Complete each chemical service by normalizing the pH with a finishing rinse. Postpone any further chemical service until the hair is reconditioned. Schedule the client for between-service conditioning.
14. Give a patch test 24 to 48 hours prior to any application of aniline derivative. Apply tint only if patch test is negative. Do not apply tint if abrasions are present. Do not apply tint if metallic or compound dye is present. Do not brush hair prior to applying color. Always read and follow manufacturer's directions. Use sanitized applicator bottles, brushes, combs, and towels. Protect client's clothing by proper draping. Perform a strand test for color, breakage, and/or discoloration. Use an applicator bottle or bowl (glass or plastic) for mixing the tint. Do not mix tint before you are ready to use it; discard leftover tint. Wear gloves to protect your hands. Do not permit the color to come in contact with the client's eyes. Do not overlap during a tint retouch. Do not use water that is too hot; use lukewarm water for removing color. Use a mild shampoo. If an alkaline or harsh shampoo is used, it will strip the color. Always wash hands before and after serving a client.

Chapter 13
CHEMICAL HAIR RELAXING AND SOFT CURL PERMANENT

(Answers to Questions on Page 384)

1. chemical hair relaxer, neutralizer, and a petroleum cream
2. a) sodium hydroxide b) ammonium thioglycolate
3. a) processing b) neutralizing c) conditioning
4. Follow the manufacturer's instructions.
5. a chemical blow out
6. a) scalp examination b) hair analysis c) strand test
7. soft curl permanent waving
8. a soft curl permanent
9. reconditioning treatments

Chapter 14
THERMAL HAIR STRAIGHTENING (HAIR PRESSING)

(Answers to Questions on Page 396)

1. thermal hair straightening
2. temporarily straightens overly curly or unruly hair
3. soft press, medium press, and hard press
4. scalp abrasion, contagious scalp condition, scalp injury, or chemically treated hair

5. Apply 1% gentian violet jelly.
6. Test on white cloth or white paper.
7. lightened, tinted, or gray hair

Chapter 15
THE ARTISTRY OF ARTIFICIAL HAIR

(Answers to Questions on Page 417)

1. personal choice, medical reasons, fashion, and practicality
2. human hair, synthetic hair, and animal hair
3. It makes hair look longer.
4. to give a professional result when shaping, setting, and styling
5. every 2 to 4 weeks
6. on a wig block
7. Color rinses can only darken the hair.

Chapter 16
MANICURING AND PEDICURING

(Answers to Questions on Page 452)

1. The word manicure is derived from the Latin *manus* (hand) and *cura* (care), which means the care of the hands and nails.
2. a) square b) round c) oval d) pointed
3. orangewood sticks, nail file, cuticle pusher, cuticle nipper or scissors, nail brush, and emery boards
4. from corner to center
5. It keeps the hands flexible, well-groomed, and smooth.
6. electric, oil, men's, and booth manicure
7. nail wraps, sculptured nails, nail tipping, dipping, press-on, and acrylic overlays
8. Pedicuring is the care of the feet, toes, and toenails. It has become an important client service because of the shoe styles that expose various parts of the heel and toes. Foot care not only improves personal appearance, it also adds to the comfort of the feet.

Chapter 17
THE NAIL AND ITS DISORDERS

(Answers to Questions on Page 464)

1. The normal, healthy nail is firm and flexible and appears to be slightly pink in color.
2. Onyx is the technical term for the nail.
3. The nail is composed mainly of keratin, a protein substance that forms the base of all horny tissue.
4. The nail consists of three parts: nail body, nail root, and free edge.
5. cuticle, eponychium, hyponychium, perionychium, nail walls, nail grooves, and mantle
6. The matrix is the part of the nail bed that extends beneath the nail root and contains nerves, lymph, and blood vessels to nourish the nail.
7. Any nail disease that shows signs of infection or inflammation (redness, pain, swelling, or pus) must not be treated in a beauty salon.

Chapter 18
THEORY OF MASSAGE

(Answers to Questions on Page 473)

1. Massage is used to exercise facial muscles, maintain muscle tone, and stimulate circulation.
2. Massage involves the application of external manipulations to the head and body.
3. The origin of a muscle is the fixed attachment of one end of that muscle to a bone or tissue.
4. The insertion is the attachment of the opposite end of the muscle to another muscle or to a movable bone or joint.
5. Direction of movement is generally from the insertion of a muscle toward its origin.
6. a) The skin and all its structures are nourished. b) The skin is rendered soft and pliable. c) The circulation of the blood is increased. d) The activity of the skin glands is stimulated. e) The muscle fiber is stimulated and strengthened. f) The nerves are smoothed and rested. g) Pain is sometimes relieved.
7. a) effleurage b) petrissage c) friction d) percussion or tapotement e) vibration

Chapter 19
FACIALS

(Answers to Questions on Page 496)

1. It is a restful, stimulating experience resulting in a noticeable improvement in skin tone, texture, and appearance.
2. to determine products to use, areas that need special attention, amount of pressure for massage, if lubricating oil or cream is needed around the eyes, and equipment to use
3. For sanitary reasons you should use a spatula to remove products from their containers.
4. Dry skin is the result of an insufficient flow of sebum from the sebaceous glands.
5. Another name for blackheads is comedones.

6. Oily skin and/or blackheads are caused by a hardened mass of sebum formed in the ducts of the sebaceous glands.
7. Milia or whiteheads is a common skin disorder, caused by the formation of sebaceous matter within or under the skin.
8. Acne is a disorder of the sebaceous glands; therefore, it requires medical direction.
9. Mask facials are recommended for dry skin.
10. Pack facials are recommended for normal and oily skin.
11. A hot oil mask facial is recommended for dry, scaly skin, or skin that is inclined to wrinkle.

Chapter 20
FACIAL MAKEUP

(Answers to Questions on Page 532)

1. The main objective of a makeup application is to emphasize the client's most attractive facial features and to minimize less attractive features.
2. When applying makeup, you must take into consideration the structure of a client's face; the color of the eyes, skin, and hair; how the client wants to look; and the results you can achieve.
3. a) oval b) round c) square d) pear e) heart f) diamond g) oblong
4. Foundation provides a base for color harmony; evens out the skin color; conceals minor imperfections; and protects the skin from soil, wind, and weather.
5. Skin tones, or pigments, determine the selection of foundation color.
6. a) liquid b) cream c) dry (compact) d) brush-on powdered (loose)
7. only if it belongs to the client
8. to enhance natural lashes and make them appear thicker and longer
9. Corrective makeup is used to minimize unattractive features and accent good features.
10. a) strip eyelashes b) semi-permanent individual eyelashes (eye tabbing)

Chapter 21
THE SKIN AND ITS DISORDERS

(Answers to Questions on Page 551)

1. The skin is the largest and one of the most important organs of the body.
2. Healthy skin is slightly moist, soft, and flexible; possesses a slightly acid reaction; and is free from any disease or disorder.
3. a) epidermis b) dermis.
4. Blood and lymph supply nourishment to the skin.
5. The color of the skin, whether fair, medium, or dark, depends, in part, on the blood supply to the skin and primarily on melanin, the coloring matter that is deposited in the stratum germinativum and the papillary layers of the dermis.
6. The skin contains two types of duct glands that extract materials from the blood to form new substances: the sudoriferous, or sweat glands, and the sebaceous, or oil glands.
7. a) protection b) sensation c) heat regulation d) excretion e) secretion f) absorption
8. Dermatology is the study of the skin, its nature, structure, functions, diseases, and treatment.
9. A lesion of the skin is a structural change in the tissues caused by injury or disease.
10. Acne is a chronic inflammatory disorder of the sebaceous glands.
11. a virus infection commonly called fever blisters
12. congenital absence of melanin pigment of the body, including the skin, hair, and eyes
13. A mole is a small, brownish spot, or blemish, on the skin.

Chapter 22
REMOVING UNWANTED HAIR

(Answers to Questions on Page 564)

1. Hirsuties means hairiness, or superfluous hair. It is recognized by the growth of hair in unusual amounts or locations, as on the faces of women.
2. a) permanent b) temporary
3. The first effective technique of permanent hair removal invented was electrolysis. This technique was devised by the ophthalmologist Charles E. Michel.
4. Thermolysis is the method of hair removal using high-frequency or alternating current, developed in 1924.
5. the blend method
6. a) shaving b) tweezing c) depilatories
7. a) lower eyelids b) inside the ears c) nostrils
8. The shortwave method, also known as the thermolysis method, is the quickest method of permanent hair removal.
9. a) Test the temperature of the heated wax. b) Use caution so the wax does not contact the eyes. c) Do not use a wax depilatory under the arms, over warts, or moles, abrasions, irritated or inflamed skin.

Chapter 23
CELLS, ANATOMY, AND PHYSIOLOGY

(Answers to Questions on Page 595)

1. As the basic functional units, the cells carry on all life processes. Cells also have the ability to reproduce, providing new ones for growth and replacement of worn and injured tissues.
2. As long as cells receive an adequate supply of food, oxygen, and water; eliminate waste products; and are favored with proper temperature, they will grow and thrive.
3. Metabolism is a complex chemical process whereby the body cells are nourished and supplied with the energy needed to carry on their many activities.
4. The brain controls the body; the heart circulates the blood; the lungs supply oxygen to the blood; the liver removes toxic products of digestion; the kidneys excrete water and waste products; and the stomach and intestines aid in the digestion of food.
5. Systems are groups of organs that cooperate for a common purpose, namely the welfare of the entire body.
6. Anatomy is the study of the structure of the body and what it is made of, for example, bones, muscles, and skin.
7. Physiology is the study of the functions or activities performed by the structures of the body.
8. Histology is the study of the minute structural parts of the body, such as hair, nails, sweat glands, and oil glands.
9. to give shape and support to the body; to protect various internal structures and organs; to serve as attachments for muscles and act as levers to produce body movements; to produce various blood cells in the red bone marrow; to store various minerals, such as calcium, phosphorus, magnesium, and sodium
10. The muscular system covers, shapes, and supports the skeleton. Its function is to produce all movements of the body. The muscular system consists of over 500 muscles, large and small, comprising 40 to 50% of the weight of the human body.
11. a) to learn how to administer scalp and facial services for the client's benefit b) to know what effects these treatments have on the nerves in the skin and scalp and on the body as a whole
12. It keeps the blood moving within the circulatory system.

...blood is composed of red and white corpuscles, ...latelets, and plasma.

...colorless, watery fluid that is derived from ...f the blood, mainly by filtration through ...walls into the tissue spaces.

15. a) exocrine, or duct glands b) endocrine, or ductless glands
16. a) kidneys b) liver c) skin d) large intestine e) lungs
17. With each respiratory, or breathing, cycle an exchange of gases takes place. During inhalation, oxygen is absorbed into the blood; carbon dioxide is expelled during exhalation.
18. The digestive system changes food into soluble form, suitable for use by the cells of the body.

Chapter 24
ELECTRICITY AND LIGHT THERAPY

(Answers to Questions on Page 614)

1. Electricity is a form of energy that produces magnetic, chemical, and heat effects.
2. A conductor is a substance that permits electric current to pass through it easily.
3. A nonconductor or insulator is a substance that resists the passage of an electric current, such as rubber, silk, dry wood, glass, cement, or asbestos.
4. Direct current (DC) is a constant, even-flowing current, traveling in one direction. It produces a chemical reaction.
5. Alternating current (AC) is a rapid and interrupted current, flowing first in one direction and then in the opposite direction. It produces a mechanical action.
6. It is a constant and direct current, reduced to a safe, low-voltage level. Chemical changes are produced when this current is used.
7. The positive pole produces acidic reactions. The negative pole produces alkaline reactions.
8. The positive pole: a) closes the pores b) soothes the nerves c) decreases blood supply.
9. The negative pole: a) opens the pores b) stimulates the nerves c) increases blood supply.
10. if it causes pain or discomfort; if the face is very florid; and if the client has many gold-filled teeth, high blood pressure, broken capillaries, or pustular conditions of the skin

Chapter 25
CHEMISTRY

(Answers to Questions on Page 652)

1. A basic knowledge of modern chemistry is an essential requirement for an intelligent understanding of the multitude of products and cosmetics currently used in the salon.
2. Organic chemistry is the branch of chemistry that deals with all substances in which carbon is present.

Inorganic chemistry is the branch of chemistry that deals with all substances that do not contain carbon.

3. a) solids b) liquids c) gases
4. A physical change refers to a change in the form of a substance, without the formation of any new substance. For example, ice, a solid substance, melts at a certain temperature and becomes a liquid.
5. A chemical change is one in which a new substance or substances are formed, having properties different from the original substances. For example, when you mix hydrogen peroxide into a para dye, a chemical change occurs.
6. The pH of a substance is a chemical measure of its acidity or alkalinity.
7. a) anionic b) cationic c) nonionic d) ampholytic
8. They are the composition of numerous parallel fibers of hard keratin in the cortex.
9. a) salt bonds called S bonds b) hydrogen bonds called H bonds c) disulfide bonds called S-S bonds
10. Permanent waving lotion causes the cuticle of the hair to swell and the imbrications to open, allowing the solution to penetrate into the cortex. The solution breaks the disulfide bonds found within the cortex.
11. The primary intermediates are composed of aromatic (fragrant) compounds obtained almost exclusively from coal. They are synthetic organic ingredients that when mixed with an oxidizer work together to create artificial color. The couplers are ingredients added to obtain a variety of colors. When you mix oxidation tints with the oxidizing agent (hydrogen peroxide), an oxidation-reduction reaction occurs at an alkaline pH, which causes the cuticle to swell.
12. a) powders b) solutions c) suspensions d) emulsions e) ointments f) soaps
13. It is no longer used as a skin sanitizer because of current classification as a hazardous chemical due to its ability to kill living tissue.
14. Depilatories contain detergents to strip the sebum from the hair and adhesives to hold the chemicals to the hair shaft for the 5 to 10 minutes necessary to remove the hair.
15. a) cleansing cream b) wrinkle treatments c) moisturizers d) massage cream
16. Astringents are designed to remove oil accumulation on the skin.
17. Many foundations contain barrier agents, such as UV inhibitors, cellulose derivatives, and silicone.

Chapter 26 THE SALON BUSINESS

(Answers to Questions un Page 672)

1. When planning to open a salon, give careful consideration to every aspect of running a business, including location, written agreements, business regulations, laws, insurance, salon operation, record keeping, and salon policies.
2. A salon can be owned and operated by an individual, a partnership, or a corporation.
3. They are used to determine income, expenses, profit, or loss; to assess the value of the salon for prospective buyers; to arrange a bank loan or financing; for reports on income tax, Social Security, unemployment and disability insurance, accidents, and for percentage payments of gross income required in some leases.
4. a) consumption supplies b) retail supplies
5. Since the reception area is the first thing clients see, it should be attractive, appealing, and comfortable.
6. Good telephone habits and techniques make it possible for the salon owner and cosmetologist to increase business and improve relationships with clients and suppliers.
7. a) Be familiar with the merits and benefits of each service and product. b) Adapt your approach and technique to meet the needs of each client. c) Be self-confident. d) Generate interest and desire, which are the steps leading to a sale. e) Never misrepresent your service or product. f) Use tact when selling to a client. g) Don't underestimate the client or the client's intelligence. h) To sell a product or service, deliver a sales talk in a relaxed, friendly manner and, if possible, demonstrate its use. i) Recognize the right psychological moment to close any sale. Once the client has offered to buy, quit selling—don't oversell, except to praise the client for the purchase and assure her that she will be happy with it.
8. all activities that promote a favorable impression on the public
9. a pleased client

Recommended Reading

FOR THE STUDENT

Basic Cosmetology

Hayden, Thomas, and James Williams. *Milady's Black Cosmetology.* 0-87350-377-5.

Texto General de Cosmetologia. 1-56253-474-2.

Basic Cosmetology: Supplements

FLASH! Cosmetology Terminology/Computerized Flashcards. 1-56253-372-X.

Milady's Cosmetology Fundamentals CD ROM. 1-56253-461-0.

Milady's Cosmetology Word Puzzles. 1-56253-059-3.

Milady's Standard Practical Workbook, 2000. 1-56253-469-6.

Milady's Standard Theory Workbook, 2000. 1-56253-468-8.

Preparing for the State Boards: Review Questions for Cosmetology. 1-56253-019-4.

Revision del Examen de Estado de Cosmetologia, 2000. 1-56253-475-0.

Smart Tutor/Smart Tester PC Package. 1-56253-272-3.

State Exam Review for Cosmetology, 2000. 1-56253-472-6.

Business/Career

Battersby, Mark E. *Tax and Financial Primer.* 1-56253-215-4.

Bergant, Kathleen Ann. *Communication Skills for Cosmetologists.* 1-56253-087-9. Audio Tape, 1-56253-342-8.

Capellini, Steve. *Massage Therapy Career Guide for Hands-on Success.* 1-56253-382-7.

Cotter, Louise, and Frances London DuBose. *The Transition: How to Become a Salon Professional.* 1-56253-263-4.

Dunlap, Kathi. *Adding it Up: Math for Your Cosmetology Career.* 1-56253-062-3.

Edgerton, Leslie. *Managing Your Business.* 1-56253-084-4. Audio Tape, 1-56253-305-3.

_____. *You and Your Clients: Milady's Human Relations for Cosmetology.* 1-56253-058-5. Audio Tape, 1-56253-304-5.

_____ and Glen R. Allie, CPA. *SalonOvations' Guide to Becoming a Financially Solvent Salon.* 1-56253-211-1.

Foley, Mark D. *The Motivated Salon.* 1-56253-320-7.

Gambino, Henry J. *Esthetician's Guide to Business Management.* 1-56253-127-1. Audio Tape, 1-56253-303-7.

_____. *Marketing and Advertising for the Salon.* 1-56253-262-6.

_____. *Salons and Computers: A Starter's Guide for Success.* 1-56253-354-1.

Harper, Victoria. *Professional By Choice: Milady's Career Development Guide.* 1-56253-148-4. Audio Tape, 1-56253-302-9.

Hoffman, Lee. *Keep 'em Coming Back: SalonOvations' Guide to Salon Promotion and Client Retention.* 1-56253-182-4. Audio Tape, 1-56253-308-8.

_____. *Salon Dialogue for Successful Results.* 1-56253-322-3.

Kilmer, Beverly. *Staffing Policies and Procedures.* 1-56253-314-2.

Lamb, Catherine. *Life Management Skills.* 1-56253-252-9.

Mataya, Geri. *The Salon Biz.* 1-56253-048-8. Audio Tape, 1-56253-301-0.

Maurer, Gretchen. *The Business of Bridal Beauty.* 1-56253-338-X.

Milady's 1998-1999 Guide to Cosmetology Licensing. 1-56253-446-7.

Morehouse, Jayne. *Public Relations for the Salon.* 1-56253-271-5.

Oppenheim, Robert. *101 Salon Promotions.* 1-56253-358-4.

Phillips, Carol. *In The Bag: Selling in the Salon.* 1-56253-236-7. Audio Tape, 1-56253-341-X.

Spear, J. Elaine. *Salon Client Care: How to Maximize Your Potential for Success.* 1-56253-349-5.

Tezak, Edward. *Salon Management for Cosmetology Students*, 4th Edition. 1-56253-065-8.

Wiggins, Joanne L. *Milady's Guide to Owning and Operating a Nail Salon.* 1-56253-201-4. Audio Tape, 1-56253-306-1.

Esthetics

Gambino, Henry J. *Modern Esthetics: A Scientific Source for Estheticians.* 1-56253-043-7. Audio Tape, 1-56253-344-4.

Gerson, Joel. *Milady's Standard Textbook for Professional Estheticians*, 8th Edition, 1999. 1-56253-359-2.

Gior, Fino. *Modern Electrology.* 0-87350-413-5.

Lees, Mark. *Milady's Skin Care Reference Guide.* 1-56253-071-2.

Mix, Godfrey. *The Salon Professional's Guide to Foot Care.* 1-56253-332-0.

Place, Stan Campbell. *The Art and Science of Professional Makeup.* 0-87350-361-9.

Poignard, Renee. *Waxing Made Easy: A Step-by-Step Guide.* 1-56253-171-9.

Rayner, Victoria. *Clinical Cosmetology: A Medical Approach to Esthetics Procedures.* 1-56253-056-9.

Schorr, Lia. *SalonOvations' Advanced Skin Care Handbook.* 1-56253-045-3.

Taylor, Pamela. *Makeup Techniques.* 1-56253-142-5.

Thrower, Angelo P. *Black Skin Care for the Practicing Professional.* 1-56253-352-5.

Warfield, Susanne S. *The Esthetician's Guide to Working with Physicians.* 1-56253-311-8.

Haircoloring

Cotter, Louise. *Hair Coloring Techniques.* 1-56253-116-6.

Rangl, Deb. *Milady's Standard Hair Coloring Manual and Activities Book.* 1-56253-356-8.

Sollock, Tom. *Corrective Hair Coloring: A Hands-on Approach.* 1-56253-083-6.

Spencer, Patricia. *Hair Coloring: A Hands-on Approach.* 0-87350-393-7.

Warren, Roxy. *Haircoloring in Plain English.* 1-56253-357-6.

Haircutting/Hairstyling

Bailey, Diane Carol, and Elizabeth Anthony. *Natural Hair Care and Braiding.* 1-56253-316-9.

Cotter, Louise. *Beautiful Black Styles.* 1-56253-222-7.

_____. *Milady's for Men Only: Styling and Techniques.* 1-56253-203-0.

_____, and Beverly Getschel. *SalonOvations' Children's Styles.* 1-56253-310-X.

_____ and Sara Ringler. *Mature Elegance: Styles and Techniques for Mature Clients.* 1-56253-339-8

Jones, Jamie Rines. *Braids and Updos Made Easy.* 1-56253-318-5.

_____. *Long Hair System.* 0-82738-730-x.

Lela's Braiding Gallery. 1-56253-441-6.

Milady's Standard System of Salon Skills: Hairdressing. Student Package. 1-56253-398-3.

The Multicultural Client: Cuts, Styles, and Chemical Services. 1-56253-178-6.

Scali-Sheahan, Maura. *Milady's Standard Textbook of Professional Barber-Styling,* 3rd edition. 1-56253-366-5.

_____. *Milady's 18 Men's Styles.* 1-56253-177-8.

Young, Kenneth. *Milady's 28 Black Styles.* 1-56253-042-9.

_____. *Milady's 28 Styles.* 1-56253-070-4.

_____. *Milady's Haircutting: Men's, Women's and Children's Cuts.* 1-56253-103-4.

_____. *Milady's Hairstyling: Men's, Women's and Children's Styles.* 1-56253-154-9.

_____. *Milady's Razor Cutting.* 1-56253-180-8.

Massage

Beck, Mark F. *Milady's Theory and Practice of Therapeutic Massage,* 3rd Edition, 1999. 1-56253-404-1 (HC), 1-56253-536-6 (SC).

Nails

Anthony, Elizabeth. *Airbrushing for Nails.* 1-56253-270-7.

Arte y Ciencia de la Tecnologia de las Unas, 1997 edition. 1-56253-331-2.

Bigan, Tammy. *Nail Art and Design.* 1-56253-118-2.

_____. *TechNails: Extensions, Wraps and Nail Art.* 0-87350-382-1.

Milady's Art and Science of Nail Technology, 1997 edition. 1-56253-326-6.

Peters, Vicki. *Nail Q and A Book.* 1-56253-266-9.

Schoon, Douglas D. *Milady's Nail Structure and Product Chemistry.* 1-56253-239-1.

Tumblety, Susan. *30 Nail Designs.* 1-56253-268-5.

Permanent Waving

Ekstrom, Candi, and Louise Cotter. *Perm Waving Styles.* 1-56253-312-6.

Padgett, Mark E. *A Contemporary Approach to Permanent Waving.* 1-56253-101-8.

Zotos Creative Designers. *Milady's Perm Techniques.* 1-56253-172-7.

Videos

Jones, Jamie Rines. *Braids and Updos Video Series:*
Advanced Braiding Made Easy. 0-87350-241-8.
Braiding Made Easy. 0-87350-650-2.
French Braiding Made Easy. 0-87350-459-3.
More Updos Made Easy. 1-56253-379-7.
Ribbon Braiding Made Easy. 1-56253-377-0.
Updos Made Easy. 1-56253-378-9.

Hair Coloring Video Package. 0-87350-659-6.

Milady's Hair Structure and Chemistry Simplified Video Package. 0-87350-669-3.

Nail Technology Video Series, 2nd edition. 1-56253-407-6.

Permanent Waving Video Package. 0-87350-977-3.

Restructuring Over-Curly Hair. 0-87350-953-6.

FOR THE INSTRUCTOR

Competency-Based Curriculum for Cosmetology. 1-56253-014-3.

The Creative Teacher: Instructor's Guide. 1-56253-015-1.

Duncan, Rosalyn. *Who's Training the Teacher?* 7 Audio Tapes. 0-87350-239-6.

Howe, Linda J. *Milady's Professional Instructor for Cosmetology, Barber-Styling, and Nail Technology.* 1-56253-073-9.

Johnson, Michele. *Management Tools for Cosmetology Education: Worksheets to Organize Your Program.* 0-87350-396-1.

Milady's Standard Computerized Testmaker and Testbank. 1-56253-408-4.

Milady's Standard Textbook of Cosmetology Course Management Guide. 1-56253-471-8.

Milady's Standard System of Salon Skills: Hairdressing. Image Library. CD-ROM. 1-56253-559-5.

Milady's Standard System of Salon Skills: Hairdressing. Instructor's Package. 1-56253-401-7.

Milady's Standard System of Salon Skills: Hairdressing. Leader's Manual. 1-56253-399-1.

Milady's Standard Textbook of Cosmetology Audio Tape Series. 1-56253-269-3.

Nighswander, James K. and A. Dan Whitley. *On Becoming a Cosmetology Teacher: A Training Program for Instructors of Cosmetology.* 1-56253-086-0.

Nizetich, Andre. *Milady's Teaching Hair Coloring: A Step-By-Step Guide to Building Props.* 1-56253-072-0.

Padgett, Mark E. *A Contemporary Approach to Permanent Waving Course Guide* 1-56253-309-6.

Spencer, Patricia. *Hair Coloring: A Hands-on Approach Curriculum Guide.* 1-56253-060-7.

Videos

Milady's Standard Textbook of Cosmetology Video Series. 1-56253-470-X.

Miller, Erica. *Facial Treatment Video TapesProfessional Education Series.* 1-56253-392-4.

Professional Skin Care Techniques Video Package, 1990 Edition. 0-87350-891-2.

FOR REFERENCE

Balhorn, Linda A. *The Professional Model's Handbook.* 0-87350-376-7.

Chesky, Sheldon R., Isabel Cristina, and Richard B. Rosenberg. *Playing It Safe: Milady's Guide to Decontamination, Sterilization and Personal Protection.* 1-56253-179-4.

Hess, Shelley. *SalonOvations' Guide to Aromatherapy.* 1-56253-313-4.

_____. *The Professional's Reflexology Handbook.* 1-56253-334-7.

Michalun, Natalia. *Milady's Skin Care and Cosmetic Ingredients Dictionary.* 1-56253-125-5.

Miller, Erica. *Day Spa Operations.* 1-56253-255-3.

_____. *Day Spa Techniques.* 1-56253-261-8.

_____. *Shiatsu Massage.* 1-56253-264-2.

Myllymaki, Theodora J., and James Akerson. *A Comprehensive Guide to Cosmetic Sources.* 1-56253-102-6.

Schoon, Douglas. *HIV/AIDS and Hepatitis: Everything You Need to Know to Protect Yourself and Others.* 1-56253-175-1.

SalonOvations' Cosmetology Dictionary. 1-56253-214-6.

Scali-Sheahan, Maura. *Milady's Human Anatomy and Physiology Workbook.* 1-56253-157-3.

Schoon, Douglas D. *Hair Structure and Chemistry Simplified,* revised edition. 1-56253-122-0.

Ventura, Judy. *Milady's Salon Receptionist's Handbook.* 1-56253-044-5. Audio Tape, 1-56253-307-X.

Glossary/Index

F

APPROXIMATE CONVERSIONS TO METRIC MEASURES

Symbol	When You Know	Multiply by	To Find	Symbol
LENGTH (speed)				
in	inches	2.5	centimeters	cm
ft	feet	30	centimeters	cm
MASS (weight)				
oz	ounces	28	grams	g
lb	pounds	0.45	kilograms	kg
	short tons (2000 lb)	0.9	tonnes	t
VOLUME				
tsp	teaspoon	5	milliliters	ml
tbsp	tablespoon	15	milliliters	ml
fl oz	fluid ounces	30	milliliters	ml
c	cups	0.24	liters	l
pt	pints	0.47	liters	l
qt	quarts	0.95	liters	l
gal	gallons	3.8	liters	l
TEMPERATURE (exact)				
°F	Fahrenheit temperature	5/9 after subtracting 32	Celcius temperature	°C